Staying Healthy with Nutrition

21ST-Century Edition

THE COMPLETE GUIDE TO DIET AND NUTRITIONAL MEDICINE

Elson M. Haas, MD
with Buck Levin, PhD, RD

CELESTIAL ARTS
Berkeley

Cover and text design by Betsy Stromberg
Cover art by Mohammad Rezaiian

Watercress Salad with Pollution Solution Dressing from *Airola Diet and Cookbook* (Phoenix, AZ: Health Plus Publishers, 1981) © 1981 by Paavo Airola. Reprinted with permission of the publisher.

Banana-Yogurt Freeze from *Fast Vegetarian Feasts*, rev. ed. (New York: Dolphin Books, 1986) © 1986 by Martha Rose Shulman, Reprinted with permission of the publisher.

Tofu Mayonnaise and Tofu Sour Cream from *New Laurel's Kitchen*, 2nd ed. (Berkeley, CA: Ten Speed Press, 1986) © 1976, 1986 by the Blue Mountain Center of Meditation, Inc. Reprinted with permission of the publisher.

Sesame Squash Butter, Sweet Carrot Butter, and Wheat-free Pie Crust from *Self-Healing Cookbook* (Grass Valley, CA: Earthtones Press, 1987) © by Kristina Turner. Reprinted with permission of the publisher.

Low-fat, Low-salt Vinaigrette from *Stress, Diet, and Your Health* (New York: Henry Holt and Co., 1982) © 1982 by Dean Ornish, MD. Reprinted with permission of the publisher.

Library of Congress Cataloging-in-Publication Data

Haas, Elson M., 1947-
    Staying healthy with nutrition : the complete guide to diet & nutritional medicine / Elson M. Haas with Buck Levin.— 21st century ed.
        p. ; cm.
    Rev. and updated of Staying healthy with nutrition / Elson M. Haas. c1992.
    Includes bibliographical references and index.
    1. Nutrition. 2. Diet therapy.
    [DNLM: 1. Nutrition—United States—Popular Works. 2. Cookery—United States—Popular Works. 3. Diet—United States—Popular Works. 4. Food—United States—Popular Works. 5. Health Promotion—United States—Popular Works. 6. Life Style—United States—Popular Works. QU 145 H14s 2006] I. Levin, Buck. II. Title.

QP141.H183 2006
613.2—dc22

2005037354

Printed in the United States of America
978-1-58761-179-7

12 11 10 9 8 7

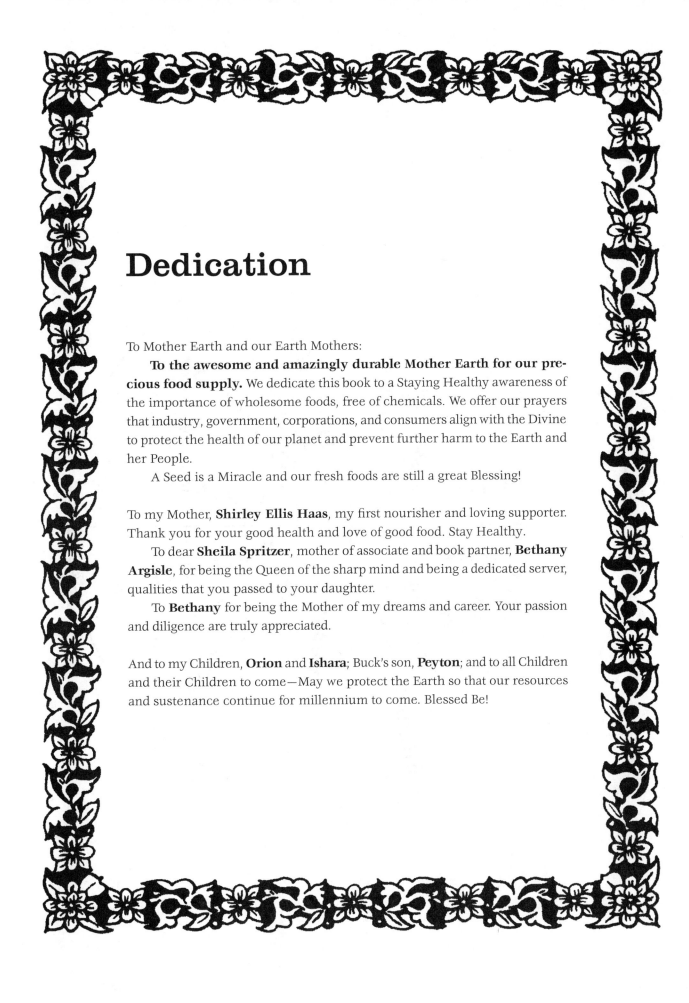

Dedication

To Mother Earth and our Earth Mothers:

To the awesome and amazingly durable Mother Earth for our precious food supply. We dedicate this book to a Staying Healthy awareness of the importance of wholesome foods, free of chemicals. We offer our prayers that industry, government, corporations, and consumers align with the Divine to protect the health of our planet and prevent further harm to the Earth and her People.

A Seed is a Miracle and our fresh foods are still a great Blessing!

To my Mother, **Shirley Ellis Haas**, my first nourisher and loving supporter. Thank you for your good health and love of good food. Stay Healthy.

To dear **Sheila Spritzer**, mother of associate and book partner, **Bethany Argisle**, for being the Queen of the sharp mind and being a dedicated server, qualities that you passed to your daughter.

To **Bethany** for being the Mother of my dreams and career. Your passion and diligence are truly appreciated.

And to my Children, **Orion** and **Ishara**; Buck's son, **Peyton**; and to all Children and their Children to come—May we protect the Earth so that our resources and sustenance continue for millennium to come. Blessed Be!

Nutrition Wheel

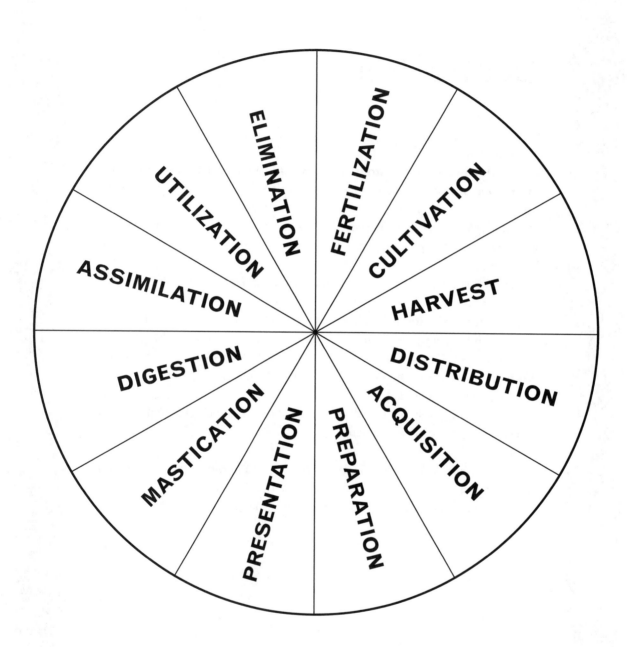

Contents

Part One

THE BUILDING BLOCKS

Acknowledgments

First I want to truly acknowledge **Bethany Argisle** for her continued grand efforts and results on my behalf in the current run of 30 years of our "blendship." Thank you, Bethany, for your inspiration and work as a creator and conceptual designer, supporter, and friend, and for your great guidance in my career as author and teacher, and reacher for good health through good nutrition. You have been there with all the book's changes and updates, making them great. Thank you so much.

— To **Buck Levin**, PhD, for your thorough review and useful additions to the original text, for your depth of knowledge in all things nutritional, and for the full references you have provided for the students using this book to understand more fully the concepts contained herein.

— To **Windy Ferges** for your consistent and conscientious work in overseeing this immense project with all the people and timetables involved. Your editorial skills in this book project were invaluable. Thank you.

— To **Jo Ann Deck**, Celestial Arts publisher, and the whole team at my longtime publishing supporter, especially **Julie Bennett** as chief editor and **Betsy Stromberg** as book designer.

— To **David Hinds**—the original guide at Celestial Arts—for supporting and bringing forth that original big baby book of *Staying Healthy with Nutrition*, and in keeping it all in one text. And to **Hal Kramer**, who first opened the door at Celestial Arts (the company you started) way back in 1979.

— To **Neil Murray** for your brilliance and professionalism in overseeing the design and organization of the first edition of *Staying Healthy with Nutrition*, and your clear insights and great design on my first book, *Staying Healthy with the Seasons*.

— To **Eleonora Manzolini** for your writing and recipe ideas in chapter 14, for your wonderful devotion to great natural cuisine. It is a real joy to work with you.

— To **Jeffrey H. Reinhardt**, nutritional biochemist and mind of minds, for your in-depth work in reviewing my original manuscript for accuracy.

— To **Evelyn Brown** for your amazing ability to read my writing, and for typing the original handwritten manuscript, which was years of work. Bless you!

— To **Dr. Ed Bauman** for your review of the fasting and detoxification sections and your support of nutrition education at your school, Bauman College.

— To **Clayton College for Natural Health** and all the devoted staff for your support and continued use of *Staying Healthy with Nutrition* as your course text.

— To **Mohammad Rezaiian** for your incredible talent and the beautiful painting you did, which we used a part of for this book's cover. You made all those fruits and vegetables come to life.

—Elson

Preface

I would like to say that I've never met a meal I didn't remember, although there have been a few I wouldn't mind forgetting. After digesting and assimilating the many thousands of cuisine concoctions consumed, I have metabolized them into the nearly 1,000 pages you have before you. I hope you'll like the flavor of this book. Please though, don't try to eat it all in one meal. Take your time, chew well, let it digest and assimilate—then you'll be able to use it for energy and health now and beyond.

I am quite proud of *Staying Healthy with Nutrition*. It was a labor of love and loads of work that took many years with my original book team of Bethany Argisle and Neil Murray, plus the supportive folks at Celestial Arts, led at that time by David Hinds. David believed the world was ready for a large nutrition text with the alternative and progressive slant to include the wide use of nutritional supplements and detoxification. Well, he was right!

Staying Healthy with Nutrition has been well received and widely used by individuals, health and medical practitioners, and schools that teach nutrition. As an example, Clayton College for Natural Health, Bauman College, and many others have used this book as part of their basic nutrition courses in providing degrees and certifications in nutrition. Taking this into account—along with the great changes, studies, and new knowledge in nutritional medicine—it was imperative to create an updated edition of this tome with the latest in research.

When I first wrote (by hand, as the world and I were in the computer transition) this text, I didn't have the wherewithal to track and share all the references I utilized. I knew this was a weakness for the scientifically minded and university courses, yet I wanted to not put off the layperson by being too formal or scientific. I am the doctor who makes things understandable to the average person. However, the transition to integrate science with user-friendliness became the new goal. A quick story will tell you how this happened.

A couple of years after the original publication, I received a call from Dr. Buck Levin, who was a professor at Bastyr University, a naturopathic school in Seattle. He was using the book for his nutrition course and loved the writing style and information. He said, "If you ever want to update this with all the current references, let me know." He even offered to have his current class, circa 1994, work on it with him as a class project. Dr. Levin is a scientist with a PhD in nutrition. So, to make a short story even shorter—years later when my publisher and I were ready to update this book, I called Buck to help in the transformation. He happily agreed, yet neither of us realized, at that time, how much work it would be. Thank you Dr. Buck for your efforts and endurance—and the great job!

There were many other players in the mix to complete this book (see the acknowledgements). Special thanks to Bethany Argisle and Neil Murray for the original 6 years of effort to lay the groundwork and design, charts, and so on, that make the base of *Staying Healthy with Nutrition*.

And thanks to all you readers who are interested in learning about nutrition and its vital importance in creating good health. Clearly the world needs a better diet—the Western world needs to get away from junk and chemicals, do some detoxification, and find better balance, while the poor nations need better nourishment to correct deficiency and end starvation. I pray we shall all work together to appreciate and care for our Mother Earth and nourish all of us better in return for that care.

I love good food and I know you will too.
ENJOY!

—Elson M. Haas, MD

Message from Dr. Buck Levin

Staying Healthy with Nutrition is a book with a payoff. In several different ways, it will pay you to read this book. First of all, *Staying Healthy* will sort out a wide range of information and make this information much easier for you to understand. Second, it will not only teach you how to apply this information in your own life, but it will also inspire you to do so. You will be able to grab onto each one of its nearly 1,000 pages and take the information inward, into the nooks and crannies of your personal life. If you will adopt the principles in this book, you will very likely become healthier and better nourished. But I hope you won't.

Or more exactly, I hope you won't settle for this inward kind of journey. What I'm hoping is that you'll also go outward. Outward into the not-you world that has nothing to do with the impact of magnesium on your cardiovascular system and in fact may offer you no personal payoff whatsoever. I even hope that you will change the name of the book in your mind from *Staying Healthy with Nutrition* to *Staying With: The Myth of Nutrition.* The reason is simple. Nourishment is mythic—not mythic in the sense of "make-believe" or "illusionary," but mythic in the sense "beyond all worldly proportions." All of us know that nutrients come from food, and we know just as clearly that food comes from the Earth. But we don't take that last part seriously, as part of our intrinsic responsibility when it comes to eating. The fact of the matter is, we cannot make food. We can only find it (and in some instances cultivate it, although we seem to botch that up a good bit of the time). Where we find food is right where it belongs, at home in its spot, some unique niche in an ecosystem where soil and seasons and climate and geography come together in some amazingly cooperative way. As my 11-year-old son Peyton would say, "That's massive dude."

It's this massiveness we've got to embrace if we want to take part in the nourishment. Food cannot be extracted from the Earth. That approach might work in business, where profit can be extracted out of a situation in a predatory way that seizes upon volatility and lack of constraints (volume constraints, speed constraints, ethical constraints). But this approach doesn't work with food. Food comes to us with earthly constraints. The only way for us to profit from food is to safeguard the Earth's potential for producing it, and that potential involves every ocean, every river, every landmass, every cubic meter of air. Carrots in a zip-lock bag and styrofoam-boxed burgers won't work because there is no "where" to put the plastic and the styrofoam once we're done. Damming up rivers for crop irrigation won't work because hydrology cycles are part of the Earth's food production potential. Nothing will work except an unbounded kindness on our part for everything natural, a "staying with" the world even when it's inconvenient and doesn't pay. The myth of nutrition is a myth of connection between our inward health and most distant reaches of the Earth. We break this connection whenever we live in an isolationist, separatist, exclusionary, exploitative, and extractive way, and we restore it by being inclusive, accommodating, integrative, and considerate. When all is said and done, nourishment is about the connection—not the payoff.

How to Use This Book

When first creating this book many meals ago, I knew that it was special in the sense that it was not available anywhere else. I personally change my nutritional plan each time I read it as it has heaps of knowledge to offer many types of folks.

Since the first publication many printings ago, I have become more aware of the planet being our plate. We in the Western world have so many choices in what we feed ourselves that the spark to make better choices is a valuable key to health, and Dr. Elson and team surely give us that guidance.

In the design of this book, which I had my hands and heart in, the logos that were originally inspired by my first computers in 1992 are a way of thinking, a pictographic communications system, which are meant to aid you and me, the readers and eaters, to target and clarify the various areas of information. The logos are your visual guides to the topics. Follow the subjects throughout the text and reread as you need. Check out the running heads, the part introductions, and make sure that you learn at least one thing regularly, whether you are a student of nutrition, a teacher of others, or just have a daily date with the meal on your plate.

This book is a great nutritional reference book and has been updated to include the latest scientific references, which were not readily available or very extensive when the first edition was written. So many more studies providing even more knowledge are in this new edition to connect you even deeper, if you so choose. However, we can also Stay Healthy by simply sitting in the garden, learning and listening to Nature and our own inner rhythm renewal so we can be sensitive to our choices, and be willing to change with the seasons of age, weather, and availability.

We know that you will be able to design your own personal program, your healthy diet and supplement plan, which can change with age and from season to season. You will learn more in this tome about supplements, chemical additives, and many other specific areas, such as phytonutrients, nutrient-rich seaweeds, and organics, plus many new items found in the natural food stores and your own garden.

This brick in the temple of healing is a guide for you and those you influence, especially our planet plate, the Earth. Stay healthy and keep healing!

My Body Tiz of Me
Health Is My Victory
—Bethany Argisle

Staying Healthy with Nutrition is many books in one. In writing it, I asked, what does the medical/nutrition-oriented consumer need to know? There are countless books on specific nutrition topics; there are also nutrition textbooks, mostly for dieticians, which are not as helpful to the general public. And I want a book that deals with the evolution of progressive nutrition that is provided in the natural food industry and the growing natural medicine movement, and is what many consumers may look to for wise guidance. I also want this book to work for nutrition students looking at nutrition as a career, and for medical students and doctors and all practitioners to have this knowledge as a basis for their practices. I believe that this new edition can work in all of these arenas.

Thus, with the need for an investigative and complete guide to nutrition clearly present, we have chosen to provide you with this reference book. *Staying Healthy with Nutrition* is unique and incorporates information from literally hundreds of previous books on a multitude of nutritional topics. It also supports a modern philosophy, a personal and planetary one to support the Earth healthfully as she supports all of us with good foods. And I appreciate Ms. Argisle for her support in bending our ears to the voice of our precious Mother Earth.

Even though this is a large book, I feel that we have it organized in a user-friendly fashion, with clear headings and guidelines. The chapter organization and table of contents will make it simple to find your areas of interest. The diet plan I suggest provides the ideal eating approach I believe offers the best health to most, and includes sample recipes, which are all in one section, found in part 3. The discussion of specific health problems and the nutritional support guidelines for different eras of our life are separated into individual sections, with Life Stage Programs in chapter 15 and Medical Treatment Programs in chapter 17.

Staying Healthy with Nutrition is in part a nutritional biochemistry text, a food and diet book, and a nutritional medicine guide. The dietary and supplement applications are very advanced, and the seasonal, natural way of eating is, I think, the healthiest diet there is.

Staying Healthy with Nutrition is to date THE most COMPLETE GUIDE TO DIET AND NUTRITIONAL MEDICINE. We hope you really savor it and make use of its nutrients harmoniously and healthfully for us all.

—Elson M. Haas, MD

STAYING HEALTHY WITH NUTRITION CAN BE USED IN A VARIETY OF WAYS

1. A reference guide that can be entered through

- The table of contents
- The index
- Or, open it and see where you land

For example, if you have a specific topic, concern, or condition you wish to look up, check the table of contents for the general topic, or for more specific interests, check the index to see if you can pinpoint the exact information location in the nutritional constellation. Having found your topic, you may discover other areas of interest to which you can then progress.

2. Textbook

Designed as a course in basic nutrition that proceeds to nutritional medicine, it can be read and studied in the order presented. For example, we begin with building blocks, then progress through foods and diets, followed by the ideal diet and a specific seasonal diet plan, and then move to part 4, with many examples of nutritional application, thus providing the individual experience.

3. Scientific text

Since the original publication of this tome, many scientific studies have emphasized the value of both diets and nutritional supplements. Therefore, *Staying Healthy with Nutrition* is now enhanced to provide supportive scientific studies to back up much of the information presented. This was done with the expertise of Dr. Buck Levin, my industrious cohort in this update and new 21st-Century Edition. In the appendices, you will find many hundreds of reference articles divided into the book's related chapters, allowing you to explore the scientific literature.

4. Special-interest manual

If the environment is of special interest to you or you wish to review certain food additives at the store or in your own cupboard, you can look them up (see chapter 11).

If you feel that your diet needs some minor or major adjustments, you may seek inspiration and guidance in how to change your food choices. Furthermore, you may choose to follow the specific seasonal diets (see chapter 14) during a specific time cycle, such as a year.

Enjoy the journey of learning more about the important foods and water that you put into your body, that you feed your family and friends, or that you guide others in helping them improve their nutrition.

General Book Disclaimers

There are many nutritional suggestions and special supplement programs contained in this book. It is written mostly to inform those of you interested in the various aspects of nutrition and lifestyle as they relate to both health and disease. Furthermore, my intention here is to assist you to act as a nutritional guide for yourself and others seeking educational support.

This new text is brought to you in the most up-to-date state based on my extensive experience and Dr. Buck Levin's vast knowledge of the latest nutritional research. Yet, this is a very active field of interest these days and I am sure that there is a great deal more to learn and add to our current information. I could continue updating this book, and especially part 4, for all of my life. You may choose to keep abreast of the latest nutritional news from the various multimedia communications. I hope you do, and apply it wisely to your daily life.

The suggestions in this book (again, especially part 4) are not meant to replace your doctor/practitioner, nor am I suggesting any of it as medical treatment. Please use this book as the educational tool it is meant to be to help you to enhance your life. If you use this compendium to design your own individual treatment program, you do so at your own risk and with your conscience at peace with your nutritional adventures. Please see an appropriately trained (and healthy example) professional if you have any questions about your health, have medical concerns, or need guidance for your life.

Good Luck and Wise Choices!

—Elson M. Haas, MD

Dear Reader,
If you have adjusted your nutritional program because of this book and have any observable results, please inform us.

Preventive Medical Center of Marin
25 Mitchell Blvd., Suite 8
San Rafael, CA 94903
www.elsonhaas.com

Write to   Dr. Elson M. Haas
c/o Celestial Arts
P.O. Box 7123
Berkeley, CA 94707
www.tenspeed.com

> The doctor of the future will give no medicines, but will
> interest his patients in the care of the human frame,
> in diet, and in the causes of disease.
> —Thomas Edison
>
> ✳
>
> The best medicines are resting and fasting.
> —Benjamin Franklin
>
> ✳
>
> Let food be your medicine.
> —Hippocrates

These quotes might do well to be on the walls of medical schools, doctors' offices, and hospitals everywhere. Nutrition has been an important part of medicine since before the time of Hippocrates; ingesting special foods and herbs as well as participating in seasonal fasting and particular diets were part of the medical care of the ancient Greeks. Continuing in that tradition, true health for us today begins in our gardens and orchards, in our markets and kitchens, and is a result of our food choices and habits. Although technology has created many advanced medical, herbal, and nutritional products, it has brought us new problems as well. A good diet and lifestyle are still the best medicine and safeguards for health.

Introduction

Staying Healthy with Nutrition was first published in 1992, based on my studies and experiences in a nutrition-oriented medical practice. What has changed since then in the field of nutritional medicine? A great deal of scientific research has been published, and nutritional and herbal supplements have advanced with many new products and formulas—store shelves are filled with them. With the plethora of choices now available, the consumer must ask, "But what is right for me?" I felt an update to the 1992 tome was vital, particularly because many students use the book in their health education studies. Readers now have the most up-to-date information available in this 21st-century edition of *Staying Healthy with Nutrition.* For a sense of this incredible expansion, see chapter 7, Special Supplements, which documents a number of new products and research.

Other new information in nutritional medicine involves the identification and important functions of *phytonutrients* as the healing components of foods and plants. See chapter 8, Foods, for each food's specific phytonutrients. The study of nutrition as a career and a practice has increased since the early 1990s with a fresh breed of nutrition practitioners who are now trained with a different focus than were the more conventional registered dietitians (RDs). The revised edition addresses the public's interest in an innovative national "nutrition certification" that guides people in the areas of a whole foods diet and the use of supplements (that is, with non-RDA nutrients, which is typically not the focus of RDs). The general public must know how to access nutritional care for themselves, their families, and the planet.

CLINICAL PRACTICE

Before the 1980s, I studied extensively and worked more with the philosopher-physician's understanding of disease and healing, researching and applying the natural therapeutic approaches of traditional Chinese medicine, herbology, body therapies, guided imagery, and other inner-healing processes in my practice. Today, I still incorporate all of these modalities into my health-oriented family medicine practice, but during the past two decades I have focused my attention more on the rapidly advancing field of nutritional medicine. Nutrition has become an area of great interest to the general population. Diet—what we eat—has been and continues to be a primary part of my practice as well as my own personal challenge. Over the years, I have made vast improvements in my own habits and food choices. **Since Western medicine does not always focus on health and preventing disease, people seek empowerment in caring for their personal health and that of their families; nutrition is a basic component of preventive medicine, and it can be effective in corrective medicine for many common health problems.**

My first book, *Staying Healthy with the Seasons* (Celestial Arts, 1981 and 2003), deals mainly with the overall concepts and guidelines for a healthy approach to nutrition and lifestyle within the cycles of life. My knowledge and practice have evolved since then toward more scientific nutrition. I test people for nutritional deficiency and toxicity and use individualized programs of foods as well as nutritional and herbal supplementation within an overall approach to health care I call "Integrated Medicine." This balance in lifestyle addresses concerns about exercise, proper sleep, managing stress, and keeping body structure aligned and energy flowing, in a framework of maintaining a healthy attitude toward life and a love for one's body. This requires motivation and a simple program that people can incorporate into their daily lives and goals. It takes a conscious effort to pay attention and to learn what works for each of us individually, especially regarding foods and supplements. Every day I see that this work pays off in great dividends and that we can deposit ever more into our "health bank accounts."

My medical clinic provides patient-centered or cooperative medicine, offering a multidisciplinary blend of services within the context of a general practice. My colleagues, staff, and I are involved in our patients' attempts to make a difference in health outcomes, although each person is ultimately the only one who can create and maintain his or her own health. We deal with as many levels and concerns as individuals bring with them. We directly involve patients in decision-making when that is relevant; inform and educate them in instances when they are not so informed; and work together to achieve the clearest approach and best results for their state of disease and healthy evolution.

Our clinic combines a wide range of laboratory evaluations and potential therapeutic approaches to achieve an advanced synthesis of medical practice, especially for disease prevention and support of health. Treatment options include both pharmaceutical and natural medicines (including nutritional supplements, homeopathic remedies, and herbal products), dietary changes, bioidentical hormone support, acupuncture, osteopathic care and massage therapy, stress management, and hypnotherapy. **I believe that medical care should provide a full spectrum of services—from crisis intervention and evaluation and treatment of illness to therapies and education that help people to grow in their daily lives and learn to stay healthy.**

I call this type of medical practice "NOW Medicine," the new modern medicine. I am currently writing a book on the subject, with the NOW standing for "Integrating Natural, Oriental, and Western Medicines while Caring for Yourself in an Evolving Healthcare System." Yes, that is a bit long for a book subtitle, but this is the next crucial area to tackle for those of us who care about putting health over disease and peace over war, as well as reducing the pollution and damage to Earth and the human body. We need to protect the food supply and keep it cleaner. We need to protect ourselves from the invasion of genetically modified (GM) foods.

NUTRITIONAL MEDICINE

It is my intention in this edition of *Staying Healthy with Nutrition* to investigate and substantiate the significance of food and nutrients as an integral and accepted part of the world of medicine and individual medical practice. I examine the emerging politics of food cultivation and what it takes to maintain healthy elements of clean air and water, rich and nutritious soil, and a sun that keeps shining. Supportive nutrition and our alignment with Nature are basic components of health, and certainly factors in disease when they are not present. A reasonable knowledge of nutritional biochemistry helps in the application of therapies that relieve many symptoms relating to or resulting from improper dietary habits and the resulting inefficient body functions. With the proper construction of a diet and lifestyle plan, we can help rebuild a patient's health (or our own) before and after illness or surgery.

Medical schools and doctors have typically been oriented to treating disease with drugs and surgery, and many health-care practitioners do not yet view foods as "powerful medicine." Although nutrition plays a more important part in preventive medicine than it does in the treatment of disease, an understanding of the body's functioning at the nutritional level can indeed help in the treatment of a variety of problems. Clearly we now realize that diet plays a crucial part in how the body looks and feels and whether it stays healthy. Generally, these effects—both good and bad—come over time, years, and decades. We can change our body and health as well as our energy and vitality with different diets. I explore these concepts in this new edition.

Nutritional medicine is an emerging and fast-growing field; it is also as ancient as medicine and healing itself, however. It is a specialty much like other medical specialties and should be considered as such. Every practitioner should understand and follow the basics of nutritional application in health care. There is still a great deal to learn about nutrition and how it relates to illness and health, and how it relates to each individual's needs, but this is true of all specialties.

The morning of April 15, 2005, the secretary of the Department of Health and Human Services, Tommy Thompson, was interviewed on Fox News and presented a message that I have been saying for many years. To paraphrase, we are spending way too much money fixing people to get them back to health (and I use that term loosely for most Americans) and nowhere near the money we should be spending on prevention. People need to be educated in how to care for themselves with nutrition, exercise, and stress management. Furthermore, medical students and doctors need to be taught how to address and teach these areas of health in their practices and bring back the *docere*, the teaching doctor.

Until we can learn everything, it makes sense that each practitioner must be aware of the limits of his or her knowledge and its applications. If, when treating or screening patients, we do not have sufficient or appropriate knowledge to help them completely, we should look for another doctor or practitioner to assist or advise us on further treatment. My own policy is to maintain an extensive referral list of helpful health-care practitioners. It is also the responsibility of patients to know something about their nutrition and to be concerned with the healthful feeding of themselves and their families. Patients must be willing to keep discovering and readjusting their own balance over time, even season to season, through various life stages and lifestyles.

MEDICAL AND NUTRITIONAL TRAINING

In my opinion, doctors have not been well trained in nutrition, and I aim to contribute to the improvement of this condition. In my own 4 years of study at a highly ranked medical school 35 years ago, I had fewer than 10 hours of nutritional education—about the same amount as in grade school—and the information presented was not much more advanced. The "four food group" idea of a balanced diet and concern over the significant and symptomatic vitamin/mineral deficiencies (citing scurvy, beriberi, and rickets as examples) were the major focus. There was a separate study of biochemistry, but very little discussion of its practical application to nutritional physiology. Some information was given about the relevance of the metabolism of specific vitamins and minerals, although there was little understanding of how diet could affect health or disease.

When I was in medical school, there was a great deal less information available as compared to today on the relationship of diet to such major diseases as cancer, cardiovascular disease, diabetes, and obesity. Yet even with today's knowledge, nutritional education is still belittled as secondary paramedical information in most medical centers. Understanding the link between diet and disease, and being able to use nutritional counseling and therapies within a medical practice, is so vital to the health-care component of medicine that it should be required knowledge for every medical school graduate and practitioner.

At my thirtieth medical school reunion in Ann Arbor, Michigan, I was quite pleased with the reception I received from my classmates and colleagues. As one of the only members of the class of 1972 to explore health and healing incorporating nutrition and natural medicine, I had stepped outside the box. Being my first reunion, and having achieved some success in my field with my well-known clinic and books, the discussions I had with doctors were quite inspiring. Many were interested in hearing about my health-care approach, as most of them (indeed, almost all Western physicians) spend much of their time dealing with disease and people in crisis.

At dinner I happened to sit next to the dean, Allen Lichter, also a classmate of mine. We spoke about nutritional education for medical students. I was surprised to hear that things had not changed all that much since the 1970s, yet Allen was very interested in adding deeper study in health and nutrition into the curriculum. He had just finished his interviews with the graduating class and had asked what they felt was a weakness in their program; the graduates had overwhelmingly answered that they had not learned enough about diet and nutrition. The subject is obviously important to all of us, including doctors themselves. Because so many patients today eat special diets and take nutritional supplements, it makes sense that the practitioners are better equipped to care for such patients when they are informed about the many aspects of health care, especially the nutritional part.

Doctors in training are typically still simply informed that there are nutritionists (RDs) who are

> Concepts of nutrition and its relationship to health and disease are rarely given the attention they deserve in the medical education of today. And so much of the disease we see today is related in meaningful ways to our dietary choices. The wave of type 2 diabetes we are encountering is a classic example, and there are many others. Once an illness is diagnosed, concepts of the proper diet both to help the underlying illness and to facilitate the success of treatment are often glossed over quickly. Efforts to make nutrition education more readily available as well as efforts to perform more nutrition-related research are things we should strongly support.
>
> —Allen S. Lichter, MD
> Dean, University of Michigan Medical School

trained to help them devise diets for sick people who need to change and/or limit their food intake to control their diseases. These dietitians are trained primarily within the disease model in medicine to help people manage such chronic problems as diabetes, heart disease, and malnutrition. The idea of a more natural nutrition, however—based on the benefits of organically grown whole foods and free of the risks associated with highly processed junk foods—is primarily absent from dietitian training. So is the importance of detoxification and nutritional supplementation. In that conventional model, there is a limited emphasis on a balanced diet and on chemicals in our foods.

The basic components of the RD's practice have been to provide diabetes-controlling diets (by reducing simple sugars and refined carbohydrates while increasing protein and fiber); to encourage weight loss (by restricting calories); to lower high blood pressure (by reducing salt intake); and to manage heart disease (by lowering cholesterol levels through decreased intake of total dietary fat, saturated fat, and dietary cholesterol). This all makes sense and is important, of course. However, there is much more involved beyond just assisting doctors in the control of diseases after they have already occurred. For the most part, doctors and dietitians have neither taken the time to study and incorporate various special diets (such as vegetarianism and fasting therapy), nor have they been willing to accept these diets or the power that specific nutrients have in the prevention and treatment of medical problems. The common belief is, if it hasn't had double-blind studies or been accepted in the medical community for at least a decade, then it must be a fad.

I am happy to say, however, that this attitude has been changing in recent decades with more RDs studying and incorporating nutrition and supplements into their practices. Just look at the knowledge and support of my collaborator on this book, Dr. Buck Levin, who is a PhD-level nutritionist and RD. He exemplifies the new model and embraces the importance of this advancing field of nutritional medicine.

There is a new breed of nutritionists who deal only with the healthy parts of nutritional therapies. This can be likened to the difference between Western-oriented doctors (who practice only Western medicine, with the naming and treating of diseases) and alternative or integrated practitioners (who really work to understand what in people's lives contribute to their ills). These practitioners provide support and guidance in correcting the causes, when that is possible. It is clear to me from my experience that when a doctor and patient work together on health care, there is much less need for disease care—that is, preventive medicine and practice really works.

SCIENCE AND NUTRITION

This book integrates experience, intuition, and research, simplifying an enormous amount of nutritional information—all designed to inspire you to apply this in positive and ongoing ways in your own life. I have deliberately avoided the regular use of footnotes and related bibliography in the text to keep the material simple, flowing, and easy to digest. All of that documentation is available in the back matter, however. With the input of Dr. Buck Levin, *Staying Healthy with Nutrition* now has the most current references, documenting the most current studies, to back up the information provided throughout the book. See the long list of references, citing scientific studies as well as books, listed in the back matter under "Bibliography." The references are divided into the various chapters of this book.

Further research and the interpretation of many scientific studies still have a long way to go. Just because someone finds something to be "true" in a particular study does not make it so. This is part of the learning process, which must involve both the seen and the unseen, the proven and the yet-to-be proven. In many instances, two research groups conducting similar studies come to opposite conclusions, depending on such issues as the economic support for the study and the consciousness of the researchers. So many factors must be incorporated to make a study valid in both scientific and experiential ways. Much of the nutritional scientific dilemma involves differences of interpretation between the "provers" and the "experiencers." I, however, believe that experience comes first, then proof, at least in regard to nutrition.

Some of the material discussed in this book, as in much of the current nutritional marketplace, is still experience waiting to be validated and accepted by the hard-core scientists and the well-designed studies.

But the cutting edge would not exist in innovative medical care if we waited for the provers to accept everything before change is implemented. For example, look at the many native and indigenous cultures throughout the world that have had their own ways of knowing for centuries. Most pharmaceutical and natural remedies vary in effect from person to person. In this way, medicine is always partly experimental or, more accurately, experiential. The information and understanding included in *Staying Healthy with Nutrition* come from my own personal explorations as well as 30 years of practice, combined with the knowledge and experience of many researchers, colleagues, and patients. The practice of good medicine is thus both a science and an art. The first level of good medical care is to do no harm and then, to serve and support people in making positive changes toward better self-care in creating lifestyle balance and, subsequently, optimal health. As technology and nutrition merge, as I discuss throughout this book, we shall continue to experience advances in medical care and the quality of life.

NEW MEDICINE

Happily, as the years pass, there are changes in attitudes and in the application of medical practice, however slow they may be. Out of the will to survive, the high and rising cost of medical care, and the potential help offered from food and supplement products, people have become more concerned and empowered in maintaining their own personal health—and nutrition clearly plays a huge role here. As people are able to maintain better health because they know more, they will need to take fewer drugs throughout their lives or have fewer operations to correct problems that interfere with their lives. Clearly, economics come into play. If the majority of doctors and hospitals make money by treating sick people, and if proper nutrition and other healthy living habits—such as regular exercise, stress management, and positive choices—help prevent disease, then it would be ludicrous for physicians to promote these ideas for fear of financial ruin. Of course this is an overstatement, although I believe it is one aspect of the overall attitude of the medical establishment.

As more people ask their doctors about nutrition, vitamin supplements, detoxification and fasting programs, or the latest herb they heard about, more doctors will attempt to learn about these areas or to add knowledgeable staff to their facilities. These interested and motivated patients will seek out the ever-growing number of doctors and other practitioners to assist them in their journey toward more healthful living programs and more natural therapies. (And then we need to convince insurance companies to cover these health practices as they commonly do medical procedures.) There will always be sick people, from those who abuse themselves to those who are aging, who wish to have and do need medical care. Yet as people become healthier, the medical profession will need to include more doctors who are educators and supporters of health. After all, the word *doctor* comes from the Latin *docere,* meaning "to teach." Ideally your physician becomes a teammate who supports you in your approach to health care or treats you in the most effective and hopefully least toxic way possible. This is the best type of doctor-patient relationship, one of cooperation and mutual respect.

A great deal of knowledge and experience has surfaced in the field of nutrition since this book was first published. An incredible amount of research is now being done on the effects of different diets and various supplements on health and disease. As I mentioned earlier, many new practitioners are calling themselves "nutritionists," and more companies are making very exacting and advanced products for dietary support and nutritional therapeutics (see appendix B for a contact list of these companies). In recent years, many disorders have been described—such as premenstrual syndrome, candida/yeast problems, viral illnesses, chronic fatigue and immune disorders, and food allergy/sensitivity reactions—that have instigated the development of innovative nutritional programs and products. I discuss many of these trends, discoveries, and nutritional programs in this book.

BASIC WESTERN NUTRITION

The public's basic knowledge of and focus on nutrition have also created a major shift in recent years. People's idea of the balanced diet has changed from the archaic "four food group" approach to meals (containing a meat, a dairy food, a cereal grain, and fruits and vegetables) to a more natural diet that is lower in fat, protein, and refined carbohydrates. The newer pyramids of healthier nutrition suggest such a diet. These offer some improvement in the educational basis of a healthy diet. Whole foods, unprocessed and without chemical additives, as Nature itself presents them to lucky us, are again becoming the mainstay of the "new American diet." But, of course, as Nature is continually polluted, so are our food supply and our health.

Dietary habits, the ways people eat, have also changed over the years. Choosing nourishing foods is becoming a top priority for many of us concerned with achieving and maintaining optimum health. Meals are becoming simpler, containing fewer foods. Many people follow the basic principles of food combining—eating foods in certain combinations for best digestion and absorption. The time of day when food is consumed, the setting, how we feel when eating, and how the food is prepared are all very important as well.

So, reader and fellow eater, let us each take the time to ask ourselves what the best diet is to help us improve and perpetuate our health. Poor nutrition is advertised and available everywhere, and restraint has not been the strongest attribute of the stereotypical American "I want it all now" public. But when we are guided and conditioned early in life about good nutrition, we will make the appropriate and healthful choices as we grow. If we learn to nurture and harvest our gardens, the Earth will continue to nourish us in return with wholesome foods.

A healthy diet most obviously involves common sense. The body sends us messages to change the diet to attune to its real needs; the internal biofeedback system is superb when we cooperate with it rather than override it. Yet many of us follow our desires and taste buds, eating the richer, sweeter, or saltier foods that industry promotes and packaged/processed nutrition provides. It may not seem to matter a great deal in the short term that we follow our passions/addictions rather than our common sense. But this *does* affect how we feel and function now, and it *does* make a difference over the long term, both in our health and in our economy.

THE WEIGHT CHALLENGE— A KEY ISSUE IN WESTERN NUTRITION

It is no secret that the average American is overweight. To many people, the word *diet* means a special program developed to lose those extra pounds that we carry around, followed only until we lose the weight and can then go back to eating the foods that produced the extra fat in the first place. The condition of the body, including one's weight, is an end result of how a person lives: a reflection of the food a person eats and his or her activity level. Therefore, when we wish to change our weight permanently, we must change our lifestyle. Usually this means eating less and exercising more—a dynamic duo that really cannot fail (unless one has a preexisting or particularly limiting condition).

Specifically, this means eating fewer of the richer foods and the sugary and flour foods for which so many of us have developed a special taste; this often requires reprogramming ourselves to find less fattening and caloric foods to replace our bad habits. Eating and weight also have a lot to do with one's emotions, psychological nature, and fear of creativity and change. In my own life, for example, I have tended to stuff myself to hold back feelings (and creativity) trying to flood from my subconscious. I have realized over the years that permanent dietary and weight change do not come easily, but usually take some level of personal transformation, psychological and emotional expression, and new creative outlets—which for me include writing such health books as this one.

Many of us, very early in life, develop body shapes, dietary habits, and specific eating patterns that become deeply ingrained. Family tradition and individual upbringing influence all of us. The early connection between love, emotional bonding, or acceptance with eating and food are common to most cultures, yet the connection is particularly strong in American Jewish and Italian American families, both of which possess a higher-than-average incidence of obesity. Chronic obesity contributes to many major illnesses and disease patterns, such as high blood pressure, heart disease, diabetes, and cancer—and then increased stress and health-care costs.

It is possible that we inherit some disease through inherited eating habits. When attempting to change diet and weight, these deeper patterns are the most difficult to recognize and transform, but they must be dealt with to bring about significant and lasting change. Uprooting unhealthy dietary habits and choices can bring a great deal of stress to traditional family relationships, however. When we cannot eat with our parents and other relatives because of dietary differences, for example, the hardships become especially clear. I experienced this difficulty during my years of nutritional radicalism when I was eating a special vegetarian diet to overcome my overweight issues. The issues of excess consumption and many poor eating and emotional habits were rampant in my family.

MY PERSONAL WEIGHT CHALLENGE

I have struggled with my weight since becoming heavy as a child from eating the average American diet, and plenty of it, during the 1950s and 1960s. I began "dieting" to lose weight at age 13. Yet success didn't come until my later twenties, when I met and began working with my courageous cohort Bethany Argisle, who became an inspiration and provided unwavering support for me to change. Her energy and passion was (and is) more powerful than the force of my eating patterns and addictions, especially when she would place herself between me and the refrigerator, and the telephone. When I would find myself ready to munch and chat when frustration of the inner creative process would arise, Bethany would say, "Go back to your desk and write. We'll eat later." I knew she was serving the higher good and that my task was to align with it.

My weight loss and the other positive health changes that resulted from that hard work became an inspiration for family members, patients, and readers of *Staying Healthy with the Seasons*. For 30 years now, Bethany has been my ally, my career guide and cheerleader, as well as a hands-on coworker for my books, newsletters, and radio shows. She still reviews much of my writing and offers advice to make it all easier for general readers to grasp. Our original publisher at Celestial Arts, David Hinds, deemed Bethany the "queen of user-friendly," and David himself (who passed on too soon) was instrumental in making the first edition of *Staying Healthy with Nutrition* happen.

Following my weight balance in the late 1970s, my new healthy lifestyle highlighted the new way I was eating (natural wholesome foods) compared with how the general public was eating (more refined, packaged, and heavily advertised products). During the 1980s and through today, however, the public's awareness of nutrition has grown. My family's diet, which was excessive and a cause for being overweight, has become healthier. My own dietary patterns also have become less restrictive and more balanced, enough so that I can eat the same meal as my family while at home or, on occasion, at a suitable wholesome restaurant. And I have continued my seasonal and annual detoxification programs over many years, including literally thousands of people in this process several times a year with January (New Year's) and September (autumn) detox groups as well as March and April spring cleansing programs. The positive results we achieve together are so rewarding for both me and my patients, and especially the class participants.

DIET, DISEASE, AND SEASONAL CYCLES

The information available in recent years regarding the relationship of diet to disease has affected the nutritional trends of the American consumer, especially since it concerns the incidence of common chronic and deadly diseases, such as cancer and cardiovascular disease. The 1988 *Surgeon General's Report on Nutrition and Health* put out the new message nationally, and the trend has continued with the great amount of nutritional studies, the new food pyramids, and the recent focus on the growing, rampant obesity in the United States in both adults and children. **The message is loud and clear: Dietary choices influence disease and health in a major way.**

I have a theory that the body has three basic metabolic functions. These are *building* or tonification, *cleansing* or detoxification, and *maintenance* or balance. Maintenance is the main function, but occasionally the body clicks into a detoxification or purification cycle when it must eliminate previous buildup. The bowels become more active and the secreting cells and the mucous membranes work more; mucus may flow out of the body, from the sinuses and nose, for example, often appearing as the result of a cold or allergies. When we continue to eat a congesting or highly processed diet of meat, milk products, breads, or too many foods at once, the condition may worsen. When we listen to the body and drink more liquids and eat lightly, emphasizing the cleansing fruits and vegetables, we may support the detoxification period and feel better.

If the body is in a building or toning cycle, however, and we are not feeding it the fuel and specific nutrients it needs, we may feel a lack of energy and not develop the strength required for future activity. This and other theories presented in this book have evolved into appropriate diets for each cycle. The yearly cycle of diet—introduced in my first book, *Staying Healthy with the Seasons*—is dealt with more thoroughly here in chapters 12 through 14, as well as in my book *The New Detox Diet* (Celestial Arts, 2004).

Our dietary needs change not only with the seasons of the year, but also with the seasons of our lives. For example, as children we need a wholesome, nutrient-rich, building diet to support growth. We use the extra nutrients, oils, and proteins to construct and expand tissues. In our 20s, 30s, and beyond, after we have stopped growing physically, we can get into trouble if we continue with this richer childhood diet. We need to shift to a maintenance-oriented diet of lighter, more fiber- and nutrient-rich natural foods, with occasional periods of fasting or detoxification. As we age even more, our metabolism and activity level often slow down and food requirements decrease further (the need for fresh and wholesome food never changes, however). Continuing the midlife maintenance diet into later life will probably cause weight increase. Thus, responding to our dietary needs and using the nutrients we consume appropriately, both metabolically and through some type of aerobic/fitness activity, is an important day-to-day goal. I see this issue clearly played out with athletes. During their active years, they can eat quite a full and even rich diet, and because of their physical output, their bodies can stay relatively balanced. Upon retirement, however, problems occur when former athletes continue their heavier food intake and eating habits. We all need to adapt to our life changes as well as to the seasons.

> The greatest discovery of any generation is that human beings can alter their lives by altering the attitudes of their minds.
>
> —Albert Schweitzer

As I mentioned earlier, psychological and emotional states also have a great deal to do with how well the body utilizes our nutrition. When we are under stress, we may not digest and absorb our nutrients as well and, at the same time, we may need higher amounts of many vitamins and minerals. Additional supplements may be necessary. The appetite is often a reflection of inner contentment. Many people override their appetite mechanism through regular eating and do not really experience hunger. When we are emotionally upset, feeling insecure or depressed, for example, we may lose our appetite. This is the appropriate response, since the body does not process food well during these times. Not eating allows us to go within more easily to explore our feelings, or lets us express our emotions more freely. Being aware of the need for nourishment via hunger and then relaxing and preparing the body to receive wholesome food in a comfortable setting are important prerequisites for healthy eating. Most people I see do not take the time or make the proper space to eat their food, don't chew thoroughly, and eat too much and too many foods at a time.

Reader, I know that your journey through *Staying Healthy with Nutrition* will inspire you to use nutrition wisely to obtain and maintain your optimum health. I also hope this book inspires other doctors and practitioners toward greater awareness and application of nutrition in their practices. Overall, my goal is to help each of us become our own nutritional doctor in order to best care for ourselves, our family and friends, and the Earth—the source of all real nutrition. Knowledge is the key. Open the door and explore the realms of your being. Yearn for and learn to "hu-manifest" the life that you are meant to bring forth. Feeding yourself well, naturally, wholesomely, and in balance will provide all the nutrients that you need to nourish your complete self.

When we shift our attitudes, we can change our entire lives. When I was in the midst of my first cleanse in 1975, for example, I felt so good that I told myself, "This is how I want to feel, and I will do what it takes to continue to feel this way. It matters what I put into my mouth; it becomes who I am and what I think and do. Therefore, I am going to treat myself with love and feed myself more natural, vital foods." I said all that, and did it as well. It was the beginning of a health change that still rewards me 30 years later. That is a blessing.

So, love yourself and care for your body with good foods and exercise. It is the only body you have, and if you treat it right, give it what it needs, in return it will care for you for life.

Blessings of health. Rise and shine, and embrace the Divine in You!

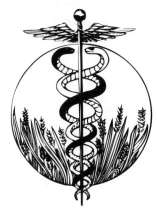

Part 1

The Building Blocks

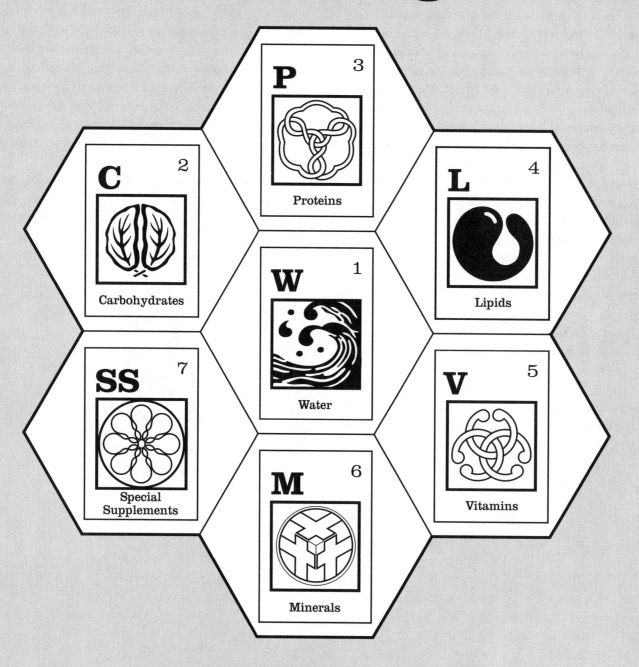

The human body needs food to function. Food is our body's fuel—our source of energy. We need food and its nutrients to maintain life and promote cell and tissue growth. The building blocks of our diet provide our sources for energy, biochemical support, and the medium in which our nutrients can function. These essentials for life include the macronutrients—*carbohydrates, proteins,* and *fats;* the micronutrients—*vitamins* and *minerals,* so important to our body chemistry; and *water*—the solvent for all soluble ingredients in the blood and cells. Water makes up by far the largest percentage of the body's volume. We get all these essential nutrients from fruits, vegetables, grains, legumes, nuts and seeds, dairy foods, and meats—the basic food groups that comprise our diet.

On the desk in my office, my purified drinking water
is in a special gold-amber bottle engraved with the slogan
"Nectar of the Golden Life of Health and Vitality."
I believe **water** to be that substance.

Chapter 1

Water

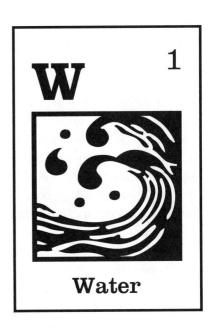

Water

ater is the medium in which all other nutrients are found. Three simple molecules—2 hydrogen and 1 oxygen—bind together to form 1 molecule of water, the most abundant and important substance both on Earth and in the human body. The hydrogen and oxygen atoms in water are never alone, however. Water is the universal solvent, as most other substances on Earth dissolve in water in varying degrees. In a mountain stream or in our bloodstream, minerals and other substances are always naturally present. Pure (100%) water does not exist naturally on our planet. There is no place that is just water, like distilled water; there are always minerals and other substances contained. The planet's natural water varies in mineral content, as does the water found within the human body. The adult body is at least 60% water, but this percentage is even higher before birth. As late as 32 weeks of gestation, the fetus is more than 80% water and is surrounded by the oceanlike water of amniotic fluid. The fetus continuously swallows this fluid for nourishment—each day about 250 milliliters for every kilogram of body weight (the equivalent for an adult of about 5 gallons per day). Without this constant swallowing of water and nutrients, the fetus would become malnourished and the digestive system itself could not be properly formed.

Water is the primary component of all the bodily fluids—blood, lymph, digestive juices, urine, tears, and sweat. Water is involved in almost every bodily function: circulation, digestion, absorption, and elimination of wastes, to name a few. Water carries the electrolytes, mineral salts that help convey electrical currents in the body; the major minerals that make up these salts are calcium, chloride, magnesium, potassium, and sodium. Water requirements vary greatly from person to person. The climate in which we live, our activity level, and our diet all influence our individual needs for water.

WATER AND HEALING

Anything that nourishes can heal, but among all nutrients—perhaps all substances of any kind—water is unsurpassed in its ability to heal. We turn to water for healing (and feelings) in all dimensions of our lives—from hot tubs to hydrotherapy, from bathing to baptism—and the mere sight of water, a mountain lake or ocean tide, can ease the pain of psychological wounds.

The pain of physical wounds is also healed through water. When we're injured, our bloodstream carries repair substances to the injury site. About 81% of that bloodstream is water. When toxic substances from the environment make their way inside our bodies, our urine (95% water) or our sweat (99% water) usually carries the toxins back out. Skin wounds heal most quickly in a wet environment, because water accelerates re-epithelialization (the making of new skin) and the rate of wound contraction. Hyaluronan, the well-researched glycosaminoglycan in skin, is believed to promote skin healing by increasing skin hydration.

In these and countless other ways, water is fundamental to life. Without clean water, we cannot experience optimum health, but by practically every public health standard issued during the past 50 years, humans have not experienced optimum health. One of the reasons for this fact is simple: **the Earth's water is in crisis.** *Crisis*—from the Greek word *krisis,* meaning "turning point" or "point of decision"—is exactly the right word to describe our present-day relationship with water, both nutritionally and ecologically. The resolution of this crisis is so fundamental to our personal health and the health of our planet that we must look more closely at water than we look at any other nutrient. What is happening to our water is simple: it is Drying Up, Getting Diverted, and Becoming Toxic.

Drying Up

On average, we need about 12 cups worth of water each day to stay hydrated. These cups don't have to come from our drinking water, however. They can include the water our food contains, as well as the water that is released when our food digests. In the United States, we average about 4 cups of water from a day's food, and the breakdown of this food provides us with an additional cup. But we actually need to drink the remaining 7 cups! According to Wirthlin Worldwide, a market research company, 20% of us drink no water at all, and 42% of us consume a mere 2 glasses or fewer. At the same time, we are consuming, on average, 1.8 cups of coffee, 1.3 cups of soda, 1.2 cups of milk, and 1.1 cups of juice a day.

Without enough water, we basically dry ourselves out (the technical term is *dehydration*). In the medical research it is linked to a long list of chronic health problems, including adult-onset diabetes, arthritis, asthma, back pain, cataracts, chronic fatigue syndrome, colitis, depression, heartburn, high blood pressure, high cholesterol, kidney stones, lupus, migraine, multiple sclerosis, and muscular dystrophy. Even 3 to 4 cups a day is not enough to lower risk for these problems. We need to increase our water intake!

Eerily similar to the health crisis in our own bodies, where dehydration is increasing our risk of chronic disease, we are experiencing a crisis with the water in our environment. There is a fascinating and probably not accidental set of events going on in many communities, as some bodies of water in the United States are drying up. Many rivers no longer reach their destination, having been diverted for irrigation or dammed up for generation of hydroelectric power. Chronic environmental problems—like decrease in salmon runs up the Columbia River in the Pacific Northwest—are riddling the country. According to the International Rivers Network based in Berkeley, California, over 77% of all river discharge in North America is affected by dams. The reservoir of water created by a large dam can trap almost all of the sediment in a river. When the dynamic flow of this sediment is lost, wildlife habitats downstream lose their ecological balance. Currently, 40 different species of freshwater fish in North America are endangered—largely as a result of this process.

Getting Diverted

All water needs to get where it was originally designed to go, and in the case of humans, that means directly into our bodies and not detoured as a result of drinking soda pop or coffee. Most people don't realize it, but coffee typically upsets our water balance, even though it consists mostly of water. Coffee is a diuretic and can actually cause us to excrete more water than it contains. Soda pop, with so much concentrated sugar, can also upset our water balance. When the highly sugar-concentrated water in soda pop enters our digestive system, it can cause the body to "steal" water from elsewhere to dilute the soda pop and make it less concentrated. This soda pop problem is referred to as *hyperosmotic load.*

Cutting back on coffee and pop are not the only steps we can take to improve our water status, however. We could also take some environmental steps by helping water reach its natural destination. Water likes to move down (from mountain snowpacks to lowland watersheds) and further down (through soil and rock and to groundwater and underground aquifers). When water passes through limestone, it picks up calcium. When it passes through dolomite, it picks up magnesium. If we leave water alone—rather than diverting it into reservoirs or damming its flow—it will typically become more mineralized and more supportive of our health. Studies in Sweden have shown that if everyone in that country were to drink water with the highest naturally occurring magnesium levels, death from heart attacks would drop by about 19%. In fact, increases in water magnesium as small as 6 mg (milligrams) per liter might be able to reduce deaths from ischemic heart disease by 10%. Similar studies in Poland and South Africa have come up with comparable conclusions. A 1-quart bottle of highly mineralized springwater can contain well over 75% of the recommended daily allowance (RDA) for magnesium. By comparison, tap water in most U.S. cities contains fewer than 10 mg per quart, or about 3% of the RDA.

Becoming Toxic

Some toxins, like MTBE (methyl tertiary butyl ether), have been placed there "accidentally." MTBE is the gasoline additive used in the United States since the 1980s to enhance octane and cut air pollution. Scientists at the U.S. Geological Survey have estimated that as many as 250,000 underground tanks used to store gasoline may have accidentally leaked MTBE into nearby soil and groundwater, contaminating as many as 9,000 community wells in 31 states. MTBE is one of several hundred substances that are now accidentally present as water percolates through the Earth.

Alongside these toxic substances that have accidentally found their way into soil and groundwater are substances we have put there intentionally. For example, a total of about 150 million tons of solid waste is deposited in our country's 7,500 municipal landfills each year. Treated sewage sludge used as agricultural fertilizer, municipal waste incineration, volatile organic compounds (VOCs) released into the air by manufacturing plants—all of these deliberate and legally sanctioned practices create a toxic pathway for water.

The U.S. Environmental Protection Agency (EPA) currently monitors about 80 toxic substances found in our drinking water. These substances include chlorination by-products like trihalomethanes (THMs), heavy metals like cadmium, pesticides like alachlor, and plastics like styrene. Because water contaminants can originate from a wide variety of sources, the exact combination and level of toxins found in water differs from region to region and depends on manufacturing and other pollution-related activities. Municipal wastewater-treatment plants, land-based disposal of treated sewage sludge, agricultural use of treated sewage sludge as a fertilizer, sewage sludge incineration, open lagoon treatment of toxic waste, and municipal waste incineration are included in the list of practices that can contaminate our drinking water. For example, water in the Mississippi River—the longest river in the United States—gets a daily dose of cadmium, mercury, and lead from a large wastewater treatment facility in St. Paul, Minnesota. Freshwater regions like the Great Lakes also get daily toxic input from industrial activities along the shoreline. This toxic input includes asbestos, dioxins, pesticides, and polychlorinated biphenyls (PCBs). The PCBs in the Great Lakes exceed international agreements for the region.

Although water purification plants that process water for human consumption take steps to minimize toxins, toxic compounds are present at potentially health-damaging levels in municipal drinking water nationwide. Over 1,100 potentially toxic compounds have been identified in drinking water across the United States. A 2001 survey of 374 communities in 12 states found the pesticide atrazine, a reproductive and immune system toxin, to be present in 96% of all water supplies tested. Drinking water in almost 30% of these communities contained at least 5 pesticides.

When water picks up toxins, the EPA has a special word for it: "impaired" (that is, the water cannot be used for the full range or purposes for which we might want to use it). The EPA estimates that 85% of all river miles and 68% of all lake acreage in the United States are currently impaired. It might be unhealthy for fishing, or swimming, or drinking. And exactly what counts as "fit for drinking" is unfortunately a matter of much debate. Toxic substances found in municipal drinking water across the United States have been indirectly linked to many chronic, degenerative diseases, including Alzheimer's, asthma, most forms of cancer, infertility, Parkinson's, and rheumatoid arthritis.

I use the word *indirectly* here because contaminated water has not been shown to directly cause disease in some simple, straightforward way. In fact, toxic substances found in drinking water may *never* be shown to *directly* cause disease, for three reasons. First, contaminants in a single glass of water are present in very small amounts, and a lifelong study would be needed to measure the effects over one's lifetime. Second, water toxins work behind the scenes, compromising our health at a largely invisible cellular level. They disrupt the energy-producing mechanisms inside our cells, they disturb chemical signals that are sent across our cell membranes, and they drain our nutrient supplies by asking our livers to work overtime. I am convinced that the negative impact of contaminated water is real, even if it is difficult to prove. We need to drink water that contains as few toxins as possible.

OUR DRINKING WATER

Fortunately, awareness of the urgent need to address water pollution is growing, both nationally and internationally, and healing our waters and providing safe and tasty drinking water are becoming a major industry in the way of filtered water systems, international springwaters, designer water, flavored waters, juice waters, and more, including nutrient-enhanced waters, making a market splash. This chapter offers a synergistic collation of the most current, usable information on water safety and toxicity. Much water information is purported to be fact by business interests, yet scientific study is lacking at this time. Surely this will change, so look for upcoming data on this crucial subject.

Because water is a basic life need, a "life force" if you will, the government and the people should spend more energy and dollars researching how to keep it safe for human consumption. My concern is that our governments will wait too long to correct the current water problems, much like modern Western medicine focuses on end-stage disease rather than on preventive medicine (although this is changing in some circles). Keeping people well and learning more about the

factors that affect their well-being must be a primary goal. Healing and maintaining the environment, keeping our basic elements (water, air, and food) clean and wholesome, is a good place to start!

Drinking water has become an issue of concern. Many water tests have shown that tap water is not totally safe. We need to ask what role drinking tap water plays in our health. What is its subtle effect on biochemical processes in our body, and what is its relationship to symptoms of illness or chronic disease? Not enough research has come out to date showing how tap water and its contents influence our health. The water supply in many U.S. cities has a high sodium level, which has been correlated with an increased likelihood of high blood pressure and subsequent cardiovascular disease. Soft water, in which a high level of sodium has replaced such biologically important minerals as calcium and magnesium, has also been implicated in reducing our resistance to heart disease.

With the trend toward using pure and natural products in personal health care, city tap water has come to be considered by many a processed, unnatural substance, containing potentially hazardous chemical additives. No wonder bottled water has become a huge industry in the past decade! In 2003, bottled water (of all kinds) was one of the fastest growing segments of the U.S. beverage market. More than 6.4 billion gallons were sold at a wholesale market value of more than $8.3 billion. These sales represented a 7.5% increase from the 2002 level, and the sixth straight year of surging growth in this sector.

For the most part, city water is heavily chlorinated to kill germs and fluoridated to prevent tooth decay; some cities add calcium hydroxide or other alkaline substances to change the pH (acidity) of the water so it does not corrode pipes. Chlorine and other additives used to treat water can react with other organic chemicals to produce chlorinated hydrocarbons that may act as carcinogens. For example, chloramines, including chloroform and other trihalomethanes, are formed in water from chlorine and such organic matter as ammonia or decaying leaves. Water pipes may contribute chemicals or metals such as copper or lead.

The EPA currently oversees implementation of the Safe Drinking Water Act (SDWA) of 1974—the nation's primary law for regulating safety of tap water. As part of its responsibility, the EPA monitors groundwater throughout the United States and has special enforcement powers to protect areas in which a single underground aquifer serves as the primary source of drinking water. Under the SDWA, the EPA monitors levels of approximately 100 potential toxins in drinking water. It also establishes safety ranges for each of these toxins.

CHOOSING YOUR DRINKING WATER

I urge people to use purified drinking water and to avoid the faucet. I personally have not drunk tap water in more than 20 years; instead, I have used well water or springwater collected from mountain or underground sources (unfortunately these waters can be contaminated also) or, more recently, home-filtered tap water using a reverse osmosis (RO) system (see page 21). But lately there have even been questions regarding the purity of bottled waters and the effectiveness of filters. What is the right thing to do? Clearly, scientific research and the marketing information of companies selling bottled water and the various water cleaners may differ. After all, advertising has a big influence on our nutrition in general and certainly has been (and continues to be) a hindrance that must be overcome to achieve a healthier diet and lifestyle. The government can only protect the consumer from gross misrepresentation and not subtle interpretation of "facts."

Let's look at our drinking water choices before we decide what the right thing to do is. Because water is second in importance only to air for sustaining life, we *do* want to do the best we can with the current knowledge and inner guidance we have, without being too fanatical. Taste and smell can help us assess if our water is good for us. However, the presence of negative health factors may not alter taste or smell. Because of space limitations, there is much technical information I cannot include in this discussion; thus my goal is to give you the basics about drinking water so you can at least ask yourself what is best for you. The first step of good nutrition is to know the origin, processing, and contents of anything we take into our bodies. Now let's talk about the many sources of water available.

Possible Contaminants in Our Drinking Water (Municipal and Well Water)

Microorganisms (bacteria, viruses, parasites)

Disinfectants (chlorine, chloramines)

Disinfectant by-products (bromates, chlorites, trihalomethanes)

Inorganic chemicals (heavy metals, asbestos, nitrates, nitrites)

Organic chemicals (solvents, pesticides, plastics, resins)

Radionucleotides (radium, uranium)

Tap Water

Most tap water comes from groundwater or from surface reservoirs formed from rivers, streams, and lakes. Groundwater refers to the subterranean reservoirs that hold much of the Earth's water and supply nearly all the rural drinking water and about half of city water supplies. The water from these sources goes through local treatment plants, many of which use an old process of settling tanks, filtration through sand and gravel, and then chemicals to clean up the water so it is fit for human consumption.

All of the categories I listed in the table of possible contaminants (adjacent) contain drinking water toxins that are currently monitored by the EPA using National Primary Drinking Water Standards. Maximum allowable contamination levels (or MCLs) are currently in place for about 80 toxic substances present in our tap water. The MCLs constitute mandatory standards, and a public water system is not allowed to exceed these standards without legal penalty. In addition to the MCLs, a second set of standards called the Secondary Drinking Water Standards, established in 1992, help ensure the safety of tap water. However, compliance with these secondary standards is voluntary, not mandatory, and substances regulated under these secondary standards are not regarded by the EPA as posing a significant health risk. The position of the EPA on these secondary substances—including aluminum and fluoride—remains open to question, because several have been well-researched and show significant health risks for some individuals. Both sets of standards are available online at www.epa.gov/water/laws.html.

Contaminants found in surface water and groundwater are also routinely monitored by the U.S. Geological Survey (USGS), which operates a Toxic Substances Hydrology Program (http://toxics.usgs.gov) and a National Water Quality Laboratory (http://nwql.usgs.gov). Pesticides, VOCs, arsenic, bacteria, and radionucleotides are among the potential toxins monitored in surface water and groundwater by the USGS.

In 2002 the Environmental Working Group (EWG), a not-for-profit environmental research organization based in Washington, D.C., completed a study on tap water quality in 42 states and found repeated violations of Primary Drinking Water Standards. Among other findings, the EWG determined that:

- More than 16 million people in 1,258 communities had been served tap water containing chlorination by-products like chloramines or THM at levels exceeding the MCLs for 12 consecutive months.

- Although large cities like Philadelphia, Pittsburgh, San Francisco, and Washington, D.C., served above-MCL contaminated tap water, more than 1,100 smaller towns with populations under 10,000 also served tap water contaminated with chlorination by-products.

- In the case of some contaminants, like THM, levels found in tap water were more than 5 times the maximum allowable level.

In a 1995 study of 26 U.S. communities on the East Coast and in the Midwest, pesticides used in the nonorganic production of corn were found to be routinely present in public drinking water. The pesticide atrazine, for example, was found in 25 out of 26 drinking water systems surveyed. In 5 of the 25 communities, atrazine levels exceeded the MCL standard, 5 or more different pesticides were found in 11 out of 26 water supplies.

One area I am especially concerned about with respect to tap water is toxic fertilizers. The recycling of industrial waste into fertilizers exposes soil and groundwater to a wide variety of toxins. The numbers here are mind-boggling. Between 1990 and 1995, 270 million

pounds of industrial waste were shipped either directly to farms or to fertilizer manufacturers across the United States; 80 million tons came from the steel industry alone. The California Public Interest Research Group (CALPIRG) Charitable Trust tested 29 fertilizers from 12 states in 1998 and found all 29 to contain potentially toxic metals, including aluminum, cadmium, lead, mercury, and uranium. Astonishing as it may be, heavy metals in fertilizer are not regulated with respect to health impact, although they are regulated with respect to land disposal as a way of preventing leakage from lined landfills. The study found 20 of 29 fertilizers to contain metals in excess of land disposal restriction levels. This problem is going to get worse, and we need to take action now to protect our tap water.

Many minerals and chemicals are used for "purification," including chlorine, alum or sodium aluminum salts, soda, ash, phosphates, calcium hydroxide, and activated carbon. Yet this process may not clear all of the many environmental pollutants, which can include fertilizers and insecticides, chemicals and wastes from industry, and air pollutants such as lead or radon. Toxic organic chemicals and petroleum spills can also pollute large amounts of water. Because much of this pollution affects groundwater as well as surface waters, most municipal or artesian well drinking waters are at risk and deserve our concern.

A January 1990 *Consumer Reports* analysis suggested that the three drinking water pollutants of most concern were lead, radon, and nitrates. Every year, the Agency for Toxic Substances and Disease Registry (ATSDR) publishes a list of the most hazardous toxins in U.S. soils, water, and air. In 2003, this list was headed up by arsenic, lead, mercury, vinyl chloride, and PCBs (polychlorinated biphenyls). Of these five substances, we are particularly likely to be exposed to arsenic and lead through drinking water. And although much further down on the ATSDR list, two other substances of particular concern are radon and nitrates.

Lead may contaminate the water of more than 40 million Americans. It occurs mainly from corrosion of water pipes, from lead solder in plumbing, and from lead in brass faucets. The possibility of contamination is of greatest concern to people living in homes more than 30 years old, whose pipes contain more lead, and for families with young children, who are more sensitive to lead toxicity (see chapter 6, Minerals, for further discussion on this topic). Testing for lead is relatively easy and inexpensive. Reverse osmosis will remove lead; solid carbon filters may also remove it to some degree.

Mercury and **arsenic** also contaminate our waters. Mercury is the more serious concern since it is toxic; some naturally-occurring arsenic is tolerated by the human body. Mercury consumption via fish is now common. Most people who consume ocean fish several times weekly have elevated levels of mercury. Since mercury is a toxin to the nervous system, this is a potential problem, although each person seems to handle mercury loads differently. (For a more thorough discussion of mercury see page 241 in chapter 6, Minerals).

Radon, a radioactive gas, is a by-product of uranium and is found in the Earth's crust. High radon gas levels are associated with an increased risk of lung cancer. This carcinogenic element can be present in any home in levels high enough to cause concern, but it is more likely to be found in Arizona, in North Carolina, and in the northeastern United States. Groundwater and water that comes from wells have a higher incidence of contamination. Municipal waters that come from lakes, rivers, and reservoirs are usually low in radon. When present in the water, radon can be released into the air when someone is showering, laundering, or washing dishes. Radon in the air at home can be tested with several new devices available on the market. If present in the water in high amounts, radon can be removed with carbon filtration, but this system must be attached to the home's entire water system.

Nitrates are present mostly in groundwater sources that have agricultural contamination; these waters may also then have higher amounts of toxic pesticides and herbicides. High nitrate levels are of greatest risk to infants and seriously ill people. Nitrates are converted to nitrites by certain intestinal bacteria; these nitrites may alter the hemoglobin molecule, converting it to methemoglobin, which cannot carry oxygen. In rural communities, pregnant women and families with infants should test their water for nitrates. If it is present in high amounts, either reverse osmosis or distillation systems will help to clear the nitrate molecules.

Other major concerns in drinking water are the chemicals that are released into our waters by industry and the agricultural chemical pesticides, herbicides, and fertilizers that run off into local waters. These organic chemicals are more toxic and carcinogenic at lower levels than many other contaminants. The THMs formed in chlorinated water are also a carcinogenic concern.

With all these possible health threats, however, the government would like us to believe that we should have no concerns about our drinking water. Clearly, tap water consumption usually does not cause immediate or significant health problems unless it is contaminated with infectious organisms. Millions of people drink water from this source every day, although many avoid drinking it straight because of the taste. More research studying the relationship of drinking water to chronic disease needs to be done. Until we know more about tap water (and even well water) and its long-range effects on well-being, it is better to be careful and not drink it. Unless we've been able to analyze the tap water (and even well water) that we are planning to drink, it is best to avoid it whenever we can make water of known quality available. It may be worthwhile to analyze questionable water for toxic chemicals and metals, as well as to analyze mineral content, hardness, and pH. Several U.S. companies analyze water, including Water Test in New Hampshire, National Testing Labs in Ohio, and Suburban Water Testing Labs in Pennsylvania. They all have toll-free 800 numbers.

Ever since 1998 and the first airing of the PBS television special "The Poisoning of America," we've been aware of the clear dangers associated with our water. Although some countries have concerns about infectious water, that problem is minimal for Americans. Our woes are problems of modern technology—toxic chemical wastes, farming wastes, and heavy metals. Yet technology can also help us correct these difficulties. We have made some progress with filtration, purification, and distillation through more chemicals and water units, but we still have a ways to go. I believe we can do better. I also believe it is going to take a half century or more to clean up our waters and counteract the destruction we've done to our planet. Thus, the next two or three generations will need to be the "dismantlers," the cleanup generation. Let us hope this process is successful.

Well Water

Well water comes primarily from groundwater supplies and can vary greatly in its mineral content. Some is very low in most minerals, while other well water is a rich source of such beneficial nutritional minerals as iron, zinc, selenium, magnesium, or calcium. Unfortunately, groundwater may also contain toxic heavy metals or such agricultural and industrial chemical pollutants as pesticides, herbicides, radon, asbestos, or hydrocarbons (gasoline by-products). If your water source is a well, have the water analyzed for bacteria, mineral content, and organic chemical pollutants. With a clean bill of health, go ahead and use this potentially nutritious water freely.

Springwater

Springwater is the "natural" water found in surface or underground springs. Some companies retrieve and bottle this water. Other than being disinfected (chlorine may be used to this end), springwater is not processed. It tastes very different from tap water and, to me, is a refreshing drink. The mineral content depends on the region from which the water is taken and on whether it is surface or underground water (surface springwater is relatively low in minerals). For example, the lakes, streams, and springwater from the southeastern and northwestern regions of the United States are relatively low in minerals, and this "soft" water may increase the incidence of cardiovascular disease. The Midwest, in contrast, has high-mineral underground waters, and the farm people who drink this unchlorinated well water have a lower cardiovascular disease rate. Of course, there may be other lifestyle factors that contribute to this finding.

Just as groundwater can be polluted, springwater can also be contaminated. It is a good idea to have springwater checked out or to get full reports or summaries of tests from companies selling springwater. Ideally, these are independent lab reports performed yearly. Also, find out if the water is bottled at the source or transported and then treated and bottled. (Water bottled at the source is preferable.) Although springwater can be costly, it is high on the list of drinkable waters.

Some water experts suggest that three ideal characteristics of drinking water are total dissolved solids of about 300 parts per million (ppm), hardness (containing at least 170 mg/l of calcium carbonate), and an alkaline pH (over 7.0), to reduce leaching of metals from pipes. Springwater and well waters may fit into these categories.

Mineral Water

Most waters are mineral waters—that is, they contain minerals. In California, the standard for bottled mineral water is more than 500 ppm of dissolved minerals. Underground bubbly water, called "natural sparkling water," usually contains lots of minerals as well as carbon dioxide (CO_2). Many companies bottling this "mineral" water must inject carbon dioxide back into the water, however, because it is easily lost between the ground and the bottle. Seltzer is any water that is carbonated with carbon dioxide; it is usually filtered tap water. Club soda is essentially the same, although it usually has more minerals added, particularly magnesium sulfate, potassium sulfate, and sodium bicarbonate. These types of waters can also be polluted, although any bottled carbonated water would be free of microorganisms, as they cannot live in that environment. Generally, though, they should be checked out for mineral levels and chemicals if you consume them in any quantity. I do not recommend large amounts of these carbonated waters, however. The carbon dioxide can get into the blood and affect the acid-alkaline balance, although the body usually handles this easily through respiration or kidney filtration.

Filtered Water

Filtration, or purification, involves the removal of extraneous matter—be it chemicals, metals, or bacteria—from water. Legally, anything called a "purifier" must remove 99.75% of incoming bacteria. Americans are purchasing about 2 million home filtering systems annually, and there are a great many models and types from which to choose, including carbon filters, both granulated and solid, and reverse osmosis. (Distillation will be discussed on page 22.) All filters that are placed at or near the faucet are referred to as point-of-use (POU) filters, as opposed to point-of-entry (POE) filters. It is a good idea to educate yourself about water filtration before purchasing a home unit. In the long run, home filters/purifiers are the least expensive and safest way to obtain safe, good-tasting drinking water.

Activated carbon (AC) is the most common type of filter. Carbon, used for centuries as a filtering substance, is "activated" by exposing it to chemicals at high temperatures and steam in the absence of oxygen. That gives the carbon a large surface on which to attach and absorb contaminants. Most carbon filtration units mechanically and biomagnetically (ionically) filter the water and remove the unpleasant appearance, odor, and taste by cleaning it of bacteria, parasites, most viruses, chlorine, and the heavier minerals and particulate matter. However, carbon is best at removing organic chemicals and chlorine and isn't perfect for all microorganisms and metals. Basically, these systems will filter out any particles or organisms over 0.04 microns, or whatever the size of the filter pores. The filters can collect bacteria and sediment, however; as a result, there is some concern that they may breed bacteria and dump it back into the water. **Hot water should not be run through carbon filters because it can cause contaminant release.** Carbon is excellent at trapping the larger molecules, chemicals, and larger microorganisms; it is not good at removing inorganic minerals, including fluoride bound strongly to sodium or calcium, the way it is added to municipal waters. Despite these limitations, solid carbon filtration is believed to be relatively effective (although this point is still controversial) at removing many of the toxic minerals with higher molecular weights, such as lead or mercury.

The two main types of carbon filters are granulated carbon and solid carbon block filters. The granulated carbon filter has air spaces between the carbon particles to trap bacteria and remove it from the water; but the bacteria can multiply within the air spaces. Silver is used in most granulated filters to assist in killing the bacteria. These silver-impregnated filters help reduce the bacterial growth within the filter, but there are concerns about ineffectiveness and silver toxicity. Although granulated carbon filters are economical, their use is short-lived and their safety is definitely questionable. For these reasons, I do not recommend them.

The **solid carbon block** (with its surrounding filter) alleviates the concern of microorganism con-

tamination. Not only can the filtering surface area of this denser carbon bed clean much more water but, because there is very little oxygen or supply nutrients within the filter, the germs will not thrive. To be safe, however, if the filter is not used for a day or longer, let the water run through it for 10 to 20 seconds before drinking. Research has demonstrated that these units also trap more chemicals, organic pollutants, radon, and asbestos than the looser granulated carbon filters. Some companies that sell solid carbon block water filters are Multi-Pure, Ametek, Omnipure, and Amway.

A key factor in determining what microorganisms are filtered out by a solid carbon block filter is the filter's micron rating. A highly efficient carbon block filter would have a rating of no greater than 1 micron, for example, and can filter out microorganisms 1 micron (micrometer) or greater, including *Giardia lamblia*, *Cyptosporidium parvum, Entamoeba histolytica,* and *Toxoplasma gondii.* Asbestos is also removed mechanically from filtered water by a 1 micron–rated solid carbon block. An activated carbon block removes most chemicals by adsorption (by electromagnetically attracting the chemicals to the block itself) as opposed to mechanically (by forcing the chemicals through small openings). Chemicals removed in this way usually include chloramines, chlordanes, lead, mercury, MTBE, PCBs, toxaphene, and VOCs like toluene and xylene.

Carbon filters are rated by volume of water treated, because they can hold only a limited amount of sediment. They should be changed regularly to avoid dumping more bacteria and chemicals back into the drinking water and because the filtration slows down when they near the end of their effectiveness. A carbon filter may clean roughly 400 to 1,000 gallons, and each unit may vary depending on the amount of sediment in the incoming water. For best results, a unit should probably be changed at about 75% of its maximum capacity. Figure your average daily usage and mark the time for change on your calendar. Activated carbon filters and purifiers, although they are more expensive than using tap water, are usually less expensive than distillers or units that use reverse osmosis.

Some authorities believe **reverse osmosis** (RO) is the best way to purify water. Under pressure, usually from the tap, water flows through special membranes with microporous holes the size of a water molecule.

These pores allow water molecules to pass through while rejecting the larger inorganic and organic materials. RO filters can remove much smaller particles than carbon block filters because of their microporous holes. For example, although a carbon block filter rated at 1 micron could remove particles 1 micron or greater, an RO filter could remove particles as small as 0.009 micron, about 100 times smaller.

RO units usually have two or three filtering mechanisms. First is a sedimentation filter, which merely allows particulate matter to settle. Then comes the RO filter. It is followed by a carbon filter that removes contaminants that cannot reliably be removed by the RO filter, including VOCs (like solvent residues) and THMs. With this system, nearly 100% of the organic material is removed, along with almost all the minerals. RO systems that use thin film composite (TFC) membranes also need carbon block prefilters, because the free chlorine found in tap water, which can deteriorate the TFC membrane, must be removed before the water is passed through the RO filter.

RO units range from small home units to those of industrial size. Home units can make from 3 to 10 gallons a day. They are energy efficient, as they require only tap water pressure, yet they are not water efficient. Until recently, these units were very expensive, but now there are good units available at competitive prices, about $300 to $700. Because the life of the RO filter is usually about 5 years, the price per gallon of water is approximately 20 to 30 cents. The carbon filter (and possibly the RO membrane) in this type of system should be replaced every year or so, and this is relatively inexpensive. Disadvantages of RO units include their bulky size, the limitation of water production determined by the size of the holding tank (usually 1 to 2 gallons), and the time involved to prepare the water for drinking (often 3 to 6 hours per gallon). The units produce many gallons of "wastewater" per gallon of drinking water because only 10% to 25% of the incoming water goes through the unit; waste can run between 2 and 30 gallons daily depending on the unit's efficiency. This is not ideal in arid climates, although this wastewater can be collected for other uses, such as watering gardens and plants.

RO units may not clear all bacteria and chemicals, but the addition of carbon filtration or purification makes them efficient. On the other hand, RO units remove almost all minerals (high-calcium waters may clog their filters), which many authorities feel are an important component in our drinking water. (Earlier in this chapter, I gave the example of naturally occurring magnesium in groundwater and mentioned research studies showing prevention of heart disease with consumption of magnesium-rich water.) Concern over the same hazard of leaching body minerals by drinking distilled water exclusively is not yet well-founded scientifically, although people drinking only these waters while fasting run the risk of depleting themselves more rapidly. Deionized water, however—different from RO or distilled—should not be used for drinking, as it can deplete body minerals more readily.

Distilled Water

The distillation process involves vaporizing water (turning it into steam) in one chamber and then condensing it into liquid in a separate chamber. This removes most minerals, organisms, and chemicals from the water. Chemicals that have a higher boiling point than water, however—like the VOC xylene—will not be removed by distillation. There is also some concern that certain volatile organic chemicals will vaporize and recondense into the second chamber's water; therefore, distillation should be preceded by solid carbon filtration. There is also concern that heating water to 212 degrees Fahrenheit before drinking it changes the water so it has a different biochemical effect in the body. Home distillers are fairly expensive and require electrical energy; furthermore, it takes significant time for the water to be distilled, usually 5 hours or more per gallon, so this limits the amount available for use.

Distilled water contains no minerals (as mentioned earlier, distillation takes out everything except volatile chemicals). Therefore, when consumed, it tends to attract minerals (and toxins) to balance with the other body fluids. The regular consumption of distilled water, especially by someone who may already be slightly deficient, can cause mineral deficiencies. Fasting for long periods exclusively on distilled water to pull out toxins is not recommended because of the potential mineral depletions it can create. However, when doing extractions (as in making herbal teas), distilled water may help bring out the most in the medicinal properties of the herbs. Also, during detoxification diets, distilled water may be suggested because it may be more effective for this process, having a stronger "magnetic" charge to pull out toxins.

A note on demineralized water: Many nutritional advocates, mostly the elders, recommend drinking demineralized water because they believe that the inorganic minerals contained naturally in some waters are not usable by the human body, and that these naturally dissolved inorganic minerals may even cause problems. This is simply not true; many of the minerals we acquire are in the inorganic or salt state and are not part of organic tissues. They can still be assimilated and used by the body. The mineral levels in water, however, are not anywhere near sufficient to satisfy body needs. Cooking foods in demineralized water pulls more minerals from them, whereas using water containing natural minerals will lessen this loss and possibly even improve food values. Furthermore, many of the dissolved solids—such as the trace minerals selenium, zinc, or silica—found in natural waters are associated with lower cancer rates in the people who consume them than in people who consume treated or demineralized water. Many of the cultures in which people live long healthy lives are located in regions with mineral-rich mountain waters. These waters have always tasted the best and felt the best to me when I have had the opportunity to drink them. I believe that the naturally occurring earth minerals contained in our water are beneficial to our health.

SO, WHAT DO WE DRINK?

Water is the substance we need most. Because good drinking water is so important to health, we should know what the water we drink contains. Water contamination is inescapable; if there is any question about the water we drink, we can have it checked for bacteria count, mineral content, and the presence of a wide number of chemical pollutants. If there is concern, we should find a filtration or purification system that makes the water safe or find another source of drinking water.

In the past, I believed that the prime choice of drinking water was the Earth's uncontaminated natural springs or wells (these may be extinct). Especially if this water comes from the area where we live, it puts us in harmony with our environment and often provides important minerals (although it should be checked for abnormally high mineral content). Because of our current pollution problems, however, it may be essential for all of us to purify our drinking water. Most of us who live in cities provided with municipal tap water from treatment plants must take appropriate steps to make our water the best it can be. Bottled water is expensive and may come in polyethylene containers, which raise their own health questions, such as plastic-toxin contamination, which is worsened by sun exposure over time. Besides, bottled water is often chlorinated and may have been in the containers for months, if not longer.

I believe that we need to create a cost-effective and water-efficient system to protect us from water pollution. Current technology is advancing, and it seems both solid carbon block and reverse osmosis technologies offer a reliable means of obtaining clean water. Solid carbon alone can help clear most bacteria, chlorine, and the majority of the chemical pollutants that infiltrate our water. At my office, we have an RO system for serving our patients water and herbal teas; at home I use a Multi-Pure stainless steel unit hooked up to our kitchen faucet, enabling my family to have purified water for drinking, cooking, and washing food (including our sprouts). This type of system is the most economical for the quality of water it delivers. Of course, it is more expensive than drinking tap water, but we have decided that it is worth the $5 to $10 a month it costs over time to know that our water is free of bacteria, chlorine, most toxic chemicals, and most heavy metals.

Solid carbon may actually be the best system for removing chemicals. An added advantage of solid carbon block filters over reverse osmosis and distillation, besides lower cost per gallon of water and easier accessibility, is that these systems leave the natural trace minerals that our bodies can use. However, if nitrate levels are high or if we want fluoride removed, reverse osmosis is necessary. Although some manufacturers offer special adsorbent resins, like activated alumina, to remove fluoride from water without having to resort to reverse osmosis, these resins may raise health questions of their own. We should remember that solid carbon block filters are very different from carbon granule filters (often silver impregnated), which can harbor bacteria and then release them, and chemicals, back into the water in even greater concentrations.

To review, the three common, most effective home treatment systems are solid carbon block filters, reverse osmosis, and distillation. Purchasing pre-bottled water is an unnecessary expense, and in many cases, the water is not as good and definitely not as fresh as water purified at home. All three systems will remove chlorine (although in RO it's the prefiller that does this), bacteria, metals, and chemicals, although I have some concern about volatile chemicals left after distillation. (Distilled water should be prefiltered by solid carbon.) Because solid carbon filtration is more economical in time, water use, and dollars—and very good at removing chemicals—this may be the best process for urban residents unless you want the added fluoride taken out. Solid carbon will not remove the fluoride ions, which are strongly bonded to sodium or calcium. Natural springwater or well water

Water Systems Analysis: What Works?					
	SOURCE		**PURIFICATION**		
CONTENTS	**Tap Water**	**Well or Spring**	**Solid Carbon**	**Reverse Osmosis**	**Distillation**
Chlorine	yes	not unless treated used also	removed unless carbon	not removed	removed
Fluoride	if added	natural or if treated	not removed	removed	removed
Bacteria	unlikely	possibly	most likely removed	removed	removed
Parasites	possibly	possibly	removed	removed	removed
Pesticides	yes	likely	removed	removed	removed
Solvents	likely	possibly	removed	not removed unless carbon used also	not removed (including VOCs)*
Heavy Metals	some	likely	possibly removed	removed	removed
Basic Minerals	some	likely	not removed	removed	removed
RESOURCE FACTORS					
Electricity Used	no	probably	no	no	yes
Wastes Water	no	no	no	yes	some

*VOCs like xylene can have higher boiling points than water and are not removed by distillation. Many VOCs are also not readily removed by reverse osmosis.

that is tested and clean may be the best choice for people living in the country. (See more on water quality and contamination in chapter 11, Food and the Earth.)

Traveler's Water

In the United States and much of the Westernized world, the greatest concern is contamination of water by pesticides and herbicides used in agriculture; by chemicals, such as hydrocarbons, from industry; and by the chlorine and other agents added to kill existing and potential germs in the water. When traveling to developing countries and other areas that do not treat their water, or when hiking or camping in natural areas in the United States, we may need to take measures to make the water safe from microorganisms.

There are always potential dangers from microbial contamination in water or food. Awareness and safety measures are important. Untreated water may harbor bacteria or parasites most commonly, or viruses on occasion. U.S. mountain rivers and streams or lake waters may contain giardia *(Giardia lamblia)* or parasitic amoeba, campylobacter or other bacteria, metals, chemicals, or radioactivity. Common organisms that may cause intestinal infection in developing countries (or in contaminated food or water in the United States) include salmonella, shigella, *Escherichia coli* (E. coli), giardia, amoebas, and cryptosporidium. Contracting hepatitis from water may also be a slight concern, but foods are a more common transmitter of infectious hepatitis.

We have a few options when traveling: First, we may carry our own water, although this is limited to short trips or when camping with a vehicle. We may also avoid drinking water totally as some try, for example, when traveling to Mexico or South America. Drinking bottled carbonated beverages such as waters, sodas, or beer usually keeps us safe from germs, as they cannot exist in the high carbon dioxide levels. But food might be washed or ice cubes made with contaminated water. Overall, there are three ways to clean water to make it safer: treating by heat, chemicals, or filtration. At sea level, boiling water for 1 minute will kill bacteria and parasites; boil 10 minutes to destroy viruses. For every 1,000 feet of elevation, add 1 minute

to the boiling time to clean the water of possible germs. So in the mountains, at 10,000 feet, water must be boiled for 10 to 20 minutes, depending on your concerns. Little heating coils or stoves may be used, but overall this process may be cumbersome, especially when larger amounts of water are needed.

Chemical treatment may be simplest and the least expensive, yet it has drawbacks—most people do not like the taste and some people might experience side effects or reactions. Both chlorine and iodine have been used effectively for this purpose. Halazone tablets release chlorine into the water. Five tablets per quart will effectively kill almost all microorganisms, but the taste is not to my liking. In my opinion iodine as 2% liquid is preferable—use 10 drops per quart and let it sit for 30 minutes to kill the germs. Globaline is a crystalline iodine. One tablet can be added to a quart of water and will work in 10 minutes. Generally, I believe that chemical treatment is a last resort for water purification.

The goal at home or when traveling is to have germ-free water without undesirable chemicals or chlorine. Filtration is the best way to do this. I have already discussed home filters, and there are also filters designed for travel and camping. These are small units that have pumps so lake or river waters can be used. In the past 10 years, the number of states reporting cases of giardiasis to the CDC (Centers for Disease Control) has almost doubled from 23 to 43. An outbreak of giardiasis can even be contracted by drinking the crystal clear, good-tasting mountain stream waters in the United States; even wilderness packers need to carry some type of water purification. With the difficulty of boiling at higher altitudes and the bad taste of chemically treated water, filtration is the best way to go for backpacking, especially if large amounts of water are needed.

Most hand filters are granulated carbon, often with silver added. Although these are not ideal for home use, they are simplest for travel. They will take out some chemicals, but our biggest concern is microorganisms. Here the pore size of the filter, which should be clearly stated in the product information, is the crucial factor in determining what germs will be removed.

The pore size of available filters ranges from 0.2 to 2.0 microns. They all will remove parasites, some will

Micron Sizes of Relevant Organisms	
Organism	**Size in microns**
Giardia lamblia	10–20
Amoebas	10–50
Cryptosporidium	2–5
Campylobacter bacteria	0.2–0.3
Cytomegalo virus (CMV) and Herpes virus	0.15–0.2
Retrovirus (AIDS)	0.1–0.12
Hepatitis viruses	0.025–0.04

remove bacteria, but most will not take out viruses. In drinking water our biggest concerns are from parasites and bacteria; viruses, more unlikely to survive in water, are really a lesser concern. The Katadyn unit, claiming a pore size of 0.2 microns, may remove some viruses as well. It is the most expensive of the travel-pump units. Most of the available travel filters can clean about 1 to 2 pints per minute. If the water is dirty or turbid, use a prefilter such as a coffee filter or clean cotton bandana, for example, before pumping. Pre-filtering extends the life of the carbon filter.

WATER REQUIREMENTS

Water is essential for all life, and drinking the right amount is important to achieving optimum health. All the beverages we drink—teas, coffee, sodas, beer—are basically water that contains other ingredients as well. Drinking good water is still the best way, I believe, to obtain our fluid requirements.

The amount of water we need is based on a number of factors—our size; our activity level, which influences the amount of fluid we lose through sweat; the climate or temperature (higher environmental temperatures increase our fluid losses); and our diet. Special circumstances in which increased amounts of water may be needed include fever, diarrhea, kidney disease, or any situation where excessive fluid losses occur through normal body elimination processes.

We lose water daily through our skin, urine, bowels, and lungs (as water vapor in the air). About half of our water losses can be replaced with the water con-

tent in our food. The remaining half requires specific fluid intake, primarily from drinking good water. Caffeinated beverages, such as coffee, tea, cocoa, or colas, and alcoholic beverages do not count as the same volume of water because they act as diuretics in the body, increasing fluid losses from the kidneys. The average human requirement is about 3 quarts of water per day, including food and beverages. An inactive person in a cool climate may need less, while an athlete training in the desert will need much more. People who eat a lot of fruits and vegetables, which are high in water content, will require less drinking water than people who consume proportionally more meats and fats, which are more concentrated and require additional water to help utilize them. In addition to a healthy diet containing fresh fruits and vegetables, I recommend that the average person consume at least 1.5 to 2 quarts of water daily.

Water is best consumed at several intervals throughout the day—1 or 2 glasses upon awakening and also about an hour before each meal. Water should not be drunk with or just after meals, as it can dilute digestive juices and reduce food digestion and nutrient assimilation. Some people like to drink 1 or 2 glasses in the evening to help flush out their system overnight, even though this may result in getting up during the night to urinate. It is important to drink water to avoid problems such as constipation and dry skin. Drinking enough contaminant-free water is likely our most significant nutritional health factor. Water will keep us current, clean, and flowing through life.

THE FUTURE OF WATER

Writing this chapter on water was a difficult task. There is so much opinion, misinformation, and proprietary hype that companies use to sell their water or their filter systems. I have distilled the best I could with what I believe. I know there are concerns with public utility water and the Earth's natural resources. Yet, what's the best way to clean it up? What's the most efficient way to filter water at home and ensure drinking safety? And what about all the new "scientific" waters, such as alkaline and "ionic" waters for better body balance (we want to be more alkaline) or microclusters and M-water, which propose to hold together in different molecular balance to be better utilized? What water will allow us to hydrate our cells and tissues better? I see all of this being explored more scientifically in the coming years. Since water is second only to air as our most important substance and body component, we really need to know the truth about it and how to make it work right in our body.

Titan, Saturn's largest moon, and Europa, a moon in Jupiter's collection first noticed by Galileo about 400 years ago, may each contain more water than all oceans on earth combined. That's why scientists have started using the word "extraterrestrial" to describe water. We should have been using that word long ago.

Water is out of this world when it comes to nutritional magic, and we're going to find ourselves more and more dazzled by the miracles of water. What comes out of the tap we will end up calling "bath water"—at best. And water that has percolated down through healthy soil, water without the pesticides and heavy metals, "real water," will refresh us in a way we can hardly imagine. On account of its mineral content alone, truly natural and pure, fresh water shall take its place along with the most touted foods and supplements as the key for prevention of heart disease and hypertension, and the key to optimal health.

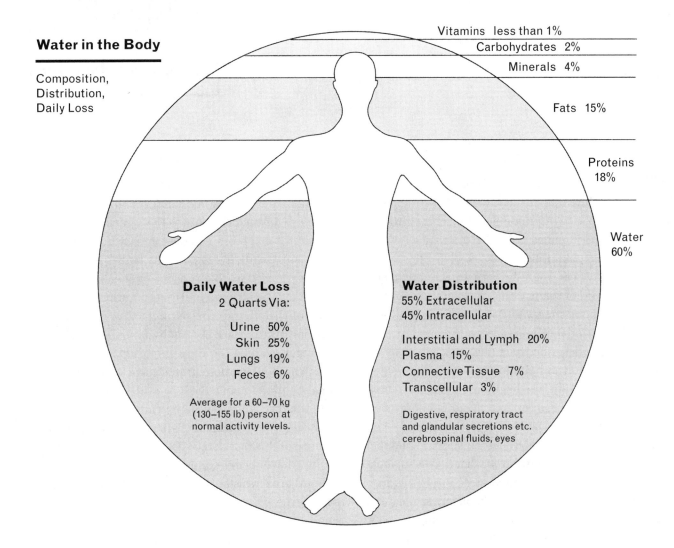

Water in the Body

Composition, Distribution, Daily Loss

Vitamins less than 1%
Carbohydrates 2%
Minerals 4%
Fats 15%
Proteins 18%
Water 60%

Daily Water Loss
2 Quarts Via:

Urine 50%
Skin 25%
Lungs 19%
Feces 6%

Average for a 60–70 kg (130–155 lb) person at normal activity levels.

Water Distribution
55% Extracellular
45% Intracellular

Interstitial and Lymph 20%
Plasma 15%
Connective Tissue 7%
Transcellular 3%

Digestive, respiratory tract and glandular secretions etc. cerebrospinal fluids, eyes

Chapter 2

Carbohydrates

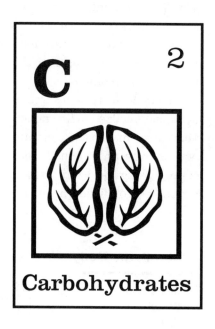

Carbohydrates

arbohydrates—along with proteins and fats—constitute one of the three basic components of food, and our understanding of their role in health and nutrition has expanded dramatically since this book was first published in 1992. Nutrition as we know it today was actually born in the late 1800s, when the world of science was completely caught up in the concept of energy and humankind's ability to harness it. During the exact same time when nutrition was first being described as a field of science (1898), the diesel engine was being patented and the second industrial revolution was beginning to spread across Europe. The idea of an engine needing energy permeated the newfound science of nutrition, and when nutritional scientists began searching for the fuel that kept bodies running, they found what they were looking for in the form of carbohydrates.

Carbohydrates are organic molecules, meaning they contain carbon and come from living sources. They are composed of carbon (C), hydrogen (H), and oxygen (O), thus the abbreviation CHO, in a 1:2:1 ratio. The basic relationship is that of carbon coupled with water molecules. You can see this relationship in the word *carbohydrate*—"carbo" and "hydrate," hydrated (or watered) carbon. There are many different kinds of carbohydrates, but some can serve as a quick source of energy for the body. It was the "quick energy" carbohydrates that prompted the forebearers of nutrition to recognize carbohydrates as the body's chief source of energy—the fuel that runs its engine.

Today, the idea of a fuel that can provide the body with a quick energy source is only one of the ways that nutritionists think about carbohydrates. In fact, it may no longer even be the most important one. Two discoveries about carbohydrates have changed nutritional thinking about their role in health. First has been the discovery that many carbohydrates are not easily digested (and they are important precisely because of this fact). Since about 1990, more than 100 studies have been conducted on what has been referred to as "resistant starch"—a small but significant percentage of starch that resists breakdown in the small intestine and consistently reaches the large intestine, where it is scooped up by bacteria.

Similar in function to resistant starch are the oligosaccharides, short sugar chains containing 3 to 20 sugars each. More than 125 studies have looked at the relationship between oligosaccharides, diet, and health, and special emphasis has been given to oligosaccharides containing fructose (fruit sugar), perhaps one of the most famous members of the carbohydrate family. As a group, the fructo-oligosaccharides (FOSs) behave just like resistant starch, making their way through the small intestine and ending up as food for bacteria in the large intestine.

The discovery of resistant starch and oligosaccharides changed the nutritional perception of carbohydrates, because these members of the carbohydrate family do not provide fuel for the body so much as stability for the digestive system. But a second area of research changed our thinking about carbohydrates even more. That area of research was called glycobiology. Scientists at the Glycobiology Institute at the University of Oxford in England were credited with creation of the term *glycobiology* in 1988. This term was (and still is) used to refer to the field of science that examines the role of carbohydrates in living creatures.

Glycobiologists have single-handedly revolutionized thinking about carbohydrates because they have learned that many carbohydrates function in the body not as fuel but as communication devices. For example, sugars that are found on the surface of our cells enable our cells to recognize and interact with each other. Sugars on the surface of our red blood cells help determine our blood type and are the basis for determining appropriate and inappropriate blood donors. The oligosaccharide branch of the carbohydrate family plays a critical role in immune function, and many carbohydrate structures turn out to be tumor—and antitumor—associated. When carbohydrates were first recognized as a body fuel, these other critical functions were unknown.

The communication function of carbohydrates has led to some fascinating discoveries about food. For example, mushrooms that have been part of Chinese and Japanese diets throughout the history of those cultures have been shown to contain carbohydrates that improve communication between immune cells and make immunotherapy for conditions like cancer more effective. Reishi, shiitake, and maitake mushrooms have been extensively studied in this regard, and carbohydrate extracts from these mushrooms have been used to support individuals diagnosed with colon cancer, stomach cancer, ulcerative colitis, and HIV infec-

tion. The best studied of the carbohydrates in this context is a polysaccharide called lentinan (technically referred to as a 1,3-beta-glucan and found in shiitake mushrooms).

In general, **carbohydrates come to us from plant (versus animal) foods, because carbohydrates are produced by photosynthesis in plants.** The carbohydrates are the primary source of energy in Nature's plant foods—fruits, vegetables, grains, legumes, and tubers. These foods play an important role in the functioning of internal organs, the nervous system, and muscles. They are the best source of energy for endurance athletics because they provide both an immediate and a time-released energy source as they are digested easily and then consistently metabolized in the bloodstream. Animal foods contain carbohydrates because animals (like humans) store carbohydrates in their muscles, and muscles are usually the part of the animal that we eat. But the broad diversity of carbohydrates that are needed to optimally support health can only be found in the plant world.

Carbohydrates play an important role in helping to regulate the metabolism of their fellow macronutrients—namely, protein and fat. Moreover, the balance between these three food components helps determine the robustness of our immune response, bone and tissue growth, joint fluidity, and rate of healing following injury. The ratio of carbohydrate to protein in a person's diet has been a topic of particular interest in nutrition research. We know that an excessively low ratio of carbohydrate to protein shifts our body's metabolism into a ketogenic state. Ketogenesis is a natural but also specialized process in which our bodies respond to stress or starvation by increasing the reliance on fat as a fuel. There is also some evidence that a diet too low in carbohydrates can make one of our hormones (insulin) less effective, therefore destabilizing our blood sugar levels.

At the other end of the carbohydrate-protein spectrum, an excessively high ratio of carbohydrate to protein has also been found to be problematic. At least some kinds of high-carbohydrate diets have been shown to have equally destabilizing effects on blood sugar and to raise certain fat levels (especially triglycerides) in the blood. This diet also appears to be the major factor in obesity issues. Many issues involving

Carbohydrates by Scientific Subcategory

Monosaccharides	Disaccharides
Glucose	Sucrose
Fructose	Lactose
Mannose	Maltose
Ribose	Trehalose
Dextrose	
Xylose	**Sugar Alcohols**
Fucose	Sorbitol
	Mannitol
Oligosaccharides	Dulcitol
Raffinose	Xylitol
Stachyose	Inositol
Verbascose	
Fructans	**Hemicelluloses**
Kestose	Pectins
Bifurcose	Xylans
Nystose	Xyloglucans
	Galactomannans
	Beta-glucans
Starches	Gums
Amyloses	Mucilages
Amylopectins	Glucomannans
Celluloses	
Glucans	

carbohydrate to protein ratios remain unresolved, however, and continue to be investigated. Researchers in Zurich, Switzerland, for example, have determined that high-carbohydrate meals in the morning have a detrimental effect on cognitive performance in comparison to high-protein or balanced meals.

Carbohydrates are scientifically classified according to their structure, and two basic types of carbohydrates are found in most plant foods: free sugars and polysaccharides. Under the heading "free sugars" can be found four subcategories of carbohydrates: monosaccharides, which consist of a single sugar; disaccharides, which consist of two sugars hooked together; oligosaccharides, which consist of several sugars hooked together; and, finally, sugar alcohols, which are typically either monosaccharides or disaccharides with a special chemical group attached to them.

Under the polysaccharide heading are two subcategories: starches and nonstarches. In both of these subcategories are found many sugars connected either in a long chain or in a treelike formation with many branches. Within the nonstarch polysaccharides, there is a further subdivision that has become important in nutrition research: the subdivision of celluloses and hemicelluloses. All of the polysaccharides share one feature in common: unlike the "free sugars" (monosaccharides, disaccharides, oligosaccharides, and sugar alcohols), the polysaccharides usually require more digestive activity before their components can participate fully in the body's metabolic processes.

SIMPLE SUGARS

The basic unit of the simple sugars (monosaccharides) is 1 hexose (containing 6 carbon atoms) or pentose (5 carbon atoms) molecule. These simple sugars are easily and quickly digested and used by the body. They have the same chemical makeup but vary in structure. The disaccharides, such as table sugar or milk sugar, require some enzymatic breakdown but are easily converted into monosaccharides for digestion. The following are the common basic free sugars.

Monosaccharides

Glucose is the metabolized form of "sugar" in the body. It is found in some fruits, such as grapes. It can also be hydrolyzed from starch, cane sugar (sucrose), milk sugar (lactose), and malt syrup (maltose). Dextrose is another name for glucose in the food industry. Glucose is carried in the blood and is the principal sugar used by the tissues and cells for energy. Glucose can be measured by the blood sugar test, which reads the current concentration of glucose in the serum or plasma. A high glucose level can signal a diabetic condition; low blood sugar is called *hypoglycemia*. Both of these abnormalities can become chronic and even life-threatening. The adrenal and pancreatic hormones adrenaline and insulin are very important in sugar metabolism. High-sugar and refined-carbohydrate diets, stress, and lack of exercise can generate elevated glucose levels in both blood and tissue. **Pregnancy is also a stress on carbohydrate metabolism because of its high metabolic demands.**

Fructose is found in most fruits and fruit juices, as well as in honey and some vegetables. Fructose is sweeter than cane sugar and is absorbed directly into the blood. Cane sugar (sucrose) is metabolized into fructose and glucose. Fructose can be changed to glucose in the liver or in the small intestine for a quick source of energy.

Galactose comes from the metabolism of the milk sugar lactose, which breaks down into galactose and glucose. Galactose is converted to glucose in the liver and is synthesized in the mammary glands to make the lactose of mother's milk. In some instances, a specific genetic defect may cause an individual to have an intolerance to this monosaccharide. For example, some children have a genetic mutation called the Duarte variant and produce only 17% of the amount of a specific enzyme (galactose-1-phosphate uridyltransferase) that they need to successfully metabolize galactose. Avoiding high concentrations of galactose in the diet is important for these children.

Xylose is a pentose that has not been well studied in food. However, the sugar alcohol made from xylose—xylitol—is widely used in the food-processing industry as a bulk sweetener that does not promote tooth decay. Although xylitol is a naturally occurring carbohydrate in some fruits, vegetables, and mushrooms, most of the xylitol used in the food industry comes from the wood fiber in birch trees. (For this reason, xylitol is sometimes called "birch sugar.") Persistent diarrhea in infants who consume formula or processed foods containing xylose or xylitol can sometimes be linked to xylose or xylitol intolerance.

Fucose is a hexose, which like xylose has not been well-studied in food. However, one type of kelp (the sea vegetable *Fucus vesiculosus,* also known as bladderwrack) contains especially high concentrations of this carbohydrate. As with xylose intolerance, fucose intolerance has been associated with persistent infantile diarrhea, and in this case, it is possible for the infant to have a specific genetic defect that causes a fucose-metabolizing enzyme (fuculokinase) to be deficient.

Even though some of the monosaccharide carbohydrates have been associated with food allergy and intolerance, this connection is much more common with the disaccharide carbohydrates, which are described next.

Disaccharides

Disaccharides can be hydrolyzed into two monosaccharides with the addition of a water molecule and the help of an enzyme. In most cases, the name of the enzyme that helps break the disaccharide into two monosaccharides is similar to the name of the disaccharide itself. Lactase is the enzyme that breaks down lactose, sucrase breaks down sucrose, and maltase breaks down maltose. The disaccharides are all water soluble and will crystallize when dehydrated.

Lactose (milk sugar), the sugar of mother's breast milk, is the only sugar of animal origin. It is composed of 1 molecule each of glucose and galactose. As mentioned earlier, lactose is broken down by the enzyme lactase, which may be especially deficient or absent in some ethnic groups, leading to problems with milk digestion. An estimated 50 to 60 million people in the United States are lactose intolerant, including more than half of all African Americans, Asian Americans, Native Americans, and Latinos or people of Hispanic origin.

It is also interesting to note that human milk, which is the best source of nourishment for a newborn, contains more lactose than cow's milk, which many mothers use in the form of formula. Human milk is also rich in the enzyme lactase, however, so the breastfeeding infant gets both the lactose and the lactase to digest it from the mother. This process is particularly important for development of the infant's nervous system, because many of the nerves must be wrapped in a special sheath (the myelin sheath) and galactose (one of the two monosaccharides in lactose) is a primary building block for this sheath. Cow's milk, on the other hand, is much lower in lactase, thus infants fed cow's milk formula are at a nutritional disadvantage because their livers do not yet have the capacity to make this enzyme.

Sucrose ("white sugar") is found in sugar cane and sugar beets, maple syrup, molasses, sorghum, and pineapple. Sucrose is composed of 1 molecule each of fructose and glucose. Sucrose is sweet and can be metabolized in the body. Its crystalline form, table sugar, is used excessively in Western society, not only as a sweetener on food and in beverages but also in cooking and hidden in the preparation of many other common foods and condiments, such as ketchup, mayonnaise, salad dressings, and baby foods. Addiction to sucrose begins early and is supported by millions of dollars of advertising. The average American consumes well over 100 pounds of sucrose a year, and this particular disaccharide is responsible for a wide variety of problems. It has been implicated in obesity, tooth decay, diabetes, and many psychological and emotional problems, including premenstrual syndrome and stress/burnout syndromes. Like lactose intolerance, although not as well researched, sucrose intolerance is also a problem for some people. Some of the research on fibromyalgia, for example, has shown sucrose intolerance to be more likely in conjunction with sensitivity to environmental toxins. Using less sugar would be a boost to anyone's health.

Maltose (malt sugar) is a short chain of two glucose molecules. It is produced during the breakdown of starches in many cereal grains. Maltose is present in beers, malted snacks, and some breakfast cereals and is the sweetener of many crackers (read product labels for this information). In most individuals, maltose is easily broken down into glucose molecules for quick use by the body. Just like lactose intolerance and sucrose intolerance, however, maltose intolerance exists and, particularly in children, shows up as maltosuria (too much maltose in the urine) due to deficiency of an enzyme (maltase) that is needed to digest this disaccharide.

Oligosaccharides

All carbohydrates falling into this subcategory contain between 3 and 20 sugar units and are found in a variety of foods (mostly plant foods). The oligosaccharides are unique among all the carbohydrates because of their special way of supporting our immune function. Many of the oligosaccharides cannot be digested in the small intestine, and when they reach the large intestine, they serve as dinner for many of the "friendly" bacteria that help keep the large intestine free from disease. In particular, oligosaccharides help enhance the growth of lactic acid–producing bacteria, including *Bifidobacterium* and *Lactobacillus*. Relatively

short oligosaccharides, especially those containing the monosaccharide fructose, appear to be especially good at this process. These especially supportive fructose-containing oligosaccharide (FOS) carbohydrates include kestose, neokestose, nystose, bifurcose, neo-bifurcose, and fructosyinystose. All of them are found in onions, burdock root, and asparagus, and some are found in garlic, chives, rye, Jerusalem artichoke, and banana. The presence of immunosupportive oligosaccharides in human milk (versus cow's milk) has also been confirmed in nutritional research studies.

Polysaccharides

The second large, umbrella group of carbohydrates—in contrast to the free sugars—is polysaccharides. They typically contain several hundred sugars (monosaccharides) but range greatly in size from several dozen to several thousand sugar units. Unlike the free sugars, which are often readily available for absorption into the body, polysaccharides must usually undergo substantial digestion before they can be absorbed. Most of this digesting is done through the use of water and enzymes (including the well-known amylases). Because of their size, structure, and requirements for digestion, polysaccharides are also called complex carbohydrates.

Within the polysaccharide division of the carbohydrates there are two major subdivisions: starches and nonstarches. Carbohydrates in each group play important roles in our nourishment.

Starches

Starches can provide a more consistent blood sugar level than the simple sugars, provided that they fall near the bottom of a special carbohydrate-rating system called the glycemic index. (I will talk more about the glycemic index later in this chapter, on pages 35–37). In the traditional diet, a high percentage of foods consumed included the complex carbohydrates of potatoes (whole and baked, with skins), vegetable roots, and such whole grains as wheat, rice, and corn. This was much healthier than the present-day preference for high-sugar and refined-flour diets, which are associated with degenerative tissue disease and aging.

There are several types of starches. If the polysaccharide chains are shorter and branched, the starch is amylopectin—the most common one found in foods. Amylose has long chains of glucose molecules, which are easily separated by the enzyme amylase. Glycogen is the animal-source starch contained in muscle and liver. It is similar in structure to amylopectin and can be broken down to release glucose for energy needs or be formed from extra glucose and stored in the liver. Both amylopectin and amylose contain only one kind of simple sugar, the monosaccharide glucose. Glycogen is really the form in which glucose is stored in our body. Dextrins are partially digested starches that are formed in the breakdown of starch.

Nonstarch Polysaccharides

Some of the polysaccharides found in food are not structured like amylose or amylopectin, and these polysaccharides are called the *nonstarch polysaccharides*. Within this category are two unique groups: the celluloses and hemicelluloses.

Celluloses. Celluose is the main component in the walls of all plant cells. Like the starches, it contains only glucose sugars, but they are connected differently. The unique structure of cellulose makes it particularly strong (a perfect material for holding the plant up!) and also resistant to breakdown by water (hydrolysis). Although fungi and ruminant animals like cows and horses can digest cellulose, humans cannot, and this nonstarch polysaccharide acts like a bulking agent in the stool. In some cases, it also serves as a fuel for friendly bacteria living in the lower part of the large intestine. Most vegetables and fruits contain cellulose.

Hemicelluloses. Having talked about celluloses, it might seem a little too technical to bring in a group of carbohydrates that sound almost identical to the celluloses. But even though their name makes it sound like the difference wouldn't interest anyone except a chemist, hemicelluloses are on the cutting edge of nutrition because they can support our immune system, boost detoxification processes in our liver, help balance our blood sugar, and lower our cholesterol. Unlike celluloses, which are sturdy and hard to break down, hemicelluloses are delicate and easily broken down in acidic fluids. They are found in nearly all types of foods and also play an important role as added ingredients in processed foods. In chemical terms, they are a complicated group of carbohydrates and

include the following subgroups: pectins, xylans, glucans, galactomannans, glucomannans, gums, and mucilages.

In processed foods, the most widely used hemicelluloses are the gums, including xanthan gum, guar gum, locust bean gum, and gum arabic. Recent studies on guar gum, for example, indicate that this hemicellulose can help stabilize blood sugar, regulate appetite and rate of stomach emptying, and improve bowel function in people with irritable bowel syndrome.

Another well-known hemicellulose is pectin—the substance used to thicken gelatin products. Pectin used to be regarded as a single substance found in apple pulp and the rinds of citrus fruits, but scientists now know it is a much more diverse group of substances. Currently, two types of pectins seem most important from a health standpoint: the rhamnogalacturonans and arabinogalactans. Both types of pectin appear to enhance immune function. Rhamnogalacturonans are found in root vegetables like potatoes and beets, as well as in corn, flax, pumpkin, and yellow mustard. In some animal studies, rhamnogalacturonans are associated with increased ability to detoxify lead. Arabinogalactans have been found in coffee beans (from which they were originally named), as well as soybeans, runner beans, raspberries, lupin (a grain legume like peas or lentils), and American ginseng *(Panax ginseng).*

In addition to gums and pectins, there is a final group of hemicelluloses that is getting more and more attention in nutrition research. This group includes the xylans, beta-glucans, galactomannans, and glucomannans. As a group, the glucomannans and galactomannans have been determined to have cholesterol-lowering activity and to help stabilize blood sugar. Aloe vera juice—sometimes used as a bowel detoxifier or to help heal the lining of the stomach—contains large amounts of glucomannans and may rely on these carbohydrates for some of its healing properties. Galactomannans have been found in fenugreek, a widely used spice in Indian cuisine, and in the gum portion of many legumes, including acacia bean and locust bean. Mushrooms and grains are the best-studied sources of the beta-glucans. All of the following mushroom types have been determined to contain these unique hemicelluloses: yellow morels, reishis, maitakes, shiitakes, and *Cordyceps.* In the grain world, oats, barley, rice, and sorghum have also been shown to contain beta-glucans. The beta-glucans found in these foods help support immune function and are currently of special interest for their anti-tumor properties.

FIBER

Unlike the terms *monosaccharide, oligosaccharide,* and *polysaccharide,* the term *fiber* has never found a universally accepted definition in the world of nutrition. Many variations of this term, including *total fiber, dietary fiber,* and *crude fiber* continue to surface in many nutrition books, as does the term *roughage,* which is usually used as a synonym for *fiber.* Crude fiber is not usually a very helpful way of looking at fiber when it comes to nutrition. This term is used to describe what is left of a food after the food has been treated with a mixture of 1.25% sulfuric acid and sodium hydroxide. (Do not do this to your food!) Crude fiber is always an underestimate of the food's fiber content. Dietary fiber is usually defined as the combination of plant polysaccharides that are resistant to digestion (namely, the celluloses and hemicelluloses discussed earlier) plus lignins. (Lignins are not true carbohydrates, but they are considered part of the dietary fiber group.) Dietary fiber is also commonly broken down into soluble and insoluble fiber, and the term *total fiber,* which is used synonymously with *dietary fiber,* usually means the total of insoluble fiber plus soluble fiber.

Fiber is exclusively a plant nutrient. Plants need fiber for structural support. Animals have bones and muscles instead, so fiber is not a significant part of their composition. Whenever we increase our intake of plants in comparison to animal foods, we are increasing our fiber intake. Whenever we head more in an animal food direction, we are decreasing our dietary fiber. Countries with the most food processing and the highest percentage of animal food intake (such as the United States) have the least consumption of dietary fiber. Americans get 10 to 15 grams of dietary fiber a day. Countries with the least food processing and the least animal food intake have the greatest consumption of dietary fiber. In some African countries, for example, daily fiber intake can reach 75 to 100 grams a day. Low-fiber diets are associated with constipation,

gastrointestinal disorders, diverticulosis, and colon cancer, while a high-fiber diet may prevent these problems. Fiber in the diet may also reduce the risk of appendicitis.

The hemicelluloses discussed earlier are not only found as naturally occurring parts of food, but are also used in supplemental form to help offset diets that are low in fiber or to provide additional bulk to the stool and speed transit time through the bowels. Psyllium seed husks are a good example of a hemicellulose that is used in this way. Other fibers used in the diet include both agar and alginate (derived from seaweed) and carrageenan, which comes from the Irish moss plant. All indigestible polysaccharides, they are used in food preparation and in cosmetics for their smooth, gelatinous consistency. Carrageenan is used commonly with dairy products such as yogurt to create a smooth consistency. Agar is used to bring a gelatinous quality to foods and desserts. Alginate can bind up minerals and metals, such as cadmium, mercury, lead, and arsenic, in the intestines and has been found useful in detoxification programs.

Several other high-fiber substances that have some use in the diet have been shown in preliminary research to help reduce cholesterol levels because of their ability to hinder fat absorption from the intestines. Konjar root flour from Japan has been shown to have some influence in moderating diabetes, in lowering cholesterol levels, and in weight control. Chitin—technically an amino sugar rather than a strict carbohydrate—is also interesting as a dietary fiber. Chitin is a naturally occurring substance found in crab, shrimp, and oyster shells, and a processing derivative of chitin called *chitosan* has been used to lower cholesterol levels, dress soft tissue and bone wounds, and deliver anti-inflammatory drugs. (For further discussion of the health aspects of fiber, see the beginning of chapter 8, Foods.)

REQUIREMENTS

In 2002, for the first time in its history, the National Academy of Sciences (NAS) established public health recommendations for carbohydrate intake. A recommended dietary allowance (RDA) of 130 grams of carbohydrate per day was set by the Institute of Medicine (IOM) at the NAS, based on selected types of research involving digestion, absorption, and use of carbohydrates in the body. The IOM recognized that between 200 and 330 grams of carbohydrate per day was the customary intake for men, and between 180 and 230 grams for women. No recommendation was made for intake of different types of carbohydrates, including both starches and sugars, although the IOM did suggest that no more than 25% of total calories come from added sugars. If a person ate 1,800 calories of food per day, this 25% would mean 450 calories worth of added sugar, or 112 grams of added sugar. This amount seems extremely high to me, because it represents more than 9 tablespoons of added sugar. I would like to see the recommendation point more in the vicinity of 1 tablespoon. The IOM also recommended adequate intake (AI) levels for total fiber of 25 grams for women 19 to 50 and 38 grams for men in this age range.

Unfortunately, these recommendations for carbohydrate aren't very helpful. There is a huge difference between 130 grams per day (the RDA minimum) and over 300 grams (the top of the customary range for men). And without specific guidelines for sugars versus starches, it is not clear exactly how a person is supposed to proceed. So here's my perspective: On the one hand, carbohydrates are one of the best sources of energy and are simple for the body to use. Moreover, many of the carbohydrate foods contain essential vitamins and minerals as well as the dietary fiber necessary for colon health and proper elimination.

On the other hand, people can live with greatly reduced carbohydrate intake; in fact, in many weight-loss programs, carbohydrate consumption is severely limited. It is wise in these cases, however, to consume supplemental fiber. Also, some people have a tendency to overeat carbohydrate foods, even to become "carb addicts," and with this, weight may increase. Obesity is associated most frequently with carbohydrate overindulgence. Allergies and emotional shifts, including "carbohydrate depression," have also been associated with sensitivity to overconsumption of this macronutrient.

Peoples in different cultures consume varying amounts of carbohydrates. Native or traditional diets may be quite high in carbohydrates, while in cold climates, as with the Eskimo culture, people may consume few carbohydrates. The average American diet includes about 40% to 50% carbohydrates. Unfor-

tunately, however, about half of that is from the refined and processed flours and sugars in breads, candies, cookies, and cakes. These foods deplete the body of many B vitamins and of minerals such as chromium. A recent estimate has indicated that 19% of all calories in the U.S. diet come from highly processed, bleached wheat flour. And according to the U.S. Department of Agriculture in its 1994–96 Continuing Survey of Food Intakes by Individuals (CFSII), the average U.S. adult consumes 20 teaspoons of added sugar each day. In addition to the already mentioned diseases of obesity and tooth decay, it is possible that this type of diet (high in simple and refined sugars, high in fats, and low in complex carbohydrates) may be influencing the incidence of diabetes, high blood pressure, heart disease, anemia, skin problems, kidney disease, and cancer.

Two areas of research have become critical for understanding the relationship between carbohydrates and health, and can help clarify what we should eat when it comes to carbohydrates. The first involves research on a carbohydrate rating system called the *glycemic index*, and the second focuses on a common metabolic problem called *insulin resistance*.

Since the early 1970s, researchers have been investigating the factors that influence rate of digestion and absorption of dietary carbohydrates. What researchers quickly realized was that identical amounts of carbohydrate-containing foods that seemed very similar did not affect blood sugar in the same way. Using a standardized rating system, researchers began to rank all carbohydrate-containing foods according to their effect on blood sugar. If a food was digested and absorbed quickly and raised blood sugar quickly, it was given a high rating (usually between 100 and 150 points). If a food moved slowly, and barely raised blood sugar, it was assigned a low rating (usually between 10 and 60 points). Many of the results were surprising. For example, ice creams received lower ratings than potatoes, and some cookies got lower ratings than corn chips. The rating system was quickly named the glycemic index, and it continues to be a topic of great interest in nutrition.

Over the past few decades, researchers have drawn several conclusions about carbohydrates based on the glycemic index. First, it is clear that evening meals influence blood sugar responses on the following morning after breakfast, and that the impact of carbohydrates on blood sugar is not limited to any single moment in digestion. Second, high-fiber foods and whole foods have lower glycemic index scores than low-fiber and highly processed foods. Finally, the impact of processing on grain products is particularly dramatic when it comes to the glycemic index: for example, whole-grain wheat can jump from 93 in its natural, unrefined, unprocessed form to 131 in a baguette.

The take-away conclusion from the glycemic index is clear: when we aim to maintain stable blood sugar levels, we need to emphasize natural, high-fiber, unrefined, unprocessed carbohydrates (particularly when it comes to grains), and we need to pay attention to this throughout the day.

A medical researcher at Stanford University, Gerald Reaven, began in the mid-1960s to look at the mechanisms of blood sugar balance in the body. What he discovered has revolutionized scientists' understanding of blood sugar balance, changing the thinking about the role of dietary carbohydrates. When we measure our blood sugar, most of us get results that place us in a normal range, indicating that we are not having problems controlling our blood sugar. (If we had blood sugars outside of a normal range, we would

---

A Glycemic Index of Foods

Grains, Breads, Cereals, and Vegetables (Minimize because They Trigger Insulin)

White bread, baked potatoes: 95

Instant rice: 90

Cooked carrots: 85

French fries, pretzels, rice cakes: 80

Corn flakes, corn-on-the cob, frozen or canned corn: 75

Plain bagels, crackers, graham crackers: 75

White flour products, puffed wheat, sweetened cereals: 75

White rice, taco shells, beets: 70

Spaghetti: 60

Sweeteners, Fruits, and Dairy Products (Minimize)

Maltose: 105–150

Glucose: 100

Raisins: 95

Honey, refined sugar: 75

Watermelon, dried apricots: 70

Pineapple: 65

Ice cream, ripe bananas: 60

Foods That Do Not Overtrigger Insulin (Those below 55)

Oatmeal, brown rice, wild rice: 55

Sweet potatoes, popcorn, pita bread: 55

Yams: 50

Pinto beans, lima beans: 50

Green beans, green peas: 45

Black beans, kidney beans, butter beans: 30

Nuts: 15–30

Artichokes: 25

Asparagus: 20

Tomatoes: 15

Green vegetables: 15

Other Foods That Do Not Overtrigger Insulin (Those below 55)

Mango, kiwi, grapes: 50

Pears: 45

Peaches, plums, apples, oranges: 40

Yogurt, with fruit: 35+

Milk, whole: 30+

Milk, skimmed: 30

Cherries, grapefruit: 25

Yogurt, plain, no sweetener: 15

The glycemic index relates to how quickly the sugars in foods are absorbed into the bloodstream, where foods with the higher numbers are absorbed more quickly and the lower less quickly. This is important when we are watching our carbohydrate and sugar intake because we are overweight, have diabetic risks, or are just sugar sensitive, yet it is important for everyone. The simplest guidance here has us think about a traffic light. Foods in the green zone (under 55) can be eaten more freely, while the yellow ranges from 55–80 and should be eaten with caution. Avoid the red-zone foods over 80.

be diagnosed with a blood sugar problem like diabetes, hyperglycemia, impaired glucose tolerance, or hypoglycemia).

What Reaven discovered, over 40 years of research, was that normal blood sugar levels can be extremely misleading. One of the ways humans regulate blood sugar is by release of a hormone called *insulin*. The pancreas is responsible for secreting this hormone, especially when there are large amounts of simple sugars in a meal. The sugars from food are quickly absorbed into the bloodstream. The pancreas takes note and puts out insulin, which helps the sugar move from the bloodstream up into cells. In this way, insulin helps prevent blood sugar levels from remaining too high.

What Reaven discovered was that many individuals have to put out far too much insulin to keep their blood sugar normal. One person might need to make two or three times as much insulin as another to regulate blood sugar. And if a person has to overproduce insulin to stabilize blood sugar, that person runs the risk of eventually being unable to lower blood sugar levels, regardless of the amount of insulin produced. Such a person is said to be insulin resistant, meaning that his or her metabolism is resistant to the normal affects of insulin and that normal insulin secretion doesn't work to stabilize blood sugars.

Astonishingly, Reaven estimated that 50% of all obese individuals in the United States (who are *not* diagnosed with diabetes or glucose intolerance) are in fact insulin resistant. In addition, 25% of all nonobese individuals (who are *not* diagnosed with diabetes or glucose intolerance) have this metabolic problem. High-carbohydrate diets—in some instances, even high-fiber, high-carbohydrate diets—tend to heighten the problems caused by insulin resistance. In terms of diet, higher protein and high-quality fat content appear to improve blood sugar balance in insulin-resistant individuals.

My conclusion from all of the research is as follows: First, we shouldn't be sticklers about the exact amount of carbohydrates in our diet. There is room for variation here. Second, we should never eat a high-carbohydrate diet (55% to 70% carbohydrate foods) unless we are simultaneously eating low on the glycemic index scale and consuming foods high in fiber content. This means no high-carbohydrate diets unless carbohydrate-containing foods are whole, unrefined, and high fiber. Third, we should be especially careful with the quality

of the grains we eat and lean more toward roots and leafy vegetables. Fourth, if moderately high levels (50% to 60% carbohydrate foods) do not seem to be working for us, or if we are obese, experimenting with a lower carbohydrate balance, in the range of 40% to 50% carbohydrate foods, seems worthwhile. In every case, we need to emphasize the quality of our carbohydrate-containing foods.

Whenever we find ourselves heading off toward the sugars and simpler carbohydrates, we could also do ourselves much good by adding some protein- or fat-containing foods to go along with our simple carbs. Some chicken or avocado mixed in with our bowl of rice, or some almond butter spread onto our rice cake, or some almonds with our apple or when drinking fruit juice would go a long way in helping us offset the unwanted consequences of excess simple carbs.

CARBOHYDRATE DIGESTION AND METABOLISM

Carbohydrates—sugars and starches—are broken down in the gastrointestinal tract by various enzymes for absorption into the blood. The disaccharides (lactose, sucrose, and maltose) are converted into monosaccharides (glucose, fructose, and galactose). The polysaccharides (starches) are converted by salivary amylase in the mouth into dextrin, a shorter-chain starch; then the dextrins are reduced to maltose by pancreatic amylase released into the small intestine. The maltose is further broken down into glucose by maltase enzymes at the intestinal lining. Also in the small intestine, sucrose is changed into glucose and fructose by the enzyme sucrase, while lactase converts lactose (the milk sugar) into glucose and galactose. The monosaccharides (the simple sugars)—such as glucose, galactose, and fructose—are the end products of carbohydrate digestion and are all absorbed into the bloodstream through the intestinal lining. The blood circulates to the liver, where fructose and galactose are easily converted into glucose, the fuel the body uses for energy.

A healthy liver regulates the use of glucose by allowing certain levels to circulate in the blood for use by the cells of the body. If the carbohydrate intake is higher than immediately needed, the liver will normally convert extra glucose into glycogen, a highly branched polysaccharide, and this glycogen can be stored in the liver or in the muscles. At a later time, if energy is needed when there are no dietary carbohydrates available, the liver will convert glycogen back to glucose and return it to the bloodstream, while the muscles may use the muscle glycogen directly for energy.

If we consume higher levels of carbohydrates than are immediately needed or can be converted to glycogen (that is, if there are already sufficient storage sources), the liver will convert the excess glucose into fatty acids and then triglycerides that can be stored as body fat, a process termed *lipogenesis*. If carbohydrates are consumed in high quantities on a regular basis by a person with a sedentary lifestyle, weight gain occurs. Fat is a reserve source of energy. With decreased carbohydrate intake and increased activity levels, fat reserves are converted back to fatty acids for body fuel, a process called *lipolysis*. This generally produces weight loss.

Even when there is little or no intake of carbohydrates, the body attempts to maintain a steady blood sugar level through many mechanisms. Glucose is used by the liver as a source of energy to help synthesize a variety of essential substances. Insulin, a pancreatic hormone, regulates blood sugar levels by stimulating glucose uptake by the cells. Activity and exercise also can reduce blood sugar by increasing tissue glucose needs. A number of hormones influence the production of glucose when the body, and especially the brain, needs more energy. Epinephrine (adrenaline) stimulates glycogen breakdown and raises blood sugar. Steroids enhance conversion of fats and proteins into glucose, and adrenocorticotrophic hormone can interfere with insulin activity. Glucagon is produced in the pancreas and can raise blood sugar, while thyroid hormone may increase intestinal absorption of glucose as it attempts to stimulate metabolism.

As in any long-term relationship, researchers have come full circle with carbohydrates in nutrition since the mid-1980s. After putting them up on a pedestal and increasing them to 60% to 70% of our total diet in the 1980s and early 1990s, we began to start running in the opposite direction in the late 1990s after discovering that high-carbohydrate diets are not always the best choice for blood sugar regulation, weight management, and even for everyday vitality. Since about 2000, there has been an immense increase in the popularity of low-carbohydrate diets, along with some impressive research involving carbohydrate reduction and blood sugar regulation. But there have also been studies talking about carbohydrates in ways nutritionists never expected. Twenty years ago, no one dreamed of treating this group of macronutrients like a key player in detoxification or in support of immune function. To maintain a healthy relationship with carbohydrates, we need to accept both realities. Many of us are going to benefit by lowering our overall carbs (especially our simple carbs) and, at the same time, by increasing our intake of high-fiber, low-glycemic-index carbs, with their immune and detox-supporting properties.

Carbohydrate Digestion and Metabolism Chart

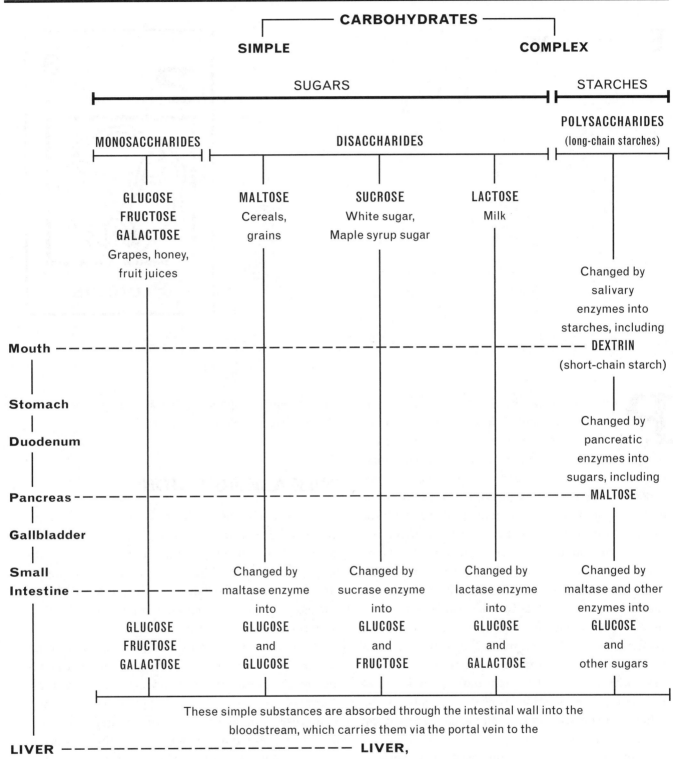

CARBOHYDRATES

SIMPLE   **COMPLEX**

SUGARS   STARCHES

MONOSACCHARIDES	DISACCHARIDES			POLYSACCHARIDES (long-chain starches)
GLUCOSE **FRUCTOSE** **GALACTOSE** Grapes, honey, fruit juices	**MALTOSE** Cereals, grains	**SUCROSE** White sugar, Maple syrup sugar	**LACTOSE** Milk	

Mouth — DEXTRIN

(Polysaccharides: Changed by salivary enzymes into starches, including DEXTRIN (short-chain starch))

Stomach

Duodenum

Changed by pancreatic enzymes into sugars, including

Pancreas — MALTOSE

Gallbladder

Small Intestine — — — — —

GLUCOSE FRUCTOSE GALACTOSE	Changed by maltase enzyme into GLUCOSE and GLUCOSE	Changed by sucrase enzyme into GLUCOSE and FRUCTOSE	Changed by lactase enzyme into GLUCOSE and GALACTOSE	Changed by maltase and other enzymes into GLUCOSE and other sugars

These simple substances are absorbed through the intestinal wall into the bloodstream, which carries them via the portal vein to the

LIVER — — — — — — — — — — — — — — — — — — **LIVER,**

the principal regulator of carbohydrate metabolism

39

Chapter 3

Proteins

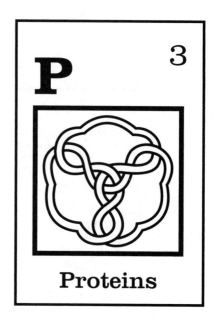

Proteins

Protein is an essential part of nutrition, second only to water in the body's physical composition. Protein makes up about 20% of our body weight and is a primary component of our muscles, hair, nails, skin, eyes, and internal organs—especially the heart (muscle) and brain. Our immune defense system requires protein, particularly for the formation of antibodies that help fight infections. Hemoglobin, our oxygen-carrying red-blood-cell molecule, is a protein, as are many hormones that regulate our metabolism, such as thyroid hormone and insulin. Biochemical deficiency can occur when there is a lack of enzymes, the protein molecules that catalyze chemical reactions in the body. Protein is needed for growth and the maintenance of body tissues; it is vitally important during childhood or pregnancy and lactation. However, despite its significance to our diet and optimum health, we can eat too much protein.

Protein molecules are composed of carbon, oxygen, hydrogen, and nitrogen, while fats and carbohydrates are made up only of carbon, oxygen, and hydrogen. All three macronutrients—proteins, fats, and carbohydrates—are organic (meaning that they contain carbon) components that are part of the Earth's living tissues of plants and animals.

THE AMINO ACIDS

Proteins are complex molecules comprised of combinations of 22 naturally occurring amino acids. Amino acids can be thought of as the building blocks of protein. Proteins, each with a unique amino acid sequence and 3-dimensional structure, exist in many different forms, including long chains, branched molecules, spheres, sheets, or helixes.

When scientists study amino acids, they shine light through them. Amino acids that move light counterclockwise (toward the left) are called *L-amino acids.* *D-amino acids* move light in the opposite direction—clockwise, or to the right. The way amino acids move light is not important in and of itself, but it turns out that very few naturally occurring amino acids move light to the right. In our body, only serine and aspartic acid are known to occur in both the L and D forms. With the possible exception of these two amino acids, it is best to supplement with the naturally occurring

L form. This L form is preferable even though the body is capable of converting between the D form and the L form in the case of some amino acids. Twenty main L-amino acids, as well as some other minor ones, are required to build bodily proteins. It is also worth noting that many scientists are using a new lettering system for amino acids. In this new system, L is called S and the D form is called R.

Few ideas have gotten nutritionists as side-tracked as the idea of amino acids being either "essential" or "nonessential." (Note: The words *indispensable* and *dispensable* are often used in place of *essential* and *nonessential*.) Nutritionists have traditionally regarded all amino acids that can potentially be produced in the body as nonessential amino acids. The argument has been that if the body has the ability to make an amino acid, it is not essential for a person to consume that amino acid in his or her diet. The amino acid should therefore be considered nonessential. Conversely, all amino acids that the body cannot possibly make (under any circumstance) have traditionally been classified as essential—that is, required as part of the diet. Most nutritionists who analyze diets only evaluate essential amino acids (presented in the table below) and do not consider nonessential amino acids *at all*.

The problem with this traditional approach is simple: just because the body is *capable in principle* of producing an amino acid (or anything else for that matter) doesn't mean it is *actually doing so* at any given moment. For example, glycine is an amino acid that the body has the potential to make (and for this reason, it has been traditionally classified as nonessential). The body makes glycine by taking another amino acid (serine) and transforming it with the help of an enzyme (serine hydroxymethyltranferase) and a vitamin (pyridoxal phosphate, a form of vitamin B6). If a person is deficient in vitamin B6, the body cannot convert serine into glycine. In this situation, it becomes extremely important for that person to consume glycine in his or her diet. In other words, under circumstances of vitamin B6 deficiency, glycine becomes an essential amino acid.

What's true for glycine is true for all nonessential amino acids. Under certain circumstances, they can become quite essential. Similarly, recent research has made it clear that essential amino acids don't always need to be eaten on a daily basis. A meal, or even an entire day's worth of meals, could be lacking in some

essential amino acid and still be nutritious if the individual consuming these meals is healthy and has adequate body pools of amino acids. For these reasons, a small but increasing number of nutritionists and other health-care professionals have abandoned the terms *essential* and *nonessential* and instead used the term *conditionally essential* to refer to all amino acids. This approach to amino acids asks that nutritionally oriented practitioners be continuously aware of the body and how it is functioning in order to decide about individual amino acid requirements.

The table below summarizes my personal approach to this issue. It makes sense to think of nine of our body's amino acids as essential. We almost always need to obtain these amino acids from food. Conversely, there are six amino acids we seldom require from food; it makes sense to think of these as nonessential, even though I recognize the need to supplement with them under certain circumstances. Finally, there are nine amino acids that lie in the middle of the spectrum. Our need for these nine can easily change from month to month, depending on our current metabolic state. For example, our toxic exposure can greatly increase our need for these conditionally essential

Essential, Nonessential, and Conditionally Essential Amino Acids

Essential	Nonessential	Conditionally Essential
Histidine	Alanine	Arginine
Isoleucine	Asparagine	Carnitine*
Leucine	Aspartic acid	Citrulline*
Lysine	Glutamic acid	Cysteine
Methionine	Homocysteine	Glutamine
Phenylalanine	Serine	Glycine
Threonine		Ornithine*
Tryptophan		Proline
Valine		Taurine*
		Tyrosine

*Amino acids not found in body proteins

Source: Adapted from Institute of Medicine, *Dietary Reference Intakes for Energy, Carbohydrate, Fiber, Fat, Fatty Acids, Cholesterol, Protein, and Amino Acids (Macronutrients)*. Washington, D.C.: National Academy of Sciences, National Academy Press, 2005.

amino acids, as can our use of prescription medications. I therefore suggest classifying these nine amino acids as conditionally essential, with the key condition being our body's *functional* status.

Looking at the body's functional status is also the best way to understand what has happened to protein and amino acids within the field of nutrition over the past 25 years. Up until that time, protein was generally regarded as a part of food that was primarily designed to support body structure. By *structure* nutritional scientists were thinking about things like muscles, connective tissue (collagen), hair, and fingernails. All of these structures are composed primarily of protein, and chronic protein deficiency tended to show up in the weakening or damaging of these structures. Protein was also known to form the structural basis for smaller and less permanent body components, including hormones and enzymes. Since about 1980, however, the focus on structure in protein nutrition has significantly widened to encompass new roles for protein in the area of communication, information processing, and cell signaling.

Research on this recently discovered relationship between protein and communication has also led to fresh thoughts about amino acids and their role in the diet. While surprising at first, it has become quite clear that individual amino acids—not yet formed into proteins at all—can carry messages from nerve to nerve in many regions of the nervous system. Amino acids that function in this way are called *neurotransmitters*. At this moment in amino acid research, scientists know that aspartic acid, glutamic acid, gamma-aminobutyric acid (GABA), glycine, taurine, and histamine all act as neurotransmitters. It is also likely that serine acts in this way, and there is a possibility for arginine as well.

Amino acids also carry information in other ways. They can combine to form *dipeptides* (each containing 2 amino acids) or *oligopeptides* (each containing 3 to 20 amino acids). Dipeptides are found in most plants and animals but are particularly interesting in human digestion. When proteins or their building blocks (amino acids) get actively transported from our intestines up into our cells, there is a definite "pecking order" with dipeptides at the top. In other words, dipeptides are more actively absorbed than any other form of protein or amino acid. Dipeptides get absorbed

more readily than single amino acids, and single amino acids get absorbed more readily than oligopeptides or proteins. Exactly why dipeptides have special privileges is not clear, but their unique communications functions may be involved.

In chemistry, any compound that contains a ring structure is called a *cyclic compound*. When a dipeptide contains a ring structure, it is called a *cyclic dipeptide*. Cyclic dipeptides have been the subject of increasing research since about 1999, primarily in relationship to cancer, where they appear to have antitumor effects by altering genetic communication.

Longer amino acid strings (oligopeptides) have also been shown to impact communications processes, although not at the genetic level. Messages within the cell body appear to be partly regulated by oligopeptides, as do certain physiological processes, including stimulation of lymph flow. (Lymph is the clear fluid that circulates around the body in its own special system of tubes, and it helps replenish the blood and fight infection.) Before leaving the topic of dipeptides and oligopeptides, I want to mention 1 further role played by these molecules. They clearly function as antibiotics. Some appear to have primarily antibacterial properties, and others, antifungal.

There are two key messages in this new research on amino acids: first, they are in our bodies not only to provide structure but also to establish communication between individual cells and entire organ systems, and second, they may turn out to be equally or even more important than proteins when it comes to our nourishment. The relatively new trend in nutritional medicine called *amino acid therapy* is a perfect example of this new focus on amino aids. Since 1998, about two dozen research studies on amino acid supplementation have been published in peer-reviewed journals, with particular focus on the role of branched-chain amino acids (leucine, isoleucine, and valine) in aging, kidney failure, and exercise performance. As an important accompaniment to supplementation of amino acids, some laboratories can run an amino acid profile to decipher the exact amino acid balance, or rather imbalance, that correlates with many disease states. It is clear from my own experience and that of many other doctors and nutritionists that amino acid analysis and therapy has great possibilities in medicine and, as research continues, can be an important addition to medical care in the future.

The following section offers individual discussions of each amino acid, along with their roles in body function and clinical uses where applicable. Amino acids are obviously most abundant in protein foods, yet all foods contain some. Such animal foods as beef, pork, lamb, chicken, turkey, eggs, milk, and cheese are known as *complete proteins* and usually contain all eight essential amino acids. Many vegetable proteins contain adequate levels of several of the essential amino acids but may be low in one or two; grains and their germ coverings, legumes, nuts and seeds, and some vegetables fit into this category. The important topic of protein complementarity—that is, combining different vegetable proteins to acquire all of the essential amino acids—is also discussed, as are specific protein functions and requirements, following the individual amino acids.

Essential Amino Acids

The essential amino acids discussed next warrant a more in-depth review of their common uses, dosages, and success levels in therapy. **When taking any individual amino acid in the amount suggested, limit its use to 6 to 8 weeks and then take a 2- to 3-week break before starting again, unless stated otherwise.** This will avoid, as with B vitamin therapy, an imbalance of any amino acid whose absorption may be inhibited by a higher intake of others. Another way to avoid a possible amino acid imbalance is to take a basic amino acid mixture that contains all the amino acids, essential and nonessential, along with the specific appropriate ones, as demonstrated in many of the programs in part 4 of this book, Nutritional Application: 32 Special Diets and Supplement Programs.

Ile **Isoleucine,** available in most food sources, is particularly high in many fish and meats, in cheeses, and relatively high in wheat germ and most seeds and nuts. L-isoleucine is a branched amino acid found in high concentrations in our muscle tissues. It is used in the body to produce certain biochemical compounds that help in energy production and has been found experimentally to reduce twitching and tremors in animals. The branched-chain amino acids—isoleucine, leucine, and valine—have been used as supplements for bodybuilding (that is, the building of muscle).

Leu **Leucine** is also readily available in good concentrations in animal protein foods (poultry and red meats) and dairy products; wheat germ and oats also contain leucine. It is essential for growth, as it stimulates protein synthesis in muscle. **Leucine can be used as a fuel source to produce energy, as can isoleucine and valine, the other branched-chain amino acids.** Although this use can occur at any time, it is especially important during periods of fasting or starvation. A leucine deficiency can cause a biochemical malfunction producing hypoglycemia in infants. Leucine is also helpful in healing wounds of the skin and bones.

Amino Acids Commonly Used in Clinical Practice

Amino Acid	Uses
L-tryptophan (or as 5-HTP)	Sleep, anxiety
L-lysine	*Herpes simplex* treatment and prevention
DL-phenylalanine	Pain
L-carnitine	Weight loss, cardiovascular disease, chronic fatigue
L-arginine/L-ornithine	Bodybuilding, cancer treatment
L-cysteine	Oxidative stress, detoxification
L-taurine	Depression, convulsions, detoxification
L-glutamine	Alcohol and sugar cravings and addictions, intestinal support
L-tyrosine	Depression and fatigue

Lysine is found in most protein food sources but is not as readily available from the grain cereals or peanuts. Lysine is particularly high in fish, meats, and dairy products and higher than most other amino acids in wheat germ, legumes, and many fruits and vegetables. Among lysine's many functions, it is concentrated in muscle tissue and helps in the absorption of calcium from the intestinal tract, the promotion of bone growth, and the formation of collagen. Collagen is an important body protein that is the basic matrix of the connective tissues, skin, cartilage, and bone. Vitamin C is needed to convert lysine into hydroxylysine, which is then incorporated into collagen. Lysine is also metabolized by transaminase enzymes in the liver; its metabolism depends on vitamins B_6, B_3, B_2, and C and on iron and glutamic acid. Dietary needs for lysine are estimated to be 750 to 1,000 mg daily. A deficiency may contribute to reduced growth and immunity, along with an increase in urinary calcium. This latter fact suggests that adequate lysine may help prevent osteoporosis through better absorption and use of calcium.

Lysine has recently become popular in the prevention and treatment of *Herpes simplex* infections. Although research has been somewhat contradictory, most studies have claimed good success, particularly for cold sores (herpes type 1). Nearly 80% of patients studied believed that taking 1 to 2 grams of L-lysine each day helped them reduce outbreaks and symptoms. The percentage was lower for genital herpes (type 2), a finding that my clinical experience supports. For people who seem to respond to lysine treatment, recent research suggests that an effective dose is 1,500 mg a day (usually 500 mg

Food Types and Their Lysine-to-Arginine Ratios

Type of Food	High Lysine	High Arginine	Lysine-to-Arginine Ratio
yogurt	yes	no	3:1
cheeses	yes	no	2.5:1
butter	yes	no	2.25:1
cow's milk	yes	no	2:1
avocado	yes	moderate	1.5:1
fish	yes	moderate	1.5:1
chicken	yes	yes	1.5:1
beef	yes	yes	1.3:1
egg	moderate	moderate	1:1
cocoa	moderate	moderate	1:1
oats, wheat	moderate	moderate	1:1
spinach	no	no	1:1
corn	no	no	1:1
carrots	no	no	1:1
banana	no	no	1:1
sesame seeds	no	yes	1:2.2
flaxseeds	no	yes	1:2.2
pumpkin seeds	no	yes	1:2.2
pecans	no	yes	1:2.4
sunflower seeds	no	yes	1:2.5
cashews	no	yes	1:4.4
almonds	no	yes	1:4.5
Brazil nuts	no	yes	1:4.8
walnuts	no	yes	1:5.4

Seeds and nuts may vary significantly in their lysine:arginine ratio.

3 times daily) during an infection and 500 mg daily when no symptoms are present. **Please remember, though, that recurrent herpes outbreaks can be a complex problem relating to stress, weakened immunity, a diet too high in acid-forming foods, and nutritional deficiencies, and that lysine therapy is not a substitute for dealing with these factors.**

Another aspect of herpes infections involves the ratio of lysine to arginine in the diet. A higher lysine-to-arginine ratio seems to help many patients reduce the incidence of herpes outbreaks. Animal proteins provide higher ratios, almost always greater than 1:1 and often as high as 3:1. Plant proteins provide lower ratios, usually 1:1 or lower. The table below gives examples of food types and their lysine-to-arginine ratios.

In herpes prevention and treatment, avoiding arginine-rich foods and eating more lysine-rich foods may be helpful. Lysine has little or no toxicity. Not uncommonly, when one stops therapy for herpes, he or she has an outbreak. Lysine is fairly safe, although I think that no amino acid should be used over a long time without a break or without supporting the diet with the other amino acids as well. Interestingly, research has suggested that therapy using L-lysine and L-arginine together is useful and possibly even better than the arginine-ornithine combination in stimulating growth hormone, muscle building, weight loss, and immune support. A dosage of 500 mg twice daily, or 1,000 to 1,500 mg taken before bed, of each amino acid would help in these functions.

Met **Methionine** is of concern mainly because it is the limiting, or the least abundant, amino acid in many foods (see the following section "Food, Protein, and Complementarity" on page 57) particularly low in most legumes, soybeans, and peanuts. Although it is higher in dairy foods, eggs, fish, and meats, it is still present in lower concentration in many of these foods than are the other essential amino acids. **Vegetarians can obtain a fairly good proportion of methionine in the protein content of many nuts and seeds, as well as corn, rice, and other grains, which are naturally lower in tryptophan and lysine.**

Methionine is one of the sulfur-containing amino acids (cysteine and taurine are others) and is important for many bodily functions. Through its supply of sulfur, it helps prevent problems of the skin and nails.

It acts as a lipotropic agent (others are inositol and choline) to prevent excess fat buildup in the liver and the body, is helpful in relieving or preventing fatigue, and may be useful in some cases of allergy because it reduces histamine release. It also may help lower an elevated serum copper level. Methionine works as an antioxidant (a free-radical deactivator) through conversion to L-cysteine to help neutralize toxins. L-cysteine is used more often than methionine as an antioxidant, however, because it seems to be better tolerated and has a wider range of protection.

Phe **Phenylalanine** is a ringed amino acid that is readily available in most food sources, particularly meats and milk products, with lower levels found in oats and wheat germ. It is essential for many bodily functions. Phenylalanine is the precursor of the amino acid tyrosine, which cannot be reconverted, so phenylalanine is essential in the diet. As a precursor of tyrosine, phenylalanine can form norepinephrine in the brain in addition to such other catecholamines as epinephrine, dopamine, and tyramine. Norepinephrine is an important neurotransmitter (that is, it conveys chemoelectric information at nerve synapses) and is apparently important for memory, alertness, and learning. Phenylalanine metabolism requires pyridoxine (B6), niacin (B3), vitamin C, copper, iron, folate, and S-adenosylmethionine (SAM). This amino acid is part of some psychoactive drugs as well as such body chemicals as acetylcholine, melanotropin, vasopressin, cholecystokinins, and the enkephalins and endorphins.

Phenylalanine has been used for treatment of depression in the D-, L-, or DL- forms, probably because it forms tyrosine, an excitatory neurotransmitter. Eric Braverman, in *The Healing Nutrients Within,* suggest that L-phenylalanine works best in bipolar disorders (with manic and depressive states) in doses of 500 mg twice daily up to 2 to 3 grams daily, along with 100 mg of vitamin B6 twice daily, whereas D- and DL-phenylalanine work better for affective depression (lack of positive attitude or emotional enthusiasm for life). Phenylalanine is better absorbed than tyrosine and produces fewer headaches, so may be more useful in depression than L-tyrosine. Both DL- and D-phenylalanine are helpful pain relievers in certain musculoskeletal problems, and this is currently their primary use.

Aspartame, the nutrient sweetener (most commonly marketed under the brand name NutraSweet), is synthesized from the combination of aspartic acid and phenylalanine. Although aspartame (in the form of NutraSweet) was added to the federal government's Generally Recognized as Safe (GRAS) list of food additives in 1983, there continue to be questions about its safety. These questions are not limited to its consumption by individuals with PKU (the hereditary problem with phenylalanine metabolism) or pregnant women. John Olney, an MD in the Psychiatry Department at Washington University School of Medicine in Saint Louis, Missouri, has raised questions about the relationship between certain types of brain cancers (glioblastomas) and consumption of aspartame. He has also found evidence of toxic compounds (called *N-nitro compounds*) being formed in the stomach from aspartame. I also believe that for some sensitive individuals aspartame acts as a nervous system irritant and adversely affects energy and mood.

I have used phenylalanine, in particular, for patients with pain problems, most commonly back pain due to muscular or ligamentous irritation, although it may be helpful for any type of pain. It probably works for this purpose because of its function of increasing endorphins in the brain, but it is not really a treatment for the *cause* of the pain, such as inflammation or spasms. The endorphins are thought to provide a more positive outlook on life, to enhance alertness, and to improve vitality. (This may be why phenylalanine works for depression.) Endorphins are the mysterious substances released when we exercise or when we experience positive emotions. They are also thought to make us less sensitive to or aware of pain. DL-phenylalanine blocks the enkephalinase enzymes that break down the endorphins and enkephalins, the natural pain relievers and mood elevators. This substance does not work all the time, however, nor is it a complete therapy; the underlying cause of the pain or depression should be discovered.

Some pain problems for which phenylalanine may be helpful are low back pain, neck pain, osteoarthritis, rheumatoid arthritis, menstrual cramps, and headaches, particularly migraines. **But patients suffering from migraines may have elevated phenylalanine levels, in which case supplementation would not help. L-tryptophan may work better in these patients.** On

a trial basis, to see whether it will be helpful for pain, DL-phenylalanine can be taken in a dose of about 500 to 750 mg 2 to 3 times daily. It really has no common side effects other than occasional headache or jitteriness. However, its catecholamine effect may raise blood pressure in some people, so this should be watched. Phenylalanine therapy is not recommended for long-term use; as with the other amino acids, it should not be taken for more than 3 weeks at a time without a break or without the support of the other amino acids.

Thr

Threonine is somewhat low in corn and some grains, although it is not the limiting amino acid in these foods (that is, the lowest relative to making a complete protein). There are good levels of threonine in most animal foods, dairy foods, and eggs and moderate levels in wheat germ, many nuts, beans, and seeds, as well as some vegetables. Threonine is an important constituent in many body proteins and is necessary for the formation of tooth enamel protein, elastin, and collagen. Newborns have threonine in high amounts, and requirements seem to decrease with age yet increase with stress. Threonine also has a minor role (a greater one when choline is deficient) as a lipotropic in controlling fat buildup in the liver.

Threonine has a mild glucose-sparing effect and is a precursor of the amino acids glycine and serine. **Threonine is one of the immune-stimulating nutrients (cysteine, lysine, alanine, and aspartic acid are others), as it promotes thymus growth and activity.** A deficiency of threonine in rats has been associated with a weakened cellular response and antibody formation. One gram of threonine twice daily may also be helpful in some cases of depression.

Trp

Tryptophan is the least plentiful essential amino acid in corn, many cereal grains, and legumes. The dietary intake of tryptophan in general is lower than most other amino acids. It is not particularly high in any foods but is readily available in animal foods, eggs, dairy products, and some nuts and seeds. It is also present in the casein component of milk. I do not support the story that tryptophan itself is the disease culprit it has been made out to be since 1989, when the U.S. Food and Drug Administration (FDA) first took action to limit the availability of tryptophan within the United States (see sidebar below). However, L-tryptophan (and 5-hydroxytryptophan, or 5-HTP is again available through doctors supplied by compounding pharmacists, and it is quite useful in the treatment of insomnia and depression.

Functionally, tryptophan is important, and it has been used effectively for a variety of medical problems. Vitamin B6, vitamin C, folic acid, and magnesium are needed to metabolize tryptophan. **It is the precursor for a vital neurotransmitter, serotonin, which influences moods and sleep; serotonin levels are directly related to tryptophan intake.** Because other amino acids, such as tyrosine and phenylalanine, compete for absorption with tryptophan, tryptophan must often be taken as a supplement to increase its blood levels. It also acts differently than other amino acids, as it can exist free in the blood and can be carried by protein. In a sense, tryptophan is an essential vitamin because it is the precursor of vitamin B3 (niacin); a deficiency of tryptophan, combined with inadequate dietary niacin, can cause the symptoms of pellagra: dermatitis, diarrhea, dementia, and death (the four Ds; see the section on "Vitamin B3 (Niacin)" on page 115 in chapter 5, Vitamins). Low tryptophan levels are found in many patients with dementia and may have subclinical or subtle psychological effects.

Tryptophan has been used effectively to treat insomnia in many people. Serotonin is needed in the brain to induce and maintain sleep. Usually, 1 to 2 grams of L-tryptophan (the desired form) are needed to increase blood levels sufficiently to induce sleep. However, the lowest dose that works to aid sleep (often as little as 500 mg) should be maintained. It can be repeated if the person wakes in the middle of the night. As an initial treatment, I suggest 1 gram of L-tryptophan taken 30 to 45 minutes before bed, which reduces the time it takes to fall asleep (the sleep latency period). Some formulas contain vitamin B6 and niacinamide, which improve tryptophan utilization. If 1 gram is insufficient, increase the dose by 500 mg each night, up to a total of 3,000 mg, and add calcium (300–600 mg) and magnesium (200–400 mg) to your good-night supplements. Tryptophan works better for acute insomnia than for chronic sleep problems. **Patients with asthma or systemic lupus erythematosus should not take tryptophan.** Generally, side effects are negligible, and tryptophan does not distort sleep patterns until more than 10 grams are taken.

Tryptophan also has an antidepressant effect and is particularly effective in manic depression and depression associated with menopause. Many depressed patients have low levels of tryptophan. Tryptophan can be a useful and safe pain reliever. It has been shown most helpful for dental pain, headaches (migraines in particular), and cancer pain, often in conjunction with aspirin or acetaminophen. Tryptophan appears to increase the pain threshold. It may help treat anorexia by increasing the appetite. Because it is the precursor of niacin, tryptophan supplementation may help to lower cholesterol and blood fat levels. Other possible uses for L-tryptophan include parkinsonism, epilepsy, and schizophrenia, and with further research, scientists may find that this important amino acid might provide help with other medical conditions.

Exactly what happened with tryptophan supplements in 1989? The tryptophan controversy started out with an outbreak of eosinophilia-myalgia syndrome in which about 500 cases were reported to the Centers for Disease Control in Atlanta, Georgia, and a total of 37 deaths were eventually reported. Certain blood cells called *eosinophils* had reached high levels in these individuals, causing problems because of the high levels of histamine and other inflammatory substances contained in these cells. The consumption of tryptophan supplements manufactured by 6 Japanese companies was initially associated with the outbreak. However, many observers believed that inadequate purification of the tryptophan through altered filtration processes and the use of genetically modified bacteria by a single company were the only factors that could definitively be linked with the outbreak. In other words, the problems seemed associated with supplement contamination due to faulty manufacturing, not to tryptophan supplementation itself. At the time of this writing, the FDA continues to restrict import of tryptophan supplements into the United States but does not expressly prohibit the sale of this amino acid in supplement form. Tryptophan is currently available through doctors and compounding pharmacists (those pharmacists that make up medicines from primary compounds).

Valine is found in substantial quantities in most foods and is an essential part of many proteins. It is perhaps most famous in the area of nutritional biochemistry for its appearance in sickle-cell disease. In this disease, a single amino acid in the hemoglobin protein (glutamic acid) is replaced by valine in the protein chain. This replacement of glutamic acid by valine alters the shape of the hemoglobin protein and prevents the red blood cell that contains it from carrying oxygen successfully. Although there is no direct evidence as of yet, valine substitution (for another amino acid in a protein) may be a process that is at work in other genetic alterations, including alterations in cancer-causing genes. The potential antitumor properties of valine are currently being investigated in this regard.

Other functions of valine are not really known, although it is thought to be somewhat helpful in treating addictions. A deficiency may affect the myelin covering of nerves. Valine can be metabolized to produce energy, which spares glucose. Like leucine and isoleucine, valine is a branched-chain amino acid with similar metabolic pathways. A potentially deadly hereditary disease, commonly called the "maple syrup urine disease," blocks the metabolism of these three amino acids. In children affected with this disease, keto acids are dumped into the urine, making it smell like maple syrup. The amino acid deficiencies that result cause seizures, problems with the nervous system, and a failure to thrive. Valine supplementation may be helpful in muscle building (along with isoleucine and leucine) and in treating liver and gallbladder disease.

Conditionally Essential Amino Acids

Arginine is usually synthesized by adults in amounts sufficient to maintain the body proteins, but additional dietary arginine is needed during periods of growth, as in childhood or during pregnancy, and possibly during times of stress. Arginine is present in most proteins, including meats, nuts, milk, cheese, and eggs. In particular, nuts and seeds have a high arginine-to-lysine ratio. These foods have been noted to increase the frequency of *Herpes simplex* attacks (both cold sores and genital lesions) in patients infected with this virus. (Eating foods high in lysine, L-lysine supplementation, or both may help

treat such outbreaks; see the earlier section in this chapter on lysine, on page 44.) Arginine deficiencies can exist in human beings and may occur during times of high protein demand; with trauma, low protein intake, or malnutrition; or from excess lysine intake, which may compete with arginine. Arginine deficiency can result in hair loss, constipation, a delay in the healing of wounds, and liver disease.

Arginine has several important functions. It is essential to the metabolism of ammonia that is generated from protein breakdown. It is also needed to transport the nitrogen used in muscle metabolism. Arginine is one of the bodybuilding amino acids and also influences several hormone functions. L-arginine has been shown to stimulate the pituitary gland to produce and secrete human growth hormone in young males, at a dose of more than 3 grams daily. Human growth hormone helps in muscle building, leading to increased muscle strength and tone, and enhances fat metabolism (increases the burning of fats), which may help with weight loss. Growth hormone in general seems to increase metabolism and energy. L-arginine has a positive effect on the immune system, mainly by stimulating thymus activity, and also helps the body heal from wounds. Some research has shown that high doses of L-arginine may increase male fertility by increasing sperm production and motility.

Arginine is also interesting in its relationship to a highly reactive gas, nitric oxide, found throughout the body. Arginine is the primary substance used as a foundation (substrate) for forming nitric oxide. Whenever the body activates the enzyme nitric oxide synthase to convert excess arginine into citrulline (another amino acid), nitric oxide is created in the process. This activity occurs primarily in the liver and is part of the body's nitrogen cycling process. The encouragement of nitric oxide formation by high levels of liver arginine has been explored by some researchers as a method of helping to regulate blood pressure and to improve male impotence, because both require increased relaxation of blood vessels and nitric oxide can produce that effect.

L-arginine has several other possible uses. The most common use, in part promoted by Pearson and Shaw's book *Life Extension,* is as a growth hormone stimulant. Bodybuilders supplement L-arginine along with L-ornithine for its muscle-building effects. Recent

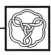

research has suggested that L-arginine and L-lysine together have a similar effect, possibly at lower dosages. L-arginine supplementation, at a dosage of 4 grams daily, has been successful in improving fertility in men by increasing low sperm count and motility. Arginine has been shown to help speed wound healing in rats, possibly by aiding collagen formation. Other possible uses for L-arginine as seen in animals are to improve decreased liver functions, to lower cholesterol levels, and to inhibit the growth of certain tumors (it may also stimulate the growth of certain tumors, however).

L-arginine, available in 500 mg capsules, is usually well tolerated in doses as high as 3 to 6 grams, although such side effects as diarrhea, nausea, and, rarely, ataxia (unsteadiness) may occur in some people. Dosages of less than 2 grams daily are usually handled without problems. A dosage of 3 to 4 grams daily is needed for the growth hormone effect. L-arginine and L-ornithine, or L-arginine and L-lysine, can be supplemented at 500 to 1,000 mg of each twice daily, or 1,000 to 1,500 mg of each before bed. To improve male fertility, a dosage of 2 grams twice daily is suggested. Children and teenagers should avoid supplementation of L-arginine for growth stimulation or body-building. **People with diabetes must be careful because of arginine's effect on insulin and carbohydrate metabolism.** Supplementation should not be done continuously for a long period. I suggest that it be used for 2 to 3 weeks, followed by a break of 1 to 2 weeks. A balanced amino acid supplement can also be used.

Cys **Cysteine** and **cystine** are sulfur-containing amino acids that are synthesized in the liver and are involved in multiple metabolic pathways. Cysteine is formed from homocysteine, which comes from the essential amino acid methionine. The process of making cysteine from methionine is complex and requires multiple enzymatic steps, vitamins, and other amino acids. Because of this complexity, there is a greater risk of functional deficiency for cysteine than for many other amino acids. Cysteine can be converted to cystine and taurine. Cystine itself is a disulfide, containing two cysteine molecules. Cysteine is contained in a variety of foods, found mainly as cystine in poultry, yogurt, oats, and wheat germ, or in the sulfur foods that contain methionine and cysteine,

such as egg yolks, red peppers, garlic, onions, broccoli, and brussels sprouts.

In recent years, findings about cysteine and its many functions in the body have been exciting. It can be used to help treat a variety of problems. **Perhaps most important has been the discovery that cysteine is required for formation of glutathione, a tripeptide that also contains the amino acids glycine and glutamic acid.** Glutathione's chemical name is gamma-glutamylcysteinylglycine, abbreviated as GSH (referring to its chemically reduced form) or GSSG (referring to its chemically oxidized form). It is difficult to overestimate the importance of glutathione in our biochemical health, or the role of cysteine in supporting it. Glutathione has been discussed in more than 27,000 research studies since 1994 and has been the main focus in more than a third of those studies. Several hundred of these studies have focused on cysteine and its relationship to glutathione. In volume alone, this number of studies is greater than work on any other nutrient since 1994. In its acetylated form, N-acetyl-cysteine (NAC), cysteine appears to support glutathione metabolism in some cases better than glutathione itself. Cysteine also appears to be a common rate-limiting factor in the formation of glutathione. This means that when glutathione is not available, the holdup is often lack of cysteine.

Why is the cysteine-glutathione connection so important? Glutathione turns out to be a critical regulator of cell health; it is absolutely essential for maintaining electrochemical balance in many cells. It functions as a detoxifying agent in the kidneys and is required for elimination of many environmental toxins, including fungicides, herbicides, nitrosamines, dyes, solvents, plastics, detergents, and insecticides. Glutathione is also required genetically, for synthesis and repair of DNA, as well as for neutralization of free radicals that can damage healthy cells. Immune function, nerve function, and cell signaling functions are also heavily influenced by glutathione. Within the immune function category, wound healing, especially healing from skin wounds, appears to depend on glutathione availability.

Because of its ability to help rid the body of toxic substances, glutathione is cancer preventing, and it is often found to be deficient in cases of cancer. For example, liver cancer and cirrhosis of the liver following alcohol abuse are situations characterized by glutathione deficiency. Some of the cancer-protective effects of glutathione are related to its ability to chelate heavy metals. *Chelate* simply means "to latch onto" (the word *chela* in Greek means "claw"), and that is what glutathione often does with heavy metals, including cadmium, mercury, and lead. By latching onto these metals, glutathione can help prevent their toxic effects from occurring.

Two enzymes are especially important for understanding the healing properties of glutathione: glutathione peroxidase (GPO) and glutathoine-S-transferase (GST). GPO contains 8 molecules of glutathione and 4 selenium atoms, and it allows the body to convert reactive oxygen molecules (called peroxides, including hydrogen peroxide) into water. GPO is especially important in protecting cell membranes and blood vessel linings from the damaging effects of peroxides. GSTs are actually an entire family of enzymes that play much the same role as GPO: they protect cells from toxic damage by combining those toxins with glutathione and allowing for their excretion from the body. High-vegetable diets and, in particular, vegetable

diets containing frequent servings of such sulfur-rich foods as onions, garlic, broccoli, and cabbage help support GST function.

The blood vessel protection provided by glutathione appears to be provided by cysteine as well. A team of medical doctors in Prague has succeeded in lessening the damage caused by heart attack through N-acetyl-cysteine (NAC) supplementation following the initial event. The dose used in this research was 100 mg of NAC for every kilogram of body weight.

Both cysteine and glutathione levels appear to decrease with aging, and for this reason, it is logical to think about them as antiaging nutrients that are necessary to keep our bodies detoxified and protected from oxygen and free-radical damage. Increased cysteine intake may be helpful in actually increasing one's life span and can be beneficial in those inflammatory problems caused by free radicals, such as arthritis and vascular irritation. Basically, it is used in amounts commonly ranging from 250 to 750 mg daily, often taken in several portions throughout the day along with 3 times the vitamin C to prevent crystallization of excess cystine.

Possible Uses of L-Cysteine

Air pollution

Asthma

Cancer prevention and treatment (decreases toxicity of offending agents)

Cataract (best in prevention)

Exposure to chemicals

Hair loss

Infection (immune support, detoxifier)

Mental illness

Metal toxicity or exposure (lead, mercury, cadmium)

Post–heart attack

Psoriasis (aids skin healing)

Rheumatoid arthritis

Smokers*

Smoker's cough/bronchitis

Surgery or injury (aids wound healing)

---

* Protects alveoli from smoke damage, along with beta-carotene, zinc, and selenium. NAC, n-acetyl-cysteine, is a good product choice in this case

---

Gly **Glycine** can be formed from choline in the liver or kidney and from the amino acids threonine and serine. It can be converted back to serine in the fasting state. **Glycine is one of the few amino acids that helps spare glucose for energy by improving glycogen storage.** It is important in brain metabolism, where it acts as a neurotransmitter and has a calming effect. Glycine is a simple amino acid needed for the synthesis of the hemoglobin molecule, collagen, and glutathione. It can also be converted to creatine, which is used to make DNA and RNA. Glycine is useful in healing wounds (taken orally or in a cream) and treating manic psychological states or problems of muscle spasticity. When the blood fats or uric acid levels are high, it helps to clear or utilize these substances. Glycine may also be helpful in reducing gastric acidity; in higher doses, 4 to 8 grams, it stimulates growth hormone release. It is also used as a mild sweetener in foods or drugs.

More recently discovered is the role of glycine in detoxification, especially by the liver, and especially in relationship to particular types of toxins. The liver attaches glycine to certain toxins as a way of making them more water soluble and available for excretion out of the body. The most commonly used food additive worldwide (sodium benzoate) must get detoxified in this way (that is, by getting linked up with glycine, or "glycinated"). Another commonly encountered substance that requires glycination is aspirin. Chemically known as *acetylsalicylic acid*, aspirin belongs to the salicylate family of molecules, and this entire family must be detoxified in the liver using glycine and the glycination process. For individuals who are sensitive to dietary salicylates, adequate glycine intake is especially important.

Dimethylglycine (DMG) is a popular substance in today's nutritional products. It is also a corollary for vitamin B15, pangamic acid. DMG is an intermediary of cell metabolism, mainly from glycine and choline. As a precursor to glycine, some of DMG's effects may be attributed to simple glycine, particularly in regard to its neuroinhibitory effect in such problems as epilepsy. DMG seems to be able to increase the immune antibody response and to improve physical energy and has been used in the treatment of infections, immune suppression, fatigue, and poor endurance. Some people experience good results, while others do not. More research is needed to properly understand dimethylglycine's role in clinical medicine.

 Histidine must also be obtained from diet during childhood and growth periods. It may be needed in malnourished or injured individuals or whenever there is need for tissue formation or repair. Histidine is found in most animal and vegetable proteins, particularly pork, poultry, cheese, and wheat germ. Histidine is involved in a wide range of metabolic processes involving blood cell production (it is present in hemoglobin) and in the production of histamine, which is involved in many allergic and inflammatory reactions. Histidine has been used supplementally in the treatment of allergic disorders, peptic ulcers, anemia, and cardiovascular disease, as it has a hypotensive effect (that is, it lowers blood pressure) through the autonomic nervous system. Some cases of arthritis have improved with a supplemented dosage of 1,000 to 1,500 mg taken 3 times daily. Histidine also acts as a metal chelating agent—that is, it can bind itself to metals—and when bound to minerals such as zinc or copper in supplements, it improves their absorption.

Proline is one of the main amino acids of collagen and is helpful to bone, skin, and cartilage formation. Proline can be formed from glutamine or the amino acid ornithine. In foods, it is found readily in dairy products and eggs, with some levels found in meats or wheat germ. Proline is helpful in maintaining joints and tendons, in tissue repair after injury, or for any type of wound healing. Recent research has implicated proline in two other health-related areas with far-reaching implications. First is the discovery that amino acid chains rich in proline are the molecules that many mammals (and insects) use to help prevent bacterial infection from gram-negative bacteria. Researchers don't know yet whether proline has infection-preventing properties in humans. Second is the recognition that some signaling processes used by cells to send messages back and forth are partly regulated by proline. Once again, exactly where this new area of research will lead is not yet known.

Traditionally "Nonessential" Amino Acids and Related Nutrients

The amino acids that our bodies normally makes and that are found in body proteins have traditionally been referred to as "nonessential." (There are other important amino acids that are not found in proteins, which include carnitine, citrulline, ornithine, and taurine.) As discussed earlier, however, just because the body is *capable in principle* of producing an amino acid doesn't mean it is *actually doing so* at any given moment. For this reason, these "nonessential" amino acids may actually become essential under specific circumstances. With that in mind, let us explore some of the functions and possible supplementary uses of these nonessential amino acids.

 Alanine is an important part of human muscle tissue and is readily found in protein foods, including beef, pork, turkey, and cheese, as well as in wheat germ, oats, yogurt, and avocado. Alanine plays a unique role in blending muscle and liver chemistry through what is called the glucose-alanine cycle. The cycle operates as follows: Working muscles need a fuel source, and some of that fuel comes in the form of glucose that is produced in the liver. As muscles work, however, amino acids get broken down, and the nitrogen in the amino acids needs some place to go. The working muscles get rid of their excess nitrogen by creating alanine (from a molecule called *pyruvate*, which serves as an attachment spot for the nitrogen). Alanine carries the nitrogen back to the liver, where it can be converted into urea and eventually excreted in the urine. **The balance between pyruvate, glucose, and alanine is important in helping to regulate blood sugar, and it is not surprising that alanine deficiency has been seen in hypoglycemia.** Alanine supplementation may be helpful in treating this condition.

Alanine stimulates lymphocyte production and may help people who have immune suppression. Alanine plays a definite role in brain metabolism, although this role is not entirely clear. It is possible that alanine may act like a neurotransmitter and may directly carry messages between nerves. There is other evidence, however, to suggest that alanine's role is limited to that of a nitrogen shuttle—much like its role in muscle-liver metabolism. In the case of the brain, however, alanine is thought to act as a nitrogen shuttle between nerves and other brain cells called *astrocytes*. In either case, the presence of alanine in the brain appears to help prevent overexcitation and, as with taurine, may be helpful in prevention of epileptic seizures. Alanine is a big part of the cell walls of many bacteria, including *Streptococcus faecium,* a normal intestinal bacterium. Beta-alanine, a variant of natural L-alanine, is not a constituent of proteins but is part of pantothenic acid, vitamin B5.

Asp **Aspartic acid,** readily available in protein foods, is active in many body processes, including the formation of ammonia and urea and their disposal from the body. It is found in high levels throughout the human body, especially in the brain, where it performs an excitatory function. This excitatory function involves a special receptor found on several kinds of cells, including nerve cells, called the *N-methyl-D-asparate (NMDA) receptor.* NMDA receptors have been a topic of intensive research since 1980 and are known to play a key role in the biochemistry of many mental health problems. Depression, anxiety, schizophrenia, and even memory lapse have been linked with changes in NMDA receptor activity. More recently, these receptors have been studied to determine their possible connection to chronic fatigue syndrome as well as Alzheimer's, Parkinson's, and Huntington's diseases. In general, excessive intake of aspartic acid (or glutamic acid) can risk excessive triggering of NMDA receptors and cause overstimulation of the nervous system. Because of this overstimulation effect, aspartic acid is often referred to as an "excitatory amino acid," as is its companion amino acid, glutamic acid. Just as problematic as overstimulation, however, is understimulation of the nervous system by deficient intake of the excitatory amino acids, including aspartate.

Aspartic acid has been found in increased levels in people with epilepsy and in decreased amounts in some cases of depression. Aspartic acid also can help form the ribonucleotides that assist production of DNA and RNA, and it aids energy production from carbohydrate metabolism. Aspartic acid can help protect the liver from some drug toxicity and the body from radiation; it may also increase resistance to fatigue. Aspartic acid is employed to form such mineral salts as potassium, calcium, or magnesium aspartate. Because aspartates are easily absorbed, they can actively transport these minerals across the intestinal lining into the blood and cells, where they can be used for their particular functions, such as energy production or bone metabolism. Asparagine, formed from aspartic acid, aids the metabolic function of the cells of the brain and the nervous system by releasing energy as it reverts back to aspartic acid.

Glu **Glutamic acid** (glutamate), together with aspartic acid, is classified as both an acidic and an excitatory amino acid (because of its ability to stimulate the nervous system). Interestingly, however, glutamic acid is quite readily converted into GABA (gamma-aminobutyric acid), and GABA does not stimulate the nervous system but actually inhibits it. GABA has been used in the treatment of epilepsy, high blood pressure, and anxiety, as it helps in relaxation. GABA may also enhance the sex drive and reduce nighttime urination.

Glutamic acid can also be readily converted into glutamine, an amino acid that is best known for its healing ability in the small intestine and its support of muscle metabolism. Glutamic acid can be made inside the body through a variety of metabolic pathways.

Glutamine is the most direct amino acid source for making glutamate, but other amino acids (including arginine, ornithine, and proline) can also indirectly be converted into glutamate. (Another common source is the organic acid alpha-ketoglutarate). Glutamic acid is abundant in both animal and vegetable proteins and is found in high concentrations in the human brain. Glutamic acid helps transport potassium into the spinal fluid and, as mentioned earlier, is itself an excitatory neurotransmitter. Glutamic acid thus has been used in the treatment of fatigue, parkinsonism, schizophrenia, mental retardation, muscular dystrophy, and alcoholism. Supplemented as L-glutamine, it penetrates the blood-brain barrier and can be used as a brain fuel. **Research has shown that L-glutamine, in a dose of 500 mg 4 times daily, decreases the craving for alcohol.** This amino acid is now commonly used in alcoholism clinics. L-glutamine also seems to reduce the craving for sugar and carbohydrates and so may be helpful for some people in dealing with obesity or sugar abuse. It may also help in the healing of ulcers.

Monosodium glutamate (MSG) is a single sodium salt of glutamic acid. This seaweed extract, now commonly produced chemically through fermentation of sugar or molasses, is included on the FDA's GRAS list as a food additive and is widely used as a flavor enhancer. In fact, about 85 million pounds of MSG are added to the overall U.S. food supply each year. Because glutamate and aspartate can stimulate the nervous system, some people experience nerve-related symptoms like numbness or tingling from relatively small doses of MSG. (A small dose usually means about $\frac{1}{8}$ teaspoon per serving.)

It is interesting to note that the amount of free glutamate in food (glutamate not bound up inside a larger protein) has increased since about 1994, primarily because of the use of protein hydrosylates in processed food. Up to 40% of the protein in protein hydrolysates can consist of glutamate and aspartate— a disproportionally high amount of these excitatory amino acids. In some processed foods containing protein hydrolysates, there are up to 1,500 mg of glutamate per serving—as much or more than the amount of MSG that gets added to other foods. Exactly how this increased exposure to glutamate impacts our health is not clear. However, what is clear is the overactivation of NMDA receptors by glutamate and aspartate in a variety of health problems, including chronic fatigue syndrome and several autoimmune conditions. It is also worth mentioning in this context that our understanding of the brain, and its susceptibility to glutamate excess, has changed since the mid-1990s. Scientists used to think that the blood-brain barrier regulated flow of glutamate into all areas of the brain and protected the brain from excess. We now know that there are regions of the brain, called the *circumventricular organs* (CVOs) that do not enjoy the protection of the blood-brain barrier and are more susceptible to glutamate and aspartate excess.

Hcy **Homocysteine** is an intermediary metabolite of the amino acid methionine. It's been the focus of more than 2,000 research studies since the mid-1990s but was first systematically investigated by Kilmer McCully, an MD currently on the medical faculty of Brown University, beginning in the late 1960s. Kilmer found out that homocysteine played a normal role in many body processes, including cell and tissue growth, bone growth, and insulin formation. In some of its effects, homocysteine appeared to act like growth hormone. Metabolizing homocysteine, however, requires adequate supplies of three vitamins: vitamin B6, vitamin B12, and folate. When these vitamins became deficient, homocysteine can't be effectively converted into other compounds, including the amino acids methionine and cysteine. Buildup of homocysteine in the blood (called *hyperhomocysteinemia*) was discovered to increase the formation of plaques on the blood vessel walls and eventual clogging and hardening of the blood vessels (a condition commonly referred to as *atherosclerosis*). Individuals with high homocysteine levels could often be identified by urine tests, which showed homocystinuria— that is, an increased presence of homocystine (a double molecule of homocysteine).

Hydroxylysine is closely related to lysine and is important in the formation of collagen, which makes up the white, fibrous connective tissue and is part of the skin, bones, and cartilage. Hydroxylysine is found in gelatin and in the digestive enzymes trypsin and chymotrypsin. Researchers are taking a close look at hydroxylysine as a marker for bone health because blood levels of this amino acid appear to predict bone formation much better than other laboratory measurements. Some forms of hydroxylysine in our connective tissue cannot be made without the help of manganese.

Hydroxyproline is also an important component of collagen. Hydroxyproline is converted from proline (discussed in the next section) by hydroxylation only after proline gets into the amino acid chains that form body proteins.

Ser **Serine** can be made in the tissue from glycine (or threonine), so it is nonessential, but its production requires adequate amounts of B3, B6, and folic acid. All cell membranes contain serine in a special form (phosphatidylserine), but the membranes of brain cells are particularly dependant on this form of serine for their flexibility. Serine is also a constituent of brain proteins, including nerve coverings. It is important in metabolism of purines and pyrimidines (part of the nucleic acids RNA and DNA), in the formation of cell membranes, and in creatine (part of muscle) synthesis. Serine is an important component of the SAM cycle (S-adnosylmethionine, is referred to as SAM in the research literature and as SAM-e in the natural products industry). This is a special metabolic process that is required in many critical areas of metabolism, including detoxification, gene regulation, and hormone production. Serine has recently become a subject of fascination for neurobiologists, because along with aspartate, it is one of the two amino acids naturally found in the D- form within the body. The implications of D-serine for health are not clear, but this unique form may be involved in serine's relationship to nervous system activity.

At this point, it appears possible that serine acts directly as a neurotransmitter as well as a modifier of other nerve-messaging processes. Recent research has also indicated a role for serine in the regulation of cell cycles and, in particular, the deliberate, programmed ending of the cell's life span, called *apoptosis*. Outside of the body, serine is known to have natural moisturizing properties and has been used in skin creams. Serine is readily found in meats and dairy products, wheat gluten, peanuts, and soy products—many foods that can cause allergy. There is some concern that elevated serine levels (especially in sausage and lunch meats) can cause immune suppression and psychological symptoms, such as is seen in cerebral allergies.

Tyr **Tyrosine** is easily made in the body from phenylalanine and is important to general metabolism, as it is a direct precursor of both adrenaline (epinephrine) as well as norepinephrine, dopamine, and thyroid hormones—all stimulants to metabolism and the nervous system. Folic acid, niacin, vitamin C, copper, and S-adenosylmethionine are needed to support tyrosine metabolism into these and other important substances, which also include melanin, estrogen molecules, and the enkephalins (natural pain relievers). Tyrosine may stimulate growth hormone and can act as a mild appetite suppressant. It may also be useful in the control of anxiety or depression. Tyrosine is known as the "antidepressant" amino acid. It has a mild antioxidant effect, binding up free radicals (unstable molecules) that can cause damage to the cells and tissues, and is useful for smokers, people with stressful lives, or those exposed to chemicals and radiation.

L-tyrosine has also been used, usually in a dose of 1 to 2 grams a day, for low sex drive, Parkinson's disease, and in programs for drug problems or weight loss. As an antidepressant, 500 to 1,000 mg of L-tyrosine can be taken 2 or 3 times daily. Because tyrosine has a more stimulating antidepressant effect, taking 1,000 to 1,500 mg of L-tryptophan (which is more tranquilizing) at night for sleep may be a good therapeutic combination to help in mild to moderate depression.

Amino Acids Not Found in Body Proteins

Many other amino acids are found in Nature and in food that, although not building blocks of human protein tissue, can be important and helpful in metabolic functions. Some of these amino acids are similar to or are by-products of the previously discussed amino acids, such as asparagine (a variant of aspartic acid) or ornithine (available from arginine); others are separate in structure and functions. Some common ones are discussed in this section.

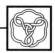

Car **Carnitine** has only recently been noted as an important amino acid (the L- form only) essential to our health. It is found in the diet and can also be made by the body, mainly in the liver and kidneys, from lysine with the help of vitamin C, pyridoxine, niacin, iron, and methionine. Carnitine is found mainly in the red meats (thus, the name) with some levels found in fish, poultry, and milk products and less in tempeh (fermented soybeans), wheat, and avocados. Carnitine is stored primarily in the skeletal muscles and heart, where it is needed to transform fatty acids into energy for muscular activity. It is also concentrated in sperm and in the brain. Carnitine is used to transport fatty acids into cells and across the mitochondrial membranes into the cellular energy factories, the mitochondria. It also increases the rate at which the liver oxidizes (uses) fats, an energy-generating process.

L-carnitine is the active form and can be taken as a safe supplement with positive benefits. **With carnitine's effect on fatty acids and energy production, especially in the heart and muscles, it is known as a nutrient that protects us from cardiovascular disease.** It has been shown to reduce blood triglycerides and cholesterol levels by increasing fat utilization; at the same time, carnitine can raise the HDL (high-density lipoprotein) portion of the cholesterol, which reduces cardiovascular disease risk. L-carnitine also helps with weight loss, usually improves our exercise capacities (possibly through the oxidation of amino acids), and may possibly enhance our muscle building and endurance. These latter two aspects may be a result of the weight loss and better exercise. Many athletes have noted improved endurance with L-carnitine supplementation. In some studies, L-carnitine has been shown to improve the symptoms of angina, reducing pain and allowing more activity. It also may lessen the risk of fatty deposits in the liver associated with alcohol abuse.

Deficiencies of carnitine have been noted, more so recently with people who avoid red meats in their diet. These deficiencies occur most often in vegetarians and during pregnancy or lactation. Vegetarians, though, often have low-fat diets and otherwise reduced cardiovascular disease risk. Deficiencies may increase symptoms of fatigue, angina, muscle weakness, or confusion. More research is needed to clarify and verify these deficiency states, as well as to establish whether the metabolic benefits of L-carnitine are clearly separate from correcting that deficiency.

The dosage of L-carnitine (not D- or DL-carnitine) suggested to improve fat metabolism and muscular performance is 1,000 to 2,000 mg daily, usually divided into 2 doses. This is basically safe and can be taken over an extended period, although it probably should be stopped for 1 week each month, until its long-term safety as a supplement is more clearly established. The *Physician's Desk Reference* has recommended L-carnitine in the treatment of ischemic heart disease and hyperlipid states (specifically, type IV hyperlipidemia) in a dosage of 600 to 1,200 mg 3 times daily. **Carnitine is not recommended for people with active liver or kidney disease or with diabetes.** However, it is definitely recommended for people with such heart problems as ischemia or arrhythmia or with increased cardiovascular risk (such as high blood fats), and for people with problems of poor endurance, muscle weakness, or obesity. I am excited about the uses of L-carnitine and look forward to more positive research in the future.

Possible Uses of L-Carnitine

Alcohol abuse

Angina pectoris

Atherosclerosis

Cardiac arrhythmias

Elevated cholesterol and/or triglyceride levels

General fatigue

Hypothyroidism

Immune suppression

Ischemic heart disease

Low HDL cholesterol

Male infertility

Muscle diseases

Muscle weakness

Overweight

Poor endurance

Pregnancy

Cit **Citrulline** can be made in the body from ornithine by the addition of carbon dioxide and ammonia and can also be converted in the body to arginine. The conversion back and forth between citrulline and arginine can involve an intermediate step where another amino acid, ornithine, is made, or it can occur more directly through activation of the enzyme nitric oxide synthase (NOS). This second path, through NOS, is the subject of extensive research, not because of the conversions between citrulline and arginine but because of the by-product of the reaction. When arginine is converted into citrulline, a molecule of nitric oxide (NO) gas is produced. When citrulline is converted back into arginine, nitric oxide is not made. For this reason, high levels of citrulline can lower NO production. Because body levels of NO help regulate muscle tension and other key physiological processes, there may eventually be recommendations for citrulline intake based on this set of events. Citrulline also promotes the detoxification of ammonia (nitrogen) in the blood and is sometimes helpful in problems of fatigue. In addition, it is thought to stimulate the immune defense system.

Gamma-aminobutyric acid (GABA) is an inhibitory neurotransmitter formed from glutamine. It is discussed earlier, under glutamic acid, on page 52.

Gth **Glutathione** (Gth also known as Gsh) is actually a tripeptide composed of 3 amino acids—cysteine, glutamic acid, and glycine. It is discussed earlier, under cysteine, on page 49. Because of cost and actual usability, GTH itself is not usually taken as a supplement (although it is available as such); rather, it is obtained from L-cysteine or L-methionine (not the D- forms). Because L-cysteine is handled better and is a more direct precursor of GTH, it is supplemented in amounts of 500 mg daily (250 mg twice daily) up to 2 to 3 grams daily. Vitamin C is usually recommended by many authors in doses at least three times that of L-cysteine to facilitate the function of L-cysteine. In general, patients should not take more than 1 gram daily of L-cysteine without being monitored by a physician. Although not all the research supports this method of generating glutathione, apparently it is currently the best way to increase glutathione levels in the body. Up to 200 to 300 mcg daily of extra selenium is also given for its

Possible Uses of Glutathione (as L-cysteine)	
Alcoholism	Drug use
Antioxidant	Metal toxicity
Cancer	Post–heart attack
Cataracts	Radiation exposure
Chemical exposure	Skin problems
Cigarette smoke exposure	Stroke and brain injury
Diabetes	Ulcers

antioxidant support, usually along with vitamin E, but not with vitamin C. Vitamin C may increase the conversion of selenite, a common form of supplemental selenium, to its more toxic form, elemental selenium.

Orn **Ornithine** can be made from arginine, and in turn it can proceed to form citrulline, arginine, and eventually glutamic acid, proline, and hydroxyproline. With arginine, ornithine is useful in nitrogen (ammonia) metabolism. It has been described as a stimulant for growth hormone release and is thought to help build the immune system, promote wound healing, and support liver regeneration. People who are poorly nourished or who lack protein in their diet may be deficient. Ornithine is usually supplemented along with arginine, as they have similar actions. The most common use is in bodybuilders as a growth hormone stimulant. A dose of 1,500 to 2,500 mg twice daily is required for this type of effect. Side effects might include insomnia.

Tau **Taurine**, a lesser known amino acid, is not part of our muscle protein yet is important in metabolism, especially in the brain. It is essential in newborns, as their bodies cannot make it. Adults can produce sulfur-containing taurine from cysteine with the help of pyridoxine, B6. It is possible that if not enough taurine is made in the body, especially if cysteine or B6 is deficient, it might be further required in the diet. In foods, it is high in meats and fish proteins, and especially in shellfish, like oysters and clams.

Taurine functions in such electrically active tissues as the brain and heart to help stabilize cell

membranes. It also has functions in the gallbladder, eyes, and blood vessels and appears to have some antioxidant and detoxifying activity. Taurine aids the movement of potassium, sodium, calcium, and magnesium in and out of cells and thus helps generate nerve impulses. Zinc seems to support this effect of taurine. Taurine is found in the central nervous system, skeletal muscle, and heart; it is very concentrated in the brain and high in the heart tissues. This amino acid also appears to serve as a sulfur "sink." In other words, whenever there is surplus sulfur in the body, not needed at the moment but helpful to keep in reserve, the body incorporates this sulfur into taurine for future use.

Taurine is an inhibitory neurotransmitter, and its main use has been to help treat epilepsy and other excitable brain states, where it functions as a mild sedative. Research shows low taurine levels at seizure sites and its anticonvulsant effect comes from its ability to stabilize nerve cell membranes, which prevents the erratic firing of nerve cells. Doses for this effect are 500 mg 3 times daily.

The cardiovascular dosage of taurine is higher. In Japan, for example, taurine therapy is used in the treatment of ischemic heart disease with supplements of 5 to 6 grams daily in 3 divided doses. Low taurine and magnesium levels have been found in patients after heart attacks. Taurine has potential in the treatment of arrhythmias, especially arrhythmias secondary to ischemia. People with congestive heart failure have also responded to a dosage of 2 grams 3 times daily with improved cardiac and respiratory function. Other possible cardiovascular uses of taurine include for hypertension, possibly related to effects in the renin-angiotensin system of the kidneys, and in patients with high cholesterol levels. Taurine helps gallbladder function by forming taurocholate from bile acids; taurocholate helps increase cholesterol elimination in the bile.

Other possible uses for taurine include improving immune suppression (by sparing L-cysteine), visual problems and eye disease, cirrhosis and liver failure, depression, and male infertility because of low sperm motility. It is also used as a supplement for newborns and new mothers. Overall, the dosage used may range from 500 mg to 5 to 6 grams, with the higher amounts needed for the cardiovascular problems and possibly epilepsy. Possible symptoms of toxicity from taurine supplementation include diarrhea and peptic ulcers.

FOOD, PROTEIN, AND COMPLEMENTARITY

The importance of balancing the diet to get sufficient levels of all the essential amino acids cannot be overstated. It is essential to health. This is why a diet containing a variety of wholesome foods is important. Certain foods have one or two amino acids that are in lower proportions than the others, and if these foods, such as rice or corn, are a predominant part of the diet, it can mean that protein production and the significant functions that protein performs can be deficient.

Each food has a different mix of amino acids. Therefore, it is important to have an understanding of protein composition and to apply it to our diet. The meat foods (including fish and poultry), dairy foods, and eggs almost all have sufficient quantities of amino acids to sustain life; that is, they are complete proteins. When we eat these foods daily, we do not really need to worry about amino acid complementarity. But there are concerns that overconsumption of protein foods (particularly meat and milk) in many societies contributes to some major illnesses, so we may not wish to consume these foods daily or at all.

Vegetarians or other people on diets that limit certain foods may need to be more knowledgeable about combining food. Lacto-ovo vegetarians, who eat eggs and dairy foods—both complete proteins—need have less concern than the pure vegetarian, or vegan. Of the essential amino acids, lysine, methionine, and tryptophan are most often deficient. They are present in all vegetable proteins but at lower levels than other amino acids. Because they are not all low in the same foods, it is not as difficult as many think to obtain a good protein balance from vegetables, grains, nuts, and legumes. The simplest idea is to eat grains with some beans or seeds, for example, millet and aduki beans or brown rice and sunflower seeds. Other complete-protein combinations of vegetable sources include soybeans and rice or soybeans with sesame, corn, wheat, or rye; peanuts with grain or coconut; grain with legumes or leafy greens; beans and corn or rice; and peas and wheat.

The *Nutrition Almanac,* in its fifth edition by Lavon Dunne, has a food-by-food breakdown of amino acid content that is helpful in creating a diet to achieve proper protein intake. The time frame in which food combining must take place has been a subject of controversy since the mid-1980s. Originally, many recommendations called for protein combining at each and every meal. In other words, the bean-rice combination would have to take place at a single dinner; it would not be possible to eat only rice in the morning or beans in the afternoon and expect the body to integrate things together. More recent research, however, indicates that protein combining is not necessary on a meal-by-meal basis and, in fact, many not even be necessary over the course of an entire day. It appears that intake of all needed amino acids can occur over a 1- to 2-day period without compromising the body's ability to make proteins. Of course, this time frame only applies to healthy people who have adequate body stores of proteins and amino acids and who are eating whole, nourishing foods throughout the week. It is still a good idea to pay attention to the protein quality of your foods.

What happens if an amino acid is deficient in our diet? Under this circumstance, the body will continue to make proteins. Most amino acids necessary to make the proteins will be available from existing cellular supplies. But the deficient amino acid will not. Instead of being able to obtain this deficient amino acid from existing supplies, the body will have to break down muscle proteins to obtain it. If over a period of 1 to 2 days we consume all of the necessary amino acids by eating a balanced and complete selection of protein-containing foods, these muscle proteins will be replaced. If not, we will experience net protein loss, thus the importance of consuming all the amino acids through a daily intake of 45 to 60 grams of "balanced" protein in forms that are easily digested and assimilated.

Many methods have been devised to measure the quality of protein foods. Some of these look at the food alone, before it has been eaten and digested within the body. Other methods look at both the food and its interaction with the body. Because I believe the interactive measures give a truer picture of protein quality, I will only mention two measurements that fall into this second category. The first is biological value (BV). This measurement of protein quality looks at the amount of nitrogen that is released from the protein and absorbed into the body. (Nitrogen is a great indicator of protein status, because it is not found in the two other major classes of macronutrients—namely, carbohydrate and fat.)

The second measurement is called net protein utilization (NPU). NPU is measured in exactly the same way as BV, except that in addition to looking at the percentage of absorbable nitrogen, NPU also looks at the digestibility of the food proteins. The digestibility of eggs, milks, meats, and cheeses, for example, is scored as 100 on the NPU scale. So is that of peanut butter. For corn, however, this number is 89, and for beans, only 82. Remember that these numbers are not based on actual protein content of the food, but on how readily the foods are digested and how efficiently the body can use the proteins. The lower digestibility of certain protein-containing foods does not mean we should not eat them, however. It only means that we should take steps to improve their digestibility or that we use the principles of protein combining to ensure adequate amino acid variety and quantity despite the slightly lower digestibility of certain plant foods. For example, soaking beans for slightly longer periods of time and adding a sea vegetable like kombu to the cooking water can improve their digestibility. See more about protein complementarity in chapter 9, Diets, in the discussion under "Lacto-ovo Vegetarian" on page 359.

DIGESTION AND METABOLISM

Proteins are first broken down in the stomach by hydrochloric acid, pepsin, and proteases into peptides (amino acid chains) by splitting peptide bonds between the amino acid protein chains. The role of the stomach in protein digestion was often viewed as a minor part of the overall process until recent years, when it became more clear that lack of acid secretion by the stomach could compromise the entire protein digestion process by failing to open the protein structure in such a way that enzymes could gain access to the amino acids in the protein chains. In the United States, lack of stomach acid (called *hypochlorhydria*) is a common problem, often linked to the use of antacids. Decreased stomach acid secretion is also associated with chronic stress, poor diet with excessive food intake and poor food combining, and aging, particularly after 60.

In the first part of the small intestine (the duodenum), the pancreatic enzyme trypsin continues the conversion of the polypeptides into dipeptides (2 amino acids) and tripeptides (3 amino acids). Farther along the small intestine, amino peptidases, including dipeptidases, reduce the polypephdes to single amino acids. These individual amino acid molecules are then absorbed into the bloodstream through the intestinal wall and carried to the liver through the portal vein circulation.

The liver is the main site and regulator of amino acid metabolism, which may also take place throughout the body. Proteins are made and broken down daily. About 60% to 70% of amino acids available in the body are recycled from old tissue proteins. These recycled amino acids are called *endogenous amino acids*; new ones from the diet are termed *exogenous*. Each cell has the capability of building its needed proteins from either or both sources of amino acids. Protein synthesis is a fairly complex though well-documented process that is described in detail in most biochemistry texts. DNA (deoxyribonucleic acid) controls and guides protein formation with the assistance of RNA (ribonucleic acid) through a duplication and replication process. Each protein has a specific sequence of amino acids used in the genetic code in our DNA.

Most of the amino acids, probably three-fourths, are used to form body proteins such as enzymes, hormones, antibodies, and the tissue proteins like muscle. Some amino acids are metabolized into other tissue substances, such as melanin (pigmentation hormone), epinephrine, creatine, niacin, choline, and so on. Most often protein is synthesized at the site in which it is to be used. Every day, protein is made (this process is called *anabolism*) and broken down (this is called *catabolism*). This daily process determines the body's balance of nitrogen (found only in proteins, not fats or carbohydrates). With an increase in protein intake, the body will have a positive nitrogen balance and growth can occur. If we have deficient protein intake, the body will have a negative nitrogen balance. Most of our lives we want to have a neutral nitrogen balance. The average healthy adult synthesizes about 250 to 350 grams of protein daily (this number may also be much higher). Depending on protein and amino acid intake, our activity level, and protein utilization, we can move into positive or negative nitrogen balance and either build more protein or lose some, which influences body weight, shape, and tone. Excess protein can be turned into fat and stored in the body as potential fuel or as glycogen in the liver. A protein deficiency can cause weight loss and a wide variety of functional problems.

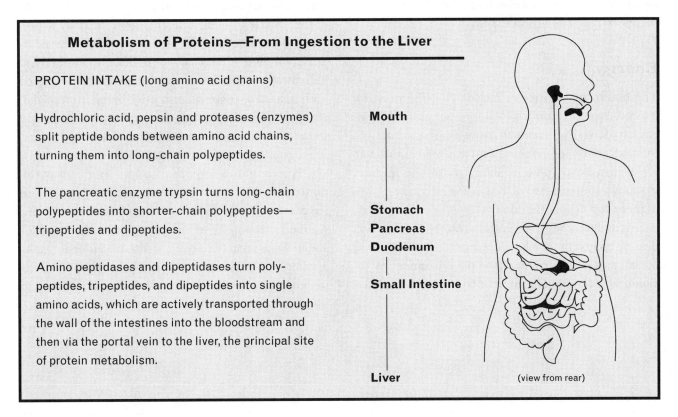

Metabolism of Proteins—From Ingestion to the Liver

PROTEIN INTAKE (long amino acid chains)

Hydrochloric acid, pepsin and proteases (enzymes) split peptide bonds between amino acid chains, turning them into long-chain polypeptides.

The pancreatic enzyme trypsin turns long-chain polypeptides into shorter-chain polypeptides—tripeptides and dipeptides.

Amino peptidases and dipeptidases turn polypeptides, tripeptides, and dipeptides into single amino acids, which are actively transported through the wall of the intestines into the bloodstream and then via the portal vein to the liver, the principal site of protein metabolism.

Mouth

Stomach
Pancreas
Duodenum

Small Intestine

Liver   (view from rear)

PROTEIN FUNCTIONS

Proteins play a wider range of functions than any other bodily component. They form all of the enzymes that spark our metabolism and many of the hormones that regulate our body chemistry. Antibodies that help neutralize bacteria, transport molecules that move minerals around our body, and structures that provide tissue with protective strength (like fingernails or bone collagen) are all composed of protein. Even the contraction of our muscles depends on protein.

Growth and Maintenance

We must have a constant supply of amino acids to build the proteins that create our body tissues. This is especially true in fetal formation during pregnancy as well as in growing children, but we are all constantly rebuilding new tissue throughout our lives. Hair and nails are growing, and the cells in the body become worn out and need replacement, requiring amino acids. Red blood cells last about a month, as do skin cells, while cells that line our intestinal tract are replaced almost twice weekly. During times of healing, during illness, and after surgery, injuries, burns, or blood loss, we require more protein production to assist in bringing back the body's strength through regeneration of cells and tissues.

Energy

The body's main priority is satisfying the need for energy. Protein supplies 4 calories per gram, as does carbohydrate. The body will first use carbohydrate and then fats for energy; if these sources are low, however, it will burn dietary protein. Should the diet be deficient in energy sources, we will break down tissue proteins to meet our needs. We do not store extra amino acids (as we do fat) other than in tissue proteins, so we will destroy body protein when fuel is needed, usually after our fat stores are depleted (see the upcoming discussion under Protein Requirements).

Building Important Substances

Enzymes are protein catalysts that stimulate biochemical reactions. There are literally thousands of different enzymes within a single cell that help join together or separate a wide variety of substances.

Hemoglobin, an iron-bearing protein that is the key component of the red blood cell, is the molecule that carries oxygen to the tissues of the body.

Hormones have a dynamic effect on our metabolism. The primary protein hormones are insulin, which regulates our blood sugar levels, and thyroid hormone (really an amino acid, tyrosine with iodine), which controls our metabolic rate.

Antibodies are proteins formed as a response to the stimulus of something foreign (usually a protein) that enters the body. These foreign proteins (antigens) can be bacteria, viruses, fungi, pollens, or protein from a food. The body will produce a specific antibody to bind with the foreign antigen and inactivate it. Different invaders require different proteins that are specific for them, and thus the body must be in constant surveillance and preparedness for production of new antibodies. Proteins are a big part of our immunity.

The immune response is the basis for using immunizations to create immunity to disease through recognition and response to an antigen. Giving a small dose of the disease-causing antigen allows the body to produce the antibody. Our immune system has near-perfect memory, so once we produce an antibody, it will always be available. Should we be contaminated with a polio or tetanus germ after being immunized, we would rapidly produce the antibody to deactivate the germs and not be infected. Thus, our protein-making capacities must always be available.

This immune response, so important for maintaining health, can also cause problems, as when we react to tissue transplants or blood transfusions. Antibody responses to antigens can be the basis for some allergic reactions. We can also misguidedly make antibodies to our own tissues, a process called *autoimmunity*, which may lead to a number of serious and difficult-to-treat problems.

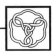

Fluid and Salt Balance

Proteins inside cells help keep the correct amount of water in the cells. Most proteins do not move in and out of cells, as can water, and large protein molecules attract water. The proteins in plasma help maintain the blood volume as well. When overall protein concentrations are low, fluid imbalances can occur. Proteins also help maintain the normal sodium and potassium balance, which is essential to life. Sodium is concentrated outside the cells, while potassium is mainly inside, a situation necessary for normal muscle and nerve cell function. Proteins push sodium out of the cell and potassium into it, thus aiding the heart, lungs, and nervous system to function optimally.

Acid-Alkaline Balance

Proteins can help normalize the acid-alkaline balance by acting as buffers. The body constantly produces acids and bases from chemical reactions. Proteins help in the elimination of excess hydrogen ions, which are part of acids. In this way, the pH (the acid-alkaline balance of the blood) is kept near constant at about 7.4.

PROTEIN REQUIREMENTS

There are definitely specific requirements for proteins, although the exact amount is somewhat questionable. The recommended dietary allowance (RDA) of protein according to U.S. government standards is 0.8 gram per kilogram (1 kilogram equals 2.2 pounds) of ideal body weight for adult males and females 19 years and older. Ideal body weight is used in the calculation because amino acids are less extensively needed by fat cells, and more critical in the lean body mass. So an adult male who should weigh about 154 pounds, or 70 kilograms, requires 70 times 0.8, or 56 grams of protein daily. A female whose ideal weight is 110 pounds, or 50 kilograms, needs 40 grams a day. The RDA increases by 25 grams during pregnancy, and also by 25 grams per day during all months of lactation. During growth, different amounts are needed. For example, 1.52 grams of protein are needed per kilogram of body weight each day in the first 6 months of life, and 1.2 grams per kilogram for the next 6 months.

These requirements are based on maintaining a positive nitrogen balance in children and an even-to-positive nitrogen balance in adults. Protein is the nitrogen-containing nutrient. As it is broken down for

---

Protein Recommendations

AGE	RDA
Infants, 0–6 months	1.52 grams for each kilogram of body weight*
Infants, 7–12 months	11 grams
Children, 1–3 years	13 grams
Children, 4–8 years	19 grams
Males and females, 9–13 years	34 grams
Males, 14–18 years	52 grams
Females, 14–18 years	46 grams
Males, 19 and older	56 grams
Females, 19 and older	46 grams
Pregnancy and Lactation	Women should add an additional 25 grams to their age-group requirement.

* This recommendation is an Adequate Intake (AI) recommendation rather than a Recommended Dietary Allowance (RDA). To determine weight in kilograms, divide weight in pounds (lbs) by 2.2.

Source: Institute of Medicine, *Dietary Reference Intakes for Energy, Carbohydrate, Fiber, Fat, Fatty Acids, Cholesterol, Protein, and Amino Acids (Macronutrients)*. Washington, D.C. The National Academies Press, 2005.

excretion, dietary nitrogen is used so that protein formation can continue. In the healthy adult, nitrogen equilibrium (or "zero balance") is the ideal, while a positive nitrogen balance is needed during times of illness and healing. In children, when growth is occurring regularly, a positive nitrogen balance is necessary, as it is in pregnancy.

As discussed on page 57 under "Food, Protein, and Complementarity," the protein requirements are also based on the protein quality, as measured by the BV. Protein is also measured by the way it supports growth. This measurement, called the *protein efficiency ratio* (PER), is determined by feeding an animal a particular protein food and measuring its growth. The reference protein for determining the BV of foods is that of eggs (ovalbumin), the food with the highest BV at 94% (although mother's milk is valued at 100%). Next are fish at 75% to 90%, whole grain rice at 86% (although polished rice can drop as low as 64%), legumes at 58% to 73%, and meats and poultry at 75% to 85%. Corn, a less complete protein than some of the others mentioned here, has a BV of approximately 60%.

Protein Excess

There is definite concern that the industrialized countries are overconsuming protein, especially from meat and dairy foods. Because nearly 700 million people in the world are protein deficient, it seems ludicrous that Americans and people in other well-to-do countries consume so much. But we could be paying the price!

The RDA protein standards may be highly overestimated, and many people consume well over these guidelines, even between 100 to 200 grams daily. The World Health Organization more conservatively puts our protein needs at about half of the U.S. government minimum levels, or 0.45 grams of protein per kilogram of ideal body weight. Interestingly, the overestimation of protein needs has been acknowledged by the U.S. government itself. As early as 1953, government scientists drafting the recommended dietary allowance (RDA) for protein wrote that "the protein allowance for artificially fed infants may well be overly generous." Similarly, in 1958, they described the requirements for the first 6 months of life as "undoubtedly in excess of the minimum requirements." By 1974, this same RDA-setting committee was stating "nor is there evidence that intakes double or triple the recommended allowances are harmful. In fact, protein intakes that exceed the RDA are often desirable, since low protein diets contain only small amounts of animal products and thus tend to be unpalatable."

A solution to overestimation of protein needs and excessive protein consumption may be to focus more on individual amino acid requirements than protein per se. With a few important exceptions, our bodies do not need large, unbroken proteins. We need shorter amino acid strings like oligopeptides, dipeptides, and individual amino acids. When we recommend 50 grams of protein in a daily diet, a large part of this recommendation is based on the underlying assumption that 50 grams of protein will get us all of the oligopeptides, dipeptides, and individual amino acids that we need. Whether we get all of the protein components we need from 50 grams of protein foods depends on the *quality* of those foods. **That is, the quality of our protein is just as important as the quantity.**

In many cuisines throughout the world, staple foods (like rice) have low protein quality. As mentioned earlier, in the case of rice, the least plentiful and limiting amino acid is lysine. But cultural wisdom, passed on throughout generations, has overcome this lysine limitation of rice by using spices and seasonings along with the rice that are relatively rich in lysine. In Indian cuisine, for example, a basmati rice dish may be seasoned with fenugreek, mustard seed, and turmeric—three spices that are relatively high in lysine. Although no spice or seasoning could provide anywhere near the 50 grams-per-day protein requirement, even small amounts of these spices, in the range of 1/5 of a teaspoon, could provide close to the daily requirement for a single amino acid like lysine, because this requirement is somewhere in the range of 750 mg per day.

Researchers are learning more and more about the role of particular amino acids in contributing to specific health problems. For example, we now know that the branched-chain amino acids (leucine, isoleucine, and valine) are the only amino acids that can be transported into the mitochondria (the aerobic energy-producing powerhouses of the cells) to assist with energy production. Health problems like chronic fatigue syndrome, fibromyalgia, and myofascial pain syndrome often involve mitochondrial dysfunction, and in these cases, it may make sense to think about

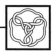

foods and supplements that are particularly rich in branched-chain amino acids, rather than foods and supplements that are merely protein-rich.

The Western world definitely has less deficiency disease than parts of the developing world, such as Africa, the Near and Far East, and Central and South America. But we also have a far greater incidence of chronic and degenerative diseases, such as arthritis, diabetes, cardiovascular disease, and cancer. All of these problems have dietary correlations, some of which are shown in specific studies, but many that, in my opinion, will be discovered in future years with research into the nutritional components of disease. Eventually, through knowledge and behavior, we need to find the right balance in our diet.

Protein Deficiency

With all the technology and the wealth of resources the modern world possesses, much of the world's population is impoverished and near starvation. Thousands of children and adults die daily from lack of nourishing food, and protein is of key importance. In areas where meats and milk products are not plentiful and where often only a few food sources are available, such as rice, wheat, corn, or potatoes, people are not getting the complete balance of amino acids and protein needed to sustain the body. They go into negative nitrogen balance and begin to experience weight loss, fluid retention, weakness, hair loss, and the inability to heal wounds.

The name for protein deficiency disease is *kwashiorkor*, a Ghanaian word for "the evil spirit that infects the child." Protein deficiency is a wasting disease that in its severe state leads to death. It is curable, of course, with consumption of complete protein foods or supplements. Marasmus, another protein deficiency disease associated with calorie or food deficiency, comes from a starvation diet and results in complete loss of energy and tissue wasting. Also called *protein-calorie malnutrition* (PCM), it is the world's most widespread and correctable malnutrition problem, killing millions yearly.

The Western world's example of protein deficiency is mirrored in the alcoholic, who obtains a large portion of his or her calorie intake from carbohydrates in the form of ethyl alcohol. Food and protein consumption may be minimal. Malnutrition and fat accumulation in the liver lead to rapidly advancing demise unless alcohol is reduced and nutrition is increased. Cirrhosis, scarring, and malnutrition of the liver is one of the top-ten degenerative diseases leading to death in the United States.

There has been worldwide concern over hunger, malnutrition, and starvation for some time. It certainly seems that humanity's primary responsibility is to find a way to feed all the people adequately. After all, on an individual or family level, food, shelter, and clothing should come before fancy cars, exclusive restaurants, and trips to the Caribbean. Donations to hunger projects, attending fundraising music concerts, and helping to raise money ourselves are short-term ways to feed some hungry people, but there are other approaches too. On a global level, higher precedence is given today to using land for grazing meat-rendering animals than for growing grain for direct human consumption. Many acres of grain and plant proteins are used to feed a small number of cattle and still more grain is used to feed poultry. This grain could feed many more people than can the meat of dead chickens! A reduction in animal meat production and an increased emphasis on vegetable and grain foods would help feed the impoverished everywhere. Yet perhaps the most important contribution we can make toward reducing hunger and starvation in the world is by helping and teaching people to plant and harvest their own food sources.

Lipids—Fats and Oils

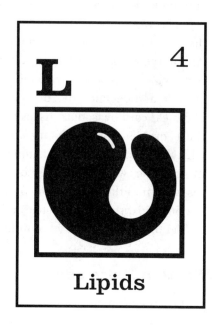

L ⁴

Lipids

Fats, or lipids, are the third main class of macro-nutrients necessary in human nutrition. The lipids are found primarily in meats, dairy foods, nuts, and seeds—at least, these are the most visible and concentrated sources—but most foods contain some fat. In addition to nuts and seeds, some of the richer vegetable sources of dietary fat are soybeans, olives, peanuts, and avocados. Fats are an important component of our diet, and at least a minimum intake is essential. **Many problems are associated with excessive intake of dietary fat, however, including obesity, cardiovascular disease, and some forms of cancer.**

The traditional view of fats has focused on their role as energy-storage compounds. Fats definitely function in this way. In nutrition, energy is usually measured in terms of calories, and ounce for ounce, fats contain more calories than any other component of food. An ounce of pure fat—for example, an ounce of pure oil, like sunflower seed oil—contains about 240 calories. An ounce of pure starch (like cornstarch) or an ounce of pure protein (like soy protein powder) contains about 100 calories. Fat packs more than twice the amount of calories as protein or carbohydrate. For this reason, when the problem is insufficient energy,

fat is the solution. Nuts and seeds need their self-contained fat to allow for germination and sprouting in the spring. Hibernating animals need it for energy throughout the winter. In the human-made world, we've also depended (too much!) on fat-based fuel for our cars, in the form of refined oil (petroleum) products.

The role of fat as an energy-storage substance is only one of its important roles. Fats are also required to transport other nutrients, such as vitamins A, D, E, and K—the fat-soluble vitamins. Fats are an essential component of the cell membrane, and internal fatty tissues protect the vital organs from trauma and temperature change by providing padding and insulation. Fatty tissue, in fact, even helps regulate body temperature. When we look at fat in energy storage, it's *quantity* that is most important. If we store up too much fat, we become obese and unhealthy. If we store up too little, we become malnourished and unhealthy. However, when we look at fat as a cell membrane component, or a transport mechanism, fat *quantity* becomes much less important than fat *quality*. This fat quality concept is relatively new in the world of nutrition. For many years, nutritionists have spoken about *saturated fat, unsaturated fat,* and *polyunsaturated fat,* but these three categories are a small part of the overall picture when it comes to fat quality. Understanding fat quality requires us to look much more closely at certain aspects of fat, and the first place we need to look is at certain fat components called *fatty acids.*

In terms of chemistry, fatty acids are essentially like chains consisting of links. (In the case of fatty acids, the links are made of carbon atoms.) They can be short, medium, or long, depending on the number of links that they contain. Short-chain fatty acids (SCFAs) contain 2 to 5 "links," or carbon atoms. The exact number is still debated. The key SCFAs are acetic acid (2 carbons), propionic acid (3 carbons), butyric acid (4 carbons), and valeric acid (5 carbons). Medium-chain fatty acids (MCFAs) are slightly larger, containing 6 to 12 fatty acids. (Once again, not everyone agrees on the number.) The most important MCFAs are caproic acid (6 carbons), caprylic acid (8 carbons), capric acid (10 carbons), and lauric acid (12 carbons). These MCFAs are well-known in the nutrition world as components of medium-chain triglyceride (MCT) oil, which has been used for more than 50 years by health-care practitioners to help people who have difficulty absorbing fat. The MCFAs in MCT oil can help with this problem, because MCFAs, unlike longer-

chain fats, can be absorbed directly from the digestive tract and don't have to follow the normal and more complicated pathway involving the lymphatic system and the liver. It is the shorter MCFAs, especially caprylic and capric acid, that seem most responsible for the clinical effectiveness of MCT oil, and the longest MCFA, lauric acid, seems not only less helpful but actually capable of raising total cholesterol and LDL (low-density lipoprotein) cholesterol levels—an unwanted health consequence for most people.

Long-chain fatty acids (LCFAs) begin with myristic acid (14 carbons) and include the well-studied fatty acids palmitic acid (16 carbons) and stearic acid (18 carbons). Palmitic acid, like the name suggests, is especially concentrated in the fat contained in palm kernels from the oil palm tree *(Elaeis oleifera).* Palmitic acid is also found in animal sources like cows or pigs, which are often used in the food-processing industry. Palmitic acid is found in a wide range of processed foods because it is used in combination with other substances to act as an emulsifier and antifoam agent. Relationships between these three types of saturated fats are summarized in the chart at left.

Up until now, all of the information about fatty acids in this chapter has involved their size, and more specifically, their length. SCFAs, MCFAs, and LCFAs are ways of classifying fatty acids according to their length. Our bodies need all three kinds of fatty acids to remain healthy. Yet there is another equally important feature that must be determined for all fatty acids, regardless of how long they are: their degree of saturation. Just like a sponge can be saturated with water (H_2O), fatty acids can also be saturated, only not with H_2O, but with H (hydrogen). Just like a saturated sponge is holding all of the water it can possibly hold, a saturated fatty acid is holding all of the hydrogen it can possibly hold. If it isn't, it is called *unsaturated.* **To remain healthy, our bodies need fatty acids not only of all three lengths (SCFAs, MCFAs, and LCFAs), but also of both types (saturated and unsaturated).**

When a fatty acid is fully saturated, it interacts the *least* with other molecules in the body, and it provides the most stable structure. Saturated fats are helpful structurally because they help stabilize cell membranes, and they are not very susceptible to damage because they are primarily inert and noninteractive. Unsaturated fatty acids are much more interactive

Saturated Fatty Acids

Types of Saturated Fatty Acid	Key Saturated Fatty Acids	Length of Saturated Fatty Acid
Short Chain	acetic acid	2 carbons
	propionic acid	3 carbons
	butyric acid	4 carbons
	valeric acid	5 carbons
Medium Chain	caproic acid	6 carbons
	caprylic acid	8 carbons
	capric acid	10 carbons
	lauric acid	12 cabons
Long Chain	myristic acid	14 carbons
	palmitic acid	16 carbons
	stearic acid	18 carbons

and susceptible to damage, but they are critical in the body because they provide flexibility to cell membranes and allow the cells to stay in dynamic communication with their surroundings. The delicacy of unsaturated fatty acids means that we have to take much greater care with the foods that contain them than we do with other types of fats. Some of the steps that are possible to prevent oxidation (damage) are refrigeration, storage in airtight green or brown glass containers, minimal opening, and even addition of antioxidants (like vitamin E). Some of the differences between saturated and unsaturated fats are easy to spot just by looking. Saturated fats are usually hard at room temperature. For example, lard, suet, and butter are common saturated animal fats, recognized as "solid" foods. In contrast, most of the unsaturated vegetable oils—including sunflower, safflower, canola (rapeseed), and soy—are liquid at room temperature and recognizable as liquids.

The saturated/unsaturated aspect of fatty acids has one further complication. When it comes to saturation, a fatty acid is either saturated or not. Everything is black and white, with no in-between. Unsaturation is a different matter, however, because there are *degrees* of unsaturation. If there is only one spot in the fatty acid where hydrogen atoms have been removed, the unsaturated fatty acid is called a *monounsaturated fatty acid* (MUFA). If there are multiple spots where hydrogens have been removed, the unsaturated fatty acid is called a *polyunsaturated fatty acid* (PUFA). All unsaturated fatty acids are either MUFAs or PUFAs. In general, the more spots where hydrogen atoms have been removed, the greater the flexibility and also the susceptibility to damage of the fatty acid. Relationships

Unsaturated Fatty Acids				
Type of Unsaturated Fatty Acid	**Key Unsaturated Fatty Acids**	**Length of Unsaturated Fatty Acid**	**Number of Double Bonds**	**Best Sources**
Monounsaturated	oleic acid	18 carbons	1 double bond	olive oil, canola oil
Polyunsaturated Omega-6s	linoleic acid	18 carbons	2 double bonds	safflower oil, sunflower oil, sesame oil, grapeseed oil
	gamma-linolenic acid	18 carbons	3 double bonds	borage oil, evening primrose oil, black currant oil, human milk, some fungi
	arachidonic acid	20 carbons	4 double bonds	beef fat, egg yolk
Polyunsaturated Omega-3s	alpha-linolenic acid	18 carbons	3 double bonds	flaxseed, pumpkin seed, hemp seed, walnut
	eicosapentaenoic acid (EPA)	20 carbons	5 double bonds	fish oil
	docosahexaenoic acid (DHA)	22 carbons	6 double bonds	fish oil

between the different types of unsaturated fatty acids, together with plant oils in which they are readily found, are presented in the chart on the opposite page.

The double-bond spots on a polyunsaturated fatty acid where hydrogens have been removed act like "hot spots" on the fatty acid. They contain twice as much energy as any other spot on the molecule, and they are quick to interact with other kinds of molecules (called radicals) and also when faced with other kinds of energy shifts. Light, heat, and oxygen all provide just the right kind of energy shift to trigger these hot spots. Through this process, the PUFA becomes damaged and can no longer function as needed. The overall process of PUFA damage from light, heat, oxygen, or radicals is called *lipid peroxidation*. In the food industry, antioxidants like BHA (butylated hydroxyanisole) or BHT (butylated hydroxytoluene) are often added to plant oils to help prevent lipid peroxidation. More natural ways to accomplish the same goal involve the addition of vitamin E, beta-carotene, or extracts from the antioxidant herbs sage, rosemary, or thyme.

In the food industry, the balance between saturated and unsaturated has gotten totally out of hand because of problems with the shelf life of nationally distributed, PUFA-containing products, which are too delicate to be processed, shipped, and shelved for long periods of time. To remedy this problem, the food industry has adopted a shelf-life extension process called *hydrogenation*. During this process, a canister of hydrogen gas is positioned below a vat of oil, and under controlled circumstances, the hydrogen gas is allowed to bubble up into the oil. In this way, some of the oil can be convinced to soak up more hydrogen and unsaturated fatty acids can be transformed into saturated ones. This transformation produces a semi-solid fat that is less likely to go rancid. The business benefit, of course, is a less delicate product with a longer shelf life. But the health cost is significant.

Hydrogenation not only lowers the quality of the oil by removing some of its delicate unsaturated fatty acids, it actually converts some of the unsaturated fatty acids into a new form (called *trans fat*) that increases blood cholesterol and LDL cholesterol, as well as the risk of atherosclerosis (hardening of the arteries). A recent study has also raised the possibility of delay in infant development because of the mother's excess intake of trans-fatty acids. Since trans-fatty acids can cross over to the baby before birth via the placenta or after birth via breastfeeding, a mother's intake of trans-fatty acids can be as important as a child's. Many fat-containing products state on the label "contains one or more of the following partially hydrogenated oils." This statement is a red flag pointing to the presence of altered PUFAs and trans-fatty acids in the product.

Research on fatty acids since the mid-1980s has radically changed our understanding of fats in the diet and taught us that one size does *not* fit all when it comes to health and fat. All saturated fat is clearly not created equal; for example, when saturated fat is short-chain, it offers important health benefits that are lacking in the long-chain version. Intake of butter was once considered problematic by many health-care practitioners because of its high saturated fat content. But today researchers know that the intake of butyric acid, a short fatty acid that constitutes about 10% to 15% of all fat found in butter, has clearly been associated with reduction of cancer risk and in some cases with reduction of tumor advancement. Although this benefit of short-chain saturated fat is not a mandate to eat butter without restraint, it points out that butter is not all bad and that saturated fat is not all the same. Butter is likely to be a better choice than most margarines, which contain hydrogenated oils and trans fats and lack the SCFA butyric acid. Similarly, stearic acid, a long-chain saturated fatty acid, was once thought to be exclusively problematic in increasing risk of heart disease, but it now appears that it doesn't have this one-sided, negative impact.

There is a final aspect of fatty acid chemistry that is critical to our nourishment and health. As described earlier, all long-chain PUFAs have multiple hot spots (a double-bonded set of carbons that stores higher amounts of energy and is chemically reactive). *Where* these hot spots are located makes a big difference to our health. When the hot spots begin 3 links down the chain, the fatty acids are called *omega-3 fatty acids*. When the hot spots begin 6 links down the chain, the fatty acids are called *omega-6 fatty acids*. Most of the PUFAs in our cell membranes are either omega-6s or omega-3s. (There are also some omega-9 fatty acids, where the first hot spot is found 9 links down the chain, but this type is less common). Omega-3 and omega-6 fatty acids have been the subject of intense research since the mid-1990s, and it is now clear that our balance of omega-6 to omega-3 affects our health as much as any other aspect of dietary fat. In other words, it is just as important for us to get the right balance of omega-6s and omega-3s as it is to have the right amount of saturated and unsaturated fat, or to have the correct amount of total fat.

There are two essential fatty acids (EFAs) that we must consume in food: linoleic acid (LA), an omega-6 fatty acid; and alpha-linolenic acid (ALA or NLA), an omega-3. EFAs are important for normal growth, especially of the blood vessels and nerves, and to keep the skin and other tissues youthful and supple as a result of their lubricating quality. The EFAs are also sometimes collectively referred to as "vitamin F." Deficiency of vitamin F can lead to dryness, scaliness, or eczema of the skin, as well as to reductions in the oil-soluble vitamins A, D, E, and K. Also, if there is deficient fat intake during growth periods, retarding in the growing process may occur.

In the typical U.S. diet, it is much easier for us to get the omega-6 EFA (linoleic acid) than the omega-3 EFA (alpha-linolenic acid). Most plant oils (including canola, corn, peanut, poppy seed, safflower, sesame, soy, sunflower, and walnut) contain plenty of this omega-6 fatty acid, as do oat germ, wheat germ, and rice bran. With alpha-linolenic acid, however, the story is quite different. Some alpha-linolenic is found in wheat germ, walnuts, and canola oil, but many of the rich sources of this omega-3 EFA are rare in the U.S. diet. These sources include flaxseed and flax oil, fenugreek seed/oil, chia seed/oil, pumpkin seed/oil, and certain sea vegetables. Some cold-water fish— including salmon, halibut, cod, trout, and mackerel— contain small amounts of this EFA. These fish are well-known in the nutrition world for their high omega-3 EFA content, but two other omega-3 fatty acids (eicosapentaenoic acid, or EPA, and docosahexaenoic acid, or DHA) are also found in these fish. Neither EPA nor DHA are considered EFAs, because both can be made from alpha-linolenic acid inside our bodies. (For more on EPA and DHA see chapter 7, Special Supplements.)

What counts as the "right" amount of omega-6s and omega-3s is still a matter of debate. In the United States, our diet has been estimated to contain about 10 to 20 times as much omega-6 as omega-3. In other words, the ratio of omega-6 to omega-3 is somewhere

between 10:1 and 20:1. All researchers agree that this ratio is far too high. Although some studies point to a desirable ratio of approximately 1:1, the majority of studies support a ratio somewhere between 2:1 and 4:1. In other words, a diet that provides at least twice the amount of omega-6s as omega-3s, but no more than 4 times as much, is preferred. The best-researched recommendations in this area have come from the Workshop on the Essentiality of and Recommended Dietary Intakes for Omega-6 and Omega-3 Fatty Acids, held at the National Institutes of Health in 1999. This workshop, headed by Artemis Simopoulos, MD, a leading expert in this area, concluded that at least 2%, and no more than 3% of total calories should come from linoleic acid, the omega-6 EFA, and that 1% of total calories should come from alpha-linolenic acid, the omega-3 EFA. The workshop also recommended that 0.1% of total calories come from the omega-3 fatty acid EPA, as well as 0.1% from the omega-3 fatty acid DHA. Although I doubt that this kind of fixed, pinpoint recommendation will hold up over time, it is a good starting point given the absence of public health recommendations about fat quality.

Because the ratio of omega-6s to omega-3s helps determine the flexibility of cell membranes, nearly all chemical communication throughout the body depends at least in part on the correct balance between omega-6s and omega-3s. Within this context, it is difficult to imagine any health problem that *isn't* partly related to the ratio of omega-6 to omega-3. Since the mid-1990s, study after study has validated this perspective. The balance between omega-6 and omega-3 EFAs has been linked to risk of noninsulin-dependent diabetes, obesity and likelihood of weight loss, coronary heart disease, chronic inflammation, and heart transplant success. Healthy genetic processes also appear to depend on this balance. The basic goal in the United States in this regard is to replace some of our omega-6 fatty acids with omega-3s. We would make some good headway toward this goal if we ate cold-water fish in place of some chicken, pork, or beef. We would also do well to swap foods high in omega-6s, like peanuts, with foods higher in omega-3s, like walnuts, sesame seeds, flaxseeds, and pumpkin seeds.

EFAs in dietary fat have a special relationship to inflammation. In Latin, the prefix *eico* means "20," and in our bodies there is a special group of regulatory molecules called *eicosanoids,* all containing 20 carbon atoms and made directly from omega-6 and omega-3 fatty acids. The four most common types of eicosanoids are prostaglandins, prostacyclins, leukotrienes, and thromboxanes. All of these molecules help regulate a wide range of chemical events in our bodies, including inflammation. Prostaglandins D_2, E_2, and F_2 are all made from the omega-6 fatty acid called *arachidonic acid* and are part of the series 2 prostaglandins (PGE2s). The PGE2s are often referred to as *pro-inflammatory* regulators: they encourage our bodies to engage in an inflammatory response in which the blood vessels constrict, the blood platelets clump together, and the body reacts as if to protect itself from physical injury (like a wound) or chemical injury (like an infection). If our bodies are really experiencing a physical or chemical injury, this response is welcomed as a natural part of the healing process. Under certain circumstances, however, the series 2 prostaglandins can trigger chronic inflammatory responses that are unwanted (that is, they are not occurring in the face of physical or chemical injury).

On the other side of the equation are prostaglandins that act in an anti-inflammatory capacity, relaxing the blood vessels and preventing the blood platelets from clumping together. The series 1 prostaglandins (including PGF_1, PGG_1, and PGH_1) generally belong to this group, as do the series 3 prostaglandins (PGF_3, PGG_3, and PGH_3). Neither series 1 nor series 3 prostaglandins are made from arachidonic acid. Series 1 molecules are made from DGLA (dihomogamma-linolenic acid), an omega-6 fatty acid that comes *before* arachidonic acid in the body's metabolic processing sequence. Series 3 molecules are not made from omega-6s at all, but rather, from omega-3s. EPA, the omega-3 PUFA described earlier in this chapter (and discussed at more length in chapter 7), is the fatty acid from which series 3 prostaglandins are made. Excessive levels of series 2 prostaglandins have been found in atopic dermatitis (skin hypersensitivity), glomerulonephritis (kidney inflammation), and colitis (inflammation in the large intestine). There may be more complexity to this PGE2-inflammation relationship, however, that will be uncovered in future research. Already, there are some indications that under certain circumstances PGE2s can help *reduce* inflammation, as appears to occur in inflammation of the lungs' airways, including some situations involving asthma.

CLASSIFICATION AND BIOCHEMISTRY

Lipids—the general name for fats, taken from the Greek word *lipos* (meaning "fat")—are a diverse group of substances that include fatty acids but also much more. About the only thing that all lipids have in common is the fact that they do not dissolve in water. Although I have discussed fatty acids in detail, they are actually only one type of lipid. Other types of lipids include phospholipids, which are found in all cell membranes; sphingolipids, also found in cell membranes and considered a subdivision of phospholipids; sphingomyelins, critical in the outer coating of most nerve cells; and steroids/sterols, including cholesterol. As a key lipid, cholesterol is also the basis for formation of many hormones and vitamins in the body, including estrogens, androgens, progesterone, cortisone, and vitamin D.

Fats, like carbohydrates, are composed of carbon, hydrogen, and oxygen; however, some phospholipids also contain nitrogen and phosphorus. The common property of all fats is that they are insoluble in water and dissolve only in fat solvents. Tissue lipids (found in normal tissues such as liver or muscle and surrounding or covering the abdominal organs) make up about 10% to 15% of the average adult's weight; total body fat consists of all the tissue lipids (subcutaneous fat) plus the stored fat (known as *brown fat*), which varies with weight and diet. Although we should keep our fat levels down, dietary fat is a high-energy food source. It also helps our cells communicate and preserve their identity, our nerves send messages, our glands make hormones, and our bodies transport vitamins and other substances where they are needed. Fat also gives food a special flavor and aroma to which many people are attracted.

Triglycerides and Fatty Acids

Triglycerides comprise about 95% of the lipids in food and in our bodies. They are the storage form of fat when we eat calories in excess of our energy needs. Burning up stored fat allows us to live without food for periods of time, as I have done during my many fasts, and bears do during winter. All triglycerides have a similar structure, being composed of three fatty acids attached to a glycerol molecule. Glycerol is a short-chain carbohydrate molecule that is soluble in water, and when triglycerides are metabolized, the glycerol can be converted to glucose.

The kind of food we eat partly determines which three fatty acids are attached onto a glycerol molecule to form a triglyceride. For example, if we routinely eat beef or pork fat, a fatty acid found especially in those fats, arachidonic acid (an omega-6 PUFA), will get attached more frequently to our triglycerides as the second of three fatty acids. Along with the other two fatty acids in the triglyceride, this fatty acid will also get stored more often in our body fat. When we eventually need to tap into our fat stores for energy, our bodies may end up releasing too much of this one particular type of fatty acid (arachidonic acid), and our risk of experiencing an unwanted inflammatory response may increase. (As discussed on page 69, arachidonic acid is an omega-6 fatty acid that is uniquely involved in inflammatory responses.) Conversely, when we increase sources of omega-3 fatty acids in our diet, we end up storing up more of those fatty acids in our triglycerides. Although our bodies can make modifications within the omega-3 and omega-6 families, we can't change 6s into 3s or 3s into 6s, so the type of fats we store are closely related to the fats we eat.

Phospholipids

In the same way that triglycerides take center stage when it comes to the storage of fats and fatty acids, phospholipids take center stage when it comes to cell membranes and their fatty acid composition. Phospholipids are almost identical to triglycerides. They contain a glycerol backbone, just like triglycerides, and there are three molecules attached to this backbone (just like triglycerides). Whereas triglycerides have three fatty acids, however, phospholipids only have two. In phospholipids, the third attached molecule isn't a fatty acid but a phosphorus-containing molecule. The most common of these molecules is phosphatidylcholine (PC), also called lecithin; the next most common ones are phosphatidylinositol (PI) and phosphatidylserine (PS). Choline (a part of PC) and inositol (a part of PI) both belong to the B vitamin family, and serine (a part of PS) is an amino acid.

The relationship of nutrition to aging, and particularly the cognitive problems that can be associated with aging, has been an active area of research since the mid-1990s. Phospholipids appear to play a key role in these events. Also in the areas of atherosclerosis and alcoholism, phospholipid changes and supplementation with phospholipid components are the topic of ongoing study. Particularly interesting here is the relationship between our nervous system, the omega-3 fatty acid DHA, and phosphatidylserine. In certain areas of the brain, more than 35% of all phospholipids have DHA attached as their middle fatty acid. (The only phospholipids with more DHA are found in the photoreceptors of the eye, where up to 60% of the middle fatty acid positions may be filled with DHA). Many of these high-DHA phospholipids also have phosphatidylserine attached to their glycerol backbones in the third position. Adequate supplies of DHA and PS appear to be critical in maintaining healthy nerve function in parts of the brain, and there is some evidence that supplementation with DHA or PS can help reduce some age-related cognitive problems. There is also some evidence that PS supplementation can help blunt the release of cortisol in people experiencing stress and thereby lessen the stress response.

Lecithin (phosphatidylcholine) is the best studied of the phospholipids, most likely because of its long-time status as a legal food additive found on the FDA's Generally Recognized as Safe (GRAS) list. The word itself comes from the Greek *lekithos,* meaning "egg yolk," which is the most concentrated, widely eaten dietary source of lecithin. For economic reasons, however, few lecithin supplements or food additives are derived from egg yolk. Most are derived from soybeans, which are also a significant (and cheaper) source. It is worth pointing out here that even though *lecithin* is another word for *phosphatidylcholine* in the world of chemistry, in the world of food processing and sometimes in the world of dietary supplements, lecithin is not pure phosphatidylcholine but actually a complicated mixture of several phospholipids, glycolipids, carbohydrates, and triglycerides. If a consumer is purchasing a lecithin supplement, it is worth making sure that the supplement has at least been standardized for phosphatidylcholine content, usually in the 10% to 20% range. Pure PC supplements are also available.

Foods Classified by Types of Fats

Saturated Fats	Monounsaturated Fats	Polyunsaturated Fats		
FOODS THAT MAY CONTAIN OVER 25% SATURATED FAT	FOODS THAT CONTAIN OVER 50% MONO- UNSATURATED FATS	FOODS THAT CONTAIN OVER 50% TOTAL POLYUNSATURATED FATS	OMEGA-6 (PERCENTAGE OF TOTAL FAT)	OMEGA-3 (PERCENTAGE OF TOTAL FAT)
Beef	Olive oil	Soybean oil	51%	7%
Pork	Canola oil	Safflower oil	74%	trace
Lamb	Almond oil	Sunflower oil (high linoleic)	69%	trace
Poultry	Avocado	Corn oil	61%	1%
Coconut oil	Macadamia nut	Sesame oil*	42%	trace
Milk	Cashew nut	Peanut oil**	34%	trace
Butter		Rice bran oil***	38%	2%
Cheese		Wheat germ oil	55%	7%
		Grapeseed oil	70%	trace
		Flaxseed oil	13%	54%
		Pumpkin seed oil	43%	5–15%
		Walnut oil	53%	3–5%
		Chia seed oil	19%	57%
		Poppyseed oil	62–68%	trace

* Sesame oil contains about 40% monounsaturated fat, 42% omega 6 fat, and 8% saturated fat.
** Peanut oil contains about 48% monounsaturated fat, 34% omega 6 fat, and 18% saturated fat.
*** Rice bran oil contains about 40% monounsaturated fat, 38% omega 6 fat, 2% omega 3 fat, and 20% saturated fat.

Lecithin is an emulsifier and helps fats interact with other nutrients like proteins and starches. For this reason, it has been widely used as a food additive in margarine, shortening, chocolate, ice cream, and processed baked goods like breads, rolls, and cake mixes. It is not clear exactly how intake of lecithin-containing processed foods impacts our body's phospholipids (although the use of lecithin as a food additive has been shown to be a significant source of our dietary choline). But it is clear that lecithin supplementation can lower LDL cholesterol while preserving HDL (high-density lipoprotein) cholesterol, thus decreasing our risk of heart disease. The ability of supplemental lecithin to activate the enzyme LCAT (lecithin-cholesterol acyltransferase) is likely to explain one of the ways that lecithin provides us with this health benefit.

Closely related to the phospholipids, yet unique in terms of their function, are the class of lipids referred to as *sphingolipids*. (The prefix *sphingo* comes from the Greek word *sphingein*, which means "to bind tight." Although logical at the time, the name doesn't really apply to our current understanding of these lipids.) In certain areas of the nervous system, including certain areas of the brain (like the hippocampus), sphingolipids are exceptionally important in helping to form the nerve cells. One specific sphingolipid, called *sphingomyelin,* has been the topic of extensive research in this area, and chemical events surrounding sphingomyelin appear to be critical in the regulation of nerve function. Sphingomyelin is found in the membranes of many nerve cells and helps regulate chemical signals that move in and out of the nerves. The nerve cell can also break sphingomyelin apart into two molecules—ceramide and phosphorylcholine. The exact role of ceramide in nerve signaling is not clear, but this molecule is also found in skeletal muscle cells, where we know that it helps regulate the uptake of glucose by partially counteracting the influence of insulin. We also know that the buildup of ceramide encourages cells to enter

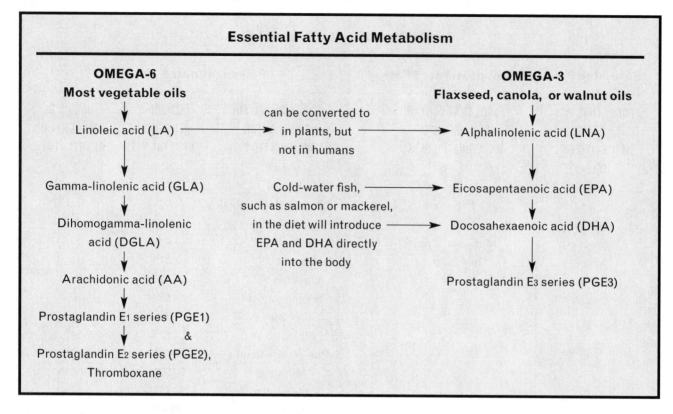

Essential Fatty Acid Metabolism

OMEGA-6
Most vegetable oils

OMEGA-3
Flaxseed, canola, or walnut oils

Linoleic acid (LA) ──── can be converted to in plants, but not in humans ────► Alphalinolenic acid (LNA)

Gamma-linolenic acid (GLA)

Cold-water fish, ────► Eicosapentaenoic acid (EPA)

Dihomogamma-linolenic acid (DGLA)

such as salmon or mackerel, in the diet will introduce ────► Docosahexaenoic acid (DHA)

EPA and DHA directly into the body

Arachidonic acid (AA)

Prostaglandin E₃ series (PGE3)

Prostaglandin E₁ series (PGE1)
&
Prostaglandin E₂ series (PGE2),
Thromboxane

into their programmed death cycle (apoptosis), which allows their components to be recycled and helps make room for new cell formation.

Sterols/Cholesterol

Sterols, the third primary category of lipids, include cholesterol, phytosterols (plant sterols), and some of the steroid hormones. **Cholesterol, the best known of the sterols, is the precursor of the bile acids and the sex hormones.** Manufactured in the body, primarily in the liver, although all tissues of the body except the brain can make it, cholesterol is present in almost all cells and is particularly high in the liver, brain and nervous tissue, and the blood. Cholesterol, like lecithin, is also available in foods, such as egg yolk, meats, and other animal fats, including milk products. Cholesterol is not present in any plant foods and cannot be produced by any plants, although it is found in the membranes of some bacteria.

Cholesterol has been implicated in occlusive cardiovascular disease, causing plaque and obstruction of the arteries. The cholesterol in foods, however, is not really the villain. It is the oxidized cholesterol in the blood that causes the trouble, and the level of this is more a function of total dietary fat intake and genetically determined aspects of cholesterol metabolism than of the amount of cholesterol in our food.

Blood cholesterol levels have been a controversy in nutrition ever since publication by the Framingham Heart Study in Massachusetts. The focus at that time was on the transport system used to carry cholesterol around the body. The LDL transport system was viewed as carrying cholesterol out from the liver to the rest of the body, and the HDL system was seen as working in the opposite direction, bringing cholesterol back to the liver from other tissues and organs. HDL became the "good guy," because it could lower our cholesterol by bringing it back to the liver for eventual elimination from the body. LDL was seen as the "bad guy," because it was depositing more cholesterol throughout the body. Researchers have since changed their thinking about HDL and LDL. Today LDL is less the bad guy, and HDL is still a good guy, but not for the reasons we originally thought. The disease-preventing effects of HDL don't appear to be connected with its liver transport of cholesterol, but instead with its ability to calm the immune system and reduce inflammation. A key point here is the continuing need for us to increase our HDL levels and maintain or lower our total cholesterol.

Unfortunately, cutting down on our total cholesterol intake cannot help us increase our HDL levels. Getting more exercise can do that, as can increasing our dietary fiber intake and our intake of plant foods, especially vegetables. Here we run into another interesting twist in the research. Decreased intake of animal foods and animal fats has always been part of our health focus, but primarily as a means of lowering total cholesterol. Now researchers have realized that it may not be the drop in total cholesterol that is important, but the ability of increased plant fiber and plant phytonutrients to reduce inflammation and oxidation and protect the body from overactivation of the immune system.

DIGESTION AND METABOLISM

Because of their viscosity and insolubility in water, fats and oils require our bodies to take special care to digest and transport them to the cells and organs. The chewing process is the first act of digestion to help separate the fats. In the stomach, gastric lipase has a minimal effect in beginning the breakdown of fats; other enzymes and hydrochloric acid do more to digest protein and carbohydrates and free the lipids from the food. Fats and oils are less dense than water; unless they are emulsified, they rise and pool at the top of the gastric contents and so are acted upon last, thus taking the longest to digest and in some ways slowing the digestion. Fatty meals seem to satisfy us longer as they cause the stomach to empty more slowly.

When the fats move into the small intestine, their main place of digestion, bile is secreted from the gallbladder (bile is made by the liver and concentrated in the gallbladder). Bile first emulsifies the fats—that is, it breaks down the fat globules into smaller groups of molecules so the other enzymes can actually work on the individual triglycerides to release the fatty acids. Pancreatic lipase is the main enzyme that splits the triglycerides into diglycerides and monoglycerides, which are ultimately hydrolyzed into their components, fatty acids and glycerol.

When the digestive system is working well, up to 95% of dietary fats are absorbed into the body. (Some are excreted through the colon.) Many of the fatty acids then need be altered in order to be absorbed and transported to the liver, the principal site of fat metabolism. The short-chained and medium-chained fatty acids, up to 12 carbons in length, are more hydrophilic (attracted to water) and can be absorbed directly through the cell membranes of the small intestine villi, the small protrusions into the intestinal lumen lined by epithelial cells and filled with capillaries; the villi increase the absorption surface of the small intestine. Within the villi, these short- and medium-chained fatty acids are picked up in the capillaries and transported through the bloodstream to the liver.

The longer-chained fatty acids, with 14 carbons or more, and the mono- and diglycerides must be reconverted to triglycerides in the intestinal wall. These triglycerides are then surrounded with a protective protein coat (like rain gear) to be transported to the liver. These become large transporter molecules, the chylomicrons, which first go into the lymph circulation before entering the blood to go to the liver. Very low-density lipoproteins (VLDLs) also carry some of the triglyceride molecules. Phospholipids and cholesterol are also incorporated into chylomicrons in order to get to the liver. After a fatty meal, the blood may be filled with chylomicrons, and the blood serum may have a milky appearance. Chylomicrons are the intestines' way of packaging fat for delivery to other parts of the body.

In the multifunctional liver, the chylomicrons are separated and the fats may be dismantled and reassembled into other needed fats. Lipids can also combine with proteins to make lipoproteins, with phosphate to make phospholipids, or with carbohydrates to form glycolipids. In the blood, free fatty acids, the active lipids for cell use, are bound to albumin, a protein. The other fats, such as cholesterol, are bound mainly to the high- and low-density lipoproteins. Each cell can take the triglycerides out of the lipoproteins and use the fatty acids for energy. Excess fat in the body is often stored in the fat cells. **The adult human has a set number of fat cells, which enlarge to accommodate the increased triglyceride stores; for example, an obese person's fat cells may be many times larger than a thin person's.** These fat cells are formed at specific times of growth, such as infancy and adolescence. So later in life, when we work to lose or gain weight, we are just shrinking or expanding our existing cells. And these fat cells are in a constant state of metabolism; they do not just sit there as many people think.

Metabolism of Fats and Oils

FROM INGESTION TO THE LIVER

Mouth	Chewing begins to separate fats.
Stomach Pancreas Duodenum	Hydrochloric acid begins to break down fats and separate lipids from foods so that pancreatic lipase can begin splitting the fats.
Gallbladder	Bile emulsifies fats, breaking them down further so that enzymes can act on individual triglycerides to release fatty acids. Pancreatic lipase splits triglycerides into diglycerides, monoglycerides, and fatty acids.
Small Intestine	Diglycerides and monoglycerides are then hydrolyzed into their components: Fatty Acids and Glycerol Shorter-chain fatty acids (up to 12 carbons) are attracted to water and are absorbed directly through the intestinal wall. Longer-chain fatty acids, diglycerides, and monoglycerides are reconverted into triglycerides to be transported through the intestinal wall with the help of glycerol. The bloodstream then carries them to the liver.
Liver ——	The Principal Site of Fat Metabolism

FUNCTIONS

Lipids perform many life-supporting functions in each cell of our body. They are part of every cell membrane and every organ and tissue. The fatty acids keep our cells strong to protect against invasion by microorganisms or damage by chemicals. Fats are important to our nervous system as well as in the manufacture of the steroid and sex hormones and the important hormonelike prostaglandins. Cholesterol is responsible for some of these functions that support the health of the brain, nervous system, liver, blood, and skin.

Besides the fact that fats add a lot of the flavor to the foods that many of us are used to and savor—such as buttery treats, gravies, and juicy meats—fats serve three primary functions in the body. They are first and foremost a ready energy source, contributing 9 calories for every gram of fat used, more than 4,000 calories per pound of fat. That is a lot of potential energy we are carrying, both from dietary intake of those fatty foods and in the stored fat of our body. This stored fat helps give the body its curves and can be used for fuel during times of reduced food intake. Second, fats in the body also act as a protective blanket shielding the organs from trauma and cold. The fat deposits surround and hold in place important organs such as the heart and kidneys. Fat below the skin helps prevent heat loss and protect against external temperature changes.

Third, the lipids are an integral part of the cell membranes. Every body cell and thus every tissue and organ is dependent on lipids in the body for its health. Fats are needed for absorption of vitamins A, D, E, and K, and by assisting in vitamin D absorption, they help calcium get into the body, especially to the bones and teeth. The cell membrane function of fats also includes an important signaling component. *Signaling* is the general term used to describe each cell's way of communicating chemically with the rest of the body. The specialized forms of membrane lipids—phospholipids, sphingolipids, and glycosphinglipids—all help cells carry out signaling tasks and stay in communication with their surroundings.

REQUIREMENTS, DEFICIENCY, AND EXCESS

In 2002, for the first time in its history, the National Academy of Sciences, through its Institute of Medicine (IOM), issued public health recommendations for intake of dietary fat. Unfortunately, from my perspective, those recommendations seem excessively broad, excessively political, and too far from the research findings to be helpful to most people. First, the IOM came up with a new category called acceptable macronutrient distribution ranges (AMDRs) to provide numbers for recommended intake. As of 2002, the AMDR for total fat intake was set at 20% to 35% of total caloric intake. If a person ate 2,000 calories of food a day, the AMDR for that person would be 400 to 700 calories from fat, or 44 to 78 grams of fat. Although the top of this range is still below what the average American eats, the range is too broad to give us true direction and likely too high, and the guideline fails to address the question of fat quality. The IOM did not set a tolerable upper limit for total fat because it found "no defined intake level of at which an adverse effect occurs."

The IOM provided no recommendation for saturated fat intake because it recognized no known role for saturated fat in the prevention of disease. It also refused to set an upper limit for saturated fat intake, "because any incremental increase in saturated fatty acid intake increased CHD [coronary heart disease] risk." Neither position makes sense to me, because intake of short-chain saturated fatty acids (SCFAs like butyric acid) has been shown to be protective of the intestinal tract and risk reducing for colon cancer, and there is clearly a level above which intake of long-chain saturated fats increases risk of heart disease, somewhere in the vicinity of 8% to 10% of total calories.

The IOM used median intake (the midpoint of what is actually eaten by U.S. adults) to set guidelines for intake of the omega-6 EFA (linoleic acid) and the omega-3 EFA (alpha-linolenic acid). The amount that is actually eaten turns out to be 17 grams a day in the case of linoleic acid, and 1.6 grams a day in the case of alpha-linolenic acid for men and 1.1 grams a day for women. The IOM found that omega-3 fatty acid deficiency "is nonexistent in healthy individuals" based on these median intakes of 1.6 and 1.1 grams. As described on page 68, however, an inappropriate ratio of omega-6 to omega-3 has been associated with a wide range of health problems. The IOM recommendation essentially guarantees an unhealthy ratio of omega-6 to omega-3, at least as high as 8:1 and potentially as high as 15:1. I think the research supports a ratio of 4:1 or less. I'd also like to support the recommendations of the NIH's 1999 Workshop on the Essentiality of and Recommended Dietary Intakes for Omega-6 and Omega-3 Fatty Acids (described on page 68) for intake of the omega-6 fatty acid linoleic acid at 2% of total calories (and no more than 3% of total calories); the omega-3 fatty acid alpha-linolenic acid at 1% of total calories; and the omega-3 fatty acids EPA and DHA at a minimum of 0.1% each. Those guidelines would be a good start for improvement of fat quality, are consistent with nutritional research, and serve public health far better than the IOM version.

As with saturated fat, the IOM refused to set a recommended guideline or an upper limit for intake of trans-fatty acids. Their reasoning was precisely the same as that for saturated fat. No recommendation was provided because there was "no known benefit to human health," and no upper limit was set because "any incremental increase in *trans*-fatty acid intake increases CHD [coronary heart disease] risk." The IOM further pointed out that "because trans-fatty acids are unavoidable in ordinary, nonvegan diets, consuming 0 percent of energy would require significant changes in dietary intake." I would like to think that the choice here is not really all or nothing, and that most people would want to minimize their trans-fatty acid intake as much as possible by reducing their intake of processed foods that contain partially hydrogenated oils.

The IOM total fat recommendation of 20% to 35% of total calories would be acceptable, with the following stipulations: Everyone needs to find his or her own place in the recommended range and take in the amount of food necessary to maintain optimum weight and not supply any excess body weight. Many individualized factors might come into play here; for example, climate and body temperature are important factors in determining fat requirements. If a person gets cold easily, he or she may need more fat in the diet, provided his or her weight and thyroid are normal.

In most Western cultures, as in American society, the real concern is over an excess intake of fat and overeating in general. Although we have made little progress in terms of fat *quality* since the mid-1980s, we have made some progress in terms of fat *quantity*. Instead of averaging about 120 grams of total fat a day— as we did when the first edition of this book was published in 1992—Americans now average about 75 grams. However, included in this 75 grams are 26 grams of saturated fat (mostly from meats and hydrogenated oils), and about 15 grams of polyunsaturated fat, nearly all omega-6. This total fat intake puts us at about 34% calories from fat—still too high, but a step in the right direction.

The American Heart Association Eating Plan for Healthy Americans, released in 2000, provided the following guidelines for food intake related to fat:

- Include fat-free and low-fat milk products, fish, legumes (beans), skinless poultry and lean meats.

- Choose fats and oils with 2 grams or fewer saturated fat per tablespoon, such as liquid and tub margarines, canola oil, and olive oil.

- Limit foods high in saturated fat, trans fat, and/or cholesterol, such as full-fat milk products, fatty meats, tropical oils, and partially hydrogenated vegetable oils. Instead choose foods low in saturated fat, trans fat, and cholesterol, such as cold-pressed plant oils like olive oil or canola oil, and nuts or seeds, including almonds, cashews, pumpkin seeds and sesame seeds.

I support these recommendations and feel particularly strongly about focusing on minimally processed plant fats and inclusion of sufficient omega-3 fats to balance the ratio of omega-6 to omega-3. I would also like to see:

- More plant protein sources, including nuts, seeds, and legumes (dried peas and beans).

- More broiling, baking, and steaming of foods instead of frying.

- More vegetables, including green leafy vegetables and root vegetables, and replacement of processed grains with whole grains.

- Reduced total fat consumption from about 40% to 30% of calorie intake.

- Reduced long-chain saturated fat intake to about 10% of total calories.

DIETARY FAT AND DISEASE

A topic of great concern in modern nutritional medicine is the correlation between increased dietary fat intake and disease. Research continues regarding the relationship between disease and cholesterol and the types of fats consumed. We now know that two aspects of diet must be considered: first, the total amount of fat intake—that is, the percentage of the total diet consisting of fats and oils, both saturated and unsaturated fats (monounsaturated or polyunsaturated); and second, the types of fats consumed. Long-chain saturated and hydrogenated fats seem to be worse in regard to increasing cholesterol and causing vascular congestive problems than the vegetable-source unsaturated ones, which may actually improve cholesterol by reducing the LDL to HDL ratio and decreasing total cholesterol. Fried foods seem to be more difficult for the body to process as well. Finally, omega-3 fats from cold-water fish, nuts, seeds, and the germs and brans of grains seem essential.

Of the diseases related to increased fat intake, number one is atherosclerosis. Clogging, or atherosclerosis, of the coronary arteries (the blood vessels that nourish the heart muscle itself with blood) is the disease process causing the most deaths in the Western "affluent diet" cultures. Clogging vital arteries with plaque (consisting of fat, mucopolysaccharides, calcium, platelets, and smooth muscle cells) decreases the delivery of life-supporting blood to the tissues and is related to a variety of other diseases. Narrowing and stiffness of blood vessels resulting from arterial plaque leads to high blood pressure, or hypertension, which forces the heart to work harder to get the blood to the body. This constant extra effort can lead to enlargement of the heart, general heart disease, and congestive heart failure. Coronary artery disease leads to the physical limitations associated with angina pectoris and is the primary cause for the big business of coronary artery bypass surgery.

I want to further delineate the role of fats in cardiovascular diseases. Saturated fats and hydrogenated vegetable oils, which contain high amounts of saturated fats in place of their once polyunsaturated oils, both raise serum cholesterol. The liver makes cholesterol from the very shortest of all short-chain saturated fats, acetic acid. A number of factors can increase the risk of cardiovascular disease, including elevated homocysteine (derived from the amino acid cysteine and often elevated because of a lack of B complex vitamins and other nutrients), elevated serum cholesterol, smoking, and high blood pressure. Anyone who smokes, has high blood pressure, and has a serum cholesterol level of more than 250, especially with a high LDL to HDL ratio, is almost certain to close off his or her arteries relatively rapidly.

Other risk factors for the cardiovascular diseases include stress, obesity, gender (the female hormone estrogen is protective for women), heredity (for heart disease or for higher cholesterol levels), lack of exercise, and elevated blood triglyceride levels. We are in a position to reduce most of these risk factors by changing our lifestyles and dietary habits, and doing so will significantly reduce our chances of developing blood vessel and heart disease. Obesity is much more likely in people who eat a high-fat diet, which is often a high-calorie diet, because each gram of fat contains 9 calories instead of the 4 calories in each gram of protein or carbohydrate. With obesity comes an increased risk of all the previously mentioned diseases, such as atherosclerosis, hypertension, and certain cancers, besides a variety of other problems, including adult-onset diabetes. Overall, the best way to lower risks of cardiovascular disease is to reduce long-chain saturated fat intake, consume adequate amounts of B vitamins and antioxidant nutrients, keep the blood pressure and blood sugar normal, not smoke, and exercise regularly.

In a nutshell, what has the past decade taught us about nutrition and heart disease? First, quality is just as important as quantity. A moderate amount of low-quality fat (like hydrogenated oil or beef fat) seems just as problematic as, or even more problematic than, a large amount of high-quality fat (like organic walnuts or pumpkin seeds). By today's research standards, however, "low-fat" isn't good enough. The fat that remains must be *high quality*. Second, getting this high-quality fat into our mouths is not enough. When it comes to our health, the journey of fat only *begins* in the mouth. We have to think about the whole process, what happens to fat once it is inside, to lower our risk of heart disease. Heart disease is not only about "bad fats" getting inside us; it is also about acceptable fats getting sabotaged during their journey around the body.

As fat is transported around, other food nutrients protect it. The molecules that carry our fat need constant protection—primarily from oxygen damage (oxidation) that can be partly prevented with a meal plan that contains plenty of antioxidant nutrients like vitamin C, vitamin E, carotenoids, and flavonoids. Poor control over our blood sugar can also contribute to problems with fat metabolism, so we need plenty of plant fiber in our diet to help keep our sugars stable. Fat can't move around safely in our blood vessels unless the walls of those vessels are sturdy and flexible. They lose some of their resilience when our homocysteine levels get too high, but we can help prevent this possibility by keeping our intake of B complex vitamins at an optimal level. Green leafy vegetables and whole grains are some of our best B vitamin sources, and so they too can play a role in allowing for safe passage of fat through our blood vessels. We need to eat high-quality fat to get the process started off successfully. We need to eat a high-quality diet to keep it on track.

With regard to nutrition and cancer (our second most prevalent deadly adult disease), it is likely that more than 50% of cancer occurrences are related at least in part to diet. The Hunza tribes of Pakistan, who are known for their longevity and have the lowest known cancer rates, eat an exclusively natural, chemical-free diet of foods they grow themselves. **High animal protein intake and low dietary fiber consumption are two important factors increasing cancer incidence, but another factor that is increasingly being shown to be the most significant is high intake of fats, particularly the saturated animal fats.** Many chemicals in foods, used as preservatives or from herbicides and pesticides, may be carcinogenic in the body, especially in the gastrointestinal tract, and many of these chemicals are stored in animal fats. Artificial red dyes, cyclamate, nitrites and nitrates in processed meats, as well as saccharin have all been implicated in cancer.

Two major types of cancer are associated with excessive dietary fat intake. The first, cancer of the colon and rectum, is the most common cancer in men and women combined. The other, cancer of the breast, is the most common major cancer in women. Both cancers can be deadly, especially if they are not diagnosed early, and both are associated with a high-fat, low-fiber diet. There is also an association between prostate cancer in men and uterine and ovarian cancer in women with high dietary fat consumption, particularly saturated fats found in animal foods.

The theory of how fat can cause cancer in the colon and rectum is based on the fact that fats in the diet cause release of bile acids from the gallbladder and liver into the intestine to help emulsify the fats. High-fat diets stimulate increased bile acid levels in the colon. Fat in the diet also weakens the metabolism of the normal colon bacteria that, when functioning optimally, may help protect the colon lining from carcinogens. These altered microflora interact with the bile acids to potentially create compounds that may cause cancer. An increased fiber content, even in a higher-fat diet, seems to be protective by increasing bowel motility, by diluting these carcinogenic substances through bulking action, and by improving bacterial detoxification functions.

More than 100,000 new cases of colon cancer are diagnosed each year. The high-fat diet increases the incidence of this cancer, which, if diagnosed early, can usually be cured through major surgery—a drastic measure that could be prevented. The high-fat diet is also commonly associated with a higher fried-food component and lower fiber content, two other important dietary factors in carcinogenesis in the colon. Numerous studies have shown the relationship of dietary fat to colon cancer. Research with the Seventh-day Adventists, who eat a vegetarian diet, reveals that their incidence of colon cancer is much lower than average. They usually consume a diet higher in fiber and lower in fat than the average American. A study of the Mormon high-fiber diet has more clearly isolated dietary fats as the main connection to colon cancer incidence. Other nutritional qualities of the fruit and vegetable fiber foods seem to help inhibit cancer formation as well. Vitamins C and E, beta-carotene, and selenium, plus the plant sterols and antioxidant phenolic compounds like bioflavonoids from such foods as berries and citrus fruits, all seem to be beneficial factors. The cruciferous vegetables, such as broccoli and cabbage, seem to have other factors, such as sulfhydryl-containing molecules, besides the fiber that may protect against the development of cancer.

The American Institute for Preventive Medicine's Cancer Risk Factors

RISK FACTORS FOR CANCER

- Exposure to the sun's ultraviolet rays, nuclear radiation, X-rays, and radon.
- Use of tobacco and/or alcohol (for some cancers).
- Use of certain medicines such as diethylstilbestrol (DES), a synthetic estrogen.
- Polluted air and water.
- Dietary factors such as a high-fat diet, specific food preservatives (namely, nitrates and nitrites), charbroiling and grilling meats.
- Exposure to a variety of chemicals such as asbestos, benzenes, VC (vinyl chloride), wood dust, some ingredients of cigarette smoke, and so on.

LIFESTYLE RISKS

- Do not smoke, use tobacco products, or inhale second-hand smoke.
- Limit your exposure to known carcinogens such as asbestos, radon, and other workplace chemicals as well as pesticides and herbicides. Have X-rays only when necessary.
- Limit your exposure to the sun's ultraviolet (UV) rays, sun lamps, and tanning booths. Protect your skin from the sun's UV rays with sunscreen (applied frequently and containing a sun protection factor [SPF] of 15 or higher) and protective clothing (sun hats, long sleeves, and so on).
- Reduce stress. Emotional stress may weaken the immune system, which is relied on to fight off stray cancer cells.

Source: American Institute for Preventive Medicine, Farmington Hills, Michigan, 2002.

Cancer of the breast and a high-fat diet have been shown to be related for some time. It is thought that saturated fats generate more cholesterol and higher estrogen levels in women. This theory supports the dietary fat and breast cancer relationship as estrogen is particularly related to increased incidence of female breast cancer. Although the dietary fat and breast cancer question is not conclusively answered, it is generally agreed that, regarding this disease, a low-fat, high-complex-carbohydrate diet minimizing alcohol, cigarettes, and preserved and chemical foods is still the best way to live to help prevent breast cancer. Countries such as Japan, whose people traditionally eat a low-fat diet, have a much lower incidence of breast cancer than countries where the population eats higher quantities of animal fat, such as Australia, New Zealand, the United States, and the countries of western Europe. Japanese people who eat more westernized diets or who move to a country in which a Western diet is consumed have a higher incidence of breast cancer. In the United States, Seventh-Day Adventist women on a vegetarian diet exhibit a lower incidence of this disease.

Not all recent studies correlate higher cancer incidence solely with total fat intake, however. There is some question as to whether certain fats are more significant than others. Milk fat and dairy foods have been implicated in several studies. The strongest correlation for breast cancer has been with the intake of the trans-fatty acids that are created when vegetable oils are hydrogenated to make margarine and solid vegetable shortening. There is even some concern with the polyunsaturated fats. Because they are less stable, they can go through peroxidation, which can lead to the formation of epoxides that may be cancer causing. This is especially true when these fats are heated. (Vitamin E and beta-carotene are two antioxidants that protect against the peroxidation process.) Because of this, I suggest using polyunsaturates moderately, along with some monosaturates, such as olive oil, which are more stable, while cutting down on saturated fats.

CANCER PREVENTION

Although there are no single, independent causes of cancer, many different factors are known to contribute to cancer risk. Many of these factors fall into the categories of nutrition and diet.

The specific cancer-preventive diet put out in 1997 by the American Cancer Society's Medical and Scientific Committee includes the following suggestions:

- Avoid obesity. Obese people have higher incidences of many cancers, particularly of the breast, colon, stomach, gallbladder, and uterus.

- Reduce total fat intake. Dietary fat is mainly associated with increased risk of colon, breast, and prostate cancer. It also adds to obesity, another risk.

- Eat more high-fiber foods, particularly fresh fruit and vegetables and whole grains. This is not conclusive, but it does seem that these nutrient-rich, low-calorie, and low-fat foods reduce the likelihood of cancer through a variety of means.

- Include in the diet those foods that are rich in vitamin A and vitamin C. Beta-carotene, the precursor of vitamin A, is found in many fruits and vegetables, such as carrots, spinach, tomatoes, apricots, peaches, and melons. This nutrient is thought to help reduce carcinogenesis. Vitamin C, found in high amounts in citrus fruits and many vegetables, may also prevent cancer. It interferes with production of nitrosamine, a carcinogen formed from dietary nitrites in preserved foods.

- Include such cruciferous vegetables as broccoli, brussels sprouts, cabbage, and cauliflower in the diet. Their actions are not known exactly, but these foods are thought to help prevent cancer.

- Minimize the consumption of alcoholic beverages. Alcohol increases the risks for certain cancers, which are even more liable to occur in those who smoke.

- Avoid the consumption of salt-cured, smoked, and nitrate-treated foods. Nitrates and nitrites can form nitrosamine, a carcinogen, in the digestive tract. Also, the smoking of foods can cause fats to be converted to polycyclic aromatic hydrocarbons, which are carcinogenic.

MORE ON CANCER PREVENTION

Additional cancer-preventive diet guidelines put out in 1997 by the American Institute for Cancer Research includes the suggestions on the following two-page chart. Also in chapter 16, you may refer to "Cancer Prevention" and "Cardiovascular Disease prevention."

Food Supply, Eating, and Related Factors to Cancer

1. Food supply and eating
Populations to consume nutritionally adequate and varied diets, based primarily on foods of plant origin. *Choose predominantly plant-based diets rich in a variety of vegetables and fruits, pulses (legumes), and minimally processed starchy staple foods.*

2. Maintaining body weight
Populations to maintain average body mass indexes (BMI) throughout adult life within the range BMI 21–23, so that individual BMI be maintained between 18.5 and 25.[a] *Avoid being underweight or overweight and limit weight gain during adulthood to fewer than 5 kg (11 pounds).*

3. Maintaining physical activity
Populations to maintain, throughout life, an active lifestyle equivalent to a physical activity level (PAL) of at least 1.75, with opportunities for vigorous physical activity. *If occupational activity is low or moderate, take an hour's brisk walk or similar exercise daily, and also exercise vigorously for a total of at least one hour in a week.[b]*

FOODS AND DRINKS

4. Vegetables and fruits
Promote year-round consumption of a variety of vegetables and fruits, providing 7% or more total energy. *Eat 400–800 grams (15–30 ounces) or five or more portions (servings) a day of a variety of vegetables and fruits, all year round.[c, d]*

5. Other plant foods[e]
A variety of starchy or protein-rich foods of plant origin, preferably minimally processed, to provide 45% to 60% total energy. Refined sugar to provide less than 10% total energy. *Eat 600–800 grams (20–30 ounces) or more than seven portions (servings) a day of a variety of cereals (grains), pulses (legumes), roots, tubers, and plantains.[c, f] Prefer minimally processed foods. Limit consumption of refined sugar.*

6. Alcoholic drinks
Consumption of alcohol is not recommended. Excessive consumption of alcohol to be discouraged. For those who drink alcohol, restrict it to less than 5% total energy for men and less than 2.5% total energy for women. *Alcohol consumption is not recommended. If consumed at all, limit alcoholic drinks to less than two drinks a day for men and one for women.[g,h,i]*

7. Meat
If eaten at all, red meat to provide less than 10% percent total energy. *If eaten at all, limit intake of red meat to fewer than 80 grams (3 ounces) daily. It is preferable to choose fish, poultry, or meat from nondomesticated animals in place of red meat.[c,j]*

8. Total fats and oils
Total fats and oils to provide 15% to no more than 30% total energy. *Limit consumption of fatty foods, particularly those of animal origin. Choose modest amounts of appropriate vegetable oils.[k]*

FOOD PROCESSING

9. Salt and salting
Salt from all sources should amount to fewer than 6 grams a day (0.25 ounces) for adults. *Limit consumption of salted foods and use of cooking and table salt. Use herbs and spices to season foods.[l]*

10. Storage
Store perishable food in ways that minimize fungal contamination. *Do not eat food that, as a result of prolonged storage at ambient temperatures, is liable to contamination with mycotoxins.*

11. Preservation
Perishable food, if not consumed promptly, to be kept frozen or chilled. *Use refrigeration and other appropriate methods to preserve perishable food as purchased and at home.*

12. Additives and residues

Establish and monitor the enforcement of safety limits for food additives, pesticides and their residues, and other chemical contaminants in the food supply. *When levels of additives, contaminants, and other residues are properly regulated, their presence in food and drink is not known to be harmful. However, unregulated or improper use can be a health hazard, and this applies particularly in economically developing countries.*

13. Preparation

When meat and fish are eaten, encourage relatively low temperature cooking. *Do not eat charred food. For meat and fish eaters, avoid burning of meat juices. Consume the following only occasionally: meat and fish grilled (broiled) in direct flame; cured and smoked meats.*

DIETARY SUPPLEMENTS

14. Dietary supplements

Community dietary patterns to be consistent with reduction of cancer risk without the use of dietary supplements. *For those who follow the recommendations presented here, dietary supplements are probably unnecessary, and possibly unhelpful, for reducing cancer risk.*[m]

TOBACCO

Tobacco

Discourage production, promotion, and use of tobacco in any form. *Do not smoke or chew tobacco.*

Data in this list has been compiled from information found in "Food, Nutrition, and the Prevention of Cancer: a global perspective," World Cancer Research Fund/American Institute for Cancer Research, Washington, DC, 1997.

a. The advice to individuals is equivalent to maintaining BMI between 18.5 and 25.0. In affluent, less physically active societies, lower average BMI levels may be desirable. For calculations of BMI for people of different heights and weights, see Figure 8.1.1 of the report.

b. For equivalents of brisk walking and for types of vigorous exercise, see Table 8.1.1. of the report.

c. Calculated on the basis of 2,000 kcal (8.4 MJ) daily energy intake, 80 grams per portion. Different bases for total energy intake and for portion sizes will produce different goals—for example, children's servings to be appropriately smaller.

d. Pulses (legumes) and starchy vegetables and fruits (tubers, starchy roots, and plantains) are not included. (See Recommendation 5.)

e. This recommendation is consistent with and generally supported by, but not primarily derived from, the data on cancer. (See chapter 8.3 of the report.)

f. In societies where diets are based on cereals, such as rice or millet, the weight of starchy and protein-rich foods may be higher, say up to 1,000 grams per day as served. Set portion (serving) sizes are not a meaningful concept in many societies, and those whose diets are cereal-based consume larger, rather than more frequent, portions.

g. Pregnant women, children, and adolescents should not drink alcohol.

h. A drink is defined as 250 ml (one small glass) of beer, 100 ml (one glass) of wine, 25 ml (one measure) of spirits, or equivalent.

i. This recommendation is designed to take into account evidence that modest alcohol intake is protective against coronary heart disease. (See chapter 8.3 of the report.)

j. "Red meat" refers to beef, lamb, and pork, as well as to products made from these meats. It does not refer to poultry or fish, or to game or meat from nondomesticated animals or birds, consumption of any or all of which is preferable to consumption of red meat.

k. The vegetable oils should be predominantly monounsaturated with minimum hydrogenation. This point relates to the prevention of cardiovascular disease. (See chapter 8.3 of the report.)

l. Children to consume fewer than 3 grams per 1,000 kcal. Salt supplies may be iodized (to prevent thyroid disorders).

m. This recommendation is made in the context of cancer prevention. (See chapter 8.3 of the report.)

CARDIOVASCULAR DISEASE PREVENTION

There's not a single example of cardiovascular disease—from atherosclerosis and high blood pressure to heart attack and stroke—that isn't partly preventable through changes in diet. This area of chronic disease is almost legendary in the research world for connecting nutritional changes with reduced cardiovascular risk. **Suggestions for reducing cardiovascular diseases include the following:**

- Reduce the amount of total fats in the diet from more than 40% of total calories (the current average) to approximately 20% to 35% or lower.

- Specifically reduce long-chain saturated fat intake by reducing consumption of red meats and full-fat milk products, such as cheeses and butter.

- Reduce intake of hydrogenated fat (also saturated fat), found in cooking oils, margarine, and other processed foods.

- Raise the ratio of polyunsaturated fats to saturated fats in the diet by maintaining or slightly increasing the dietary intake of polyunsaturated fats found in vegetable oils such as sunflower, canola, and sesame oil and in most seeds and nuts. These also contain high amounts of the essential fatty acids, which are important to

healthy body function. Within this group, make a special effort to increase the omega-3 foods, including walnuts, flaxseeds, and pumpkin seeds.

- Eat more cold-water fish (at least twice weekly), rather than red meats, for the omega-3 fatty acid content.

- Keep the blood pressure under control, do not smoke, and exercise regularly.

- See more on cardiovascular disease and prevention in chapter 16.

Dietary Guidelines for Preventing Cardiovascular Disease

Healthy food habits can help you reduce three risk factors for heart attack and stroke—high blood cholesterol, high blood pressure, and excess body weight. We have adapted the American Heart Association Eating Plan for Healthy Americans and these basic dietary guidelines, released in October 2000:

- Eat a variety of fruits and vegetables. Choose 5 or more servings per day.
- Eat a variety of grain products, primarily whole grains. Choose 6 or more servings per day.
- Eat fish at least twice a week, particularly fatty fish.
- Include legumes (beans), and some fat-free and low-fat milk products, skinless poultry, and lean meats.
- Choose quality fats and oils low in saturated fats, such as olive, coconut, sunflower, corn, and soybean oils.
- Limit your intake of foods high in calories or low in nutrition. This includes foods with a lot of added sugar like soft drinks, candy, and baked goods.
- Limit foods high in saturated fat, trans fat, and/or cholesterol, such as full-fat milk products, fatty meats, tropical oils, partially hydrogenated vegetable oils, and egg yolks.
- Eat less than 6 grams of salt (sodium chloride) per day.

- If you drink alcohol, have no more than 1 drink per day if you're a woman or 2 per day if you're a man.
- To maintain your weight, balance the number of calories you eat with the number you use each day.
- Get enough physical activity to keep fit, and balance the calories you burn with the calories you eat.

Following these guidelines will help you achieve and maintain a healthy eating pattern. The benefits include a healthy body weight, a desirable blood cholesterol level and a normal blood pressure. Every meal doesn't have to meet all the guidelines. It's important to apply the guidelines to your overall eating pattern over a period of several days. However, be aware that dietary excesses that raise blood cholesterol drive cholesterol to fatty buildups in arteries. It's much harder for the cholesterol to come out of the artery, so you don't quite "make up" for the excess by an equivalent period of healthy eating.

These guidelines may do more than improve your heart health. They may reduce your risk for other chronic health problems, including type 2 diabetes, osteoporosis (bone loss), and some forms of cancer.

Dietary Guidelines for Healthy American Adults, American Heart Association, October 2000.

Chapter 5

Vitamins

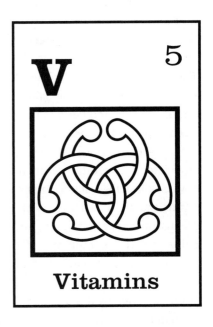

V 5

Vitamins

itamins are one of two groups of substances classified as micronutrients (the other is minerals) that are essential in human nutrition. Vitamins are organic, meaning they contain the element carbon and are found in plant and animal substances in small amounts. We obtain them by eating the plants and animals that make them. Most vitamins cannot be manufactured in our bodies; exceptions are some of the B vitamins, which can be made by our intestinal bacteria, and occasional biochemical conversions from a precursor to the active form of the required vitamin, as when beta-carotene is converted to vitamin A. **Vitamins, however, are not sources of energy (calories). We obtain our energy from the macronutrients— carbohydrates, proteins, and fats.** In fact, vitamins help to convert these macronutrients to more bioavailable, or metabolically useful, forms. Vitamins function principally as coenzymes (in collaboration with enzymes) for a variety of metabolic reactions and biochemical mechanisms within our many bodily systems. Each enzyme is specific to one biochemical reaction. **Enzymes are catalysts—that is, they speed up specific chemical reactions that would proceed very slowly, if at all, without vitamins.**

Vitamins themselves are not part of our body tissues; they are not building blocks but helpers in metabolism. We cannot live on vitamins but need food that provides energy and helps form the actual tissues of our body. In fact, we need food and certain minerals to best absorb any vitamin supplements we take. **Vitamins are essential for growth, vitality, and health and are helpful in digestion, elimination, and resistance to disease.** Depletions or deficiencies can lead to a variety of both specific nutritional disorders and general health problems, according to what vitamin is lacking in the diet.

Historically, vitamins were discovered primarily through the deficiency diseases caused by their absence in the diet. Many vitamins were discovered in naturally occurring human experiments and in laboratory studies using rats, mice, or birds fed specific diets lacking certain essential foods. It was not until the early 1900s, however, that Sir Frederick Galen Hopkins published a paper suggesting that there were some "accessory nutrients" needed in the human diet in small quantities to maintain good health. In 1911, the first vitamin was isolated from rice polishings (this vitamin was thiamin). It was found to be an amine (containing nitrogen) and thus was termed *vitamine*—that is, "amine essential for life." Other vitamins were ultimately discovered that were not amines, and the term was converted to its current form, *vitamin*.

Back in the 1500s, records were first made of nature's vitamin experiments and vitamin deficiency disease. The British Royal Navy during Queen Elizabeth's reign was fed a diet of dried or salted meat or fish, biscuits, butter, cheese, and beer. Many men developed a serious and painful disease, and more than 10,000 died during a 20-year period. The disease, named *scurvy*, was associated with rotten gums and tooth loss, painful jaws, swollen legs, aches and pains, and easy bruising. When the men were fed raw potatoes, watercress, raisins, or scurvy grass—all sources of vitamin C—their pains and other symptoms of the disease reversed rapidly. Likewise, beriberi, now known to be a thiamin deficiency, was in the late 1800s a debilitating and potentially deadly disease among Japanese sailors who ate a diet deficient in whole-grain foods; contributing particularly to this disease was the processing that removed the outer covering of rice. Dietary adjustment was helpful in curing this disease. The simple addition of wheat aboard sailing vessels was enough to shift the prevalence of this problem on sailing vessels, although it took much longer for broad cultural trends to shift. When rats were experimentally fed only proteins, starches, sugars, and fats—without milk products or vegetables—their eyes were affected and they failed to grow. Vitamin A was then isolated from milk, butter, liver, and egg yolks, and this substance was shown to reverse the eye problem and promote growth in the rats. There are many more stories regarding experiments and discoveries of specific vitamins. Various experiments have determined the U.S. government's development of the commonly quoted recommended dietary allowances (RDAs), which are discussed in this chapter.

Vitamins are usually classified into two categories: those that are water soluble and those that are fat soluble. They are further categorized by letters, groups, and individual chemical names.

Water-soluble vitamins include mainly the many B vitamins and vitamin C. They are most likely to be lost when foods are cooked, because they are especially sensitive to heat. But water-soluble vitamins can also be lost from raw foods because they can also be sensi-

tive to air, light, and the passage of time. The more time that passes between harvest and eating, the more likely the loss of water-soluble vitamins, so it is good to consume produce that is fresh and locally grown. Commonly found in the vegetable foods, these vitamins are contained less so in most animal sources. The water-soluble vitamins are not stored in the body to a very large degree, so they are needed regularly in our diets; this makes them much less potentially toxic than the fat-soluble vitamins, which are stored when taken in higher dosages. Most of the water-soluble vitamins act in the body as coenzymes in combination with an inactive protein to make an active enzyme.

Fat-soluble vitamins are vitamins A, D, E, and K, which are found in the lipid component of both vegetable- and animal-source foods (the source varies for each vitamin). Grains, seeds, and nuts contain vitamin E, and many vegetables contain vitamin A or, more commonly, its precursor beta-carotene. These fat-soluble vitamins can be stored in the body tissues, so we can function for longer periods of time without obtaining them from the diet than we can without the water-soluble ones. For this reason, toxic levels can occur more easily from regular increased intake of these vitamins, especially vitamin A; vitamins D and K can also cause problems when taken in high dosages. Toxicity is less likely with vitamin E, because it is used readily by the body as an antioxidant to help protect against the harmful by-products of metabolism and against outside pollutants. Vitamin A adds cellular protection as well as resistance to infection, while vitamin D aids in absorption of calcium from the gut and thus is important to skeletal health. Vitamin K helps make factors crucial to blood clotting to prevent bleeding.

DIETARY REFERENCE INTAKES (DRIs)

RDAs are the most widely adopted and most widely criticized nutritional guidelines in the United States. These guidelines were first established in 1941 by the National Academy of Sciences, a private, not-for-profit agency partly funded by the federal government and by private companies. Development of the most recent 1997 dietary guidelines for calcium, for example, was partly funded by the National Dairy Council.

Criticism of the RDAs has involved three major components: their failure to account for individual differences, their failure to address disease prevention, and their failure to address optimal nourishment. Until 1998, when the National Academy of Sciences (NAS) began its major overhaul of public dietary guidelines in the form of the dietary reference intakes (DRIs), this organization never pretended that it was trying to accomplish either of these first two objectives. The NAS did not see itself as issuing guidelines for us to make personal decisions about nutrition, and as late as 1995 asked that its guidelines "be applied to population groups rather than to individuals." The NAS also purposely steered clear of disease prevention. It offered the RDAs

Dietary Reference Intakes (DRIs) Table*

DRIs	Definition and Notes	Concepts Illustrated by the Figure
Estimated Average Requirements (EARs)	• data-based, statistically relevant estimate of the average daily nutrient intake level that will meet the requirement of half of the healthy individuals in a given life stage and gender group	The EAR is the intake at which the risk of inadequacy is 50% to an individual.
Recommended Dietary Allowances (RDAs)	• the average daily nutrient intake level sufficient to meet the nutrient requirement of nearly all (97% to 98%) healthy individuals in a particular life stage and gender group • calculated from the EAR	The RDA is the intake at which the risk of inadequacy to the individual is very small (only 2% to 3%).
Adequate Intakes (AIs)	• a recommended average daily nutrient intake level based on observed or experimentally determined approximations or estimates of nutrient intake, by a group (or groups) of apparently healthy people, that are assumed to be adequate • set when insufficient data exist to determine an EAR, and thus an RDA • indicates that more research is needed to determine the mean and distribution of requirements for the specific nutrient	The AI does not bear a consistent relationship to the EAR or the RDA because it is set without being able to estimate the requirement, and as such, cannot be placed on the figure.
Tolerable Upper Intake Levels (ULs)	• the highest average daily nutrient intake level likely to pose no risk of adverse health effects to almost all individuals in the general population	At intakes between the RDA and the UL, the risks of inadequacy and of excess to the individual are both close to zero. At intakes above the UL, the potential risk of adverse effects to the individual increases. Little is known about the shape of the risk curve, so the proportion of the population experiencing adverse effects at any specific intake above the UL cannot be estimated accurately.

The chart was produced by the Office of Nutrition Policy and Promotion, Health Canada. Their website is: http://www.hc-sc.gc.ca/hpfb-dgpsa/onpp-bppn/contactus_e.html

as guidelines for groups of people who were *already healthy.* "Already healthy" assumed no diagnosed disease and no risk of disease. Beginning in 1996, however, the NAS began to change its position, and along with this change came a major overhaul of the RDAs.

The NAS has established three new categories of dietary guidelines to work alongside the RDAs, and it has placed all three categories, as well as the RDAs themselves, under a new umbrella heading called *dietary reference intakes* (DRIs). In other words, as of 1997, the RDAs are now a subdivision of the DRIs. The three additional categories of recommendations are as follows: adequate intakes, estimated average requirements, and tolerable upper intake levels. The chart on page 85 provides the technical clarifications of these terms.

As of 2003, DRIs of some kind (including at least one of the four types of guidelines just defined) have been established for about 50 nutrients. Some nutrients no longer have RDAs, and some have all four types of guidelines. In every instance, however, there is a systematic relationship between AIs, EARs, and RDAs.

Adequate intake (AI) recommendations are the starting point for the NAS and require the least scientific evidence. The AIs can be based on experimental approximations and can only tentatively be used in setting nutritional goals. For example, the AI for calcium intake in newborn to 6-month-old infants (210 mg of calcium per day) is based on the average calcium intake of exclusively breast-fed infants but not on any measurement of infant health or physical function. There is no longer any RDA for calcium, infants or otherwise.

Estimated average requirements (EARs) are dietary guidelines that fall a step between AIs and RDAs. These guidelines indicate the amount of a nutrient that would have to be consumed in order for half of the individuals within any particular group to meet their nutrient requirement. The EAR for vitamin E in 1- to 3-year olds, for example, is 5 mg per day. It takes more scientific research to establish an EAR than an AI.

Recommended dietary allowances (RDAs) are dietary guidelines that the NAS expects to meet the daily nutrient requirements of 97% to 98% of all individuals within a specific age-gender group and, as of 1997, the RDAs are "intended primarily for use as a goal for daily intake by individuals." The RDAs also

attempt to take into account disease prevention. For example, research involving prevention of heart disease was considered by the NAS when establishing the RDAs for vitamin E.

The last puzzle piece in this confusing new set of guidelines is the **tolerable upper intake level (UL),** set for most of the revised nutrients. The UL is described as the maximum amount of a nutrient that an individual can consume each day without increasing the risk of a health problem. For women 31 to 50, for example, the UL for calcium is 2.5 grams, 2.5 times the AI of 1.0 gram.

What do I make of this new and confusing set of guidelines? It is clear that the NAS felt some political pressure to address disease prevention and individual needs in its guidelines. I am glad to see these issues addressed in the DRIs. But the NAS has still missed the boat, because even within this new DRI framework, dietary recommendations have nothing to do with maintaining vitality for a given individual. Nor is it likely that they are the amounts needed during recovery from serious disease or even minor sicknesses. And what about possible increased needs during times of extra stress or if we drink a lot of alcohol or coffee, or eat sugar, all of which could deplete some vitamins or create extra needs? And what are our requirements if we are on a special diet or are planning to have surgery? No one knows for certain the answers to these questions, but many doctors and other people do not go by the DRIs in these situations. We recognize them as the minimum, not the optimum. And even these minimum levels may not be provided by diet alone, so many people take additional supplements for insurance against deficiency problems. But vitamin advertisers and nutritional magazines promote all kinds of supplements. Consumers must be aware of this and gain knowledge to make healthy choices.

In this chapter, I look at the optimum levels of each nutrient, explain what each can do at these levels, explore potential deficiency problems, and list the food sources from which each nutrient can be obtained. Providing knowledgeable use of diet and nutritional supplements for each individual is my goal. In the discussions of individual vitamins, I provide the specific DRIs, including those for children, adults, and the elderly when they are different, and special requirements during times when health is below normal. I also provide optimum intake levels of the various vitamins. Vitamin levels for the fat-soluble nutrients A, D, E, and K, as well as the water-soluble vitamins, are given is in either milligrams (mg) or micrograms (mcg).

OTHER NUTRITIONAL SUPPLEMENT TERMS

Natural. Vitamins are considered natural when they are extracted exclusively from food sources and contain the specific mix of nutrients found in nature. Often this mix includes other enzymes, catalysts, or minerals to aid the body's use of the vitamins. **Yeast, liver, corn, soy, rosehips, and alfalfa are common sources from which vitamins and minerals are extracted. People who are allergic or sensitive to any of these foods may be reacting to the other ingredients but not to the vitamins themselves.** The amounts of individual nutrients in purely natural vitamins are usually not very high, and thus many higher-dose vitamins contain a combination of natural and synthetic vitamins. It is also important to note that in terms of nutritional labeling, there is no legal definition of *natural*, and products bearing this label may or may not meet the criteria just described.

Synthetic. When vitamins are made chemically in the laboratory, rather than extracted from foods, they are termed *synthetic*. The amounts of these vitamins can range from low to very high. Although synthetic vitamins are able to perform the same functions and chemical reactions in the body as natural vitamins (because they have the same chemical structure), many people, especially those who are sensitive to chemicals, do not tolerate them as well. Synthetic vitamin products are more likely than those from natural sources to contain binders and fillers that might cause allergic reactions or gastrointestinal distress.

Organic. Scientifically speaking, all vitamins are organic in that they contain carbon, but as with the term *natural*, the health industry uses this term differently. Here, *organic* means that foods or supplements come from pesticide- and herbicide-free plant sources or naturally raised animals. In the body, nutrients can also be "organically" bound into tissues—for example, iron in the hemoglobin of the red blood cell.

The agricultural term *organic* means that foods are grown without the addition of chemicals to the soil or the food. When vitamins are naturally derived from organically grown food, they can truly be called *organic* vitamins. As you can see, the term has become quite confusing. Fortunately, however, there has been at least one clarifying event in the world of organics, since the U.S. Congress passed the Organic Foods Production Act (OFPA) of 1990 and provided the country with preliminary standards for determining whether foods qualify as organic. A finalized and fully detailed version of this act became law in 2001. I discuss these new federal standards in detail in chapter 11, Food and the Earth.

Inorganic. Vitamins are organic and minerals are inorganic—that is, they do not contain carbon. Within the agricultural meaning of the term, though, almost all nutritional supplements are *inorganic* (meaning "nonorganic") in the sense that they are chemically manufactured or extracted from foods grown with chemicals.

Chelated. When minerals are bound to another molecule to enhance absorption from the digestive tract, they are said to be *chelated*. (The verb *chelate* comes from the Greek word *chela,* meaning "claw".) This organic molecule must have a special chemical arrangement and a special electrochemical charge to hold the mineral. Many minerals, such as iron, calcium, zinc, and chromium, are more readily absorbed when they are chelated because they have less competition for active absorption sites. Examples of chelated minerals are iron fumarate, calcium aspartate, and zinc citrate.

Time-release. In order to sustain blood and body levels of the water-soluble vitamins over a longer period of time, they may be manufactured in micropellets within the vitamin pill. These micropellets are digested and absorbed into the body more slowly—that is, time-released—usually over an 8- to 12-hour period.

Orthomolecular medicine. Treating each individual's medical problems with the appropriate level, or right amount, of each nutrient, usually higher levels of the various vitamins and minerals than the RDAs, is termed *orthomolecular medicine*. The term was coined by Nobel Prize–winning chemist Linus Pauling in 1968, using the prefix *ortho* meaning "right" and *molecular* meaning "molecules." The objective of orthomolecular medicine is to achieve a balanced metabolism by having the appropriate nutrient or biochemical molecule in the appropriate location at the appropriate time.

Orthomolecular psychiatry. This is a type of orthomolecular medicine where the large doses of vitamins and minerals are used in conjunction with therapy for psychiatric conditions, such as depression and schizophrenia.

Megavitamin therapy. This is a simplistic extension of the orthomolecular approach, using dosages many times the RDAs to prevent problems, treat certain biological symptoms and potential genetic and nutritional deficiencies, and obtain optimum health. Megavitamin therapy has been advocated by many people, including Linus Pauling, pioneering authors like Adelle Davis, research biochemists like Richard Passwater, pharmacologists like Carl Pfeiffer, and pioneers in life extension like Durk Pearson and Sandy Shaw.

VITAMIN AVAILABILITY

Vitamins are available in a variety of forms: tablets, capsules, powders, and liquids. **Tablets** are most common because of their convenience and longer shelf life. However, they usually have fillers, binders, or coatings to keep them more stable. Vitamins without these unnecessary additives may be more beneficial. In addition, tablets may be overly compacted by the manufacturer and fail to digest properly once swallowed.

Capsules, which are also easy to take and probably more easily digested and absorbed than tablets, are used for powdered formulas and the fat-soluble vitamins. Capsules may be opened easily and the contents can be sprinkled on foods, as powders, or applied to the skin, as with vitamin A or E oil. Most capsules are made from beef or pork gelatin. Although an expensive vegetable gelatin has been developed, it is not really used yet in vitamin manufacturing. True vegetarian vitamins must be put into tablets or powdered; the powders and liquids are potentially the purest.

Powdered vitamins, usually mixed with water or juice, are suggested because of their rapid absorbability, but they are not always as convenient or palatable as tablets and capsules. They are especially helpful for people who have trouble swallowing pills, who have weak digestion, or who need higher levels of particular nutrients, most commonly vitamin C.

Liquid vitamins are most often used for infants and children and have the same advantages as powders for adults. However, many are colored and sweetened, often artificially, as are the common children's chewables. With vitamin supplements, as with foods, reading labels may help us determine their origins and the manufacturing policies. Many liquid injectable vitamins are available for use in treating certain illnesses. These can be used in the hospital, doctor's office, or, occasionally, at home for intramuscular injection. B complex and vitamin B_{12} injections are commonly given. Intravenous vitamins are used by some doctors in the clinical setting. Homeopathic medicines often come in liquids or disolvable tablets. Herbs are commonly found in liquid extracts, both in alcohol and alcohol free, which often incorporates glycerin, a natural sweetener.

WHO NEEDS VITAMINS?

Vitamin supplements to our diet can be used as a preventive approach to maintain or improve health, characterized as a basic state of vitality and involvement—a multileveled relationship—with life. Vitamins may also be used in the primary treatment or in the support of other treatments for a variety of symptoms, short-term illnesses, and chronic diseases. Nutritional supplements are increasingly being used by nutritionists, physicians, and individuals as treatment for a multitude of problems. And many times they are helpful. Another positive benefit is that vitamins rarely ever make matters worse, although they may have many side effects, including diarrhea or other detoxification symptoms.

In this chapter, I also describe the use of supplements as medical treatment for specific problems under each individual nutrient. Programs for specific illnesses and lifestyles are detailed in part 4 of this book, Nutritional Application: 32 Special Diets and Supplement Programs. Often, when people refer to *vitamins,* they do not mean the specific essential vitamins, such as A, B, and C, but the more general idea of taking vitamins, which alludes to the minerals and other nutritional pills as well. In the following discussion, *vitamins* refers to the general concept of taking nutritional supplements.

Does everyone need vitamin supplements? Although I do not believe that the average, basically healthy individual who has a sensible, balanced diet and low-stress lifestyle needs to take supplements regularly, there are times in a healthy person's life when certain supplements or a general high-level nutritional program will be helpful on a daily, monthly, or yearly basis. Certain people taking vitamins will notice a big change in health or energy, particularly if they have been deficient in the elements they are supplementing. With an adequate level of the basic micronutrients—that is, a multivitamin/mineral—most active people will notice a difference. So when a healthy person is under more stress, or during times of change or early illness, or if symptoms or illnesses are coming more frequently, a specific supplement program may be helpful. These individual nutritional programs can be designed, either to build up, to balance, or to detoxify the body, as the situation requires.

Those of us who lead busy, active lives, drive cars in traffic regularly, live in the city, work at busy or stressful jobs, or do not necessarily eat as well as we could may benefit from a daily basic regimen of nutritional supplements. This is really the "insurance" concept of vitamin use: we take supplements to make sure we do not become deficient in any nutrient and to balance out the effects of a stressful lifestyle so we will not break down and become ill. This works for a lot of people. Stress is a reason to take supplements. Illness, especially recovering and rebuilding from illness, is another reason to make sure we are getting our basic nutrient needs. Supplements, of course, do not replace a good diet. But often when we are ill, we do not feel much like eating or our digestion and absorption functions are not working optimally. After injury or before and after surgery, extra nutritional supplements may be helpful in supporting rapid healing. Minimally, vitamin A, vitamin C, and zinc can help tissue repair and very likely lessen the chance of infection after injuries or surgery. A full supplement program may be even more helpful. With proper application of supplements and observation, many surgeons would be impressed with general recovery and wound healing in their patients taking additional vitamins before and after surgery.

People who are dieting or go on special or limited diets because of allergies, a desire to lose weight, or from personal preference would do well to cover themselves with a basic general supplement program to ensure that all their essential micronutrient requirements are met. With unexplained weight loss, there may be a need for additional nutrient intake, as well as finding out the cause of the weight loss. Fatigue also has a variety of causes, but often a combination of nutrient supplements with a well-balanced diet and stress reduction may be helpful in restoring and enhancing energy.

During all life transitions, it is wise to take additional supplements. During childhood, especially for children who do not eat a balanced diet or who consume sugar foods, which deplete body nutrients, an extra daily multivitamin/mineral is a good idea. For elderly people, whose digestive systems are not always working optimally and some of whose nutrient needs may be increased, especially for such minerals as calcium, magnesium, and potassium, extra supplementation may help with continued vitality and health. **For many children or elders, more easily digested and absorbed supplements, such as a liquid or powdered vitamin/mineral combination, may be advantageous.**

Sugar is a nutrient-depleting substance, devoid of its own nutrients. Those who have consumed lots of sugary foods or crave and eat refined sugar products need additional supplements for two reasons. First, they may replace any depleted nutrients from the generally poor diet. Second, such supplements as the B vitamins, vitamin C, the amino acid glutamine, and chromium and other minerals may help to balance out the fluctuating blood sugar and reduce food cravings, especially for sweets. For example, one of my patients claims that when she takes calcium and magnesium, her intense craving for chocolate is reduced. Cravings for sugary sweets, especially for chocolate, often occur around the menses and during pregnancy.

Those who smoke may also get some protection by taking nutritional supplements. Regular smoking of tobacco causes a lot of potential problems in the body, many of which result from inhalation of tars and other chemicals that lead to increased formation of free-radicals (unstable, irritating molecules). General supplementation plus specific antioxidant therapy, which helps bind these potentially damaging free radicals, may reduce some harmful effects of smoking. **Vitamin A or beta-carotene, vitamin C, vitamin E and selenium, and L-cysteine all have this antioxidant effect, and all may be required in higher amounts in smokers.**

Regular alcohol use and abuse may also generate depletion of bodily nutrients. In extreme cases, an alcoholic can become malnourished when not consuming a proper diet and can suffer a number of vitamin and mineral deficiencies, as well as have problems with carbohydrate metabolism and maintaining blood sugar levels and with fat accumulation in the liver. **A balanced diet and a supplement program including the B vitamins, beta-carotene, and minerals can give a little insurance against the effects of alcohol abuse.** Extra minerals and fluids can help counteract the dehydrating effects of alcohol and may reduce the morning-after doldrums.

Of course, if we all created our own healthy, balanced lifestyle and were not the victims of a busy, high-tech society, we would likely be able to obtain our needed nutrients completely from our fresh, homegrown vital foods. Breathing clean air and drinking fresh, noncontaminated water are additional bonuses to our health. But for most of us, our high-demand, fast-paced, stressful lifestyle places extra requirements on our bodies, and we need the additional support and protection that supplementation can give us. Even our natural fruits, vegetables, and whole grains may not be nourishing us in the way they used to because of the depletion of soil minerals and the additional stress on our bodies caused by chemical and pesticide exposure. Let's face it, with all the changes and stresses that society is experiencing, we need all the help we can get—and nutritional support is an important ally.

SPECIAL SUGGESTIONS

Because vitamins and minerals are essential constituents of vegetable and animal foods, my first and most important suggestion is that they need to be viewed as food supplements—that is, they are digested and assimilated best when taken with or following food. **The B vitamins, vitamin C, and the minerals, all of which are water-soluble, especially need to be dissolved and digested with food before they can be assimilated and thereby used by the body. The fat-soluble vitamins can be utilized, as is often suggested, when taken alone either in the morning before breakfast or at bedtime.** They also can be taken after meals of fat-containing foods. Emulsified, water-dispersed forms of vitamins E and A, for example, which can be taken along with the other vitamins, are also available.

Some authorities suggest taking all vitamins on an empty stomach because that way the body has a better chance to absorb them, although I would separate the oil-soluble and water-soluble vitamins. No studies yet demonstrate comparative blood levels of vitamins taken with or without food consumption. On the basis of my experience and sense, however, I suggest consuming vitamins with food, usually after meals. Most healthy people with good digestive tracts handle this well. Sensitive people may need to isolate individual nutrients. People whose stomachs become upset when taking supplements or those with weak digestive systems notice that they do better taking supplements either with food or with digestive supplements, such as enzymes or hydrochloric acid.

In general, I do not suggest big, time-release "horse pills." Our digestion, especially hydrochloric acid output, needs to be very efficient to use them. Young, healthy people seem to do fairly well with these pills, but during illness or other weakened states or in elderly people, I do not think this type of multiple is useful. Too many times I have received reports from radiologists who have seen whole pills in the intestines.

I also usually suggest simple, easy-to-absorb supplements and powdered formulas whenever possible, either in capsules or as straight powder to mix in water or juice. Their percentage of bioavailability is higher, I believe, than that of tablets. To obtain increased blood levels of vitamin C, for example, I suggest either a concentrated ascorbic acid powder or a mineralized (with calcium, magnesium, and potassium, for example) vitamin C powder to be taken every couple of hours throughout the day, because vitamin C is used rapidly in the body.

For people who have energy problems, such as fatigue, hyperactivity, or insomnia, I will often separate the supplement plan so they take their B vitamins early in the day with breakfast and lunch and their minerals, such as calcium and magnesium, later in the day and before bed. The B vitamins tend to be stimulating, while the minerals tend to be relaxing and balancing to muscles and the nervous system.

I like to plan nutrient programs with patients after doing a diet review and measuring the blood levels of minerals or vitamins, as well as food antibody levels to assess immune reactions to common foods, so my suggestions can be tailored to the individual's needs. (See Appendix A, Laboratories, and Clinical Nutrition Tests.) Then, at a later time, we can repeat certain tests to see whether the supplements have helped in achieving the appropriate balance. When people are on nutritional supplements, I prefer to meet with them every few months, accompanied with all their bottles of whatever, to review their program. The patient might have read an article or talked to a friend and then added a new supplement. I feel that it is important to change programs occasionally and not get too rigid in the plan. Even if everything is working well, reassessment and change, at least every 6 months to a year, is a good idea. Often, certain nutrients are not really needed in the same amounts or a new supplement might be appropriate. Too often, people find supplements that work and may take them for years without checking to see if their biochemistry is balanced. Overall, I encourage individuals to learn and understand what they are doing nutritionally and to adopt some type of process for self-evaluation and listening to their body to make healthy choices at appropriate times.

Establishing a proper individual nutritional supplement program is a fine art. If we focus on a particular nutrient and take higher amounts of it, we may become deficient in other nutrients that have a similar process of absorption into the blood. The B vitamins are absorbed fairly well, so this is less a concern for them, although I still do not suggest supplementing just one. The main concern is for the different minerals that tend to compete for absorption sites—taking a high amount of 1 may limit utilization of the others. If we take a lot of zinc, for example, we may absorb more zinc into our body, but then we may not absorb as much copper, manganese, or magnesium out of our food if we are not supplementing

them also. Giving all our nutrients a "fair chance" will let the body's natural wisdom work more easily over time.

My main medical goal is to guide people in developing the skills to become their own best doctor and thus be able to make more informed, conscious choices.

THE INDIVIDUAL VITAMINS

Following is a detailed discussion of each of the currently known vitamins. I have listed them in two groups: the fat-soluble vitamins, alphabetically, and then the more numerous water-soluble ones. For each vitamin, after a general description of what the vitamin is, how the body handles it, and its special features, the discussion is organized into the following categories:

- **General Information.** Introduction to each vitamin.

- **Sources.** The best food sources for the vitamin.

- **Functions.** What the vitamin does in the body.

- **Uses.** How we can use the vitamin in treatment or prevention of disease.

- **Deficiency and toxicity.** What can happen if we do not receive sufficient amounts of it, and what problems are caused by too much of the vitamin.

- **Requirements.** Ranging from the nontherapeutic, general dietary recommendations, or DRIs, for each vitamin to the therapeutic and safe maximum dosages and, wherever appropriate, what forms are available and which is best used by the body. I use the term *dosage* loosely to describe the suggested amount, not to infer a likeness to pharmaceutical prescriptions. *Intake levels* or *requirements* are more accurate terms.

FAT-SOLUBLE VITAMINS

   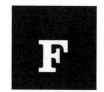

Vitamin A   Vitamin D   Vitamin E   Vitamin F— Essential Fatty Acids   Vitamin K

The fat-soluble vitamins are vitamin A (retinol and beta-carotene), vitamin D, vitamin E, vitamin F (the essential fatty acids), and vitamin K. Note: Potential problems of toxicity may occur with overuse of these fat-soluble vitamins, more so than with higher intakes of the water-soluble vitamins, because oil-based nutrients are more readily stored in our body tissues. The range between efficacy and toxicity, especially for vitamins A and D, is much closer than for most other essential nutrients. Thus caution is advised in supplementing higher amounts than those suggested in the following discussions of these fat-soluble vitamins.

Vitamin A

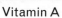 Vitamin A has the unique distinction of being the first vitamin officially named, thereby earning it the letter A as its identifying mark. It also has the distinction of being much more complicated than researchers originally thought in 1913, the year it was discovered. At that time, the focus was on what we now call *preformed* vitamin A, or retinol. One of the main functions of retinol is easy to remember, because its name is adopted from the term *retina,* the location in the eye where preformed vitamin A plays one of its most important roles. The rods of the eye, which are located within the retina, contain rhodopsin, a pigment also known as "visual purple." This pigment enables the rods to detect small amounts of light, and the pigment itself cannot be made without preformed vitamin A. More specifically, it is retinal—a special chemical form of retinol called the *aldehyde* form—that is required for synthesis of the rhodopsin pigment.

Since the discovery of retinol, however, the research focus has shifted to include a broader group of sub-

stances known as *provitamin A*. These substances are all members of the carotenoid family of pigments, mostly visible to us as the oranges and yellows of vegetables and fruits. About 600 carotenoids have been identified by plant scientists, and as many as 50 are suspected to qualify as provitamin A compounds. (The *provitamin A* label simply means that these carotenoids can be converted into retinol.) At this point in nutritional research, the best studied of the provitamin A carotenoids are alpha-carotene, beta-cryptoxanthin, and beta-carotene, with beta-carotene leading the way by thousands of studies.

Although the division between preformed and provitamin A has been a fascinating development in vitamin chemistry over the past century, it has also made vitamin A the messiest of all vitamins when it comes to dosage and measurement. Vitamin A used to be measured exclusively in terms of international units (IUs), and IUs still appear on food and supplement labels. They do not measure the physical amount of vitamin A that is present, but rather the level of chemical activity belonging to the vitamin A. The RDAs for vitamin A—along with other public health recommendations—no longer use IUs as the form of measurement for this vitamin. Beginning in 2000, RDAs for vitamin A began to be expressed in terms of micrograms of retinol equivalents (mcg REs). This new unit of measurement for vitamin A brought in an actual physical amount (mcg) but also allowed a chemical activity factor (retinol equivalents) to be maintained. When converting between IUs and mcg REs, 1 mcg RE is equal to 3.33 IU.

Vitamin A is absorbed primarily from the small intestine. **Absorption of this fat-soluble vitamin is reduced with alcohol use, with vitamin E deficiency, with cortisone medication, and with exces-**

sive iron intake or the use of mineral oil, as well as with exercise. As a fat-soluble vitamin, vitamin A can be stored in the body and used when there is decreased intake. About 90% of the storable vitamin A is in the liver; it is also stored in the kidneys, lungs, eyes, and fat tissue. In addition to reducing absorption, alcohol use also depletes liver stores. The storage of vitamin A is decreased during times of stress or illness unless intake is increased. The body needs the mineral zinc to help release stores of vitamin A for use. I believe that vitamin A is needed at a level of at least 5,000 IU (or 1,500 mcg RE) a day, although this may vary due to many factors. Deficiencies of vitamin A are still fairly common worldwide and cause many difficulties. Analysis of the average American diet reveals that it provides about 3,300 IU (1,000 mcg RE) of vitamin A daily, so the many problems of vitamin A deficiency, such as visual changes, skin dryness, and increased infections, are more common than most people realize.

Sources. The two forms of vitamin A come from different food sources. Preformed A (retinol) is the main animal-source vitamin A. It is found in highest concentrations in all kinds of liver and fish liver oil, which is a common source for supplements. Egg yolks and milk products, such as whole milk, cream, and butter, are also good sources of vitamin A. Provitamin A, mainly in the form of beta-carotene, is found in a wide variety of yellow- and orange-colored fruits and vegetables, as well as leafy green vegetables. Beta-carotene is actually a double molecule of vitamin A. It may be converted to vitamin A in the upper intestine before absorption; beta-carotene can also be converted to vitamin A in the liver. People with diabetes, low thyroid activity, and who use a lot of polyunsaturated fatty acids (PUFAs) without antioxidants such as vitamin E have lowered ability to convert beta-carotene to A. Assimilation of vitamin A and the carotenes is helped by the presence of bile salts and fatty acids in the intestine.

Functions. Vitamin A performs many important functions in the human body. The following are the most common.

Eyesight. Vitamin A is needed for the formation of rhodopsin, or visual purple, which allows us to see at night. As mentioned earlier, it is actually retinal—an aldehyde form of retinol—that is required for synthesis of the rhodopsin pigment. When vitamin A is lack-

---

Beta-Carotene Sources

Leafy and Green Vegetables	Other Vegetables
Asparagus	Carrots
Broccoli	Pumpkin
Brussels sprouts	Red cabbage
Kale	Sweet potatoes
Lettuce	Winter squash
Mustard greens	Yams
Parsley	**Fruits**
Seaweed (nori)	Apricots
Spinach	Cantaloupe
	Cherries
	Mango
	Papaya
	Peaches
	Watermelon

---

ing, there is a lag period in regenerating visual purple and a resulting inability to see well at night, termed *night blindness*. Vitamin A also helps maintain the health of the cornea, the eye covering. Vitamin A deficiency may allow irritation or inflammation of the eye tissue to occur more easily.

Growth and tissue healing. This vitamin is involved in laying down new cells, including bone cells, during growth and promoting healthy teeth. The exact mechanisms by which vitamin A supports cell growth are not clear, but we know that retinoic acid is required for the production of many glycoproteins, and that these glycoproteins help control the process by which cells attach to each other and form new tissue. After tissue injury or surgery, vitamin A is needed for repair of the tissues and to help protect the tissues from infection.

Healthy skin. Vitamin A stimulates growth of the base layer of the skin cells. It helps the cells differentiate normally (progress from less to more mature cell forms) and gives them their structural integrity. It does this for both the external skin cells and the body's inner skin, the mucous membrane linings of the nose, eyes, intestinal tract, respiratory lining, and bladder. By this function, it also helps protect these areas from cancer cell development. By moisturizing the mucous lining cells, which helps proper secretion, and by maintaining their structural integrity, vitamin A helps the body fight off infectious agents and environmental pollutants. The epithelial tissues protected include the linings of the lungs, nose, throat, stomach, intestines, vagina, bladder, and urinary tract, as well as the eyes and skin.

Antioxidation. Vitamin A helps protect the body (particularly cell membranes and tissue linings) from the irritating effects of free radicals (unstable molecules) by neutralizing them. Beta-carotene also protects the tissues from the toxic singlet oxygen radical. This function usually requires an amount higher than the RDA dose, perhaps 10,000 to 20,000 IU per day or more. Through its antioxidant effects, vitamin A and beta-carotene help protect the body from the irritating effects of smoke and other pollutants and may also be helpful in preventing problems like ulcers and atherosclerosis and its attendant complications, such as high blood pressure and stroke.

Lowering cancer risk and supporting immune function. As just discussed, vitamin A helps maintain the structural integrity of cells and the healthy functioning of the mucous linings. It also helps with proper cell differentiation of the surface cells. But support of proper cell differentiation is only one of the ways in which vitamin A helps reduce cancer risk. This vitamin always plays an important role in support of overall immune system activity. In its preformed, retinol form, vitamin A has been shown to optimize the function of white blood cells, to enhance recognition of food antigens (allergy-triggering substances) by antibodies (immune cells made by our body in response to allergy-triggering substances), and also to block the activity of certain viruses. The beta-carotene form of vitamin A has also been shown to enhance immune system function, although the exact mechanisms for this health benefit are not yet clear. In these ways, vitamin A seems to prevent the development of cancer, and a number of studies have shown reduced lung and colon cancer rates in people with higher intakes of beta-carotene.

Regulating genetic processes. The role of vitamin A in the regulation of genetic processes is only beginning to be understood. Researchers know, however, that many cell types have retinoic acid receptors (RARs) on their nuclear membranes and that the

binding of retinoic acid to these receptors alters genetic processes.

Uses. With the many functions performed by vitamin A, it has a variety of uses in basic tissue and health maintenance, in clinical treatment for a number of problems (some of which may be vitamin A deficiency symptoms), and in the prevention of many illnesses and diseases. Vitamin A works better when there are sufficient body levels of zinc and an adequate intake of protein.

Infections. Vitamin A helps in many cases to protect tissues during infections and promote rapid recovery, primarily through its support of the health of the skin and mucous lining barriers and its stimulation of mucus production. It also appears to improve antibody response and white blood cell functions. In these ways, vitamin A may be even more helpful in the prevention of infections. By keeping the mucous membranes healthy, it helps protect against the irritating effects of smoke and pollution.

Eye problems. Vitamin A is often suggested for a variety of eye problems. Night blindness may be an early sign of vitamin A deficiency, but vitamin A functions in many ways to support the health of the eye tissue. It has been used in the treatment of conjunctivitis, blurred vision, nearsightedness, cataracts, and glaucoma, but there is no hard scientific evidence, other than anecdotal, that vitamin A works for these conditions.

Skin problems. Because of its beneficial effects on the skin, vitamin A is used to treat a variety of skin problems, both by local application to rashes, boils, skin ulcers, and so on, and by increased intake to help the skin's internal healing process. It may have some effect in psoriasis and in periodontal disease. Vitamin A can be supplemented for all kinds of wound healing, including before and after surgery. Its use in healing acne has been controversial, with some studies showing very good results and other studies showing no demonstrable effects. The amount used is usually about 75,000 to 100,000 IU per day, as 25,000 to 30,000 IU 3 times daily or 50,000 IU twice daily, with doses up to 300,000 IU per day having better success. Used with 800 IU of vitamin E daily (which need not be taken at the same time as an A supplement), the vitamin E promotes the activity of vitamin A. Taking 100,000 IU of vitamin A may help alleviate severe acne in many cases. **Of course, with these**

higher doses of vitamin A, some signs of toxicity, such as frontal headaches, can develop and should be watched. If these occur, decreasing the amount of vitamin A will usually alleviate the headaches. Retin-A, a pharmaceutical derivative of vitamin A, appears to help reduce wrinkles (and acne) by restoring skin tissue when applied topically.

Cancer prevention. By its influence in maintaining the cell integrity of the skin and the mucous membrane linings, as in the lungs, the digestive system, and the urinary and genital tracts, and by its support of proper cell differentiation, vitamin A as beta-carotene has been shown to be helpful in lowering lung cancer risks. It is likely, because of its effects on epithelial cell membranes, that adequate beta-carotene intake will reduce risk of many other cancers. Likewise, a deficiency of vitamin A, beta-carotene, or both increases the risk of cancers.

It is important to note that two long-term research studies, involving thousands of participants, have shown *increased* risk of lung cancer and in some cases heart disease following beta-carotene supplementation. Because the subjects of these studies were long-term, heavy smokers, often with routine consumption of alcohol, it is not clear whether any of the results can be generalized to nonsmokers or nondrinkers. I believe some aspects of the studies actually show cancer-protective effects of beta-carotene, but the authors of the studies did not focus on these aspects when publishing their work. The studies do seem to make it clear, however, that you can't smoke 20 cigarettes a day for 36 years (the average in one of the studies) and expect a vitamin supplement to fix it. We have to take better care of ourselves than that.

Pollution protection. The antioxidant function of vitamin A helps to protect the body tissues from the irritating effects of stress, smoke, air pollution, and chemical exposure.

Other uses. Vitamin A has also been tried with some success in treating a variety of other problems, including asthma, fibrocystic breast disease, plantar warts, sebaceous cysts, ulcers, and premenstrual syndrome. In fibrocystic problems, one small study showed a reduction in breast pain and lumps with 150,000 IU daily, used under medical supervision.

Reproductive health is an additional area where beta-carotene may hold special promise. Researchers do not yet know the exact function of this vitamin in female reproduction, but the corpus luteum (a hormone-secreting structure that forms in the ovary following ovulation) has a higher concentration of beta-carotene than any other organ in the body. In animals, increased consumption of beta-carotene is associated with increased ovarian function and hormonal output.

Deficiency and toxicity. A number of difficulties can arise from a deficiency of vitamin A, many of which are based on impairments in the biochemical functions that this important nutrient performs. It is estimated that approximately 25% of Americans get less than half of the RDA for vitamin A in their diets. This commonly occurs in those who avoid the carotene-containing fruits and vegetables or when the diet is filled with processed foods that are depleted of vitamins. **The fruits and vegetables are really the most important food groups for intake of the many vitamins and minerals, as well as for fiber and water content.** The elderly, teenagers, and alcoholics are the three groups most commonly deficient in vitamin A. Worldwide, vitamin A deficiency is even more common than it is in the United States, likely from the even greater lack of fresh foods available and consumed.

Night blindness is probably one of the first signs of vitamin A deficiency. Lack of general eye tissue health and vitality may occur, as can impaired vision, irritated, reddened, or dry eyes, and eyes that tire easily; in severe deficiency states, corneal ulcers may develop. Supplemental vitamin A or beta-carotene will usually correct these problems; the RDA of vitamin A will prevent night blindness and these other eye problems.

Perhaps of greater significance, vitamin A and beta-carotene deficiencies may decrease our protection against infectious agents and the internal process of carcinogenesis. A depletion or deficiency of vitamin A reduces both T lymphocyte (cellular immunity) and B lymphocyte (antibody production) responses; severe vitamin A deficiency has been shown to cause atrophy of the thymus and spleen, both immunologically important organs, and to reduce the number of circulating lymphocytes. Low dietary levels of vitamin A have been associated with an increased risk of many cancers, including breast, cervical, lung, prostate, laryngeal, and stomach cancers; beta-carotene deficiency has also clearly been seen in patients with cancers of the cervix or lungs.

Vitamin A deficiency also affects the skin. Dry, bumpy skin may occur, especially on the backs of the arms. Because vitamin A promotes skin growth, moisture retention, and proper cell differentiation, a deficiency causes decreased skin tone and rapid aging of the skin and a variety of blemishes, acne, or boils. Vitamin A supports the mucus-secreting cells of the internal mucous membranes, and mucus protects these membranes from infection and irritants. When vitamin A is deficient, these internal epithelial cells secrete a protein (keratin) commonly found externally in hair and nails. This keratinization process makes the epithelial cells harder and dryer and thus less protecting.

Vitamin A along with adequate protein intake generates healthy hair. With a lack of A, the hair may lack luster and dandruff is more likely because of the loss of scalp skin moisture. Bone softness or abnormal menstruation may also develop from vitamin A deficiency. Fatigue and insomnia are also possible, as are a decrease in the appetite and some loss of smell and taste. When vitamin A is deficient, vitamin C seems to be lost more rapidly from the body. In addition to the lowered immune function and increased infection rate associated with vitamin A deficiency, periodontal disease, kidney stone formation, ear problems, and acne may occur more frequently.

A number of toxicity symptoms and difficulties may occur when we take too much vitamin A. Because it is stored in the body and is not readily excreted, toxicity may occur from mildly increased doses beginning at 14,000 IU for children and 25,000 IU for adults per day over an extended time, 1 or 2 months, or from very high doses (330,000 IU for children and 660,000 IU for adults, as evaluated in research) over a shorter period. However, I usually use less than this for fear of toxicity, although I rarely have seen it. In my practice, when I intervene with high-dose vitamin A in acute illness, I usually limit my intervention to 30,000 IU 3 times a day for 3 days, and then I decrease the amounts over the next 5 days or so, such as 20,000 IU twice daily for 2 days and then 10,000 IU twice a day for 5 to 7 days. It appears that the "burst" of vitamin A helps the body fight off infections from both viruses and bacteria.

Animal liver meats have the highest concentrations of vitamin A; beef liver has about 15,000 IU per ounce, while polar bear liver has much higher concentrations and has been known to cause vitamin A toxicity from one serving. It is highly unlikely that one would get vitamin A toxicity from the diet alone (without lots of liver), because we receive much of it in the form of beta-carotene, which must then be converted to active vitamin A. **The synthetic vitamin A supplements, such as the palmitate or acetate forms, have a greater potential to produce toxic symptoms; high amounts of fish liver oil (like cod liver oil) may produce side effects as well.** The levels that cause symptoms vary from person to person, just as the proper optimum dosage

---

DRIs for Vitamin A

In 2000, the National Academy of Sciences established the following AI levels for consumption of vitamin A by infants:

Age	AI Level
Males and females, 0–6 months	1,333 IU (400 mcg RE)
Males and females, 7–12 months	1,666 IU (500 mcg RE)

For children and adults, the following RDAs were established:

Age	RDA
Males and females, 1–3 years	1,000 IU (300 mcg RE)
Males and females, 4–8 years	1,333 IU (400 mcg RE)
Males and females, 9–13 years	2,000 IU (600 mcg RE)
Males and females, 14 years and older	3,000 IU (900 mcg RE)

Finally, for pregnant and lactating women, the following EARs were established:

Age	EAR
Pregnant women	1,767 IU (530 mcg RE)
Lactating women, 18 years or younger	2,933 IU (880 mcg RE)
Lactating women, 19 years or older	3,000 IU (900 mcg RE)

does. When we are under high levels of stress, with illness or trauma, if we smoke or live in a polluted environment, or if we are pregnant or nursing, our vitamin A requirements are higher. When there is depletion or deficiency of vitamin A, higher amounts can be taken for up to a month without the usual risks of toxicity.

The only problem that may arise from high amounts of beta-carotene, as can occur with a high intake of yellow and orange fruits and vegetables and the leafy greens, is an orange-yellow discoloring of the skin. This condition, called *carotenodermia* or *carotenosis* occurs occasionally when people drink large amounts of carrot juice daily over time. It is of no real consequence and will clear when there is a reduction in carotene intake. Carotenosis can be differentiated from jaundice somewhat by the color and also by the fact that the white parts of the eyes do not turn color as they do with jaundice.

Too much preformed vitamin A (retinol) intake, however, can lead to slight swelling of the brain and resulting pressure headaches, which may be described as the feeling of a tight band around the forehead. Nausea and vomiting may also occur, as can irritability, dizziness, abdominal pain, and hair loss. Itchy, flaky, or dry skin can also result from too much vitamin A. Anorexia (loss of appetite) and resulting weight loss, liver enlargement, menstrual problems, bone abnormalities or stunted growth, and dry or bleeding lips may also occur. There may be an increased risk of birth defects in pregnant women taking high amounts of vitamin A, say, more than 400 IU per pound of body weight. **To be safe, I suggest that pregnant women limit their preformed vitamin A to 10,000 IU total, with no more than 5,000 IU coming from supplements.**

In 2000, because of the toxicity risks listed for vitamin A, the National Academy of Sciences set the following tolerable upper limit (UL) guidelines for daily vitamin A intake.

Before leaving the question of vitamin A toxicity, I want to tell you about a flurry of recent studies linking excess vitamin A to increased risk of bone fracture. There is plenty to take seriously here, because the studies involve not only supplements but foods themselves, and the amounts of vitamin A involved can be as small as 1,750 IU (about 500 mcg, or 1 good serving of calf's liver). First, you should know that all of the research involves retinol (the animal version of vitamin A) not beta-carotene (the plant version), so carrot juice drinkers have nothing to worry about. Second, until we get to the 500 to 1,000 mcg (1,666–3,333 IU) intake level, there appears to be no increased risk. So we would easily have room for a poached egg with its 100 mcg of retinol. With a retinol-rich food like calf's liver, however, or a retinol-rich supplement like cod liver oil, we might want to exercise a little more caution. In some studies, every 1,000 mcg increase in retinol intake over a baseline level of 1,000 mcg has been shown to increase risk of bone fracture by 68%. I believe there are still plenty of good reasons for taking retinol-containing supplements—including cod liver oil—but we need to factor this new information about fracture risk into our decision-making process when doing so.

Requirements. The RDA—that is, the minimum dietary or supplemental amount to prevent vitamin A deficiency—is approximately 3,000 IU per day for the adult. About 10,000 IU of beta-carotene will probably convert to about 3,000 IU of vitamin A in the body. Approximately two medium-sized carrots will give us

ULs for Vitamin A	
Age	**ULs**
Males and Females, 3 years or younger	600 mcg (2,000 IU)
Males and Females, 4–8 years	900 mcg (3,000 IU)
Males and Females, 9–14 years	1,700 mcg (5,666 IU)
Males and Females, 14–18 years	2,800 mcg (9,332 IU)
Males and Females, 19 years and older	3,000 mcg (10,000 IU)
Pregnant or lactating women, 18 years or younger	2,800 mcg (9,332 IU)
Pregnant or lactating women, 19 years or older	3,000 mcg (10,000 IU)

that daily amount. Because this vitamin is fat soluble and stored in the body, daily sources are not absolutely necessary. Requirements depend on body weight, however, so larger people need more vitamin A. **Needs are also increased with illness, infection, trauma, anxiety or stress, pregnancy, lactation, and alcohol use or smoking.**

Approximately 5,000 to 10,000 IU should be the average adult intake and is a safe amount to consume. The lower RDA amount of 3,000 IU will prevent most deficiency symptoms, such as night blindness, but for vitamin A's antioxidant properties, I recommend these higher amounts. About 10,000 to 20,000 additional IU of beta-carotene and other carotenoids may also be helpful for those of us with some level of anxiety and stress. If vitamins C and E are also used, slightly lower amounts of A are needed, because C and E help prevent the loss of stored vitamin A.

The upper intake, including diet and supplemental vitamin A, ranges from 50,000 to 100,000 IU per day for short periods of 1 or 2 weeks. These amounts often produce some side effects over time, however. If no body deficiency or increased body needs of vitamin A are present, amounts as low as 20,000 IU may sometimes cause problems. Infants and children can run into difficulty with doses as low as 10,000 to 15,000 IU given over time, depending on their size. This is why it is important to know our food sources and supplement levels of preformed vitamin A (not beta-carotene, which is safe at higher levels), so that we can find the right amounts for each of us and our family members.

Vitamin D (Calciferol)

D Vitamin D refers to several related fat-soluble vitamin variants, all of which are sterol (cholesterol-like) substances. No vitamin requires more whole-body participation than vitamin D. The skin, bloodstream, liver, and kidneys all contribute to the formation of fully active vitamin D. The process starts with the skin cells and sunlight. Vitamin D is known as the "sunshine" vitamin because it is actually manufactured in the human skin when in contact with the ultraviolet light in the sun's rays. The sunlight interacts with 7-dehydrocholesterol (a form of cholesterol) to form cholecalciferol, which is then transferred to the liver or kidneys and converted to

25-hydroxycholecalciferol, one form of vitamin D. This form of vitamin D is also called *calcidiol*. It is not the most active form of the vitamin, however. The calcidiol formed in the liver must be sent further to the kidneys for conversion into the most fully active form of vitamin D, called 125-dihydroxycholecalciferol. This form is also called *calcitriol*, or vitamin D3, and is considered by some researchers to be the only truly active form of vitamin D. Wintertime, clouds, smog, and darkly pigmented skin reduce the body's production of the "sunshine" vitamin.

This fat-soluble vitamin, when ingested, is absorbed through the intestinal walls with other fats with the aid of bile. Mineral oil binds vitamin D in the gut and reduces its absorption. From the blood, calciferol is taken mainly to the liver, where it is used or stored. It is interesting to note here that a special protein, alpha-2 globulin vitamin D binding protein (DBP), is made by the liver specifically for the purpose of carrying vitamin D around the bloodstream. Because of its unique relationship to vitamin D, lack of DBP or malformation of this protein can result in vitamin D deficiency. Vitamin D is stored not only in the liver, but also in the skin, brain, spleen, and bones. Vitamin D intake must be more finely tuned in regard to the right therapeutic level than most other vitamins, and it is considered by many authorities to be the most potentially toxic vitamin. **Symptoms of vitamin D toxicity can easily occur when vitamin D is taken in large amounts or with excessive sun exposure.** (It is possible that part of sun-poisoning symptoms are due to vitamin D toxicity.)

Sources. Although dietary supplements are available containing plant-derived as well as animal-derived vitamin D, there is a difference between these two sources. Plants do not have cholesterol, the initial building block for vitamin D3 (calcitriol). Instead, they have a similar steroid molecule called *ergosterol*. When sunlight hits the plant leaf, it converts ergosterol into ergocalciferol in exactly the same way as sunlight on our skin converts 7-dehydrocholesterol into cholecalciferol. However, the ergocalciferol derived from plants, also called vitamin D2, does not appear to have all of the same functions as the cholesterol-based vitamin D3. For this reason, the animal-derived forms of vitamin D, which can be converted by the body into fully active D3, may be the most desirable supplementation forms. Various forms of D3, or natural vitamin D, are found in fish liver oil, which is the traditional source of both A and D. Cod liver oil is a commonly used source. Egg yolks, butter, and liver have some D, as do the oily fish, such as mackerel, salmon, sardines, and herring. Most homogenized milk and some breakfast cereals are fortified with synthetic vitamin D to give children, particularly, sufficient amounts. The plant foods are fairly low in D2, with mushrooms and dark leafy greens containing some. Strict vegetarians who do not get adequate exposure to sunlight need to be concerned about getting their 400 IU of vitamin D daily.

Functions. Vitamin D helps to regulate calcium metabolism and normal calcification of the bones in the body, as well as influencing the body's use of the mineral phosphorus (calcium and phosphorus, together with other minerals, make up our bones). Vitamin D3 helps increase the absorption of calcium from the gut, decreases excretion from the kidneys, stimulates resorption of calcium and phosphorus from bone, helps put these minerals into teeth, and helps to maintain normal blood levels of calcium and phosphorus. With these functions, vitamin D is closely tied to the work of the parathyroid glands. Vitamin D is most important in regulating calcium metabolism in the body. Even with adequate calcium and phosphorus intake, if our vitamin D intake is low, we will have poor calcification of our bones, whereas with good vitamin D intake, we will have better calcification even with low calcium and phosphorus intake.

This function is especially important in menopausal women, for whom many doctors prescribe straight calcium without vitamin D, which is not likely to do much good unless they are sunbathing, an activity that doctors no longer recommend. **Actually, taking calcium, magnesium, and vitamin D all together is probably ideal for best bone health.** Phosphorus is usually readily available in adequate amounts in most diets. Because of its regulation of calcium and phosphorus metabolism, vitamin D is also important in the growth of children, especially for healthy bones and teeth. It is helpful in maintaining the nervous system, heart function, and for normal blood clotting—all of which are affected by calcium levels.

Vitamin D works together with parathyroid hormone for calcium metabolism. Functionally, vitamin D is actually more like a hormone than a vitamin; it is produced in one part of the body (the skin) and released into the blood to affect other tissues (the bones). There is a feedback system with the parathyroid to produce active vitamin D3 when the body needs it, and this vitamin is closely related structurally to the body hormones estrogen and cortisone. Again, vitamin D regulates bone formation. If D is low, blood levels of calcium and phosphorus decrease, and the body pulls these minerals from the bones. This creates demineralized, weak bones, a condition called *osteomalacia* (loss of bone mineral), or adult rickets. Osteoporosis involves loss of bone mass (minerals and proteins together). The decreased level of calcium in the blood also affects the heart and nervous system. Because of its ability in certain tissues, like bone, to actively regulate cell division, cell growth, and cell numbers, I would suggest that a role for vitamin D in prevention and treatment of various cancers may also be on the horizon. Look for future research in this area.

Uses. Vitamin D works best with adequate calcium and phosphorus intake. It is supplied primarily to prevent or to cure rickets, the vitamin D deficiency disease. It also is used to maintain healthy bones and dentition, as D is helpful in preventing tooth decay and gum problems. Calciferol supplementation may be used to aid the healing of fractures, osteoporosis, and other bone problems.

Taking vitamin D with vitamin A has been shown in some studies to reduce the incidence of colds. It has also been used in the treatment of diabetes, cataracts, visual problems, allergies, sciatica pain, and skin problems. Some success in treating myopia (nearsightedness) and conjunctivitis has been had with high doses of vitamin D. Vitamins A and D together have helped muscle spasms, especially when related to anxiety states. A and D have been used in the treatment of asthma and arthritis as well. Menopausal symptoms such as hot flashes and depression have been helped by the use of calcium and vitamin D together. Other than the use in menopause, however, these other applications of vitamin D have not been very common in recent years. Medically, high vitamin D supplementation is used to treat hypocalcemia (low blood calcium) secondary to such problems as hypoparathyroidism, which may occur after thyroid surgery.

Deficiency and toxicity. There are some toxicity problems related to hypervitaminosis D. These usually occur with doses of more than 1,000 to 1,500 IU daily for a month or longer in adults, more than 400 IU daily in infants, or more than 600 IU daily in children. These are not exact numbers, of course, and may vary between individuals, time of year, and specific needs; however, it is wise to be careful with supplemental vitamin D. The National Academy of Sciences set tolerable upper intake levels for vitamin D in 1997 as follows: infants, a maximum of 1,000 IU per day; children and adults, 2,000 IU maximum per day; and pregnant and lactating women, 2,000 IU maximum per day. I personally think the combination 1,000 IU D and 25,000 IU A formulas are potential trouble if taken at all regularly. If some people have poor fat digestion and assimilation, however, they may handle higher amounts of oral vitamin D. A final note on vitamin D formulas is that many people regard the plant-derived form (ergocalciferol, D2) as a safer form than the animal-derived one (calcitriol, D3). This assumption is not correct. Because both forms are fat-soluble, both can pose a risk.

Excessive thirst, diarrhea, nausea, weakness, and headaches are the milder symptoms of vitamin D toxicity. There are also increased levels of calcium and phosphorus in the blood and urine, and abnormal calcification of soft tissues may occur. There is some suggestion that excess vitamin D speeds the atherosclerosis process. Most symptoms decrease and clear up after excessive doses of vitamin D are discontinued. Toxic doses of vitamin D can be made by the skin through prolonged sun exposure, especially before the body has adapted through pigmentation (tanning), which protects the deeper layers where the vitamin D is synthesized. I have personally wondered if the weakness, nausea, dizziness, or headaches from sun exposure may be related to vitamin D toxicity.

Most people do not take very large amounts of supplemental vitamin D but make sufficient amounts through the skin from sun exposure. There is more concern with toxicity from products fortified with vitamin D, especially milk. This synthetic, irradiated ergocalciferol (D2) has decreased the incidence of rickets, but it may be contributing to calcification of the arteries (atherosclerosis) from infancy through old age. The added 400 IU per quart of milk is about 15 times

the amount normally found in milk and may increase the amount of calcium in the circulation, which could be a problem.

Beginning in 2004, with the publication of almost 400 peer-reviewed studies, vitamin D deficiency re-emerged into the research spotlight as a major potential problem in the United States. Many different forms of chronic pain, chronic kidney disease, Crohn's disease, hyperparathyroidism, osteoporosis, osteopenia, osteomalacia, and rickets during adolescence in minority populations have all shown strong links with this deficiency. Based on much of the new research involving population blood levels of vitamin D, David Hanley, MD at the University of Calgary in Alberta, Canada, has concluded that virtually 100% of all Canadians are vitamin D deficient during some part of the year when sunlight exposure is scarce. Individuals in long-term care facilities are especially susceptible to vitamin D deficiency when less ambulatory and not apt to be out in the fresh air.

In addition, the skin production of vitamin D appears to decrease significantly along with aging. The sun's action on the skin to produce vitamin D is inhibited by pollution, clouds, clothing, window glass, skin pigmentation, and sunscreens. There is still some debate about the relationship between sunscreen use and vitamin D deficiency, even though most studies show decreased photoproduction of vitamin D in our skin cells when sunscreens are used. Sunscreen protection factor (SPF) ratings are based on the sunscreen's ability to block ultraviolet B (UVB) radiation from the sun. UVBs are the only wavelengths of light that can activate vitamin D in our skin cells.

The decreased absorption of calcium, along with the retention of phosphorus that usually accompanies it, leads to poor mineralization of bone and the inability of the bones to handle stress. This problem, called *osteomalacia,* is manifested by poor calcification and soft bones. Vitamin D deficiency in the elderly increases general bone loss and osteoporosis. Supplementing this vitamin improves calcium absorption and reduces bone loss. In children, the bone disorder from vitamin D deficiency is rickets. It is characterized by soft skull bones and fragility of other bones, with bowing of the legs, spinal curvature, and an increase in the size of the joints, such as the wrists, ankles, and knees. Muscular development may be

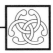

diminished as well. Because of low calcium availability, the teeth may have poor structure, and there may be muscle spasms from a problem called *tetany*, which causes tingling and weakness of the areas affected. Nearsightedness (myopia) and loss of hearing may develop from vitamin D deficiency because of the vitamin's influence on the eye muscles and from loss of calcium in the ear bones. Furthermore, one of the current theories of multiple sclerosis is that it may be influenced by low vitamin D levels in puberty.

Requirements. Vitamin D is best utilized by the body with vitamin A. Most of our calciferol needs are met with some vitamin D in foods and regular sunlight exposure. If we live in smoggy cities or where tall buildings block the sunlight, we may need more vitamin D. Those who have darkly pigmented skin, work nights, or cover their bodies with lots of clothes, as do members of some religious orders, probably need more vitamin D than the avid sunbather. In winter, we usually require more D from supplements; exactly how much remains under debate.

In 1997, the National Academy of Sciences revised the dietary guidelines for vitamin D. In its revision, the NAS decided that there was not enough research evidence to set specific RDAs and instead issued AI levels. (I explained the details about these levels earlier in this chapter, on pages 84–86). The current AIs for vitamin D are set as follows:

AI Levels for Vitamin D	
Age	**AI Level**
Infants and children	5 mcg (200 IU)
Teenagers	5 mcg (200 IU)
Males and females, up to 50 years	5 mcg (200 IU)
Males and females, 51–70 years	10 mcg (400 IU)
Males and females, older than 70 years	15 mcg (600 IU)
Pregnant and lactating women	5 mcg (200 IU)

The NAS chose to issue its vitamin D recommendations in microgram amounts, not in international units, but I have included the IU numbers because many people are still most familiar with them. In the case of vitamin D, 1 mcg is equivalent to 40 IU. In general, it is wise for adults to limit any supplemented vitamin D to the 400 IU per day commonly found in multivitamins and to limit use of vitamin D–fortified milk for a variety of reasons.

Vitamin E (Tocopherols)

Vitamin E is a light yellow oil, a fat-soluble vitamin, that is actually two families of compounds, the tocopherols and tocotrienols, both found in nature. Alpha-tocopherol is the most common and the most active of the eight currently described tocopherols—alpha, beta, gamma, delta, epsilon, zeta, eta, and theta. (Only four of these forms—alpha, beta, gamma, and delta—have been determined to have vitamin activity). D-alpha tocopherol is the most potent form, more active than the synthetic dl-alpha tocopherol. (The tocopherols are also sometimes referred to as *tocols*, a more chemistry-based name that refers to the chemical presence of saturated side chains.) Although researchers understand a little less about the tocotrienols at this point, alpha, beta, gamma, and delta tocotrienol have all been identified and are believed to have their own unique functions. (Chemically speaking, the tocotrienols are sometimes just referred to as *trienols* and are identifiable by their unsaturated side chains.)

Vitamin E was discovered in 1922 during experiments on rats. When fed a purified diet devoid of vitamin E, the rats became infertile, but adding wheat germ oil to their diet restored their fertility. Later, the oil-based substance was isolated and called the "antisterility" vitamin. (*Tokos* and *phero* are the Greek words for "offspring" and "to bear," respectively, so *tocopherol* literally means "to bear children.") Although there is no isolated deficiency disease in humans, vitamin E is well accepted as an essential vitamin by researchers and the general public alike. There is some question, however, as to whether vitamin E is needed for fertility. At the time of this writing, there is no clear evidence that it enhances fertility if there is not a specific deficiency prior to its use. Many people, especially men, take vitamin E with some claimed success regarding sexuality and vitality. Much of this effect, however, may be a result of the antioxidant function and improved circulation and oxygenation.

Alpha-tocopherol is basically stable in heat and in acids; other forms are lost in heat, with storage or freezing, or when oxidized by exposure to the air. All vitamin Es are slightly unstable in alkali and are readily used up when in contact with polyunsaturated oils or rancid fats and oils, which are protected from oxidative destruction by vitamin E. Frying in oil, the processing and milling of foods, the bleaching of flours, and cooking remove much of the vitamin E content of whole foods. Because of this, the average American diet today contains much less natural vitamin E than it did 50 years ago. During the refinement and purification of vegetable oils, vitamin E is lost; the vitamin E–rich by-products of this process are used to make some of the E used in supplements.

Vitamin E is absorbed from the intestines, along with fat and bile salts, first into the lymph and then into the blood, which carries it to the liver to be used or stored. Vitamin E is not stored in the body as effectively as the other fat-soluble vitamins, A, D, and K. More than half of any excesses may be lost in the feces, but some vitamin E is stored in the fatty tissues and the liver, and to a lesser degree, in the heart, muscles, testes, uterus, adrenal and pituitary glands, and blood. Vitamin E is partially absorbed through the skin when used as an ointment or oil application. Intestinal absorption, however, is reduced somewhat with chlorine, inorganic iron, and mineral oil. Unsaturated oils and estrogen also deplete vitamin E, increasing the body's demand for it.

Sources. Vitamin E, as its various tocopherol forms, is found in both plant and animal foods. In general, the animal sources of E are fairly poor, with some being found in butter, egg yolk, milk fat, and liver. **The best sources of vitamin E are the oil components of all grains, seeds, and nuts, which contain tocopherol.** It was first isolated from wheat germ oil, which is still a commonly used, rich source of vitamin E. The protective covering or germ part of the grains is what contains the E, which is lost easily in the milling of flour or in the refinement of grains. For the vitamin E to be preserved, extraction of the oils from nuts and seeds must be done naturally, as by cold-pressing, rather than by heat or chemical extraction, which is used commonly in food processing. Because of these forms of processing, the average American diet has lost many of its natural sources of tocopherols,

and intake is typically very low. When whole-grain wheat is commercially processed into flour, for example, close to 50% of its original vitamin E can be lost if the bran and the germ that contain the E are processed out. Some researchers believe that nearly half of the U.S. population that is now getting less than 75% of the RDA for vitamin E would in fact be getting more than 100% of this vitamin if whole wheat products were consumed in place of highly processed wheat flour products.

The cold-pressed vegetable oils are the best sources of vitamin E, and these are most healthfully used in their raw form in salad dressings and sauces rather than in cooking, because most are polyunsaturated oils, which are adversely affected by heating. With refined or cooked polyunsaturates, more vitamin E is needed to prevent oxidation, which could lead to formation of free radicals—unstable molecules that can lead to cellular and tissue irritation and damage. Free radical–induced changes occurring at the cellular level are the primary processes leading to many chronic degenerative diseases. The vitamin E content of most foods is related to the content of linoleic and linolenic acids, the most essential fatty acids (see chapter 4, Lipids—Fats and Oils). Also, the content of active alpha-tocopherol varies among the different foods and oils. Safflower oil is one of the best sources, with about 90% of the E being the alpha variety. Corn oil has only about 10% alpha-tocopherol. Some other foods that contain significant amounts of vitamin E are soybeans, some margarines and shortenings made from vegetable oils, and a few vegetables, such as uncooked green peas, spinach, asparagus, kale, and cucumber; tomato and celery also have a little E.

Functions. The primary function of vitamin E is as an antioxidant, which is important in our present-day society with widespread pollution, processed food diets, and chemical exposure. Vitamin E helps reduce oxidation of lipid membranes and the unsaturated fatty acids and prevents the breakdown of other nutrients by oxygen. Some scientists compare the function of vitamin E on the cell membrane to a lightening rod nullifying the damage that occurs if lightening strikes. This function of vitamin E is also performed and enhanced by other antioxidants, such as vitamin C, beta-carotene, glutathione (L-cysteine), coenzyme Q, and the mineral selenium. In fact, there is a direct recycling process for vitamin E that requires the immediate presence of beta-carotene, vitamin C, flavonoids, and coenzyme Q to work.

Oxidation in the body of such substances as fat molecules, particularly from polyunsaturated fats, and from eating other oxidized fats such as hydrogenated oils and rancid oils, causes the genesis of free radicals, which leads to chronic inflammation, especially in the vascular lining. Excess free-radical formation comes from a variety of chemical reactions in the body and is the biochemical basis of many diseases, such as atherosclerosis, heart disease, hypertension, arthritis, senility, and probably even cancer. Without vitamin E, cell membranes, active enzyme sites, and DNA are less protected from free-radical damage. Oxidation by circulating peroxides and superoxides (2 types of free radicals) is also reduced by such enzymes as glutathione peroxidase and superoxide dismutase. These antioxidant enzymes also protect, by indirect mechanisms, the polyunsaturated fatty acids and vitamin A from oxidative destruction. Fried foods have more oxidized fat by-products, which increase the requirement for vitamin E, but they do not contain any E. This is partly why fried foods are so dangerous when consumed on a regular basis.

As an antioxidant, vitamin E specifically helps to stabilize cell membranes and protect the tissues of the skin, eyes, liver, breasts, and testes, which are more sensitive to oxidation. It protects the lungs from oxidative damage from environmental substances. Vitamin E also helps maintain biological activity of vitamin A, another important oil-soluble vitamin. Vitamin E protects the unsaturated fatty acids in the body and prevents the oxidation of some hormones, such as those released from the pituitary and adrenal glands. Free-radical formation and oxidation are tied to cancer development, so the family of nutritional antioxidants may help in preventing tumor growth. More definitive research is needed in regard to this important function.

In simple terms, vitamin E's key function is to modify and stabilize blood fats so that the blood vessels, the heart, and the entire body are more protected from free-radical-induced injury. Vitamin E also has some anticlotting (antithrombotic) properties and protects the red blood cells' mem-branes from oxidative damage. Because it helps heart and muscle cell respiration by improving their functioning with less oxygen, vitamin E may help improve stamina and endurance and reduce cardiovascular disease (CVD) risk, especially in those with already existing CVD. Vitamin E has recently been shown to reduce platelet aggregation and platelet adhesiveness to collagen, even more so than aspirin. These platelet functions are linked to an increased risk of atherosclerosis and cardiovascular disease, especially in high-risk groups. Vitamin E has also been shown to neutralize free radicals generated during surgery, particularly cardiopulmonary bypass surgery. In addition, it protects against the toxicity of some of the gases used in anesthesia.

Uses. There is quite an extensive list of uses for this popular nutrient, most commonly in the middle-aged and older populations. And there are many positive effects. Some of these claims are backed by good research, and more investigation is being done on vitamin E by medical and nutritional scientists. There is hope that the results of this research will enable us to better understand its mechanisms and apply them most effectively to prevent and treat our industrial-age medical conditions.

The antioxidant function gives vitamin E a variety of uses. The protection of cells and tissues against oxidation and injury from unstable molecules, pollution, and fats may be the basis for the prevention of aging and many chronic diseases. The many claims about vitamin E's role in preventing premature aging and promoting longevity are major areas of investigation. Aging, tissue degeneration, and skin changes may be brought about by the damage that free radicals cause to cells unprotected by antioxidant nutrients in the body. Cancer and heart and vascular disease may be created in this way, and vitamin E therapy may help reduce the risks of these major illnesses. Decreased blood clotting and increased tissue oxygenation may help reduce symptoms of heart and vascular limitations, such as angina pectoris, arterial spasm, and intermittent claudication (leg pain with walking because of the insufficiency of blood and oxygen, for which vitamin E has clearly been helpful). In both congenital and rheumatic heart diseases, vitamin E may help reduce symptoms caused by impaired tissue oxygenation.

Possible Uses of Vitamin E

Oral Vitamin E
Anemia
Autoimmune diseases
Cancer
Cataract prevention
Cerebral thrombosis prevention
Dermatitis
Diabetes
Fibrocystic breast disease
Herpes infection
Impotence
Intermittent claudication
Menopause
Menstrual pain
Miscarriage prevention
Muscle cramps
Osteoarthritis
Peptic ulcers
Periodontal disease
Premenstrual syndrome
Protects against toxic effects of smoke, alcohol,
    ozone, estrogen, and Adriamycin
Shingles
Surgery, especially cardiovascular
Vascular fragility
Viral disease
Wound healing

Topical Vitamin E
Dermatitis
Herpes infections
Lupus rash
Skin ulcers
Wound healing

Vitamin E may be of help in the prevention of atherosclerosis. Its antioxidant effect reduces thrombin formation and thus helps decrease blood clotting, and it also appears to minimize platelet (blood-clotting component) aggregation and stickiness, aspects that either generate or perpetuate the atherosclerotic process. Vitamin E was thought to raise HDL ("good") cholesterol levels, especially when they were low;

however, recent research suggests it has only a very mild effect, if any, in this regard. Vitamins A and E together can help to decrease cholesterol and general fat accumulation. To assist in healing and to minimize clotting, tocopherol is a useful nutrient before and after surgery, but it is limited to dosages of 200 to 300 IU per day (higher amounts may actually suppress the healing process).

Also, before and after surgery, vitamin E neutralizes free-radical formation and thus reduces possible problems from that. Recently, this antioxidant effect of vitamin E was shown in cardiopulmonary bypass surgery. In regard to its healing powers, vitamin E is used most commonly both internally and externally to assist in the repair of skin lesions, ulcers, burns, abrasions, and dry skin and to heal or diminish the scars caused from injury or surgery. (Vitamin A also appears to work in this regard, possibly even better than E in some instances where skin and tissue healing are needed.) Decreasing scars internally may be important in resolving damage from inflammation of blood vessels and may reduce the potential for clotting and thrombophlebitis. Vitamin E, with the help of vitamins C and P (bioflavonoids), may be useful in preventing progression of varicose veins, more so than treating them once they have occurred.

Research on vitamin E has also shown relief from menstrual pains as well as various menstrual disorders. Many problems that accompany menopause—headaches, hot flashes, vaginal itching because of dryness—may be reduced with the use of supplemental vitamin E. When birth control pills are used, the tocopherols may help protect the body from the pills' possible side effects. **Estrogen may decrease the effect of vitamin E, so more is needed when estrogen therapy is used.** Vitamin E has been used both topically and orally with some success in the treatment of fibrocystic breast disease, or cystic mastitis, likely due to its protective mechanisms against estrogen, which seems to potentiate this disease.

Vitamin E's antioxidant functions also help to protect our cell membranes and lung tissue from pollution, particularly from ozone (O_3) and nitrogen dioxide (NO_2) in the air. Research in rats clearly showed their ability to tolerate increased ozone levels and to survive much longer with vitamin E. In addition, with vitamin E there is some cardiac protection from the effects of smoke and alcohol, as well as protection against the cardiotoxic effects of Adriamycin, an anticancer drug.

Vitamin E has been used to enhance immunity in the treatment of viral illness and to reduce the neurologic pain from shingles, a viral infection of the nerves and skin. It is helpful in preventing eye problems, such as poor vision or cataracts, that may be due to oxidation of fatty tissues and free-radical formation leading to areas of inflammatory damage. Headaches may sometimes be helped with tocopherol treatment, depending on the cause. Various kidney and liver diseases and muscular dystrophy have all been treated with vitamin E, although more immediate inflammatory problems—as in bursitis, gout, and arthritis—seem to benefit more. Leg cramps and circulatory problems associated with diabetes may be helped with vitamin E treatment. For various skin rashes, including those of lupus erythematosus, vitamin E usually along with vitamin A may be of some help.

Deficiency and toxicity. Vitamin E is not stored as readily as are the other fat-soluble vitamins. Excess intake is usually eliminated in the urine and feces, and most doses clear the body within a few days. For these reasons, toxicity from vitamin E use is unlikely. In animal studies, high amounts of E have been shown to retard growth and decrease muscle tissue, decrease the red blood count, and cause poor bone calcification, although in humans these seem more likely to be signs of E deficiency. High intakes of vitamin E oil can cause nausea, diarrhea, or flatulence in some people.

Large doses of vitamin E are generally avoided for people with high blood pressure, as it has been thought to raise blood pressure, although this has not been easily reproduced experimentally. Usually, though, 400 to 600 IU daily (the nonoily, water-dispersible vitamin E succinate may be preferable for patients with hypertension) can provide some antioxidant and circulatory benefits without increasing blood pressure. It is possible that large doses of vitamin E (more than 1,200 IU) have a mild immune-suppressing effect; smaller doses seem to be immune supportive. There is also some concern about using higher doses of vitamin E in people with rheumatic heart disease and administering it to people undergoing digitalis or anticoagulant therapy, as vitamin E may increase the anticoagulant effects of these medicines. These same blood-clotting issues also make vitamin E supplementation a concern for individuals who are deficient in vitamin K. Its effects on blood clotting must be watched carefully in such cases. Vitamin E does not contribute to blood clots or abnormal lipid patterns as is sometimes thought. Primarily because of these blood-clotting issues, and in recognition of the fact that high levels of supplemental vitamin E are widely available in natural food stores, in 2000 the National Academy of Sciences set a tolerable upper limit of 1,000 mg (1,500 IU of alpha-tocopherol) for supplementation purposes only. In other words, they recommended we consume vitamin E–containing foods as desired and restrict supplements to 1,500 additional IU of vitamin E.

Vitamin E deficiency is fairly rare, with vague symptoms that are difficult to diagnose; there is no clear deficiency disease in humans as there is with deficiency of vitamin C or many of the B vitamins. Infertility as an effect of vitamin E deficiency has not been revealed as clearly in humans as it was in the rat study. It is likely that vitamin E deficiency is simply more difficult to diagnose symptomatically because of its wide range of effects on the nervous, reproductive, muscular, and circulatory systems and because other nutrients may mask vitamin E deficiencies. However, biochemically, low levels of vitamin E can be measured in the blood and have been seen in such conditions as acne, anemia, infections, some cancers, periodontal disease, cholesterol, gallstones, neuromuscular diseases, and dementias such as Alzheimer's disease. Recent research has focused on the relationship between vitamin E deficiency and nerve dysfunction near the hands and feet (called *peripheral neuropathy*). Similarly, there are links between pain, tingling, and loss of sensation in the arms, hands, legs, and feet and lack of adequate circulating vitamin E.

Deficiencies are more of a concern in premature babies, because there is no maternal-fetal vitamin E transfer; vitamin E depletion may appear in newborns fed on cow's milk (which contains no vitamin E) instead of breast milk (which contains some if the mother's diet is healthy). Deficiency is also more likely in adults with gastrointestinal disease, with poor fat digestion and metabolism, or with pancreatic insufficiency.

The first sign of vitamin E deficiency may be loss of red blood cells due to fragility caused by the loss of cell membrane protection. Oxidized polyunsaturated fatty acids may also weaken the red blood cell membranes and cause rupture. The generalized decrease in cell and tissue protection from free-radical molecules may lead to abnormal fat deposits in muscles, muscle wasting, and problems in the kidneys and liver because of the circulating dead cells and toxins released. Men may have changes in the testicular tissue with vitamin E deficiency.

With increased oxidation, there is an increased requirement for vitamin E. Vitamin E deficiency may lead to free-radical effects on the unsaturated fatty acids, inhibiting their functions in the health of cell membranes and tissues. Pituitary and adrenal function may be lowered, as these glands may suffer from the cumulative effects of oxidation. Degenerative changes produced by deficiency of vitamin E may not be corrected by vitamin E therapy.

There is some question as to whether tocopherol deficiency reduces the ability to carry pregnancy to term and increases the likelihood of premature birth or causes problems in infants. Is it related to increased heart disease or atherosclerosis or even cancer? Surely, there is a lot more to learn about vitamin E.

Requirements. The amount of vitamin E required depends on body size and the amount of polyunsaturated fats in the diet, because vitamin E is needed to protect these fats from oxidation. More is needed when any refined oils, fried foods, or rancid oils are consumed. Supplemental estrogen or estrogen imbalance in women increases the need for vitamin E, as does air pollution. And vitamin E should not be taken with iron, especially inorganic iron, such as ferrous sulfate or the iron added to food products, as iron depletes vitamin E absorption in the small intestine. Chlorine, ferric chloride, and rancid oils also deplete or destroy vitamin E. Selenium, another important antioxidant, however, may increase the potency of vitamin E.

Even though the RDA for vitamin E is quite low, many people do not consume this in their diet alone. In fact, half of all U.S. adults currently get less than two-thirds of the RDA for vitamin E. For the d-alpha tocopheral form of this vitamin, 1 mg equals 1.49 IU. The different forms of vitamin E have various potencies, with d-alpha the most active and most prevalent in nature. Vitamin E extraction, purity, and activity also vary. The best forms, in my opinion, are those that contain the natural, unesterified d-alpha tocopherol along with the other naturally occurring tocopherols

---

AI Levels and RDAs for Vitamin E

In 2000, the National Academy of Sciences established the following AI levels for infant intake of vitamin E:

Age	AI Level
Males and females, 0–6 months	4 mg (6 IU)
Males and females, 7–12 months	5 mg (7.5 IU)

In the same year, the National Academy of Sciences established the following RDAs for vitamin E for children and adults:

Age	RDA
Males and females, 1–3 years	6 mg (9 IU)
Males and females, 4–8 years	7 mg (10.5 IU)
Males and females, 9–13 years	11 mg (16 IU)
Males and females, 14 years and older	15 mg (22 IU)
Pregnant females, 18 years and older	15 mg (22 IU)
Lactating females, 18 years and older	19 mg (28 IU)

(beta, gamma, and delta) as well as the naturally occurring tocotrienols. This type of E is not easy to find because it is more difficult and costly to produce.

The vitamin E palmitates and acetates are synthetic water-dispersible forms of vitamin E that have a good level of activity and are often easier to take, as they can be taken with other vitamins. Vitamin E oil is taken ideally in the morning before breakfast or at night before bed. It can also be taken after meals containing some fat. Approximately 400 to 600 IU is used preventively, whereas for therapeutic effects, between 800 and 1,600 IU daily is suggested. **With therapeutic uses of vitamin E, it is best to start with a low level and gradually increase it.** Levels over 1,600 IU a day are not recommended unless there is close medical supervision.

Vitamin F (The Essential Fatty Acids)

F Not that far back in the history of nutrition, the essential fatty acids were referred to as "vitamin F" and classified alongside the other fat-soluble vitamins. Like other vitamins, the fatty acids were a subject of constant debate as to their essential or nonessential nature—that is, whether we needed to obtain them from our daily food. Today these debates still continue to some degree, but the fatty acids are seldom categorized as vitamins. I discuss the current debates and provide my own perspective on fatty acids in chapter 4, Lipids—Fats and Oils.

Vitamin K

K This group of three related substances is the last of the fat-soluble vitamins, completing the family that also includes vitamins A, D, and E. This nutrient, both found in nature and made in the body, helps blood clotting, or coagulation. Phylloquinone, the natural vitamin K found in alfalfa and other foods, was discovered in Denmark and named *vitamin K* for the Danish word *koagulation.* Food-source phylloquinone is termed K1, while the menaquinone produced by intestinal bacteria is labeled vitamin K2. A synthetic compound with the basic structure of the quinones is menadione, or vitamin K3. It has twice the activity of the natural Ks and is used therapeutically in people who may not use natural vitamin K well, such as those with decreased bile acid secretion.

All vitamin K variants are fat soluble and stable to heat. Alkalis, strong acids, radiation, and oxidizing agents can destroy vitamin K. It is absorbed from the upper small intestine with the help of bile or bile salts and pancreatic juices and then carried to the liver for the synthesis of prothrombin, a key blood-clotting factor. High intake (as with supplementation) of vitamin E or calcium may reduce vitamin K absorption. Vitamin K is stored in small amounts; most is excreted after therapeutic doses. Yogurt, kefir, and acidophilus milk may help to increase the functioning of the intestinal bacterial flora and therefore contribute to vitamin K production. Antibiotics that reduce these bacteria will diminish vitamin K synthesis in the colon. Rancid oils and fats, X-rays, radiation, aspirin, air pollution, and freezing of foods all destroy vitamin K.

Mineral oil binds with K and rapidly eliminates it from the intestines.

Sources. Vitamin K is found in both natural plant and animal sources. Good supplies are found in the dark leafy greens, most green plants, alfalfa, and kelp. Blackstrap molasses and the polyunsaturated oils, such as safflower, also contain some vitamin K. In animal-source foods, K is found in liver, milk, yogurt, egg yolks, and fish liver oils. The best source for humans is that made by the intestinal bacteria. It is important for the production of many nutrients that we keep our "friendly" colon bacteria active and doing their job; to aid this process we should minimize our use of oral antibiotics, avoid excess sugars and processed foods, and occasionally evaluate and treat any abnormal organisms interfering in our colon, such as yeasts or parasites.

Functions. Vitamin K is necessary for normal blood clotting. It is required for the synthesis of prothrombin and other proteins (factors IX, VII, and X) involved in blood coagulation. Vitamin K also helps prothrombin convert to thrombin with the aid of potassium and calcium; thrombin is the important factor needed for the conversion of fibrinogen to the active fibrin clot. The relationship between vitamin K and protein synthesis may turn out to be much broader than these coagulation-related proteins, however. In chemical terms, the role of vitamin K involves a process called *carboxylation;* these clotting-related proteins are not the only proteins in the body that get carboxylated. Expect more vitamin K–protein relationships as the research unfolds.

Coumarin, which comes from sweet clover, acts as an anticoagulant by competing with vitamin K at its active sites. Coumarin or synthetic dicumarol is used medically primarily as an oral anticoagulant to decrease prothrombin. The salicylates, such as aspirin, increase the need for vitamin K.

Uses. Vitamin K is used commonly by physicians in the treatment of clinical problems. **It should not be taken routinely without the ability to monitor its effects on blood clotting.** Its most regular application in Western medicine is when newborns are injected with it to prevent hemorrhage and other minor bleeding problems. Vitamin K is not transferred from the mother, nor are there colon bacteria to make it in newborns because the gastrointestinal tract is usually sterile for a few days after birth. The production of vitamin K and therefore prothrombin usually begins by the fourth day of life, giving babies their ability to clot blood when necessary.

Vitamin K is also sometimes given by injection to women before labor (a deficiency can occur during pregnancy) or to patients before or after surgery to prevent hemorrhage. Higher doses of vitamin K than are needed by the body do not cause excessive blood clotting, so this is not a concern. Additional K is given at times to women with heavy menstrual flow, to help relieve menstrual pain, or to reduce the nausea and vomiting of pregnancy. It is also used to promote blood clotting in people with liver disease, jaundice, or malabsorption problems. Those people who bruise easily or whose blood clots slowly after injury sometimes benefit from supplemental vitamin K, as do some sufferers of rheumatoid arthritis, where K may reduce irritation in the synovial linings of the joints.

An occasional use of vitamin K that can be lifesaving is the treatment of people who have taken too much of the anticoagulant Coumadin. People with strokes, heart attacks, thrombophlebitis, or pulmonary embolism or who are at risk of having problems related to abnormal blood clotting may receive this type of anticoagulant therapy. As described previously, the coumarol medications reduce blood clotting by competing with vitamin K sites and reducing prothrombin formation. If bleeding problems occur in patients on Coumadin therapy, an injection of vitamin K may help correct it rapidly.

Vitamin K is also used at times as a preservative in foods; it helps control fermentation. If vitamin K deficiency is suspected, it is usually wise to consume more foods high in this vitamin before using supplements.

Deficiency and toxicity. Toxicity rarely occurs from vitamin K from its natural sources—that is, from foods or from production by the intestinal bacteria—but toxic side effects are more likely from the synthetic vitamin K used in medical treatment. Natural vitamins K1 and K2 are easily stored or eliminated, whereas menadione (K3) can build up in the blood and cause some toxicity. Hemolytic anemia, a reduction in red blood cells due to destruction, is a possible problem. This usually increases the bilirubin, a breakdown product of hemoglobin in the blood, more of a problem in infants, who have a harder time handling high levels of biliru-

AI Levels for Vitamin K	
In 2002, the National Academy of Sciences, for the first time in its history, set the following AI guidelines for vitamin K:	
Age	**AI Level**
Males and females, 0–6 months	2.0 mcg
Males and females, 7–12 months	2.5 mcg
Males and females, 1–3 years	30 mcg
Males and females, 4–8 years	55 mcg
Males, 9–13 years	60 mcg
Males, 14–18 years	75 mcg
Males, 19 years and older	120 mcg
Females, 9–13 years	30 mcg
Females, 14–18 years	75 mcg
Females, 19 years and older	90 mcg
Pregnant women, 18 years and younger	75 mcg
Pregnant women, 19 years and older	90 mcg
Lactating women, 18 years and younger	75 mcg
Lactating women, 19 years and older	90 mcg

bin. Symptoms of adult toxicity may include flushing, sweating, or a feeling of chest constriction, although such problems are rare. Because of insufficient evidence concerning toxicity problems with vitamin K, the National Academy of Sciences in 2002 decided not to set tolerable upper limits for this vitamin.

Deficiency of vitamin K is also uncommon. It is more likely with poor intestinal absorption, low dietary intake, or decreased production in the intestines, or when the liver is not able to use vitamin K (which may be caused by either a genetic condition or liver disease). Deficiency of vitamin K is also more common in those with sprue or celiac disease (intestinal malabsorption problems), colitis, or ileitis, or after bowel surgery. I mentioned that for a few days the newborn baby is at risk of bleeding because of lack of vitamin K; vitamin K deficiency may also be a problem in the elderly, when the diet is poor or when antibiotic use or other factors decrease intestinal bacterial production. The problems that may occur from vitamin K deficiency involve abnormal bleeding, as in nosebleeds and internal hemorrhage, which can be severe if it occurs in the brain or internal organs. Miscarriage may occur secondary to bleeding problems from vitamin K deficiency in pregnancy. Fortunately, this is uncommon.

Requirements. An average diet will usually provide close to the AI, the suggested minimum, although 100 to 300 mcg daily may be optimal. Absorption may vary from person to person, estimated from 20% to 60% of intake. Overall, suggested needs are about 2 mcg per kilogram (2.2 pounds) of body weight.

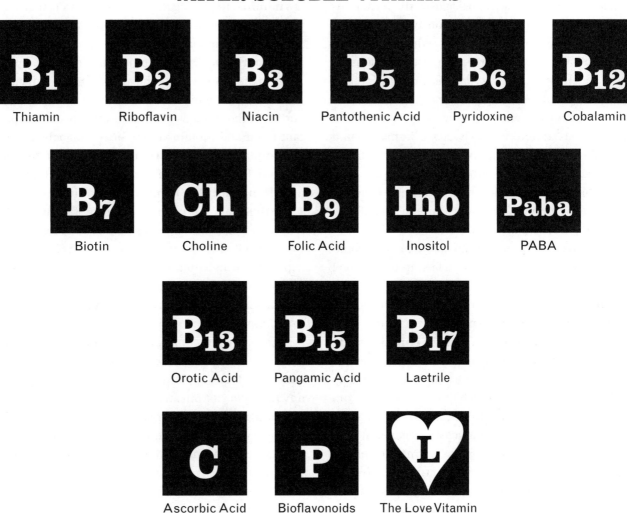

WATER-SOLUBLE VITAMINS

| B₁ Thiamin | B₂ Riboflavin | B₃ Niacin | B₅ Pantothenic Acid | B₆ Pyridoxine | B₁₂ Cobalamin |

| B₇ Biotin | Ch Choline | B₉ Folic Acid | Ino Inositol | Paba PABA |

| B₁₃ Orotic Acid | B₁₅ Pangamic Acid | B₁₇ Laetrile |

| C Ascorbic Acid | P Bioflavonoids | L The Love Vitamin |

B COMPLEX VITAMINS

Here I provide a brief overview of the whole B vitamin group before dealing with each individually. They are all water soluble and are not stored very well in the body. Thus they are needed daily through diet or supplement to support their many functions. Deficiencies of one or more of the B vitamins may occur fairly eas-

ily, especially during times of fasting or dieting for weight loss or with diets that include substantial amounts of refined and processed food, sugar, or alcohol. As a group they are named the B complex vitamins because they are commonly found together in foods and have similar coenzyme functions, often needing each other to perform best. Some of the B vitamins can also be made in the body by inhabitant microorganisms, primarily in the large intestine. Bacteria, yeasts, fungi, and molds are all capable of producing B vitamins.

These vitamins are fairly easily digested from food or supplements and then absorbed into the blood, mainly from the small intestine. When the amount of Bs taken exceeds the body's needs, the excess is easily excreted in the urine, giving it a dark yellow color. Excesses of certain B vitamins, such as thiamin (B1), are also eliminated in perspiration. Because there are many deficiencies and no known toxicities of the B vitamins, taking modest excesses is of no concern and may be helpful to many people. However, taking huge quantities is probably not needed under most conditions.

A general note about B vitamins: for many of these vitamins, special chemical forms (known as *active forms*) are needed for the vitamins to work. Vitamin B1, for example, has several uniquely active forms, thiamin monophosphate and thiamin pyrophosphate. For vitamin B6, a uniquely active form is pyridoxal-5-phosphate (P5P). Sometimes individuals can have ample B vitamin intake but still appear deficient because their bodies are unable to produce these active forms.

Sources. The B vitamins are found in many foods, and they often occur together. In fact, in nature, no B vitamin is found in isolation. Heating, cooking, acid, and alkali affect each vitamin differently, so check the sections in this chapter on individual Bs for this information. **The richest natural source containing the largest number of B vitamins is brewer's yeast, or nutritional yeast.** I'll talk more about yeast in chapter 11, Food and the Earth, when I review some common food additives. Products labeled as brewer's yeast, nutritional yeast, and torula yeast are generally better B vitamin sources than products simply labeled as baker's yeast. Yeast is a common source used to make B vitamin supplements. This is not necessarily an ideal food for many people, however, because sensitivities to yeast may cause digestive tract problems or allergies. Different yeasts may also vary in their concentrations of specific B vitamins.

The germ and bran of cereal grains are good sources of these vitamins, as are some beans, peas, and nuts. Milk and many leafy green vegetables may also supply small amounts of B vitamins. Liver is an excellent source of the B complex vitamins. Other meats, such as beef, are fairly low, except for B12, which is found mainly in animal foods (although not produced

there). Check the discussion of each individual B vitamin for its best sources. And remember, many B vitamins are produced by human intestinal bacteria. The ability of intestinal bacteria to produce B vitamins depends heavily on diet, but at this point, it appears that most healthy mixes of food will support healthy B vitamin production by bacteria. **Such antibiotics as sulfa drugs and tetracyclines, which kill the intestinal bacterial flora, also lower our potential to produce B vitamins.** Replacing the lactobacillus intestinal bacteria after taking antibiotics is important in maintaining the health and microbial ecosystem in the colon.

Functions. The B vitamins are catalytic spark plugs in the human body; they function as coenzymes to catalyze many biochemical reactions, such as converting carbohydrates to glucose, and they are important in fat and protein/amino acid metabolism. **The B complex vitamins are also important for the normal functioning of the nervous system and are often helpful in bringing relaxation or energy to individuals who are stressed or fatigued.** The health of the skin, hair, eyes, and liver is influenced by the B vitamins, as is that of the mucosal linings, especially in and around the mouth. The general muscle tone of the gastrointestinal tract is enhanced with proper levels of B vitamins, allowing the bowels to function most efficiently.

Uses. The functions of the B vitamins are so interrelated that it is suggested they be taken combined in B complex food supplements. They are usually part of any multiple vitamin and are often taken in increased amounts for problems of stress, fatigue, anxiety and nervousness, insomnia, and hyperactivity. B vitamins are also used for many kinds of skin problems, especially dry or itchy dermatitis rashes or cracks at the corners of the mouth. Some cases of vitiligo may be helped by B complex supplements, including higher amounts of para-aminobenzoic acid (PABA). Premenstrual and menopausal problems may be helped with additional B complex vitamins. Treatment of alcoholism and withdrawal from alcohol may be aided by taking large amounts of the B vitamins.

A wide range of various B vitamin deficiency symptoms can be treated with supplemental Bs. The natural food extract supplements are often preferred over the synthetic B complex because they seem to work more harmoniously and are more easily tolerated;

in addition, it is likely that there are other enzymes, cofactors, and possibly even undiscovered B vitamins within the natural supplements.

Deficiency and toxicity. There are basically no real toxicity problems with any of the B vitamins, even in large amounts, because the body readily eliminates the excesses. In fact, because of their safety track record, the National Academy of Sciences has chosen not to set tolerable upper limits for most of the B vitamins. (Exceptions have been made for vitamins B3, B6, choline, and folate, but mostly to warn consumers against imbalanced, extremely high-dose supplementation.) There may be, of course, some subtle problems from taking high-dose individual B vitamins for too long. One such problem is that this may cause a depletion of other Bs. Therefore, it is best to take a complete B complex supplement whenever taking any individual B vitamin regularly in higher amounts.

At least thirteen B vitamins are regularly found in food. But some may be lacking in many Americans' diets because of the consumption of refined flour products, sugar, coffee, and alcohol, which can deplete B vitamins. Deficiency symptoms include fatigue, irritability, nervousness, depression, insomnia, loss of appetite, sore (burning) mouth or tongue, and cracks at the corners of the mouth. Some deficiencies may also reduce immune functions or estrogen metabolism; other potential problems, to name a few, are anemia, especially from vitamin B12 or folic acid deficiency, constipation, neuritis, skin problems, acne, hair loss, early graying of the hair, increased serum cholesterol, and weakness of the legs.

Requirements. The daily amount required for each of the B vitamins varies, and the RDA is not very high for any of them. (For specific values, see the separate discussions of the various Bs.) The overall recommended minimums may be too low, however, and most people who take B vitamins take much higher amounts than the RDA. Because the body does not store much of the B complex vitamins and because many commonly consumed substances such as sugar, coffee, and alcohol deplete B vitamins in the body, the B vitamins should be taken daily. B vitamins are needed for growth, so increased amounts are suggested for children and for pregnant or breastfeeding women. Stress, infections, and high-carbohydrate diets also may cause greater requirements of B vitamin supplements.

Vitamin B1 (Thiamin or Thiamine)

Although not accepted by the American Medical Association in the late 1930s under the name *vitamin B1,* this vitamin was in fact the first of the B family to be chemically identified and recognized for its unique metabolic function. Its odor and flavor are similar to those of yeast. Thiamin can be destroyed by the cooking process, especially by boiling or moist heat, but less by dry heat, such as baking. It is also depleted by use of sugar, coffee, tannin from black teas, nicotine, and alcohol. Like most other B vitamins, thiamin is needed in regular supply, although after its absorption from the upper and lower small intestine, some B1 is stored in the liver, heart, and kidneys. Most excess thiamin is eliminated in the urine; some seems to be excreted through perspiration as well.

Sources. There are a number of food sources for thiamin; however, they may not be the everyday fare for many people. Good sources of vitamin B1 include the germ and bran of wheat, rice husks (the outer covering), and the outer portion of other grains. With the milling of grains and use of refined flours and white, or polished rice, many of us are no longer getting the nourishment of thiamin that is available when we eat wholesome, unprocessed foods. In addition to whole wheat or enriched wheat flour and brown rice, other good sources are brewer's yeast and blackstrap molasses. Oats and millet have modest amounts, as do many vegetables (such as spinach and cauliflower), most nuts, sunflower seeds, and legumes (such as peanuts, peas, and beans). Brazil nuts, pecans, and pine nuts are also moderate sources. Of the fruits, avocado is the highest in vitamin B1. Pork has a high amount of this B vitamin. Many dried fruits contain some thiamin, although the sulfur dioxide often added as a preservative seems to destroy this vitamin.

Functions. Thiamin helps a great many bodily functions, acting as the coenzyme thiamin pyrophosphate (TPP). (TPP can also be called TDP, which stands for thiamin diphosphate.) It has a key metabolic role in the cellular production of energy, mainly in glucose metabolism. Thiamin is also needed to metabolize ethanol, converting it to carbon dioxide and water. B1 helps in the initial steps of fatty acid and sterol production. In this way, thiamin helps convert carbohydrate to fat for storage of potential energy.

Thiamin is important to the health of the nerves and nervous system for at least two reasons. First is its role in the synthesis of acetylcholine (via the production of acetyl CoA), an important neurotransmitter. This particular neurotransmitter carries messages between the nerves and the muscles, and it is especially important for helping ensure proper muscle tone. When thiamin is deficient, it becomes more difficult for us to maintain proper muscle tone. If this difficulty is experienced in the heart muscle, compromised heart function can be the result. It is conceivable that adequate thiamin levels may help prevent the accumulation of fatty deposits in the arteries and thereby reduce the progression of atherosclerosis.

Second is the role of thiamin in the development of the fatlike covering around most of our nerves. This covering is called the *myelin sheath*. When vitamin B1 is deficient, this covering may not form properly, or if already formed, may start to degenerate or become damaged. For this reason, with a lack of vitamin B1, the nerves are more sensitive to inflammation. (Vitamin B12 is also important in the formation of nerve coverings.) In addition, thiamin is linked to individual learning capacity and to growth in children.

Uses. Vitamin B1 is, of course, used to treat any of the symptoms of its deficiency or its deficiency disease beriberi. It is used in the treatment of fatigue, irritability, low morale, and depression, as well as to prevent air- or seasickness. It seems to help the nerves, heart, and muscular system function well. By aiding hydrochloric acid production, thiamin may help digestion or reduce nausea, and it can remedy constipation by increasing intestinal muscle tone. Thiamin is used commonly to improve healing after dental (or often any) surgery.

Increased thiamin intake may be suggested for numerous mental illnesses and problems that affect the nerves. These include alcoholism, multiple sclerosis, Bell's palsy (a facial nerve paralysis), and neuritis. Treatment with thiamin, for example, has been helpful in decreasing the sensory neuropathy that accompanies diabetes and in lessening the pain of trigeminal neuralgia. Thiamin also has a mild diuretic effect and is supportive of heart function, so it is suggested in the treatment program for many cardiovascular problems.

Because thiamin is eliminated through the skin somewhat, doses of more than 50 to 100 mg per day may help repel insects such as flies and mosquitoes from those with "sweet blood." Other uses for increased thiamin include treatment of stress and muscle tension, diarrhea, fever and infections, cramps, and headaches.

Deficiency and toxicity. There is no known toxicity in humans from thiamin taken orally. People have taken hundreds of milligrams daily without any harmful effect, although some may become more stimulated than others. Research on high-dose thiamin treatments is fairly strong, because very high doses have been used in the treatment of maple sugar urine disease (MSUD) and because thiamin has been given intravenously in the treatment of alcoholism. Thiamin injections, however, have occasionally been associated with trauma or edema.

Prolonged restriction of thiamin intake may produce a wide variety of symptoms, particularly affecting the general disposition, nervous system, gastrointestinal tract, and heart. With thiamin deficiency, as with deficiency of most any essential nutrient, symptoms range from mild to moderate depletion disorders to the serious disease state that RDA amounts usually prevent.

Beriberi is the name given to the disease caused by thiamin deficiency. There are three basic expressions of beriberi—namely childhood, wet, and dry beriberi. The name itself comes from the Sinhalese word *beri* meaning "weakness," and muscle weakness is in fact a common symptom of the disease. Childhood beriberi stunts the growth process, and in infants a high-pitched scream and a rapid heartbeat are associated with the disease. Wet beriberi is the classic form with edema (swelling) in the feet and legs, spreading to the body, and associated decreased function of the heart. Dry beriberi is not accompanied by swelling but seems to be manifested by weight loss, muscle wasting, and nerve degeneration. Another thiamin deficiency disease involves degeneration of the brain and affects the general orientation, attitude, and ability to walk. This has been termed the Wernicke-Korsakoff syndrome and is usually seen in people who have been addicted to alcohol for many years.

These severe problems can and do lead to death when they are not corrected with dietary change or supplemental thiamin. Before vitamin B1 was discovered, this affected many people who ate a diet consisting mainly of polished rice. Today, deficiency of this vitamin is still quite common. Although it does not usually lead to beriberi, a number of symptoms can result from a depletion of levels of thiamin in the body. A low-B1 diet consisting of polished rice or unenriched white flour is not often the culprit in our culture. The diet that contributes to deficiency today, especially among teenagers, is high in colas, sweets, fast foods, and many other empty-calorie foods. This diet can also lead to skin problems and symptoms of neurosis, almost like a Jekyll-and-Hyde disposition.

With a deficiency of thiamin, carbohydrate digestion and the metabolism of glucose are diminished. There is a buildup of pyruvic acid in the blood, which can lead to decreased oxygen utilization and therefore mental deficiency and even difficulty breathing. Although B1 is needed for alcohol metabolism, alcohol abuse is often associated with a poor diet and poor B1 absorption. The poor perceptions, mental states, and nerve problems that come with alcoholism may be associated with thiamin deficiency.

The first symptoms of thiamin deficiency may be fatigue and instability, followed by confusion, loss of memory, depression, clumsiness, insomnia, gastrointestinal disturbances, abdominal pain, constipation, slow heart rate, and burning chest pains. As the condition progresses, there may be problems of irregular heart rhythm, prickling sensation in the legs, loss of vibratory sensation, and tender and atrophied muscles. The optic nerve may become inflamed and the vision will be affected.

Generally, with low vitamin B1 levels, the central nervous system—the brain and nerves—does not function optimally. The gastrointestinal and cardiovascular systems are also influenced greatly. B1 levels have been shown to be low in many elderly people, especially those who experience senility, neuroses, and schizophrenia. Society might do well to question how much of the degeneration and disease of old age may be a result of withering digestion and assimilation, leading to deficiencies of various vitamins and other necessary nutrients.

Requirements. Thiamin needs are based on many factors. Given good health, we need about 0.5 mg per 1,000 calories consumed, because B1 is required for energy metabolism. Thus needs are based on body weight, calorie consumption, and the amount of vita-

min B1 synthesized by intestinal bacteria, which can vary greatly from person to person. Thiamin needs are also increased with higher stress levels, with fever or diarrhea, and during and after surgery. Those who smoke, drink alcohol, consume caffeine or tannin from coffee or tea, or who are pregnant, lactating, or taking birth control pills all need more thiamin, possibly much more than the RDA, for optimum health.

Thiamin is needed in the diet or in supplements daily. There are some stores in the heart, liver, and kidneys; however, these do not last very long. The minimum B1 intake for those who are healthy is at least 2 mg per day. A good insurance level of thiamin is probably 10 mg a day, although even higher levels may be useful in some situations. When we do not eat optimally, have any substance abuse habits (especially alcohol abuse), or are under stress, increased levels of thiamin are recommended. An example is the B complex "50" products—that is, 50 mg of B1 along with that amount of most of the other B vitamins—suggested as a daily regimen. The upper intake levels of thiamin should not be much more than 200 to 300 mg daily. Often B1, B2 (riboflavin), and B6 (pyridoxine) are formulated together in equal amounts within a B complex supplement. Many people feel a difference in energy and vitality when they take higher amounts of the B vitamins. (Note: Riboflavin taken for any length of time is best limited to 50 mg daily. See discussion below.)

AI Levels and RDAs for Vitamin B1

Set in 1998 by the National Academy of Sciences, the RDAs for B1 are as follows:

Age	AI/RDA
Infants, 0–6 months	200 mcg (AI)
Infants, 7–12 months	300 mcg (AI)
Children, 1–3 years	500 mcg (RDA)
Children, 4–8 years	600 mcg (RDA)
Males, 9–13 years	900 mcg (RDA)
Males, 14 years and older	1.2 mg (RDA)
Females, 9–13 years	900 mcg (RDA)
Females, 14 years and older	1.1 mg (RDA)
Pregnant females of any age	1.4 mg (RDA)
Lactating females of any age	1.5 mg (RDA)

Vitamin B₂ (Riboflavin)

B₂ This vitamin is an orange-yellow crystal that is more stable than thiamin. (The yellow aspect of this vitamin is actually how it got its name: the word *flavus* in Latin means "yellow"). B₂ is stable to heat, acid, and oxidation. It is sensitive to light, however, especially ultraviolet light, as in sunlight. So foods containing even moderate amounts of riboflavin—for example, milk—need to be protected from sunlight. Only a little of the B₂ in foods is lost in the cooking water. B₂ is easily absorbed from the small intestine into the blood, which transports it to the tissues. **Excess intake is eliminated in the urine, which can give it a yellow-green fluorescent glow, commonly seen after taking 50 mg or 100 mg B-complex supplements.** Riboflavin is not stored in the body, except for a small quantity in the liver and kidneys, so it is needed regularly in the diet.

Intestinal bacteria produce varying amounts of riboflavin; this poses some questions regarding different people's needs for B₂ and may minimize the degree of riboflavin deficiency, even with diets low in riboflavin intake. Although there are many deficiency symptoms possible with low levels of B₂ in the body, no specific serious deficiency disease is noted for riboflavin, as there is for vitamins B₁ and B₃ (niacin). Riboflavin-5-phosphate, a form of riboflavin, may be more readily assimilated by some people.

Sources. Riboflavin is found in many of the foods that contain other B vitamins, but it is not found in high amounts in many foods. For this reason, dietary deficiency is fairly common, and supplementation may help prevent problems. Brewer's yeast is the richest natural source of vitamin B₂. Liver, tongue, and other organ meats are also excellent sources. Oily fish, such as mackerel, trout, eel, herring, and shad, have substantial levels of riboflavin too. Nori seaweed is also a fine source. Milk products have some riboflavin, as do eggs, shellfish, millet, wild rice, dried peas, beans, and some seeds, such as sunflower. Other foods with moderate amounts of riboflavin are dark leafy green vegetables (such as asparagus, collards, broccoli, and spinach), whole or enriched grain products, mushrooms, and avocados. Lower levels of vitamin B₂ are found in cabbage, carrots, cucumbers, apples, figs, berries, grapes, and tropical fruits.

Functions. Riboflavin functions as the precursor or building block for two coenzymes that are important in energy production. Flavin mononucleotide (FMN) and flavin adenine dinucleotide (FAD) are the two coenzymes that act as hydrogen carriers to help make energy as adenosine triphosphate (ATP) through the metabolism of carbohydrates and fats. Riboflavin is also instrumental in cell respiration, helping each cell use oxygen most efficiently; is helpful in maintaining good vision and healthy hair, skin, and nails; and is necessary for normal cell growth.

Two other functions of riboflavin stand out in the research literature. First is its relationship to its fellow B vitamins niacin (vitamin B₃) and pyridoxine (B₆). One of the ways the body can make niacin is through conversion from the amino acid tryptophan. This conversion process requires riboflavin. The most bioactive form of B₆, pyridoxal phosphate (PLP), also requires riboflavin for its production. Recycling of glutathione is the second of these standout functions. Glutathione is a small, proteinlike molecule that is critical in preventing oxygen-based damage to structures throughout the body. Like many "antioxidant" molecules, glutathione must be continuously recycled, and riboflavin allows this recycling to take place.

Uses. Supplemental riboflavin is commonly used to treat and help prevent visual problems, eye fatigue, and cataracts. It seems to help with burning eyes, excess tearing, and decreased vision resulting from eye strain. Riboflavin is also used for many kinds of stress conditions, fatigue, and vitality or growth problems. For people with allergies and chemical sensitivities, riboflavin-5-phosphate may be more readily assimilated than riboflavin. Riboflavin is given for skin difficulties such as acne, dermatitis, eczema, and skin ulcers. B₂ is also used in the treatment of alcohol problems, ulcers, digestive difficulties, and leg cramps, and supplementing it may be advantageous for prevention of or during treatment of cancer. There is not much published research to support these common uses, however. Several promising studies have looked at the benefits of high-dose riboflavin (200–400 mg) in treatment of headaches, especially migraines. Look for future research in this area.

Deficiency and toxicity. There are no known toxic reactions to riboflavin, although high doses may cause losses, mainly from the urine, of other B vitamins. The lack of documented toxic effects was a key factor in the decision of the National Academy of Sciences to set no tolerable upper limit for riboflavin intake when it established riboflavin guidelines in 1998. Like most of the B vitamins, deficiency is a much greater concern. Some authorities claim that riboflavin (B2) deficiency is the most common nutrient deficiency in America. But because of its production by intestinal bacteria, it may not cause symptoms as severe as other vitamin deficiencies. Insufficient levels of riboflavin can occur when people follow diets that do not include such riboflavin-rich foods as liver, yeast, and vegetables; with special diets for weight loss, ulcers, or treatment of diabetes; or in the diets of people who have bad eating habits and consume mostly refined foods and fast foods. Rather, **riboflavin deficiency is more commonly seen in persons with alcohol problems, in the elderly and the poor, and in depressed patients.**

Symptoms of vitamin B2 deficiency include sensitivity or inflammation of the mucous membranes of the mouth; cracks or sores at the corners of the mouth, called *cheilosis;* a red, sore tongue; eye redness or sensitivity to light, burning eyes, eye fatigue, or a dry, sandy feeling of the eyes; fatigue and/or dizziness; dermatitis with a dry yet greasy or oily scaling; nervous tissue damage; and retarded growth in infants and children. Cataracts may occur more frequently with B2 deficiency. Hair loss, weight loss, a general lack of vitality, and digestive problems are also possible with depletion or deficiency states of vitamin B2; these problems may begin when daily intake is 0.6 mg or less.

Recent research has also shown that heavy exercise can increase the need for riboflavin. Particularly in women training for athletic events, the need for riboflavin may be increased by 10 to 15 times the normal amount. Individuals in this group would also be at special risk of deficiency.

Requirements. The RDA of vitamin B2 is based on weight, state of metabolism and growth, and protein and calorie intake. Riboflavin is related closely to energy metabolism. There are only small tissue reserves, and these may be lost when daily intake is lower than 1.2 mg. **Women who take estrogen or birth control pills, people on such antibiotics as sulfa, and those under stress need additional amounts of riboflavin.** The use of tricyclic anti-

depressants like amitriptyline (Elavil) or doxepin (Sinequan) also decreases availability of this vitamin. Specific amounts must be determined for each individual. Riboflavin may be taken in amounts between 25 and 50 mg. Many B vitamin supplements offer 100 mg a day of riboflavin, which may be excessive; 10 mg daily is considered a good insurance level.

AI Levels and RDAs for Vitamin B2

The RDAs for B2, set in 1998 by the Institute of Medicine at the National Academy of Sciences, are as follows:

Age	AI/RDA
Infants, 0–6 months	300 mcg (AI)
Infants, 7–12 months	400 mcg (AI)
Children, 1–3 years	500 mcg (RDA)
Children, 4–8 years	600 mcg (RDA)
Males, 9–13 years	900 mcg (RDA)
Males, 14 years and older	1.3 mg (RDA)
Females, 9–13 years	900 mcg (RDA)
Females, 14–18 years	1.0 mg (RDA)
Females, 19 years and older	1.1 mg (RDA)
Pregnant females of any age	1.4 mg (RDA)
Lactating females of any age	1.6 mg (RDA)

Vitamin B3 (Niacin)

B3 The name *B3* is commonly used to refer to two different compounds, nicotinic acid and niacinamide. B3 was first isolated during oxidation of nicotine from tobacco and was thus given the name nicotinic acid vitamin, shortened to niacin. It is not, however, the same as or even closely related to the molecule nicotine. Niacin, as nicotinic acid or niacinamide, is converted in the body to the active forms nicotinamide adenine dinucleotide (NAD) and a phosphorylated form (NADP). Niacin is one of the most stable of the B vitamins. It is resistant to the effects of heat, light, air, acid, and alkali. A white crystalline substance that is soluble in both water and alcohol, niacin and niacinamide are both readily absorbed from the small intestine. Small amounts may be stored in the liver, but most of the excess is excreted in the urine.

Another important fact about vitamin B3 is that it can be manufactured from the amino acid tryptophan, which is essential (that is, needed in the diet). So niacin is not truly essential in the diet when enough protein containing adequate tryptophan and other nutrients are consumed. When niacin is not present in sufficient amounts, extra protein is needed. Also, when we are deficient in such nutrients as vitamins B1, B2, and B6, vitamin C, and iron, we cannot easily convert tryptophan to niacin. (B2 is especially important in this regard.) Many foods that are low in tryptophan are also low in niacin or, as in corn, the niacin is not readily available. Corn is low in tryptophan and its niacin is bound, so it must receive special treatment. Native Americans knew this and would soak corn in ash water before or after grinding to release the niacin. Even when they subsisted almost solely on corn, they did not experience the serious niacin deficiency disease called *pellagra*, the disease of the "three Ds"—diarrhea, dermatitis, and dementia. During the American Civil War, poor white farm workers in the South subsisted on "quick cornmeal," the poorly prepared white people's version, and pellagra was epidemic until the discovery that it was a dietary deficiency disease. Pellagra historically has been a problem of corn eaters, whereas beriberi has been a disease most correlated with rice-eating cultures.

Sources. Only small to moderate amounts of vitamin B3 occur in foods as pure niacin; other niacin is converted from the amino acid tryptophan, as just discussed. The best sources of vitamin B3 are liver and other organ meats, poultry, fish, and peanuts, all of which have both niacin and tryptophan. Among the fish, tuna, salmon, and halibut are among the richest sources. Yeast, dried beans and peas, wheat germ, whole grains, avocados, dates, figs, and prunes are pretty good sources of niacin. Milk and eggs are good because of their levels of tryptophan. Although B3 is stable, the milling and processing of whole grains can remove up to 90% of the niacin. Thus manufacturers will often enrich their products by adding niacin.

Functions. Niacin acts as part of two coenzymes, NAD and NADP, that are involved in more than 50 different metabolic reactions in the human body. They play a key role in glycolysis (that is, extracting energy from carbohydrates and glucose), are important in

fatty acid synthesis and in the deamination (nitrogen removal) of amino acids, are needed in the formation of red blood cells and steroids, and are helpful in the metabolism of some drugs and toxicants. Thus niacin is a vital precursor for the coenzymes that supply energy to body cells. Basically, the coenzymes of niacin help break down and utilize proteins, fats, and carbohydrates. Vitamin B3 also stimulates circulation, reduces cholesterol levels in the blood of some people, and is important to healthy activity of the nervous system and normal brain function. Niacin supports the health of tissues of the skin, tongue, and digestive tract. In addition, this important vitamin is needed for the synthesis of the sex hormones, such as estrogen, progesterone, and testosterone, as well as other corticosteroids.

Niacin, taken orally as nicotinic acid, can produce redness, warmth, and itching over areas of the skin; this **niacin flush** usually occurs when doses of 50 mg or more are taken and is a result of the release of histamine by the cells, which causes vasodilation. This reaction is harmless; it may even be helpful by enhancing blood flow to the flushed areas, and it lasts only 10 to 20 minutes. When these larger doses of niacin are taken regularly, however, this reaction no longer occurs because stores of histamine are reduced. Many people feel benefit from this flush, but if it is not enjoyable, supplements that contain vitamin B3 in the form of niacinamide or nicotinamide can be used, as they will not produce this reaction. (Note: When vitamin B3 is used to lower cholesterol levels, the nicotinic acid form must be used, as the niacinamide form does not work for this purpose.)

Recent vitamin research has expanded our understanding of niacin in two important ways. First, a key component of the genetic material in our cells, deoxyribose nucleic acid (DNA), requires B3 for its production. Without a sufficient supply of niacin, the risk of genetic damage has been shown to clearly increase. Similarly, this connection between DNA and B3 points to the importance of B3 availability in prevention of cancers. The stabilizing of our blood sugar, through regulation of insulin activity, is a second quickly expanding area of niacin research. It is not yet known exactly how niacin is involved in insulin metabolism, but some researchers support the idea of a glucose tolerance factor (GTF) that includes vitamin B3.

During the mid-1990s, niacin became a fairly popular supplement for individuals with high cholesterol levels, because of the ability of high-dose niacin (in the form of nicotinic acid, with a dose range of 1–3 grams per day) to decrease LDL cholesterol. Some studies actually showed reduced mortality from atherosclerosis following high-dose niacin supplementation. **More recently, however, researchers have discovered that high-dose niacin can also increase our blood homocysteine levels—a very unwanted event for anyone at risk of cardiovascular disease.** These increases in homocysteine are associated with as little as 1 gram of niacin per day. Although very early in its testing and research, there is an alternative form of niacin, called inositol hexaniacinate, that may be just as effective in reducing LDL cholesterol without raising homocysteine levels. Expect to hear more about this form of B3 in years ahead.

Uses. Niacin is used to support a variety of metabolic functions and to treat a number of conditions. Many niacin deficiency symptoms can be treated by adjusting the diet and by supplementing B3 tablets along with other B complex vitamins. Many uses of niacin are based primarily on positive clinical experience and are not as well supported by medical research, although more studies are being done.

Niacin helps increase energy through improving food utilization and has been used beneficially for treating fatigue, irritability, and such digestive disorders as diarrhea, constipation, and indigestion. It may also stimulate extra hydrochloric acid production. Niacin, mainly as nicotinic acid, helps in the regulation of blood sugar, particularly in people with hypoglycemia problems, and provides a greater ability to handle stress. It is helpful in treating anxiety and possibly depression. B3 has been used for various skin reactions and acne, as well as for problems of the teeth and gums. Niacin has many other common uses. It is sometimes helpful in the treatment of migraine-type headaches or arthritis, probably in both cases through stimulation of blood flow in the capillaries. This vitamin has also been used to stimulate the sex drive and enhance sexual experience, to help detoxify the body, and to protect it from certain toxins and pollutants. For most of these problems (as well as for the cardiovascular-related ones mentioned below) the preference is to take the flushing form of niacin, or nicotinic acid—not niacinamide.

Nicotinic acid works rapidly, particularly in its beneficial effects on the cardiovascular system. It stimulates circulation and for this reason may be helpful in treating leg cramps caused by circulatory deficiency; headaches, especially the migraine type; and Mánière's syndrome, associated with hearing loss and vêrtigô. Nicotinic acid also helps reduce blood pressure and acts as an agent to lower serum cholesterol. Treatment with about 2 grams a day of nicotinic acid has produced significant reductions in both blood cholesterol and triglyceride levels. To lower the LDL component and raise the "good" HDL cholesterol, people usually take 50 to 100 mg twice daily and then increase the amount slowly over 2 or 3 weeks to 1,500 to 2,500 mg. Generally, for those with high cholesterol levels, it has been used to help reduce the risk for atherosclerosis. Because of its vascular stimulation and effects of lowering cholesterol and blood pressure, vitamin B3 has been used preventively for such serious secondary problems of cardiovascular disease as myocardial infarctions (heart attacks) and strokes. Also, some neurologic problems, such as Bell's palsy and trigeminal neuralgia, have been helped by niacin supplementation. In osteoarthritis, to help reduce joint pain and improve mobility, niacinamide has been used in amounts beginning at 500 mg twice daily and increasing to 1,000 mg 3 times a day, along with 100 mg daily of B complex.

Niacin has been an important boon to the field of orthomolecular psychiatry for its use in a variety of mental disorders. It was initially well demonstrated to be helpful for the neuroses and psychoses described as the "dementia of pellagra," the niacin deficiency disease. Since then, it has been used in high amounts, well over 100 mg per day and often more than 1,000 mg a day (and up to 6,000 mg), to treat a wide variety of psychological symptoms, including senility, alcoholism, drug problems, depression, and schizophrenia. Niacin has been helpful in reversing the hallucinatory experience, delusional thinking, or wide mood and energy shifts of some psychological disturbances. Although this therapy has its skeptics, as do all applications of nutritional medicine, some studies show promising results in treatment of schizophrenia with niacin and other supplements. Other studies show little or no effect. More research is definitely needed.

People on high blood pressure medicines and those who have ulcers, gout, or diabetes should be careful taking higher-dose supplements of niacin because of its effect of lowering blood pressure, its acidity, its liver toxicity, its potential to raise uric acid levels, and its effect in raising blood sugar—although niacin has been shown to have a positive effect on glucose tolerance (it is part of glucose tolerance factor) and thereby on diabetes as well. Exercise and niacin are helpful for people with adult diabetes through their positive effects on blood sugar and cholesterol.

Deficiency and toxicity. As with the other B vitamins, there are really no toxic effects from even high doses of niacin, although the so-called niacin flush previously described may be uncomfortable for some. With the use of high-dose niacin in recent years, however, the occasional person has experienced some minor problems, such as irritation of the gastrointestinal (GI) tract or the liver, which subsides with decreased intake of niacin. In addition, some people taking niacin experience sedation rather than stimulation. The risk of flush and mild GI and liver symptoms prompted the National Academy of Sciences in 1998 to set a tolerable upper limit specifically for niacin supplements. The limit is 35 mg and applies to all adults. A relatively new form of niacin, inositol hexaniacinate, may be helpful for reducing LDL cholesterol without raising homocysteine levels or causing niacin flush. Given the availability of this alternative form for niacin, and given the successful experience of many practitioners in increasing niacin doses carefully over time to minimize unwanted reactions, I believe there is still a place for doses of niacin higher than 35 mg in treatment of some health problems, but it would be wise to use caution in this area.

As discussed earlier, niacin deficiency problems—primarily pellagra—have been much more common than niacin toxicity. For a long time pellagra was a serious and fatal problem, characterized by the "3 Ds"—dermatitis, diarrhea, and dementia. The fourth D was death. One of the first signs of niacin deficiency is the skin's sensitivity to light; the skin becomes rough, thick, and dry (*pellagra* means "skin that is rough" in Italian). The skin then becomes darkly pigmented, especially in areas of the body prone to be hot and sweaty or those exposed to sun. The first stage of this condition is extreme redness and sensitivity of those exposed areas; it was from this symptom that the term *redneck,* describing the bright red necks of eighteenth- and nineteenth-century niacin-deficient fieldworkers, came into being.

In general, niacin deficiency affects every cell, especially in those systems with rapid turnover, such as the skin, the GI tract, and the nervous system. Other than photosensitivity, the first signs of niacin deficiency are noted as decreased energy production and problems with maintaining healthy functioning of the skin and intestines. These symptoms include weakness and general fatigue, anorexia, indigestion, and skin eruptions. These can progress to other problems, such as a sore, red tongue, canker sores, nausea, vomiting, tender gums, bad breath, and diarrhea. The neurological symptoms may begin with irritability, insomnia, and headaches and then progress to tremors, extreme anxiety, depression—all the way to full-blown psychosis. The skin will worsen, as will the diarrhea and inflammation of the mouth and intestinal tract. There will be a lack of stomach acid production (achlorhydria) and a decrease in fat digestion and thus lower availability from food absorption of the fat-soluble vitamins A, D, and E. Death could occur, usually from convulsions, if the niacin deficiency is not corrected.

Niacin deficiency symptoms can be seen in diets with niacin intake below 7.5 mg per day, but often this is not the only deficiency; vitamin B_1, vitamin B_2, and other B vitamins as well as protein and iron may be low. To treat pellagra and niacin deficiency disorders, vitamin B_3 supplements should be taken along with good protein intake to obtain adequate levels of the amino acid tryptophan. About 50% of daily niacin comes from the conversion in our livers of tryptophan to niacin with the help of pyridoxine (vitamin B_6).

Requirements. Many food charts list only sources that actually contain niacin and do not take into account tryptophan conversion into niacin. Approximately 60 mg of tryptophan can generate 1 mg of niacin. But tryptophan is available for conversion only when there are more than sufficient quantities in the diet to synthesize the necessary proteins as tryptophan is used in our body with the other essential amino acids to produce protein. Niacin needs are based on calorie intake. Adults need about 6.6 mg per 1,000 calories, and no less than 13 mg per day.

AI Levels and RDAs for Vitamin B3

Set in 1998 by the National Academy of Sciences, the RDAs for B3 are as follows:

Age	AI/RDA
Infants, 0–6 months	2 mg (AI)
Infants, 7–12 months	4 mg (AI)
Children, 1–3 years	6 mg (RDA)
Children, 4–8 years	8 mg (RDA)
Males, 9–13 years	12 mg (RDA)
Males, 14 years and older	16 mg (RDA)
Females, 9–13 years	12 mg (RDA)
Females, 14 years and older	14 mg (RDA)
Pregnant females of any age	18 mg (RDA)
Lactating females of any age	17 mg(RDA)

Niacin needs are increased during pregnancy, lactation, and growth periods, as well as after physical exercise. **Athletes require more B3 than less active people. Stress, illness, and tissue injury also increase the body's need for niacin.** People who eat a lot of sugar or refined, processed foods require more niacin as well. Realistically, 25 to 50 mg per day is an adequate intake of niacin if minimum protein requirements are met. On the average, many supplements provide at least 50 to 100 mg per day of niacin or niacinamide, which is a good insurance level. For treatment of the variety of conditions just described, higher amounts of niacin may be needed to be helpful, and levels up to 2 to 3 grams a day are not uncommon as a therapeutic dose. The other B vitamins should also be supplied so as to not create an imbalanced metabolic condition.

Vitamin B5 (Pantothenic Acid)

B5 Vitamin B5, another of the B complex vitamins, is a yellow viscous oil found usually as the calcium or sodium salt—that is, calcium pantothenate. It is present in all living cells and is important to metabolism, where it functions as part of the molecule called coenzyme A (CoA). Pantothenic acid is found in yeasts, molds, bacteria, and plant and animal cells, as well as in human blood plasma and lymph fluid. B5 is stable to moist heat and oxidation or reduction (adding or subtracting an electron), although

it is easily destroyed by acids (such as vinegar) or alkalis (such as baking soda) and by dry heat. More than half of the pantothenic acid in wheat is lost during milling, and about one-third is degraded in meat during cooking. In many whole foods, vitamin B5 is readily available.

Sources. The name *pantothenic acid* comes from the Greek word *pantos,* meaning "everywhere," referring to its wide availability in foods. It is easily accessible in the diet, and deficiency is uncommon, except in those with a highly processed diet, because much of the available vitamin B5 activity is lost during refinement of foods. Good sources of pantothenic acid include organ meats, brewer's yeast, egg yolks, fish, chicken, whole-grain cereals, cheese, peanuts, dried beans, and a variety of vegetables, such as sweet potatoes, green peas, cauliflower, mushrooms, and avocados. Vitamin B5 is also made by the bacterial flora of human intestines, another source for this important metabolic assistant or coenzyme.

Functions. Pantothenic acid as coenzyme A is closely involved in adrenal cortex function and has come to be known as the "antistress" vitamin. It supports the adrenal glands to increase production of cortisone and other adrenal hormones to help counteract stress and enhance metabolism. Through this mechanism, pantothenic acid is also thought to help prevent aging and wrinkles. It is generally important to healthy skin and nerves. Through its adrenal support, vitamin B5 may reduce potentially toxic effects of antibiotics and radiation. In the coenzyme, pantothenic acid is important in cellular metabolism of carbohydrates and fats to release energy and also supports the synthesis of acetylcholine, an important neurotransmitter agent that works throughout the body in a variety of neuromuscular reactions. Coenzyme A is vital in the synthesis of fatty acids, cholesterol, steroids, sphingosines, and phospholipids. It also helps synthesize porphyrin, which is connected to hemoglobin.

In future research, expect more attention to this vitamin in relationship to fat metabolism. Not only does pantothenate (the acetyl CoA form of the vitamin) help provide fat with its chemical structure, but it also helps deliver these fat precursors where they need to go. Pantothenate accomplishes this task by enabling the activity of a special transport molecule, acyl carrier protein (ACP).

Uses. Pantothenic acid, found in multiple sources, is used in a wide variety of conditions. **Again, it is known as the "antistress" vitamin and is used to relieve fatigue and stress as well as the many problems induced by stress through its support of the adrenal glands.** Allergies, headaches, arthritis, psoriasis, insomnia, asthma, and infections have all been treated with some effectiveness using vitamin B5, possibly through its adrenal support and adequate production of adrenocorticosteroids.

Vitamin B5 has also been used after surgery when there is paralysis of the GI tract to stimulate GI peristalsis. It has been helpful in many cases for people who grind their teeth at night, a problem called *bruxism*. Other conditions treated by this vitamin are such nerve disorders as neuritis, epilepsy, and multiple sclerosis, as well as various levels of mental illness and alcoholism. Of course, the effectiveness may vary according to the amount supplemented, the length of time used, and individual responsiveness. Sound research to support the use of pantothenic acid in many of these treatments or for its energy-enhancing or antiaging effects is lacking, although some research has shown positive results from the use of calcium pantothenate in reducing arthritis symptoms of joint pain and stiffness.

Deficiency and toxicity. As with other B vitamins, there are no specific toxic effects from high doses of pantothenic acid. More than 1,000 mg daily has been taken for over 6 months with no side effects; when 1,500 mg or more is taken daily for several weeks, some people experience a superficial sensitivity in their teeth and mild diarrhea. (In fact, in much lower doses of about 500 mg, pantothenate has been used to treat constipation.) However, it is possible that if B5 is taken without other B vitamins, it may create metabolic imbalance. This overall lack of evidence for toxicity is the reason that the National Academy of Sciences declined to set a tolerable upper limit for pantothenate in its 1998 public health recommendations.

Fatigue is probably the earliest and most common symptom of pantothenic acid deficiency, although it is an unlikely vitamin deficiency because of the availability of B5 in many foods, plus the fact that it is also produced by intestinal bacteria. A diet high in refined and processed foods or a reduction or destruction of intestinal flora, most commonly by antibiotic use, can lead to a vitamin B5 deficiency. Teenagers are more likely to experience a deficiency, because their diets often include high amounts of fast foods, sugars, and refined flours (all low in B vitamins). And the problem may be compounded because the acne often associated with this type of diet is commonly treated with tetracycline antibiotics, which reduce the intestinal bacteria and thereby the production of pantothenic acid in the colon. Poor digestion can also increase the risk of pantothenate deficiency, because this vitamin is found in food mostly in its CoA form and has to be released from this form through proper digestion in order to be absorbed.

Studies of pantothenic acid deficiency in rats showed increased graying of the fur, decreased growth, and, in the extreme, hemorrhage and destruction of the adrenal glands. In humans, the decreased adrenal function caused by B5 deficiency can lead to a variety of metabolic problems. Fatigue is most likely; there may also be physical and mental depression, a decrease in hydrochloric acid production and other digestive symptoms, some loss of nerve function, and problems in blood sugar metabolism, with symptoms of hypoglycemia (low blood sugar) being the most common. Pantothenic acid affects the function of cells in all systems, and a deficiency may reduce immunity—both cellular and antibody responses. Other symptoms of B5 deficiency include vomiting, abdominal cramps, skin problems, tachycardia, insomnia, tingling of the hands and feet, muscle cramps, recurrent upper respiratory infections, and worsening of allergy symptoms.

AI Levels for Vitamin B5

The AI levels for B5, set in 1998 by the Institute of Medicine at the National Academy of Sciences, are as follows:

Age	AI Level
Infants, 0–6 months	1.7 mg
Infants, 7–12 months	1.8 mg
Children, 1–3 years	2 mg
Children, 4–8 years	3 mg
Males, 9–13 years	4 mg
Males, 14 years and older	5 mg
Females, 9–13 years	4 mg
Females, 14 years and older	5 mg
Pregnant females of any age	6 mg
Lactating females of any age	7 mg

Many other sources feel the minimum needs are more likely to be about 25 to 50 mg, and 50 to 100 mg is probably a good insurance range. Therapeutic ranges are more like 250 to 500 mg daily and even higher, taken, of course, along with the other B complex vitamins. Individual needs vary according to food intake, degree of stress, and whether one is pregnant or lactating. Those people who eat a diet of processed foods, have a stressful lifestyle, or have allergies require higher amounts of pantothenic acid. For all of these problems, 250 to 500 mg taken twice daily is a safe and beneficial amount.

Vitamin B6 (Pyridoxine)

B6 Vitamin B6 (pyridoxine and pyridoxal-5-phosphate [P5P], the active coenzyme form of vitamin B6) is an important B vitamin, especially for women. It seems to be connected somehow to hormone balance and water shifts in women. B6 is actually three related compounds, all of which are found in food—pyridoxine, pyridoxal, and pyridoxamine. Once inside the body, each of these three forms often gets a phosphorus group attached, creating pyridoxine phosphate, pyridoxal phosphate, or pyridoxamine phosphate. Pyridoxal phosphate is the predominant biologically active form; in vitamin supplements, however, pyridoxine is the form used because it is the least expensive to produce commercially. Vitamin B6 is stable in acid, somewhat less stable in alkali, and fairly easily destroyed with ultraviolet light, such as sunlight, and during the processing of food. It is also lost in cooking or with improper food storage.

Pyridoxine is absorbed readily from the small intestine and used throughout the body in a multitude of functions. Fasting and reducing diets usually deplete the vitamin B6 supply unless it is supplemented. Usually within 8 hours, much of the excess is excreted through the urine; some B6 is stored in muscle. It is also produced by the intestinal bacteria.

Sources. Vitamin B6 in its several forms is widely available in nature, although not many foods have very high amounts. Because it is lost in cooking and in the refining or processing of foods, it is not the easiest B vitamin to obtain in sufficient amounts from the diet, especially if we eat a lot of processed food, as it is not replaced in such enriched flour products as cereals and pastries. The best sources of vitamin B6 are meats, particularly organ meats, such as liver, and whole grains, especially wheat. Wheat germ is one of the richest sources. Besides meat, good protein sources of B6 include fish, poultry, egg yolk, soybeans and other dried beans, peanuts, and walnuts. Vegetable and fruit sources include bananas, prunes, potatoes, cauliflower, cabbage, collard, turnip, mustard greens, garlic, mushrooms, spinach, bell peppers, and avocados. Raw sugar cane has a good amount, while refined sugar has none; whole wheat flour contains about 100 mcg pyridoxine per ounce (wheat germ and wheat flakes have much more), while refined wheat flour has almost none, and even whole wheat bread has lost nearly all of its vitamin B6.

Functions. Pyridoxine and its coenzyme form, P5P, have a wide variety of metabolic functions in the body, especially in amino acid metabolism and in the central nervous system, where it supports production of gamma-aminobutyric acid (GABA). Many reactions, including the conversion of tryptophan to niacin and arachidonic acid to prostaglandin E2, require vitamin B6. The pyridoxal group is important in the utilization of all food sources for energy and in facilitating the release of glycogen (stored energy) from the liver and muscles. It helps as well in antibody and red blood cell production (hemoglobin synthesis) and in the synthesis and functioning of both DNA and RNA. By helping maintain the balance of sodium and potassium in the body, B6 aids fluid balance regulation and the electrical functioning of the nerves, heart, and musculoskeletal system; B6 is needed to help maintain a normal intracellular magnesium level, which is also important for these functions. The neurotransmitters norepinephrine and acetylcholine and the allergy regulator histamine are all important body chemicals that depend on P5P in their metabolism. **Also, the brain needs it to convert tryptophan to serotonin, another important antidepressant neurotransmitter.**

Pyridoxine is especially important in regard to protein metabolism. Many amino acid reactions depend on vitamin B6 to help in the transport of amino acids across the intestinal mucosa into the blood and from the blood into cells. By itself and with other enzymes, P5P helps build amino acids, break them down, and change one to another; it is especially related to the production and metabolism of choline, methionine, serine, cysteine, tryptophan, and niacin.

The role of B6 in tryptophan, cysteine, and methionine metabolism underscores its importance in sulfur metabolism, because each of these amino acids contains an atom of sulfur. This sulfur connection makes B6 a strong candidate for consideration in support of the body's detoxification processes, because sulfur compounds are frequently required to detoxify pesticides, additives, and heavy metals. B6 is connected with detox in a second way, because it is equally important in helping to recycle chemical groups called *methyl groups*. Like sulfur, methyl groups are required for the processing of literally hundreds of toxins.

The body has a high requirement for vitamin B6 during pregnancy. It is important for maintaining the mother's hormonal and fluid balance and for the baby's developing nervous system. Pyridoxine may somehow be related to the development and health of the myelin covering of the nerves, which allows them to conduct impulses properly.

Uses. With its many functions, there is also a wide range of clinical uses of vitamin B6, clearly being most helpful when symptoms and diseases are related to a pyridoxine/P5P depletion or deficiency. Recently there has been widespread use of higher doses of B6, usually from 50 to 200 mg per day (although some studies use 500 mg per day of pyridoxine in time-release form) for premenstrual symptoms, especially water retention, which can lead to breast soreness and emotional tension. Pyridoxine has been very helpful in this role, probably because of its diuretic effect through its influence on sodium-potassium balance and its mysterious influence on the hormonal system. B6 also helps with the acne that often develops premenstrually, as well as with dysmenorrhea, or menstrual pain; magnesium is usually used as well in all of these menstrual problems. In pregnancy, B6 has been helpful to many women for controlling the nausea and vomiting of morning sickness, which some authorities feel is highly related to vitamin B6 deficiency.

As an example, Linda B., a 33-year-old wife and mother of two, came to see me complaining of premenstrual irritability along with severe breast swelling and pain, all of which interfered with her life. She began a simple supplement regimen that included 50 mg of vitamin B6 3 times daily. She felt remarkably better during her next two menstrual cycles. Follow-up care included some diet shifts, weight loss, and a continued supplement program. Linda began feeling better throughout the month, and her well-being has continued for years. My office still receives thank-you notes from her.

It seems that whenever there are increased levels of estrogen in the body, more B6 is required. This occurs not only in pregnancy but also for women who take birth control pills and those postmenopausal women on estrogen treatment as well. It is likely that some of the emotional symptoms experienced by many women on the pill—such as fatigue, mood swings, depression, and loss of sex drive—may be related to a deficiency of B6 and thereby helped by supplementa-

---

Possible Clinical Uses of Vitamin B6

Acne, especially premenstrual	Chemical and radiation protection	Kidney stones (mainly calcium oxalate)*	Schizophrenia
Allergies	Depression	Learning disabilities	Seborrheic dermatitis (topical)
Anxiety	Drug use	MSG reactions	Sickle-cell anemia
Any effect from improper amino acid metabolism*	Dysmenorrhea	Muscle fatigue	Stress ulcers
	Epilepsy	Muscle pain*	Toxemia of pregnancy
	Estrogen therapy*	Nausea associated with pregnancy*	Water retention*
Asthma	Fatigue*		
Atherosclerosis	Female infertility	Neuritis	
Autism	Hyperkinesis	Other anemias	
Birth control pills*	Immune suppression	Parkinsonism	
Carpal tunnel syndrome*	Joint pain	Premenstrual syndrome*	*Important uses

tion. The connection of pyridoxine with estrogen may be related to metabolic processing of estrogen in the liver, which usually attaches a sulfur-group to estrogen for transport or excretion. As mentioned previously, B6 is a key player when it comes to sulfur metabolism.

Vitamin B6 is used for people with stress conditions, fatigue, headaches, nervous disorders, anemia, and low blood sugar or diabetes, and in men for prostatitis, low sex drive, or hair loss. P5P is occasionally used in formulas or as an individual supplement for certain conditions. As the active coenzyme of pyridoxine, P5P can go more directly into the metabolic cycles and does not have to be converted; thus it may be more helpful than pyridoxine alone in such problems as fatigue, allergies, viral disease, chemical sensitivities, mental illness, and cancer. Pyridoxine supplementation is also used for a variety of skin problems—dandruff, eczema, dermatitis, and psoriasis. Regarding the nervous system, B6 has been supportive in cases of epilepsy, Parkinson's disease, multiple sclerosis, and neuritis. Vitamin B6 therapy, from 100 to 300 mg daily for 8 to 12 weeks, reduces carpal tunnel syndrome and in most patients increases the ability to use the hands.

Pyridoxine is a natural diuretic and is often helpful in overweight individuals, in those who retain fluids, and as an adjunct to blood pressure control. Vitamin B6 (along with magnesium) has received some note regarding preventing the formation of kidney stones or the recurrence of stones in those who have had them. Fairly high therapeutic doses of the vitamin in the range of 250 to 500 mg per day have been used in some of these studies, and the duration of treatment needed for positive results has been fairly long-term. In one study, about 18 months were required for the impact of B6 to take place.

A combination of B6 and magnesium helps in some hyperactive kids and those with fits or problems of autism. Pyridoxine in fairly large doses will stimulate dream activity as well as reduce the potential toxicity of barbiturate drugs, carbon monoxide, some other chemicals, and irradiation. These benefits are undoubtedly related to B6's sulfur and methyl detox involvements.

Pyridoxine, probably more than the other B vitamins except folic acid, is supportive of healthy immune function. B6 deficiency can produce immune weakness, and B6 treatment may be helpful against infections and cancer. Recent studies have shown that pyridoxine can

inhibit the growth of some cancer cells, specifically mouse and human melanoma cells. Further research with B6 will likely find an even wider range of uses. Vitamin B6 works best when taken with magnesium, zinc, riboflavin, and brewer's yeast or the other B vitamins.

Deficiency and toxicity. There is basically no toxicity with pyridoxine at reasonable daily dosages, although there has been some recent concern about this. Regular oral intake of 200 mg and intravenous doses of 200 mg have shown no side effects. Usually the toxic doses are much higher, between 2 and 5 grams. Some recent reports in the medical literature show that regular usage of more than 2,000 mg per day, which some women have taken, are correlated with episodes of peripheral neuritis. Although the experience of weakness or tingling in the arms or legs has been transient and mostly correctable by decreasing the B6 dosage, this warrants some concern about excessive use of B6, especially long-term use. Because part of the neuropathy problem comes from the liver's inability to convert all of the pyridoxine to active P5P, this concern can be lessened by supplementing some of the B6 as P5P (as I have done in many of my programs), especially when the B6 dose exceeds 200 mg per day. In addition, using increased amounts of magnesium with the higher levels of vitamin B6 will reduce the occurrence of peripheral neuritis. The mere fact of an association between peripheral neuritis and high-dose pyridoxine was sufficient, however, for the National Academy of Sciences to act in 1998 to set a tolerable upper limit on intake of B6 for adults of 100 mg.

Deficiency, as usual, is a bigger concern with B6, as it is with all the B vitamins. So many functions are performed by pyridoxine that its deficiency affects the whole body. Most of these deficiency symptoms are fairly vague. Muscle weakness, nervousness, irritability,

---

B6 Deficiency Concerns

Alcoholism	Elderly
Asthma	Immune suppression
Birth control pills	Malabsorption
Cervical cancer	Multiple sclerosis
Crohn's disease	Peptic ulcer
Depression	Pregnancy

and depression are not uncommon. Many of the symptoms are similar to those of both niacin and ribo-flavin deficiencies; depression is common in all of them.

Metabolically, pyridoxine deficiency has a dramatic effect on amino acid metabolism, with a decreased synthesis of niacin from tryptophan, a decrease in neuro-transmitter chemicals, and a decrease in hemoglobin production. Fatigue, nervous system symptoms, and anemia are all influenced by deficiency. Further nerve-related problems include paresthesia, incoordination, confusion, insomnia, hyperactivity, and, more severely, neuritis, electroencephalogram (EEG) changes, and convulsions. Other problems of pyridoxine deficiency include visual disturbances as well as dermatitis or cracks and sores at the corners of the mouth and eyes.

There is special concern about deficiency during pregnancy, when vitamin B6 needs are higher, as it may cause water retention and the nausea and vomiting of morning sickness and has been correlated with a higher incidence of common problems of later pregnancy, such as toxemia (preeclampsia, high blood pressure, edema, and hyperreflexes) and eclampsia (those same symptoms plus seizures). B6 deficiency in later pregnancy can be associated with birthing difficulties. There is also an increased likelihood of diabetic and blood sugar problems in pregnancy when vitamin B6 is deficient.

Overall, vitamin B6 deficiency can cause a variety of nervous symptoms, skin problems, and amino acid/protein metabolic abnormalities. These can lead to the more common expressions—headache, dizziness, inability to concentrate, irritability and epileptic-type activity, labile depression, and weakness. Water retention is common. Nausea, vomiting, and dry skin, especially extensive dandruff and a cracked, sore mouth and tongue, are also more likely with B6 deficiency.

Requirements. As mentioned, the need for vitamin B6 increases in a variety of situations. During pregnancy and lactation and with use of birth control pills or estrogen, higher levels are required. For those who eat a high-sugar or heavily processed-food diet or a high-protein diet, requirements for B6 are greater and deficiencies or depletion are more common. When there is cardiac failure, radiation use, or impairment of the digestive system, needs for vitamin B6 are increased. As part of the typical aging process, one's needs also increase. Smokers are at increased risk of pyridoxine deficiency.

Drugs that influence needs for B6 are oral contraceptives, isoniazid (for tuberculosis), hydralazine, furosemide, and reserpine (all for high blood pressure), amphetamines, asthma-related drugs like theophylline, and some antibiotics, including gentamycin. More B6 is utilized with an increased intake of the amino acid methionine. Adequate magnesium in the body is important to B6 functions.

A safe, basic intake for vitamin B6 is probably 10 to 15 mg per day, although much higher daily amounts are easily tolerated. B6 should also be taken along with other B vitamins to prevent metabolic imbalance. For therapeutic purposes, amounts between 50 and 100 mg (P5P usually comes in this quantity) are most common, and up to 200 to 500 mg per day in time-release forms is used for some conditions, such as premenstrual problems and depression. With the current questions about neurologic side effects associated with megadoses of vitamin B6, particularly as pyridoxine hydrochloride, I suggest limiting regular daily intake to 500 mg daily or 1,000 mg for a short course of treatment, such as 1 to 2 weeks; also, take some additional magnesium, 200 to 300 mg, which may help reduce any neurologic concerns.

AI Levels and RDAs for Vitamin B6

B6 intake, although based on many factors, is determined primarily by protein intake, because it is so important to protein metabolism. In 2000, the National Academy of Sciences established the following RDAs:

Age	AI/RDA
Infants, 0–6 months	100 mcg (AI)
Infants, 7–12 months	300 mcg (AI)
Children, 1–3 years	500 mcg (RDA)
Children, 4–8 years	600 mcg (RDA)
Males, 9–13 years	1.0 mg (RDA)
Males, 14–50 years	1.3 mg (RDA)
Males, older than 50 years	1.5 mg (RDA)
Females, 9–13 years	1.0 mg (RDA)
Females, 14–50	1.2 mg (RDA)
Females, older than 50 years	1.5 mg (RDA)
Pregnant females of any age	1.9 mg (RDA)
Lactating females of any age	2.0 mg (RDA)

Vitamin B₁₂ (Cobalamin)

B₁₂ Vitamin B12 is called the "red vitamin," as it is a red crystalline compound. It is the only vitamin that contains an essential mineral—namely, cobalt. Cobalt is thereby needed to make B12 and so is essential for health. B12 is also unique in that it is required in much tinier amounts than the other B vitamins. Only 3 to 4 mcg are needed at minimum; however, higher levels, up to 1 mg, are often used therapeutically.

Vitamin B12 is a complex molecule. Besides cobalt, it also contains carbon, oxygen, phosphorus, and nitrogen atoms in a unique kind of ring structure called a *corrin ring*. Cobalamin is stable to heat, sensitive in heated acid or alkali solution, slightly sensitive to light, and destroyed by oxidizing and reducing agents and by some heavy metals. It was first isolated in 1926 as the factor that treated a feared disease, pernicious anemia—termed *pernicious* because it could be fatal, most often from neurologic degeneration. But the substance cobalamin when given orally (liver was used as the cure, as it contains high amounts of B12) did not cure all of the people with the disease, and some people still developed pernicious anemia. It was later found that a mucoprotein enzyme produced by the stomach (by the parietal cells that also make hydrochloric acid) was also needed for vitamin B12 to be absorbed into the body from the intestines. This enzyme has been termed the *intrinsic factor,* while vitamin B12 is the *extrinsic factor.*

In numerous research studies, suspected deficiency of cobalamin has actually turned out to be deficiency of the intrinsic factor. Aging, stress, and problems with the stomach or stomach surgery weaken the body's ability to produce the intrinsic factor; also, some people appear to have a genetic predisposition that makes them more prone to pernicious anemia. **Hydrochloric acid helps absorption of B12; if acid production is weak, the absorption is lessened.** Calcium and thyroid hormone assist as well. Aging more likely lessens some of the many factors needed for ideal absorption of B12, so deficiency symptoms are more common in older people.

Cobalamin is absorbed primarily from the last part of the small intestine, the ileum. In the blood, it is bound to a protein globulin to be carried to the various tissues. The body actually stores vitamin B12, so any deficiencies may take several years to develop. The highest concentrations of B12 are found in the liver, heart, kidney, pancreas, brain, testes, blood, and bone marrow—all active metabolic tissues. The red vitamin is important to the blood, and about 5 mcg circulate daily between the digestive tract and the liver.

Cobalamin is made in nature by microbial synthesis, produced by bacteria in the intestinal tracts of animals and stored in their tissues. Certain yeasts, molds, and algae can also produce this vitamin. Some B12 is made during fermentation of foods as well. Cobalamin is the naturally occurring vitamin B12, while cyanocobalamin, as B12 is often known, is actually the commercial variety of B12 and contains a cyanide molecule attached to the cobalt. B12 is not synthesized but, like penicillin, must be grown in bacteria or molds and then processed. Other forms of B12 include hydroxycobalamin (technically, B12A), aquacobalamin (B12B), and nitrocobalamin (B12C).

Sources. B12 is found in significant amounts only in animal protein foods. Fermented foods, including tempeh and miso, may contain small amounts of this vitamin, depending on the method of fermentation. B12 is also manufactured by bacteria in the human intestines, but it is not known how much we can naturally absorb and use from that source. In general, digestion and absorption must be good for adequate B12 to be obtained. Many laxatives and overuse of antacids can reduce absorption and deplete stores of B12.

Our primary food sources of vitamin B12 include meat, most fish (especially the oily ones like trout, herring, and mackerel), crab, scallops, shrimp, oysters, eggs (the yolk), and milk products, especially live-culture yogurt. Such organ meats as liver, heart, and kidney are particularly high in B12. The vegan—that is, the strict vegetarian who consumes no animal-source foods—is not getting the necessary vitamin B12 from diet (although tempeh, a fermented soybean product, and some sprouts may contain some vitamin B12); thus vegans will often need an additional supplement (which absorbs well) or periodic injections.

Functions. Although vitamin B12 apparently does not have as many functions as some of the other B vitamins, it does have some important ones. It is essential for the metabolism of the nerve tissue and necessary for the health of the entire nervous system.

The outer wrapping of most nerves (the myelin sheath) does not appear to form properly under conditions of B12 deficiency. Vitamin B12 stimulates growth and increases appetite in children. Cobalamin, along with iron, folic acid, copper, protein, and vitamins C and B6, is needed for the formation of normal red blood cells. When this vitamin is deficient, the cells become oversized and poorly shaped (the condition of pernicious anemia referred to on page 125).

Vitamin B12 is the "energy" vitamin, as it often increases the energy level, whether obtained from eating the B12 foods or from supplemental use. There may be several reasons for this. Cobalamin stimulates the body's utilization of proteins, fats, and carbohydrates. It also helps iron function better and is important for the synthesis of DNA and RNA, as well as for the production of choline, another B vitamin, and methionine, an amino acid.

Uses. Vitamin B12 is also known as the "longevity" vitamin, possibly because it helps the energy level and activity of the nervous system in the elderly. B12 injections (the main therapeutic use of this vitamin) have been a common practice of many doctors for the treatment of fatigue, and in my experience, it works often. However, it would only be a "cure" when the tiredness is a result of B12 deficiency. There are many reasons for fatigue. As we age, our digestion and absorption are not usually as finely tuned as when we were young, particularly when we eat and live the way most of us do. **And vitamin B12, even though it is needed in such small doses, is one of the most difficult vitamins to acquire through diet and to metabolize.** The "red vitamin" is the main "anti-fatigue" vitamin; often given along with folic acid, it helps boost energy and prevents most anemia, provided there is good iron absorption and hydrochloric acid production. Medically speaking, it is wise to check patients with fatigue for anemia and to measure vitamin B12 and folic acid levels before embarking on a treatment regimen.

Given intramuscularly, usually in doses of 500 to 1,000 mcg (0.5–1.0 mg), B12 is used 1 to 3 times weekly for a period of time to both boost energy and, in adults, to help with appetite suppression in weight loss programs. These amounts also replenish the B12 stores. It has a mild diuretic effect as well and may be used premenstrually to diminish water retention symptoms. In the treatment of pernicious anemia and the earlier symptoms of B12 deficiency, injections of cobalamin or its variants are usually necessary because most everyone with deficiency has poor absorption. **It is difficult to become B12 deficient from diet alone, unless someone has been on a strict vegan diet for years and does not take additional supplements.** In any anemia, it is wise to supplement B12, because it helps the red blood cells develop to a point where protein, folic acid, iron, and vitamin C can then complete their maturation so that they can better carry oxygen and energy to all of the cells.

Vitamin B12 will stimulate growth in many malnourished children. In older people, it has helped with boosting energy levels as well as treating psychological symptoms, including senile psychosis. B12 has also been used to help treat osteoarthritis and osteoporosis and for neuralgias, such as Bell's palsy, trigeminal neuralgia, or diabetic neuropathy. It has likewise been used in the treatment of hepatitis, shingles, asthma and other allergies, allergic dermatitis, hives, eczema, and bursitis. Cobalamin has been used for many other symptoms besides fatigue, including nervousness and irritability, insomnia, memory problems, depression, and poor balance. Vitamin B12 is something to keep in mind when we are not "feeling our health."

Deficiency and toxicity. There have been no known toxic effects from megadoses of vitamin B12. Thousands of times more than the RDA have been injected both intravenously and intramuscularly without any ill consequences—on the contrary, there is often some benefit. Vitamin B12 deficiency usually results from a combination of factors. The restricted diet of some vegetarians or that of people in poor nations can be very limited in B12. Because the absorption into the body is so finely tuned, depletion and deficiency occur even more commonly from poor digestion and assimilation, or from deficient production of intrinsic factor. That is why it is so important to be aware of B12 and use some sort of supplementation once a deficiency has been diagnosed. Vitamin B12 blood levels, along with folic acid levels, are the most common vitamin tests performed by doctors. As we age, it is more likely that we may become B12 deficient. Also, alcoholics and people with malabsorption or dementia may have low B12 levels. Because the body stores vitamin B12, it may take several years to become deficient with dietary restriction or a decrease in the intrinsic factor.

With B12 deficiency, the body forms large, immature red blood cells, resulting in a megaloblastic anemia. Pernicious anemia refers to the deficiency in blood cells as well as the myriad of psychological and nerve symptoms. The anemia usually generates more fatigue and weakness. Menstrual problems, even amenorrhea (lack of menstrual flow), may also occur in B12-deficient women.

The strict vegetarian is of more concern than the average meat- and dairy-eating person. B12 is not found in the vegetable kingdom other than in foods fermented by certain bacteria (most fermented foods have some vitamin B12). However, in vegetarians there is usually a high folic acid intake, and because folic acid and B12 work similarly in the body, a B12 deficiency may be masked for a period of time before more pronounced symptoms may occur. If B12 is deficient in an animal eater, then we pretty much know there is a problem in absorption of the vitamin.

Most problems of B12 deficiency affect the blood, energy level, state of mind, and nervous system. Often, subtle symptoms may start with the nervous system. As mentioned earlier, B12 nourishes the myelin sheaths over the nerves, which help maintain the normal electrical conductivity through the nerves. Soreness or weakness of the arms or legs, decreased sensory perceptions, difficulty in walking or speaking, neuritis, a diminished reflex response, or limb jerking may result from B12 deficiency. Psychological symptoms may include mood changes, with mental slowness being one of the first symptoms.

The problems related to the nervous system caused by vitamin B12 deficiency can lead to permanent damage, not correctable by B12 supplementation. This irreversible nerve damage may occur when the B12 deficiency effect on the red blood cells is masked by adequate levels of folic acid, as just discussed. More severe pernicious anemia can cause a red, sensitive tongue, referred to as "strawberry tongue," which may even ulcerate, and nerve or brain and spinal cord degeneration, which can cause weakness, numbness, tingling, shooting pains, and sensory hallucinations. Paranoid symptoms may even occur. In the early part of the twentieth century, pernicious anemia was often a fatal disease.

RDAs for Vitamin B12	
Set in 1998 by the National Academy of Sciences, the RDAs for B12 are as follows:	
Age	**RDA**
Infants, 0–6 months	400 pcg
Infants, 7–12 months	500 pcg
Children, 1–3 years	900 pcg
Children, 4–8 years	1.2 mcg
Males, 9–13 years	1.8 mcg
Males, 14 years and older	2.4 mcg
Females, 9–13 years	1.8 mcg
Females, 14 years and older	2.4 mcg
Pregnant females of any age	2.6 mcg
Lactating females of any age	2.8 mcg

Requirements. Vitamin B12 is essential but required only in minute amounts, measured not in milligrams like most other vitamins, but in micrograms, a thousand times smaller.

From 10 to 20 mcg daily is a good insurance level, although some people may need increased amounts with higher protein intake. Vitamin B12 is often taken in higher doses, 500 to 1,000 mcg per day, to relieve fatigue. Injections in these amounts are used to treat a variety of low-energy and mental symptoms previously described as well as during some weight loss programs. When there is fatigue or anemia, it is a good idea to get the blood level of B12 checked by a doctor. It may lead to a very simple and successful treatment.

OTHER B VITAMINS

I include here other important B vitamins that are known primarily by their chemical names. These are biotin, choline, folic acid, inositol, and para-aminobenzoic acid (PABA). Biotin, choline, and inositol are often thought of together because of their similar functions. Folic acid is closely related to amino acid metabolism and maturation of blood cells and vitamin B12, and folic acid deficiency is possibly among the more common deficiencies of the B vitamin family. PABA is popularly used to promote healthy hair and as a sunscreen to protect the skin from burning. In general, these vitamins are commonly found in those foods that contain other B vitamins, such as brewer's yeast, liver, wheat germ, and whole grains. Folic acid is also abundant in the dark green leafy vegetables. Deficiencies of these important nutrients, like those of other B vitamins, can affect the skin, nervous system, and mental and physical energy levels and attitudes.

After discussion of these five essential B vitamins, I mention three other substances—orotic acid, pangamic acid, and amygdalin or laetrile. These are not B vitamins in the strict sense nor are they essential, but they have become known as vitamins B13, B15, and B17, respectively.

Biotin

B7 A fairly recently designated B vitamin, biotin was discovered by the deficiency symptoms created through consuming large amounts of raw eggs (about 30% of the diet). Avidin, a protein and carbohydrate molecule in the egg white, binds with biotin in the stomach and decreases its absorption. Cooking destroys the avidin, so the only concern about this interaction is with raw egg consumption. Otherwise, biotin is one of the most stable of the B vitamins.

Sources. Many foods contain biotin, but most have only trace amounts. It is hard to obtain enough from diet alone. Luckily, our friendly intestinal bacteria (lactobacillus) produce biotin. This vitamin is also found in egg yolks, liver, brewer's yeast, unpolished rice, peanuts, almonds, carrots, tomato, chard, onion, cabbage, and milk.

Functions. The biotin coenzymes participate in the metabolism of fat. Biotin is needed for fat production and in the synthesis of fatty acids. **These roles make biotin particularly important for formation of new tissue, especially skin tissue, because skin cells die and are replaced very rapidly.** Biotin also helps incorporate amino acids into protein and facilitates the synthesis of the pyrimidines, part of nucleic acids, and therefore it helps in the formation of DNA and RNA.

Uses. A common use of biotin is to help normalize fat metabolism and utilization in weight-reduction programs and to help reduce blood sugar in diabetic patients, with a dosage of between 200 and 400 mcg per day. Biotin has also been widely used to prevent or slow the progression of graying hair or baldness. However, this may work only when these symptoms are related to biotin deficiency, but because of the nutrient and protein support of biotin, the vitamin may indeed have some hair-stimulating effect. The use of biotin in relation to the scalp is not limited to adults. In infants, the most common biotin deficiency-related symptom is cradle cap, an inflammatory condition in which crusty whitish/yellowish patches appear around the infant's scalp, head, and eyebrows as well as behind the ears.

Biotin is often used for such problems as dermatitis or eczema, especially in infants, most often with appropriate intake of other B vitamins, such as riboflavin, niacin, and pyridoxine, and vitamin A. It has also been used to treat muscle pains, although skin and hair are the main focus of supplementation. More recently, biotin has been used for diabetics and those with an overgrowth of intestinal yeast.

Deficiency and toxicity. There is no known toxicity with biotin, even in high amounts. Excesses are easily eliminated in the urine. For these reasons, there is also no tolerable upper limit for biotin in the dietary guidelines issued by the National Academy of Sciences. Deficiency symptoms are also uncommon. Unless we are on a raw-egg diet or have taken a lot of antibiotics, especially sulfa, which diminish the biotin-producing intestinal bacteria, we are usually secure against a biotin deficiency.

Symptoms that have been seen with biotin deficiency include dry and flaky skin, loss of energy, insomnia, increases in cholesterol, sensitivity to touch, inflamed eyes, hair loss, muscle weakness, muscle cramps, lack of coordination, loss of appetite, nausea or vomiting, depression, and impaired fat metabolism. Several enzymes depend on biotin to function properly. Without them, we cannot utilize our foods as well.

Biotin deficiency is sometimes seen in babies when a biotin-deficient formula is used or there is some problem with intestinal biotin synthesis. If this occurs, hair loss, muscle weakness, irritated eyes, and a scaly rash may result. In some studies in juveniles, biotin deficiency was seen to result in hair loss and occasional balding. With more advanced biotin deficiency in people of all ages, elevation in cholesterol, anemia, or changes in the electrocardiogram may occur.

Requirements. Public health guidelines for biotin intake have dropped sharply since the mid-1990s, from recommended ranges in hundreds of micrograms to the present-day guidelines. The jury may still be out on optimal intake for this vitamin, but doses in the 100 to 200 mcg range may provide a good safety margin.

AI Levels for Biotin

The AI levels for biotin, set in 1998 by the Institute of Medicine at the National Academy of Sciences, are as follows:

Age	AI Level
Males and females, 0–6 months	5 mcg
Males and females, 7–12 months	6 mcg
Males and females, 1–3 years	8 mcg
Males and females, 4–8 years	12 mcg
Males, 9–13 years	20 mcg
Males, 14–18 years	25 mcg
Males, 19 years and older	30 mcg
Females, 9–13 years	20 mcg
Females, 14–18 years	25 mcg
Females, 19 years and older	30 mcg
Pregnant females of any age	30 mcg
Lactating females of any age	35 mcg

Choline

 Choline is the newest official member of the B vitamin family, receiving public health guidelines for the first time in 1998. Choline has several unique connections to fat, and its name reflects this fact—*chole* in Greek means "bile," and bile is the liver's unique fluid for processing fat. Choline is also nestled into the fat layers of the membranes of every cell in the body, and it modifies membrane fats to give them greater flexibility in sustaining the cells. Because it helps with the utilization of fats in the body, choline is often referred to as one of the "lipotropic" B vitamins. This vitamin is widely available in food but is sensitive to water and may be destroyed by cooking, food processing, improper food storage, and the intake

of various drugs, including alcohol, estrogen, and sulfa antibiotics.

Choline is easily absorbed from the intestines and is one of the only vitamins that crosses the blood-brain barrier into the spinal fluid to be involved directly in brain chemical metabolism. Choline is sometimes referred to as the "memory" vitamin, as it is an important part of the neurotransmitter acetylcholine. Its incorporation into this neurotransmitter has also made it especially valuable in improvement of nerve-muscle function. Choline has been used experimentally to help improve movement and coordination in neurodegenerative diseases like Parkinson's and Alzheimer's, for example.

Sources. Choline is present in all living cells and is widely distributed in plants and animals. Humans can synthesize choline from the amino acid glycine. The highest amount of choline is present in lecithin, usually obtained from soybeans. Other good sources include egg yolk, brewer's yeast, wheat germ, fish, peanuts, some leafy greens, and liver and other organ meats. Peanuts, potatoes, cauliflower, lentils, oats, sesame seeds, and flaxseeds also contain this B vitamin. In addition, choline is probably manufactured by intestinal bacteria.

Functions. Choline as phosphatidylcholine is a basic component of soy lecithin and in that form helps in the emulsification of fats and cholesterol in the body, by helping form smaller fat globules in the blood and aiding the transport of fats through the smaller vasculature and in and out of the cells. Choline is combined with fatty acids, glycerol, and phosphate to make lecithin, an important part of cell membranes. (For more on lecithin, see page 70 in chapter 4, Lipids—Fats and Oils.)

Choline is also an integral part of the neurotransmitter acetylcholine. Its availability preserves the integrity of the electrical transmission across the gaps between nerves, and this helps the flow of electrical energy within the nervous system. It is also important to the health of the myelin sheaths covering the nerve fibers. Choline helps the liver and gallbladder function and is vital to brain chemistry, as it seems to aid thinking capacity and memory.

Choline's unique chemistry also makes it important in the body's detoxification system. This vitamin is called a *trimethylated* molecule because it contains three methyl groups. The liver needs this supply of methyl groups to neutralize many toxins. Methyl groups like those supplied by choline also play a key role in regulating the activity of our genes.

Uses. There are a great many uses for this important B vitamin. Choline may be helpful in the treatment of nerve conduction problems, memory deficiencies, muscle twitching, heart palpitations, and Alzheimer's disease, where it seems to help brain function and slow the progression of the disease. Evidence has been mixed, however, as to effectiveness of phosphatidylcholine/lecithin treatment for Alzheimer's disease; it has certainly not been shown to be a great panacea.

Choline has also been used for many kinds of liver and kidney problems, especially hepatitis and cirrhosis, by improving emulsification, transport, and utilization of fat. It may actually help with general body detoxification by "decongesting" the liver of excess fats. Choline has been helpful in reducing some side effects of the phenothiazine drugs, which may cause abnormal facial muscle twitching and spasms, a syndrome called *tardive dyskinesia*. It probably works by increasing acetylcholine function, thus promoting the transmission functions at nerve synapses. Recently, purified egg lecithin, which contains choline, has been used in the treatment of AIDS.

Other possible uses for choline are for headaches, dizziness, insomnia, constipation, glaucoma and other eye problems, abnormal ear noises such as tinnitus (ringing), hypoglycemia, and alcohol problems. Choline may be helpful for fatigue. Some athletes have benefited from choline supplementation. **With high cholesterol and high blood pressure, both important factors in cardiovascular disease, phosphatidylcholine (lecithin) may be helpful in reducing the progression of atherosclerosis.** It seems to be effective as a fat and cholesterol emulsifier, and supplementation has been shown to reduce some gallstones. Choline has also been used with some benefit in stroke patients.

Deficiency and toxicity. High doses of choline in the 10 to 15 gram range have been linked in nutrition research to vomiting, sweating, increased salivation, and unusual body odor. Most of these effects appear to be due to choline's nerve stimulation potential. High doses could also aggravate epileptic conditions for this same reason. The body odor symptom

appears to involve increased presence of trimethylamine, a breakdown product of choline. In some research studies, 5 to 10 gram doses of this vitamin have also been associated with loss of blood pressure and faintness or dizziness. For these reasons, the National Academy of Sciences established a tolerable upper limit for choline of 3.5 grams per day.

Mild deficiency of choline has been linked to fatigue, insomnia, poor ability of the kidneys to concentrate urine, and memory problems. Moderate deficiency has been indirectly linked to coronary heart disease and other heart-related problems because of the link between choline and homocysteine. Because choline is needed to convert homocysteine into other substances, choline deficiency can leave too much homocysteine in the bloodstream. When choline is depleted, fat metabolism and utilization may be decreased, conceivably leading to fat accumulations. However, the main concern could involve loss of cell membrane integrity and the effects on the myelin covering of the nerves.

Requirements. Choline is often supplemented at 500 mg along with the same amount of inositol because both are necessary for membrane integrity. Soy lecithin is the most common source for choline supplementation. One capsule of lecithin contains about 40 to 50 mg of choline, while a tablespoon (5 grams) of lecithin has about 500 mg of choline.

AI Levels for Choline

In 1998, the National Academy of Sciences established AI levels for choline as follows:

Age	AI Level
Infants, 0–6 months	125 mg
Infants, 7–12 months	150 mg
Children, 1–3 years	200 mg
Children, 4–8 years	250 mg
Males, 9–13 years	375 mg
Males, 14 years and older	550 mg
Females, 9–13 years	375 mg
Females, 14–18 years	400 mg
Females, 19 years and older	425 mg
Pregnant females of any age	450 mg
Lactating females of any age	550 mg

Therapeutic amounts of choline are usually in the 500 to 1,000 mg area. More than this may produce some side effects and is likely not needed, although some experiments have used higher amounts. It is best taken with other B vitamins. If large amounts of lecithin are taken, more calcium is usually needed to balance the phosphorus contained in the lecithin. Additional choline may be needed when higher amounts of niacin, such as 1 to 3 grams daily, are taken to lower cholesterol levels. Recently, high-quality, concentrated phosphatidylcholine capsules have become available for specific use of this nutrient in place of the more variable lecithin. Prevention of liver damage was the main criterion used in establishment of recommended levels.

Folic Acid (Folacin or Folate)

 Folic acid is another of the key water-soluble B vitamins. It received its name from the Latin word *folium,* meaning "foliage," because **folic acid is found in nature's leafy green vegetables, such as spinach, kale, and beet greens.** Folacin, a derivative of folic acid, is a dull yellow crystalline substance made up chemically of a pteridine molecule, PABA, and glutamic acid. It is actually a vitamin within a vitamin, with PABA as part of its structure. Folic acid is sensitive and easily destroyed in a variety of ways— by light, heat, any type of cooking, or an acid pH below 4. It can even be lost from foods when they are stored at room temperature for long periods. The potency of this B vitamin is diminished in most food processing and food preparation.

When folic acid is consumed, it is actively transported into the blood from the gastrointestinal tract, where it acts as a coenzyme for a multitude of functions and often is converted to its active form, tetrahydrofolic acid (THFA), in the presence of the niacin coenzyme (NADP) and vitamin C. In the body, folic acid is found mainly as methyl folate, and vitamin B12 is needed to convert it back to the active THFA form. Extra folic acid is stored in the liver, enough for 6 to 9 months of body use before deficiency symptoms might develop.

Folic acid was discovered in 1931 as a "cure" for the anemia of pregnancy. Eating extra yeast also seemed to relieve the symptoms of pernicious anemia, but the neurological symptoms of this disease either were not resolved or appeared later on, confirming some doctors' feelings that there were two different problems involved. In 1945, folic acid was isolated from spinach; we now know that B12 and folic acid produce two similar deficiency problems. B12 deficiency may lead to progressive and irreversible neurological damage, whereas a lack of folic acid will not, but taking a lot of folic acid may cover up the B12 anemia and other symptoms until it is too late for effective treatment with vitamin B12. Therefore, vitamin tablets of folic acid with over 400 mcg have been taken off the market and are available by prescription only. If megaloblastic anemia occurs (enlarged red blood cells), both folic acid and vitamin B12 levels should be checked to assure proper treatment and follow-up.

Sources. The best source of folic acid is foliage, the green leafy vegetables. These include spinach, kale, beet greens and even beets, chard, asparagus, and broccoli. Other sources are liver, kidney, and brewer's yeast. Starchy vegetables containing some folacin are corn, lima beans, garbanzo beans (chickpeas), green peas, sweet potatoes, artichokes, okra, and parsnips. Bean sprouts—such as lentil, mung, and soy—are particularly good, as are wheat germ or wheat flakes and soy flour. Whole wheat bread, other natural, whole-grain baked goods, and milk also have some folic acid. And many fruits have folic acid, such as oranges, cantaloupe, pineapple, banana, and many berries, including loganberries, boysenberries, and strawberries.

Remember, folic acid is available from fresh, unprocessed food, which is why it is so commonly deficient in our culture's processed-food diet. Luckily, though, it is easily absorbed, used, and stored by the body. It is also manufactured by intestinal bacteria, so if colon flora is healthy, we have another good source of folic acid.

Functions. Folic acid—or more specifically, its coenzyme tetrahydrofolic acid (THFA)—has functions similar to those of cobalamin, vitamin B12. Folic acid aids in red blood cell production by carrying the carbon molecule to the larger heme molecule, which is the iron-containing part of hemoglobin (the oxygen-carrying molecule of the red blood cells). With B12 and vitamin C, THFA helps in the breakdown and utilization of protein. With B12, it assists in many amino acid conversions, such as the methylation of methionine, serine, histidine, and even the B vitamin choline. Folic acid is also used in the formation of the nucleic acids for RNA and DNA. Actually, the anemia that results from folic acid deficiency comes from the lack of THFA and decreased synthesis of the purines and pyrimidines that make up the DNA. So folic acid has a fundamental role in the growth and reproduction of all cells.

Because folic acid is important to the division of cells in the body, it is even more essential during times of growth, such as pregnancy, a period of rapid cell multiplication. If there is a deficiency of folic acid, there is decreased nucleic acid synthesis and cell division is hampered. This deficiency can lead to low birth weight or growth problems in infants.

The relationship of folate to brain function and development may turn out to be one of the most critical examples of this vitamin's central place in nutrition. By helping to maintain the body's supply of methyl groups, folate allows for proper balancing of brain neurotransmitter levels, including the levels of catecholamines (like epinephrine and norepinephrine). Folate also lets us maintain supplies of tetrahydrobiopterin, a folatelike molecule that is needed for production of other brain neurotransmitters like serotonin. These multiple connections between folate and the brain are one reason why it has been the subject of recent research on Down's syndrome, where it appears to be both deficient and important as a treatment consideration.

In addition to these brain and nervous system connections, folate also plays a critical role in the development of an infant's nervous system. The likelihood of neural tube defects in infants—including the problems of anencephaly, encephalocele, and spina bifida—is increased by folate deficiency. In these neural tube problems, the brain may be underdeveloped, the skull incompletely formed, or spine malformed. Beginning in 1998, the government has required fortification of all enriched cereal grain products with folate as a way to help increase folate intake for women of childbearing age. Studies so far suggest that this approach has worked to some degree.

Folate supplementation has also been shown to be capable of reducing high blood levels of homocysteine. This relationships between folate and homocysteine is important because elevated homocysteine

is a primary risk factor for many forms of cardiovascular disease. More important research developments are expected in this area.

Uses. Folic acid is, of course, used to restore its deficiencies and treat the problems resulting from them. People who are stressed or fatigued or who have any loss of adrenal gland function may benefit from additional folic acid. Those who drink alcohol or take high amounts of vitamin C also require more of this vitamin. Also, epileptics on drug therapy require more folic acid, which may help them by improving mood and mental capacities. In patients with psoriasis, folate is used rapidly by the skin, thus it is needed in increased amounts. The elderly as well as teenagers on poor diets who eat no vegetables are often helped by folic acid supplementation.

With increased estrogen, as in pregnancy or when taking birth control pills, folic acid supplementation helps prevent deficiency symptoms. More is also required during lactation to support mother and baby. Folic acid is often used when there are any menstrual problems. Restless leg syndrome, which is characterized by creeping, irritating sensations in the legs and occurs most commonly in later pregnancy, is often

---

Clinical Uses of Folic Acid

Acne	Immune weakness
Alcoholism	Infection
Anemia	Lactation
Atherosclerosis	Neuropathy
Birth control pills	Organic brain
Canker sores	syndrome
Cervical cancer	Osteoporosis
Cervical dysplasia	Periodontal
Dementia	problems
Depression	Poor appetite
Diarrhea	Pregnancy
Down's syndrome	Restless leg
Elderly	syndrome
Estrogen	Seborrheic
supplementation	dermatitis
Fatigue	Skin ulcers
Gingivitis	Viral hepatitis
Gout	

helped by increasing folic acid, as it may specifically be a deficiency problem.

With both folic acid deficiency anemia and pernicious anemia, folic acid is usually supplemented along with vitamin B12. The fatigue, easy bruising, and inflammation of the tongue that may go along with anemia are often helped as well. Treatment of various blood diseases, osteoporosis, and atherosclerosis has been supported with folic acid. There is some suggestion that it helps in ischemia, with reports of improved blood flow to the eyes and improved vision in those with circulatory deficits.

Folic acid has been used for chronic diarrhea or malabsorption problems and to stimulate a depressed appetite. It may also be helpful in some cases of depression, dementia and brain disorders, epilepsy, or neuropathies, especially when deficient. Folic acid supports healthy skin and may help in healing skin ulcers, particularly of the leg, or seborrheic dermatitis. Usually a 1 mg tablet daily or an oral folate solution may be helpful in treating gingivitis or other periodontal diseases. It has been suggested and used with varying results, usually along with PABA and pantothenic acid, to prevent the graying of hair. Higher doses may have some use in healing dysplasia (precancerous cell changes) of the cervix, which is often associated with lowered folate levels. Further research is needed to substantiate some of these uses.

Deficiency and toxicity. Folic acid deficiency may still be one of the most common vitamin deficiencies. It is more likely to be a problem in the elderly, in alcoholics, in psychiatric patients, in epileptics, in women on birth control pills, and with those taking such drug therapies as the sulfa antibiotics and tetracyclines that deplete folic acid–producing bacteria in the colon. Pregnancy is a time for concern about sufficient folic acid intake (the RDA doubles during pregnancy). Also, those eating the standard American diet that is high in fats, meats, white flour, white sugar, and desserts may develop folic acid deficiency. Eating some fresh or lightly cooked vegetables daily will allow us to maintain normal folate levels.

There are no specific toxic symptoms from folic acid intake, at least up to 1 mg daily. At doses in the 2 to 5 mg range, supplemental folate can sometimes trigger some of the same mild symptoms it is ordinarily taken to prevent, including insomnia, irritability, general malaise, and sometimes intestinal irregularity. The possibility of these symptoms prompted the National Academy of Sciences in 1998 to set a tolerable upper limit for folate of 1 mg for adults. This limit applies only to folate supplements. In my clinical experience, it seems a little strict, and folate doses of 3 to 10 mg and even more would not be a problem for most people. However, excess folic acid in the face of a B12 deficiency, when B12 is not supplemented and absorbed, may lead to serious consequences. Folic acid will mask the B12-related anemia and early symptoms of B12 deficiency by helping the synthesis of DNA and red blood cell production, but folic acid has no effect on the myelin sheath covering the nerves, so nerve damage may occur where folic acid covers up a B12 deficiency. Higher doses of folate may also depress B12 levels. In recent research where higher levels (15 mg daily) of folate have been used, some side effects developed after a month of treatment. These included gastrointestinal symptoms, insomnia, irritability, and malaise.

Folic acid deficiency generates a picture similar to that of a B12 deficiency—anemia, fatigue, irritability, anorexia, weight loss, headache, sore and inflamed tongue, diarrhea, heart palpitations, forgetfulness, hostility, and a feeling of paranoia. Often, the mental symptoms occur before the anemia, with poor memory (possibly from decreased RNA synthesis), general apathy, withdrawal, irritability, and a decrease in basic mental powers.

Folic acid–deficiency anemia is not correctable with iron, and as it progresses, it appears very different from iron-deficiency anemia. The blood shows large, irregular red blood cells, while low iron causes small red blood cells. In pregnancy, this megaloblastic anemia is of great concern. Folic acid deficiency is common during pregnancy, when the requirements are at least double those for the nonpregnant state. Because folic acid stores in the liver can last several months, deficiency symptoms are more likely in later pregnancy. The fetus can readily draw on the folic acid of the mother, and deficiencies can cause problems in both. The mother's folacin-deficiency mental symptoms of indifference, lack of motivation, withdrawal, or depression may be passed over as hormonal. The anemia may likewise not be considered a matter for concern. Serious problems can result from a major deficiency.

Toxemia of pregnancy, premature birth, and hemorrhage are all possible in addition to the mother's anemia. The fetus could develop birth deformities, brain damage, or show poor growth as a child; thus it is important to supplement folic acid during pregnancy.

In general, folic acid deficiencies can result from:

- Inadequate nutrition, particularly lack of fresh fruits and vegetables

- Poor absorption, as in malabsorption, with intestinal problems, with pellagra, or after stomach or intestinal surgery

- Metabolic problems, such as those created by alcohol, smoking, or drug use

- Excessive demands by tissues, as with stress, illness, or pregnancy

Requirements. Many factors increase the minimum requirement for folic acid. But one out of five people in the United States get under 50% of the RDA for folate. This reveals why disorders involving folic acid deficiency are so common. Between 180 and 200 mcg of folic acid are needed daily to maintain the tissue stores of folate. As mentioned, during pregnancy, times of stress or illness, or with alcohol use, the demands are increased, and a 200 mcg daily intake is not sufficient for supporting folic acid functions and maintaining tissue stores. Birth control pills may reduce absorption of this vitamin by 50%. Other drugs, including the sulfa antibiotics, phenobarbital, and antiepileptic drugs such as Dilantin and Mysoline, may also interfere with absorption or metabolism. Cholesterol-lowering drugs (like cholestyramine), biguanide drugs (like buformin, phenformin, or metformin used in the treatment of diabetes), and potassium-sparing diuretics (like triamterene) can also deplete folate supplies. Consumption of more than 2,000 mg of vitamin C per day also increases the need for folic acid. Anyone in these situations needs supplements of folic acid.

Most vitamin formulas contain 400 mcg of folic acid. Higher amounts, such as 1 mg, 1.5 mg, or even 10 mg, are available only by prescription because of the concern of masking vitamin B12 deficiency. Some doctors describe impressive results in many patients, especially the elderly, with injections of 1,000 mcg of

B12 and 10 mg of folic acid. The suggested therapeutic dosages for most uses of folic acid or treating deficiency problems is about 1 mg twice daily; it may take several months for this vitamin therapy to correct the deficiency and replenish stores of folic acid. Some studies are researching folic acid doses of 5 to 15 mg and even up to 60 mg daily.

AI Levels and RDAs for Folic Acid

The RDAs for folic acid, set in 1998 by the Institute of Medicine at the National Academy of Sciences, are as follows:

Age	AI/RDA
Infants, 0–6 months	65 mcg (AI)
Infants, 7–12 months	80 mcg (AI)
Children, 1–3 years	150 mcg (RDA)
Children, 4–8 years	200 mcg (RDA)
Males, 9–13 years	300 mcg (RDA)
Males, 14 years and older	400 mcg (RDA)
Females, 9–13 years	300 mcg (RDA)
Females, 14 years and older	400 mcg (RDA)
Pregnant females of any age	600 mcg (RDA)
Lactating females of any age	500 mcg (RDA)

Inositol

 Inositol, also part of the B vitamin complex, is closely associated with choline. Like choline, inositol (as phosphatidylinositol) is also found in lecithin, although in lesser amounts than choline, and acts as a lipotropic agent (milder than choline) in the body, helping to emulsify fats. The body can produce its own inositol from glucose, so it is not really essential. We have high stores of inositol; its concentration in the body is second-highest of the B vitamins, surpassed only by niacin.

Sources. Inositol is present in both plants and animals. It is part of phospholipids in animals; in plants, it is contained in phytic acid, which can bind calcium and iron. It is not totally clear how inositol is produced by the body; it may be made by intestinal bacteria. It is stored in the body but drinking lots of coffee can deplete these stores. Inositol is found in whole, unprocessed grains, citrus fruits (except lemons), can-

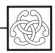

taloupe, brewer's yeast, unrefined molasses, and liver. It is also available in wheat germ, lima beans, raisins, peanuts, cabbage, and some nuts. And, of course, lecithin is a good source.

Functions. Inositol, as phosphatidylinositol, has its primary function in cell membrane structure and integrity. Other functions of phosphatidylinositol are not well researched, but its role in brain nutrition is emerging as perhaps the most critical. Chemical signaling between brain cells clearly becomes impaired when inositol is deficient, and the effectiveness of some psychiatric drugs like lithium may well depend on inositol status. Inositol is especially important for the cells of the bone marrow, eye tissue, and intestines. In addition, it may have something to do with hair growth.

Uses. Although inositol has been used to treat and prevent progression of atherosclerosis throughout the body and to help reduce cholesterol, there is no good evidence from human studies that inositol lowers cholesterol and protects against cardiovascular disease. As a mild lipotropic agent, though, it is commonly used by overweight people to help with weight loss, and it may help in redistributing body fat. Exercise helps, too, of course.

Inositol helps promote healthy hair and skin. It has been used to treat eczema, and it may help the hair, especially if there is an inositol deficiency. For sleep, 500 mg of inositol before bed has a mild anti-anxiety effect (perhaps a placebo) as well as possibly helping to utilize fat and cholesterol during sleep. Inositol has also had some success therapeutically in improving the nerve function in diabetic patients with pain and numbness due to nerve degeneration. Generally, diabetic people should take extra inositol. People with multiple sclerosis may also receive some benefit with inositol supplementation, as there seems to be a higher percentage of inositol deficiency in nerve cell membranes in those patients.

Deficiency and toxicity. There is no known toxicity with inositol even in amounts of 50 grams, which is much higher than normal use. Deficiencies are also uncommon, because inositol is so available in foods and the body also makes it. Caffeine, however, can produce an inositol deficiency. Some problems that have been associated with low levels of inositol in the body are eczema, constipation, eye problems, hair

loss, and elevations of cholesterol. There may also be a greater propensity for fatty plaques to form in the heart and arteries and more likelihood for cardiovascular disease.

Requirements. There is no specific RDA for inositol, because it can be made in our bodies. We usually obtain it readily from food in an amount of about 1 gram daily. A therapeutic dosage is usually about 500 mg; however, it should be taken with choline and other B vitamins and mainly as lecithin, which contains the natural balance of phospholipids. **I generally do not recommend taking separate inositol capsules. Needs are increased with regular coffee consumption of more than 2 cups daily.** Soy lecithin contains about 40 mg of phosphatidylinositol per capsule.

Para-Aminobenzoic Acid (PABA)

 Para-aminobenzoic acid (PABA) is also a member of the B vitamins and is part of the folic acid molecule. PABA itself is readily available in food and is made by intestinal bacteria. It is known specifically for its nourishment to hair and its usefulness as a sunscreen.

Sources. PABA is found in liver, brewer's yeast, wheat germ, and whole grains such as rice, as well as in eggs and molasses. It is stored in body tissues and is also synthesized by the natural bacterial flora in our intestines.

Functions. As part of the coenzyme tetrahydrofolic acid, PABA aids in the metabolism and utilization of amino acids and is also supportive of blood cells, particularly the red blood cells. PABA supports folic acid production by the intestinal bacteria. PABA is important to skin, hair pigment, and intestinal health. Used as a sunscreen, it also can protect against the development of sunburn and skin cancer from excess ultraviolet light exposure.

Uses. Although PABA has been much used in attempts to stimulate hair growth and to turn gray hair back to its natural color, it has not had wide success in such uses. It may work in some cases that are related to a PABA deficiency. If graying of hair is caused by vitamin deficiency, it is likely a deficiency of a combination of vitamins, mostly the various Bs. PABA is usually used along with biotin, pantothenic acid, and folic acid in the restoration of hair, often with vitamin E as well. PABA is also used to reduce aging of the skin and lessen wrinkles. Vitiligo, a skin depigmenting condition, which could result from deficient hydrochloric acid, vitamin C, or pantothenic acid, may be helped somewhat by PABA, both orally and as a cream. PABA ointment is used commonly to prevent and treat sunburns and, with vitamin E, is often applied to other burns.

Deficiency and toxicity. It is possible that high doses of PABA can be somewhat irritating to the liver; in addition, nausea and vomiting have occurred, as have anorexia, fever, skin rash, and even vitiligo. Deficiency problems are not very common; they occur more frequently with the use of sulfa drugs or other antibiotics that alter the functioning of intestinal bacteria and therefore the production of PABA. General fatigue, irritability, depression, nervousness, graying hair, headache, and constipation or other digestive symptoms may occur. Several patients have told me that they are sensitive to PABA in vitamin formulas and thus cannot take them (most vitamin combinations contain PABA). I do not know what this reaction is unless it is some allergy to the PABA molecule.

Requirements. No RDA is listed for PABA. It is available in supplements of 50 to 1,000 mg. Up to 1,000 mg is used therapeutically in a time-released capsule, although the common treatment amount is usually about 50 to 100 mg 3 times daily. If we take antibiotics, we might increase our intake of PABA for a while, although PABA taken with sulfa antibiotics may reduce their effectiveness. A therapeutic approach used by some authorities to attempt to restore normal hair color is 1,000 mg, time-released, daily for 6 days a week, taken with 400 mcg of folic acid.

Vitamin B13 (Orotic Acid)

 I mention orotic acid here only for the sake of completeness. It is not really recognized as a vitamin, but it may be an accessory nutrient. Actually, there is not much information about orotic acid. It has been used recently as orotate salts combined with such minerals as calcium, magnesium, and potassium. This is based on work by German doctor Hans Nieper. Nieper's work has included treatment of multiple sclerosis and other chronic diseases with these mineral orotates. His experience concluded that orotate salts were active transporters of these minerals into the blood from the gastrointestinal tract. The salts then separate from the mineral in the blood, allowing the mineral to be used and leaving orotic acid available. Some recent research has verified the fact that orotic acid helps fix magnesium, and for this reason it may be involved in many magnesium-related events. These events include maintaining proper heart rhythm, protecting the heart from excessive response to stress, and allowing blood vessels to dilate when necessary. Because magnesium plays such a critical role in relaxing the muscles around the intestine, the use of orotic acid to help treat certain gastrointestinal diseases may also turn out to be important.

Orotic acid is found in a few natural food sources—for example, milk products and some root vegetables, such as carrots, beets, and Jerusalem artichokes. Orotic acid is a nucleic acid precursor and is needed for DNA and RNA synthesis. The body can make orotic acid for this purpose from its amino acid pool. As long as protein nutrition is adequate, the body can carry on nucleic acid synthesis. Neither toxicity nor deficiency of orotic acid are likely a concern.

Vitamin B15 (Pangamic Acid)

Pangamic acid is still a fairly controversial "vitamin." The quotation marks suggest that we are not sure whether it is in fact a vitamin. Pangamic acid has not yet been shown to be essential in the diet (by definition, vitamins must be supplied from external sources), and no symptoms or deficiency diseases are clearly revealed when consumption is restricted. The FDA has been concerned about the wide range of medical conditions it treats, primarily in other countries, and therefore pangamic acid is not readily available to the U.S. consumer. Because most of the information about pangamic acid is dated and is mainly from European and Soviet research, I discuss this substance here mainly for completeness.

Russia has been the most enthusiastic about pangamic acid, feeling that it is an important nutrient with physiological actions that can treat a multitude of symptoms and diseases. Russian scientists have shown that pangamic acid supplementation can reduce the buildup of lactic acid in athletes and thereby lessen muscle fatigue and increase endurance. It is used regularly and commonly in Russia for many problems, including alcoholism and drug addiction; mental problems such as those of aging and senility, minimal brain damage in children, autism, and schizophrenia; heart disease and high blood pressure; diabetes; skin diseases; liver disease; and chemical poisonings.

Because the FDA has taken pangamic acid products off the market, some people have used dimethyl glycine (DMG) as a substitute as it is thought to increase pangamic acid production in the body. DMG combines with gluconic acid to form pangamic acid. Researchers think that DMG is the active component of pangamic acid.

Sources. Pangamic acid was first isolated in 1951 by Drs. Ernest Krebs, Sr. and Jr., from apricot kernels, along with laetrile, termed vitamin B17. At that time, as today, they were not sure whether it was essential to life. Pangamic acid is also found in brewer's yeast, pumpkin and sunflower seeds, and beef blood, as well as in such whole grains as brown rice. Water and direct sunlight may reduce the potency and availability of B15 in these foods.

Functions. Pangamic acid is mainly a methyl donor, which helps in the formation of certain amino acids such as methionine. It may play a role in the oxidation of glucose and in cell respiration. By this function, it may reduce hypoxia (deficient oxygen) in cardiac and other muscles. Like vitamin E, it acts as an antioxidant, helping to lengthen cell life through its protection from oxidation. Pangamic acid is also thought to offer mild stimulation to the endocrine and nervous systems, and by enhancing liver function, it may help in the detoxification process.

Uses. Although many of these uses are not proven, there have been reports of pangamic acid or DMG providing some benefits for a wide range of symptoms, diseases, and metabolic problems. It may be useful for such symptoms as headaches, angina and musculoskeletal chest pain, shortness of breath, insomnia, and general stress—to be used, of course, only after specific medical conditions are ruled out. B15 has also been shown to lower blood cholesterol, so it could provide some nutritional support for those with high serum cholesterol or cardiovascular problems or be used to reduce heart and blood vessel dis-

ease risks. It may also help improve circulation and general oxygenation of cells and tissues, so it may be used with any decreased cardiac or brain functions. Pangamic acid may be helpful in general for atherosclerosis and hypertension, America's most common diseases.

In Europe, vitamin B15 has been used to treat premature aging because of both its circulatory stimulus and its antioxidant effect. It is felt to be a helpful protectant from pollutants, especially carbon monoxide. Pangamic acid (and possibly DMG) support for anyone living in a large polluted city or with a high-stress lifestyle could be a wave of the future. In Russia, a big use of pangamic acid has been for treating those with alcohol problems, possibly reducing the craving. It has been reported to diminish hangover symptoms when alcohol has been abused. B15 has also been used to treat fatigue, as well as asthma and rheumatism, and it may even have some antiallergic properties. Some child psychiatrists have reported good results using pangamic acid in disturbed children; it may help by stimulating speaking ability and other mental functions. B15 may also be useful in problems of autism. More studies regarding all claims of the benefits of pangamic acid must be done, of course, to see which ones may be valid. But as of now, it certainly is a "vitamin" or supplemental nutrient with potential health benefits and research interest.

Deficiency and toxicity. There are no known toxic effects from even high amounts of pangamic acid; 50 to 100 mg (and even more) taken 3 times daily has revealed no side effects. There are reports of initial mild nausea with use of pangamates at high levels, but this only lasts a few days. There is limited information about deficiencies of pangamic acid. There are no clear problems when it is absent in the diet, although some diminished circulatory and oxygenation functions are possible. Decreased cell respiration—that is, decreased oxygen use by cells—may influence many other cellular functions that may lead to effects on the heart.

Requirements. There is no RDA for pangamic acid because at the time of this writing it is not legal to distribute B15 in the United States, although it was used as a supplement for some time in the 1970s. The most common form of pangamic acid was once calcium pangamate, but currently it is dimethyl glycine

(DMG), which may even be the active component that has been hailed in the Soviet Union. When used, pangamic acid or DMG is often taken with vitamin A and vitamin E. A common amount of DMG is 50 to 100 mg taken twice daily, usually with breakfast and dinner. This level of intake may improve general energy levels and support the immune system. It is also thought to reduce cravings for alcohol; thus it may be helpful in moderating chronic alcohol problems.

Vitamin B17 (Laetrile)

Vitamin B17, also known as *laetrile* and *amygdalin*, is another controversial "vitamin," as its source, the apricot kernel, becomes a focus of increasing interest. B17 was also discovered by Dr. Ernest T. Krebs Sr., who thought it a vitamin essential to health. Krebs first tried amygdalin therapeutically. Amygdalin is not digested in the stomach by hydrochloric acid but passes into the small intestine, where it is acted on by enzymes that split it into various compounds, which are then absorbed. Laetrile is a nitriloside compound composed of 4 molecules: 2 sugars, 1 benzaldehyde, and 1 cyanide. Using laetrile—alternately known as amygdalin, B17, or nitriloside—as a treatment for cancer is now illegal in the United States. Some people seeking such treatment go to Mexico or other laetrile-supportive countries.

Arguments against laetrile as a therapy cite concerns about possible cyanide toxicity as well as studies that show it is not effective as a cancer treatment. Studies cannot be completely objective, however, especially on a subject as complex as cancer, which is influenced by so many factors. The proponents of laetrile claim that cyanide is a natural molecule found in food and is not toxic in normal doses; laetrile treatment itself is not known to have any side effects in usual dosages. But obviously, considering Western medicine's use of chemotherapy, radiation, and surgery, side effects are not the main concern when treating a life-threatening disease. The proof in any treatment is ultimately whether it works.

Sources. Laetrile is found primarily in apricot kernels and comprises about 2% to 3% of the kernel. It is also available in the kernels of other fruits, such as plums, cherries, peaches, nectarines, and apples. Almonds are a second major food source of laetrile.

The fruit kernels or seeds generally have other nutrients as well—some protein, unsaturated fatty acids, and various minerals. B17 is not found with other B vitamins in yeasts. Many plants also contain some B17, with the sprouting seeds, especially mung bean sprouts, containing the highest amount.

Functions. The specific theoretical function of laetrile is its effect on cancer cells. Normal cells have an enzyme, rhodanese, that inactivates the cyanide molecule of the laetrile compound. Cancer cells do not possess this enzyme. In fact, they have an enzyme, beta-glucosidase, that releases the cyanide, which then poisons the cancer cells.

Uses. The main use for laetrile is in the treatment of cancer, particularly to reduce tumor size and further spread, and to alleviate the sometimes severe pains of the cancerous process. As I stated, more well-designed research needs to be done to determine whether this compound in its natural form is effective. Other uses reported for laetrile have been in the treatment of high blood pressure and rheumatism.

Deficiency and toxicity. There are no known problems caused by not consuming this "vitamin," other than, theoretically, a deficiency could increase the likelihood of developing cancer. There are, however, concerns over toxicity, because of the cyanide within the compound or possibly from other metabolic effects. Usually, treatment amounts are limited to 1 gram to reduce potential side effects, which initially are most likely gastrointestinal in nature. Toxicity of cyanide may be related to the functional status of a person's rhodanese enzymes. Toxicity of this molecule must be researched further.

Requirements. This nutrient is not required for optimum health as far as we know; in fact, distribution of it is against the law in the United States. When used, laetrile is administered at 250 to 1,000 mg daily. Higher amounts—up to 3 grams per day—have been used, but divided into several smaller dosages, each usually limited to 1 gram. If the source is whole apricot kernels, the quantity is usually about 10 to 20 kernels a day; 1 to 2 cups of fresh mung bean sprouts may provide an equivalent amount. If apricot kernels are blended or pulverized, it is suggested that they be consumed immediately.

Vitamin C (Ascorbic Acid)

C Vitamin C is an important essential nutrient—that is, we must obtain it from diet. It is found only in the fruit and vegetable foods and is highest in fresh, uncooked foods. Vitamin C is among the least stable vitamins, and cooking can destroy much of this water-soluble vitamin in foods. In recent years, the C of this much publicized vitamin has stood for *controversy*. With scientist Linus Pauling and others claiming that vitamin C has the potential to prevent and treat the common cold, flus, and cancer—all of which plague our society—concern has arisen in the medical establishment about these claims and the megadose requirements needed to achieve the hoped-for results. Some studies suggest that these claims have some validity; however, there is more personal testimony from avid users of ascorbic acid than there is irrefutable evidence. There has also been some recent research that disproves the claims about treatment and prevention of colds and cancer with vitamin C. In most cases, studies show vitamin C to be ineffective used in lower dosages than Pauling recommended. Overall, however, vitamin C research is heavily weighted to the positive side for its use in the treatment of many conditions.

The C also stands for *citrus*, where this vitamin is found. It could also stand for *collagen,* the protein cement that is formed with ascorbic acid as a required cofactor. Many foods contain vitamin C, and many important functions are mediated by it as well. Vitamin C is a weak acid and is stable in weak acids. Such alkalis as baking soda, however, destroy ascorbic acid. It is also easily oxidized in air and sensitive to heat and light. **Because it is contained in the watery part of fruits and vegetables, it is easily lost during cooking in water.** Loss is minimized when such vegetables as broccoli or brussels sprouts are cooked over water in a double boiler instead of directly in water. The mineral copper, present in the water or in the cookware, also diminishes the vitamin C content of foods.

Ascorbic acid was not isolated from lemons until 1932, although the scourge of scurvy, the vitamin C deficiency disease, has been present for thousands of years. It was first written about circa 1500 B.C. and then described by Aristotle in 450 B.C. as a syndrome characterized by lack of energy, gum inflammation,

tooth decay, and bleeding problems. In the 1700s, high percentages of sailors with the British navy and other fleets died from scurvy until researcher James Lind discovered that lemon juice could cure and also prevent this devastating and deadly disease. The ships then carried British West Indies limes for the sailors to consume daily to maintain health, and thus these sailors became known as "limeys." Other world cultures discovered their own sources of vitamin C. Powdered rose hips, acerola cherries, or spruce needles were consumed regularly, usually as teas, to prevent the scurvy disease.

In earlier times, humans consumed large amounts of vitamin C in their fresh and wholesome native diet, as apes (which also don't make vitamin C) still do. Most other animals, except guinea pigs, produce ascorbic acid in the liver from glucose, and in relative amounts much higher than we get from our diets today. For this reason, Pauling and others feel that the body needs somewhere between 2,000 and 9,000 mg of vitamin C daily. These amounts seem a little high to me, given the basic food values of vitamin C. Some authorities feel we need 600 to 1,200 mg daily based on extrapolations from the historical human diet. These levels can be obtained by eating sufficient fresh food; a diet that includes foods with high levels of vitamin C can provide several grams or more per day.

Ascorbic acid is readily absorbed from the intestines, ideally about 80% to 90% of that ingested. It is used by the body in about 2 hours and is then usually out of the blood within 3 to 4 hours. For this reason, it is suggested that vitamin C supplements be taken at 4-hour intervals rather than once a day; or it may be taken as time-released ascorbic acid. Vitamin C is used up even more rapidly under stressful conditions, with alcohol use, and with smoking. **The vitamin C blood levels of smokers are much lower than those of nonsmokers given the same intakes.** Other situations and substances that reduce absorption or increase utilization include fever, viral illness, antibiotics, cortisone, aspirin and other pain medicines, environmental toxins (such as DDT, petroleum products, or carbon monoxide), and exposure to heavy metals such as lead, mercury, or cadmium. Sulfa antibiotics increase elimination of vitamin C from the body by 2 to 3 times.

Some ascorbic acid is stored in the body, where it seems to concentrate in the organs of higher metabolic activity. These include the adrenal glands (about 30 mg), the pituitary, the brain, the eyes (especially the retinas), the ovaries, and the testes—a total of about 30 mg per pound of body weight. We likely need at least 200 mg a day through diet to maintain body stores—much more if we smoke, drink alcohol, are under stress, have allergies, are elderly, or have diabetes.

Vitamin C is a complex and important vitamin. The recommended amounts vary more widely than those for any other nutrient, ranging from the 60 mg or so to prevent deficiency up to 50 to 100 grams in treatments of various conditions, mainly viral illnesses. People commonly take 2 or 3 grams daily for maintenance and cold prevention. Even without any overt health problems, vitamin C requirements may vary as much as threefold or fourfold between one person and another. C is also the most commonly supplemented vitamin among the general public, either because of its good effects or the popular press.

Sources. The best-known sources of vitamin C are the citrus fruits—oranges, lemons, limes, tangerines, and grapefruits. The fruits with the highest natural concentrations are citrus fruits, rose hips, and acerola cherries, followed by papayas, cantaloupes, and strawberries. Good vegetable sources include red and green peppers (the best), broccoli, brussels sprouts, tomatoes, asparagus, parsley, dark leafy greens, and cabbage. There is not much available in whole grains, seeds, and beans; however, when these are sprouted, their vitamin C content shoots up. Sprouts, then, are good foods for winter and early spring, when other fresh fruits and vegetables are not as available. Animal foods contain almost no vitamin C; although fish, if eaten raw, has enough to prevent deficiency symptoms.

Natural vitamin C supplements are usually made from rose hips, acerola cherries, peppers, or citrus fruits. C can be synthesized from corn syrup, which is high in dextrose, much as it is made from glucose in most other animals' bodies. Synthetic ascorbic acid, although it can be concentrated for higher doses than natural extracts, is still usually made from food sources. Sago palm is another fairly new source of vitamin C supplements. It is used primarily as a lower allergenic source than the corn-extracted ascorbic acid.

Functions. One important function of vitamin C is in the formation and maintenance of collagen, the basis of connective tissue, which is found in skin, ligaments, cartilage, vertebral disks, joint linings, capillary walls, and the bones and teeth. **Collagen, and thus vitamin C, is needed to give support and shape to the body, to help wounds heal, and to maintain healthy blood vessels.** Specifically, ascorbic acid works as a coenzyme to convert proline and lysine to hydroxyproline and hydroxylysine, both important to the collagen structure.

Vitamin C also aids the metabolism of tyrosine, folic acid, and tryptophan. Tryptophan is converted in the presence of ascorbic acid to 5-hydroxytryptophan, which forms serotonin, an important brain chemical. Vitamin C also helps folic acid convert to its active form, tetrahydrofolic acid, and tyrosine needs ascorbic acid to form the neurotransmitter substances dopamine and epinephrine. C stimulates adrenal function and the release of norepinephrine and epinephrine (adrenaline), the stress hormones; however, prolonged stress depletes vitamin C in the adrenals and decreases the blood levels. Ascorbic acid also helps thyroid hormone production, and it aids in cholesterol metabolism, increasing its elimination and thereby assisting in lowering blood cholesterol.

C is an antioxidant vitamin, meaning it helps prevent oxidation of water-soluble molecules that could otherwise create free radicals, which may generate cellular injury and disease. The recycling of vitamin C back and forth between its reduced (ascorbate) and oxidized (ascorbyl radical) form is essential in maintaining the body's supply of vitamin E. C also indirectly protects vitamin A as well as some of the B vitamins, such as riboflavin, thiamin, folic acid, and pantothenic acid, from oxidation. Ascorbic acid acts as a detoxifier and may reduce the side effects of such drugs as cortisone, aspirin, and insulin; it may also reduce the toxicity of the heavy metals lead, mercury, and arsenic.

Vitamin C has been shown through continued research to stimulate the immune system; through this function, along with its antioxidant function, it may help in the prevention and treatment of infections and other diseases. Ascorbic acid may activate neutrophils, the most prevalent white blood cells, which work on the frontline defense in more hand-to-hand combat than other white blood cells. It also seems to increase production of lymphocytes, the white cells important in antibody production and in coordinating the cellular immune functions. In this way, C may be helpful against bacterial, viral, and fungal diseases. In higher amounts, ascorbic acid may actually increase interferon production and thus activate the immune response to viruses; it may also decrease the production of histamine, thereby reducing immediate allergy potential. Further research must be done for more definitive knowledge about vitamin C's actions in the prevention and treatment of disease.

When vitamin C gets broken down, it can readily be converted into three other molecules: lyxonic acid, threonic acid, and oxalic acid. These molecules have their own separate functions and roles to play in body chemistry. Our individual vitamin C requirements may be partly related to the levels of these C-derived substances in our metabolism.

Uses. There are a great many clinical and nutritional uses for ascorbic acid in its variety of available supplements. C for the common cold is indeed used widely; its use in the treatment of cancer is more controversial, probably because of the seriousness of the disease and the political environment within the medical system—anything nutritional or alternative in regard to cancer therapy is often looked upon with skepticism by orthodox physicians. For the prevention of cancer, however, there is reason for more optimism about the usefulness of vitamin C (as well as the other antioxidant nutrients—vitamin E, selenium, beta-carotene, and zinc) because of its effect in preventing the formation of free radicals (caused mainly by the oxidation of fats), which play a role in the genesis of disease.

Given the functions of vitamin C alone, it has a wide range of clinical uses. For the prevention and treatment of the common cold and flu syndrome, vitamin C produces a positive immunological response to help fight bacteria and viruses. Its support of the adrenal function and role in the production of the adrenal hormones epinephrine and norepinephrine can help the body handle infections and stress of all kinds. Because of this adrenal-augmenting response, as well as thyroid support provided by stimulating production of thyroxine (T4) hormone, vitamin C may help with problems of fatigue and slow metabolism. It also helps counteract the side effects of cortisone drug therapy and may counteract the decreased cellular immunity experienced during the course of treatment with these commonly used immune-suppressive drugs.

Because of ascorbic acid's role in immunity, its antioxidant effect, the adrenal support it provides, and probably its ability to make tissues healthy through its formation and maintenance of collagen, vitamin C is used to treat a wide range of viral, bacterial, and fungal infections and inflammatory problems of all kinds. I have used vitamin C successfully in many viral conditions, including colds, flus, hepatitis, *Herpes simplex* infections, mononucleosis, measles, and shingles. Recently, vitamin C has been shown in some studies to enhance the production and activity of interferon, an antiviral substance produced by our bodies. To affect these conditions, the vitamin C dosage is usually fairly high, at least 5 to 10 grams per day, but it is possible that much smaller doses are as effective. Vitamin C is also used to treat problems due to general inflammation from microorganisms, irritants, and decreased resistance; these problems may include cystitis, bronchitis, prostatitis, bursitis, both osteo- and rheumatoid arthritis, and some chronic skin problems (dermatitis). With arthritis, there is some suggestion that increased ascorbic acid may improve the integrity of membranes in joints. In gouty arthritis, vitamin C improves the elimination of uric acid (the irritant) through the kidneys. **Ascorbic acid has also been helpful for relief of back pain and pain from inflamed vertebral disks, as well as the inflammatory pain that is sometimes associated with rigorous exercise.** In asthma, vitamin C may relieve the bronchospasm caused by noxious stimuli or when this tight-chested feeling is experienced during exercise.

Vitamin C's vital function in helping produce and maintain healthy collagen allows it to support the body cells and tissues and bring more rapid healing to injured or aging tissues. Therefore, it is used by many physicians for problems of rapid aging, burns, fracture healing, bedsores and other skin ulcers, and to speed wound healing after injury or surgery. Peptic ulcers also appear to heal more rapidly with vitamin C therapy. The pre- and postsurgical use of vitamin C supplementation can have great benefits. With its collagen function, adrenal support, and immune response support, it helps the body defend against infection, supports tissue health and healing, and improves the ability to handle the stress of surgery. Vitamin A and zinc are the other important pre- and postsurgical nutrients shown by research to reduce hospitalization time and increase healing rates, thereby preventing a number of potential complications.

Vitamin C is also used to aid those withdrawing from drug addictions to such substances as narcotics and alcohol as well as to nicotine, caffeine, and even sugar, three common addictions and abuses. High-level ascorbic acid may decrease withdrawal symptoms from these substances and increase the appetite and feeling of well-being. For this reason, it may be helpful in some depression and other mental problems associated with detoxification during withdrawal. Vitamin C also may reduce the effects of pollution, likely through its antioxidant effect, its detoxifying help, and its adrenal and immune support; specifically, it may participate in protecting us from smog, carbon monoxide, lead, mercury, and cadmium.

Vitamin C is a natural laxative and may help with constipation problems. In fact, the main side effect of too much C intake is diarrhea. For iron-deficiency anemia, vitamin C helps the absorption of iron (especially the nonheme or vegetable-source iron) from the gastrointestinal tract. In diabetes, it is commonly used to improve the utilization of blood sugar and thereby reduce it, but there is no clear evidence that regular C usage alone can prevent diabetes. There are some preliminary reports that ascorbic acid may help prevent cataract formation (probably through its antioxidant effect) and may be helpful in the prevention and treatment of glaucoma, as well as certain cases of male infertility caused from the clumping together of sperm, which decreases sperm function.

Vitamin C has a probable role in the prevention and treatment of atherosclerosis and thereby in reducing the risks of heart disease and its devastating results. It has been shown to reduce platelet aggregation, a factor important in reducing the formation of plaque and clots. Ascorbic acid has a triglyceride- and cholesterol-reducing effect and, more important, may help to raise the "good" HDL. This action needs further investigation, although the research is supportive so far. It is also vital to the prevention of scurvy, which really takes very little C, about 10 mg per day. Nutrition research studies make it clear that our vitamin C supplies become more depleted in the normal course of aging. For this reason, the risk of deficiency may be increased in later life, regardless of our state of health.

To adequately explore the cancer and vitamin C issue, the debate deserves a book by itself; thus I will not discuss it at length here. Suffice it to say, however, if we closely analyze the functions that C performs in the body (antioxidant, immune support, interferon, tissue health and healing), along with the still mysterious influences of higher-dose ascorbic acid intake, we can see how vitamin C may have a positive influence in fighting and preventing cancer, still the greatest medical dilemma in the twenty-first century.

Deficiency and toxicity. For most purposes, vitamin C or ascorbic acid in its many forms of use is nontoxic. It is not stored appreciably in the body, and most excess amounts are eliminated rapidly through the urine. However, amounts over 10 grams a day that some people use and some doctors prescribe are associated with some side effects, although none that are serious. Diarrhea is the most common and usually the first sign that the body's tissue fluids have been saturated with ascorbic acid. Most people will not experience this with under 5 to 10 grams a day, the

Clinical Uses of Vitamin C

Anemia	Glaucoma
Arthritis	Gout
Asthma	Hepatitis
Atherosclerosis	Herpes infections
Bruising	High cholesterol
Bursitis	levels
Cancer prevention	High triglyceride
Cataract prevention	levels
Cervical dysplasia	Hypertension
Chemical exposure	Immune suppression
Colds	Infertility
Depression	Peptic ulcer
Diabetes	Periodontal disease
Fatigue	Skin ulcers
Flu	Surgery recovery
Gallbladder disease	Varicose veins
Gingivitis	

amount that is felt to correlate with the body's need and use. Other side effects include nausea, dysuria (burning with urination), and skin sensitivities (sometimes sensitivity to touch or just a mild irritation). Hemolysis (breakage) of red blood cells may also occur with very high amounts of vitamin C. With any of these symptoms, it is wise to decrease intake.

There is some concern that higher levels of vitamin C intake may cause kidney stones, specifically calcium oxalate stones, because of increased oxalic acid clearance through the kidneys due to C metabolism. This is a rare case, if it does exist, and I personally have not seen, nor do I know any doctors who have seen, kidney stone occurrence with people taking vitamin C. In addition, there is no research evidence supporting this possibility. In fact, a recent study not only found evidence lacking in this area, but actually suggested a protective effect. In that study, the Harvard Prospective Health Professional Follow-Up Study, groups with the greatest vitamin C intake (greater than 1,500 mg per day) had a lower risk of kidney stones than groups with the least intake.

Only people who are prone to kidney stones or gout should give this any thought. If there is concern, supplementing magnesium in amounts between half and equal to that of calcium intake (which should be done anyway with calcium supplementation) would reduce that risk, at least for calcium-based stones. I usually suggest using a buffered vitamin C preparation with calcium and magnesium, which alleviates this concern.

As far as deficiency problems go, the once fairly common disease of scurvy is rare these days. Early symptoms of scurvy or vitamin C deficiency are more likely in formula-fed infants with little or no C intake or in teenagers or the elderly who do not eat any fresh fruits and vegetables. There is also a phenomenon (questioned by some clinicians as being a legitimate concern) called "rebound scurvy" that occurs when babies are born to mothers who take higher doses of C (at least 2–3 grams). Because vitamin C crosses the placenta, the babies get used to higher vitamin C levels in utero, and after birth they feel relatively deficient unless breastfed with the mother taking the same amount of vitamin C as during her pregnancy. This so-called rebound scurvy is not a serious problem and can be completely avoided if the newborn baby is breastfed and the mother continues her previous level of C intake, or if liquid vitamin C is provided for the infant until his or her body adjusts to lesser amounts of the vitamin. **Smokers with poor diets and people with inflammatory bowel disease more often have lower vitamin C blood levels.** Other people commonly found to be low in ascorbic acid include alcoholics, psychiatric patients, and patients with fatigue.

The symptoms of scurvy are produced primarily by the effects of the lack of ascorbic acid on collagen formation, causing reduced health of the tissues. The first signs of depletion may be related to vitamin C's other functions as well, where deficiency could lead to poor resistance to infection and very slow wound healing. Easy bruising and tiny hemorrhages (called *petechiae*) in the skin, general weakness, loss of appetite, and poor digestion may also occur. With worse deficiency, nosebleeds, sore and bleeding gums, anemia, joint tenderness and swelling, mouth ulcers, loose teeth, and shortness of breath could be experienced. During growth periods, there could be reduced growth, especially of the bones. The decrease in collagen may lead to bone brittleness, making the bones more fragile. The development and health of the teeth and gums are also affected. In breastfeeding women, lactation may be reduced. With the elderly, vitamin C deficiency could enhance symptoms of senility. The bleeding that comes from capillary wall fragility may lead to clotting and increased risk of strokes and heart attacks.

Requirements. We need only about 10 to 20 mg to prevent scurvy, and there is more than that in a single portion of most fruits or vegetables. Infants need 35 mg. About 50 mg between ages 1 and 14 and 60 mg afterward are the suggested minimums. Realistically, between 100 and 150 mg daily is a minimum dosage for most people. It is interesting to note that vitamin C is the most commonly supplemented nutrient by registered dietitians, and they average about 250 mg in their supplementation.

Vitamin C needs, however, are increased with all kinds of stress, both internal (emotional) and external (environmental). Smoking decreases C levels and increases minimum needs to about 200 mg per day. Birth control pills, estrogen for menopause, cortisone use, and aspirin also increase ascorbic acid requirements. Both nicotine and estrogen seem to increase blood levels of copper, and copper inactivates

AI Levels and RDAs for Vitamin C	
In 2000, the National Academy of Sciences established the following RDAs for C:	
Age	**AI/RDA**
Infants, 0–6 months	40 mg (AI)
Infants, 7–12 months	50 mg (AI)
Children, 1–3 years	15 mg (RDA)
Children, 4–8 years	25 mg (RDA)
Males, 9–13 years	45 mg (RDA)
Males, 14–18 years	75 mg (RDA)
Males, 19 years and older	90 mg (RDA)
Females, 9–13 years	45 mg (RDA)
Females, 14–18 years	65 mg (RDA)
Females, 19 years and older	75 mg (RDA)
Pregnant females, 18 years and younger	80 mg (RDA)
Pregnant females, 19 years and older	85 mg (RDA)
Lactating females, 18 years and younger	115 mg (RDA)
Lactating females, 19 years and older	120 mg (RDA)

vitamin C. In general, though, absorption of C from the intestines is good. Vitamin C (as ascorbic acid) taken with iron helps the absorption of iron (and many minerals) and is important in treating anemia, but the iron decreases absorption of the ascorbic acid. Overall, it is probably best to take vitamin C as it is found in nature, along with the vitamin P constituents (which I discuss on pages 145–146 of this chapter)—the bioflavonoids, rutin, and hesperidin. These may have a synergistic influence on the functions of C, although there is no conclusive research on humans to support this theory.

Vitamin C is the most commonly consumed nutrient supplement and is available in tablets, both fast-acting and time-released, in chewable tablets, in powders and effervescents, and in liquid form. It is available as ascorbic acid, L-ascorbic acid, and various mineral ascorbate salts, such as sodium or calcium ascorbate. One of my favorite formulas, which was developed by antioxidant researcher and supplement formulation expert Stephen Levine at Nutricology (Allergy Research Group) in Alameda, California, is a

buffered powder made from corn or cassava that contains 2,135 mg of vitamin C per teaspoon, along with 405 mg of calcium, 215 mg of magnesium, and 90 mg of potassium. It gets into the body quickly and is very easy on and often soothing to the stomach and intestinal lining. The potassium-magnesium combination can be helpful for fatigue.

Vitamin C works rapidly, so the total amount we take over the day should be divided into multiple doses (4 to 6) or taken as a time-released tablet a couple of times a day. When increasing or decreasing vitamin C intake, it is best to do so slowly because our body systems become accustomed to certain levels.

My basic suggestion for vitamin C use is about 2 to 4 grams per day with a typical active and healthy city lifestyle. Based on previous levels in our native diets, Dr. Linus Pauling feels that the optimum daily levels of C are between 2,500 and 9,000 mg. Clearly, requirements for vitamin C vary and may be higher according to state of health, age (needs increase with years), weight, activity and energy levels, and general metabolism. Stress, illness, and injuries further increase the requirements for ascorbic acid. Many authorities suggest that we take at least 500 mg of C daily to meet basic body needs.

During times of specific illnesses, especially viral infections, doctors who use megadose vitamin C treatment suggest at least 20 to 40 grams daily, some of it intravenously. Vitamin C has been used safely and effectively in dosages of 10 grams or more dripped slowly (over 30 to 60 minutes) into the blood to reach optimum tissue levels before excretion, so as to bathe the cells in C. Some doctors prescribe what is called "bowel tolerance" daily intake of vitamin C—that is, increasing the oral dose until diarrhea results and then cutting back. This level can vary greatly from a few grams to 100 grams or more. The claim is that the body knows what it needs and will respond by changing the water balance in the colon when it has had enough. Although family physician Robert Cathcart has used C this way in his practice for years to treat many problems, with claimed good success, I do not have the experience to make an adequate conclusion. This practice does, however, add further mystery to the vitamin C controversy. More research is definitely needed regarding ascorbic acid, and new discoveries will likely be made in the coming years.

Vitamin P (Bioflavonoids)

P A good number of these are the water-soluble companions of ascorbic acid, usually found in the same foods. Vitamin P includes a number of components that work together—citrin, hesperidin, rutin, flavones, flavonols, and catechin and quercetin, which are also discussed in chapter 7, Special Supplements. Their association with vitamin C is the reason that natural forms of C are more effective than are synthetic ascorbic acids without the bioflavonoids in the equivalent amounts.

Vitamin P was first discovered in 1936 by Hungarian scientist Dr. Albert Szent-Györgyi, who found it within the white of the rind in citrus fruits. It is contained mainly in the edible pulp of the fruits rather than in the strained juices. The letter P was given to this group of nutrients because they improve the capillary lining's permeability and integrity—that is, the passage of oxygen, carbon dioxide, and nutrients through the capillary walls. The bioflavonoids are easily absorbed from the intestinal tract, as is vitamin C. Some is stored in the body, although most of the excess is eliminated in the urine and perspiration.

Sources. A primary source of bioflavonoids is citrus fruit—lemons, grapefruits, oranges, and, to a lesser extent, limes. Rose hips, apricots, cherries, grapes, black currants, plums, blackberries, and papayas are other fruit sources of vitamin P. Green pepper, broccoli, and tomatoes are some good vegetable sources of bioflavonoids. The buckwheat plant, both leaf and grain, is also a particularly good source of bioflavonoids, especially the rutin component.

Functions. The bioflavonoids are helpful in the absorption of vitamin C and protect the multifunctional vitamin C molecule from oxidation, thereby improving and prolonging its functioning. Therefore, the bioflavonoids are indirectly, and possibly directly, involved in maintaining the health of the collagen that holds the cells together by forming the basement membranes of cells, tissues, and cartilage.

The main known function of the bioflavonoids is to increase the strength of the capillaries and to regulate their permeability (the so-called P factor). The capillaries link the arteries to the veins. They deliver oxygen and nutrients to the organs, tissues, and cells and then pick up carbon dioxide and waste and carry them through the veins and back to the heart. By its support of the capillaries, vitamin P helps to prevent hemorrhage and rupture of these tiny vessels, which could lead to easy bruising. Also, capillary strength may help protect us from infection, particularly viral problems. Bioflavonoids can reduce the amount of histamine released from cells; quercetin is definitely strong in this function. Because of their histamine-inhibiting effects, flavonoids can be accurately described as anti-inflammatory compounds.

Flavonoids can also act directly as antibiotics. In the case of both bacteria and viruses, some flavonoids are able to disrupt the function of these microorganisms and thereby prevent or treat infection. The antiviral function of some flavonoids has been demonstrated with the HIV virus, and HSV-1, a *Herpes simplex* virus.

Uses. A primary use of the bioflavonoids is to provide synergy in the utilization of vitamin C; therefore they contribute to many vitamin C applications—for example, the treatment of colds and flus. Bioflavonoids themselves are often supplemented for problems where improved capillary strength is needed, such as bleeding gums, easy bruising, and duodenal bleeding ulcers, which may be worsened by weak capillaries. The rutin component is particularly good for decreasing bleeding from weak blood vessels. In hemorrhoids, varicose veins, spontaneous abortions, excess menstrual bleeding (menorrhagia), postpartum hemorrhage, nosebleeds, the bleeding problems of diabetes, and generally during pregnancy, the bioflavonoids may be helpful in maintaining capillary health and reducing bleeding concerns. For women who have repeated spontaneous abortions or premature labor, supplementing citrus bioflavonoids—for example, 200 mg 3 times daily—may be helpful in remedying these problems. Vitamin P has also been used in asthma, allergies, bursitis and arthritis, and eye problems secondary to diabetes and as protection from the harmful effects of radiation.

Deficiency and toxicity. There is no known toxicity from any of the components of the bioflavonoids. In research studies, even very high amounts (for example, 140 grams per day) fail to show toxicity effects. Deficiency symptoms are fairly unlikely, although, as with vitamin C, an increased tendency to bruise or bleed is possible with vitamin P deficiency. The protection that vitamin C gives against inflammatory problems, as in arthritis, may be lost when the bioflavonoids are not in the diet or supplemented. In my medical experience, a question arises: If people respond to bioflavonoid (or any nutrient) supplementation, does that suggest that a deficiency or depletion was present? If we consume few fresh fruits or vegetables, we are likely to have flavonoid deficiency (in the same way that we would also be likely to have vitamin C deficiency).

Requirements. There is no RDA for the bioflavonoids, perhaps because they naturally occur with vitamin C. When they are supplemented, 500 mg bioflavonoids—containing 50 mg rutin and 50 mg hesperidin—is usually taken from 1 to 3 times daily. Supplements of 125 or 250 mg of bioflavonoids are also commonly available and can be taken daily with the same frequency.

Vitamin L (aka "The Love Vitamin")

 This vitamin is commonly known as the "universal" or "love" vitamin, as coined by humanologist Bethany Argisle. One of the most important nutrients for optimum health is a daily dose (or more) of love. This vital human emotion/expression/experience is necessary for the optimal functioning of people and all of their cells, tissues, and organs. It is found in most of Nature—in foods, domestic animals, friends, and family—and is used to heal a wide variety of diseases. There are no toxic effects, but deficiency can cause a wide range of ailments.

Sources. As stated, L is found in a great variety of sources but must be developed and nurtured to be available. Fear, anger, worry, self-concern, and many other human emotions can destroy vitamin L. It is found readily in most moms and dads and is highly concentrated in grandmothers and grandfathers. Sisters and brothers may be a good source of vitamin L, although often this is covered up in early years, developed in the teens, and more available in adulthood. Massage therapy is a particularly good source of vitamin L.

Vitamin L is also found in cats, dogs, and horses; in flowers and birds; and in trees and plants. In food, it is especially found in home-cooked or other meals where vitamin L is used consciously as an ingredient. It is digested and absorbed easily and used by the body in its pure state, being eliminated almost unchanged;

in this, it is unique among the vitamins. It is also made by friendly bacteria and all positive reactions and attitudes in the body.

Functions. This vitamin acts as the "universal" vitalizing energy. Vitamin L helps to catalyze all human functions and is particularly important to heart function and the circulation of warmth and joy. Digestion is very dependent on appropriate doses of vitamin L, as is the function of the nervous system. Adrenaline, the brain endorphins (natural tranquilizers and energizers), and other hormones are enhanced by vitamin L as well. A wide variety of other bodily and life functions are dependent on vitamin L, and it is extremely important to the healing process.

Uses. The list of uses is even longer than that of the functions. Vitamin L is an important nutrient in all human relations, domestic and international. We should definitely put it in the drinking supply! It is a vital ingredient in all health practitioners, doctors, clinics, and hospitals Love is also known as the catalytic "vitamin of healing." It can pass through the healer's energy vibrations to the recipient. It should be used in all heart problems and a wide variety of medical conditions. Vitamin L is also particularly helpful in all kinds of psychological disturbances. Depression, sadness, anger, fear, worry, pain, concern over world affairs, and many stresses of life can be helped by vitamin L therapy. It is particularly important in resolving relationship difficulties. **Fear, one of the more difficult problems to treat, usually requires megadoses of vitamin L, as does greed.**

Deficiency and toxicity. There are rarely any serious problems from excess intake of vitamin L. Side effects, however, may include swooning, a strange feeling in the center of the chest, goose bumps, staring blankly into space, or singing without cause. Usually, though, amounts many times the minimum requirements offer no difficulty and are often helpful. Deficiency, as with many of the vitamins, causes a great many more problems than overdoses. Fatigue, muscle tension, increased likelihood of stress conditions, digestive upset, drug problems, and sexual aberrations are only a few of the possible effects of vitamin L deficiency. Diseases of the heart are of particular concern. Vitamin L can become deficient easily in people under great demand to perform, such as doctors, nurses, and other hospital workers, or in people

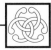

whose jobs are very cerebral, such as businesspeople, accountants, and stockbrokers.

Abrupt withdrawal from regular vitamin L use could be hazardous, as the love vitamin is somewhat addicting. People have varying sensitivities to decreases in vitamin L, and deficiency symptoms may occur easily. It is wise to replace any reductions with vitamin L from other sources (a key reason for having compassionate health practitioners). Increased amounts of vitamin L are more easily tolerated by most people, although huge increases should be taken slowly to prevent the side effects just mentioned.

Requirements. The requirements may vary from person to person, according to a wide range of factors. There are no specific RDAs for vitamin L, although infants and small children usually require fairly large doses. International hug experts advise a minimum of 4 hugs daily is needed to prevent vitamin L deficiency, 6 hugs a day for maintenance, and 10 hugs a day for growth. The whole body just works better when there is plenty of LOVE.

THE FUTURE OF VITAMINS

We might as well start thinking about vitamins like stars in a galaxy, because gone will be the days when we can count them on our fingers. The research insights of molecular medicine will prove to us beyond a shadow of a doubt that thousands of food-based substances are essential to our health, regardless of our body's ability to make them on its own. The idea that a single vitamin—like vitamin C—makes a food valuable (like orange juice or broccoli) will become a nice history exhibit in the Museum of Human Nourishment. There will be a hundred different substances in orange juice and a hundred more in broccoli that we will have a hard time calling anything but "vitamins."

Many vitamin- (and mineral-) enhanced foods and drinks will become more available—that has already started. More research on the health benefits and disease-prevention aspects of specific vitamins is forthcoming. Nutritional medicine is now part of mainstream research, and this is very exciting. Keeping ourselves healthy with the right vitamins and all essential nutrients will become a key factor in health care.

Possible Areas of Upcoming Vitamin Research

- The widespread awareness of vitamin deficiencies in modern societies with changes in food production and soil/plant health, and the effects these issues have on human nutrition.

- The effects of genetically modified foods on both a plant's ability to produce vitamins as well as enhanced capabilities of the plants, and these effects on human health, nutrition, and food allergy.

- Higher levels of vitamin D therapeutic dosages and whether people can tolerate the 2,000–6,000 IUs or more daily that practitioners are now suggesting for treatment of such problems as osteopenia and osteoporosis, cancer prevention, depression, memory loss and aging, and other areas of health support. Taking 1,000–2,000 IUs daily is now quite common.

- The use of vitamin K in the treatment of blood coagulation problems that are the basis of cardiovascular disease and subsequent heart attacks and strokes. Vitamin K usage and needs have been underestimated; K2 is the best form to use.

- Genetic testing (looking at weaknesses in the genes/genomes to measure propensities to specific diseases and dysfunctions) will be available with the knowledge of specific nutriceuticals that can counter these metabolic limitations. Some examples include cardiovascular risk, cancer potential, detoxification capabilities, and utilization of nutrients such as folic acid and other B vitamins.

- A clearer understanding of homocysteine and its relationship to cardiovascular disease and B-vitamin deficiencies, which may also relate to Alzheimer's. Methylation, an important biochemical step related to the homocysteine buildup, may be as important as antioxidants in preventing disease.

- How much vitamin L (Love) do we really need for good health?

Chapter 6

Minerals

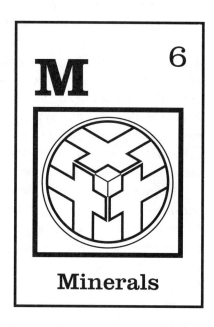

M inerals are what remain as ash when plant or animal tissues are burned or decompose completely after death. These "minerals" constitute most of what we call "elements," the basic building blocks of matter. Approximately 112 have been identified, and are listed on chemical charts called periodic tables. **Mineral elements come from the Earth and eventually return to the Earth; they can most simply be defined as chemical molecules that cannot be reduced to simpler substances.** They are the basic constituents of all matter, part of living tissue as well as existing in their inorganic form in the Earth. Approximately 4% to 5% of the body's weight is mineral matter, and most of that is in the skeleton. Minerals are also present in tissue proteins, enzymes, blood, some vitamins, and so on. If the human body were left to decompose completely, most of the organic tissues—which are made up of proteins, carbohydrates, and fats (themselves composed of carbon, oxygen, hydrogen, and nitrogen)—would break down into water (H_2O), carbon dioxide (CO_2), and nitrogen (N_2) and either evaporate into the atmosphere or enter the soil. What would be left would amount to about 5 pounds of elemental mineral ash. Of this, about 75% would be calcium and phosphorus, mostly from the bones; there would be about a teaspoon of iron, a couple of teaspoons of salt (sodium and chloride), and a little more of potassium; the rest of the ash would contain numerous other elements.

Dr. John Emsley, science writer in residence at Cambridge University, has written at length on the elemental composition of the human body and describes the body as being 61% oxygen (O), 23% carbon (C), 10% hydrogen (H), and 2% nitrogen (N). Approximately 90% of the oxygen and 70% of the hydrogen combine to make the body's water, which constitutes a little less than two-thirds of the body's weight. The remaining elements form the organic constituents—proteins, fats, and carbohydrates (by definition, organic molecules contain carbon). Much of the body's inorganic minerals is incorporated into organic matter as well.

Because all minerals originally come from and eventually return to the Earth, it is fascinating to compare this mineral composition of humans to the mineral composition of the Earth itself. Just as oxygen is the most abundant element in our bodies, so too is it the most abundant element in the Earth's crust.

(Hydrogen is also in the crust's top-10 most abundant elements.) And just as 75% of our ashes consist of calcium and magnesium, these two elements are also among the most plentiful in the Earth's crust, ranking fifth and seventh, respectively. While we are alive, we are about two-thirds water, and so is the planet—all of the oceans, when combined, account for about two-thirds of the Earth's total surface area. As humans, we are minerally in sync with the Earth, thus we have good reason to pay attention to its mineral balance as well as our own.

The main elements, each of which makes up more than 0.01% of total body weight, are termed the bulk minerals, or macrominerals. These are calcium (1.5% of body weight), phosphorus (1%), potassium (0.35%), sulfur (0.25%), sodium (0.15%), chloride (0.15%), magnesium (0.05%), and silicon (0.05%). (Silicon is not often listed as an essential element, although researchers have begun to realize its importance since the mid-1990s.) Most of the calcium and phosphorus is in the bones, but some is also present in the blood as well as in every cell. **Calcium**

Elemental Composition of the Human Body (70 kilograms = 154 pounds)

Macrominerals and Elements	Key Function	Grams
Oxygen	Cell and tissue respiration, water	43,000
Carbon	Protoplasm	12,000
Hydrogen	Water, tissue	6,300
Nitrogen	Protein tissue	2,000
Calcium	Bones and teeth	1,100
Phosphorus	Bones and teeth	750
Potassium	Intracellular electrolyte	225
Sulfur	Amino acids, hair, and skin	150
Chloride	Electrolyte	100
Sodium	Extracellular electrolyte	90
Magnesium	Metabolic electrolyte	35

Microminerals	Key Function	Milligrams
Iron	Hemoglobin, oxygen carrier	4,200
Fluoride	Bones and teeth	2,600
Zinc	Metalloenzymes	2,400
Strontium	Bone integrity	320
Copper	Enzyme cofactor	90
Silicon	Connective tissue	30
Cobalt	Vitamin B12 core	20
Vanadium	Lipid metabolism	20
Iodine	Thyroid hormones	15
Tin	Unknown	15
Selenium	Enzyme, antioxidant, detoxification	15
Manganese	Metalloenzymes	13
Nickel	Unknown	11
Molybdenum	Enzyme cofactor	8
Chromium	Glucose tolerance factor	6

* This table is adapted from Dewitt Hunter, MD, "Essential Trace Elements, an Overview," and is based on percent body weights and ppm in this text.

particularly is vital to heart and muscle function and nerve conductivity. The remaining phosphorus and most of the sulfur mix with the four primary elements to form the fats, proteins, and nucleic acids.

The next group of elements is also essential to health, although they are found only in minute amounts in the body. By definition, the trace minerals, or trace elements, constitute less than 0.01% of total body weight. Many of these are measured in micrograms (mcg) or in milligrams (mg), as are the macrominerals (1 gram = 1,000 mg; 1 mg = 1,000 mcg; thus, 1 million mcg per gram). Historically, the minerals have been measured in parts per million (ppm) of body weight (1 ppm = 1 mcg per gram).

Most of the trace elements discussed in this chapter are essential for life and health. Of these, iron is the most prevalent (60 ppm). Next is fluoride (37 ppm). There is some controversy about whether fluoride is actually essential, and although it does seem to prevent tooth decay when applied directly to the teeth or supplied in drinking water, there is clearly some danger of toxicity (fluorosis) from its regular use. Some recent, wide-scale studies have found links between the occurrence of cancer—especially bone cancer, mainly in men—and the consumption of maximally fluoridated drinking water. Zinc follows fluoride at 33 ppm; the rest of the elements are present in considerably lower concentrations. Rubidium and strontium are both measured at 4.6 ppm; neither is regarded as essential. Bromine (2.9 ppm) is possibly essential, and copper (1.2 ppm) is definitely needed by our bodies. The remaining are trace elements boron (0.7 ppm), barium (0.3), cobalt (0.3), vanadium (0.3), iodine (0.2), tin (0.2), manganese (0.2), selenium (0.2), molybdenum (0.1), arsenic (0.1), and chromium (0.09), often mentioned as an "ultra trace element." Of these, cobalt, iodine, manganese, selenium, molybdenum, and chromium are absolutely essential.

Other elements contained in the body include some of the toxic metals, which may cause harm in relatively high concentrations. These are primarily lead (1.7 ppm), aluminum (0.9), cadmium (0.7), and mercury (0.17). Through mining the Earth, humans have removed and used many of these toxic minerals, known as the heavy metals. They are now found more often in the atmosphere (for example, lead from car exhaust), in rivers, in our food sources, and in many industrial products. **Metal poisoning primarily affects the metabolic enzymes, the brain, and the nervous system, but it can affect many other bodily functions as well.** In addition to these toxic metals, some essential elements—such as copper, arsenic, iodine, selenium, chromium, and even iron and calcium—are more likely than other minerals to cause health problems when high levels are present in the body, resulting either from excessive intake or reduced ability to eliminate them.

What do minerals do for us? Like the vitamins, they do not contain calories or energy in themselves, but they assist the body in energy production. Although our bodies can manufacture some vitamins, we make no minerals. Rather, our natural minerals come from the Earth (that is, if a mineral nutrient is contained in the soil, it will be present in the food grown there and thus will be provided to us when we consume that food). Loss of topsoil, continual replanting without enriching the soil, and the farmer's use of fertilizers that contain only nitrogen, phosphorus, and potassium (all of which stimulate plant growth) and not the other important macro- and micro- (trace) minerals—all contribute to the growing problem that our food may not contain all the minerals it once did. Fruits and vegetables grown in rich, well-nourished soils obviously have more of the essential minerals necessary for our health and vitality. Recent studies on organically grown food, for example, have found routinely higher levels of minerals in organically grown foods. Although the increases have generally been found to be in a moderate range of 5% to 15%, in some cases minerals like calcium have been found to be over 50% higher in organic versus nonorganically grown foods. Spinach, cabbage, carrots, and leeks are some of the foods that have been found to have higher mineral levels when organically grown. Unfortunately, refinement and processing of foods further decrease the mineral content.

Obtaining the full spectrum of essential minerals is important. In fact, in clinical, nutritional medicine, minerals may be even more important than vitamins. **Deficiencies of many vital minerals are more common than deficiencies of vitamins because our body does not manufacture minerals (as it does vitamins) and because foods may be enriched with vitamins.** Also, minerals are harder to liberate from food complexes during digestion—thus, lower amounts are absorbed. There is also more uptake competition between minerals, and compared with vitamins, a lower percentage of minerals move passively from the gastrointestinal tract to the blood. Like vitamins, minerals are essential to our physical and mental health and are a basic part of all cells, particularly blood, nerve, and muscle cells, as well as our bones, teeth, and all soft tissue. Minerals offer us both structural and functional support. The special electrolyte minerals—sodium, potassium, and chloride—help regulate the fluid and acid-base balance of our bodies. Other minerals are part of enzymes that catalyze biochemical reactions and aid the production of energy or participate in metabolism. Some minerals also help in nerve transmission, muscle contraction, cell permeability, and blood and tissue formation.

What does it mean for a mineral to be "essential"? Like other nutrients, when our bodies cannot produce them or produces them in quantities insufficient to support the functions in which they are used, these minerals are said to be essential. In the case of minerals, of course, the body cannot "produce" them in the sense of creating them from scratch, because they are the simplest forms of matter. **In more practical terms, however, a mineral is considered essential if deficiency symptoms are seen when it is lacking in the diet and the symptoms resolve when it is resupplied.** This is easy to demonstrate with many of the body's bulk minerals, such as calcium, magnesium, sodium, and potassium; many problems arise when these minerals are not supplied in the diet. Essentiality of the trace minerals is more difficult to determine. However, recent research has shed a great deal of light on many important subtleties of the trace minerals. Chromium and selenium, for years primarily the subject of toxicity concerns, now are known to be essential to carbohydrate metabolism and blood sugar regulation. Chromium is a component of glucose tolerance factor (GTF), and selenium is important in proper immune function, heart function, and cancer prevention.

Other methods have been used to determine whether a mineral is essential to the body. If it is a necessary component of another essential nutrient, as is cobalt within vitamin B12, it is considered essential. If it is a necessary part of tissues, fluids, or an enzyme used in a metabolic or bioenergetic process, it may be

deemed essential. There are approximately 17 essential minerals. (The primary elements carbon, hydrogen, oxygen, and nitrogen, part of all living tissue and food, are not included in these 17.) **The seven macrominerals are calcium (Ca), chloride (Cl), magnesium (Mg), phosphorus (P), potassium (K), sodium (Na), and sulfur (S).**

The trace minerals that are known to be essential are chromium (Cr), cobalt (Co), copper (Cu), iodine (I), iron (Fe), manganese (Mn), molybdenum (Mo), selenium (Se), silicon (Si), and zinc (Z). Boron (B), tin (Sn), and vanadium (V) are most likely essential. Research on lithium (Li) and rubidium (Rb) indicates that they are also probably essential. Arsenic (As), barium (Ba), bromine (Br), fluoride (F), nickel (Ni), and strontium (Sr) are all possibly essential in very small amounts. Minerals probably nonessential are aluminum (Al), cadmium (Cd), gold (Au), lead (Pb), mercury (Hg), and silver (Ag). Aluminum, cadmium, lead, and mercury—possibly along with beryllium (Be), bismuth (Bi), and higher amounts of arsenic (As)—are considered to be toxic minerals. However, when things are out of balance, most minerals can have toxic effects, such as heart irregularities with potassium excess, or abnormal calcifications with calcium.

Through several mechanisms, the body fine-tunes the levels of most of the minerals to maintain optimum functioning. This process begins in the stomach, where minerals often have to be detached from food proteins as a preparation for absorption. Absorption from the gastrointestinal tract, the next step in getting the mineral into the circulation, can be a fairly complex process. The primary way to reduce mineral levels is by elimination through the kidneys with the urine or from the liver and bile or other digestive juices through the intestinal tract. The body can utilize a mineral in metabolic functions or store it in the tissues. Also, the body may control absorption of one mineral by preferentially absorbing a similar one, according to current needs. **Many of the minerals compete with each other when naturally present in the diet or when supplemented.** For example, large amounts of calcium can reduce absorption of magnesium, phosphorus, zinc, and manganese. Zinc can reduce iron, copper, and phosphorus absorption, while phosphorus when taken in excess can interfere with the absorption of a great many minerals.

Minerals are available to the body in a variety of forms. One common form is inorganic salts, such as sodium chloride or ferrous phosphate. They can also be part of organic salts or contained in plant or animal tissues, as mineral chelates, or bound to amino acids or protein molecules, as iron is in hemoglobin. *Chelation*, from the Greek word for "claw," refers to holding or "grabbing" a mineral by a special type of chemical bonding. **Many minerals are chelated by organic molecules in Nature; this is a natural process that enables a mineral to be better absorbed into the body.**

Many minerals may be found in water in their free ionic states—that is, as positively or negatively charged particles. The salts that are the major components of seawater also provide the general matrix of cellular life. The main cations (positively charged ions)—sodium, potassium, calcium, and magnesium—combine with the negatively charged anions chloride, phosphate (phosphorus and 4 oxygen atoms), and carbonate (carbon and 4 oxygen atoms). The minerals may be in solution, such as calcium, magnesium, sodium, or potassium in water, or they may be present as free metals. **The charge, or valence, of a mineral describes its balance between protons (positively charged particles) and electrons (negatively charged particles), which determines the mineral's capacity to combine and whether it acts as an acid or a base in the body.** The monovalent ions, those with 1 extra proton or electron (sodium [+], potassium [+], and chloride [–]), are absorbed more easily through the intestinal wall than the divalent ions, which have 2 extra protons, or a plus-2 charge (calcium and magnesium). The lining of the gastrointestinal tract is both electrically and ionically charged and thus may not allow other ions to pass through easily. That is why chelated minerals or mineral salts (positive and negative ions joined together) may be absorbed more easily.

Iron is a good example of the complexity of mineral absorption. Iron is found in two positive ionic forms, ferrous (2+) and ferric (3+). Ferric iron, as in iron pellets, is not very stable in nature or usable by the body, so iron supplements commonly contain ferrous forms, such as ferrous sulfate. The ferrous salts themselves vary in solubility. Vitamin C can help convert ferric ions to the more usable ferrous ones. Ferrous sulfate is potentially more irritating to the digestive tract than many other forms and may cause irritation, "gripping," and constipation. Other salts, such as ferrous gluconate or ferrous fumarate, are handled more easily by most people.

Minerals are available in water and, of course, in food when they are in the soil in which a particular food is grown. Minerals commonly found in water include calcium, magnesium, sodium, potassium, chloride, phosphates, and sulfates, and depending on the source of the water, these could include iron, zinc, or copper as well. It is wise to investigate the mineral levels of our drinking water because imbalances or toxicities could develop from regular use of water from some sources. "Soft" water, which has had most of the minerals removed, is usually higher in sodium; for most people, however, this extra amount will not cause any problems. The deliberate softening of water raises its sodium level by about 8 mg per quart—far under the thousands of milligrams that will fit comfortably into most diets. "Hard" water usually has more of the other minerals, such as calcium and magnesium, which may be helpful. The Water Quality Association of the United States defines "hard" water as water containing dissolved minerals at a level greater than 1 grain per gallon (a grain is about 65 mg).

A food's mineral content gives it the potential for being acid or alkaline in the body. (Acid and alkaline diets are further discussed on pages 503–505 in Chapter 12, The Components of a Healthy Diet.) When food decomposes or is incinerated, either an acid or a base ash is left. Thus a food can be either acid forming or alkaline forming. The body acid-base balance (pH) is slightly alkaline, so more of the diet should consist of alkaline-forming foods, primarily fruits and vegetables. Interestingly enough, these foods usually have a relatively high mineral content. Even though many people think of citrus foods as acidic, they are actually alkaline in function—that is, they create an alkaline residue. Meats, dairy foods, and most nuts, seeds, and grains decompose with an acid residue, so too much of these may throw off the body's pH.

In general, most minerals are only moderately well absorbed even when the digestive system is functioning well. With digestive difficulties, such trace minerals as chromium and zinc may be absorbed poorly, and deficiency symptoms may develop quite rapidly.

Most minerals are not destroyed by heat, but some are soluble in water and therefore are lost or leached out during the cooking process. I have already mentioned a number of factors—agricultural (modern farming), environmental (pollution and depletion), and food-processing (refined and nutritionally deficient)—that cause the loss of even more of the once-prevalent elemental substances essential to human life.

Marion Nestle (PhD, MPH, professor and chair of the Department of Nutrition and Food Studies at New York University for more than 15 years) has carefully documented the relationship between food processing, nutrient loss, and chronic disease in *Food Politics: How the Food Industry Influences Nutrition and Health.* Milling of wheat has been the subject of the most research, and the findings are listed in the table below, "Potential Mineral Loss in Food Processing." But similar losses arise with polishing rice and refining cornmeal, and with many other aspects of food handling and processing. Raw cane sugar has a wide range of trace elements, almost all of which are lost when white sugar is made; figures for these losses are also given in the table below. The molasses left after refining sugar, which is rich in minerals, is usually fed to animals; the same is true of the "mill feed" pulled out of wheat and other grains. Similar losses occur for most of the vitamins during food handling and processing.

Many minor and major problems can arise from mineral deficiencies. Well-known is osteoporosis, a loss of bone minerals due mainly to long-term, low calcium intake (and vitamin D deficiency). Low calcium and probably low magnesium levels may contribute to hypertension, as does high sodium with lower potassium levels. Magnesium deficiency has also been associated with muscular spasms and nerve-related pain and, more recently, with acute heart attacks. Low zinc or selenium levels may hinder the immune system and make us prone to infection. The list goes on.

Even though many of these minerals are essential to life, there are daily requirement intake (DRI) minimums for relatively few—calcium, chromium, copper, fluoride, iodine, iron, magnesium, manganese, molybdenum, phosphorus, and zinc. DRI minimums need to be established for many others, and the awareness of subtle, undiagnosed mineral deficiency states needs to increase. Even the minerals for which DRIs have been established need to be reevaluated; for instance, I believe that magnesium warrants much more attention and research. Further investigation into the mineral content of foods and requirements in the diet should result in a new focus not only by the federal government and the food industry but by the public as well.

All the macrominerals are needed in doses of more than 100 mg daily, with sodium requirements somewhere from 2 to 5 grams, potassium 3 to 4 grams, phosphorus about 1 to 2 grams, calcium 1 to 1.5 grams, and magnesium probably about 0.5 to 1 gram. The trace minerals are needed in much smaller amounts. To be on the safe side, daily intake of iron should probably be about 5 to 15 mg; zinc about 10 to 25 mg; manganese about 5 to 10 mg; and copper about 2 mg. Other trace minerals—such as chromium, cobalt, iodine, molybdenum, and selenium—are needed in amounts of less than 1 mg per day. (See the discussions of the individual minerals in this chapter for the specific requirements.)

The healthiest approach for assuring optimum mineral levels is to get the majority of them from wholesome foods. Eating a variety of foods, with a lot of organic, local produce and grains, is a good start. Nourishing the soil is necessary to begin to get

Potential Mineral Loss in Food Processing

Wheat Milling		Refining Sugarcane	
MINERAL	LOSS	MINERAL	LOSS
Manganese	88%	Magnesium	99%
Chromium	87%	Zinc	98%
Magnesium	80%	Chromium	93%
Sodium	78%	Manganese	93%
Potassium	77%	Cobalt	88%
Iron	76%	Copper	83%
Zinc	72%		
Phosphorus	71%		
Copper	63%		
Calcium	60%		
Molybdenum	60%		
Cobalt	50%		

Data in this table has been compiled from information found in Henry Schroeder, MD, *The Trace Elements and Man.*

these basic elements into, and then back from, the Earth. Harvesting and eating fresh vegetables from our own composted gardens would be ideal. Avoiding refined and processed foods that have poor mineral content, or high-sugar foods, caffeine, and alcohol—all of which can flush or deplete body minerals—is also a helpful habit. Eating a calcium-rich diet has been confused with drinking lots of milk, which poses potential health concerns related to fat intake. Raw nuts and seeds, whole grains, and leafy greens can provide adequate amounts of calcium. If we orient ourselves to the healthiest of diets, we will assure ourselves the basics of good mineral nutrition.

THE MACROMINERALS

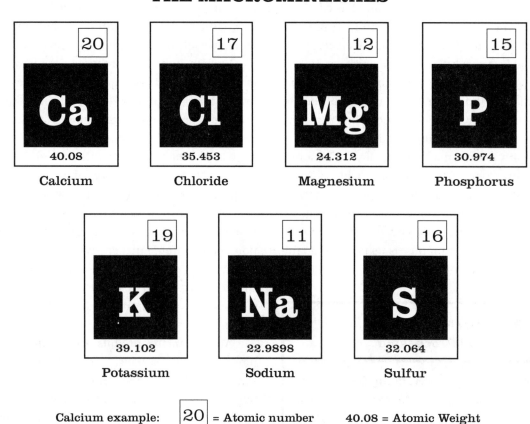

20	17	12	15
Ca	**Cl**	**Mg**	**P**
40.08	35.453	24.312	30.974
Calcium	Chloride	Magnesium	Phosphorus

19	11	16
K	**Na**	**S**
39.102	22.9898	32.064
Potassium	Sodium	Sulfur

Calcium example: | 20 | = Atomic number   40.08 = Atomic Weight

Calcium

Ca Calcium is the most abundant mineral in the human body and among the most important. This mineral constitutes about 1.5% to 2.0% of our body weight. Almost all (98%) of our approximately 3 pounds of calcium is contained in our bones, about 1% is in our teeth, and the rest is in the other tissues and the circulation. Calcium and magnesium are earth alkali minerals found in the Earth's crust, usually as salts that are fairly insoluble. (The word *calcium* comes from the Latin *calc,* meaning "lime," as in limestone, a calcium carbonate substance.) Dolomite, a calcium-magnesium earth mineral combination that is a little more soluble and usable by the body than some other forms, is a commonly used calcium supplement. When purchasing this form, however, **make sure the product has been certified as lead free, because many clays that serve as the source for dolomite have been found to contain this heavy metal.**

Many other nutrients, vitamin D, and certain hormones are important to calcium absorption, function, and metabolism. Phosphorus as well as calcium is needed for normal bones, as are magnesium, silicon, strontium, possibly boron, and the protein matrix—all part of our bone structure. The ratio of calcium to phosphorus in our bones is about 2.5:1; the best proportions of these minerals in the diet for proper metabolism are currently under question. **Calcium works with magnesium in its functions in the blood, nerves, muscles, and tissues, particularly in regulating heart and muscle contraction and nerve conduction.** Vitamin D is needed for much calcium (and phosphorus) to be absorbed from the digestive tract. Along with parathyroid hormone and calcitonin, secreted by the thyroid, vitamin D helps maintain normal blood calcium levels.

Maintaining a balanced blood calcium level is essential to life, especially for cardiac function. A normal blood calcium level is about 10 mg percent—that is, about 10 mg per 100 milliliters (ml) of blood. Of that, approximately 5.5 mg are in ionic form as Ca^{++}, about 4 mg are bound to carrier proteins, and about 0.5 mg is combined with phosphate or citrate. If there is not enough calcium in the diet to maintain sufficient amounts of calcium in the blood, the parathyroid glands will release more parathyroid hormone (PTH), which will then draw calcium out of the bones as well as increase intestinal absorption of available calcium. So even though most of the body's calcium is in the bones, the blood and cellular concentrations of this mineral are maintained first. This is why, with nearly 30% of people in the United States eating calcium-deficient diets, osteoporosis (a loss of bone substance) is so prevalent.

Elderly people usually have less calcium in their diets, and calcium deficiency particularly affects postmenopausal women. But low dietary calcium is only one factor in the huge and complex topic of calcium bioavailability from foods, calcium absorption, and osteoporosis. Many factors are involved in making calcium available for its many essential functions. Vitamin D is, of course, most essential to calcium absorption, although this may be less necessary when the calcium chelates, such as calcium aspartate or calcium citrate, are used. Clinical studies are necessary to see which calcium supplements are readily transported into the body and how vitamin D may affect them. Many doctors do not consider this impor-

tant absorption issue and prescribe calcium from an oyster shell, dolomite, or bonemeal (ground cattle bones) source as a supplement. Frequently, calcium lactate or calcium carbonate pills (such as Tums)—which are more alkaline and slowly absorbed—are prescribed without suggesting additional vitamin D and magnesium, so important for calcium balance and metabolism. A woman who needs more calcium could be taking an extra gram a day without really getting much of it into her blood or bones.

In general, calcium absorption becomes less efficient as we age. During infancy and childhood, 50% to 70% of the calcium ingested may be absorbed, whereas an adult might use only 30% to 50% of dietary calcium in his or her body. It is likely this is based on natural body needs. Various factors can improve calcium absorption. Besides vitamin D, vitamins A and C can also help support normal membrane transport of calcium. Protein intake helps absorption of calcium, but too much protein may reduce it. Some dietary fat may also help absorption, but high fat may reduce it. Lactose helps calcium absorption, and because of this as well as the protein-fat combination, the calcium content of milk is a reliable source of easily assimilated calcium. For other reasons, however, milk is not an ideal food for many people, especially the homogenized variety fortified with synthetic vitamin D, making milk a less-than-perfect (and definitely not the only) source of calcium. Nonfat milk does not improve calcium absorption and, in fact, may decrease it.

Gastric hydrochloric acid helps calcium absorption. The duodenum is the main location for absorption of calcium because farther down the small intestine the local environment becomes too alkaline. A fast-moving intestinal tract can reduce calcium absorption. Exercise has been shown to improve absorption, and lack of exercise can lessen it. Stress also can diminish calcium absorption, possibly through its effect on stomach acid levels, digestion, and intestinal motility. Although calcium in the diet improves the absorption of the important vitamin B12, too much of it may interfere with the absorption of the competing minerals magnesium, zinc, iron, and manganese.

Many dietary factors also reduce calcium absorption. Foods that are high in oxalic acid—such as spinach, rhubarb, chard, and chocolate—can interfere with calcium absorption by forming insoluble salts in the gut. Phytic acid, or phytates, found in whole grain foods or foods rich in fiber, may reduce the absorption of calcium and other minerals as well. Protein, fat, and acid foods may help calcium absorption, but high-protein diets may increase calcium elimination through the intestines. Calcium absorption is sensitive and requires energy to transport it into the body. Calcium is often chelated with proteins or amino acids (specifically, glutamic or aspartic acid) to make it more absorbable.

Factors Affecting Calcium Absorption

Increased by:

Body needs—growth, pregnancy, lactation

Vitamin D

Milk lactose

Acid environment—hydrochloric acid, citric acid, ascorbic acid (vitamin C)

Protein intake and amino acids such as lysine and glycine

Fat intake

Exercise

Phosphorus balance

Decreased by:

High fat intake

High phosphorus intake

High protein intake

Hypochlorhydria (low stomach acid)

Gastrointestinal problems

Lack of exercise

Oxalic acid foods (beet greens, chard, spinach, rhubarb, cocoa)

Phytic acid foods (whole grains)

Stress

Vitamin D deficiency

Because of the many complex factors affecting calcium absorption, anywhere from 30% to 80% may end up being excreted. Some may be eliminated in the feces. The kidneys also control calcium blood levels through their filtering and reabsorption functions. Excess salt intake can lead to increased calcium losses in the urine. Sugar intake may reduce the reabsorption

of calcium and magnesium and cause more to be eliminated (see the table at left, "Factors Affecting Calcium Absorption," for a summary). Overall, we need good sources of calcium in our diets, good nutritional habits, and a diet that promotes healthy gastrointestinal function. **Taking calcium and magnesium at bedtime or between meals, when the stomach may be more acidic, is often helpful for better absorption.** Regular exercise, good nutrition, and lots of vegetables are important basics for ensuring adequate calcium levels and for good health in general.

Sources. Calcium is found in many foods but is in high amounts in only a few. Milk should be considered a good source of calcium; it also contains protein and fat and has a good balance of magnesium and phosphorus (a balanced calcium-phosphorus ratio is important). The lactose in milk helps calcium absorption, but about 70% of African Americans and 6% of Caucasians are lactose-intolerant—that is, drinking milk makes them sick. An 8-ounce glass of whole milk contains about 300 mg of calcium. Most other milk products—yogurt, most cheeses, and buttermilk, for example—also provide good supplies of calcium.

Many green, leafy vegetables are good sources of calcium, but some contain oxalic acid, so their calcium is not easily absorbed. Spinach, chard, and beet greens are not particularly good sources of calcium, whereas broccoli, cauliflower, and many peas and beans offer better supplies. (Pinto, adzuki, and soybeans are excellent sources of calcium.) Many nuts (particularly almonds, Brazil nuts, and hazelnuts) and seeds (such as sunflower and sesame) contain good amounts of calcium. Although their phosphorus content is about double that of their calcium, this is much more of a concern with meats, which often contain 20 to 30 times as much phosphorus as calcium. Molasses (both black-strap and Barbados) is fairly high in calcium, while some fruits (such as citrus, figs, raisins, and dried apricots) have modest amounts.

When the diet is high in phosphorus, we can lose extra calcium through the urine, resulting in calcium being pulled out of the bones. Phosphorus is plentiful in meat foods and is of particular concern in soft drinks that have added phosphoric acid (phosphate). This phosphorus-calcium imbalance may lead to kidney stones and other calcification problems as well as to increased atherosclerotic plaque.

This issue is fairly complex and is under investigation. It is currently felt that the best calcium-phosphorus ratio in the diet is about 1:1.

Sunlight increases the manufacture of vitamin D in the body and is like having an extra calcium source because vitamin D improves absorption of any available dietary calcium. Calcium supplements could be taken in the first couple of hours after sunbathing to improve utilization.

Dolomite and bonemeal are good sources of calcium and magnesium. In recent years, however, both of these natural sources have been found to be contaminated with lead and other heavy metal toxins. It is probably wise not to take these supplements in large amounts or over prolonged periods of time unless they are tested for contamination. This same rule applies to oyster shell calcium, which is another commonly available form. Calcium found in hard water may also be an important source for maintaining body levels.

Functions. Calcium has some important life-supporting functions; the best known is the development and maintenance of bones and teeth. The body's need for calcium is critical during the growth years of infancy and childhood, but it is also important lifelong to keep the bones healthy. Exercise, vitamin D, and many other nutrients, such as phosphorus and magnesium, are also needed to maintain the skeleton. Bones are primarily calcium phosphate and a protein matrix. Tooth enamel is the hardest substance in the body, made up of 99% minerals, primarily calcium. Bones are not only the most basic physical support structures, they are the main reservoir for calcium. Most minerals are in a state of dynamic activity and function, and even the calcium in bones is being added to and removed depending on the calcium balance in the body. The bones provide calcium to the blood and other tissues when we are not getting sufficient amounts from our diet. Vitamin D, parathyroid hormone, and calcitonin are responsible for maintaining this balance.

Circulating calcium also performs many other vital functions. Ionized calcium (Ca^{++}) is needed for muscle contraction, as in muscular activity and in regulating the heartbeat. **Heart function is mediated by several minerals: calcium stimulates contraction, magnesium supports the relaxation phase, and sodium and potassium are also important in generating the electrical impulse.** Exercise can improve the circulation of calcium as well as that of all the other nutrients and thereby help the tone and function of the muscles, the heart, and the nervous system, where calcium is important in nerve transmission. Calcium ions influence nerve and cell membranes and the release of neurotransmitters. Calcium activates some enzyme systems, such as choline acetylase, which helps generate acetylcholine, an important neurotransmitter. Norepinephrine and serotonin are also affected by calcium. Calcium is said to be

Calcium Sources		
Food	**Portion**	**Calcium (mg)**
Swiss cheese	2 oz	530
Jack cheese	2 oz	420
Cheddar cheese	2 oz	400
Other cheeses	2 oz	300–400
Yogurt	6 oz	300
Broccoli, cooked	2 stalks	250
Sardines (with bones)	2 oz	240
Goat's milk	6 oz	240
Cow's milk	6 oz	225
Collard greens, cooked	6 oz	225
Turnip greens, cooked	6 oz	220
Almonds	3 oz	210
Brazil nuts	3 oz	160
Soybeans, cooked	6 oz	150
Molasses, blackstrap	1 tablespoon	130
Corn tortillas (4, with lime)	2 oz	125
Carob flour	2 oz	110
Tofu	3 oz	110
Dried figs	3 oz	100
Dried apricots	3 oz	80
Parsley	1 1/2 oz	80
Kelp	1/4 oz	80
Sunflower seeds	2 oz	80
Sesame seeds	2 oz	75

calming to the nerves, as higher concentrations tend to decrease nerve irritability.

Calcium has also come under increasing scrutiny in nervous system research because of its potential role in excitotoxicity. The problem here involves too much calcium rushing into the nerve cell and causing the cell to become overexcited and excessively exposed to oxygen damage. Fingers currently seem to be pointing not at calcium directly, but at toxins and other molecules that open the calcium floodgates. In addition, it appears that higher magnesium levels would help fight this phenomenon, because magnesium is able to nestle itself into the middle of the calcium channels and prevent too much calcium from rushing into the cells. Calcium is also necessary in cell division, where it is needed to activate prothrombin, which helps convert fibrinogen to fibrin and is essential to blood coagulation.

Uses. Because of calcium deficiency and osteoporosis, calcium is one of the minerals most commonly prescribed by medical doctors (potassium is the other one). Osteoporosis is more common in the elderly population and occurs four times as often in women as in men. It can also occur at younger ages with chronic dietary insufficiency of calcium or with early menopause. Good evidence shows that there is a relationship between decreased calcium intake and osteoporosis; lack of exercise also increases bone loss. Moderate daily exercise as well as supplementing calcium and vitamin D helps restore a positive calcium balance. In other words, the best way to combat osteoporosis is to prevent it with regular exercise, a calcium-rich diet not too high in phosphorus, and calcium supplements. Exercise can actually stimulate bone renewal by improving bone uptake of calcium and other minerals.

With respect to osteoporosis, I believe we may have partly missed the boat by not paying enough attention to other bone minerals and nonmineral nutrients. For example, we know that supplementation with magnesium and boron (and manganese) alongside of calcium can improve bone health in some situations, and that vitamin K is critical to bone support. Protein intake is important, because of the role played by collagen in bone tissue. There is also some positive research on supplementation with MCHC (microcrystalline hydroxyapatite)—a whole bone supplement

usually made from calf bone that contains minerals, proteins, and other nutrients as contained in the bones of that animal. **Overall, be aware of the sources of calcium you are using.**

Osteoporosis (the term literally means "porous bones") is actually a loss of bone mass as the result of the loss of both minerals and protein; this differs slightly from osteomalacia, the bone problem seen in adults with vitamin D deficiency, which involves a softening of bones due to mineral loss alone. Rickets is the childhood equivalent of osteomalacia and is also caused by vitamin D deficiency. Extra calcium can help alleviate these problems somewhat, but the body needs supplemental vitamin D to get appreciable levels of calcium into the blood, tissues, and bones. Osteopenia refers to milder bone loss than osteoporosis.

Calcium is still the primary substance used in the prevention and treatment of osteoporosis, although estrogen used in menopausal hormone replacement therapy can reduce the likelihood of this disease in women. Because osteoporosis is found mainly in menopausal and postmenopausal woman, calcium is commonly seen as a treatment for problems of menopause. It does, in fact, reduce a number of the potential symptoms. Calcium not only helps the bones, especially when supplemented with magnesium and vitamin D, it may also reduce the headaches, irritability, insomnia, and depression sometimes associated with menopause.

It is likely that a high percentage—as much as 70% to 90%—of bone fractures in people older than 60 are due to osteoporosis. These fractures are often more serious than an average fracture because demineralized bones shatter when they break and take longer to heal. Because osteoporotic fractures usually occur in the elderly and are so disabling, about 1 in 6 people dies within 3 months after sustaining such a fracture. Almost 8 million fractures annually in the United States are related to this prevalent nutritional deficiency disease. By helping to retard osteoporosis, calcium can prevent some fractures.

Osteoporosis is most common in elderly white women with a history of borderline calcium intake. **Calcium is often drained from the bones during pregnancy and nursing and becomes hard to replace in later years,** especially with reduced consumption of milk products and a lower calcium intake in general. Calcium supplementation can be helpful in reducing leg cramps of pregnancy and fatigue and depression after delivery. Children's leg cramps, from "growing pains" or muscle cramps, both of which are common problems possibly associated with natural overexertion, are usually reduced by giving them calcium and magnesium. Calcium supplements tend to stimulate retention of calcium and decrease urinary excretion.

Calcium is often helpful for menstrual problems, particularly menstrual cramps, irritability or apprehension, and muscle cramps that occur around menstruation. Premenstrual syndrome (PMS), first identified in the 1930s but not recognized as a genuine health problem until the early 1960s, is often helped in part with additional calcium, although magnesium supplementation may be even more important (see "Premenstrual Syndrome" on page 719, chapter 17, Medical Treatment Programs). In some cases, however, *reducing* calcium intake can be helpful. Generally, muscle cramps or leg and foot cramps can be helped by calcium and vitamin D. Also, some cases of hyperkinesis in children, when associated with calcium deficiency, may be helped by supplementation.

Other problems related to bone health affect the mouth, jawbone, and teeth. In some cases, calcium may be helpful for problems of loose teeth, gingivitis (gum inflammation), and periodontal disease. Usually 1,000 mg of calcium supplemented in the diet along with a dietary intake of phosphorus ranging from 1,000 to 2,000 mg is suggested.

Calcium is often used to reduce heart irregularity; along with magnesium, it helps regulate heart contraction and relaxation. Through increasing contractility, calcium can help in congestive heart failure. Additional calcium may protect us from the toxicity of cadmium, rubidium, or mercury exposure by competing for absorption. Proper calcium intake may reduce the incidence of colon and rectal cancers through forming insoluble soaps with some mild carcinogens produced in the body, including bile acids and free, ionized fatty acids. A good calcium-to-phosphorus ratio in the diet also reduces the risk of cancer in the large intestine.

Deficiency and toxicity. Excessive intakes of calcium (more than 3,000 mg per day) may result in elevated blood calcium levels, a condition known as hypercalcemia. If blood levels of phosphorous are low at the same time as calcium levels are high, hypercalcemia can lead to soft tissue calcification. This condition involves the unwanted accumulation of calcium in cells other than bone. In general, a high calcium intake for brief periods does not cause any problems, as excesses are usually eliminated in the urine and intestines. **With magnesium deficiency, though, high amounts of calcium or vitamin D can lead to calcification of the soft tissues or to kidney stone formation.** It is possible that prolonged high amounts of calcium (higher than a 2:1 calcium- to-phosphorus ratio) and supplemental vitamin D can lead to abnormal calcification of long bones in children or to hypercalcemia and soft tissue calcification in adults as well as to a decrease in bone strength. Also, if the parathyroid glands are not functioning well, calcium can accumulate and cause problems. For all of these reasons, in 1997 the Institute of Medicine set a tolerable upper intake level (UL) for calcium of 2,500 mg per day.

Calcium itself is thought to be one of the concerns in atherosclerosis, forming part of the plaque laid down in the arteries. Guy Abraham, MD, who is known for his work in premenstrual syndrome, expressed a concern over routine calcium supplementation as he feels it exacerbates the degenerative process in the blood vessels, kidneys, and other organs and tissues. It is possible that these problems of calcium excess are not specifically related to dietary calcium but rather to calcium's metabolism in relationship to the endocrine system. More research is clearly needed in this area. This potential toxicity concern makes me realize that it is important to be aware of calcium metabolism and individual needs and to not just blindly supplement it.

Still, though, calcium deficiency is a more common concern in the United States than is excess calcium. This is especially true for the elderly, for alcoholics, for pregnant women, and for people with gastrointestinal disease. **The standard American diet of minimal fresh foods and higher amounts of refined, processed foods does not meet the optimum calcium requirements; part of this problem is because of high phosphorus levels in the diet.** Phosphorus is found in most foods, but soft drinks, diet sodas, meats, eggs, and processed foods such as lunch meats and cheese spreads contain especially high amounts. The ideal dietary phosphorus-to-calcium ratio is about 1:1. The ratio in the average American diet is often greater than 2:1, however, and sometimes even 4:1 or 5:1. At those levels, excess calcium is removed from bone and eliminated, blood levels are reduced, and there is bone demineralization. A diet high in phosphorus and low in calcium has been shown to cause bone loss and increase tissue calcification.

The skeletal system suffers most from calcium deficiency. Teeth minerals are more stable, although there is a possibility of poor dentition with insufficient calcium. Tooth loss, periodontal disease, and gingivitis can be problems, especially with a high phosphorus intake, particularly from soft drinks. All kinds of bone problems can occur with prolonged calcium deficiency, which causes a decrease in bone mass. Rickets in children, osteomalacia in adults, and osteoporosis can occur when calcium is withdrawn from bones faster than it is deposited. Although there must be loss in bone mass of almost 40% before it is visible by X-ray, the problem may be detected earlier through diet history or blood and nutritional tests.

Calcium deficiency in the blood can cause a wide range of other symptoms, such as toxemia of pregnancy, anxiety, hyperkinesis, otosclerosis, and alcoholism. One theory about multiple sclerosis correlates it with calcium and vitamin D deficiency in puberty. Mild calcium deficiency can cause nerve sensitivity, paresthesias, muscle twitching, brittle nails, irritability, palpitations, insomnia, confusion, or a feeling of chronic depression. As it progresses, leg and foot or other muscle cramps, heart palpitations, numbness, tingling, and, finally, tetany (the sustained contraction of some muscles causing severe pain) may all occur. **Evidence shows that drinking soft water, which is high in sodium and low in calcium, can lead to increases in cardiovascular disease.** Hard water supplies extra calcium and magnesium, which may protect the heart.

Requirements. Because absorption of calcium is so variable, it is difficult to determine the right amount of calcium for all people. Many factors regarding absorption come into play. And the body can adapt to lower levels of calcium, even as low as 200 mg per day, and still maintain calcium balance, although this

adjustment usually needs to be started in childhood. In most Western cultures, with average absorption rates ranging from 30% to 50%, even the 1,000 mg AI may not be enough to prevent osteoporosis and other calcium deficiency problems. According to the USDA's Continuing Surveys of Food Intake by Individuals, 25% of the population is getting less than 600 mg of calcium per day, and 50% is getting less than 900 mg. An additional concern is that absorption usually decreases with age and with excessive use of antacids. But, luckily, humans are adaptable. Lower intake may lead to greater absorption efficiency, and higher intake usually leads to more elimination in the urine and feces. The body may naturally guide us to calcium foods that we can use.

The AIs for calcium, shown in the table below, are based on a fairly complicated formula that is specific to each age-gender group listed. In pregnancy and during nursing, 1.5 grams per day of calcium are suggested, especially in the last 2 months of pregnancy, when more than half of the baby's calcium needs are supplied. The calcium intake suggested for postmenopausal women has recently been changed to 1.5 grams per day for women not undergoing hor-

---

Adequate Intake Levels for Calcium

In 1998, the Institute of Medicine at the National Academy of Sciences issued the following new AI levels for calcium:

Age	AI Level
Males and females, 0–6 months	210 mg
Males and females, 7–12 months	270 mg
Males and females, 1–3 years	500 mg
Males and females, 4–8 years	800 mg
Adolescents, 9–13 years	1,300 mg
Adolescents, 14–18 years	1,300 mg
Adults, 19–50 years	1,000 mg
Adults, older than 51 years	1,200 mg
Postmenopausal women not taking hormone replacement therapy	1,500 mg
Pregnancy and lactation, younger than 18 years	1,300 mg
Pregnancy and lactation, older than 18 years	1,000 mg

mone replacement therapy, with some additional magnesium and vitamin D because of higher elimination and decreased absorption.

People with high-protein, high-phosphorus, or high-fat diets need even more calcium. When we increase calcium, we should also increase our magnesium intake, keeping it at about one-half the calcium supply. Magnesium helps calcium stay more soluble and thereby may reduce the risk of kidney stone formation and other calcifications. For phosphorus, an intake of about 800 to 1,000 mg is recommended when the calcium intake is 1,000 to 1,200 mg.

Calcium is not absorbed well in an alkaline environment because it is less soluble. It is best taken between meals or in the absence of foods, when the stomach is more acidic. Taking calcium with vitamin D and extra hydrochloric acid also increases absorption. Supplements of calcium or of calcium and magnesium are often taken at night before bed to help absorption and to prevent the extra loss of body calcium that can occur during the night. And calcium with magnesium is a good evening tranquilizer. Other ideas for maximizing use of dietary calcium are spreading out calcium intake in balanced portions throughout the day; consuming protein, vitamin D, and vitamin C foods or supplements; adding more calcium-rich foods to the diet, especially in place of junk foods or phosphorus-rich soda pops; and taking supplemental calcium as part of a total mineral balance with magnesium, zinc, and manganese, for example. Recently, the trace mineral boron has been shown to help in calcium utilization and bone health.

The form in which calcium is supplied is also important. Bonemeal and dolomite are good natural calcium and magnesium sources. They do not contain vitamin D but are still reasonably absorbable, although less so than other forms. There is some concern over lead and other toxic metals contaminating both dolomite and bonemeal. Oyster shell calcium is subject to this same toxicity concern. **The form that I most highly recommend is aspartate or citrate salts of calcium, which are probably the most absorbable.** Calcium aspartates are between 50% and 90% absorbable, which will likely place us in a positive calcium balance—exactly where we wish to be. Chelated calcium with amino acids are also easily absorbed. Calcium gluconate is the next choice, followed by calcium carbonate and calcium lactate, which are absorbable sources.

Chlorine/Chloride

 The element chlorine itself is a poisonous gas that is soluble in water; in Nature and in our body, it exists primarily as the chloride anion, the negatively charged ion that joins with cations such as sodium to make salt (sodium chloride) and with hydrogen to make stomach acid (hydrochloric acid). Chloride makes up about 0.15% of our body weight and is found mainly in the extracellular fluid, along with sodium. Less than 15% of the body chloride is found inside the cells, with the highest amounts within the red blood cells. **As one of the mineral electrolytes, chloride works closely with sodium and water to help the distribution of body fluids.** Chloride is easily absorbed from the small intestine. It is eliminated through the kidneys, which can also retain chloride as part of their finely controlled regulation of acid-base balance. Chloride is also found along with sodium in perspiration. Heavy sweating can cause the loss of large amounts of sodium chloride as well as some potassium.

Chlorine gas is used by many water-treatment plants as an agent to kill microorganisms in the water. It has been a great public health addition for eradicating disease in contaminated areas. But is it overused? Some scientists and practitioners are concerned with the levels of residual chlorine in drinking water because excess chlorine is thought to combine with certain organic water pollutants to form toxic chemicals and carcinogens (for more on this discussion, see chapter 1, Water, pages 15–16).

Sources. Chloride is obtained primarily from salt, such as standard table salt or sea salt. It is also contained in most foods, especially vegetables. Seaweeds (such as dulse and kelp), olives, rye, lettuce, tomatoes, and celery are some examples of good chloride-containing foods. Potassium chloride (KCl) is also found in foods or in the form of "salt substitute."

Functions. Chloride travels primarily with sodium and water and helps generate the osmotic pressure of body fluids. It is an important constituent of stomach hydrochloric acid (HCl), the key digestive acid. Chloride is also needed to maintain the body's acid-base balance. The kidneys excrete or retain chloride mainly as sodium chloride, depending on whether they are trying to increase or decrease body acid levels. Chloride may also be helpful in allowing the liver to clear waste products.

Until the mid-1990s or so, chloride research was somewhat limited. But since that time, enormous changes in the science of genetics have paved the way for new research about chloride and chronic disease. Researchers know now that chloride channels help many cells in the body release large molecules. For example, release of digestive enzymes from the pancreas is partly regulated by chloride channels, and defects in these channels are a direct cause of pancreatic inflammation. Chloride channels also help explain the classic symptom of cystic fibrosis—"salty sweat"—because genetic defects in chloride channel mechanisms prevent normal distribution of chloride in body fluids. In the years ahead, we are going to see other chronic diseases involving different organ systems becoming associated with chloride channel problems, and chloride is going to attract more attention in nutrition research.

Uses. Chloride is commonly used as sodium chloride, such as in salt tablets, to help replace the sodium and chloride lost in perspiration on hot days or with exercise. Chlorine is used in treating drinking water, swimming pools, hot tubs, and so on, to kill bacteria and other microorganisms.

Deficiency and toxicity. From a dietary standpoint, neither problem is very common nor worthy of much concern. Large amounts of chloride intake (more than 15 grams per day), usually in salt, may cause some problems with fluid retention and altered acid-base balance (although the main problem lies with the sodium). Chlorine itself, as gas or liquid, can be very irritating and toxic, and chlorine-containing pesticide residues are a real problem when it comes to nonorganically grown foods. There is also some concern about chloroform, a volatile liquid that can be formed spontaneously from chlorinated water and can have toxic effects. Domestic activities, like taking a hot shower, appear to be one of our main sources of chloroform exposure, and this exposure would obviously not be possible were it not for the chlorination of our drinking water. (There are dechlorinator attachments for showerheads to remove this concern.) Chlo-

ride deficiency can arise from diarrhea, vomiting, or sweating. It can lead to metabolic alkalosis (body fluids becoming too alkaline), low fluid volume, and urinary potassium loss. This can cause further problems in acid-base balance. Infant formulas without chloride can cause some of these problems, which are alleviated when chloride is given.

Requirements. Chloride is readily available in the normal food supply and there is no recommended dietary allowance (RDA). Infants probably need about 0.5 to 1 gram daily. The amount increases with age; adults needs are in the range of 1.7 to 5 grams daily, but many people consume much more because of the salt content in their diet.

Magnesium

 Magnesium is an important essential macro-mineral, even though there are only several ounces in the body (0.05% of body weight). It is involved in several hundred enzymatic reactions, many of which contribute to production of energy and cardiovascular function. The great amount of research on magnesium done since the mid-1990s has resulted in major changes in our knowledge. Decreases in magnesium intake have been more prevalent in the American diet with additions of supplemental vitamin D and calcium, dietary phosphorus, and refined or processed carbohydrate foods. **Drinking soft water decreases magnesium intake, while diuretic drugs cause magnesium loss, as do alcohol, caffeine, and sugar.** Decreased blood and tissue levels of magnesium have been shown to be related to high blood pressure, kidney stones, heart disease, and, particularly, heart attacks due to coronary artery spasm (magnesium helps relax and dilate coronary arteries). Studies have indicated that a decreased concentration of magnesium is found in the heart and blood of heart attack victims, although it is not clear whether this is a cause or a result of the problem. Magnesium's role in alleviating PMS has made big news as well.

Magnesium, like calcium, is an earth alkali mineral. The word *magnesium* comes from the name of the Greek city Magnesia, where large deposits of magnesium carbonate ($MgCO_3$) were found. This "salt" was first used as a laxative; magnesium carbonate and magnesium sulfate are still used in this way. Magnesium is the "iron" of the plant world—as iron is to hemoglobin, magnesium is to chlorophyll, the "blood" pigment of plants. The central atom of the chlorophyll structure is magnesium.

About 65% of our magnesium is contained in the bones and teeth. As with calcium, the bones act as a reservoir for magnesium in times of need. The remaining 35% of magnesium is contained in the blood, fluids, and other tissues; there is a high concentration, actually higher than in the blood, in the brain. Magnesium is also present in significant amounts in the heart. Most of it, like potassium, is inside the cells.

The process of digestion and absorption of magnesium is similar to that of calcium. The suggested ratio of intake of these two vital nutrients is about 2:1, calcium to magnesium. Magnesium also requires an acidic stomach environment for best absorption, so taking it between meals or at bedtime is recommended. Meals high in protein or fat, a diet high in phosphorus or calcium (calcium and magnesium can compete), or alcohol use may decrease magnesium absorption. It is possible that some of the hangover symptoms related to alcohol are in part due to magnesium depletion. Taking this mineral with some thiamine (B1) and drinking extra water can help prevent hangover symptoms.

Usually, about 40% to 50% of the magnesium we consume is absorbed, although this may vary from 25% to 75% depending on stomach acid levels, body needs, dietary habits, and the exact form of magnesium. Stress may increase magnesium excretion, the resulting temporary magnesium depletion may make the heart more sensitive to electrical abnormalities and vascular spasm, which could lead to cardiac ischemia. The kidneys can excrete or conserve magnesium according to body needs. The intestines can also eliminate excess magnesium in the feces. Otherwise, magnesium absorption is generally affected by the factors shown in the table "Factors Affecting Calcium Absorption," on page 156 in this chapter).

Sources. Almost all of our magnesium supplies come from the vegetable kingdom, although seafood has fairly high amounts. As a component of chlorophyll, this mineral is important to plant photosynthesis; therefore, the dark green vegetables are good sources of magnesium. Most nuts, seeds, and legumes have high amounts of magnesium; soy products, especially soy flour and tofu, and such nuts as almonds, pecans, cashews, and Brazil nuts are good examples. The whole grains, particularly wheat (especially the bran and germ), millet, and brown rice, as well as such fruits as avocado and dried apricot are other sources. Hard water can also be a valuable source of magnesium. Dolomite and bonemeal are good sources of magnesium, but as I mentioned earlier, they must be certified as free from heavy metal toxins.

Many factors affect magnesium availability from foods. One is the amount of magnesium in the soil in which the food is grown. Much magnesium can be lost in the processing and refining of foods and in the making of oils from the magnesium-rich nuts and seeds. Nearly 85% of the magnesium in grains is lost during the milling of flours. Soaking and boiling foods can leach magnesium into the water, so the "pot liquor" from cooking vegetables may be high in magnesium and other minerals. Oxalic acid in such vegetables as spinach and chard and phytic acid in some grains may form insoluble salts with magnesium, causing it to be eliminated rather than absorbed. For these reasons and those previously discussed, many people get insufficient magnesium from their diets. In fact, according to the USDA, almost one-third of the U.S. population gets under 65% of the RDA for this mineral.

Functions. Magnesium is considered the "anti-stress" mineral. It is a natural tranquilizer, as it functions to relax skeletal muscles as well as the smooth muscles of blood vessels and the gastrointestinal tract. (While calcium stimulates muscle contraction, magnesium relaxes them.) Because of its influence on the heart, magnesium is considered important in preventing coronary artery spasm, a significant cause of heart attacks. Spasms of the blood vessels lead to insufficient oxygen supply through them and pain, injury, or death of the muscle tissue that they nourish. **To function optimally, magnesium must be balanced in the body with calcium, phosphorus, potassium, and sodium chloride.** For example, with low magnesium, more calcium flows into the vascular muscle cells, which contracts them—leading to tighter vessels and higher blood pressure. Adequate magnesium levels prevent this.

Magnesium is primarily an intracellular nutrient. It activates enzymes that are important for protein and carbohydrate metabolism, and it is needed in DNA production and function. Magnesium also modulates the electrical potential across cell membranes, which allows nutrients to pass back and forth. It helps in the release of energy by transferring the key phosphate molecule to adenosine triphosphate (ATP), an energy source generated by the cytochrome system. In addition, magnesium has the ability to sit at the entrance to nerve cell calcium channels and help prevent overstimulation of the cells because of calcium flooding. For this reason, magnesium is thought of as helping to prevent excitotoxicity. Magnesium is also thought to dilate the blood vessels.

Uses. As time goes on, magnesium is recommended and used in more and more treatments. Prevention or treatment of myocardial infarctions, prevention of kidney stones, and treatment of PMS are some important recent uses. Magnesium has been used with some success in relieving certain kinds of angina and reducing the risks of coronary artery spasms, which can lead to angina or, more severely, heart attack. Deficient magnesium levels have been found in the blood and hearts of cardiac victims. Besides preventing heart attacks, magnesium has a mild effect on lowering blood pressure and so is used to treat and prevent hypertension and its effects. Magnesium supplementation can reduce many of the symptoms of mitral valve prolapse, such as palpitations or arrhythmias, and it may help in other cardiac arrhythmias, such as atrial tachycardia or fibrillation, or those caused by taking excess digitalis, a cardiac drug. It may also reduce the bronchoconstriction in asthma by relaxing the muscle around the bronchial tubes. Intravenous solutions containing magnesium and other nutrients have been used successfully to break acute asthma attacks.

Magnesium sulfate has been used specifically to lower blood pressure in pregnant women with preeclampsia, which is characterized by edema, hypertension, and hyperreflexia. These problems could become more severe and lead to seizures (then termed *eclampsia*) as well. Magnesium sulfate also acts as a mild anticonvulsant in this case. Through its nerve- and muscle-relaxing effect, magnesium may be helpful in reducing epileptic seizures caused by nerve excitability.

By increasing calcium solubility, especially in the urine, magnesium can help prevent kidney stones,

---

Problems That May Be Helped by Magnesium

Alcoholism	Hyperactivity
Angina pectoris	Hypertension
Anxiety	Insomnia
Arrhythmias	Kidney stones
Atherosclerosis	Menstrual pain
Autism	Muscle cramps
Bronchial asthma	Osteoporosis
Epilepsy	Premenstrual syndrome
Fatigue	

---

especially calcium oxalate stones. Research has shown this effect in a high percentage of people who form kidney stones regularly. Actually, it is thought that calcium oxalate stones are most likely to form in people who are magnesium deficient, so treatment of calcium oxalate stones may primarily be a question of remedying magnesium deficiency. Through this same effect, magnesium is helpful in preventing calcification of other tissues and blood vessels (and thereby atherosclerosis), as well as some problems of the teeth, including cavities. For these purposes, a daily dose of 50 mg of vitamin B6 and 200 to 300 mg of magnesium oxide is often given.

Supplementing magnesium has been shown to be helpful in alleviating many symptoms related to the menstrual period. Menstrual cramps, irritability, fatigue, depression, and water retention have been lessened with magnesium, usually given along with calcium and often with vitamin B6. Magnesium is often at its lowest level during menstruation, and many symptoms of PMS are relieved when this mineral is replenished. Supplementing magnesium in the same amount (or more) as calcium (about 500 to 1,000 mg daily) is currently recommended for premenstrual problems.

Fatigue is often reduced with magnesium (and potassium) supplementation. The many enzyme systems that require magnesium help restore normal energy levels. Because of this function and magnesium's nerve and muscle support, it may also be helpful for nervousness, anxiety, insomnia, depression, and muscle cramps. Magnesium is given as part of a treatment for autism or hyperactivity in children, usually along with vitamin B6. **Getting children and fatigued adults to eat more green vegetables and chlorophyll is often helpful for supplying additional naturally occurring magnesium.** People tend to sleep better after taking magnesium before bed. Alcoholics tend to have low magnesium levels; thus this mineral can be helpful during withdrawal and to prevent or reduce hangover symptoms. Also, a special form of magnesium, combined with malic acid as magnesium malate, is used with some success in people with chronic fatigue syndrome and fibromyalgia pains. (See "Fatigue" on page 669 in Chapter 17, Medical Treatment Programs.)

When given orally, magnesium sulfate (Epsom salts) is not absorbed but attracts water into the colon and thus acts as an effective laxative. Epsom salts in a bath are absorbed slightly and are known to be relaxing. For injuries, a concentrated solution is used as a compress to help drain toxins. Magnesium is also thought to reduce lead toxicity and its buildup, possibly through competing for absorption. Because magnesium is an alkaline mineral, it is used in several over-the-counter antacids.

Deficiency and toxicity. Toxicity due to magnesium overload is almost unknown in a nutritional context, as excesses are usually eliminated in the urine and feces. However, symptoms of magnesium toxicity can occur if calcium intake is low. These symptoms may include depression of the central nervous system, causing muscle weakness, fatigue, sleepiness, or even hyperexcitability. In extreme states, magnesium overload can cause death. Magnesium can also function as a bowel laxative, and milk of magnesia has been used for many years for precisely this reason. It is somewhat baffling to me that in 1997, however, the Institute of Medicine could have used mild, infrequent, and reversible diarrhea as its reason for setting 350 mg as the tolerable upper limit for mineral supplements containing magnesium. It is even more baffling when I think about the fact that 420 mg is the new RDA for adult men, and that 15% of all adult men in the United States get 175 mg per day or less! As long as a balance is kept with other minerals, especially calcium, I am comfortable with supplements up to approximately 1,000 mg.

Magnesium deficiency is actually fairly common. It is usually not looked for, however, and therefore not found or corrected. Deficiency is more likely in those who eat a processed-food diet; in people who cook or boil all foods, especially vegetables; in those who drink soft water; in alcoholics; and in people who eat food grown in magnesium-deficient soil, where synthetic fertilizers containing no magnesium are often used. Deficiency is also more common when magnesium absorption is decreased, such as after burns, serious injuries, or surgery, and in patients with diabetes, liver disease, or malabsorption problems. Deficiency can also occur when magnesium elimination is increased, as in people who use alcohol, caffeine, or excess sugar, or who take diuretics or birth control pills.

In the body, magnesium works closely together with vitamin D, phosphorus, and calcium. The processed food supply has given us an artificial abundance of vitamin D, in the form of fortified milk and dairy products; a surplus of phosphorus, in the form of phosphoric acid added to soft drinks; and extra calcium in everything from orange juice to pancake mix. By comparison, we do not have any "false surplus" of magnesium, and I suspect that at least part of our magnesium deficiency is due to the false elevations of these other nutrients in the highly processed food supply.

Early symptoms of magnesium deficiency can include fatigue, anorexia, irritability, insomnia, and muscle tremors or twitching. Psychological changes, such as apathy, apprehension, decreased learning ability, confusion, and poor memory may occur. Tachycardia (rapid heartbeat) and other cardiovascular changes are likely with moderate deficiency, while severe magnesium deficiency may lead to numbness, tingling, and tetany (sustained contraction) of the muscles, as well as delirium and hallucinations. Arterial spasm, specifically of the coronary arteries, is a significant recent concern with magnesium deficiency. This could lead to angina symptoms or even a heart attack. Blood pressure can rise with magnesium deficiency, while an increased likelihood of kidney stones and other tissue calcification is also possible.

Requirements. The minimum required intake for magnesium can be expressed as about 6 mg per kg (2.2 pounds) of body weight. Using this standard, a 150-pound person would need about 410 mg. Many authorities feel that the RDA should be increased by about 50%, to about 600 to 700 mg daily. An average diet usually supplies about 120 mg of magnesium per

1,000 calories, for an estimated daily intake of about 250 mg. Unless absorption is great, that is not going to produce adequate tissue levels of magnesium for most people.

Magnesium chelated with amino acids or organic acids is probably the most absorbable form. The limited research in this area points to two nonchelated forms of magnesium, magnesium oxide (4% to 15% absorption) and magnesium sulfate (25% to 40% absorption), as among the least absorbable forms, with chelated forms being better absorbed. Most estimates show the amino acid chelates of magnesium (magnesium glycinate and magnesium aspartate) and the organic acid chelates (including magnesium citrate, magnesium fumarate, magnesium gluconate, magnesium lactate, and magnesium carbonate) to be absorbed in the 75% to 98% range. By comparison, overall magnesium absorption from food appears to be about 30% to 60%.

RDAs and AI Levels for Magnesium Intake

In 1997, the Institute of Medicine set the following guidelines for magnesium intake:

Age	AI/RDA Level
Males and females, 0–6 months	30 mg (AI)
Males and females, 7–12 months	75 mg (AI)
Males and females, 1–3 years	80 mg (RDA)
Males and females, 4–8 years	130 mg (RDA)
Adolescents, 9–13 years	240 mg (RDA)
Males, 14–18 years	410 mg (RDA)
Females, 14–18 years	360 mg (RDA)
Males, 19–30 years	400 mg (RDA)
Males, 31 years and older	420 mg (RDA)
Females, 19–30 years	310 mg (RDA)
Females, 31 years and older	320 mg (RDA)
Pregnancy, younger than 18 years	400 mg (RDA)
Pregnancy, 19–30 years	350 mg (RDA)
Pregnancy, 31–50 years	360 mg (RDA)
Lactation, younger than 18 years	360 mg (RDA)
Lactation, 19–30 years	310 mg (RDA)
Lactation, 31–50 years	320 mg (RDA)

The calcium-magnesium balance is important. It is usually suggested that when people supplement with calcium, they take about half that amount in magnesium. If calcium intake is increased, magnesium should likewise be increased. Magnesium intake should also be increased when more phosphorus, vitamin D, or protein is consumed or when there is higher blood cholesterol. Postmenopausal women, as well as those on birth control pills or diuretics and those who drink alcohol, need more magnesium.

The levels of magnesium used by physicians are commonly in the range of 600 to 1,000 mg; however, the researchers in early kidney stone studies used only 200 to 300 mg of supplemental magnesium oxide. Calcium and magnesium are both alkaline minerals, so they are not taken with or after meals, as they can reduce stomach acid and are poorly absorbed when taken with food. They are absorbed better when taken between meals or on an empty stomach, especially with a little vitamin C as ascorbic acid. Many calcium-magnesium combinations are formulated with hydrochloric acid and vitamin D to aid the mineral absorption. And taking them before bedtime may be helpful in increasing utilization of both these important minerals and lead to a sleep-filled night.

Phosphorus

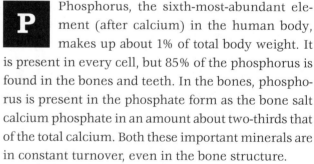 Phosphorus, the sixth-most-abundant element (after calcium) in the human body, makes up about 1% of total body weight. It is present in every cell, but 85% of the phosphorus is found in the bones and teeth. In the bones, phosphorus is present in the phosphate form as the bone salt calcium phosphate in an amount about two-thirds that of the total calcium. Both these important minerals are in constant turnover, even in the bone structure.

The body uses a variety of mechanisms to control the calcium-to-phosphorus ratio and metabolism. This ratio in the diet has been the subject of much recent interest. **The typical American diet provides too much phosphorus and not enough calcium, leading to reduced body storage of calcium; thus many of the problems of calcium deficiency may develop** (discussed on pages 159–160). Phosphorus and calcium can compete for absorption in the intestines. High consumption of meats or soft drinks increases phosphorus intake and may contribute to this imbalance. Recent research has shown clear problems with maintenance of bone health when this ratio gets too low, in the 1:3 or 1:4 range. The ideal ratio of calcium to phosphorus is somewhere between 1:1 and 1.5:1, with slightly more calcium being desirable. Phosphorus is absorbed more efficiently than calcium. Nearly 70% of phosphorus is absorbed from the intestines, although the rate depends somewhat on the levels of calcium and vitamin D and the activity of parathyroid hormone (PTH), which regulates the metabolism of phosphorus and calcium.

Most phosphorus is deposited in the bones, a little goes to the teeth, and the rest is contained in the cells and other tissues. Much is found in the red blood cells. The plasma phosphorus measures about 3.5 mg (3.5 mg of phosphorus per 100 ml of plasma), while the total blood phosphorus is 30 to 40 mg. The body level of this mineral is regulated by the kidneys, which are also influenced by PTH. Phosphorus absorption may be decreased by antacids, iron, aluminum, or magnesium, which may all form insoluble phosphates and be eliminated in the feces. Caffeine causes increased phosphorus excretion by the kidneys.

Sources. Because phosphorus is part of all cells, it is readily found in food, especially animal tissues. Most protein foods are high in phosphorus. Meats, fish, chicken, turkey, milk, cheese, and eggs all contain substantial amounts. Most red meats and poultry have much more phosphorus than calcium—between 10 and 20 times as much—whereas fish generally has about 2 or 3 times as much phosphorus as calcium. The dairy foods have a more balanced calcium-to-phosphorus ratio. Seeds and nuts also contain good levels of phosphorus (although they have less calcium), as do the whole grains, brewer's yeast, and wheat germ and bran. Most fruits and vegetables contain some phosphorus and help to balance the ratio of phosphorus to calcium in a wholesome diet.

In recent years, the increased consumption of soft drinks, which are buffered with phosphates, has been a concern. There may be up to 500 mg of phosphorus per serving of a soft drink, with essentially no calcium. In 2000, Americans spent $60 billion on carbonated soft drinks, and billions more on noncarbonated "fruit" beverages. During the same year, the average American consumed more than 53 gallons

of soft drinks. Because some people do not drink any of these beverages, quite a number of people are drinking even more than the average amount of soft drinks and thus consuming a lot of phosphorus.

Functions. Phosphorus is involved in many functions besides forming bones and teeth. Like calcium, it is found in all cells and is involved in some way in most biochemical reactions. Phosphorus is vital to energy production and exchange in a variety of ways. It provides the phosphate in adenosine triphosphate (ATP), which is the high-energy carrier molecule in the body's primary metabolic cycles. Phosphorus is important to the utilization of carbohydrates and fats for energy production and also in protein synthesis for the growth, maintenance, and repair of all tissues and cells. As inorganic phosphate in ATP, it is needed in protein synthesis and in the production of the nucleic acids in DNA and RNA, which carry the genetic code for all cells.

Phosphorus is also a component of the phospholipids, fat molecules essential to cell membranes; lecithin is the best-known phospholipid. It helps in fat emulsification and in other body functions. In the cell membranes, the phospholipids help maintain both fluidity and permeability, allowing the nutrients to pass in and out of the cells. The sphingolipids, involved in nerve conduction, also contain phosphorus. Phosphorus is combined with the B vitamins to assist their functions in the body. Furthermore, phosphoproteins are contained in many enzyme systems.

In addition to its role in these processes and in skeletal growth and tooth development, phosphorus has a number of other functions. It helps in kidney function and acts as a buffer for acid-base balance in the body. Phosphorus aids muscle contraction, including the regularity of the heartbeat, and is also supportive of proper nerve conduction. This important mineral supports the conversion of niacin and riboflavin to their active coenzyme forms. As mentioned, parathyroid hormone regulates the phosphorus blood level and helps phosphorus carry out all of its essential functions. Phosphorus also has an important role to play in genetics. The backbone of our primary genetic material, DNA, is formed out of alternating phosphorus and sugar molecules.

Uses. Phosphorus by itself is used in only a few medically significant conditions. It is not needed as frequently as calcium to balance the ratio between

Tolerable Upper Limits for Phosphorus

Age	UL
Infants, 0–6 months	not determined
Infants, 7–12 months	not determined
Children, 1–3 years	3 g
Children, 4–8 years	3 g
Males and females, 9–18 years	4 g
Males and females, 19–70 years	4 g
Males and females, older than 70 years	3 g
Pregnancy, 18 years or younger	3.5 g
Pregnancy, 19–50 years	3.5 g
Lactation, 18 years or younger	4 g
Lactation, 19–50 years	4 g

RDAs and AI Levels for Phosphorus

In 1997 the Institute of Medicine set the following dietary guidelines for phosphorus:

Age	RDA/AI Level
Infants, 0–6 months	100 mg (AI)
Infants, 7–12 months	275 mg (AI)
Children, 1–3 years	460 mg (RDA)
Children, 4–8 years	500 mg (RDA)
Males and females, 9–13 years	1,250 mg (RDA)
Males and females, 14–18 years	1,250 mg (RDA)
Males and females, 19 years and older	700 mg (RDA)
Pregnancy, 18 years or younger	1,250 mg (RDA)
Pregnancy, 19–50 years	700 mg (RDA)
Lactation, 18 years or younger	1,250 mg (RDA)
Lactation, 19–50 years	700 mg (RDA)

these two minerals. However, phosphorus has been used to treat many kinds of bone problems; it (along with calcium) helps in healing fractures by minimizing calcium loss from bones. It is used in the treatment of osteomalacia and in osteoporosis. Rickets has also been treated with phosphorus, as well as with calcium and vitamin D.

Rebalancing the calcium-to-phosphorus ratio in the diet can help reduce stress and many problems relating to calcium metabolism, arthritis being an example. Tooth and gum problems can be alleviated with dietary phosphorus, again in balance with calcium. Cancer research has revealed that cancer cells tend to lose phosphorus more readily than do normal cells, so phosphorus may be useful in the nutritional support of cancer patients; however, a high phosphorus-to-calcium intake is to be avoided.

Deficiency and toxicity. Based on problems associated with calcium metabolism, excessive depositing of calcium in body tissues (other than bone), and parathyroid hormone imbalances, in 1997 the Institute of Medicine set the following tolerable upper limits) for phosphorus intake.

A low calcium-to-phosphorus ratio in the diet can also increase the incidence of hypertension and the risk of colorectal cancer. Although research in this area is limited, the low ratio seems to be consistently problematic for pregnancy-related hypertension in women and prostate cancer in men. Problems of phosphorus deficiency are fairly uncommon, because it is so readily obtained in the diet. It is usually consumed in greater amounts than calcium and is readily absorbed. Relative deficiency of phosphorus can be caused by very high calcium intake or by taking a lot of antacids, which can bind phosphorus. Aluminum, magnesium, and iron can interfere with phosphorus absorption. Low vitamin D intake can also lead to deficient body phosphorus.

Symptoms of phosphorus deficiency may include anorexia, weakness, weight loss, irritability, anxiety, stiff joints, paresthesias, bone pain, and bone fragility. Decreased growth, poor bone and tooth development, and symptoms of rickets may occur in phosphorus-deficient children. A low calcium-to-phosphorus ratio is most likely to generate problems in adults. Osteoporosis is often brought on by high phosphorus and low calcium intake. Other adult problems include skin disease, tooth decay, and even arthritis.

Requirements. If phosphorus intake is high or body levels are increased, we may need to take more calcium to achieve a ratio in the desired range of 1:1.5 to maintain biochemical homeostasis. Phosphorus in small amounts like 100 to 200 mg is often contained in multimineral or multivitamin formulas. It is unlikely that anyone takes phosphorus as a separate supplement.

Potassium

K Potassium is a significant body mineral, important to both cellular and electrical function. It is one of the main blood minerals called *electrolytes* (the others are sodium and chloride), which means it carries a tiny electrical charge (potential). Potassium is the primary positive ion (cation) found within the cells, where 98% of the 120 grams of potassium in the body is found. The blood serum contains about 4 to 5 mg (per 100 ml) of the total potassium; the red blood cells contain 420 mg, which is why a red blood cell level is a better indication of an individual's potassium status than the commonly used serum level.

Magnesium helps maintain the potassium in the cells, but the sodium and potassium balance is as finely tuned as those of calcium and phosphorus or calcium and magnesium. Research has found that a high-sodium diet with low potassium intake influences vascular volume and tends to elevate the blood pressure. Then doctors may prescribe diuretics that can cause even more potassium loss, aggravating the underlying problems. The appropriate course is to shift to natural potassium-rich foods and away from high-salt foods, lose weight if needed, and follow an exercise program to improve cardiovascular tone and physical stamina. A natural diet high in fruits, vegetables, and whole grains is rich in potassium and low in sodium, helping to maintain normal blood pressure and sometimes lowering elevated blood pressure. The body contains more potassium than sodium, about 9 ounces to 4, but the American diet—with its reliance on fast foods, packaged convenience foods, chips, and salt—has become high in sodium (salt). Because the body's biochemical functions are based on the components found in a natural diet, special mechanisms conserve sodium, while potassium is conserved somewhat less.

Potassium is well absorbed from the small intestine, with about 90% absorption, but is one of the most soluble minerals, so it is easily lost in cooking and processing foods. Most excess potassium is eliminated in the urine; some is eliminated in the sweat. When we perspire a great deal, we should replace our fluids with orange juice or vegetable juice containing potassium rather than just taking salt tablets.

The kidneys are the chief regulators of the body's potassium, keeping the blood levels steady even with wide variation in intake. The adrenal hormone aldosterone stimulates elimination of potassium by the kidneys. **Alcohol, coffee (and other caffeine drinks), sugar, and diuretic drugs, however, cause potassium losses and can contribute to lowering the blood potassium.** This mineral is also lost with vomiting and diarrhea.

Sources. Potassium is found in a wide range of foods. Many fruits and vegetables are high in potassium and low in sodium and, as mentioned, help prevent hypertension. Most of the potassium is lost when processing or canning foods, while less is lost from freezing fruits or vegetables. Such leafy green vegetables as spinach, parsley, mustard greens, and lettuce, as well as broccoli, peas, lima beans, tomatoes, and potatoes, especially the skins, all have significant levels of potassium. Fruits that contain this mineral include oranges and other citrus fruits, bananas, apples, avocados, raisins, and apricots, particularly dried. Whole grains, wheat germ, seeds, and nuts are high-potassium foods. Such fish as flounder, salmon, sardines, and cod are rich in potassium, and many meat foods contain even more potassium than sodium, although they often have additional sodium added as salt. Mushrooms are also a good source of this mineral.

Functions. Potassium is important in the human body. **Along with sodium, it regulates the water balance and the acid-base balance in the blood and tissues.** Potassium enters the cell more readily than does sodium and instigates the brief sodium-potassium exchange across the cell membranes. In the nerve cells, this sodium-potassium flux generates the electrical potential that aids the conduction of nerve impulses. When potassium leaves the cell, it changes the membrane potential and allows the nerve impulse to progress. This electrical potential gradient, created by the *sodium-potassium pump*, helps generate muscle contractions and regulates the heartbeat.

Because of its role in muscle contraction and heartbeat, potassium is an important regulator of blood pressure. In fact, for most individuals with high blood pressure, increasing potassium intake is a much more reliable way to lower blood pressure than decreasing intake of sodium. Potassium is also important in cellular biochemical reactions and energy metabolism; it participates in the synthesis of protein from amino acids in the cell. Potassium also functions in carbohydrate metabolism; it is active in glycogen and glucose metabolism, converting glucose to glycogen, which can be stored in the liver for future energy. Potassium is important for normal growth and for building muscle.

Uses. In medicine, potassium is one of the most commonly prescribed minerals. It is also commonly measured in biochemical testing and is supplemented if it is low. Because potassium is crucial to cardiovascular and nerve functions and is lost in diuretic therapy for edema or hypertension, a prevalent American disease, it must frequently be added as a dietary supplement. As stated before, the average American diet has reversed the natural high-potassium and low-sodium intake, and a shift back to this more healthful balance can reduce some types of elevated blood pressure. Supplementing potassium can be helpful in treating hypertension specifically caused by a hyperresponse to excess sodium.

Pharmacological preparations of potassium are commonly prescribed for many of these conditions. A 10% potassium chloride solution is often given, but its taste is unpleasant. More easily used formulas are tablets that are swallowed or effervescent tablets. K-Lor, Slow-K, K-Lyte, and Kaochlor are common preparations. Time-release formulas, such as Micro-K, are also available. Potassium chloride has occasionally been helpful in treating infant colic, some cases of allergies, and headaches. During and after diarrhea, potassium replacement may be necessary, and many people feel better taking potassium during weight-loss programs. Fatigue or weakness, especially in the elderly, is often alleviated with supplemental potassium, along with magnesium. Additional potassium may be required for dehydration states after fluid losses and may be used to prevent or reduce hangover symptoms after alcohol consumption.

Deficiency and toxicity. Elevations or depletions of this important mineral can cause problems and, in the extreme, even death. Maintaining consistent levels of potassium in the blood and cells is vital to body function. Even with high intakes of potassium, the kidneys will clear any excess, and blood levels will not be increased. For elevated potassium levels (called *hyperkalemia*) to occur, there must usually be other factors involved; decrease in renal function is the most likely cause. Major infection, gastrointestinal bleeding, and rapid protein breakdown also may cause elevated potassium levels. Cardiac function is affected by hyperkalemia; electrocardiogram changes can be seen in this condition. Because the kidneys are so important as a means of clearing excess potassium, people with kidney disease need to be especially careful to avoid excessive potassium.

Deficiency of potassium is much more common, especially with aging or chronic disease. Some common problems that have been associated with low potassium levels include hypertension, congestive heart failure, cardiac arrhythmias, fatigue, and depression and other mood changes. Many factors reduce body levels of potassium. Diarrhea, vomiting, and other gastrointestinal problems may rapidly reduce potassium. Infants with diarrhea must be watched closely for low blood potassium, termed *hypokalemia*. Diabetes and renal disease may cause low as well as high potassium levels. Several drugs can cause hypokalemia—diuretic therapy is of most concern. Long-term use of laxatives, aspirin, digitalis, and cortisone may also deplete potassium. Heat waves and profuse sweating can cause potassium loss and lead to dehydration, with potassium leaving the cells, along with sodium, and being lost in the urine. This can generate some of the symptoms associated with low potassium; most people are helped rapidly with potassium supplements or potassium-rich foods. People who consume excess sodium can lose extra urinary potassium, and people who eat lots of sugar also may become low in potassium.

Fatigue is the most common symptom of chronic potassium deficiency. Early symptoms include muscle weakness, slow reflexes, and dry skin or acne; these initial problems may progress to nervous disorders, insomnia, slow or irregular heartbeat, and loss of gastrointestinal tone. A sudden loss of potassium may lead to cardiac arrhythmias. Low potassium may impair glucose metabolism and lead to elevated blood sugar. In more severe potassium deficiency, there can be serious muscle weakness, bone fragility, central nervous system changes, decreased heart rate, and even death. Potassium is the most commonly measured blood mineral in medicine, and deficiencies must be watched for carefully and treated without delay with supplemental potassium.

Requirements. There is no specific RDA for potassium, although there is an estimated safe and adequate daily dietary intake (ESADDI) range of 1.9 to 5.6 grams per day. It is thought that at least 2.5 to 3.5 grams per day are needed, or about 1.25 to 1.75 grams per 1,000 calories consumed. The average American diet includes from 2 to 6 grams per day. In cooking or canning foods, potassium is depleted but sodium is increased, as it is in most American processed foods. I suggest that we include more potassium than sodium in our diets; a ratio of about 2:1 would be ideal. When we increase sodium intake, we should also consume more potassium-rich foods or take a potassium supplement. Over-the-counter potassium supplements usually contain 99 mg per tablet. Prescription potassium is usually measured in milliequivalents (mEq); 1 mEq equals about 64 mg. About 10 to 20 mEq (640–1,280 mg) per day may be recommended as a supplement to the individual's diet.

The inorganic potassium salts are found as sulfate, chloride, oxide, or carbonate. Organic salts are potassium gluconate, fumarate, or citrate. These organic molecules are normally part of our cells and body tissues. Potassium liquids and salt substitutes containing potassium chloride (KCl) are other ways to obtain this mineral. Potassium is well absorbed, so it is available to the body in most forms.

Sodium

 Sodium is the primary positive ion found in the blood and body fluids; it is also found in every cell, although it is mainly extracellular, working closely with potassium, the primary intracellular mineral. About 60% of body sodium is in the fluids around cells (extracellular), 10% is inside the cells, and around 30% is found in the bones. Sodium is one of the electrolytes, along with potassium and chloride, and is closely tied in with the movement of water. As the saying goes, "Where sodium goes, water goes." Sodium represents about 0.15% of the body weight. Approximately 90 to 100 grams are present in the body, most of which occurs in combination with chloride as salt, or sodium chloride.

Sodium chloride is present on a large part of the Earth's surface in ocean water. In common usage, the word *salt* refers mainly to sodium chloride, but in chemistry, a salt is any combination of a positive and a negative ion in crystalline form or in solution. Sodium chloride is only 75% of the salt in seawater, which also contains potassium chloride (KCl), calcium chloride ($CaCl_2$), and calcium phosphate ($Ca(CPO_4)_2$), as well as other mineral salts.

Sodium, or salt, has been valued throughout history. The word *salt* is the source of the word *salary*, which originally referred to money paid to soldiers to buy salt. Yet this value placed on salt has possibly led to its overuse in industrial society. For millions of years, the human species lived on a natural diet containing less than 1 gram a day of sodium, and elevated blood pressure was very rare. Nowadays, 6 to 12 grams of salt a day (and even higher amounts) are consumed by people eating processed and snack foods or as salt added in cooking and preparing foods. Salt itself is 40% sodium and 60% chloride. Therefore, 5 grams of salt (about 1 teaspoon) contain approximately 2 grams of sodium.

High blood pressure is now epidemic in the United States as well as in other cultures that eat high-salt diets. Where natural foods are the only source of sodium, there is almost no hypertension. These foods contain more potassium, which is found in high amounts in plant cells as well as in human cells. There is still some controversy about the relationship between salt and high blood pressure; the sodium-to-potassium ratio may be even more important in controlling blood pressure than the actual amount of sodium. Certain people seem to be more sensitive to sodium and its effects on blood pressure, although it is not clear whether this is due to genetic or other physiologic factors. Restricting sodium may significantly help the estimated 15% to 25% of the general population that is salt sensitive. (Salt sensitivity is defined as having your blood pressure decrease by 10 points [10mm Hg, where Hg stands for the mercury in the blood pressure tube that moves down the tube 10 ml] after you have been given a trial dose of salt and then waited for your body to eliminate it.) It may also help about 30% to 50% of the people who are already diagnosed with high blood pressure, especially those who are also obese or older than 65. (This age-related aspect of salt sensitivity may be related to a decline in kidney function that can occur in later life.) Reducing salt intake among the general population, of any age, may have less effect on blood pressure. In any event, eating a low-sodium diet that is also high in potassium, magnesium, and calcium on a long-term basis may be one of the best ways to prevent hypertension.

Sodium, like potassium, is soluble and therefore is easily absorbed from the stomach and small intestine—nearly 100% of the sodium consumed gets into the body. It goes into the blood and is circulated through the kidneys, which can reabsorb or eliminate it in order to maintain stable blood sodium levels. About 90% of the sodium consumed in the average diet is in excess of body needs and must be eliminated in the urine. Therefore, urine levels reflect dietary intake. Aldosterone, a hormone made and secreted by the adrenal cortex, acts on the kidneys to regulate sodium metabolism.

Some sodium is stored in the bones and is available if needed. Sodium can be lost with excessive sweating and with vomiting or diarrhea. When this happens, we naturally crave water and salt. Should we then consume only water, we may experience *water intoxication*, wherein water goes into the cells and causes swelling, which may lead to such symptoms as headaches, weakness, loss of appetite, or poor memory. More commonly, though, we first crave salt and then become thirsty for water to dilute or, rather, balance the osmotic effects of sodium and help it to be eliminated. This is all carefully regulated by our masterful kidneys and our active adrenal glands.

Sources. Almost all foods contain some sodium, particularly as sodium chloride. It is found in high amounts in all seafood, in beef, and in poultry, and some sodium is in many vegetables, including celery, beets, carrots, and artichokes. Kelp and other sea vegetables are fairly high in sodium.

No wholesome natural food has a high salt content. It is only the Westernized diet of processed foods that has significant salt content, and many people consume these foods as their primary diet. Breads, crackers, chips, cheeses (especially the processed types), some peanut butter, and salt-cured foods such as olives and pickles may constitute a good percentage of a typical unhealthy diet. Lunchmeats and processed or cured meats, such as bacon, bologna, corned beef, and hot dogs, are particularly high in salt and other preservatives, such as nitrates and nitrites. Luckily, most people can clear excess sodium chloride from their bodies, but it creates additional work for the kidneys. After many

years, the kidneys may weaken from this chronic stress and be unable to clear the salt as well, which may lead to more problems, including high blood pressure.

Sodium can also come from nonsalt sources, such as baking soda (sodium bicarbonate), monosodium glutamate (MSG), sodium propionate, or any other ingredient listed on a package as soda or sodium "something." Soy sauce, or tamari, has high amounts of sodium as well, but the sodium is less concentrated than in crystal salt. Softened water also has extra sodium added to replace the naturally occurring magnesium and calcium that are removed. This is done because the more soluble sodium can wash clothes better and bubble more for daily cleaning and bathing, but when this water is used as a drink, it adds to the already excessive sodium levels.

Functions. Along with potassium, sodium helps to regulate the fluid balance of the body, both within and outside the cells. Through the kidneys, by buffering the blood with a balance of all the positive or negative ions present, these two minerals help control the acid-base balance as well. The high blood levels of sodium contribute to the osmolarity (concentration of solutes in solution) and thereby regulate the fluid volume of the body and blood. The shifting of sodium and potassium across the cell membranes helps to create an electrical potential (charge) that enables muscles to contract and nerve impulses to be conducted. Sodium is also important to hydrochloric acid production in the stomach and is used during the transport of amino acids from the gut into the blood.

Because sodium is needed to maintain blood fluid volume, excessive sodium can lead to increased blood volume and elevated blood pressure, especially when the kidneys do not clear it efficiently. It is easier to prevent hypertension with low salt intake than to treat it by lowering salt in the diet. Hypertension is more frequent in people who have a high salt intake, especially when there is a low level of potassium in the diet. Fresh fruits and vegetables are high in potassium and low in sodium, and research shows that increased potassium can balance out some of the effects high-sodium intake has on blood pressure. Elderly people and the African American population are more prone than other groups to elevated blood pressure. In cultures that consume low sodium diets, there is little, if any, hypertension.

Uses. There is not really a physiologic need for added salt or sodium in the diet. Our bodies tolerate and, in fact, probably do best on a much lower sodium intake than is provided by the average Westernized diet. So far more problems are caused by excess sodium—high blood pressure, premenstrual symptoms, and water retention, for example—than there are low-sodium difficulties that require treatment with sodium. Low sodium levels can, however, result from habitually avoiding sodium or from hot weather and severe perspiration; extra salt or sodium can help here. Potassium may also be needed. Preventing and treating heatstroke and leg cramps are occasional uses for sodium. It is possible that on one hand, low sodium levels can cause blurred vision, edema, and even high blood pressure or, on the other, decreased fluid volume and low blood pressure. In these situations, additional sodium may be helpful. Salt is also employed to preserve foods, protecting them from oxidation and breakdown from microorganism activity.

Deficiency and toxicity. In the case of sodium, there is more of a concern with toxicity from excesses than with deficiencies. Some people, as many as 30%, are sensitive to high levels of dietary sodium and develop hypertension from too much salt. Hypertension is only one of the problems related to excess sodium, however. Premenstrual problems may become more severe with too much salt, and toxemia of pregnancy is correlated with dietary sodium levels.

Consumption of more than 12 grams a day of salt is not uncommon; it is wise to limit salt intake to a total of about 5 grams per day, which provides about 2 grams of sodium. To reduce sodium intake, eat more potassium-rich fruits and vegetables and prepare foods without adding salt before eating.

Sodium deficiency is less common than excess sodium, as this mineral is readily available in the diet, but when it does occur, as with excessive sweating and sodium losses, deficiency can cause problems. The body can lose up to 8 grams a day of sodium through sweat; however, a loss of this amount usually requires about 2 to 3 quarts of sweat. Other causes of sodium deficiency include low intake, diarrhea or vomiting, and general malnourishment. The deficiency is usually accompanied by water loss. When sodium and water are lost together, the extracellular fluid volume is depleted, which can cause decreased blood volume, increased hematocrit (blood count), decreased blood pressure, and muscle cramps. Other symptoms include nausea and vomiting, dizziness, poor memory and impaired concentration, somnolence, and muscle weakness. Circulatory collapse and shock may also occur. Debilitating or wasting diseases, such as cancer or tuberculosis, may also produce low-sodium states.

When sodium is lost alone, water flows into the cells, causing cellular swelling and symptoms of water intoxication. These may include anorexia, fatigue, apathy, and muscle twitching. With low sodium, there is also usually poor carbohydrate metabolism. When we lose sodium through sweat, the best treatment is not just replacement with salt tablets but by drinking a salt solution prepared by adding about $1/5$ teaspoon (1 gram) of salt to 1 quart of water; this will replenish us with a concentration similar to that in perspiration. Most salt tablets contain 1 gram of salt. One tablet can be taken with 1 quart of water, or 2 or 3 tablets with 2 or 3 quarts of water to replace greater fluid losses. It is ideal to add some potassium as well, about 500 mg per quart.

High-Salt Foods to Avoid

- Salt from the shaker, in cooking or at the table
- All smoked or salted meats, such as bacon, hot dogs, bologna, and sausage
- Food from Chinese restaurants with salt, soy sauce, and MSG
- Brine-soaked foods, such as pickles, olives, and sauerkraut
- Canned and instant soups unless salt free (watch out for MSG, too)
- Salted and smoked fish and caviar
- Processed cheeses
- Commercially prepared condiments, such as ketchup, barbecue sauce, mayonnaise, salad dressings, mustard, and steak sauce
- Most ready-made gravies and sauces
- Snack foods, such as chips, salted peanuts and popcorn, pretzels, and the majority of crackers on the market
- Any foods with added soda or sodium salts, such as sodium phosphate

Requirements. There is no specific RDA for sodium. However, since the mid-1990s, several large-scale research studies have looked at the sodium problem, including the Trials of Hypertension Prevention, Phase II (TOHP II, 1997), the trial of Dietary Approaches to Stop Hypertension (DASH, 1997), and the Trial of Nonpharmacologic Interventions in the Elderly (TONE, 1998). Based on these studies, the National High Blood Pressure Education Program recommended that we eat no more than 2,400 mg of sodium, or about 6 grams of salt (sodium chloride), a day. Most public health organizations have supported this guideline, and it seems to make sense. We really need only about 0.5 gram to maintain the body's salt concentration and probably 1 to 2 grams to be safe, unless we perspire a great deal or are active exercisers.

Most people consume excess sodium. The average American diet contains about 3 to 6 grams of sodium, or about 7 to 15 grams of salt, per day. **Although salt intake is not the only cause of hypertension, it has been shown that in societies with the highest sodium use, there is a greater incidence of high blood pressure.** One way to evaluate salt intake is to break down how it comes into the diet. The average diet derives about 3 to 4 grams of naturally occurring salt in food, 4 to 5 grams from eating processed foods, and another 3 to 4 grams from salt added in cooking or at the table. That adds up to about 10 to 13 grams of sodium chloride, or approximately 4 to 5 grams of sodium per day, twice the suggested level. Higher sodium intake has evolved over the past couple of centuries as a result of habit, taste, and social customs. It is probably most helpful to limit sodium to 1 to 3 grams a day and to obtain at least as much potassium as sodium, although the ideal potassium intake is double that of sodium.

These precautions reduce the risk of sodium-sensitive hypertension and other effects of excess sodium. Potassium chloride as a salt substitute may be a helpful way to maintain this sodium-potassium balance. Eating more fresh fruits and vegetables is a good safeguard against problems with high blood pressure or diseases of the cardiovascular system.

Before leaving the subject of sodium, I would like to add a final thought on taste. Real food—organically grown, whole, and unprocessed—has real taste. Real cuisines—the ethnic cooking traditions that are passed on from generation to generation—blend tastes together in an almost magical way. When we rely on convenience, processed, nonorganic food, there is no real taste left, and then we need to add salt or MSG to artificially provide some flavor to what is basically artificial food. Returning to real food, prepared in culturally traditional ways, would in most cases be a good strategy for reducing sodium intake.

Sulfur

 Sulfur is an interesting nonmetallic element that is found mainly as part of larger compounds. It is not discussed much in nutrition books, mainly because it has not been thought to be essential—that is, sulfur deficiency does not cause any visible problems. This approach to sulfur as nonessential could not be further off the mark. This element is arguably the most critical single element in our body's detoxification processes, and in its ability to escape from oxygen-based damage.

Sulfur represents about 0.25% of our total body weight, similar to potassium. The body contains approximately 140 grams of sulfur—mainly in the proteins, although it is distributed in small amounts in all cells and tissues. Sulfur has a characteristic odor that can be smelled when hair or sheep's wool is burned. Keratin, present in the skin, hair, and nails, is particularly high in the amino acid cysteine, which is found in the keratin protein. The sulfur-sulfur bond in keratin gives it greater strength.

Sulfur is present in four amino acids: methionine, an essential amino acid; the nonessential cystine and cysteine, which can be made from methionine; and taurine. Sulfur is also present in two B vitamins, thiamin and biotin; thiamin is important to skin and biotin to hair. Sulfur is also available as various sulfates or sulfides. But overall, sulfur is most important as part of protein. The table "Important Sulfur-Containing Molecules" lists molecules that play important roles in metabolism and have sulfur as a key component.

Sulfur has been used commonly since the early 1800s. Grandma's "spring tonic" consisted mainly of sulfur and molasses. This also acted as a laxative. Sulfur has been known as the "beauty" mineral because it helps the skin stay clear and youthful. Many people are familiar with one common sulfur byproduct, and that's hydrogen sulfide gas. It is what's in onions that causes tearing. This gas can also be made by intestinal bacteria and is absorbed by the body or released as gas with a characteristic odor.

Sulfur is absorbed from the small intestine primarily as the four sulfur-containing amino acids or from sulfates in water or fruits and vegetables. Even though inorganic forms of sulfur play a critical role in our health—especially in our ability to detoxify many chemicals—it is thought that elemental sulfur alone (not combined with any other element) is not used by the human organism. Sulfur is stored in all body cells, especially the skin, hair, and nails. Excess amounts are eliminated through the urine or in the feces.

Sources. As part of four amino acids, sulfur is readily available in protein foods—meats, fish, poultry, eggs, milk, and legumes are all good sources. Egg yolks are one of the better sources of sulfur. Other foods that contain this somewhat smelly mineral are onions, garlic, cabbage, brussels sprouts, kale, collards, mustard greens, chard, broccoli, lettuce, kelp and other seaweed, and turnips. Nuts have some sulfur, as do raspberries. Complete vegetarians (those who eat no eggs or milk) and people on low-protein diets may not get sufficient amounts of sulfur; the resulting sulfur deficiency is difficult to differentiate clinically from protein deficiency, which is of much greater concern.

Functions. As part of four amino acids, sulfur performs a number of functions in enzyme reactions and protein synthesis. It is necessary for formation of collagen, the protein found in connective tissue in the body. Sulfur is also present in keratin, which is necessary for the maintenance of the skin, hair, and nails, helping to give strength, shape, and hardness to these protein tissues. Sulfur is also present in the fur and feathers of other animals. The cystine in hair gives off the sulfur smell when it is burned. Sulfur, as cystine and methionine, is part of other important body chemicals: insulin, which helps regulate carbohydrate metabolism, and heparin, an anticoagulant. Taurine is found in bile acids, used in digestion. The sulfur-containing amino acids help form other substances as well, such as biotin, coenzyme A, lipoic acid, and glutathione. The mucopolysaccharides may contain chondroitin sulfate, which is important to joint tissues.

Sulfur is important to cellular respiration, as it is needed in the oxidation-reduction reactions that help the cells utilize oxygen, which aids brain function and all cell activity. These reactions are dependent on cysteine, which also helps the liver produce bile secretions and eliminate other toxins. The connection between sulfur and detoxification is especially important. Many naturally occurring substances in the body move around while attached to sulfur. Estrogen, for example, is almost always attached to sulfur ("sulfated") when it moves through the bloodstream. When we experience an overload of potentially toxic substances, we can quite quickly create a functional sulfur deficiency because many of these toxic substances may also require sulfur in order to be detoxified and transported out of the body. In this kind of circumstance, our ability to detoxify environmental and food toxins as well as our ability to maintain healthy estrogen balance can be disrupted by sulfur deficiency. That is one of the reasons I believe this mineral is especially important.

Uses. In its elemental form, sulfur was used for many disorders during the nineteenth century. In the twentieth and twenty-first centuries, the focus is more on the sulfur-containing amino acids, used internally; or as elemental sulfur-containing ointments used for skin disorders such as eczema, dermatitis, and psoriasis. Psoriasis has been treated with oral sulfur along with zinc. Other problems of the skin or hair have been treated with additional sulfur-containing compounds.

Important Sulfur-Containing Molecules

Acetyl CoA (building block for fat synthesis)

Biotin (B complex vitamin)

Ceruloplasmin (key mineral transporter)

Cysteine (amino acid)

Glutathione (key antioxidant)

Lipoic acid (key antioxidant)

Metallothionein (key mineral transporter)

Methionine (amino acid)

Taurine (amino acid)

Taurocholic acid (component of bile)

Vitamin B_1 (thiamin)

Joint problems can often be helped by chondroitin sulfate, which is found in high amounts in the joint tissues. For centuries, arthritis sufferers have been helped by bathing in waters that contain high amounts of sulfur. Oral sulfur as sulfates in doses of 500 to 1,000 mg may also reduce symptoms in some patients. Magnesium sulfate, which is not absorbed, has been used as a laxative. Taurine, another sulfur-containing amino acid, has been used in epilepsy treatment, usually along with zinc. A physiologic form of sulfur called methylsulfonyl methane (MSM) is also available and can be helpful with a wide variety of health problems (see chapter 7, Special Supplements).

If we need additional sulfur, we can usually get it by eating 1 or 2 eggs a day or eating extra garlic or onions, as well as other sulfur foods, including broccoli, kale, chard, and other greens. There is no real cause for concern about the cholesterol in eggs if the diet is generally low in fat and the blood cholesterol level is not elevated.

Deficiency and toxicity. There is minimal reason for concern about toxicity of sulfur in the body. As explained earlier, functional deficiencies of sulfur are possible when we are exposed to a lot of toxins that cannot be detoxified without sulfur. No clearly defined symptoms exist with either state. Sulfur deficiency is more common when foods are grown in sulfur-depleted soil, with low-protein diets, or with a lack of intestinal bacteria, although none of these seems to cause any problems in regard to sulfur functions and metabolism.

Requirements. There is no specific RDA for sulfur, although the amino acids that contain them are needed to meet protein requirements. Our needs are usually easily met through diet. Current research studies point to 12.6 mg per kilogram of body weight as the average need for sulfur-containing amino acids. Translated into everyday terms, a 154-pound person would need about 880 mg of sulfur-containing amino acids (methionine, cystine, and taurine). Most of us would get this amount readily if we included sulfur foods in our diet, because we eat 50 to 75 grams of protein (or 50,000–75,000 mg) per day. Recent research studies have also shown that the ratio of sulfur-containing amino acids found in whole foods is perfectly in keeping with healthy sulfur balance, and supplementing with amino acids in order to change the ratio of cysteine to methionine, for example, is not necessary.

THE MICROMINERALS

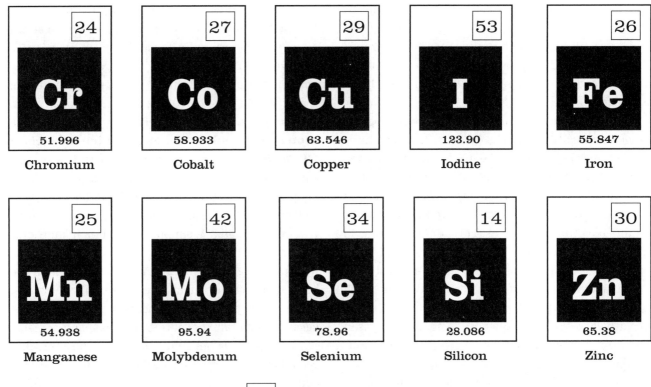

24 **Cr** 51.996 Chromium	27 **Co** 58.933 Cobalt	29 **Cu** 63.546 Copper	53 **I** 123.90 Iodine	26 **Fe** 55.847 Iron
25 **Mn** 54.938 Manganese	42 **Mo** 95.94 Molybdenum	34 **Se** 78.96 Selenium	14 **Si** 28.086 Silicon	30 **Zn** 65.38 Zinc

Chromium example: 24 = Atomic number   51.996 = Atomic Weight

Chromium

Chromium has become a subject of much interest in recent years, and we continue to learn more about it. Chromium was long thought to be a toxic mineral until it was discovered in 1957 to be the essential part of glucose tolerance factor (GTF). GTF (and thus chromium) is vital in regulating carbohydrate metabolism by enhancing insulin function for proper use of glucose in the body. Researchers are still not certain if GTF is actually a single chemical compound or if it is a group of nutrients that work closely together to support blood sugar balance. If GTF is a single compound, it most likely consists of 1 chromium molecule in the trivalent state (a +3 charge), 2 niacin molecules, and 3 amino acids—glycine, cysteine, and glutamic acid.

Trivalent chromium is the biologically active form. Hexavalent chromium (+6) is fairly unstable and is potentially toxic in the body. Chromium is not found in nature as a free metal, so it must be reduced to its elemental form to make the chrome used in the auto industry. This form is not available to the body, however, so we cannot meet our daily chromium needs by sucking on car bumpers. The chromium in the blood is in the organic active form in the trivalent state, as part of GTF or carried with a beta globulin protein.

Chromium is considered an "ultra trace mineral," because it is needed in such small quantities to perform its essential functions. The blood contains about 20 parts per billion (ppb), a fraction of a microgram. Even though it is in such small concentrations, this mineral is important to health. There are about 6 mg of chromium stored in the bodies of those who live in the United States; tissue levels of people in other countries are usually higher, which tends to be associated with a lower incidence of diabetes and atherosclerosis. There is less hardening of the arteries in people of Asian countries, who it is estimated have five times higher chromium tissue levels than Americans. People of Near Eastern countries who have about four times the average U.S. levels, and African people who have twice our chromium levels, seem to experience less diabetes than Americans. These higher tissue levels of chromium are due primarily to better soil supplies and a less refined diet. Chromium may be only one of the factors accounting for the differences in rates of diabetes and atherosclerosis between cultures, but it is probably a major one.

Chromium is a difficult mineral to absorb. Figures range from 0.5% to 3% absorption for the inorganic chromium salts often found in food. The organic complexes of chromium, such as GTF, are absorbed better, at about 10% to 20%. The kidneys clear any excess from the blood, while much of chromium intake is eliminated through the feces. This mineral is stored in many parts of the body, including muscles and fat, as well as the skin, brain, spleen, kidneys, and testes.

Tissue levels of chromium tend to decrease with age, which may be a factor in the increase of adult-onset diabetes, a disease whose incidence has risen more than sixfold since 1950. This increase may mirror the loss of chromium from our diets because of soil deficiency and the refinement of foods. Much of the chromium in whole grains and sugarcane is lost in making refined flour (40% loss) and white sugar (93% loss). In addition, there is some evidence that refined flour and sugar deplete even more chromium from the body. Reduced absorption related to aging, diets that are stressful to the digestive system, and the modern refined diet all contribute to chromium deficiency. Higher fat intake also may inhibit chromium absorption. If chromium is as important as we think it is to blood sugar metabolism, its deficiency may be in part responsible, along with the refined and processed diet, for the third leading cause of death (more than 300,000 yearly) in this country—diabetes mellitus—and this figure does not reflect other deaths that may be related to chromium deficiency, because high blood sugar levels seen in diabetes also increase the progression of atherosclerosis and cardiovascular disease, the number-one killer. Diagnosing and treating chromium deficiency is simple and should be done as early as possible, as it is much easier to prevent diabetes than to treat it.

Sources. Food refinement and the loss of topsoil through poor agricultural practices reduce the chromium level in foods. There are, however, still many good food sources. Since GTF is better absorbed than inorganic chromium, the level and activity of GTF in foods affect how well they supply us with this mineral. GTF activity may not always correspond to the actual amount of chromium in foods; however, many foods with good GTF activity also have good amounts of chromium. Hard water often contains some chromium; it may supply up to half of the daily needs of an adult.

Brewer's yeast is likely the best available source of chromium as well as having the highest GTF activity. About 2 tablespoons, or 6 tablets, per day supply most of our chromium needs; however, many people, maybe 30% to 40%, do not tolerate yeast very well and find that it causes digestive upset or bloating. If yeast is tolerated, it supplies a great many nutrients and is a low-calorie and low-fat source.

Following yeast in chromium concentration are beef, liver, whole wheat, rye, fresh chiles, oysters, onions, potatoes, tomatoes, wheat germ, green peppers, eggs, chicken, apples, butter, bananas, and spinach. Black pepper (10 ppm) and molasses (2 ppm) are other good sources of chromium, but because they are usually consumed in small quantities, it is best to have other chromium foods in the diet. In general, the whole grains, meats, shellfish, chicken, wheat germ and bran, and many vegetables, especially potato skins, are adequate sources. Beets and mushrooms may contain chromium.

Functions. Chromium is an essential mineral—that is, it is not made by the body and must be obtained from the diet. As the central part of GTF, it enhances the effect of insulin in the body. GTF is necessary for proper insulin function in the utilization of glucose and is needed in both human and animal nutrition for carbohydrate metabolism. Specifically, chromium/GTF improves the uptake of glucose into the cells so it can be metabolized to produce energy (ATP). GTF is thought to bind to the cell receptors for insulin, increasing their responsiveness to insulin and thus helping to lower the blood sugar. This function of the glucose tolerance factor prevents continued elevations of blood sugar, which can lead to diabetes. If glucose does not enter the cells, the excess circulating sugar can cause damage to the cells, the retina of the eye, and the arteries, for example. Therefore, proper control of blood sugar may help to prevent atherosclerosis and its subsequent problems.

Chromium recently has been shown to lower blood cholesterol while mildly raising HDL (high-density lipoprotein), the "good" portion of cholesterol. This lowers the risk ratio for coronary artery disease. (Exercise is a key factor in raising HDL cholesterol and reducing coronary artery disease risk. Exercise also promotes the efficiency of insulin-mediated uptake of glucose into cells.) Recent research has connected chromium to nucleic acid metabolism. Nucleic acids are the building blocks of DNA, our genetic material. The exact nature of this link between chromium and genetics is not yet known.

Uses. Chromium and GTF are used in the treatment of both hypoglycemia and diabetes mellitus, both problems of blood sugar utilization and metabolism. Preventing chromium deficiency is the key here. The earlier treatment is begun, especially with potential diabetes, the more helpful it may be. Preformed GTF is not readily available, although formulas that contain all of its components seem to work better than chromium alone, and small amounts given daily have been shown to both increase glucose tolerance and decrease blood fats, both cholesterol and triglycerides, as well as to raise HDL. Some of these formulas include chromium polynicotinate, chromium dinicotinate glycinate, or chromium yeast. Chromium alone has also been used along with niacin (also a part of GTF) in the treatment of high blood cholesterol.

Henry Schroeder, MD, who has done numerous studies with chromium, has shown that 2 mg of inorganic chromium given daily reduced cholesterol levels by about 15%. He has produced diabetes in lab animals by feeding them chromium-deficient diets. Such a diet raises not only blood sugar but blood cholesterol as well; both conditions return to normal with chromium supplementation. When Schroeder fed rats a chromium-rich diet, they showed improved longevity, along with a reduction of atherosclerotic plaque found in the blood vessels at death. Chromium is used to help reduce atherosclerosis in people, especially in those who show low chromium levels. Cultures with higher tissue levels of chromium also appear to have lower incidences of atherosclerosis and heart disease.

Deficiency and toxicity. Because of the low absorption and high excretion rates of chromium, toxicity is not at all common in humans, especially with the usual forms of chromium used for supplementation. The amount that would cause toxicity is estimated to be much more than the amount commonly supplied in supplements. The only exception to the above scenario would involve people with liver or kidney problems, who might need to limit their chromium supplementation to 200 mcg per day. The National Academy of Sciences chose not to establish a tolerable upper limit for chromium in its 2001 guidelines, but it did issue a concern for people with liver or kidney problems.

Chromium deficiency is another story, however, with an estimated 25% to 50% of the U.S. population deficient in chromium. **The United States has a greater incidence of deficiency than any other country, because of low soil levels of chromium and the loss of this mineral from refined foods, especially sugar and flours.** Deficiencies are more common in both the elderly and the young, especially teenagers who eat poor diets. Even though chromium is needed in such small amounts, it is difficult to obtain. Given these factors, and the fact that the already low chromium absorption rate decreases even further with age, chromium deficiency is of great concern. It may even be the missing link in the development of adult-onset diabetes, a serious problem increasing rapidly in our culture. Nearly 1 in 5 adult Americans now develops diabetes.

A high-fat, high-sugar diet that contains refined flour products is probably the most important risk factor for diabetes. Such a diet tends to be low in chromium content and also causes more insulin to be produced, which requires even more chromium. In addition, high simple sugars result in increased loss of chromium through the urine. Milk and other high-phosphorus foods tend to bind with chromium in the gut to make chromium phosphates that travel through the intestines and are not absorbed.

Even mild deficiencies of chromium can produce symptoms other than problems in blood sugar metabolism, such as anxiety or fatigue. Abnormal cholesterol metabolism and increased progress of atherosclerosis are associated with chromium deficiency, and deficiency may also cause decreased growth in young people and slower healing time after injuries or surgery. Most important, the low chromium levels seen in the United States are associated with a higher incidence of diabetes and arteriosclerosis. Further research is needed to confirm these associations and to determine whether correcting the chromium deficiency would actually reduce the incidence of these diseases.

Requirements. Average daily intake of chromium may be about 80 to 100 mcg, although some small studies have shown much lower average intake in the 25 to 50 mcg range. We probably need a minimum of 1 to 2 mcg going into the blood to maintain tissue levels; if only around 2% of our intake were absorbed, we would need at least 50 to 100 mcg in the daily diet. A safe dosage range for chromium supplementation is between 100 and 300 mcg. Children need somewhat less. Many vitamin or mineral supplements contain about 100 to 150 mcg of chromium. Some people take up to 1 mg (1,000 mcg) per day for short periods without problems; this is not suggested as a long-term regimen but rather to help replenish chromium stores when deficiency is present. All of the precursors to the active form of GTF are used in some formulas, but usually with chromium in lower doses, such as 50 mcg, because it is better absorbed with niacin and the amino acids glycine, cysteine, and glutamic acid. Because chromium gets carried around on the transferrin protein that also serves as the carrier molecule for iron, iron excess can also interfere with chromium metabolism and may be a reason to supplement on the high side.

AI Levels for Chromium

In 2001 the Institute of Medicine established the following AI levels for chromium:

Age	AI Level
Infants, 0–6 months	0.2 mcg
Infants, 7–12 months	5.5 mcg
Children, 1–3 years	11 mcg
Children, 4–8 years	15 mcg
Males, 9–13 years	25 mcg
Females, 9–13 years	21 mcg
Males, 14–18 years	35 mcg
Females, 14–18 years	24 mcg
Males, 19–70 years	35 mcg
Females, 19–70 years	25 mcg
Males, 71 years and older	30 mcg
Females, 71 years and older	20 mcg
Pregnancy, 18 years or younger	29 mcg
Pregnancy, 19–50 years	30 mcg
Lactation, 18 years or younger	44 mcg
Lactation, 19–50 years	45 mcg

In summary, to avoid deficiency and maintain a good intake of chromium, avoid sugar and sugar products, soda pops, candy, and presweetened breakfast cereals; avoid refined, white flour products, such as white breads and crackers; use whole wheat products, wheat germ, and/or brewer's yeast; eat whole foods; and take a general supplement that contains chromium, approximately 100 to 200 mcg daily.

Cobalt

Co Cobalt is another essential mineral needed in very small amounts in the diet. It is an integral part of vitamin B12, or cobalamin, which supports red blood cell production and the formation of myelin nerve coverings. Some authorities do not consider cobalt to be essential as a separate nutrient, because it is needed primarily as part of B12, which is itself essential. Cobalt is not easily absorbed from the digestive tract. The body level of cobalt normally measures 80 to 300 mcg. It is stored in the red blood cells and the plasma, as well as in the liver, kidneys, spleen, and pancreas.

Sources. Cobalt is available mainly as part of B12. There is some question as to whether inorganic cobalt is actually usable in the human body. The latest research in this area shows that cobalt is able to activate certain enzymes in the body, but this ability has only been demonstrated in a test tube, not in an actual person. Meat, liver, kidney, clams, oysters, and milk all contain some cobalt. Ocean fish and sea vegetables have cobalt, but land vegetables have little; some cobalt is available in legumes, spinach, cabbage, lettuce, beet greens, and figs.

Functions. As part of vitamin B12, cobalt is essential to red blood cell formation and is also helpful to other cells.

Uses. Cobalt is used to prevent anemia, particularly pernicious anemia; vitamin B12 is also beneficial in some cases of fatigue, digestive disorders, and neuromuscular problems. There are no other known uses except for the radioactive cobalt 60 used to treat certain cancers.

Deficiency and toxicity. Toxicity can occur from excess inorganic cobalt found as a food contaminant. Beer drinker's cardiomyopathy (enlarged heart) and congestive heart failure have been traced to cobalt introduced into beer during manufacturing. Increased intake may affect the thyroid or cause overproduction of red blood cells, thickened blood, and increased activity in the bone marrow. Deficiency of cobalt is not really a concern if we get enough vitamin B12. **Vegetarians need to be more concerned than others about getting enough cobalt and B12.** The soil in this country is becoming deficient in cobalt, further reducing the already low levels found in plant foods. As cobalt deficiency leads to decreased availability of B12, there is an increase of many symptoms and problems related to B12 deficiency, particularly pernicious anemia and nerve damage.

Requirements. No specific RDA is suggested for cobalt. Our needs are low, and vitamin B12 usually fulfills them. The average daily intake of cobalt is about 5 to 8 mcg. It is not usually given in supplements.

Copper

 Copper has been known to be an essential trace mineral for some time. Recently there has been some increasing concern about copper in nutrition, and it has been coming from two different directions. First, we have spent a lot of time focusing on zinc and making sure to include it in supplements, lozenges, and nutritional assessments. Only recently have we learned how closely zinc's function is tied to copper. **For some chemical reactions in the body, the ratio of zinc to copper is more important than the absolute amount of either mineral alone.** Particularly if we supplement with zinc and forget to pay attention to copper, we may create a situation where copper becomes functionally deficient. Alongside of this research about the zinc-to-copper ratio, however, there have been some equally compelling studies suggesting that copper toxicity may occur more often than previously thought. The levels here have been fairly high, however—hundreds of times the RDA—and so toxicity from food seems like a pretty remote possibility for most people. Copper is present in all body tissues. The total amount in our bodies is about 75 to 100 mg, less than that contained in a copper penny.

Copper is found in many foods in small amounts (oysters and nuts are the richest sources). The standard amount available in our diet, whether it is excessive or deficient, is a controversial topic; the naturalist in me feels that if it is in wholesome foods, it must be the right amount. **However, this mineral is present in water that flows through copper piping.** Increases in estrogen hormone levels, from taking birth control pills or during pregnancy, for example, often increase serum copper levels to more than double normal values, while levels in red blood cells, where copper is important, may actually be lower. This may contribute to some of the psychological or other symptoms seen during pregnancy or with birth control pill use. **Increased copper levels have been associated with schizophrenia, learning disabilities, and senility,** although none of these associations have been demonstrated with certainty. Depression and other mental problems, premenstrual syndrome, and hyperactivity have also been correlated with high copper levels, often in combination with low zinc levels. The most recent surveys show women averaging about 1 mg and men about 1.4 mg per day, with an additional 0.4 mg coming from nutritional supplements. Of course, these surveys do not take into account additional copper from copper pipes, or copper shifts inside the body due to medications like birth control pills.

Zinc and copper have a complementary and yet seesaw relationship in the body, competing with each other for absorption in the gut, but working together to support metabolism. Both zinc deficiency and copper toxicity have increased since the switch from zinc (galvanized) to copper water pipes. We can avoid this problem by not drinking tap water. Some studies of schizophrenics have revealed high blood copper with low urinary copper (showing that copper is being retained) and low blood zinc. In some of these cases, zinc was helpful as an antianxiety agent.

About 30% of copper intake is absorbed into the body from the stomach and upper intestine; it is fairly rapidly absorbed, usually within 15 minutes. This percent absorption does vary, however, depending on the amount of copper in our food, and can range from 12% to 71%. Copper is transferred by albumin across the gut wall and carried to the liver, where it is formed into ceruloplasmin, a copper-protein complex. About 90% of the average 100 mcg of copper in the blood is in the form of ceruloplasmin. As a balancing mechanism to minimize copper toxicities, absorption of copper is decreased when ceruloplasmin levels are adequate. A second protein, called metallothionein, can also bind copper and helps regulate the flow of copper between the liver and other organ systems. **Vitamin C, zinc, and manganese all interfere with copper absorption. Protein and fresh vegetable foods have been shown to improve copper absorption.**

About 100 mg of copper are stored in the body, with the highest concentrations in the liver and brain tissues, which account for about one-third of the total. Muscles contain approximately another third, with the remaining copper in the other tissues. At birth, a high amount is contained in the liver; by about age 10, the normal adult level of copper is reached, both in the liver and the rest of the body. Excess copper is eliminated mainly through the liver into the bile and is lost through the intestines. A minimal amount is excreted in the urine.

Sources. Copper is available in most natural foods. Some authorities believe that our average intake is higher than our actual needs, that low intakes are uncommon, and that toxicity is a potential problem. The other school of thought holds that low intake is common because soil depletion has decreased the copper level in many foods and because many people avoid natural copper-containing foods. Foods with good supplies of copper are the whole grains, particularly buckwheat and whole wheat; shellfish, such as shrimp and other seafoods; liver and other organ meats; most dried peas and beans; and nuts, such as Brazil nuts, almonds, hazelnuts, walnuts, and pecans. **Oysters have high amounts, about five times as much as other foods.** Soybeans supply copper, as do dark leafy greens, mushrooms, and some dried fruits, such as prunes. Cocoa, black pepper, and yeast are also sources. In addition to food sources, copper can come from water pipes and cookware.

Functions. Copper is important as a catalyst in the formation of hemoglobin, the oxygen-carrying molecule. Copper in the red blood cells is bound to erythrocuprein, a substance thought to have superoxide dismutase (SOD) activity, which is energy enhancing. Copper is also part of the cytochrome system for cell respiration, an energy-releasing process. It also helps oxidize vitamin C and works with C to form collagen (part of cell membranes and the supportive matrix in muscles and other tissues), especially in the bone and connective tissue. It helps the cross-linking of collagen fibers and thus supports the healing process of tissues and aids in proper bone formation. An excess of copper may increase collagen and lead to stiffer and less flexible tissues.

Copper is found in many enzymes; most important is the cytoplasmic SOD. SOD, when it is found in the main compartment of the cell, is one of the enzymes regulated by the copper-to-zinc ratio. (When it is located in the cell's aerobic energy center, called the mitochondrion, SOD is regulated by manganese instead of the zinc-to-copper ratio.) Earlier, I explained how the ceruloplasmin protein plays a key role in copper metabolism. Ceruloplasmin also acts as an enzyme (called ferroxidase I), and it is responsible for getting dietary iron ready for transport around the body. For this reason, copper should be thought of as playing a direct role in iron metabolism. Copper enzymes play a role in oxygen–free radical metabolism, and in this way have a mild anti-inflammatory effect. Copper also functions in certain amino acid conversions. Being essential in the synthesis of phospholipids, copper contributes to the integrity of the myelin sheaths covering nerves. It also aids the conversion of tyrosine to the pigment melanin, which gives hair and skin their coloring. Copper, as well as zinc, is important for converting T3 (triiodothyronine) to T4 (thyroxine), both thyroid hormones. Low copper levels may reduce thyroid functions.

Copper, like most metals, is a conductor of electricity; in the body, it helps the nervous system function. Copper is especially important in the production of adrenaline (norepinephrine) because three steps in the adrenaline-production process require copper. When we are copper deficient, our levels of adrenaline drop. It also helps control levels of histamine, which may be related to allergic and inflammatory reactions. Copper in the blood is fixed to the protein cerulosplasmin, and copper is part of the enzyme histaminase, which is involved in the metabolism of histamine.

A chemical reaction in the formation of connective tissue also depends on copper. In future research, more attention may be paid to copper with respect to arthritis and other joint problems in this context. We may also see more about copper in relationship to pain and pleasure, because our blood levels of enkephalins and endorphins are affected by copper status. The details of this relationship are not yet clear, however.

Uses. Some nutritional doctors feel that copper should not be supplemented because of the narrow line between the therapeutic and toxic doses. Copper has, however, been used in cases of anemia, vitiligo, fatigue, allergies, and stomach ulcers, where low levels of copper have been found. Whenever copper is deficient, which it can be for many reasons, it should be supplemented. Copper can be measured in the blood, both plasma and red blood cell levels, to help determine the amount of copper to be supplemented.

The use of copper bracelets in the treatment of arthritis has a long history, and wearers continue to claim positive results. The copper in the bracelets reacts with the fatty acids in the skin to form copper salts that are absorbed into the body. The copper salts may cause a blue-green stain on the skin, but this can be removed with soap and water. Recent research suggests that copper salicylate used to treat arthritis reduces symptoms more effectively than either copper or aspirin alone.

In a Danish study, arthritis patients who were treated with injections of SOD obtained relief from many of their symptoms, such as joint swelling, pain, and morning stiffness. SOD is available in tablets in the United States; however, it is not thought to be stable in the stomach and small intestine, so it may not be of any help for arthritis when taken orally. Additional research with enteric-coated tablets of active SOD may provide new insights into oral SOD treatment of arthritis and other inflammatory disorders.

Deficiency and toxicity. Copper toxicity has been the subject of great concern in recent years. High copper levels, especially when associated, as they often are, with low zinc levels, have been described in a wide variety of conditions. Whether this is incidental, a cause of these problems, or a result of them is not known for certain. Problems of copper toxicity may include stress and anxiety states, joint and muscle pains, psychological depression, mental fatigue, poor memory, lack of concentration, insomnia, manic depression, schizophrenia, senility, epilepsy, autism, hypertension, stuttering, hyperactivity in children, premenstrual syndrome, preeclampsia of pregnancy, and postpartum psychosis. Until further research clarifies the problems of copper toxicity, it is wise to check levels of copper (and zinc) in people with these conditions as well as those with alcoholism, cancer, and infectious diseases. The World Health Organization (WHO) has finally recognized copper's potential for toxicity and has established the 2 to 3 mg range as its provisional acceptable range of oral intake (AROI) upper limit.

Hair levels of copper are not very helpful in detecting increased body copper because external contamination from the fungicides and algicides used in swimming pools or hot tubs may leave copper on the hair, causing misleading test results. However, hair copper is suggestive of body state, such that if hair (or blood) copper levels are elevated, it is wise to check the 24-hour urine copper level or the blood ceruloplasmin level. Red blood cell copper levels may be a good test to measure increased copper levels as well; serum copper levels may be easier for detecting deficiency.

Symptoms of mild copper toxicity may be classified as hypochondriac or "neurotic" ones. Fatigue, irritability, nervousness, depression, and learning problems are some common symptoms. Higher levels of copper intoxication can lead to nausea, vomiting, diarrhea, liver damage, gingivitis, dermatitis, or a discoloration of the skin and hair. In their book *Trace Elements, Hair Analysis, and Nutrition,* Drs. Richard Passwater and Elmer Cranton describe a case of three women who lived together in a house with copper pipes. All presented symptoms of fatigue, irritability, muscle and joint aches, and headaches, and all had elevated copper levels. They were treated successfully with increased levels of zinc and manganese, which compete with copper for absorption and also help eliminate copper through the bile and urine. Carl Pfeiffer, MD, suggests using zinc (50 mg), manganese (3 mg), and vitamin B6 (50 mg) daily without supplemental copper to increase copper excretion. If copper levels are very high, treatment with penicillamine or chelation therapy with ethylenediaminetetraacetic acid (EDTA) may be needed. In Europe, a compound called Dimeval (di-mercapto-succinic acid) may be used to lower copper levels.

A genetic disorder called Wilson's disease affects copper metabolism and leads to low serum and hair copper with high liver and brain copper levels. This can be a serious and even fatal problem unless treated by chelating agents; penicillamine is most often used, as it binds copper in the gut and carries it out.

A low-copper diet and more zinc and manganese in the diet and as supplements also help reduce copper levels. Menkes' disease is a rare problem of copper malabsorption in infants. In this condition, which can often be fatal, decreased intestinal absorption causes copper to accumulate in the intestinal lining.

Copper deficiency has long been considered unlikely even with a suboptimal diet because it was thought to be readily available from foods. Newer surveys seem to suggest that with soil deficiency and poor diet, the average dietary intake is now less than 1 mg per day. Our bodies require more than this. As of 2000, 25% of all adults were under the 900 mcg RDA for copper. These 25% were only slightly below, however, and with consumption of drinking water from copper pipes, were probably unlikely to be deficient if in otherwise good health.

Copper deficiency is commonly found together with iron deficiency, especially with iron-deficiency anemia. Fatigue, paleness, skin sores, and edema may appear with this, as may slowed growth, hair loss, anorexia, diarrhea, and dermatitis. High zinc levels or intake can lead to lower copper levels and some symptoms of copper deficiency. The reduced function and life span of red blood cells can influence energy levels and cause weakness and labored respiration from decreased oxygen delivery. Low copper levels may also affect collagen formation and thus tissue health and healing. Reduced thyroid function, weakened immunity, cardiovascular disease, increased cholesterol, skeletal defects related to bone demineralization, and poor nerve conductivity, including irregular heart rhythms, might all result from copper depletions. Copper deficiency results in several abnormalities of the immune system, such as reduced cellular immune response, reduced activity of white blood cells, and, possibly, reduced thymus hormone production, all of which may contribute to an increased infection rate. Infants fed an all-dairy (cow's milk) diet without copper supplements may develop copper deficiency. Some children with iron deficiency show reduced levels of copper as well. It is also likely that during pregnancy copper will be deficient unless supplemented with at least 2 mg daily.

Requirements. Many nutritionists do not supplement copper at all or at least not more than 2 mg per day in a general supplement because of the con-

cern about toxicity and because excess copper can interfere with absorption of zinc. Zinc deficiency can cause a great number of problems, such as hair loss, menstrual problems, and weakened immunity. If the soil in which our food is grown is known to be high in copper, or if we drink water from copper pipes, we should probably avoid copper supplements. If we eat a diet that includes whole grains, nuts, and leafy green vegetables or eat much liver (if you eat liver, buy it from the cleanest source you can find since liver can store many toxins), we are probably obtaining sufficient levels from our diet. However, if we do supplement zinc, we should also take copper in a ratio of 15 to 30 mg zinc to 2 mg copper, unless of course, we are trying to reduce copper or correct a zinc deficiency. Likewise, if we take copper we should add zinc, unless we are treating high zinc levels or copper deficiency.

AI Levels and RDAs for Copper

In 2000, the National Academy of Sciences established the following new recommendations for copper, including AI levels for infants up to 1 year and RDAs for people older than 1 year:

Age	AI/RDA
Infants, 0–6 months	200 mcg (AI)
Infants, 7–12 months	220 mcg (AI)
Children, 1–3 years	340 mcg (RDA)
Children, 4–8 years	440 mcg (RDA)
Males and females, 9–13 years	700 mcg (RDA)
Males and females, 14–18 years	890 mcg (RDA)
Males and females, 19–70 years	900 mcg (RDA)
Males and females, 71 years and older	900 mcg (RDA)
Pregnancy, 14–50 years	1,000 mcg (RDA)
Lactation, 14–50 years	1,300 mcg (RDA)

Iodine

 Iodine is a good example of a trace mineral whose deficiency creates a disease that is easily corrected by resupplying it in the diet. Goiter, an enlargement of the thyroid gland, develops when this important metabolic gland does not have enough iodine to manufacture hormones. As it increases its cell size to try to trap more iodine, the whole gland increases in size, creating a swelling in the neck. Without supplemental iodine, a hypothyroid condition results, likely leading to fatigue and sluggishness, weight gain, and coldness of the body; at this stage, the condition may be harder to treat with iodine alone and thyroid hormone supplementation may be needed.

Goiter was first noted in the Great Lakes region; the "goiter belt" included that area and the Midwestern and Great Plains states. In the 1930s, approximately 40% of the people in Michigan had goiter, due mainly to iodine-deficient soil; glacier melting had washed away the iodine. Areas by oceans or in the vicinity of ocean breezes usually contain enough iodine to prevent goiters. In 1924, iodine was added to table salt, a substance that was already in wide use (our salt problem has been around for a long time). Iodized salt was first introduced in Michigan; by 1940, it was in general use throughout the country. Even today, however, iodine deficiency is still a problem, and many people in the United States have goiter. Cretinism, another condition caused by iodine deficiency, is characterized by mental retardation and other problems. It may be present in iodine-deficient babies or children born to women who are lacking iodine. It is a serious and nonreversible problem that should be avoided by proper iodine intake.

Iodine itself is a poisonous gas, as are the related halogens chlorine, fluorine, and bromine. However, as with chlorine, the salts or negatively charged ions of iodine (iodides) are soluble in water, and iodine is essential to life in trace amounts. Plants do not need iodine, but humans require it for the production of thyroid hormones that regulate the metabolic energy of the body and set the basal metabolic rate (BMR).

The body contains about 15 to 20 mg of iodide (the ionic form of iodine). A small percentage of this is in the muscles, 20% is in the thyroid, and the rest is in the skin and bones. Only 1% is present in the blood. The concentration of iodine in the thyroid gland is very high, more than 1,000 times that in the muscles. **Approximately one-fourth of thyroid iodine is in the two main thyroid hormones, T4 (thyroxine) and T3 (triiodothyronine). Thyroxine itself is nearly two-thirds iodine.** The remainder is in the precursor molecules of these important hormones.

Iodine is well absorbed from the stomach into the blood. About 30% goes to the thyroid gland, depending on the need. Iodine is eliminated rapidly. Most of the remaining 70% is filtered by the kidneys into the urine. Our bodies do not conserve iodine as they do iron, and we must obtain it regularly from the diet. There is recent concern that perhaps iodine is being overconsumed, especially in iodized salt. However, the incidence of goiter has been rising again so there may be factors other than iodine involved in this problem.

Interestingly, the element iodine may be almost nonexistent in the gut, because it is quickly converted into its charged form, iodide. What is interesting here is that one of the most critical "antioxidants" in the body—glutathione—also appears to be one of the common compounds that converts iodine into iodide.

Sources. The life from ocean waters provides the best source of iodine. Fish, shellfish, and sea vegetables (seaweed) are dependably rich sources. Cod, sea bass, haddock, and perch are a few examples of iodine-rich sea animals consumed by humans; kelp is the most common high-iodine sea vegetable. **Kelp in particular is rich in other minerals and low in sodium and thus is a good seasoning substitute for salt.**

The use of iodized salt has certainly reduced most iodine deficiency. It contains about 76 mcg of iodine per gram of salt. The average person consumes at least 3 grams of salt daily, exceeding the RDA for iodine of 150 mcg. Many authorities feel (and I concur) that commercial iodized salt is overused and has other drawbacks. It often contains aluminum and other unneeded chemicals and may contribute to other problems. Fast foods may be very high in iodine because of the added salt. Adding iodine to salt is part of the paternalistic thinking of the industrial age, not counting on people to learn or adapt: "Just put it in their food or water and save them from their own ignorance." There are healthier ways to obtain iodine than in table salt; eating fish, especially fresh ocean fish, is probably the best way, as it also may help reduce cholesterol and cardiovascular disease risk. Sea salt from ocean water is a natural source of iodine, although it is not nearly as high in this mineral as iodized salt. Iodized forms of sea salt are also available.

Dietary iodine content may vary widely, depending on the iodine content in the soil in which food grows. Plants grown in or animals grazed on iodine-rich soil contain substantial amounts of iodine. Milk and its products may be sources of iodine when the cows have an iodized salt lick in their pasture. Eggs may also be a good source when iodine is in the chicken feed. Bakers may add iodine to dough, so some may be present in bread. Other foods that may contain iodine, especially when the soil is good, are onions, mushrooms, lettuce, spinach, green peppers, pineapple, cantaloupe, strawberries, peanuts, cheddar cheese, and whole wheat bread. More and more, people are eating wholesome, natural foods and avoiding iodized salt, so they must eat more of the iodine-rich foods or obtain iodine from a general vitamin-mineral supplement to make sure they are getting adequate amounts.

Functions. Iodine is an essential nutrient for production of the body's thyroid hormones and therefore is required for normal thyroid function. The thyroid hormones, particularly thyroxine, which is 65% iodine, are responsible for our basal metabolic rate (BMR)—that is, the body's use of energy. Thyroid hormones are required for cell respiration and the production of energy as ATP and further increases oxygen consumption and general metabolism. The thyroid hormones, thyroxine and triiodothyronine, are also needed for normal growth and development, protein synthesis, and energy metabolism. As thyroid stimulates the energy production of the cellular mitochondria and affects our BMR, it literally influences all body functions. Nerve and bone formation, reproduction, the condition of the skin, hair, nails, and teeth, as well as our speech and mental state are all influenced by thyroid. Thyroid and thus iodine also affect cholesterol synthesis, carbohydrate absorption, and the conversion of carotene to vitamin A and of ribonucleic acids to protein.

Iodine is picked up by the thyroid and combines with the thyroid hormones and amino acid tyrosine to make the thyroid hormone precursors diiodotyrosine, diiodothyronine, and monoiodotyrosine and then the hormones T3 and T4. The mineral selenium is also required for this process. These hormones are then carried through the body by a protein called thyroid binding globulin (TBG).

Several other important roles for iodine are suggested by research, although the details here are not nearly as clear as they are for thyroid. Iodine may be important in the body as a way of helping to deactivate unwanted bacteria—similar to the way we use iodine-containing preparations as skin disinfectants or water purifiers. In this way, and perhaps others, we may end up thinking about this mineral as important in immune support.

Uses. Supplemental iodine may be helpful in correcting hypothyroidism and goiter caused by deficient iodine intake, and it may reverse many of the symptoms of cretinism if given soon after birth. Thus, **iodine's main use is really in the prevention or early treatment of its deficiency diseases.** Iodine has also been used to help increase energy level and utilization in cases of fatigue, mental sluggishness, and weight gain caused by hypothyroidism. Iodine itself will not help with weight loss if there is normal thyroid function. If weight gain results from iodine deficiency causing decreased thyroid activity, this hypothyroid condition may be improved with iodine followed by thyroid hormone supplementation.

Because of the thyroid's role in fat and cholesterol metabolism, sufficient iodine and thus normal thyroid levels are thought to help reduce atherosclerosis potential. Also, iodine and thyroid may help maintain healthy hair, skin, and nails. It is possible that iodine deficiency increases the risk of certain cancers, such as breast, ovary, and uterus. Iodine levels may be low in people with fibrocystic breast disease; in this case, supplementation to correct iodine deficiency may improve this condition by helping to modify the impact of estrogen shifts on breast tissue. There is also some evidence that the correcting of iodine deficiency can help prevent miscarriage.

Iodine solutions, such as iodine tincture or Betadine, are commonly used as antiseptics and can actually kill bacteria and fungi. Another substance, potassium iodide, has been used medicinally for skin problems and as an expectorant for bronchial congestion. Silver iodide has been used to seed clouds to bring rain, but this practice is considered ecologically unsound. Iodine supplements may help prevent uptake of radioactive iodine if that is present in the environment or in medical diagnostic procedures. If the thyroid were saturated with normal iodine, it would eliminate the radioactive molecules more rapidly.

Deficiency and toxicity. There is no significant danger of toxicity of iodine from a natural diet, although some care must be taken when supplementing iodine or using it in drug therapy. High iodine intake, however, may actually reduce thyroxine production and thyroid function. Excessive quantities of iodized salt, taking too many kelp tablets, or overuse of potassium iodide expectorants such as SSKI can cause some problems, but regular elevated intake of iodine is needed to produce toxicity. Some people have allergic reactions, mainly as skin rashes, to iodine products. Iodine supplementation may also worsen acne in some cases. Because of risks associated with supplementation or iodized foods, the National Academy of Sciences set tolerable upper limits for iodine in 2001 as follows.

Tolerable Upper Limits for Iodine	
Age	**UL**
Children, 1–3 years	900 mcg
Children, 4–8 years	300 mcg
Males and females, 9–13 years	600 mcg
Males and females, 14–18 years	900 mcg
Males and females, 19 years and older	1,100 mcg
Pregnancy and lactation,	
18 years and younger	900 mcg
Pregnancy and lactation, 19–50 years	1,100 mcg

Deficiencies of iodine have been very common, especially in areas where the soil is depleted, as discussed earlier. Several months of iodine deficiency can lead to goiter and/or hypothyroidism, decreased thyroid function leading to slower metabolism, fatigue, weight gain, sluggishness, dry hair, thick skin, poor mental functioning, decreased resistance to infection, a feeling of coldness, and a decrease in sexual energy. With decreased iodine, the thyroid cells and gland enlarge, creating a goiter, which may be noticed mainly by the swelling it causes in the base of the neck. More advanced hypothyroidism may worsen these symptoms as well as create a hyperactive, manic state and hypertension, which is paradoxical because this may occur with an overactive thyroid as well. Iodine by itself usually will not cure goiter and hypothyroidism but often will slow their progression.

Goitrogens are substances that can induce goiter, primarily by interfering with the formation and function of thyroglobulin. Some natural goitrogens are soybeans, cabbage, cauliflower, and peanuts, especially when they come from iodine-deficient soils. Millet has recently been described as having goitrogenic tendencies. Certain drugs, such as thiouracil and sulfonamides, also act as goitrogens.

Some early studies correlate low iodine levels with an increased risk of breast cancer. These low levels usually correlate with low selenium levels as well, more classically associated with cancer. A higher incidence of breast cancer has been shown to occur in the goiter belt, whereas areas with high soil levels of iodine and selenium show a lower incidence.

Requirements. In 2001, the National Academy of Sciences developed the following new DRIs for iodine. AIs were established for children up to 1 year, and RDAs were determined for people older than 1 year.

Average intake from diet ranges from 65 mcg to about 650 mcg, with midrange values between 190 and 210 mcg for women and 240 and 300 mcg for men. Much of that may come from iodized salt, which is not highly recommended; however, it is difficult to avoid salt completely in our culture because it is added to so many prepared foods and by restaurants and food preparers everywhere. A 6-ounce portion of ocean fish contains about 500 mcg of iodine, more than is contained in 1 teaspoon of salt but without the extra 2 grams of sodium. **Ideally, we can meet our iodine requirements by eating seafood, seaweed, and vegetables grown in iodine-rich soil.** A typical mineral or complete vitamin supplement will contain the RDA, 150 mcg, of iodine per day. More iodine is needed during pregnancy and lactation. People on low-salt diets may need supplemental iodine.

AI Levels and RDAs for Iodine	
Age	**AI/RDA**
Infants, 0–6 months	110 mcg (AI)
Infants, 7–12 months	130 mcg (AI)
Children, 1–8 years	90 mcg (RDA)
Males and females, 9–13 years	120 mcg (RDA)
Males and females, 14–18 years	150 mcg (RDA)
Males and females,	
19 years and older	150 mcg (RDA)
Pregnancy	220 mcg (RDA)
Lactation	290 mcg (RDA)

Iron

 Iron is a well-known trace mineral with a long history. It may well have been the first mineral to be incorporated into living tissue and is clearly an important mineral. About 5% of the mineral content of the Earth's crust is iron. **Iron is found in every cell of the body, almost all of it combined with protein.** There is a total of about 4 grams, or $^1/_{10}$ teaspoon, of iron in an average 150-pound person. The hemoglobin molecule, essential for carrying oxygen throughout our system, contains 60% to 70% of the body's iron. If we lack iron, we produce less hemoglobin and therefore supply less oxygen to our tissues. Besides being part of hemoglobin, iron is also stored in the liver, spleen, and bone marrow, which can be drawn on to supply extra iron for hemoglobin production.

Iron deficiency anemia is a well-known and all-too-common problem, even with our modern knowledge about the condition and the attention given to preventing it. The preanemia state is not easy to diagnose. Decreasing iron stores and a relative decrease in serum iron levels and protein-bound iron may cause symptoms before low tissue iron levels or anemia are measurable. **More of this important mineral is needed during growth; iron deficiency is more common in infancy, childhood, adolescence, and pregnancy.** Even the elderly may become deficient due to poorer absorption and diet. Women in their reproductive years have higher requirements and a greater problem with iron deficiency because of losses in menstrual blood. Minority and low-income people tend to have a higher incidence of problems related to low iron, primarily caused by dietary deficiency. Women in their childbearing years require at least 18 mg of iron daily, but more than 25% of them probably obtain less than this amount. Usually, when the body needs more iron, absorption improves through an increase in iron-carrying proteins in the blood called *iron transferrin*.

Iron absorption from the intestinal tract is a subtle process; poor absorption is among the main reasons, along with low-iron diets, that iron deficiency is so prevalent. **Along with calcium, which is also difficult to absorb, iron and zinc are the minerals most commonly deficient in the diet.** Average iron absorption is about 8% to 10% of intake. All vegetable sources contain the nonheme form of iron, which is poorly absorbed and utilized. Heme iron, a special formulation of iron, is found only in flesh foods, beef and liver being the best sources. Between 10% and 30% of heme iron is absorbed. Combining heme foods with nonheme foods improves the absorption of iron from the nonheme foods. This is why **complete vegetarians have trouble obtaining sufficient iron from the diet alone.** Phytates present in whole grains and oxalates found in certain vegetables may bind up some of the iron and make it unabsorbable. Meat foods improve absorption, possibly by stimulating increased stomach acid production and by the fact that the iron contained is already bound into muscle and blood tissue in the form of the iron proteins myoglobin and hemoglobin.

Iron absorption is a slow process, usually taking between 2 and 4 hours. The natural ferrous ($+2$) iron is absorbed much better than iron in the ferric ($+3$) form. Vitamin C in the gut along with iron converts any ferric iron to ferrous and thus improves absorption. Iron absorbed into the blood is usually bound to the protein transferrin and goes mainly to the bone marrow, where it can be used to make red blood cells. Some also goes to the liver and spleen. About 25% of body iron is stored bound to the protein ferritin and as the iron complex hemosiderin. Ferritin has good iron-binding capacity. A fully saturated ferritin molecule, which is actually ferric oxide surrounded by the protein apoferritin, can contain about 4,000 iron atoms. Ferritin stored in the liver, spleen, and bone marrow, for example, provides a good reserve of iron to meet body needs. Measuring serum ferritin levels is a fairly new medical test that provides a good indication of iron storage levels. A normal value is 15 to 200 mcg. A level below 15 mcg suggests depleted iron reserves. Iron toxicity may show ferritin levels in the thousands.

About three-quarters of the iron in our bodies is active. Of that, about 70% is in hemoglobin, 5% is in myoglobin (muscle-oxygenating protein), and the rest is part of iron cofactors and such enzymes as catalases, peroxidases, and the cytochromes. Some is also in transition, attached to transferrin, which transports iron to the bone marrow, liver, and other tissues for its functions in processing hemoglobin, myoglobin, and various enzymes. **Fortunately, the body conserves iron very well, although this increases the possi-**

bility of toxicity. Toxicity has not been a great concern until recently, when the possibility of liver irritation and the increased risk of heart disease in men and postmenopausal women due to the oxidant effect of iron was suggested. About 1% of red blood cells are recycled each day (their average life span is 120 days), and we use the iron from them (about 30–50 mg daily) to manufacture new cells. The recycled iron provides about 90% of the iron required to make new cells and to carry out other functions; therefore, we need only a little more for full functioning—unless, of course, there is blood loss.

Iron lost from the body must be replaced through dietary iron, but this often takes time and requires a regular source from food or supplements. A pint of blood contains about 200 mg of iron. Even though iron absorption increases with increased need, it can still take several months to completely replenish iron concentration in the blood. About 30 to 40 mg of iron is lost during an average female menstrual cycle; this is why menstruating women need a consistently higher iron intake than men, a minimum of 18 mg per day. During breastfeeding, the nursing mother loses about 1 to 2 mg per day. In pregnancy, the mother transfers 500 to 1,000 mg of iron to her growing baby, most of that (500–700 mg) during the last few months. Because there are usually less than 500 mg stored in the bone marrow and other tissues, the mother needs a regular, good dietary and supplemental intake of iron or she will become depleted and will be less able to obtain the extra oxygen she requires during pregnancy, labor, and delivery of her baby. After delivery, iron depletion could cause her to feel run-down and to have difficulty caring for her infant.

Many factors can increase iron absorption from the intestines and improve our chances of maintaining adequate body levels. Absorption improves when there is increased need for iron, as during growth periods, pregnancy, and lactation or after blood loss. Acids in the stomach, such as hydrochloric acid, and ascorbic acid (vitamin C) in the small intestine help change any ferric iron to the more easily absorbable ferrous form. Citrus fruits and many vegetables contain vitamin C and therefore help iron absorption. The animal flesh foods have the more easily absorbed heme (or blood) iron and also provide amino acids, which stimulate production of hydrochloric acid in the stomach. Cooking with an iron skillet adds iron to the food and makes more of it available for absorption. Copper, cobalt, and manganese in the diet also improve iron absorption.

Likewise, many factors can reduce the body's iron absorption. Low stomach acid or taking antacids or other alkalis diminishes iron absorption. Rapid gastric motility reduces the chance to absorb iron, which is a slow process anyway. Phosphates, found in meats and soft drinks; oxalates, in spinach, chard, and other vegetables; and phytates, in the whole grains—all can form insoluble iron complexes or salts that will not be absorbed. Soy protein is being researched, as it may also reduce iron absorption. The caffeine and tannic acid in coffee and tea lower the absorption of iron. Low copper in the gut and in the body also reduces absorption, and high calcium can compete with iron. Supplementing calcium with iron may create a more alkaline digestive medium, which further reduces iron absorption. Iron absorption usually decreases with age.

Factors Affecting Iron Absorption

Potentially Increased by:
Blood loss or iron deficiency
Body needs during growth, pregnancy, and
    lactation
Citrus fruits and vegetables
Copper, cobalt, and manganese
Hydrochloric acid
Iron cookware
Meats (heme iron)
Protein foods
Vitamin C

Potentially Decreased by:
Antacids
Calcium
Coffee and black tea
Fast gastrointestinal motility
Low copper
Low hydrochloride acid
Oxalates in leafy green vegetables
Phosphates in meats and soft drinks
Phytates in whole grains
Soy protein

Any unabsorbed iron is eliminated in the feces. Otherwise, only minute amounts are lost in the urine, sweat, nail clippings, and hair. Other than through blood loss, most body iron is retained fairly well. Normal iron loss in the average person is about 1 mg per day. When we have plenty of iron, we can say we are "in the pink." In that state, we usually will have good circulation, rosy cheeks, pink earlobes, and a pink tongue. If the tongue or the mucosal lining of the mouth is pale, we should look for anemia.

But we can also be "too pink" or red, with an excess of iron and blood cells. Accumulation of excess iron in the body (iron overload) is a much more common problem than people may think. There are many forms of iron overload disease. One form, hereditary hematomacrosis, is highly likely if a person inherits the double-gene version of this disease and possible if the single-gene version is present. About 1 out of every 200 people in the United States is believed to have the double gene, and 13% are estimated to have the single-gene version. Specific lab tests, called *serum ferritin* and *transferrin saturation,* are necessary for determining iron overload. Because iron overload can disrupt immune function and metabolic events almost anywhere in the body, symptoms can vary dramatically and can even include the same kinds of anemia that are associated with iron deficiency.

Research on iron overload has also shown that when excess iron crosses the blood-brain barrier into the brain, it may increase the severity of chronic neurodegenerative disease, like Parkinson's or Alzheimer's. For all of these reasons, we need to avoid iron excess. One group with particular concerns may be men who take iron-containing supplements, especially those who not only take these supplements but also routinely eat red meat. The reason men may be more at risk than women in this case is related to the lack of a mechanism for releasing iron in men that corresponds to menstruation in women.

Sources. Where the soil is iron deficient, the plants grown or the animals grazed there may contain relatively smaller amounts of iron, although this is not yet a major concern. The milling of grain removes about 75% of the iron present in whole grains, as much of the iron is found in the outer bran and germ. The fortified or enriched grain foods, such as cereals and breads, contain some iron (plus vitamins B_1, B_2, and

B_3), but this iron is in the poorly absorbed ferric state. Cooking in iron pots or skillets adds absorbable iron to food, but if this is done excessively over time, iron toxicity is a possibility.

Heme iron, found in meats, is generally thought to be the iron that is best absorbed, several times more absorbable than the nonheme iron found in the vegetable kingdom. This does not mean that we need to eat meats in order to get sufficient iron, although that is often recommended in cases of iron deficiency. The 18 mg of iron a day needed by a woman in the childbearing years is not always easy to obtain through diet. If we carefully selected only high-iron plant foods, we would need 1 ounce of pumpkin seeds, 2 cups of whole wheat pasta, 2 cups of steamed chard, and 1 tablespoon of blackstrap molasses to reach the 18 mg RDA for adult women. (To reach the RDA for adult men, we would need about half this much). So it is by no means impossible, but it is not always easy. In addition to beef, liver, and other organ meats that have relatively high amounts of absorbable iron, pork, lamb, chicken, and such shellfish as clams and oysters contain reasonable iron levels. Egg yolks are fairly good sources, and salmon is another great source.

Whole grains are among the overall best sources because of their germ and bran. Wheat, millet, oats, and brown rice are all iron-containing grains. The legumes—dried peas and beans—are good, especially lima beans, soybeans, kidney beans, and green peas. Nuts, such as almonds and Brazil nuts, and most seeds contain iron. Pumpkin seeds are a particularly good source. Such green leafy vegetables as spinach, chard, kale, and dandelion are also good sources, as are broccoli and asparagus. Such dried fruits as prunes, raisins, and apricots have a good amount of iron. Prune juice often gives us additional iron. Unsulfured molasses, especially blackstrap molasses, is concentrated in iron; 1 tablespoon contains about 3 mg. Tomatoes, strawberries, and many other fruits and vegetables contain some iron, so it is possible to obtain adequate amounts of iron from dietary sources without consuming a lot of meat by eating wholesome foods.

Functions. The primary function of iron in the body is the formation of hemoglobin, as it is the central core of the hemoglobin molecule, the essential oxygen-carrying component of the red blood cell

(RBC). In combination with protein, iron is carried in the blood to the bone marrow, where, with the help of copper, it forms hemoglobin. The ferritin and transferrin proteins actually hold and transport the iron. Hemoglobin carries the oxygen molecules throughout the body. Red blood cells pick up oxygen from the lungs and distribute it to the rest of the tissues, all of which need oxygen to survive. Iron's ability to change back and forth between its ferrous and ferric forms allows it to hold and release oxygen. Each hemoglobin molecule can carry four oxygen molecules. This large protein molecule makes up approximately 30% of the RBCs. Amazingly, there are some 20 trillion RBCs in the average human body (men have more than women), and about 115 million RBCs are made every minute. Approximately 90% of the iron needed to make those cells comes from recycled RBCs that are normally destroyed by the spleen at the end of their 120-day life span.

Myoglobin is similar to hemoglobin in that it is an iron-protein compound that holds oxygen and carries it into the muscles, mainly the skeletal muscles and the heart. It provides our ability to work by increasing oxygen to our muscles with increased activity. Myoglobin also acts as an oxygen reservoir in the muscle cells. So muscle performance actually depends on this function of iron, besides the basic oxygenation by hemoglobin through normal blood circulation.

Hemoglobin—and therefore iron—gives us our strength and the look of good health (that is,

Foods Most Concentrated in Iron

Food	Amount	Iron (mg)	Food	Amount	Iron (mg)
Soybeans, cooked	1 cup	8.8	Raisins	1/2 cup	2.2
Blackstrap molasses	2 tbsp	7.0	Beef tenderloin	4 oz	2.0
Lentils, cooked	1 cup	6.6	Cashews	1/4 cup	2.0
Quinoa, cooked	1 cup	6.3	Figs, dried	5 medium	2.0
Tofu	4 oz	6.1	Seitan	4 oz	2.0
Pumpkin seeds	1/4 cup	5.2	Bok choy, cooked	1 cup	1.8
Kidney beans, cooked	1 cup	5.2	Bulgur, cooked	1 cup	1.7
Venison	4 oz	5.1	Apricots, dried	10 halves	1.6
Chickpeas, cooked	1 cup	4.7	Potato	1 large	1.4
Lima beans, cooked	1 cup	4.5	Soy yogurt	6 oz	1.4
Pinto beans, cooked	1 cup	4.5	Tomato juice	8 oz	1.4
Black-eyed peas, cooked	1 cup	4.3	Veggie hot dog	1 hot dog	1.4
Swiss chard, cooked	1 cup	4.0	Almonds	1/4 cup	1.3
Tempeh	1 cup	3.8	Peas, cooked	1 cup	1.3
Black beans, cooked	1 cup	3.6	Green beans, cooked	1 cup	1.2
Bagel, enriched	3 oz	3.2	Kale, cooked	1 cup	1.2
Turnip greens, cooked	1 cup	3.2	Sesame seeds	2 tbsp	1.2
Veggie burger, commercial	1 patty	3.0	Sunflower seeds	1/4 cup	1.2
Calf's liver	4 oz	3.0	Broccoli, cooked	1 cup	1.1
Prune juice	8 oz	3.0	Brussels sprouts, cooked	1 cup	1.1
Spinach, cooked	1 cup	2.9	Millet, cooked	1 cup	1.0
Beet greens, cooked	1 cup	2.7	Prunes	5 medium	1.0
Tahini	2 tbsp	2.6	Watermelon	1/8 medium	1.0

Source: *USDA Nutrient Data Base for Standard Reference*, Release 12 (Washington, D.C.: United States Department of Agriculture, 1998).

our rosy cheeks). One of the first symptoms of low iron is weakness, fatigue, or loss of stamina. Anemia results only after longer deficiency of iron or other nutrients; then, less hemoglobin and usually fewer red blood cells are made, and our ability to carry oxygen through the body is diminished. Iron and hemoglobin also improve respiratory activity. Many of the oxygen-dependent diseases (diseases that have symptoms based on circulation and the delivery of oxygen to tissues), such as coronary artery disease and vascular insufficiency, are worsened with iron deficiency. Many other symptoms, both psychological and physical, occur when we do not have enough iron. An equally serious risk, however, is iron overload.

Iron is needed by some important enzymes for energy production and protein metabolism. The cytochrome system (a class of protein molecules that play a role in oxidative processes) depends on iron enzymes, which work within the mitochondria (energy factories) of the cells to produce energy. The iron cytochromes catalase and peroxidase also help protect our tissues and cells from oxidative damage. These enzymes contain iron locked into a heme protein molecule. Research is also being done on iron's role in the formation and health of tissue collagen and elastin and the involvement of iron in the immune system's health. When iron in the body is low, there seems to be an increased incidence of infections, possibly because of a decrease in lymphocyte proliferation and other white blood cells' ability to kill microorganisms. Iron also is helpful in the production of carnitine, a nonessential amino acid important for the oxidation and utilization of fatty acids.

Uses. Of course, the main use of iron is in the prevention and treatment of iron deficiency and iron-deficiency anemia, whether caused by blood loss, pregnancy, or a low-iron diet. When total body iron or circulating iron is low, fatigue, learning difficulties, irritability, and other subtle symptoms may occur long before actual anemia is seen. Many emotional symptoms may occur in children as well.

Iron is used routinely during pregnancy and breastfeeding to prevent iron deficiency. Because of increased iron needs during these times, it is difficult to obtain all the required iron from the diet alone. The infant usually gets enough iron but pulls stores from the mother, who could become depleted. Also, whenever there are

menstrual periods with more than normal amounts of bleeding (medically called menorrhagia), iron is often suggested as a regular supplement. Iron has also been helpful in reducing pain in some women who have difficult menstrual periods.

Sometimes fatigue, especially muscle fatigue and poor physical stamina, responds to iron supplements. Subtle oxygen-deficit respiratory problems may be helped by attaining adequate iron levels, probably because the iron provides increased hemoglobin production and improved oxygenation of the tissue. There is some question as to whether iron acts as a mild antioxidant, protecting the cells and tissues from oxidative damage, or whether it actually stimulates oxidation and can cause problems.

Deficiency and toxicity. Iron overload is a significant (and often overlooked) problem. Following a 12-hour fast, it is easy to measure the total amount of iron in your blood serum, as well as the capacity of your red blood cells to bind iron (total iron binding capacity, or TIBC). It is also easy to measure your transferrin saturation (TS) by dividing your total iron by your TIBC. Transferrin is the main protein molecule used in the body to transport iron, and saturation is an estimate of its iron-filled status. If your TS is greater than about 44%, you are at risk for iron overload.

Serum ferritin can also be measured. Ferritin is the protein on which most iron is stored. This lab test usually reports values between 5 and 150, and anything near the top of this range represents a risk of iron overload because high numbers here are telling you that the proteins for storing iron in your body are completely loaded with this mineral. In other words, if all of the molecules for transporting and storing iron are filled up with iron, and your blood levels are high, there is really no place for any additional iron to go, and your body is overloaded. Since the mid-1990s or so, an ever-increasing list of health problems have been associated with possible iron overload, including chronic fatigue, arthritic join pain, impotence, premature onset of menopause, depression, hypothyroidism, heart arrhythmia, Parkinson's disease, Alzheimer's disease, and in some cases even anemia.

Research by University of Florida Medical School pathologist Jerome Sullivan, MD, suggests that iron overload is also a factor in the development of atherosclerosis. A high-meat diet, separate iron supplements, or even the extra 18 mg of iron that is contained in the average RDA-type multivitamin is more than many people, particularly men, require. **Men lose very little iron, because the body recycles most of it; their needs are only about 10 mg daily.** Consuming much more than this may increase the risk of atherosclerosis and heart disease by an as-yet-undetermined mechanism, possibly through increased oxidation and free-radical formation. Women in the menstruating years seem to be protected from this increased risk, although they lose this protection after menopause, when their risk of heart disease rises to a level close to men's.

Exposure to cigarette smoke, as well as wood smoke, can also increase our risk of iron overload. In this case, iron ends up floating freely in our cells and bloodstream because it is unable to attach itself to our red blood cells. The reason? Carbon monoxide from the smoke latches onto our red cells first and prevents iron from attaching in its usual way. Unless the vast balance of iron in our body is attached to proteins (like transferrin, ferritin, or the heme proteins in red blood cells), it can increase our risk of health problems by triggering unwanted chemical reactions, especially formation of overly reactive molecules. Children have been known to develop acute toxicity from eating extra vitamins or finding some of their parents' ferrous sulfate or other iron supplements. Each year there are about 10 deaths reported of young children who eat more than ten 300 mg iron tablets—that is, more than 3 grams of iron—all at once.

These considerations prompted the National Academy of Sciences to set a tolerable upper limit in 2001 of 45 mg for iron intake by those 14 years and older, and 40 mg for those under 13 years. These guidelines include pregnant women as well as teenage girls who have started their menstrual cycles. Although I generally concur with the trend toward reduced iron intake given the real problem of iron overload, there are times when I believe that doses above this 45 mg level may be necessary—for example, in some situations where there is significant iron deficiency during pregnancy, or in the case of teenage girls who begin menstruation alongside of substantial iron deficiency.

The term for excess iron storage in the body is *hemosiderosis,* or *siderosis.* Here an amorphous brown

pigment called *hemosiderin* (about 35% iron as ferric hydroxide) is deposited in the liver and other tissues, which is not usually a problem unless there are excessive amounts. These increased iron stores usually come not from diet but from iron supplements or blood transfusions. Symptoms of iron toxicity include fatigue, anorexia, weight loss, headaches, dizziness, nausea, vomiting, shortness of breath, and a grayish hue to the skin. Iron has been found in increased levels in joints of patients with rheumatoid arthritis and may contribute to inflammation through increased hydroxyl free radicals. **Supplementation should be avoided by patients with arthritis unless a proven iron deficiency is present.**

In cases of full-fledged iron overload, where transferrin saturation and ferritin are very high, changes in dietary intake are not usually sufficient to bring iron back into balance. Instead, therapeutic phlebotomy (medical bloodletting) is used, where iron-overloaded blood is gradually (periodically) removed from the body under close medical supervision over a period of time that may involve many months.

Those most vulnerable to iron deficiency are infants, adolescents, pregnant or lactating women, vegetarians, people on diets, premenopausal women, and people with bleeding problems. People taking certain drugs—such as allopurinol for gout, tetracyclines, or high amounts of aspirin—may have impaired absorption of iron and thus may develop iron deficiency over time. Both iron-deficiency anemia and iron deficiency without anemia occur fairly commonly when a rapid growth period increases iron needs, which are often not met with additional dietary intake. Several studies have shown that often more than half of children ages 1 through 5, teenagers, and women ages 18 through 44 had iron intakes below the RDA.

Females need more iron than men but often consume less. Iron deficiency is particularly common in pregnancy, especially later pregnancy, when the fetus needs about 7 to 8 mg per day. Even though there is better absorption at this time than the average 10% to 20% of intake, the average diet supplies only 15 to 25 mg per day, which is not enough to meet the needs of both mother and child.

Iron-deficiency anemia is characterized as microcytic (the RBCs are small) and hypochromic (the

RBCs are pale because of decreased hemoglobin). This type of anemia can be determined by doing a complete blood count and checking the hemoglobin, hematocrit, and red blood cell count, along with the RBC indices—the MCV (mean corpuscular volume), MCH (mean corpuscular hemoglobin), and MCHC (mean corpuscular hemoglobin concentration). A doctor or lab technician can also easily see small, pale red blood cells under the microscope. Iron deficiency can occur and generate vague symptoms before clinical anemia actually occurs. This state may be assessed by checking the serum iron concentration. If this is low, it may suggest iron deficiency, usually from low intake or increased losses. Even before serum iron is low, iron saturation, serum transferrin (iron-carrying protein), total iron binding capacity (TIBC), or, more recently, the ferritin level may be measured to detect low iron stores. The body draws on these muscle and tissue stores to maintain normal serum levels.

Anemia is basically defined as a reduction in the number of red blood cells. It can also be defined as a reduced oxygen-carrying capacity of the blood. In this context, other factors besides iron, such as low copper, manganese, zinc, pyridoxine (vitamin B6), folic acid, and vitamin B12 may contribute to anemia. Vitamin B6 and zinc deficiency may mimic iron deficiency, but giving iron may lead to iron toxicity problems in these cases. **Measuring serum iron is the best way to ensure that the problem is actually iron deficiency,** and measuring B6 and zinc levels can help diagnose those hidden, though common, deficiency problems as well. So iron deficiency is but one cause of anemia. I have discussed the B6 and folic acid vitamin deficiency anemias in chapter 5, Vitamins; copper, zinc, and manganese are some minerals whose deficiency can cause other forms of anemia. Thyroid problems or lead toxicity may cause anemia as well. We also need adequate protein, calcium, and vitamins E and C to keep our red blood cells healthy. Thus many nutritionally related problems can lead to anemia; decreased production or increased destruction of RBCs and bleeding, however, are the most common causes. Overall, it is wise to diagnose and treat the definitive cause of anemia, not just give iron.

Many symptoms may arise from iron deficiency. Fatigue and lack of stamina usually arise first, caused by fewer red blood cells, low hemoglobin, and a reduced ability to hold and carry oxygen. Children who are iron deficient may experience psychological problems, learning disabilities based on hyperactivity or a decreased attention span, and even a lower IQ, besides other symptoms of anemia. Headaches, dizziness, weight loss from decreased appetite, constipation, and lowered immunity (a weakened resistance) may occur. With anemia, paleness of the skin, cheeks, lips, and tongue may occur, as can a sore tongue, canker sores in the mouth, hair loss, itching, and brittle nails. Not uncommon is a general state of apathy, irritability, and/or depression—a lack of enthusiasm for life—which can improve rapidly with iron supplementation, however. Decreased memory may also occur. In children particularly, iron deficiency may cause a strange symptom called *pica*—eating and sucking on inedible objects, such as toys, clay, or ice. This usually disappears with iron treatment. In pregnancy, morning sickness may occur more frequently with low iron, perhaps because of the relatively low oxygen distribution to cells. It can take several months for improved absorption and increased intake to catch up to needs.

In general, it is wise to discover the cause of iron deficiency. Is it from low intake? If so, the diet should be evaluated. Or is it due to poor absorption? Then check the absorption factors such as low stomach acid. Or is there some bleeding problem, especially a slow blood loss? Intestinal bleeding, as in colitis, ulcers, or even hemorrhoids, is not uncommon. Excess menstrual bleeding, often with the presence of uterine fibroids, is a common cause of iron loss in women. Parasites can cause iron deficiency anemia, as can cancer. Donating blood too frequently can lead to anemia and iron deficiency symptoms. Supplementing iron may help over time, but it is especially important to rule out any internal bleeding.

Requirements. In 2000, the National Academy of Sciences established the following AI levels for infants and RDAs for all other age categories:

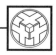

AI Levels and RDAs for Iron	
Age	**AI/RDA**
Infants, 0–6 months	0.27 mg (AI)
Infants, 7–12 months	11 mg (RDA)
Children, 1–3 years	7 mg (RDA)
Children, 4–8 years	10 mg (RDA)
Males, 9–13 years	8 mg (RDA)
Females, 9–13 years	8 mg (RDA)
Males, 14–18 years	11 mg (RDA)
Females, 14–18 years	15 mg (RDA)
Males, 19 years and older	8 mg (RDA)
Females, 19–50 years	18 mg (RDA)
Females, 51 years and older	8 mg (RDA)
Pregnancy, 14–50 years	27 mg (RDA)
Lactation, 18 years and younger	10 mg (RDA)
Lactation, 19–50 years	9 mg (RDA)

Because iron status is influenced by the type of diet consumed and by the use of oral contraceptives, the National Academy of Sciences established additional recommendations for vegetarians and for women taking oral contraceptives. These recommendations are as follows.

Special Circumstances: RDAs for Iron	
Circumstance	**RDA**
Adult men following a vegetarian diet	14.0 mg
Adult, premenopausal women following a vegetarian diet	33.0 mg
Adolescent girls following a vegetarian diet	26.0 mg
Adolescent girls taking oral contraceptives	11.4 mg
Adult, premenopausal women taking oral contraceptives	10.9 mg

Because these guidelines can be confusing, let's do a little simplifying here. Except during growth, pregnancy, lactation, and a woman's reproductive years, the iron RDA is 8 mg. So, taking 10 mg daily in supplements is the most that might be taken in men and in menopausal women. Iron needs increase with growth and development, when more red blood cells and body tissues are being made; during pregnancy, when extra iron is going to the growing fetus; and for at least several months postpartum during lactation, when losses through milk are high. Average daily intake is about 6 mg per 1,000 calories consumed, so a 2,000-calorie diet supplies about 12 mg, which is more than the amount needed by teenage boys and adult men, but less than is needed by female teens and adult women (especially during pregnancy and lactation). Luckily, when body needs increase, iron absorption improves, and we usually develop a craving or taste for iron-containing foods as part of our natural survival and health instincts.

Most people, especially women, should be aware of iron intake and absorption. Eating vitamin C–containing foods along with the high-iron foods or taking an ascorbic acid supplement, even 50 to 100 mg, improves the absorption of iron in supplements. Iron absorption from food is also increased when vitamin C is present. Protein foods improve absorption and usually have a higher iron content, so eating more of these foods, such as meats and legumes, as well as leafy greens, helps get more iron into the body.

Iron supplements are strongly recommended when there are increased requirements, as with teenagers and most women, especially with heavy or long menstrual flow and definitely during pregnancy and lactation, when iron needs may triple. Most men, however—unless there is some bleeding problem—do not require additional iron. When there is sufficient iron intake, more iron will not necessarily help; in fact, it could lead to problems associated with excess iron storage over a period of time.

The ferrous $(2+)$ forms of iron, not the ferric $(3+)$ state, are the forms to have in supplements. **Ferrous sulfate is the most commonly prescribed form of iron, although ferrous fumarate and gluconate are also prescribed by doctors.** As an example, 325 mg (5 grains) of ferrous sulfate contains about 120 mg of elemental iron. With at least a 10 percent absorption rate, that allows more than 12 mg of iron per tablet to get into the body; if these are taken several times daily in pregnancy or in anemia, as some doctors recommend, this may be excessive.

To improve iron absorption, take the iron with 250 mg of vitamin C and between meals, if tolerated. During pregnancy, the increased need also improves the percentage absorbed. Ferrous sulfate is often used because it is inexpensive and fairly assimilable for most women, although it can also be irritating to the gastrointestinal tract and cause constipation or blackening of the stools, which could cover up an intestinal bleeding problem (blood in the stool can also cause it to be black). Ferrous gluconate and fumarate are considered organic irons (as found in living tissues) and are also inexpensive and have good absorption, and they tend to cause fewer symptoms (constipation, intestinal upset) than the inorganic ferrous sulfate. The dosages are similar; 325 mg of ferrous gluconate taken 2 or 3 times daily during pregnancy or to treat iron deficiency or blood losses. These amounts should not be taken regularly as a preventive or safeguard.

The form that probably is best assimilated and easiest on the intestinal tract is the hydrolyzed protein chelate of iron—that is, chelated iron. Usually about 50 mg of chelated elemental iron taken once or twice daily satisfies most iron needs during pregnancy or with iron deficiency. This can be used until the iron and red blood cell levels are normalized. The choice of form for iron supplements is based on absorption and gentleness. In order of preference, the suggested forms are chelated iron, such as iron aspartate, ferrous succinate, and ferrous fumarate, followed by ferrous gluconate and ferrous lactate. Ferrous sulfate is commonly used but produces more symptoms than the other forms.

There is some concern about vitamin E's interaction with iron. It can bind the iron to a nonutilizable form, which then can oxidize and thus inactivate the vitamin E when the two are taken together, although this occurs more so with the ferric forms of iron. Ferrous sulfate has some interaction with E. The organic forms of iron—gluconate, aspartate, and fumarate—as well as the chelated iron have little effect on reducing vitamin E. **But, to be safe, it is best not to take vitamin E with iron; rather, vitamin D should be taken by itself at night or in the morning.**

Overall, iron is a very important mineral of which we must be constantly aware. Extra iron is not needed by everyone—and should be carefully avoid by some people—but when it is required, we must increase iron foods or take supplemental iron to prevent loss of energy and enthusiasm for life and the many other problems caused by iron deficiency.

Manganese

 Manganese, little known and often underrated by both doctors and the general public alike, is an essential mineral important to many enzyme systems in carrying out such functions as energy production, protein metabolism, bone formation, and the synthesis of L-dopamine, cholesterol, and mucopolysaccharides. The human body contains a total of about 15 to 20 mg of manganese. About half of that is in the bones, and the remainder is found in the liver, pancreas, pituitary gland, adrenal glands, and kidneys—the active metabolic organs. Manganese is present in many enzymes in body cells, particularly in the mitochondria as manganese-containing superoxide dismutase, an antioxidant enzyme.

In the food chain, most manganese is present in plant tissues, mainly in nuts, seeds, and whole grains, but in most vegetables as well, particularly the dark leafy greens. Like that of iron, our absorption of manganese is low; utilization of manganese from the diet has been estimated in the range of 15% to 30% efficiency. Absorption may be influenced by body manganese levels. Alcohol and lecithin cause slight increases in manganese absorption.

Large amounts of calcium and/or phosphorus interfere with manganese absorption. Heavy milk drinkers, meat eaters, or consumers of soda beverages may therefore need additional manganese. Magnesium, as is found in antacids, may interfere somewhat with manganese absorption. Iron definitely has a seesaw interaction with manganese; too much of either mineral interferes with absorption of the other. In other words, taking extra manganese can interfere with iron absorption and lead to deficiency, which must then be corrected by taking extra iron. Zinc, cobalt, and soy protein may also interfere with manganese absorption into the blood from the intestines. Manganese can interfere with copper absorption and can decrease copper levels. Optimal absorption of manganese occurs when it is taken in the absence of other minerals or food and in its protein-chelated form.

After absorption, manganese is transported to the liver and then to other organs, such as the kidneys, for storage. The globulin protein transmangamin carries the manganese molecules in the blood. Manganese is eliminated mainly through the feces after being excreted in the bile. The kidneys clear only a small amount. A manganese blood level (whole blood) can be measured; this level is often low in a person who eats the average American diet.

Sources. Nuts and whole grains are the best sources of manganese. Most animal foods have low levels, although egg yolks are a decent source. Seeds, legumes (peas and beans), and leafy greens (especially spinach, mustard greens, and kale) are all good sources of manganese if there is manganese in the soil in which these plants are grown. Alfalfa is high in manganese, and black teas and coffee beans have some. There is also usually some manganese in romaine lettuce and in pineapples.

A number of factors, however, can affect dietary manganese levels. Food manganese levels may vary greatly because of soil deficiencies; the leafy greens are particularly sensitive to this. **Soil mineral losses related to runoff and high-tech farming have created manganese and other mineral depletion problems.** Lime added to the soil binds manganese, and, although it may make nice greens, it results in most foods having a lower manganese content.

Also, though the whole grains (such as barley, whole wheat, millet, and oats) all have good levels of manganese, most of it is in the bran and germ, and these outer parts are often stripped away through milling and refining. Nearly 90% of manganese is lost in the refinement of wheat to white flour. Ideally, we should eat whole and unprocessed foods from healthy, balanced soil to get sufficient amounts of manganese and many other minerals.

Functions. Manganese is involved in many enzyme systems—that is, it helps to catalyze many biochemical reactions. These and its other functions, shown to be essential in animals, are still under investigation for humans, but researchers are finding out that manganese has some important roles in the human body. There are some biochemical suggestions that manganese is closer to magnesium in more than just the name. It is possible that magnesium can substitute for manganese in certain conditions when manganese is deficient.

Manganese activates the enzymes necessary for the body to use biotin, thiamin (B1), vitamin C, and choline. It is important for the digestion and utilization of food, especially proteins, through peptidase activity, and it is needed for the synthesis of cholesterol and fatty acids and in glucose metabolism. As a cofactor in glycolysis, manganese aids glucose metabolism. By activating the arginase enzyme, manganese helps form urea, the end product of protein and ammonia breakdown cleared by the kidneys. Manganese may also be important in the growth and development of normal bone structure and in the formation of mucopolysaccharides, which are needed for healthy joint membranes. Recent studies have shown manganese to activate glycosyltransferase and xylosyltransferase enzymes that are involved in bone formation. Another key enzyme activated by manganese is glutamine synthetase, which helps provide the cells of the small intestine with their primary fuel source—glutamine. This discovery may open the door for increased use of manganese with intestinal problems like inflammatory bowel disease.

Manganese may function as a protective antioxidant, especially in its +2 valence state. Divalent manganese, commonly found in the brain and other tissues as part of the enzyme superoxide dismutase (SOD), can bind oxygen free radicals, thus protecting the cell membranes and tissues from degeneration and disruption. Those areas in danger of oxidative damage are the cell membranes, nerve coverings (myelin), and tissue linings, and these are mainly protected by the antioxidant nutrients and enzymes. The manganese present in SOD is found in the mitochondria and this enzyme protects the mitochondrial membrane from destruction, especially from superoxide free radicals. Trivalent (+3) manganese may be a pro-oxidant, meaning that it may generate oxidation and unstable molecules. This role, as well as manganese's antioxidant functions, are still being researched.

Also still under study is manganese's role in the production of thyroxine, essential for thyroid function; its role in normal lactation, in bone health, and in glucose metabolism; and its importance in reproduction. Because manganese seems to be needed in cholesterol synthesis, which is important to sex hormone formation, it may be essential in normal sexuality and reproduction. The idea that manganese is important to some enzymes that seem to stimulate maternal instincts is vague and difficult to research, and there is currently no proof to support this contention.

Uses. Manganese has been used as a therapeutic nutrient, but other than preventing problems of manganese deficiency, its influence on certain disease states seems only anecdotal to date; further research will provide more evidence. The superoxide dismutase enzymes, only one of which contains manganese (others use zinc or copper), have an antiinflammatory effect in the body, and this function may be relevant to many of the possible uses suggested here. Manganese has been helpful in some cases of fatigue (possibly by enhancing certain enzymes), poor memory (by protecting brain tissue and helping oxygenation), and nervousness, irritability, or dizziness. In his book *Mental and Elemental Nutrients,* Carl Pfeiffer, MD, suggests that manganese along with zinc helps decrease copper levels by both decreasing absorption and increasing urinary losses. He feels that copper in higher than normal amounts can cause psychological problems and even some forms of schizophrenia (see the discussion on copper, on page 181). Also, by some unknown mechanism, manganese may help reduce some of the parkinsonian symptoms, such as muscle rigidity and twitching, secondary to phenothiazine drug use. Manganese supplementation may also help in some cases of epilepsy.

Whether manganese is useful in the treatment of diabetes by helping glucose metabolism or in people with osteoarthritis by stimulating mucopolysaccharide production to heal joints is still undemonstrated and questionable. It is more likely that a manganese deficiency reduces the ability to handle glucose and may thus worsen a diabetic condition. Manganese has also been tried in treatment for multiple sclerosis and myasthenia gravis. When given with B vitamins, manganese may alleviate fatigue or weakness by enhancing nerve impulses. Research has found most tumors and cancer cells to be very low in this mineral, which suggests a possibility that manganese may have a role in preventing cancer cell production and protecting against cancer growth.

Deficiency and toxicity. From a nutritional point of view, manganese may be among the least toxic minerals. There is no known natural toxicity from manganese in food or from taking reasonable amounts in supplements. In the case of water, however, there is active debate about toxicity risk, sparked by the fact that research from several villages in Greece has linked manganese in drinking water at levels of about 2 mg per liter to neuromuscular problems like those found in Parkinson's disease. Because the diet was not studied, however, the total exposure to manganese was not known. I think it is also possible for the manganese to have somehow been more available from water than from food. There is no question, however, that from an environmental standpoint, lung problems can be caused by breathing in the dust when mining the inorganic mineral or in certain occupations, like welding and battery making.

In Chile, where much manganese is mined, workers sometimes develop a strange syndrome they call *locura manganica,* or "manganese madness." The first symptoms may be anorexia, weakness, and apathy. However, there may be an initial manic phase, characterized by inappropriate laughter, increased sexuality, insomnia, and even delusions or hallucinations. Violence and other mental changes may occur. The earlier mania may shift to depression, impotence, and excessive sleeping. Parkinsonian symptoms such as tremors and muscle rigidity may also appear in the later stages. These symptoms may appear, as in Parkinson's disease, from a loss of dopamine in the brain cells. L-dopa, which converts to dopamine in the brain, is used in the treatment of manganese toxicity to reduce symptoms. Avoiding further manganese inhalation is obviously also suggested.

Partly because of the water controversy, and partly because of the known environmental health risks, the National Academy of Sciences decided in 2001 to set the following tolerable upper limits for manganese intake.

Manganese deficiency in animals has been studied extensively. In rats, manganese deficiency can lead to sterility or, if occurring during pregnancy, to poor growth in the offspring and decreased lactation in the mother. There is decreased bone growth, especially in length. Poor brain function may occur from decreases in several manganese activities. A decreased threshold for seizures has also been measured. Poor bone and cartilage health and spinal disk degeneration are possible with low manganese. The relevancy of these findings

Tolerable Upper Limits for Manganese	
Age	**UL**
Infants, 0–12 months	prohibit supplemental manganese, no guideline for food intake
Children, 1–3 years	2 mg
Children, 4–8 years	3 mg
Males and females, 9–13 years	6 mg
Males and females, 14–18 years	9 mg
Males and females, 19 years and older	11 mg
Pregnancy and lactation	9 mg

AI Levels for Manganese	
Age	**AI Level**
Infants, 0–6 months	3 mcg
Infants, 7–12 months	600 mcg
Children, 1–3 years	1.2 mg
Children, 4–8 years	1.5 mg
Males, 9–13 years	1.9 mg
Females, 9–18 years	1.6 mg
Males, 14–18 years	2.2 mg
Males, 19 years and older	2.3 mg
Females, 19 years and older	1.8 mg
Pregnancy and lactation	2.0 mg

to humans is currently only theoretical and needs further documentation.

In children, severe manganese deficiency may lead to convulsions, paralysis, or blindness. In adults, dizziness, weakness, and problems with hearing (such as hearing strange noises), are associated with manganese deficiency. In children, some of these problems result from underdevelopment of structures in the inner ear, called *otoliths*, that regulate sense of balance. Decreased strength and ataxia (unstable gait) have also been related; in addition, weight loss, irregular heartbeat, and skin problems are described by some authors.

Manganese deficiency may cause decreased glucose tolerance or decreased ability to remove excess sugar from the blood, as occurs with chromium or zinc deficiency. Low manganese levels may even cause decreased function of the pancreatic cells, and this problem might be helped by manganese supplementation. Research on this relationship between manganese and glucose tolerance and other suggested effects of manganese deficiency is at a preliminary stage, and, to my knowledge, none of these effects has yet been proved. Whether the decreased manganese levels found in cancer are indicative of a causal relationship (which implicates a role of SOD in cancer) or a result of increased nutrient use is of great interest as well.

Requirements. Adequate intake levels for manganese, set in 2000 by the Institute of Medicine at the National Academy of Sciences, are as follows.

The average diet for men contains about 2.2 mg, depending on manganese soil levels, and for women about 1.7 mg. Intakes from food may range from 1 to 9 mg per day. To be safe, we should get at least 4 to 5 mg per day. When we take extra calcium and/or phosphorus, we probably also need extra manganese. However, taking supplemental manganese may decrease iron utilization and storage, so we need to make sure we get enough iron as well.

Because dietary manganese is relatively nontoxic, even 5 to 10 mg per day is safe. Multivitamin/mineral supplements usually contain from 2 to 4 mg, but the amount may range from 1 to 9 mg. Separate manganese supplements are available in the chelated form or as manganese sulfate or gluconate. These are best absorbed when taken between meals and without other minerals, as these may interact with manganese and reduce its absorption. We should probably limit our intake of additional manganese to 10 to 15 mg per day on a regular basis. Up to 50 mg daily has been used in some research studies without negative effects, although the data here is limited.

Molybdenum

 Molybdenum, whose name may be one of the more difficult to pronounce ("muh-LIB-duh-nem"), is not generally well-known. But this mineral's importance has been discovered in recent years. It is now considered to be an essential trace mineral. It has been found to be essential in most mammals, as well as in all plants. We obtain it primarily from foods, but because it is often scarce in the Earth's crust and therefore deficient in many soils, molybdenum deficiency can be a problem. In fact, it was recently discovered that molybdenum deficiency in the soil in an area of China was responsible for the area having the highest known incidence of esophageal carcinoma over many generations. In nature, molybdenum is found as part of other metal complexes. **In the soil, it serves as a catalyst to the nitrogen-fixing process; thus decreased soil molybdenum can lead to deficient plant growth.**

The body contains minute amounts, about 9 mg, of molybdenum. It is found mainly in the liver, kidneys, adrenal glands, bones, and skin, but it is present in all tissues. It is important to several enzyme systems, most significantly that of xanthine oxidase, which supports many functions, including uric acid metabolism and mobilization of iron from the liver for body use. Molybdenum is fairly easily absorbed from the gastrointestinal tract, although it competes with copper at absorption sites. It is eliminated through the urine and the bile.

As with chromium, depletions or deficiencies of molybdenum are common, and its availability in foods is decreased through soil depletion and food technology. **This mineral has come to the nutritional forefront since the mid-1990s with the recognition of its essential nature and the concern about deficiency.**

Sources. Food levels of molybdenum depend largely on soil content. The amount in food may be increased a hundredfold with molybdenum-rich soil; in certain areas, hard water may contain some molybdenum. Soft water and refined foods contain hardly any, however. Whole grains, particularly the germ, usually have substantial amounts; oats, buckwheat, and wheat germ are some examples of grains containing molybdenum. Many vegetables and legumes are also good sources; these include lima beans, green beans, lentils, potatoes, spinach and other dark leafy greens, cauliflower, peas, and soybeans. Brewer's yeast also has some molybdenum, and liver and organ meats are often fairly high in the mineral as well.

Absorption of molybdenum seems fairly high, with studies showing about 85% from green leafy vegetables like kale, and about 55% from soybeans and other soy foods.

Functions. Molybdenum is a vital part of three important enzyme systems—xanthine oxidase, aldehyde oxidase, and sulfite oxidase—and so has a vital role in uric acid formation and iron utilization, in carbohydrate metabolism, and in sulfite detoxification. In the soil and possibly in the body, as the enzyme nitrate reductase, molybdenum can reduce the production or counteract the actions of nitrosamines, known cancer-causing chemicals, especially in the colon. Found more in molybdenum-deficient soils, nitrosamines have been associated with high rates of esophageal cancer.

Xanthine oxidase (XO) helps in the production of uric acid, an end product of protein (purine) metabolism. Although an excess of uric acid is known to cause gout, recent studies show that, in proper concentrations in the blood, it has antioxidant properties and helps protect the cells and tissues from irritation and damage caused by singlet oxygens and hydroxyl free radicals. This protection may prevent tissue wear and aging, in addition to other free-radical diseases discussed throughout this book. Thus uric acid has a new image as being an important part of balanced human function and not just a waste product. In fact, recent studies using oxygen radical absorbance capacity (ORAC) lab tests have suggested that uric acid is the number-one antioxidant molecule in the bloodstream. With its different effects, uric acid is somewhat like cholesterol in its biochemistry. As with cholesterol, it is both made in the body and obtained through the diet; some people are genetically inclined to elevated levels; and, whereas the right amount is essential to important functions, excesses can lead to problems (cholesterol appears to be much more of a concern on this count than uric acid). Xanthine oxidase may also help in the mobilization of iron from liver reserves.

Aldehyde oxidase helps in the oxidation of carbohydrates and other aldehydes, including acetaldehyde, produced from ethyl alcohol. Sulfite oxidase helps to detoxify sulfurs in the body, particularly sulfites, which are used to preserve food. These potentially toxic and harmful substances can cause nausea or diarrhea and precipitate asthma attacks in sensitive individuals. This so-called salad bar syndrome is caused by sulfite sprays used on vegetables to keep them "fresh" longer. It is possible that adequate tissue levels of molybdenum keep the sulfite oxidase activity levels high enough to counteract this chemical and reduce potential symptoms; molybdenum deficiency may be a factor in those people who are more sensitive to sulfites.

Uses. Because molybdenum's activities in humans are so newly known, it does not have wide usage. Even the uses suggested in some nutritional texts are under question and require more research. **Molybdenum may help prevent anemia by helping mobilize iron, provided there are sufficient iron stores.** The suggestions that it protects the teeth from dental caries and that it prevents sexual impotence are not yet supported by definitive research. Molybdenum deficiency may reduce uric acid formation; this was not previously thought to be a problem, but it may be important to supplement molybdenum to maintain uric acid levels in mid-normal range for the antioxidant function as well as other possible functions.

There are a handful of studies linking molybdenum supplementation to cancer prevention and treatment, with some suggestion that molybdenum can interfere with copper metabolism and, in so doing, interrupt blood vessel changes that are needed to nourish cancer cells. Adding molybdenum to the soil and diet has helped reduce the incidence of esophageal cancer in the Lin Xian area of China's Hunan Province, which had the highest incidence in the world of this deadly disease. It is unlikely, however, that lack of molybdenum in the soil and thus in the diet was a direct cause of the cancer; it was probably due to the production of nitrosamines in the soil, which could not be metabolized because of a deficiency in the plants' roots' activity of the molybdenum enzyme, nitrate reductase. Nitrates and nitrites (such as those in hot dogs, lunch meats, and other cured meats) also increase food levels of nitrates, which can lead to the formation of carcinogenic nitrosamines in the stomach. Both vitamin C, which helps detoxify nitrosamine, and nitrate reductase, which needs molybdenum to function, can help reduce the levels of this carcinogenic chemical as it has done for the Chinese esophageal cancer rates secondary to low soil molybdenum. It is also possible that molybdenum can help protect the body from nitrosamine formation after consumption of foods high in nitrates or nitrites, such as lunch meats.

Deficiency and toxicity. Molybdenum, like most trace minerals, is required in a specific narrow range of daily intake; amounts much greater than this may be toxic. Animals given large amounts experience weight loss, slow growth, anemia, or diarrhea, though these effects may be more the result of low levels of copper, a mineral with which molybdenum competes. In people who are sensitive to it, high doses of molybdenum may lead to high uric acid levels and gouty arthritis symptoms related to increased action of the enzyme xanthine oxidase.

Some animal studies also raise the possibility of reproductive and kidney problems resulting from high molybdenum intake. Based completely on animal studies, the National Academy of Sciences decided to err on the cautious side in 2001 and set tolerable upper limits for molybdenum as follows.

Tolerable Upper Limits for Molybdenum	
Age	**UL**
Infants, 0–12 months	no food recommendation, but prohibit supplements
Children, 1–3 years	300 mcg
Children, 4–8 years	600 mcg
Males and females, 9–13 years	1,100 mcg
Males and females, 14–18 years	1,700 mcg
Males and females, 19 years and older	2,000 mcg
Pregnancy and lactation, 18 years	1,700 mcg
Pregnancy and lactation, 19 years and older	2,000 mcg

Information about molybdenum deficiency is limited as well. Low soil levels of molybdenum lead to increased soil and plant levels of nitrates and nitrosamines, which increase risk of cancer, especially in the esophagus and stomach. Increased sensitivity to sulfites used in foods may be related to low molybdenum and deficient sulfite oxidase enzymes. In animals, molybdenum-deficient diets seem to produce anorexia, weight loss, and decreased life span. In humans, deficiency may lead to visual problems, rapid heart rate and breathing, and depression of consciousness. I am also concerned with the antagonism between molybdenum and tungsten. Tungsten is a naturally occurring element that belongs to the same family as molybdenum, and its extensive use as a catalyst in light bulb filaments and other electronics may end up depositing too much in our groundwater following the discard of these products. If too much tungsten ended up in our drinking water, we would be at increased risk for molybdenum deficiency.

Requirements. In 2001, the National Academy of Sciences set adequate intake levels for molybdenum for infants and RDAs for everyone else. These recommendations are as follows.

AI Levels and RDAs for Molybdenum	
Age	**AI/RDA**
Infants, 0–6 months	2 mcg (AI)
Infants, 7–12 months	3 mcg (AI)
Children, 1–3 years	17 mcg (RDA)
Children, 4–8 years	22 mcg (RDA)
Males and females, 9–13 years	34 mcg (RDA)
Males and females, 14–18 years	43 mcg (RDA)
Males and females, 19 years and older	45 mcg (RDA)
Pregnancy and lactation	50 mcg (RDA)

The amount of molybdenum provided by the average diet ranges widely, from 50 to 500 mcg a day. Studies have shown men averaging 109 to 180 mcg and women averaging 76 to 180 mcg, but within these ranges, the numbers are highly variable. A safe and sensible amount of added molybdenum is from 150 to 500 mcg for adults and 50 to 300 mcg for children over 1 year of age. A molybdenum-rich yeast may be available as an added nutrient, which usually contains a lot of other minerals and B vitamins. Sodium molybdate, which recently has come on the market, can be taken by people who want more molybdenum, although intake should be limited to 500 mcg daily. **It is probably best to take molybdenum in a general multivitamin and to take 2 to 3 mg of copper daily as well, because of the potential copper loss with molybdenum supplementation.** Further research is required, but it appears that molybdenum is important for optimum health and longevity.

Selenium

 Selenium became one of the most exciting nutrients of the 1970s and 1980s when it switched from being classified solely as a toxic mineral to being regarded as an essential one, needed in small daily amounts. **Selenium functions as a component of the enzyme glutathione peroxidase, which accounts for part of its antioxidant function and thus its important contribution to the prevention of the twenty-first-century plagues— cancer and cardiovascular disease.**

Low soil levels of selenium are associated with higher cancer rates, and soil-rich areas have below-average cancer rates for a number of body systems, particularly the breasts, colon, and lungs. Keshan disease, a form of heart disease prevalent in children and characterized by an enlarged heart and congestive heart failure, may be a direct result of selenium deficiency, as it has responded well to selenium treatment. People in Keshan, China, where the disease was discovered, treat it with the common herb astragalus, which accumulates selenium from the soil. The soil in many parts of the United States is also low in this important mineral. The western states generally have higher selenium levels than the eastern; South Dakota has the highest levels and Ohio the lowest (Ohio has more than twice South Dakota's rate of a number of common cancers). Most states with high levels of soil selenium show a decreased rate of cancer deaths. There is some concern, however, that high amounts of selenium, particularly elemental selenium and inorganic sodium selenite, may be toxic in areas where it is found in high concentrations in the water and soil, such as South Dakota.

Selenium and vitamin E work together synergistically in that they carry out antioxidant and immunostimulating functions better together than individually, but their mechanisms of action are probably not the same. Both of these nutrients are part of the "antiaging" or "longevity" group, which may be directly attributable to their antioxidant functions because tissue oxidation by free radicals may be the contributing factor to degenerative disease.

Despite its importance, there is less than 1 mg of selenium in the body, most of it in the liver, kidneys, and pancreas and, in men, in the testes and seminal vesicles. Men have a greater need for selenium, which may function in sperm production and motility. Some selenium is lost through the sperm as well as through the urine and feces. It is absorbed fairly well from the intestines, with an absorption rate of nearly 60%. When selenium is combined with amino acids, its absorption rate is higher (50% to 80%) than when it is found in its inorganic selenite form (44% to 70%).

Sources. Soil levels of selenium vary greatly from state to state and even within local regions across the United States, as well as from country to country throughout the world. So the amount of selenium in our food sources, whether consumed directly as plants or as meat from animals that have eaten the vegetation, varies according to the soil levels. Further, most selenium in foods is lost during processing, such as when making white rice or white flour. Many natural foods contain selenium, mainly an organic form that is much less toxic than sodium selenite and definitely less so than elemental selenium. Selenium may be present in some drinking water, and it is sometimes even added to drinking water where it is deficient. We may see this more in the future as a general disease-prevention measure. Mother's milk usually has several times more selenium than cow's milk. Selenium is also used in some shampoos and skin lotions, and it is possible that we absorb small amounts of selenium from these products.

Brewer's yeast and wheat germ, both regarded as so-called health foods, usually contain high concentrations of selenium. Animal sources such as liver, butter, most fish, and lamb have adequate amounts. Many vegetables, whole grains, nuts, and molasses are fairly good selenium foods. Brazil nuts have high amounts; barley, oats, whole wheat, and brown rice are also good sources; and shellfish, such as scallops, lobster, shrimp, clams, crab, and oysters are all rich in selenium. In the fish family, salmon, snapper, and halibut also have high levels. Garlic, onions, mushroom, broccoli, tomatoes, radishes, and Swiss chard may be good sources if the soil in which they are grown contains selenium. Among the spices and seasonings, mustard seeds also contain this mineral. **Therefore, if we want to make sure we get adequate amounts of selenium and other minerals, it is best to eat a varied diet of wholesome foods.**

Functions. Selenium has a variety of functions, and research is revealing new information. Many of the newly discovered functions for selenium center on a group of protein enzymes called *selenoproteins*. The best-studied of these proteins is glutathione peroxidase (GPO). **Selenium is part of a nutritional antioxidant system that protects cell membranes and intracellular structural membranes from lipid peroxidation.** It is actually the selenocysteine complex that is incorporated into GPO, an enzyme that helps prevent cellular degeneration from the common peroxidase free radicals, such as hydrogen peroxide. (Selenomethionine can be supplemented to generate the organically complexed and active selenocysteine.) GPO also aids red blood cell metabolism and has been shown to prevent chromosome damage in tissue cultures. Solidification of tissue membranes may occur through the oxidation of fatty acids. As an antioxidant, then, selenium in the form of selenocysteine prevents or slows the biochemical aging process of tissue degeneration and hardening—that is, loss of youthful elasticity. This protection of the tissues and cell membranes is enhanced by vitamin E. The antioxidant effect may also benefit the cardiovascular system and protect against cancer. We need adequate daily amounts of selenium for the maintenance of these antioxidant functions and for selenium's other cellular functions as well.

Other selenoproteins may turn out to be just as essential for our health as GPO. Worth mentioning here are thioredoxin reductase, selenoprotein N, and selenoprotein X. Thioredoxin reductase appears to function in much the same way as GPO, allowing recycling of the antioxidant molecule thioredoxin. Selenoprotein N is especially interesting in relation to rigid spine muscular dystrophy (RSMD), because the difficulty of breathing in RSMD appears to be related to deficient function of this selenoprotein, which is found in the muscles of the diaphragm. We do not know much about selenoprotein X yet, although it is likely to have far-reaching effects because it has been found in the cells of every living organism studied so far.

Selenium also appears to help stimulate antibody formation in response to vaccines. This immunostimulating effect is also enhanced by vitamin E; the presence of these two nutrients can increase antibody formation by 20 to 30 times, as shown by research. Selenium is also thought to offer protection against cardiovascular disease, possibly by its antioxidant function but possibly by another as-yet-unknown mechanism. Epidemiological studies show an increased incidence of strokes and other cardiovascular problems in many low-selenium areas.

Selenium has also been found to have an anticarcinogenic effect; its blood or tissue levels may correlate more closely with cancer risk than those of any other substance. Public health research shows this relationship in many cases; good selenium levels correlate with low cancer rates and low levels with increased cancer rates. It is not known exactly how this works other than possibly through the antioxidant function. Perhaps selenium decreases cell division or helps cell repair, or perhaps it protects against mutagenic changes in the first place.

Selenium also seems to protect us from the toxic effects of heavy metals and other substances. **People with adequate selenium intake have fewer adverse effects from cigarette smoking, alcohol, oxidized fats, and mercury and cadmium toxicity.** Aside from the likely antioxidant influence, the specific mechanism by which selenium affords this protection is not known, although the effect is confirmed by some research.

In addition, selenium may aid in protein synthesis, growth and development, and fertility, especially in the male. It has been shown to improve sperm production and motility. Thus selenium may prevent male infertility; however, we do not know whether selenium deficiency actually causes male infertility. These are only some of the conjectures about other selenium functions.

Support of the thyroid gland is another important role for selenium. For the thyroid to produce T3 (triiodothyronine, which is converted from thyroxine, or T4), the most active form of thyroid hormone, selenium is required. For this reason primarily, **selenium deficiency has been associated with low thyroid hormone production.**

Uses. A growing number of clinically effective uses of selenium have been developed, and others are being tested for possible value. As part of nutritional antioxidant therapy with vitamin E, zinc, beta-carotene, and vitamin C, selenium (as selenomethionine) will form the active selenocysteine, which may be beneficial in treating a variety of inflammatory problems, and may be helpful in most acute or degenerative diseases to moderate the inflammatory process. Its use in treating arthritis and some autoimmune problems, such as lupus erythematosus or vasculitis, shows promise but needs further study. Selenium is known to help prevent cardiovascular disease and decrease the risk of complications such as strokes and heart attacks (possibly by reducing platelet aggregation) related to the number one disease process in the United States—atherosclerosis. This use, along with selenium's confirmed ability to reduce the incidence of certain cancers, makes this trace mineral quite important.

Where selenium is abundant in the soil or when it is added to the diet, it has an anticarcinogenic effect. These conditions are associated with both decreased cancer rates and decreased cancer mortality, especially regarding the number-one female cancer, that of the breast, but also cancer of the colon/rectum, prostate, lung, ovary, bladder, pancreas, and skin. This is a wide range. In animal studies, 1 to 4 ppm of selenium added to the food or water is clearly associated with decreased cancer rates. In the United States, high breast cancer rates are associated with areas of low selenium in the soil, and human epidemiological studies confirm these findings throughout the world.

Because of selenium's immunostimulating function, it is very useful in the treatment of many immunosuppression diseases. With its antioxidant properties, selenium, especially along with vitamin E, may become a routine and powerful nutritional treatment in the medical world. Autoimmune diseases, recurrent illnesses or infections, and other inflammatory problems may be helped by restoring adequate selenium levels in the body. Selenium can help us prevent disease by increasing our resistance. In some cases, selenium promotes more rapid recovery from many basic disease processes. More controlled human studies related to specific illnesses need to be done to generate greater acceptance by the medical establishment of selenium's important role.

Selenium's postulated antiaging effect offers another possible use of the mineral; this cell membrane–protecting influence on improving tissue elasticity also needs further research. With vitamin E, selenium appears to be helpful in treating acne. Selenium sulfide used topically seems to help in certain skin conditions, such as dandruff and dermatitis, and to improve skin health. It is also a helpful treatment for the mild skin fungus tinea versicolor.

There are even more exciting possibilities for selenium's use in heart diseases. One angina study showed reduced symptoms in nearly 100% of the patients when selenium was used in a dosage of 1 mg per day with 200 IU of vitamin E, whereas the placebo group reported little benefit. Selenium supplementation helps correct the serious symptoms of Keshan disease, a cardiomyopathy (heart muscle disease with heart enlargement) associated with congestive heart failure and the resulting symptoms of body swelling, shortness of breath, and eventual circulatory collapse. This disease has been more prevalent in China, where it was first reported, but with our new knowledge, more cases are being found in other areas of the world. It may simply be a disease of selenium deficiency. The antioxidant function of selenium likely decreases vascular clogging of inflamed artery linings by soothing irritation and binding free radicals; thus selenium may play a role in reducing or preventing atherosclerosis at its initial biochemical level.

There is a disease of the joints, Kashin-Beck's disease, which is somewhat parallel to Keshan disease of the heart. Selenium deficiency has been shown to be a primary contributing cause of Kashin-Beck's disease, and a primary treatment is increasing the body's supply of this mineral.

Some evidence suggests that selenium supplementation is also helpful in reducing menopausal symptoms. In addition, it has been suggested, with vitamin E, for male impotency. Although these uses need further study, it is certainly possible that selenium can increase sexual potency and fertility by improving sperm production and motility and by protecting against oxidative damage in the testes and related organs. (Fertility, potency, and sexuality are, however, more intricate than just these physiological processes.)

As described earlier, a possible role for selenium in the treatment of underactive thyroid has also been suggested in research studies, as well as a possible role for improvement of breathing difficulty in muscular dystrophy. I am sure that researchers will find more uses for selenium in the near future.

Deficiency and toxicity. In the mid-1980s, selenium was considered a nonessential toxic mineral.

There is still justifiable concern over elemental selenium toxicity, but researchers have found that the value of inorganic selenium salts, such as sodium selenite, and organically bound selenomethionine at appropriate levels far exceeds the potential to cause problems. Selenium can actually be tolerated for short periods in higher amounts than was previously thought. Inorganic selenium, usually as sodium selenite, is the common form found in Nature and can be more toxic in the short term than the organically bound selenium in the form of selenomethionine. Although more than 1 mg per day of sodium selenite is likely to produce symptoms, the body may tolerate several milligrams daily of organic selenium without toxicity problems occurring. It is possible that the organic forms of selenium accumulate in the body, however, and may be of long-term concern. Different authorities provide varying figures for selenium intake as well as divergent viewpoints as to the question of toxicity; some sources state that toxicity is possible when 2,000 mcg (2 mg) are taken daily by people who already have total body stores of more than 2.5 mg (the normal level is 1 mg), or when water or food sources regularly contain more than 5 to 10 ppm.

Selenium is thought to interfere with sulfur compounds and even replace the sulfur in the body, as these two minerals are similar biochemically, and thus may decrease a number of enzyme actions. The complexity of these issues in regard to selenium points out the importance of individual assessment and monitoring when taking certain supplemental products. Given this evidence, and in a decision to err on the conservative side, the National Academy of Sciences set tolerable upper limits for selenium in 2000.

There is no clearly defined syndrome of selenium toxicity. Cattle that graze on selenium-rich soil have exhibited visual, muscular, and heart problems. Similar symptoms of toxicity have been found in humans living in high-selenium areas. Long-term ingestion of high amounts may cause problems with tooth enamel and strength, as higher selenium levels seem to increase tooth decay. One highly speculative theory is that selenium competes with fluoride in teeth, decreasing their strength. Other problems may include loss of hair, nails, and teeth, as well as skin inflammation, nausea, and fatigue. Some subtle symptoms that have been experienced include a garlic odor, a metallic taste, or dizziness. Acute selenium poisoning can lead to fever, anorexia, gastrointestinal symptoms, liver and kidney impairment, and even death if the levels are high enough. None of these symptoms should occur when selenium is taken in a therapeutic amount, however. There has been some fear of mutagenicity (that is, ability to cause developmental defects) of selenium in higher amounts. This might be true of the sodium selenite form, which may have both mutagenic and antimutagenic properties, depending on the amount. This theory needs further detailed study.

Tolerable Upper Limits for Selenium

Age	UL
Infants, 0–6 months	45 mcg
Infants, 7–12 months	60 mcg
Children, 1–3 years	90 mcg
Children, 4–8 years	150 mcg
Males and females, 9–13 years	280 mcg
All others, including pregnant and lactating women	400 mcg

Selenium levels are frequently low in the soils of some regions and in certain Western diets. There appears to be problems associated with selenium deficiency; however, no clearly defined selenium deficiency syndrome has been accepted, although several theories postulate such a syndrome and evidence to support them seems to be mounting. One of the problems with identification of a selenium deficiency syndrome involves the effect of selenium deficiency on the health impact of other minerals, especially some of the potentially toxic metals. There is some evidence that metals like cadmium, arsenic, silver, copper, and mercury can become more toxic in the presence of selenium deficiency.

Given selenium's many important functions and uses, its deficiency may generate increases in many of the disease states that it can prevent and treat. With selenium deficiency, there may be increased risk and rates of certain cancers, cardiovascular disease, hypertension, strokes, myocardial infarction, and kidney disease—all heavyweights along death row. Other problems possibly associated with selenium deficiency include eczema, psoriasis, rheumatoid arthritis, cataracts, cervical dysplasia, alcoholism, and infections.

Selenium absorption may be reduced with aging, and older people often consume less selenium-containing fresh and whole foods. Cataracts have been shown to contain only about one-sixth as much selenium as a normal lens; research is needed to determine whether this is a cause or a result of the cataract. Many books describe more rapid aging and decreased tissue elasticity with selenium deficiency, but this has not been confirmed with solid evidence.

Scientists need to find better ways to evaluate body levels of selenium. Blood levels are not easy to evaluate, as they are low and much selenium is stored. Hair analysis is not a very reliable method for evaluating selenium levels because so many hair products contain selenium to cure dandruff that it often is elevated. Until we find reasonably priced testing methods that correlate accurately with tissue levels and health status, it is wise to take additional selenium, unless of course one lives in a selenium-rich area.

Requirements. In 2000, the National Academy of Sciences established the following guidelines for infants, children, teens, and adults for selenium.

The usual suggested intake is between 50 and 200 mcg, which is also the range provided by the average diet of wholesome foods and water. Selenium is increasingly available in vitamin-mineral supplements and is part of all nutritional antioxidant formulas. The conservative safe amount of selenium is between 100 and 200 mcg per day for adults and about 30 to 150 mcg

AI Levels and RDAs for Selenium

Age	AI Level/RDA
Infants, 0–6 months	15 mcg (AI)
Infants, 7–12 months	20 mcg (AI)
Children, 1–3 years	20 mcg (RDA)
Children, 4–8 years	30 mcg (RDA)
Males and females, 9–13 years	40 mcg (RDA)
Males and females, 14–18 years	55 mcg (RDA)
Males and females, 19 years and older	55 mcg (RDA)
Pregnancy	60 mcg (RDA)
Lactation	70 mcg (RDA)

per day for children, depending on age. Men may need more selenium, especially when sexually active. I usually suggest no more than 200 to 400 mcg per day in supplemental form, although some people do take more. Studies have used 1 mg per day for extended periods without any adverse effects. It is likely that we need more than 100 mcg daily to support some of selenium's functions, such as its antioxidant, anticarcinogenic, and immunostimulating effects, although further research is needed to confirm this.

Some of these functions may be best performed with the help of vitamin E; the antioxidant effects of selenium and E are synergistic. There is also a concern that vitamin C may inactivate selenium in the stomach or small intestine. This is not the case with organic selenium (selenocysteine or selenomethione), but it seems that vitamin C combines with sodium selenite and may make the selenium formed by this interaction less absorbable and possibly more toxic. So for improved function, it is wise to take selenium in the absence of vitamin C and along with vitamin E.

Silicon

Si Silicon is another mineral that is not commonly written about as an essential nutrient. It is present in the soil and is actually the most abundant mineral in the Earth's crust, as carbon is the most abundant in plant and animal tissues. Silicon is very hard and is found in rock crystals such as quartz or flint. Silicon dioxide (SiO_2) is an "active" form of silicon and is used to make glass. **Silicon molecules in the tissues, such as the nails and connective tissue, give them strength and stability.** Silicon is present in bone, blood vessels, cartilage, and tendons, helping to make them strong. Silicon is important to bone formation, as it is found in active areas of calcification. It is also found in plant fibers and is probably an important part of their structure. This mineral is able to form long molecules, much the same as is carbon, and gives these complex configurations some durability and strength. It represents about 0.05% of our body weight.

Although clearly an important part of the body's structure and function, many specifics about silicon remain unknown. Studies have revealed retarded growth and poor bone development in young rats fed a silicon-deficient diet. Rabbits showed more atherosclerotic arterial plaques when fed diets low in silicon. Chicks raised on silicon-deficient diets do not form the skull or long bones properly. Rats also show numerous bone abnormalities when fed silicon-deficient diets. Silicon is clearly required for the formation of collagen, but it may also turn out to be required for the formation of proline, an important amino acid found in the collagen portion of connective tissue. I am sure that researchers will find additional information regarding silicon and its functions in coming years.

Sources. Silicon is widely available in food. It is part of plant fibers (although not of cellulose) and is found in high amounts in the hulls of wheat, oats, and rice, in sugar beet and sugarcane pulp, in alfalfa, and in the herbs horsetail, comfrey, and nettles. Horsetail *(Equisetum arvense)* is a common source used to make supplemental silica. Silicon is also present in lettuce, cucumbers, avocados, strawberries, onions, and dandelions and other dark greens. The pectin in citrus fruits and alginic acid in kelp also contain small amounts of silicon. Hard drinking water is a good source, and water ranks along with beer and coffee as a main contributor of silicon to the average U.S. diet. In fact, according to some studies, an estimated 55% of all our silicon comes from these three sources. **This mineral is lost easily in food processing, however.** Only about 2% of the original silicon is left in milled flour. Soil may also become deficient in silicon, and it is not being replaced; this loss could affect inherent plant structure.

Functions. Silicon promotes firmness and strength in the tissues. It is part of the arteries, tendons, skin, connective tissue, and eyes. Collagen contains silicon, helping hold the body tissues together. As mentioned earlier, not only might it be required to weave the amino acid proline into our connective tissue, it might also be necessary to form proline itself. Silicon is present with the chondroitin sulfates of cartilage, and it works with calcium to help restore bones. Other glycosaminoglycans in the connective tissue, including hyaluronic acid and keratin sulfate, also require silicon for their production.

Silicon is thought to radiate or transmit energy in its crystalline structure, as in quartz crystal. Some researchers think it is able to deeply penetrate the tissues and help to clear stored toxins. Silicea tissue salt, a homeopathic remedy, is described poetically as acting like a "microscopic surgeon."

Uses. Silicon is often used in herbal remedies to promote strength in the hair, skin, and nails. It helps maintain the elasticity of the skin, so it may be one of our antiaging nutrients. Other possible uses of silica or silicon that are under investigation are to reduce the risk of atherosclerosis and heart disease and to treat arthritis and other joint or cartilage problems, gastric ulcers, and other conditions where tissue repair and healing are needed. Silicon is thought to help heal fractures and may have some role in the prevention or treatment of osteoporosis.

Deficiency and toxicity. The National Academy of Sciences' 1997 report on silicon found no toxicity related to intake of food alone. It did find some evidence of kidney stone formation after several years' intake of silicon-containing antacids, however. (Some over-the-counter antacids contain magnesium trisilicate, with 5 to 10 mg of silicon per tablet.) In animal studies, excessive intake of silicon has been linked to changes in both calcium and magnesium metabolism, although it is not clear exactly how problematic these changes actually are. Given the lack of evidence for food-related toxicity, no tolerable upper limit was set for silicon.

Silicon deficiency problems are under investigation. Results of studies on animals suggest that silicon may be essential in humans. Decreased growth and deficient bone and tooth structure were found in rats with silicon-deficient diets. Silicon deficiency may increase atherosclerosis and heart disease; or it may not be a cause-and-effect relationship, but rather a result or association of these diseases. It would seem that the essential strength and stability this mineral provides to the tissues should give them protection from disease. Other research reveals that silicon levels affect physical endurance, with low tissue levels correlating with lowered stamina.

Requirements. There is no RDA for silicon because it has still not been officially determined to be essential. As of 1991, studies show adult men eating, on average, about 40 mg of silicon per day, with adult women eating about half as much, 19 mg. In most studies, the amount of silicon we consume also corresponds closely to the amount of fiber in the diet. When we eat high amounts of fiber, silicon moves up toward the 45 to 50 mg level. At the low-fiber extreme, however, it drops to 20 mg or less. **Thus, to get extra silicon, one of our best bets is to increase our fiber!** We can accomplish this goal by eating more whole grains and fresh vegetables, plus other foods containing a combination of fiber and silicon. We can also take advantage of herbs, such as horsetail capsules or alfalfa tablets.

Zinc

Think zinc! Zinc has so many important functions and potential uses that both doctors and patients should think of zinc more often for handling many day-to-day problems. **Zinc deficiency is fairly common now as a result of soil losses and losses in food processing, and this deficiency or depletion can produce a variety of symptoms.**

In 1934, zinc essentiality was first suggested. Not until the early 1960s, however, was it discovered that low intake or low body stores of zinc can cause deficiency symptoms. In recent years, since the discovery that this mineral is becoming less available in our soil and thus in our food chain, zinc has been given more attention, and increased research has produced much new information. We now know that zinc is needed in probably more than 100 enzymes and is probably involved in more body functions than any other mineral. It is important in normal growth and development, the maintenance of body tissues, sexual function, the immune system, and detoxification of chemicals and metabolic irritants. Carbohydrate metabolism is influenced by zinc, and zinc is needed in the synthesis of DNA, which aids the body's healing process. Zinc is often helpful in reducing healing time after surgery or burns, in many male prostate problems, in skin diseases, and in many other difficulties.

Zinc is found in the body in small amounts, only about 2.0 to 2.5 grams total. Of the trace minerals, it is second in concentration to iron, with 33 ppm to iron's 60 ppm. (Although fluoride is found at 37 ppm in the average human body, it is still questionable whether it is essential. This 37 ppm is also a result of the use of fluoridated water, vitamins, and stannous fluoride toothpaste.) Although zinc is the twenty-fifth most abundant element in the Earth's crust, measuring about 0.01%, it is water soluble both in soil and in food. Rains can wash zinc (as well as iodine, sulfur, and selenium) from our farming soils, as can modern agricultural techniques. When we cook food, much of the zinc may go into the water, as do other minerals and vitamins, so the cooking liquids, especially from vegetables, should be consumed as well. **More important, when foods are processed, as in the refining of grains, much of the zinc is lost, along with manganese, chromium, molybdenum, and B vitamins.** Usually only iron and sometimes vitamins B_1 and B_2 are added back in "enriched" foods (and this iron is not even in the easily usable form). Adding zinc, manganese, chromium, and more B vitamins, such as B_6, would be much better and help us avoid common deficiencies.

Zinc absorption may vary from about 12% to 59% of ingested zinc, depending mainly on body needs and stomach acid concentrations. Like iron, zinc from animal foods, where it is bound with proteins, has been shown to be better absorbed. About 70% of the zinc in an average U.S. diet comes from animal sources. When bound with the phytates or oxalates found in grains and vegetables, less zinc is absorbed. Calcium, phosphorus, copper, iron, lead, and cadmium all compete with zinc for absorption. Milk and eggs reduce zinc absorption. Fiber foods, bran, and phytates, found mainly in the outer covering of grains, may also inhibit zinc absorption. Phytic acid may combine with the zinc in the upper intestine before this mineral can be absorbed.

The zinc-cadmium relationship is interesting. Cadmium is considered a potentially toxic heavy metal. When it contaminates our food, it is found in the center of grain; zinc is found mainly in the grain covering. So eating whole grains, which have a higher amount of zinc than of cadmium, reduces any possible absorption of cadmium. With refining of grains into flour, the zinc-to-cadmium ratio is decreased, and cadmium is more likely to be absorbed and cause problems.

In the body, the 2.5 grams of zinc are stored in a variety of tissues. By far the most popular storage spots, however, are skeletal muscle and bone; 85% of all zinc ends up in those places. Zinc is most concentrated, though, in the prostate and semen, which suggests zinc's tie to male sexual function (impotence can be related to low zinc). The next most concen-

trated tissues are the heart, spleen, lungs, brain, adrenal glands, and the retina of the eye. The skin contains a high amount of zinc, but there it is less concentrated than in the organ tissues. Nails, hair, and teeth also have some zinc, and this mineral is important to those tissues as well.

Zinc is eliminated through the gastrointestinal tract in the feces. Some is also eliminated in the urine; alcohol use increases urinary losses of zinc. It is also lost in the sweat, possibly as much as 2 to 3 mg a day. This amount can increase substantially from a heavy workout with profuse sweating. Stress, burns, surgery, and weight loss all seem to increase body losses of zinc.

In evaluating body zinc status, plasma or serum zinc levels may not reflect body stores; if they are low, however, zinc is likely deficient. Low levels of zinc in the hair appear to reflect zinc deficiency, which then should be substantiated through a blood test. High levels of zinc in the hair may also be seen with zinc deficiency, although this is not as correlative as low levels. In general, the red blood cell (or white blood cell) measurement of zinc may be most indicative of the body's true status of zinc nutriture. In addition to measuring the concentration of zinc in our red blood cells, measuring the concentration of a zinc-binding protein called metallothionein may also turn out to be an excellent way of determining zinc status. There is also some indication of a gene marker for zinc status, related to this same metallothionein protein as found in the messenger RNA of other blood cells called *monocytes*.

Sources. Most animal foods contain adequate amounts of zinc. Oysters are particularly high, with more than 10 times as much as other sources; they are also high in copper and possibly in ocean-polluting chemicals and metals. Zinc is added to animal feeds to increase growth rates, so meat usually contains high amounts. Red meats (beef, lamb, and pork) and liver are fairly high; herring is good, as are egg yolks and milk products (although the zinc in eggs and milk products may not be as available to the body as that found in other sources). Other fish and poultry also contain fair zinc levels. **As with iron, the zinc in animal foods seems to be better absorbed than that in the vegetable sources, but one can reduce meat foods and eat whole grains and beans and still obtain adequate zinc.** Overall, though, in my experience it is not easy for most people eating a relatively healthy diet to obtain the minimum requirement of 15 mg daily unless they focus on zinc-containing foods.

Whole grains such as whole wheat, rye, and oats are rich in zinc and are good sources for vegetarians. Even though the mineral from these foods is utilized less well because the fiber and phytates in the grain covering bind some zinc in the gastrointestinal tract, much of the zinc in these foods is still available to the body. Nuts are fairly good sources, with pecans and Brazil nuts containing the highest zinc levels. Pumpkin seeds contain zinc and are thought to be helpful to the prostate gland. Ginger root is a good zinc source, as are mustard, chili powder, and black pepper. In general, fruits and vegetables are not good zinc sources, although peas, carrots, beets, and cabbage contain some zinc.

The zinc in grains is found mainly in the germ and bran coverings, so refining them lowers the zinc content. Approximately 80% of zinc is lost in making white flour from whole wheat. Because zinc is soluble in water, canning foods or cooking in water can cause zinc losses. Zinc losses have also been prevalent in agricultural soils, and it is therefore less available in foods grown in that soil. Chemical fertilizers also decrease zinc soil levels. The soil in nearly 30 states is deficient in zinc. Water, especially from some wells, contains zinc. Water was a better source when some of the water pipes were galvanized (containing zinc), as were some cooking pots. Now, water pipes are more commonly made of copper, which can become toxic at higher levels.

Functions. Zinc is involved in a multitude of body functions and is part of many enzyme systems. With regard to metabolism, zinc is part of alcohol dehydrogenase, which helps the liver detoxify alcohols, including ethanol (drinking alcohol), methanol, ethylene glycol, and retinol (vitamin A). Zinc is also thought to help utilize and maintain body levels of vitamin A. Through this action, zinc may help maintain healthy skin cells and thus may be helpful in generating new skin after burns or injury. By helping collagen formation, zinc may also improve wound healing. Zinc aids the skin's oil glands and so may help in acne problems.

Zinc is needed for lactate and malate dehydrogenases, both important in energy production. Zinc is a cofactor for the enzyme alkaline phosphatase, which helps contribute phosphates to bones. Zinc is also part of bone and tooth structure. Zinc is important to male sex organ function and reproductive fluids. It is in high concentration in the prostate gland as well as in the eye, liver, and muscle tissues, suggesting its functions in those areas.

Zinc in carboxypeptidase (a digestive enzyme) helps in protein digestion. Zinc is important for synthesis of nucleic acids, both DNA and RNA. The process of gene transcription, where DNA gets converted into RNA, is a process where zinc remains in the research spotlight. In fact, we are finding that zinc has some antioxidant function. As part of superoxide dismutase (SOD), it helps protect cells from free radicals. Through this antioxidant effect, zinc is also helpful in cell membrane structure and function.

Zinc has also been shown to support immune function. Zinc improves antibody response to vaccines and can improve cell-mediated immunity by helping regulate the function of the white blood cells. A somewhat higher amount of zinc has caused an increase in production of T lymphocytes, important agents in cell-mediated immunity.

Zinc is important to normal insulin activity and is also related to normal taste sensation. Zinc may have an anti-inflammatory function, especially in the joints and artery linings. It may also be involved in brain function, in maintaining acid-alkaline balance through carbonic anhydrase, another zinc-containing enzyme, and in phosphorus metabolism.

More research is needed on this important mineral. As zinc, because of its function in many enzymes, is so important to chemical detoxification and our ability to handle environmental chemicals and toxins, zinc deficiency may be an underlying factor in those people who become environmentally sensitive. This is just a single example of where further zinc research may be valuable.

Uses. Just as it has many functions, zinc has a wide variety of clinical uses. Some of these regularly show positive results; other uses have variable outcomes, and some new therapeutic trials are under way.

Zinc is used commonly to enhance wound healing. Taken before and after surgery, zinc has been shown in numerous studies to speed recovery time and reduce the incidence of postoperative complications, such as wound infections. This use has the potential to greatly cut down on hospital costs. In some studies, the hospital stay has been reduced by more than half. Zinc

Possible Uses for Zinc

Acne	Immune suppression
Alcoholism	Infections
Anorexia nervosa	Infertility
Benign prostatic	Male sexual
hypertrophy	problems
Boils	Pregnancy
Cataracts	Prostate congestion
Colds	Psoriasis
Decreased hearing	Schizophrenia
Environmental	Skin ulcers
sensitivity	Sore throats
Fatigue	Surgery recovery
Gastric ulcers	Weak muscles
Hypertension	Wound healing

may be helpful in speeding healing after burns or injury as well. This wound-healing effect is a likely result of zinc's function in DNA synthesis. The results seem to be particularly pronounced when there is zinc deficiency before the treatment. In many of the wound-healing studies, zinc dosages of 150 mg per day were used. It is possible that lower amounts, even 30 to 60 mg per day, would produce these effects.

Zinc may be useful in treating such skin problems as boils, bedsores, general dermatitis, and acne. Research on zinc and acne shows variable results, but many teenagers and others have been helped, especially when zinc deficiency was present; it is likely that other factors and nutrients are also involved in acne, however. Leg ulcers have healed more rapidly with zinc treatment in a dose of 150 mg per day. Internally, gastric ulcers have responded favorably to zinc in a similar dosage. Psoriasis is even occasionally responsive to zinc supplementation. White spots on the fingernails, which can be a result of zinc deficiency, may respond to zinc treatment. Zinc may also be helpful to general nail health, as well as skin and hair health. Cataracts also seem to be associated with zinc deficiency and have been helped by treatment.

My friendly travel agent developed a case of hoarseness that persisted for more than a month. Her otolaryngologist diagnosed chronic inflammation and had suggested long-term quietude and learning to live

with it—neither of which was a big hit. In passing (I was quite aware of the foibles of her diet), I suggested zinc lozenges. She began sucking on 3 to 4 lozenges daily, and within a week her voice was back. In this case, the $5 bottle of zinc helped more than the $70 to $100 office visit. I believe that she was zinc deficient and that the supplement helped to heal her inflamed tissue.

Zinc is used in a variety of immune problems. It is among the supportive nutrients used to treat lowered immunity. Zinc has been shown to increase T lymphocyte production and enhance other white blood cell functions. **Recent double-blind studies verify that zinc therapy is helpful in reducing the incidence and severity of colds and other infections.** Also, infections such as herpes, trichomoniasis, or AIDS may be curtailed some with zinc, especially if it is deficient. Sucking a 25 to 50 mg dissolvable zinc lozenge can provide dramatic relief in some cases of sore throat and has been shown to prevent the progression of viral flu symptoms. Individuals with allergies and environmental sensitivities may benefit from zinc supplementation. Measuring zinc status and following it during treatment may be useful in validating its positive effects.

For male prostate problems, there is no scientific evidence that zinc works, although there are a great many anecdotal accounts from men who claim to have been helped by zinc. There is good reason to think these anecdotal accounts harbor a truth, however, because several large epidemiological studies, including the Prostate Cancer Prevention Trial, involving 15,387 men, have shown preventive effects of zinc supplementation. Mild or persistent nonbacterial infections or congestion have commonly been helped by oral zinc treatments. Of course, when zinc deficiency produces such sexual symptoms as infertility, impotency, or poor sexual development, supplementation of this mineral may have great benefit. There is some suggestion that the prostate enlargement that comes with age, termed benign prostatic hypertrophy (BPH), is related to low zinc (and cadmium toxicity) and that regular zinc supplementation may prevent this common problem. More research is needed to clearly evaluate zinc's relationship to prostate and sexual health.

Zinc may also be beneficial in rheumatoid arthritis, for which it has been shown to reduce symptoms; in preventing dental caries by strengthening tooth enamel; and with symptoms of heart disease, where the zinc-to-copper ratio may be important. The use of zinc in cancer prevention and the support of patients with cancers such as Hodgkin's disease and leukemia has been the subject of some interest.

Zinc therapy can reduce cadmium toxicity from pollution or from cadmium in water or foods. Cadmium toxicity may aggravate hypertension, atherosclerosis, and heart disease and produce complications of hypertension or stroke.

Zinc with vitamin B6 has also been used in the nutritional treatment of schizophrenia and, given along with manganese, zinc has been helpful in some cases of senility. Zinc treatment may help with the loss of taste sensation that comes especially with aging, which is often due to zinc deficiency, and it may help stimulate the taste for food in patients with anorexia nervosa. Menstrual irregularity and female sexual

organ difficulties may have some relationship to zinc levels and be helped by zinc therapy, although copper may be more important for these areas.

Deficiency and toxicity. Zinc is fairly nontoxic, especially in amounts of less than 100 to 150 mg of elemental zinc daily, although this much zinc is probably not really needed and may interfere with the assimilation of other minerals. Some studies suggest a partial suppression of immune function at daily doses of 300 mg for 6 weeks. Zinc salts such as gluconate or sulfate are commonly available in 220 mg tablets or capsules, each providing 55 mg of elemental zinc. Taking one of these 2 or 3 times daily may cause some gastrointestinal irritation, nausea, or diarrhea but is more likely to have positive effects. Excessive supplementation may cause some immune suppression, premature heartbeats, dizziness, drowsiness, increased sweating, muscular incoordination, alcohol intolerance, halluci-

---

Factors Related to Zinc Deficiency

- **Diet**—low in zinc or high in copper; high in fiber, phytates, clay, alcohol, or phosphates, all of which bind zinc in the intestines and reduce absorption; food grown in low-zinc soils.
- **Aging**—when zinc absorption and intake are often reduced.
- **Pregnancy**—when zinc needs are increased.
- **Growth periods**—infancy, especially with increased copper intake levels and for those on low-zinc formulas; puberty, especially in adolescent boys.
- **Birth control pills**—use of these increases copper levels and thus reduces zinc.
- **Premenstrual symptoms**—associated with low zinc.
- **Increased copper intake**—high copper intake in water, food, or supplements reduces zinc.
- **Fasting or starvation**—causes zinc depletion and increases needs for zinc.
- **Serious illness or injury**—causes zinc depletion and increases needs due to tissue healing.
- **Hospitalization**—the stress of illness or treatment, particularly intravenous therapy without zinc supplementation.

- **Stress**—increases zinc use and needs.
- **Burns**—increases needs for tissue healing and dealing with stress.
- **Acute or chronic infections**—greater requirements from stress and for healing.
- **Surgery**—increased requirements for dealing with stress and for healing.
- **Alcoholism**—often associated with low zinc intake and higher needs; alcohol flushes zinc from the liver, causing increased losses.
- **Diuretic therapy**—may cause extra zinc losses.
- **Psoriasis**—rapid skin activity may deplete zinc.
- **Parasites**—cause zinc depletion and poor absorption.
- **Malabsorption**—from pancreatic insufficiency or after gastrointestinal surgery.
- **Cirrhosis**—zinc levels may be half of normal.
- **Renal disease**—causes increased excretion of zinc.
- **Chronic disease**—metabolic and debilitating diseases such as cancer.
- **Athletics**—increased zinc losses in sweat.
- **Cadmium toxicity**—interferes with zinc absorption and utilization.

nations, and anemia, some of which is due to copper deficiency. More than 2 grams of zinc taken in one dose will usually produce vomiting. If not, it will likely lead to other symptoms until the body clears the excess zinc. Luckily, only a certain amount of it will be absorbed.

Zinc may interfere with copper absorption, so regularly taking zinc supplements without copper can cause copper deficiency. This interferes with iron metabolism and possibly causes anemia, as copper and iron are important in red blood cell formation. We usually need supplemental copper and vitamin A to balance the effect of extra zinc. Some formulas—for example, Nutrilite's product A plus Zinc—contain vitamin A and zinc together, which improves the effect of both; additional copper, about 2 mg, might also be supplemented daily, although at another time of day than the zinc.

Other problems associated with low zinc levels are peptic ulcers, pernicious anemia, cystic fibrosis, and Down's syndrome.

There are also some questions about zinc's interactions with iron. Some studies show interference between zinc and iron in both directions when the ratio between these 2 minerals gets too lopsided. However, these findings have not been consistent and do not seem to apply that readily to food versus supplement sources of zinc and iron.

Zinc deficiency is likely more common and more complex than previously thought. In the United States, 3 out of 4 people get fewer than 15 mg per day; 1 out of 2 people get fewer than 8 mg per day. Zinc deficiency was first identified in Iran and Egypt in 1961, in male dwarfs with slow growth and poor sexual development. The unleavened bread that is a staple in the diet there is high in the phytates that bind zinc, and a type of clay used for cooking in Iran also ties up zinc. Zinc treatment was found to help these conditions, stimulating growth and sexual development.

Aging is among the main factors in zinc deficiency. However, some recent environmental changes have also contributed to the deficiency problem. Soil losses and losses due to food processing are two of the main factors in zinc depletion in foods. With the change from iron- and zinc-containing water pipes to copper ones, not only is zinc intake decreased, but the additional copper interferes further with zinc absorption. The average diet, especially one with low protein intake, supplies only 9 to 13 mg daily.

In general, both infants and adolescents have more zinc deficiency, as do the elderly and women, often because of low intake. For example, with the average American diet, a man would need to eat about 2,500 calories to obtain 11 mg of zinc (the RDA for adult men), and many men do not eat that much. Good-quality food is needed, and therefore poor people are more likely to experience zinc shortages.

The subject of our diet and zinc deficiency is an important one. The all-too-typical advanced-technology, anti-Nature diet that is high in refined grains, fat, sugar, convenience foods, and fried meats is often low in zinc and many other important trace minerals and B vitamins. **Also, strict vegetarians and consumers of much grain and little animal protein may not obtain sufficient zinc.**

There are many symptoms and decreased body functions due to zinc deficiency. It may cause slowed growth or slow sexual development in the pubertal years. Lowered resistance, fatigue, and increased susceptibility to infection may occur with zinc deficiency, which is related to a decreased cellular immune response. Sensitivity and reactions to environmental chemicals may be exaggerated in a state of zinc deficiency, as many of the important detoxification enzyme functions may be impaired.

Children with zinc deficiency may show poor appetite and slow development, have learning disabilities or poor attention span, and in later years have acne and decreased sexual development. Dwarfism and a total lack of sexual function may occur with serious zinc deficiency. Fatigue is common.

Acute deficiency may cause hair loss or thinning, dermatitis, and decreased growth. Both poor appetite and poor digestion are also experienced by adults with zinc deficiency. Loss of taste sensation may occur, as can brittleness of the nails or white spots on the nails, termed *leukonychia*. These and most other symptoms can be corrected with supplemental zinc. Sulfur may be helpful as well. Skin rashes, dry skin, and delayed healing of skin wounds or ulcers may result from zinc deficiency, and stretch marks, called *striae*, are also produced by this condition. **Zinc and copper are both needed for cross-linking of collagen, and when they are low, the skin tissue may break down.**

Zinc deficiency may cause delayed menstruation in teenage females or, in later years, cause menstrual problems. In addition to zinc, vitamin B6 often also helps correct this. **Females on birth control pills usually have elevated copper levels and need additional zinc and B6.** When zinc is further reduced by the increased copper, depression is more likely, a common side effect of birth control pill use. Morning sickness in pregnancy may result from low zinc and B6 levels, and supplementing these nutrients may help reduce symptoms.

One fascinating route for evaluating zinc deficiency involves a simple test called the zinc sulfate tally. In this test, a measured amount of zinc sulfate, in liquid form, is held in the mouth and evaluated for taste. People who are zinc deficient usually taste nothing at all. By contrast, people with good supplies of zinc usually taste something disagreeable—either a metallic or furry taste. This test is fascinating, because zinc is perhaps the most critical mineral for providing us with a sense of taste in the first place. At a simple level, the test also seems to point out that the body is smart, knows when zinc seems unnecessary, and brings out an unwanted taste as a warning flag to lower intake.

Male teenagers with low zinc have delayed or absent sexual development. Sterility may result from zinc deficiency; when it is caused by testicular degeneration, it may be irreversible. Subtle zinc deficiencies may be responsible for male growth lag in puberty. Even in sexually developed males, low zinc levels have been correlated with a decrease in testosterone levels and a lower sperm count. Prostate problems are more prevalent with zinc deficiency.

Birth defects have been associated with zinc deficiency during pregnancy in animal experiments. The offspring showed reduced growth patterns and learning disabilities. In humans, children with zinc deficiency have decreased intelligence and erratic behavior. With zinc treatment, the IQ and behavior may both improve if the problem is related to zinc deficiency.

Requirements. The RDAs for zinc, set in 1999 by the Institute of Medicine at the National Academy of Sciences, are as follows.

The average woman's diet contains only about 9 mg of zinc; the average man's contains about 13 mg. When zinc needs are considered, we likely need even more than these amounts to be sure we are meeting our requirements. Adequate amounts can be met by a

RDAs for Zinc	
Age	**RDA**
Infants, 0–6 months	2 mg
Infants, 7–12 months	3 mg
Children, 1–3 years	3 mg
Children, 4–8 years	5 mg
Males and females, 9–13 years	8 mg
Females, 14–18 years	9 mg
Males, 14–18 years	11 mg
Males, 19 years and older	11 mg
Females, 19 years and older	8 mg
Pregnancy, under 18 years	13 mg
Pregnancy, 19 years and older	11 mg
Lactation, under 18 years	14 mg
Lactation, 19 years and older	12 mg

good diet, especially with good protein and calorie intake. Vegetarians can eat more whole grains; even with some of the zinc binding to grain phytate, we still get a fair share into the body from these zinc-rich foods. Because absorption is about 30% to 40%, our total zinc body tissue needs are about 4 to 6 mg per day.

We probably need 15 to 30 mg of available (elemental) zinc daily for maintenance and probably about 30 to 60 mg for treatment, although more is sometimes used. General supplement formulas often include 15 mg of zinc. Separately, zinc gluconate and sulfate in reasonable amounts are used commonly without any side effects, although zinc gluconate is usually a little better tolerated than zinc sulfate. **The amino acid–chelated zinc is probably the best tolerated and absorbed,** but it is more expensive. Zinc sulfate tablets or capsules of 220 mg provide 55 mg of elemental zinc. A supplement labeled "zinc 25 mg as gluconate" should provide 25 mg elemental zinc. In medical treatment or research, 220 mg of zinc sulfate may be used 2 to 3 times daily, supplying about 100 to 150 mg of available zinc for absorption. This dosage is usually tolerated fairly well.

Many people also have good success with another delivery form of zinc, called zinc monomethionine. As the name suggests, this form finds zinc bound up with the amino acid methionine. Other available forms include zinc glycinate, zinc aspartate, zinc picolinate, zinc orotate, zinc succinate, and zinc citrate. All of these forms involve the chelation of zinc with an amino acid or an organic acid. Sometimes it may make sense to select a form in which the chelate is also needed—that is, zinc monomethionine might be selected when not only zinc, but also methionine is needed.

Although 30 to 60 mg of elemental zinc per day is the usual therapeutic level, more may be needed to correct zinc deficiency. Taking zinc alone 2 hours after meals or first thing in the morning increases absorption by reducing the competition with other nutrients, such as calcium and copper, or food constituents, such as the phytates and fibers in grains. With infections or burns, before or after surgery, during pregnancy, or with aging (often accompanied with lower absorption), 50 to 75 mg per day is suggested as a therapeutic dose.

When taking higher amounts of zinc, we must make sure we get adequate amounts of copper—at least 2 to 3 mg supplemented and possibly more with higher zinc intakes—so copper deficiency does not occur. The suggested zinc-to-copper ratio is about 15:1. About 200 mcg per day of selenium should also be taken to prevent depletion by supplemental zinc. Zinc may be taken with magnesium, vitamin C, and B complex vitamins, but it is best to take a regular vitamin-mineral combination with 15 to 30 mg of zinc in proper proportion to other minerals, so that deficiencies of zinc or imbalances of the other minerals do not occur.

POSSIBLY ESSENTIAL TRACE MINERALS

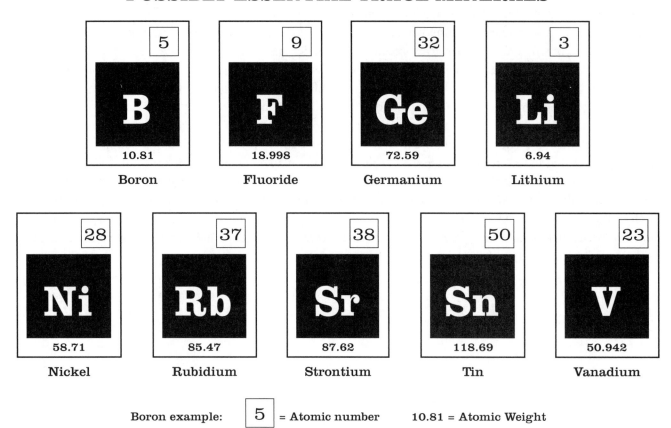

Boron example: [5] = Atomic number   10.81 = Atomic Weight

There has been a great deal of new nutritional research since the first edition of this book in 1992. Seeking understanding and knowledge of the Earth's natural elements (of which little is known) has been part of this research. Although the initial studies began in animals, oftentimes the findings have applied to humans. Many of the currently known important trace minerals were discovered through this type of investigation during the twentieth century. We, of course, have much more to learn about mineral medicine.

Relatively recently, we have found valuable uses for such minerals as boron, fluoride, lithium, rubidium, strontium, and vanadium. Nickel and tin, though usually considered mildly toxic minerals, may be required in very small amounts. Arsenic, discussed later in this chapter, is also possibly needed in modest amounts, although its toxicity is of concern (see the discussion on page 231). Germanium, an exciting mineral new to the nutritional scene, is not known to be essential, yet it may be valuable in the treatment of disease. It is discussed mainly in chapter 7, Special Supplements.

Boron

Boron has recently been making nutritional medicine news and will likely be noted as the next essential trace mineral. It appears to help maintain calcium balance, keeping bones healthy and preventing osteoporosis. The most recent research has been government sponsored, and it looks favorable regarding the positive effects from adequate boron nutriture. The level of boron needed in the diet is not known; it is probably between 3 and 5 mg daily. The highest concentration of boron in the body is in the parathyroid glands, suggesting its tie to calcium metabolism and bone health.

Boric acid has been used for decades as an astringent and antiseptic for the skin and eyes. Boric acid eye wash is probably boron's most common medicinal use. **Boric acid use is not suggested for infants and small children, however, as many are sensitive.** Excess use in anyone can lead to dry skin or gastrointestinal upset.

Sources. Boron is available in the soil and in many whole foods. Such fruits as apples, pears, and grapes are high in boron. Leafy greens, legumes, and nuts also are good sources. Avocado, peanuts, and prunes are other sources. A poor diet, high in refined foods and low in wholesome ones, likely provides insufficient boron and may lead to deficiency problems, one of which may be osteoporosis in the elderly. Meat and fish are poor sources of this mineral.

Functions. Boron physiology is not totally clear as yet. It possibly affects calcium, magnesium, and phosphorus balance and the mineral movement and makeup of the bones by regulating the hormones, mainly parathyroid, that control these functions. Boron's aid in preventing bone loss and osteoporosis is only projected at this date, and further study is needed to understand its relationship to the bones. Some of the controversy here hinges around the issue of vitamin D deficiency. Apparently, some of the changes in calcium metabolism attributed to boron alone may be changes influenced primarily by vitamin D deficiency and then exaggerated by deficiency of boron. At the least, simultaneous deficiency of these nutrients might be necessary in order for calcium balance to be disrupted.

Boron may also play a role in hypertension and arthritis via its relationship to calcium metabolism. Both of these diseases, as well as atherosclerosis, are in part related to abnormal calcium metabolism and balance. Adequate calcium (and magnesium) may help maintain normal blood pressure, while abnormal calcium deposition may increase artery plaque and joint irritation.

One role for boron may be emerging in connection with blood sugar, where animal studies are showing a need for more insulin secretion when boron is missing from the diet. A brain connection may also be unfolding, because attention span, eye-hand coordination, and short-term memory appear to be decreased when boron is deficient. More research in these areas may prove interesting.

Uses. The current suggestion is to provide adequate levels of boron (3–5 mg) in the diet to maintain healthy bones. Boron is now used in more calcium/bone-replenishing nutritional formulas. At this time, because of its low potential toxicity and possible necessity, elderly people and anyone at risk of osteoporosis should eat boron-rich foods and further supplement boron at a level of about 1 to 3 mg daily. Whether boron

is useful in the treatment of osteoporosis, arthritis, other bone diseases, or hypertension must be studied further.

Deficiency and toxicity. Boron toxicity to date is associated with excessive use or increased sensitivity to boric acid, as just mentioned. The ingestion of boric acid can lead to immediate nausea and vomiting. Later problems could be anemia, hair loss, skin eruption, and seizures. Diborane inhalation or exposure to liquid boron hydride can adversely affect the lungs and nervous system. Boron toxicity has also been associated with increased loss of vitamin B_2 through the urine. For adults 19 years and older, the tolerable upper limit (UL) set for boron by the National Academy of Sciences in 2000 is 20 mg.

Boron deficiency is apparently more of an everyday concern. It may be associated with an increased incidence of osteoporosis. Preliminary research of arthritis incidence suggests a correlation with soil boron levels. In Israel, where people have a very low rate of arthritis (less than 1%), there are high levels of boron in the soil, while Jamaica has the opposite situation—low boron soil levels and a high incidence of arthritis. Clearly, more epidemiological research is needed to isolate boron or boron deficiency as a factor in these diseases.

The deficiency and toxicity aspects of boron are interesting because of a further research discovery: Boron moves through our blood in the form of boric acid (or borate) and readily latches onto, and lets go of, a variety of other nutrients, including vitamins B_2, B_6, and a form of vitamin C called *dehydroascorbate*. Overall, boron deficiency may offer some concern, while boron toxicity may as well.

Requirements. There is no RDA for boron at this time. Probably about 1 mg daily in the diet is sufficient to prevent deficiency. In the United States, we currently average 0.75 to 1.35 mg of boron per day, and we get an extra 0.135 mg from supplements, bringing us to 0.89–1.49 mg per day on average. Researchers Curtiss Hunt, PhD, and Forrest Nielsen, PhD, of the Department of Agriculture's Human Nutrition Research Center in Grand Forks, North Dakota, say that 3 to 5 mg of boron daily can improve calcium retention, based on a 6-month study of postmenopausal women. After a low boron diet, 3 mg daily were supplemented. These boron-supplemented subjects then showed lower daily losses, nearly 50%, for both calcium and magnesium than when on the boron-deficient diet. More multi-vitamin/minerals and bone supportive supplements are currently adding 1 to 2 mg boron. It appears that this mineral is part of our nutritional picture for the future.

Fluoride

 Although fluorine as fluoride has been shown to reduce dental cavities when added to toothpaste or drinking water, there is still some question as to whether it is an essential element. In other words, if we do not have fluoride, will we develop any problems? Eating a natural diet low in refined flours and sugars along with some basic oral hygiene will maintain healthy teeth and gums.

Fluorine itself is a poisonous gas, as are the related elements chlorine and bromine. *Fluoride* is a general term that is used to describe any circumstance in which the single element fluorine has been combined together with something else. The "something else" could be another element or a more complicated molecule. Fluorine, as fluoride, is found in the Earth's crust in combination with other minerals, and is also part of seawater. Fluoride is available naturally in the diet as calcium and sodium fluoride.

Sodium fluoride is added to the drinking water of many cities to help reduce dental caries. There is some controversy as to whether fluoridation has some subtle poisoning effect or whether it is nontoxic and beneficial. **In my opinion, fluoridated water is another example of technology's treating the effect instead of correcting the cause—primarily, poor diet.**

Fluoride is probably not essential to humans, although it is helpful in strengthening the bones and teeth. In the body it is found only in trace amounts, about 2 to 3 grams, and most of that is in bones and teeth. The blood level of fluoride is about 0.3 mg per 100 ml. Fluoride has no known function other than strengthening teeth and bones.

Intestinal absorption of fluoride in its sodium fluoride, drinking-water form is very high. When fluoride is found in food, however, this absorption rate drops down from 90% to 100% to 50% to 80%. Calcium, aluminum, and perhaps other minerals may interfere somewhat with absorption by making less-soluble fluoride salts. About half of ingested fluoride, about 3 mg per day, is eliminated through the kidneys and a little

more through perspiration. The remainder is stored mainly in the bones.

Sources. Natural fluoride is present in the ocean as sodium fluoride, so most seafood contains some. People who eat large quantities of fish, such as the cultures of the Caribbean, have been shown to have stronger teeth and a lower incidence of dental cavities, the most common disease worldwide, than do others. This may be related to other factors as well, however. Gelatin and tea also contain fluoride. In fact, a study showed that school children in England were obtaining more than 1 mg of fluoride daily from tea alone (black tea, with caffeinelike molecules theophylline or theobromine plus tannic acid, not herbal teas). Most plant-source foods contain some fluoride, although the amount can vary greatly depending on soil fluoride content. Soil deficiency of fluoride is fairly common.

Fluoride is added to the drinking water of many municipalities at the concentration of 1 ppm. More than 2 ppm can cause problems, so the concentration must be finely monitored. People drinking city water who also consume fluoride-containing foods or black teas can develop fluoride problems as well, although toxicity has not been found to be appreciable with moderate amounts.

Stannous (tin) fluoride was originally used in toothpaste for protection against tooth decay. But it has been found that fluoride is more effective in this area when provided internally by drinking water than when it is applied locally, and we probably do not want too much extra tin anyway (although tin may be an essential mineral in trace amounts as well). **Overall, I do not advocate drinking fluoridated water—or any city water, for that matter** (see chapter 1, Water, for more on this issue). To be safe from chemical and toxic metal pollutants, it is better to drink filtered water. I also advocate eating a more natural diet with some seafood, which is also thought to protect against atherosclerosis and heart disease as well as to keep the teeth healthy.

Functions. Studies show that fluoride helps strengthen the crystalline structure of bones and teeth. The calcium fluoride salt forms a fluorapatite matrix, which is stronger and less soluble than other calcium salts and therefore is not as easily reabsorbed into circulation to supply calcium needs. In teeth, this fluoride salt reduces the potential for breakdown from acids in the mouth or from demineralization, minimizing tooth decay. Fluoride also helps decrease the occurrence of dental caries (cavities) by affecting bacteria in the mouth. Fluoride can stop some of these bacteria from taking in too much sugar, and as a result, these bacteria put out less acid (a breakdown product of sugar). With less acid being produced by the mouth's bacteria, the enamel of the teeth is less likely to be damaged. In bones, fluoride reduces loss of calcium and thereby may reduce osteoporosis. No other functions of fluoride are presently known, although it has been suggested to have a role in growth, in iron absorption, and in the production of red blood cells. This needs further research.

Uses. Fluoride's main use is as an additive to drinking water as well as toothpaste and mouthwash for the prevention of tooth decay. When added to water at 1 ppm, it can reduce dental caries by 30% to 50%. Fluoridated water works best, however, when its use is begun in infancy or early childhood and continued throughout childhood. Fluoride-treated water does not decrease the gum disease that may also result from poor nutrition and poor hygiene, however. As is typical of much Western medical thinking, some scientists treat the result as if it were the problem itself, rather than correcting the cause—the overuse of sugar and poor dietary habits in general—that may be causing decay even deeper in the body, a process that may take many more years to discover. On a more positive note, the use of sodium fluoride has been shown to be helpful in the treatment and possibly the prevention of osteoporosis, although the results from various studies are mixed. Epidemiologically, the incidence of osteoporosis is slightly reduced in fluoridated-water users. In older studies, bone density as well as blood pressure was improved by treatment with 50 mg of sodium fluoride (NaF), 900 mg of calcium daily, and 50,000 IU of vitamin D twice weekly. There is concern, however, that fluoride-treated bones will not give up calcium easily to the body when needed, which may contribute to calcium deficiency. It is obviously much better to prevent osteoporosis by eating calcium-rich foods; supplementing calcium, magnesium, and vitamin D; maintaining overall mineral balance; eating a healthy diet; and exercising regularly.

There is some preliminary research evidence that fluoride may help in treating otosclerosis, a loss of hearing due to deposits in the ear. Hearing loss in later years, when it is a result of osteoporosis, or loss of minerals from the tiny ear bones, may be reduced with fluoride treatment as well.

Fluoride is not generally used as a supplement in multivitamin/mineral formulas. It is added to some infants' and young children's vitamins to aid in the prevention of tooth decay. As sodium fluoride, it is occasionally prescribed medically in the prevention or treatment of dental disease.

Deficiency and toxicity. Toxicity from fluoride is definitely a potential problem. Fluoridated water must be closely monitored to keep the concentration at about 1 ppm to effectively reduce dental decay without producing side effects. At concentrations greater than 2 ppm, fluoride can cause mottling, discoloration, and pitting of the teeth, although it will still maintain tooth strength and prevent cavities. For infants and children, this discoloration of teeth occurs when fluoride intake levels reach 2 to 8 mg per kilogram of body weight. At 8 ppm to about 20 ppm, initial tissue sclerosis will occur, especially in the bones and joints, which can cause arthritic symptoms. At more than 20 ppm, much damage can occur, including decreased growth and cellular changes, especially in the metabolically active organs such as the liver, kidneys, adrenal glands, and reproductive organs. More than 50 ppm of fluoride intake can be fatal.

In terms of total fluoride intake, around 20 mg per day usually causes some tooth discoloration and bone problems. Animals consuming extra fluoride in grains, vegetables, or water have been shown to have tooth and bone lesions. Fat and carbohydrate metabolism has also been affected. There are many other concerns about fluoride toxicity, including bone malformations, cancer, and attention-deficit/hyperactivity disorder (ADHD). Since 1966, at least 40 studies have been conducted worldwide on the relationship between fluoridation and cancer. Approximately half have shown no link or have been inconclusive, with the other half showing a connection.

Sodium fluoride is less toxic than most other fluoride salts. In cases of toxicity, extra calcium binds with the fluoride, making a less soluble and less active compound. The combination of these and other circumstances prompted the National Academy of Sciences to set tolerable upper limit levels for fluoride in 1997 as follows.

Tolerable Upper Limit Levels for Fluoride	
Age	**UL**
Infants, 0–6 months	0.7 mg
Infants, 7–12 months	0.9 mg
Children, 1–3 years	1.3 mg
Children, 4–8 years	2.2 mg
Everyone 9 years and older, including pregnant and lactating women	10 mg

Fluoride deficiency is less of a concern. Low fluoride or lack of fluoride use does correlate with a higher number of dental caries, given the lack of stability and strength of the bones and teeth in general. It is possible that traces of fluoride are essential, but it is not clear whether it is a natural component of the body's tissues. **Low fluoride levels may correlate with a higher amount of bone fractures in the elderly,** but that is usually in the presence of osteoporosis.

Requirements. There is no specific RDA for fluoride. Nor is it mandatory to add fluoride to the water. Many cities do not follow this much-supported preventive measure. On a worldwide level, there has been a lot of disappointment with the use of fluoridated water. People who drink fluoridated city water get about 1 mg per day from it. Research shows that the amount in the average diet varies widely, depending on choices of foods and water use. Nonfluoridated water users take in between 0.35 mg and 1.5 mg per day, while the average city diet with fluoridated water contains about 2 to 3 mg. The suggested safe intake of fluoride (not necessarily the optimum, which researchers really do not know) is between 1.5 and 4.0 mg per day. Amounts up to 15 to 20 mg per day are probably well tolerated, although researchers do not know the long-range effects. And until they do, I discourage overuse of fluoride.

Germanium

Ge Germanium, trace mineral 32, has recently become popular after being developed into an organic germanium compound in Japan. This organo-germanium, bis-carboxyethyl germanium sesquioxide (Ge-132), has been tested and used for the treatment of a variety of medical problems that require improved oxygenation and immune function, ranging from simple viral infections to cancer. Organo-germanium is discussed in detail in chapter 7, Special Supplements. Germanium belongs to the same chemical group as silicon and has many of the same chemical properties. In animal studies, some of the problems with bone development stemming from silicon deficiency have been reversed by supplementation with germanium.

The trace mineral germanium itself may be needed in small amounts by the human body; however, research has not yet shown this. **It is found in the soil, in foods, and in many healing plants, such as aloe vera, garlic, and ginseng.** The organo-germanium currently used does not, however, release the mineral germanium to the tissues for specific action; rather, it is absorbed, acts, and is eliminated as the entire compound, Ge-132. More research is needed to clearly understand the potential importance of both elemental germanium and the Ge-132 compound.

An especially interesting group of studies on germanium involves delay and/or prevention of cataracts in diabetic mice. Organo-germanium supplements appear to help prevent attachment of sugar to proteins in the eye—a process that can lead to cataract. There is some far-reaching potential here for germanium, because attachment of sugar to proteins (called *glycation*) is a problem not only with cataracts but with many chronic health problems related to blood sugar excess.

Germanium may pose a special toxicity risk for the kidneys if supplemented in the form of germanium salts instead of organo-germanium (Ge-132), or other organic forms, including carboxyethyl germanium sesquioxide, germanium citrate, or germanium lactate. Inorganic forms may be too easily converted to gases like germanium dioxide, which can be toxic.

Lithium

Li Lithium is usually found in nature not as a metal but as lithium salts. Its name comes from *lithos,* the Greek word for "stone," as the lithium crystals are hard, beautiful rocks. Aside from hydrogen, which is present in almost all of life, lithium is the lightest element in use. It is unique among the minerals in that it is used in medical treatment of manic-depressive disorders, commonly as lithium carbonate. It is chemically similar to sodium and can displace sodium (and vice versa) in many bodily reactions. **Its involvement in sodium transport across cell membranes probably accounts for lithium's therapeutic support of people with manic disorders.** Although it has been used in this area since about 1950, its acceptance has been slow, possibly because it is a natural mineral and not as profitable for the pharmaceutical companies as synthetic drugs. Recent evidence indicates that lithium may be an essential element, needed in trace amounts (minute in comparison to the high doses used in treatment).

We have in our body only about 2 to 3 mg of lithium. Absorption from the intestine is good, about 70% to 90%. People with mania often have very good absorption of lithium. Excess lithium is eliminated in urine and feces.

Sources. Scientists do not completely understand what effect lithium in foods has or what particular foods are high in lithium. Some natural mineral waters are high in lithium, and these are said to calm the nerves, cheer the spirit, and soothe the digestion. Sugarcane and seaweed have been shown to contain lithium, as have some dairy products and smoked fish. Tobacco has some lithium, but the effect of inhaled lithium is not known.

Functions. It is not yet known what particular function of lithium may make it an essential nutrient. It is thought to stabilize serotonin transmission in the nervous system; it influences sodium transport; and it may even increase lymphocytic (white blood cell) proliferation and depress the suppressor cell activity, thus strengthening the immune system. It is clear that lithium is active in the brain, and we know that it both activates and blocks the activity of several enzymes responsible for the relay of chemical messages. In some ways lithium appears to work opposite to the B vitamin–like compound inositol, because it appears to block the transfer of messages when inositol is the messaging molecule. There is also speculation that lithium is in some way involved in cancer genesis or prevention.

Uses. Lithium's main use is in treating manic-depressive disorders, for which it is used in what could be considered megadosages. Certain depression problems, probably those sensitive to sodium transport difficulties, may be helped by lithium, even where there

is little or no manic component. Manic symptoms of insomnia, hyperactivity, talkativeness, grandiose thinking, and delusions can usually be controlled with lithium therapy. Dosages of between 600 and 1,000 mg per day are needed to obtain the appropriate blood level to treat mania. Smaller amounts of natural lithium orotate or aspartate, for example 5 to 10 mg taken twice daily, can be used to balance moods and mild versions of manic-depressive swings.

Lithium has occasionally been used in treating alcoholism, where it apparently decreases the taste for alcohol and generates a more cheerful attitude toward life. Lithium treatment does, however, produce some side effects, such as a metallic taste in the mouth, increased thirst, and more frequent urination. It is not routinely taken as a nutritional supplement but is used primarily as a medicinal drug.

Deficiency and toxicity. Deficiency of lithium is not really known. The theory that a deficiency of lithium can cause an increase in depression has not been adequately proved. **Lithium toxicity, however, is a real possibility when it is used as a medicine.** In the treatment of manic disorders, there is a fine line between therapeutic and toxic levels. Because it is cleared in the urine, anyone with kidney disease must take lithium with caution. It is given in therapeutic doses only by prescription, with blood levels followed closely by the doctor.

Lithium produces some of its symptoms by upsetting the fluid balance and mineral transport across cell membranes. Symptoms of lithium toxicity include nausea, vomiting, diarrhea, thirst, increased urination, tremors, drowsiness, confusion, delirium, and muscle weakness. Skin eruptions may also occur. With further toxicity, staggering, seizures, kidney damage, coma, and even death may occur.

Requirements. There is no specific RDA for lithium, nor is it known how much, if any, we need. Dietary studies estimate that we get about 2 mg daily. A therapeutic intake can vary from 500 to 1,500 mg daily, although usually 300 mg of lithium carbonate 3 times daily provides the blood levels needed to treat manic disorders, which may require long-term therapy. Under these circumstances, blood levels should be checked occasionally to make sure there are sufficient amounts present, and symptoms (side effects) of lithium toxicity should be watched for carefully.

Nickel

Ni Nickel has been considered a possibly essential trace mineral for several decades. We have a total of about 10 mg in our body, but we still do not know exactly what it does. Most of the nutritional research on nickel has been done with chicks and rats. It is an essential nutrient for these animals, and they suffer considerable problems with nickel deficiency.

Nickel is found in many foods and in all animal tissues, including human tissues. It appears to be relatively concentrated in the thyroid and adrenal glands and may also accumulate in hair, bone, and soft tissues, like the lungs, kidneys, and liver. Because it occurs in food and is part of the Earth's crust and not a contaminant, many scientists feel that it is probably essential to humans. But nickel is potentially toxic in its gaseous form, nickel carbonyl.

Absorption of nickel appears to vary widely according to its food source. Overall dietary absorption is less than 10%, but when nickel is added to drinking water, this percentage increases to about 50%. When added to coffee, tea, orange juice, or cow's milk, nickel is also better absorbed, at a rate of about 30% to 40%. Nickel is transported around the body in attachment to two proteins. One is albumin, a common and well-researched blood protein. About 43% of the nickel in our blood is transported by a more specialized protein, nickelplasmin. Scientists are not yet sure about the general nature of nickelplasmin, however. The kidneys can either clear excess nickel or retain it; such a control mechanism suggests essentiality.

Sources. Nickel is contained in many foods. Most beans, soybeans, lentils, and split and green peas have fairly high amounts. Nuts, such as walnuts and hazelnuts, are the best sources of nickel. Of the grains, oats have the highest content, followed by buckwheat, barley, and corn. Chocolate and cocoa are also rich sources. Many vegetables and some fruits, such as bananas and pears, have moderate amounts. Animal products and fatty foods are fairly low in nickel; of these, herring and oysters are the highest. Refined foods are also low. Interestingly, even though nickel can form a very stable complex with phytate in foods, this binding together of nickel with phytate does not appear to decrease its absorption as would be the case with other minerals, like iron.

There are external, nonfood sources of nickel also, but it is not clear how much nickel we actually absorb from these sources. Nickel is found in coins, costume jewelry, eyeglass frames, hair clips, pins, scissors, batteries, and some kitchen appliances. Regular contact with these nickel products may allow some absorption into the body. Allergic dermatitis from nickel products is not at all uncommon.

Functions. The biological function of nickel is still somewhat unclear. Nickel is found in the body in highest concentrations in the nucleic acids, particularly RNA, and is thought to be somehow involved in protein structure or function. It may activate certain enzymes related to the breakdown or utilization of glucose. Nickel may aid in prolactin production and thus be involved in human breast milk production.

Nickel clearly plays a role in helping to regulate iron metabolism and probably reduces free-radical production because it helps our cells use a particular form of iron called *ferric iron*. It is also clearly involved with copper and zinc metabolism and appears to block copper absorption while reacting in a more complicated way with zinc. Some zinc deficiency problems in animals have been lessened through nickel supplementation. In other cases, nickel supplements shifted the distribution of zinc in the body, but did not improve symptoms.

Some of the enzymes that use zinc or magnesium may be able to use nickel instead. Metabolism of the branched-chain amino acids—leucine, isoleucine, and valine—as well as certain fatty acids may require nickel. So might the function of vitamin B12, although this connection is far from certain. Most of the information about nickel comes from testing with animals, and its relevancy to humans is still not proven. More research is needed to reveal the properties of this interesting mineral in the human body.

Uses. There are presently no clear uses for nickel supplementation. Studies have shown that there are increased levels of nickel in patients following heart attacks, burns, and strokes, and with toxemia of pregnancy. Whether this is a partial cause or, as is more likely, is a result of tissue metabolism or represents some other function of nickel is not yet known. Decreased levels of nickel have been seen in psoriasis, in cirrhosis of the liver, and with kidney disease, but it has not been shown that nickel treatment helps any of these conditions.

Deficiency and toxicity. Toxicity is the main concern here—not from elemental nickel or the nickel found in foods but from inhaled nickel carbonyl, a carcinogenic gas that results from the reaction of nickel with heated carbon monoxide, from cigarette smoke, from car exhaust, and from some industrial wastes. Nickel carbonyl is toxic and can cause such symptoms as frontal headaches, nausea, vomiting, or vertigo with acute exposure. Inhaled nickel accumulates in the lungs and has been associated with increased rates of lung, nasal, and laryngeal cancers. Nickel allergy can also cause local skin or systemic reactions. The nickel in jewelry, dental materials, or prosthetic joints or heart valves may also be allergenic sources.

Despite the clear overriding concerns about nickel toxicity, there are also some lesser but still lingering questions about whole body performance (for example, rate of growth in early life) from nickel supplementation with rats. Based on these concerns, and erring on the safe side, the National Academy of Sciences decided to set tolerable upper limits for nickel in 2001 as follows.

Tolerable Upper Limits for Nickel	
Age	**UL**
Infants, 0–12 months	no level set for food, but no supplemental nickel is recommended
Children, 1–3 years	200 mcg
Children, 4–8 years	300 mcg
Males and females, 9–13 years	600 mcg
Everyone 14 years and older, including pregnant and lactating women	1,000 mcg

Nickel deficiency has not been proven to be a concern in humans, but it is definitely a problem in chicks and other small animals, where low nickel can lead to decreased growth, dermatitis, pigment changes, decreased reproduction capacities, and compromised liver function. In humans, increased sweating, such as from exercise, can cause nickel losses, and extra dietary nickel may be required to maintain its still mysterious functions.

Requirements. There is, of course, no RDA for nickel. Up to 500 mcg is probably a safe daily intake. If nickel is clearly found to be essential, the minimum requirement would likely be 50 to 100 mcg. **Nickel is easily obtainable in most diets and is not usually contained in any supplements, except for occasional trace mineral formulas.** In the United States, our average dietary intake is about 75 to 100 mcg, although a study of Canadian adults has shown a much higher average of about 200 to 400 mcg.

Rubidium

Rubidium is present in the Earth's crust, in seawater, and in the human body. The body contains about 350 mg. It has not yet been shown to be essential. Chemically, it is like potassium, and in some animals it can replace potassium in certain functions, although this does not seem to be the case in humans. Rubidium can possibly be a potassium antagonist in regard to absorption and utilization, although this needs further investigation. Rubidium is absorbed easily from the gut, at a rate of about 90%. It is found generally throughout the body, with the least amount in the bones and teeth; it is not known to concentrate in any particular tissue. Excess rubidium is eliminated mainly in the urine.

Sources. Food sources of rubidium have not yet been researched very well. Some fruits and vegetables have been found to contain about 35 ppm. Rubidium may also be found in some water sources.

Functions. There are currently no known essential functions of rubidium in humans. There are some indications, however, that rubidium may function like an antidepressant, because of its ability to increase levels of serotonin in rats. In studies with mice, rubidium has also helped decrease tumor growth, possibly by replacing potassium in cell transport mechanisms or by rubidium ions attaching to the cancer cell membranes. Rubidium may have a tranquilizing or hypnotic effect in some animals, possibly including humans. It is likely that we will hear more about this mineral in relationship to its fellow minerals, because in animal studies, interactions have already been shown with sodium, potassium, phosphorus, calcium, magnesium, iron, zinc, and copper.

Uses. There are no clear uses for rubidium as yet. Because of its possible tranquilizing effect, it could help in the treatment of nervous disorders or epilepsy. It may also turn out to be helpful as an antidepressant.

Deficiency and toxicity. There is no known deficiency or toxicity for rubidium.

Requirements. There is no RDA for rubidium. The average dietary intake may be about 1.5 mg daily.

Strontium

There is no evidence yet that strontium is an essential mineral. The body contains about 300 to 350 mg, nearly 99% of it in the bones and teeth. It closely resembles calcium chemically and can actually displace it. It forms strontium bone salts, which may actually be slightly stronger than those of calcium. So close is the relationship between strontium and calcium that this mineral is quickly becoming one of the preferred markers for measuring calcium absorption from the intestinal tract.

Radioactive strontium (Sr 90) is a hazardous by-product of nuclear fission. Taking trace amounts of strontium may possibly protect us from picking up the radioactive form when exposed to it. Generally, we do not need to worry about strontium, even if it is essential, because it is available in most diets, through the soil. This means that the strontium content in food varies geographically. Strontium absorption varies from about 20% to 40%. It is stable in the tissues, mainly the bones and teeth, and most extra strontium is eliminated in the feces.

Sources. Strontium is present in seawater and some other waters. The level of strontium in soil may vary. Strontium is found, generally in low amounts, in most foods.

Functions. Strontium may help improve the cell structure and mineral matrix of the bones and teeth, adding strength and helping to prevent tooth decay or soft bones, although it is not known if low body levels of strontium cause these problems.

Uses. There are no clear uses for supplemental strontium. The use of strontium to help bone metabolism and strength in osteoporosis has been investigated but is still questionable. Whether strontium prevents tooth decay has not been shown. As stated, trace amounts of nonradioactive strontium may be taken to reduce uptake of the radioactive form of this element.

Deficiency and toxicity. There have been no cases of known toxicity from natural strontium. In some studies involving villages in Turkey with high consumption of grains, however, the prevalence of rickets has been shown to vary according to soil content of strontium. We do not understand the nature of this connection, but because rickets is a vitamin D deficiency disease closely linked with calcium metabolism, there may end up being some strontium risks in this context. Like toxicity, deficiency of strontium has not been demonstrated, although in rat studies, strontium deficiency may correlate with decreased growth, poor calcification of the bones and teeth, and an increase in dental caries.

Requirements. There is no RDA for strontium. Food intake may supply us with about 2 mg daily.

Tin

Tin, or *stannum* in Latin, is essential in some mammals, including rats, but it has not been shown to be needed in humans. It is more often considered a mildly toxic mineral. One of the reasons its essentiality is questionable in humans is its absence in newborns and in many animals. It is present in the Earth in small amounts. Tin is most often thought of as an environmental contaminant, both as tin cans and as inhaled industrial pollution. Levels in the body, especially in the lungs, increase with age.

Primitive humans had much less tin in their bodies than modern humans. Tin has been used since the Bronze Age began more than 3,500 years ago (bronze contains copper and tin). It has been used for food storage for more than 200 years. Food does absorb tin from cans, so we ingest this tin. Luckily for us, however, it is poorly absorbed from the gastrointestinal tract, probably at levels less than 5%, making it less likely to cause toxicity. Most excess tin is excreted in the feces. Some is eliminated in sweat and even less in urine.

Sources. Tin is present in very low amounts in the soil and in foods. Canning, processing, and packaging often add some tin to food; the solder in iron or copper pipes contains tin; stannous fluoride in toothpaste may add more. Also of concern here, since the early 1990s, has been the replacement of lead capsules around bottled beverages (including wine, beer, some soft drinks, and some herbal drinks) with tin. Because we consider tin primarily a contaminant, though fairly nontoxic, we should try to avoid it. Using few canned

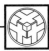

foods and avoiding toothpaste with tin are some ways to do this.

Functions. There are no known functions for tin in humans. If it has a function, it may be related to protein structure or oxidation and reduction reactions, although tin is generally a poor catalyst. Tin may interact with iron, zinc, and copper, particularly in the gut, and thus inhibit absorption of these minerals.

Uses. No uses for tin are presently known.

Deficiency and toxicity. It is clear that environmental exposure to tin dust, as has occurred during the mining of tin in China, can cause lung cancer. However, even though tin is considered a mildly toxic mineral, there are no known chronic or serious diseases from tin ingestion. Exactly how much food-based tin our bodies can process without problem is not clear. Researchers have already identified several specific enzymes that tin can disrupt, including enzymes involved with bone and red blood cell metabolism. Tin has also been shown to disrupt glutathione balance, and as mentioned earlier, to adversely affect copper, zinc, and iron status. With copper in particular, too much tin can decrease absorption. Studies in rats have also shown a slightly shortened life span with higher-level supplementation of tin. With the exception of the tin mining research, I have found no cases of acute tin exposure; chronic low-level environmental and food contamination is more likely.

Avoiding eating too much food from tin cans is probably the best we can do (oily foods seem to pick up more tin than others). In the United States, tin cans are now lacquered, which prevents some food absorption. Lacquered cans have a slight yellow coloring, while the unlacquered cans, which are more common with imported foods, are brighter metal. We can also avoid beverage bottles sealed with foil capsules, or if purchasing them, take extra care in peeling the foil away and wiping the bottle neck with a cloth. There are no known problems from tin deficiency in humans.

Requirements. There is currently no RDA or any known requirement for tin. We should avoid any large or long-term exposure. The average diet may contain about 2 mg per day, but this can vary from about 0.2 to 20 mg per day, depending on the foods ingested. Tin is not likely to be found in many supplements other than occasional trace mineral formulas, and there is no current reason to add tin to any nutritional program.

Vanadium

 Vanadium was classified as an essential trace mineral fairly recently, and it is still a little-known element. The body contains about 20 to 25 mg, distributed in small amounts throughout, some being stored in the fat tissue. Vanadium has been known to be essential in rats and chickens longer than it has in humans. Rats store vanadium primarily in their bones and teeth. We humans seem to follow suit—studies show that long-term accumulation of vanadium takes place primarily in the bones, probably because vanadium binds tightly to phosphate groups, and phosphate is highly concentrated in our bones. After bone, the liver and spleen seem to store most of this mineral. Vanadium is needed by some bacteria and can occasionally substitute for molybdenum. The ascidian worms use vanadium in their blood cells as hemovanadium, which makes green-colored blood cells.

Vanadium is present in soil, although the amount varies geographically, and its distribution is similar to that of selenium. Some studies have shown decreased rates of heart disease in vanadium- and selenium-rich areas, such as many South American countries. Modern humans get vanadium contamination through the air from burning petroleum. With age, the mineral may accumulate somewhat in the lungs, although it seems to be fairly nontoxic.

Vanadium has one of the lowest rates of absorption of all minerals studied so far. It is generally less than 5%, but the percentage may be even lower because vanadium is usually converted to vanadyl and linked to iron-containing proteins before being absorbed. In its vanadyl form, vanadium may be 3 to 5 times *less* likely to be absorbed. Because most of the vanadium in our food is not absorbed, it is eliminated via the feces. In fact, so little is the urine used as a route of elimination that in animal studies, one of the biggest problems with excess exposure to and absorption of vanadium is getting the excess excreted through the urine without causing kidney problems. The same protein that carries iron (transferrin) also carries vanadium around the bloodstream, and the same protein that stores iron (ferritin) also stores vanadium. Not much is stored, however.

Sources. Vanadium content in the vegetable kingdom varies, mostly according to soil differences. Several foods stand out for their vanadium content, however—spinach, black pepper, parsley, mushrooms, and oysters. Vanadium is generally present in low amounts in foods and probably most available in fats and vegetable oils, especially the unsaturated variety. Soy, sunflower, safflower, corn, and olive oils and the foods these oils come from all contain fair amounts of vanadium. Buckwheat, parsley, oats, rice, green beans, carrots, and cabbage also contain vanadium. Dill and radish have fairly high concentrations, while eggs have a moderate amount. Most fish are low, although oysters and herring have good levels.

Functions. Most of the research on vanadium has focused on two important roles. The first is its ability to help regulate blood sugar by mimicking the action of insulin. Unfortunately, the supplemental doses of vanadium required to improve blood sugar balance are much higher than would naturally occur in the body, and so the implications of this insulin-like activity are not clear. In addition, in some studies, vanadium does not appear to have the same helpful effects in nondiabetics as in diabetics. The second fairly well-studied role involves an energy transport system called the *sodium-potassium ATP pump*. Vanadium inhibits this pumping system, which in turn affects the passage of molecules back and forth across our cell membranes. Researchers do not yet understand the full implications of vanadium's involvement in this process, however.

Vanadium is also known to stimulate an important enzyme in the body, adenylate cyclase. This enzyme is central to chemical messaging within cells and helps regulate the flow of chemical information throughout the body. Vanadium's ability to trigger this enzyme has potentially far-reaching implications, but once again, the details are not yet known.

Uses. It is clear that insulin requirements can be reduced in type 1 diabetes with vanadium supplementation because of its insulin-like effects. Because the doses used to treat diabetes have been much higher than would normally occur in the body (about 100 mg of either vanadyl sulfate or sodium metavanadate), there has been debate about this practice.

There was some early evidence that vanadium might be helpful in prevention of heart disease and atherosclerosis, but most of the helpful impact now appears to involve better blood sugar regulation rather than direct impact on cardiovascular function. Finally, in a nonmedicinal context, vanadium has been widely used in sports nutrition to help improve body composition and increase lean body mass. Contrary to popular claims, however, there is not yet any research evidence that vanadium increases lean body mass by enhancing the movement of amino acids into muscle cells.

Deficiency and toxicity. Vanadium has been thought to be essentially nontoxic in humans, possibly because of poor absorption. However, recent studies have revealed elevated levels of vanadium in patients with mania and depression. In addition, some toxicity can occur in rats, primarily because of kidney problems in trying to eliminate the mineral. Based solely on rat-based research involving kidney problems, and without any corroborating evidence in humans, the National Academy of Science still decided to err on the safe side in 2001 and establish tolerable upper limits for vanadium. For adults 19 and older, the limit is 1.8 mg per day. For all other age groups, and for pregnant and lactating women, no limit was established. This guideline is probably not a bad idea until we learn more about food aspects of this mineral.

Vanadium is more commonly an industrial and environmental pollutant, although this has not been shown to be a concern. There is vanadium in the air—more in winter because of the burning of petroleum. Workers who clean vanadium-containing petroleum storage tanks inhale and absorb additional vanadium. The dust can be a bit irritating to the lungs, and the tongue may become somewhat green, neither of which seems to be a serious problem.

Deficiency problems of vanadium have not been clearly shown in humans, although there is a suspicion that low vanadium can increase susceptibility to blood sugar problems, heart disease, and cancer or lead to higher cholesterol and triglyceride levels. In chickens and rats, vanadium deficiency causes some problems with feather and fur growth, bone development, and reproduction.

Requirements. There is currently no RDA for vanadium. In the United States, we average only 6 to 18 mcg of vanadium per day from food. It is fascinating that we also average 9 mcg from dietary supplements—one of the few times that we may be averaging nearly as much intake of a nutrient from supplements as from our diet. Whether we are compensating for vanadium deficiency in the food supply with supplements will be a story worth following in the world of nutrition research.

TOXIC MINERALS AND HEAVY METALS

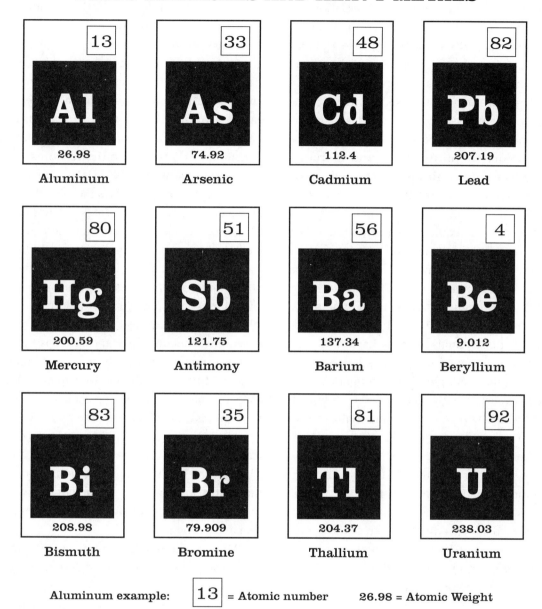

13 **Al** 26.98 Aluminum	33 **As** 74.92 Arsenic	48 **Cd** 112.4 Cadmium	82 **Pb** 207.19 Lead
80 **Hg** 200.59 Mercury	51 **Sb** 121.75 Antimony	56 **Ba** 137.34 Barium	4 **Be** 9.012 Beryllium
83 **Bi** 208.98 Bismuth	35 **Br** 79.909 Bromine	81 **Tl** 204.37 Thallium	92 **U** 238.03 Uranium

Aluminum example: 13 = Atomic number   26.98 = Atomic Weight

This discussion should be of interest to everyone, as we are all being exposed to such heavy metals as lead, mercury, and cadmium. Although not normally found in or used by the human body, these metals are becoming more widely present in the environment, leading to serious concerns. There are possibly more problems from these metals, which interfere with normal bodily function, than have been considered in most mainstream medical circles. Reviewing all of the vitamins (see chapter 5) and minerals has shown us that most every substance that is useful to the body can also be a toxin or poison. **The metals discussed in this section are known primarily—almost exclusively—for their potential toxicity in the body, although commercially they may have great advantages.**

Until the early 1970s, the medical community's concern over metal toxicity was primarily in regard to acute industrial exposure, where certain dramatic measures such as hospitalization and intravenous therapy were performed to stimulate elimination of those metals. More recently, there has been concern over lead intoxication in children from sucking or eating lead-based paint, for example, and legislation has been enacted to reduce this possible contamination, although these measures will probably have a greater effect on future generations. For most of the potentially toxic minerals, there are many common uses and possible contamination sources throughout society; our concern must be with more widespread and long-term observation of and protection from these dangers. **Arsenic, cadmium, lead, and mercury, and, more recently, aluminum are the main toxic minerals.** Beryllium, bismuth, and bromine must be considered as well. And there are other heavy and radioactive metals that could bring future difficulties.

Most of these minerals were present in the environment only in minute amounts until recent centuries, when the orientation toward industrialization and production brought about many technological advances. But technology, like medicine, has its side effects. Mining these metals from the Earth and using them in society—as leaded gasoline or silver-mercury tooth amalgam, for example—have brought all of us into regular exposure with these metals—unless, of course, we live in a completely unindustrialized environment, harder and harder to find in the twenty-first century. These toxic metals have polluted our atmosphere, our waters, our soil, and our food chain.

We cannot realistically put all the lead and cadmium, for example, back into the Earth and cover it up. We need to deal with the presence of these metals. At best, we can find better ways to evaluate them in our water, our air, our food, and our body; learn more about where we are exposed to them; and work preventively to avoid excessive exposure. Most of these heavier metals are quite stable and decompose fairly slowly, if at all, so they remain in the environment. Luckily, the human body is able to clear much of the modest amount we pick up by eliminating it through urine, sweat, and feces. Absorption of these metals is usually pretty low as well. But when our natural means of elimination are reduced or our exposure is increased, we may run into trouble.

The basic way that these heavy metals cause problems is by displacing or replacing related minerals that are required for essential body functions. For example, cadmium can replace zinc, and lead displaces calcium; when this happens, the cadmium or lead is stored in the bones or other tissues and becomes harder to clear, while the important functions of the minerals that are replaced cannot be carried out.

Blood or urine analysis is not very reliable for measuring toxic levels of most of these heavy metals, especially with long-term exposure and tissue buildup. **Hair analysis, although controversial, offers the best easily available evaluation for accumulation of heavy metals, and in many studies, hair levels do correlate fairly well with tissue stores.** The heavier the element, the more reliable is the hair analysis. Measuring these toxic minerals is probably the most useful aspect of hair analysis. A fecal (stool) test for toxic metals may be very useful at assessing the level of this problem. In the future, researchers may find even better ways to measure, treat, and prevent this dangerous heavy mineral contamination. Currently, doctors and laboratories familiar with this field can offer a more advanced, "challenge" test, whereby we have the patient consume a chelating substance such as DMSA (dimercaptosuccinic acid, actually meso-2,3-dimercaptosuccinic acid), which is fairly well tolerated, and then collect urine for 6 hours. The chelator can pull metals from the tissues, which are then excreted through the kidneys into the urine, and the metals (for example, lead, mercury, and arsenic) are measured by the lab. This test can be repeated again months later to look at the treatment progress. Some practitioners also use the oral and intravenous chelator DMPS (2,3-dimercapto-1-propane sulfonate).

Most of the available information concerns the main heavy metals—arsenic, cadmium, lead, and mercury, as well as aluminum, which is not "heavy" but still has some toxicity concerns. For each of these, a general introduction to the history of the metal and how the body handles it is provided.

- Sources of contamination

- Methods of toxicity

- Symptoms of toxicity

- Amounts leading to toxicity

- Who is susceptible?

- Treatment of toxicity

- Prevention of toxicity (exposure)

There are no known nutritional deficiencies or bodily uses of these metals, with the possible exception of arsenic, which may be both essential and toxic, so it isn't necessary to discuss requirements. The remaining heavy metals—antimony, beryllium, bismuth, bromine, thallium, and a few even more minor ones—less commonly produce toxicity problems, and here they are described only generally.

Aluminum

Aluminum has only recently been considered a problem mineral. Although it is not very toxic at normal levels, neither has it been found to be essential. **Aluminum is abundant in the Earth and in the sea. It is present in only small amounts in animal and plant tissues.** However, it is commonly ingested in foods and in medicines, such as antacids, and is used in cosmetics. Many scientists feel that because of its prevalence in the Earth and its common uses, aluminum is not actually very toxic.

Aluminum is not really a heavy metal—that is, it is not a sufficiently dense element to qualify as "heavy." **To qualify as a heavy metal, an element has to be at least five times as dense as water.** For this reason, aluminum behaves differently from metals such as lead or mercury. Recent investigations, however, implicate aluminum toxicity in Alzheimer's disease and other brain and senility syndromes. The evidence regarding aluminum's toxicity or essentiality is not conclusive as yet.

The amount of aluminum in the human body ranges between 50 and 150 mg, with an average of about 65 mg. Most of this mineral is found in the lungs, brain, kidneys, liver, and thyroid. Our daily intake of aluminum may range from 10 to 110 mg, but the body eliminates most of this in the feces and urine and some in the sweat. With decreased kidney function, more aluminum will be stored, particularly in the bones.

Sources of contamination. For most people, the greatest aluminum intake comes from food additives. Sodium aluminum phosphate is an emulsifier in processed cheese, potassium alum is used to whiten flour, and sodium silicoaluminate and/or aluminum calcium silicate are added to common table salt to help it run freely and not cake. In the average diet, 40 to 50 mg a day may come from foods.

With use of aluminum pots and pans and aluminum foil, some aluminum leaches into food, especially with such acid foods as tomatoes or rhubarb. Soft drinks are typically acidic, and when packaged in aluminum cans, can leach up to 250 ppb of aluminum. In Spain, studies on 37 fast foods and convenience foods have shown aluminum to be present in the 1 to 38 ppm range. **Cooking with fluoridated water in aluminum cookware increases the aluminum in the water and the food.** Still, the amounts we obtain in this manner are small in comparison with those from additives. Aluminum salts used in antiperspirants are the primary contaminant for some people, especially when these products are used daily. (Aerosol deodorant sprays, especially, should be avoided for environmental toxicity reasons.) Antacids containing aluminum hydroxide can be a big source if they are taken regularly or abused, as antacids sometimes are. Some children's aspirins have been found to contain aluminum as well. Also under fire most recently has been the use of aluminum in infant vaccinations, currently legal in the range of 125 to 850 mcg per dose.

Methods of toxicity. Aluminum is probably the least toxic of the minerals discussed in this section, although the concern is that it has become so pervasive and is now found in higher levels in human tissues. It is not clear how aluminum functions or interferes with activities in the human body, but this may occur through some magnesium functions. It may reduce vitamin levels or bind to DNA, and it has been correlated with weakened tissue of the gastrointestinal tract. In Alzheimer's disease, there are increased aluminum levels in the brain tissue and an increase in what are called *neurofibrillary tangles,* which tend to reduce nerve synapses and conduction.

Oral aluminum, as obtained from antacids, can bind pepsin and weaken protein digestion. It also has astringent qualities and thus can dry the tissues and mucous linings and contribute to constipation. Regular use of aluminum-containing deodorants may contribute to the clogging of underarm lymphatics and then to such breast problems as cystic disease. Ann Louise Gittleman, a prominent nutritionist, calls aluminum a "detrimental protoplasmic poison."

Symptoms of toxicity. Acute aluminum poisoning has been associated with constipation, colicky pain, anorexia, nausea and gastrointestinal irritation, skin problems, and lack of energy. Slower and longer-term increases in body aluminum may create muscle twitching, numbness, paralysis, and fatty degeneration of the liver and kidney. Aluminum toxicity is worse with reduced renal function. Aluminum may reduce the absorption of selenium and phosphorus from the gastrointestinal tract. The loss of bone matrix from aluminum toxicity can lead to osteomalacia, a softening of the bone. Skin rashes have occurred with local irritation from aluminum antiperspirants.

As hinted above, aluminum toxicity has been implicated in such brain-aging disorders as Alzheimer's disease and parkinsonism, both of which have become more prevalent as the incidence of aluminum toxicity has increased. Areas with high amounts of aluminum in the drinking water are showing an increase in the incidence of Alzheimer's disease (alum and aluminum sulfate are used to treat water in many cities). Nearly 100,000 people of the 1.5 to 2 million people with Alzheimer's are dying each year. Although increased aluminum has been measured in the brain and other body tissues in patients with Alzheimer's disease, other factors may be contributing as well. There seems to be a weakening of the blood-brain barrier in Alzheimer's disease, and this may allow a variety of brain toxins to reach the central nervous system. What is causing this breakdown of the barrier between the brain and the rest of the body is not yet clear. It is also important to examine aluminum toxicity in children with hyperactivity and learning disorders, as it has been implicated in these problems.

Amounts leading to toxicity. It is not known exactly what levels of aluminum or what other factors cause it to become a problem. With blood and hair analysis, normal ranges of aluminum may vary from lab to lab. **Hair analysis is probably one of the better ways to measure body aluminum.** The mineral analysis laboratory that I use, Doctor's Data in Chicago (see appendix A, "Laboratories and Clinical Nutrition Tests"), suggests that a reading under 15 to 20 ppm in hair is considered normal, but less than that, say under 10 to 15 ppm, is probably ideal.

Who is susceptible? Everyone has contact with aluminum; it is present in most diets. However, researchers do not yet know why and how aluminum becomes a problem, if it truly does. It appears that the elderly may have more of a problem with aluminum, if indeed it is a cause, or part of the cause, of Alzheimer's disease and other brain syndromes. **Those who eat refined foods, refined flours, baked goods, processed cheeses, and common table salt are more likely to have higher aluminum levels in their bodies.** Those who use antacids or antiperspirants that contain aluminum, or who cook with aluminum kitchenware or foil, also have more contact with this potentially toxic mineral.

Treatment of toxicity. Decreasing contact with and use of aluminum-containing substances reduces intake and allows more aluminum to leave the body. Oral chelating agents, such as DMSA and DMPS, also help to clear aluminum more rapidly. The antibiotic tetracycline is actually a mild chelator for aluminum. Calcium disodium edetate (EDTA) binds and clears aluminum from the body; this substance is fairly nontoxic and is used as the agent for chelation therapy, an intravenous treatment used to pull such metals as lead from the body and more recently used in the treatment of atherosclerosis and cardiovascular diseases. Deferoxamine, an iron chelator, also binds aluminum. In a study with Alzheimer's patients, nearly 40% showed an improvement in symptoms with deferoxamine treatment. There is some evidence that intravenous chelation with EDTA helps Alzheimer's patients. More research is needed to evaluate aluminum's involvement with this disease.

An interesting relationship is also emerging in the research literature between aluminum and silica. Silica is the common name for silicon dioxide (SiO_2), commonly found in quartz and sand. Soluble silica is also part of our diet and may play an important role in binding potential toxins like aluminum and preventing their absorption. Interestingly, however, when aluminum and Alzheimer's disease were first studied, a method used to *increase* Alzheimer's-like brain problems in rats involved administration of a substance that combined aluminum with silica. This substance, called aluminosilicate or kaolin, caused overaccumulation of certain proteins, called *beta-amyloid proteins,* in the brains of the rats. The jury is still out on the role of silica and silicon in preventing aluminum toxicity.

To evaluate toxic states of aluminum, the best testing available is hair analysis, ideally used along with blood and urine analysis. The values can be followed during treatment by a knowledgeable doctor to see whether higher amounts are being eliminated and lesser amounts retained in body tissues.

Prevention of toxicity (exposure). The best way to prevent aluminum buildup is to avoid the sources of aluminum. Eliminating foods that have aluminum additives is probably healthier overall. Not using common table salt is a positive health step as well. Some tap waters contain aluminum; this can be checked. Avoiding aluminum cookware and replacing it with stainless steel, ceramic, or glass is a good idea. Blocking skin and sweat pores with aluminum antiperspirants has always seemed strange to me; I would think it would be better to cleanse regularly, reduce stress, balance weight, and eat a wholesome diet that creates sweat that smells more like roses.

Arsenic

 Arsenic is the perfect example of a heavy metal with equally strong potential as both a toxin and a required nutrient. This heavy metal has been ranked as the number-one toxic threat to our health, but at the same time, it is a mineral with the greatest chance to be named essential for all vertebrates, including humans. Evidence for arsenic as an essential nutrient is beginning to accumulate in the area of amino acid metabolism, where arsenic appears essential for proper metabolism of both methionine and arginine. The methionine research is particularly interesting, because an enzyme whose activity is closely linked to atherosclerosis seems impaired when arsenic is deficient.

In nature, arsenic is most commonly found in an organic form, combined together with carbon compounds. These organic forms of arsenic, which include trimethylarsine, arsenocholine, and arsenobetaine, are the least toxic forms of arsenic. Inorganic forms of arsenic appear to be the most toxic forms. These include arsenate and arsenite. Of these two forms, the more toxic appears to be arsenite. However, because arsenates found in food can be converted by our bod-

ies into arsenites, and because both arsenates and arsenites are both fairly well absorbed from the digestive tract, we need to limit our intake of both forms as much as possible; for example, by selecting organically grown foods that have not been treated with arsenic-containing pesticides.

Arsenic can accumulate in the body, particularly in the skin, hair, and nails, but also in internal organs. On the average, there is about 10 to 20 mg of arsenic in the human body; higher levels may lead to problems. Arsenic can also accumulate when kidney function is decreased. Hair and blood levels are the best way to evaluate arsenic levels. They usually show increased levels when higher amounts are present in the body.

Sources of contamination. Arsenic is present in small amounts in soil and therefore is present in our food. It is present in the ocean, so there is some arsenic in most seafood, especially the filtering mollusks, such as clams, mussels, and oysters. Some arsenic is present as a contaminant in meats as well. Arsenic is also found in many fuel oils and coal, so it is added to the environment when these are burned. Weed killers and some insecticides (particularly the lead-arsenate sprays) are the main sources of contamination with arsenic. This use of arsenic is responsible for a twenty-fold increase in the level found in humans since ancient times. Treated wood products, including many found at parks and playgrounds across the country, have been injected with arsenic-containing pesticides to help prevent rot. Although legislation is under way to ban use of arsenic-containing chemicals in these products, they are still actively manufactured at this point in time.

Every year, the U.S. Agency for Toxic Substances and Disease Registry (ATSDR) puts out its CERCLA Priority List of Hazardous Substances. (CERCLA stands for the Comprehensive Environmental Response, Compensation, and Liability Act passed by Congress in 1980). **In 2001, as in many previous years, arsenic ranked as the number-one toxin of concern in the United States based on its potential to cause harm to human health.** Yet, I personally believe that mercury is the greatest modern concern because of widespread contamination of our waters. Arsenic received 1,653 points in the CERCLA rating system and was followed closely by two other heavy metals—

namely lead, which received 1,528 points, and mercury, which earned 1,503.

Methods of toxicity. We have known for a good number of years that very high doses of arsenic, as might occur occupationally near a copper smelter, can be acutely toxic. The levels here involve inhalation of several hundred milligrams, and both the nervous system and the cardiovascular system are strongly affected. Fortunately, our food never contains arsenic in this amount. Food levels of arsenic are also known to be potentially toxic. However, the mechanisms for this toxicity have only been studied in animals. Arsenic may compete with selenium and iodine and impair the metabolism of both minerals. It may also increase the formation of free radicals and damage genetic structures through this mechanism. Damage to genetic structures can result in unwanted gene mutations and can increase the risk of cancer, and researchers attribute the carcinogenicity of high-dose arsenic to this oxygen-based gene damage. None of these connections are clearly established at this point in time.

Symptoms of toxicity. Arsenic in drinking water at levels of 11 mg per liter or higher have been associated with nervous system problems, including numbness or tingling in the hands and fingers or feet and toes. Other possible effects of arsenic toxicity include hair loss, dermatitis, diarrhea and other gastrointestinal symptoms, fatigue, headaches, confusion, muscle pains, red and white blood cell problems, and liver and kidney damage. Acute arsenic exposure may cause a rapid series of symptoms. Arsine gas exposure is very toxic to the lungs and kidneys and is often fatal. Death from low-level, chronic arsenic exposure has the appearance of death from natural causes—a often used twist in murder-mystery books.

Amounts leading to toxicity. The amount of arsenic naturally present in food does not appear to pose any risk with respect to toxicity. However, "naturally present" would only apply here to an organically grown food, because once nonorganic food is considered, there is a good chance that arsenic-containing pesticides have entered into the picture. The same could be said for unfiltered water, because of contamination with environmentally released arsenic. Arsenic trioxide, for example, is used industrially and may be one of the most poisonous forms of arsenic. Arsenical pesticides are commonly used on both food and textile crops. In fact, one of the most dangerous occupations in the country with respect to arsenic toxicity is work in or near a cotton gin, because of the heavy arseno-pesticide residues on the cotton. When trying to determine whether your own arsenic exposure is safe, a hair analysis can be helpful. Below 7 to 10 ppm of arsenic in hair is a relatively safe level.

Who is susceptible? Exposure to insecticides, weed killers, contaminated meats, and fumes from the burning of arsenic-containing coals and oils may cause some toxicity problems. Miners, smelters, and vineyard workers may have a higher level of arsenic trioxide exposure and a higher incidence of lung cancer. The body does not clear trivalent arsenic as easily as it does some other toxic minerals, so buildup can occur with regular exposure, generating chronic problems. At risk are farm workers, people working around preserved wood products, people working around tobacco or constantly exposed to smoke-filled air, and, as mentioned earlier, people working in or near cotton gins.

Treatment. Chelation therapy with EDTA can clear some arsenic, but not as easily as it clears some of the other heavy metals. Dimercaprol is the treatment of choice for arsenic toxicity, but it should be given in the first 24 hours after exposure. Vitamin C protects the body somewhat from arsenic toxicity.

Prevention of toxicity (exposure). Again, avoiding sources of contamination from arsenic is all we can do.

Cadmium

 Cadmium has become a more prevalent cause for concern in recent years. It is an underground mineral that did not enter our air, food, and water in significant amounts until it was mined as part of zinc deposits. **Now there is widespread environmental contamination with cadmium.** The health risks associated with this increased exposure to cadmium have placed it thirteenth on the government's CERCLA Priority List of Hazardous Substances.

As cadmium and zinc are found together in natural deposits, so are they similar in structure and function in the human body. Cadmium may actually displace zinc in some of its important enzymatic and organ functions, especially within the cardiovascular system; thus it prevents these functions from being completed. The zinc-to-cadmium ratio is important, as cadmium toxicity and storage are greatly increased with zinc deficiency, and good levels of zinc protect against tissue damage by cadmium. The refinement of grains reduces the zinc-to-cadmium ratio, so zinc deficiency and cadmium toxicity are more likely when the diet is high in refined grains and flours. The closeness of zinc and cadmium is also reflected in cadmium production, where companies frequently "produce" cadmium from the smelting and refining of zinc concentrates. It is also reflected in the word *cadmium* itself. Originally, cadmium got its name from zinc, because in Greek, the word *kadmeia* was a name for calamine, or in chemistry terms, zinc carbonate.

Cadmium has a special relationship with manganese, because the system that transports manganese around the body also transports cadmium. There is some evidence that only manganese and cadmium share this particular transport system.

Cadmium levels in humans tend to increase with age, most likely due to chronic exposure. Like mercury and lead, two other toxic heavy metals, **cadmium can cross the placental barrier and reach the fetus (more often in mothers who smoke), as well as partially cross the blood-brain barrier and reach the brain. However, lead and mercury appear to pose more widespread and greater risks to newborns and adults than cadmium.**

We may have as much as 40 mg of cadmium in our body and probably consume at least 20 mcg daily. Levels vary according to region, as we get most of it from soil by way of food that is grown in it and water that is percolated down through it. In urban and industrial areas, the concentration of cadmium in water can reach up to 36 mcg per liter, and in food, up to about 15 mcg per ounce. Cadmium levels in the atmosphere are much higher in industrial cities.

Cadmium is not very well absorbed, with a rate of about 20%, but this is still a higher rate than that of many other minerals. Cadmium is not particularly well eliminated. Besides fecal losses, it is excreted mainly by the kidneys. This mineral is stored primarily in the liver and kidneys. As zinc has an affinity for the testes, cadmium is also stored there in higher concentrations than in other tissues. With zinc deficiency, more cadmium is stored. With aging, cadmium accumulates in the kidneys and may predispose to hypertension. As I stated, it does not get into the brain, nor does it pass into the fetus during pregnancy or the breast milk during lactation.

Sources of contamination. There are many sources from which our environment and our bodies can be contaminated with cadmium. Cigarette smoke, refined foods, water pipes, coffee and tea, burning coal, and shellfish are all definite sources. Cadmium is also a common component of alloys, used in electrical materials and the process of electroplating. In addition, it is present in ceramics, dental materials, and storage batteries, especially nickel-cadmium rechargeable batteries. Cadmium red (Red No. 108) is a widely used pigment in paints and in print media and can show up as the red in a color newspaper picture. Cadmium yellow (Yellow No. 37) is another cadmium-containing paint pigment.

During the growth of such grains as wheat and rice, cadmium (from the soil) is concentrated in the core of the kernel, while zinc is found mostly in the germ and bran coverings. With refinement, zinc is lost, increasing the cadmium ratio. **Refined flours, rice, and sugar all have relatively higher ratios of cadmium to zinc than do the whole foods.**

One pack of cigarettes contains about 20 mcg of cadmium, or about 1 mcg per cigarette. About 30% of that goes into the lungs and is absorbed, and the remaining 70% goes into the atmosphere to be inhaled by others or to contaminate the environment. With long-term smoking, the risk of cadmium toxicity is increased. Although most of it is eliminated, a little bit is stored every day. Marijuana may also concentrate cadmium, so regular smoking of cannabis may also be a risk factor for toxicity from this metal. Air pollution of cadmium comes from zinc mining and refining and from the burning of coal. Cadmium is also an industrial contaminant from the steel-making process.

Water pipes can be a source of cadmium concentration. Cadmium is often used to protect metals from corrosion. Galvanized (zinc) pipes usually contain some cadmium, as does the solder used to hold them together. Soft or acid water is corrosive and causes the metals in the pipes to break down, releasing cadmium and other minerals from them. Hard water containing calcium and magnesium salts actually coats the pipes and protects against the leaching of other minerals. So common is the presence of cadmium in drinking water that the U.S. Environmental Protection Agency established a level of 5 mcg per liter as the maximum contaminant level for this heavy metal in its National Primary Drinking Water Standards in 1994.

Soil levels of cadmium are increased by cadmium in water, by sewage contamination, by cadmium in the air, and by high-phosphate fertilizers. Coffee and tea may contain significant cadmium levels. Such root vegetables as potatoes may pick up more cadmium, and grains can concentrate cadmium. Seafood, particularly crustaceans (such as crab and lobster), and mollusks (such as clams and oysters) have higher cadmium levels, although many are also higher in zinc, balancing the cadmium.

Methods of toxicity. Although cadmium has no known useful biological functions, it competes with zinc for binding sites and can therefore interfere with some of zinc's essential functions. In this way, it may inhibit enzyme reactions and utilization of nutrients. It is worth pointing out here that water-soluble forms of cadmium, like cadmium chloride, are better absorbed and therefore more toxic than insoluble forms like cadmium sulfide. Cadmium may be a catalyst to oxidation reactions, which can generate free-radical tissue damage. This heavy metal is known to block activity of several energy-processing enzymes (including those found in a key energy-producing cycle called the *Krebs cycle*) and to disrupt the metabolism of both calcium and vitamin D. One of the far-reaching potential impacts of cadmium involves the B vitamin choline and the nervous system messenger acetylcholine. Acetylcholine is made in part from choline, and when it is broken down, choline is released. Even though cadmium does stop acetylcholine from being made, it stops it from being released within the nervous system, upsetting nerve-muscle activities. But there is a double whammy here, because cadmium also activates the enzyme cholinesterase, which breaks acetylcholine apart. The net result: Far too little acetylcholine and increased risk of neuromuscular problems.

Researchers have recently learned that cadmium can prevent cells from beginning their natural dying process. All cells have a natural dying process that is planned and regulated, and that gets initiated when things get too far out of control. Cadmium interferes with this process, called *apoptosis*, or programmed cell death.

Symptoms of toxicity. In his book *Trace Elements and Man*, Henry Schroeder, MD, the late expert in trace and toxic elements, described in detail cadmium's involvement in generating, or at least contributing to, high blood pressure. **Cadmium concentrates in the kidneys and can generate kidney tissue damage and hypertension, as well as an increased incidence of calcium kidney stones.** Initially, protein and sugar may be spilled in the urine. Some patients with high blood pressure show elevated urine cadmium levels. This hypertension is likely related to the reduced zinc-to-cadmium ratio. The cadmium effect may contribute not only to hypertension but to heart disease as well. In rat studies, higher levels of cadmium are associated with an increase in heart size, higher blood pressure, progressive atherosclerosis, and reduced kidney function. And in rats as well as in humans, cadmium toxicity is worse with zinc deficiency and reduced with higher zinc intake.

Cadmium appears to depress some immune functions, mainly by reducing host resistance to bacteria and viruses. It may also increase cancer risk, possibly for the lungs and prostate. Cadmium toxicity has been implicated in generating prostate enlargement, possibly by interfering with zinc support.

Cadmium also affects the bones. It has been known to cause bone and joint aches and pains. This syndrome, first described in Japan, where it was termed the *itai-itai* ("ouch-ouch") disease, was caused by cadmium pollution there. It was also associated with weak bones leading to deformities, especially of the spine, or to more easily broken bones. This disease was fatal in many cases.

Researchers may be seeing an increase in emphysema due to cadmium exposure. Anemia also seems to be a problem. Most of these potential cadmium toxicity problems, including its immunosuppressant actions and its precise role in cancer, hypertension, and heart and kidney disease, need to be substantiated by more research.

Amounts leading to toxicity. What level of cadmium causes toxicity is not clear; zinc levels in the body play a role in determining this. Estimates of daily cadmium exposure range from 25 to more than 200 mcg, mostly from food. About 40 to 50 mcg daily is probably a safe guess, and in published research on a worldwide basis, the range is 30 to 50 mcg. This should be handled fairly well by a normally functioning body. Below 2 ppm in hair and 0.015 ppm in whole blood are considered current normal ranges for body cadmium levels.

Who is susceptible? People who have higher exposure to cadmium are at higher risk. Industrial workers, metal workers, zinc miners, and anyone who works with zinc galvanization may accumulate more cadmium. Those who drink soft water; those who smoke or whose friends, roommates, or coworkers smoke; coffee and tea drinkers; and those who eat refined flours, sugars, and white rice are also likely to receive greater exposure to cadmium. But all of us may face a certain amount of risk; a 1992 study in the Netherlands estimated an average lifetime total intake of 435 mg for cadmium.

Treatment of toxicity. Intravenous EDTA chelation is effective in increasing cadmium elimination, although this is probably indicated only at more toxic levels. Avoiding further cadmium exposure is emphasized. **High intake of zinc as well as of calcium and selenium protects against further cadmium absorption, and adequate body levels of zinc may displace some tissue cadmium.** Iron, copper, selenium, and vitamin C have been shown to increase cadmium elimination as well, as can be measured by urine levels. Hair analysis is a good way to follow cadmium levels.

Prevention of toxicity (exposure). With good health, cadmium is probably not a problem unless there is increased exposure, zinc deficiency, or weakened kidney function. Cadmium toxicity also seems to be a little worse with lead intoxication. There are two good ways to protect against cadmium toxicity. The first is to avoid cadmium exposure and intake—primarily by minimizing smoking and exposure to cigarette smoke and avoiding refined foods, shellfish, coffee, tea, and soft water. Air contamination is usually minimal compared to that from food and water. The second way to protect against cadmium toxicity is to maintain good zinc levels by eating high-zinc foods, such as whole grains, legumes, and nuts (oysters are high in zinc but also high in cadmium). Tak-

ing additional zinc, 15 to 30 mg daily in a supplement, offers further protection against cadmium problems.

Lead

 "Get the lead out!" is a common idiom referring to a heaviness of a body that cannot quite get moving. **The heavy metal lead is the most common toxic mineral and the most abundant contaminant of our environment and our body.** (Yet, mercury problems have increased in the past decade, while lead environmental concerns have decreased.) It is among the worst and most widespread pollutants—and also among the most toxic. On the government's 2001 CERCLA Priority List of Hazardous Substances, lead ranks second, just behind arsenic and just ahead of mercury. When lead levels become too high, they can prove fatal.

Lead is found deep within the Earth. Ancient civilizations had almost no exposure to it until 4,000 or 5,000 years ago, when lead was found as a by-product of silver smelting. Since then, it has been used increasingly throughout history. In the Roman Empire, lead was widely used in water pipes and drinking and storage vessels. Many scientists and historians now feel that lead led to the downfall of the Roman Empire, with the ruling classes suffering decreased mental capacities, decreased birthrate, and shortened life span.

In the twentieth century, lead was widely used in paint, some containing a high percentage of lead. **This has been a problem especially with children, who are more sensitive to lead than adults because of their better absorption and smaller bodies.** Lead has a mildly sweet taste, and children often suck on or eat the paint chips off of houses or out of the dirt, leading to many cases of lead poisoning. In the 1920s, tetraethyl lead was added to gasoline as an antiknock, higher-octane additive. This has probably been the most widespread and pervasive source of environmental contamination from lead to date. Other common uses for lead are as seals for tin cans, in pewter, in ceramics and pottery glazes, in insecticides, and more.

In recent years, however, there has been an attempt to decrease this environmental contamination. Cars are now using unleaded gasoline. This does not, of course, eliminate the problems of carbon monoxide and burned hydrocarbons, but it will help to decrease lead exposure in the future. In 1971, Congress passed the Lead Paint Act, limiting the use of lead in paints. This will also help, but not for many years to come, because many older homes still contain leaded paints. About 85% of all homes in the United States built before 1978 contain lead-based paint. As they deteriorate, lead gets into the soil and does not degrade. In 1979, a law was passed decreasing the use of lead in food storage cans, although it is still present in some solders.

Bone analysis of very old skeletons indicates that modern humans have nearly 500 to 1,000 times more lead in our bones than did our ancient ancestors. Our total body content of lead nowadays is estimated at 125 to 200 mg. We can handle nearly 1 to 2 mg daily with normal functioning, but the margin of safety is narrow. Luckily, most people's daily exposure is less than that, about 300 to 400 mcg. Although most of this exposure is nondietary, a national study has shown our weekly intake of lead from food to average up to 63 ppb. This amount would translate into about 3 to 4 mcg per week of lead.

Lead is a neurotoxin and commonly generates abnormal brain and nerve function. It passes into the brain and can also contaminate the in utero fetus and breast milk. Most lead, though, is stored in the bones. With lead intoxication, "lead lines" are visible in the bones on X-rays. Some is also stored in the liver and soft tissues. Infants are born with very little lead in their systems, but body concentrations usually increase with age. Luckily, lead is not very well absorbed, usually between 10% and 15%, although children absorb it at a much higher rate, sometimes ranging up to 50%. Many minerals, such as calcium and iron, interfere with further lead absorption. When lead gets into the blood, it does not stay long, either going into the bones and other tissues or being eliminated. Most ingested lead leaves with the feces; that which is absorbed or inhaled will usually be cleared by the kidneys or through perspiration.

Evaluating lead exposure and measuring lead levels in humans is not easy. Blood and urine tests are not very good indicators, because lead is cleared fairly rapidly. With acute toxicity, both of these body fluids may have high measurements, but most exposure is chronic. **Hair analysis is the simplest and best test for evaluating chronic lead poisoning, which has become much more common with long-term exposure.**

Hair-test screening for lead is fairly reliable and can be done on both adults and children. Hair (and urine) levels can be remeasured to follow the progress of treatment. Increased body burdens of lead can be shown by testing with an intravenous dose of a chelating drug such as EDTA. A high level of urinary lead elimination suggests increased levels of body stores, especially in the bones. Also, because lead interferes with many red blood cell enzymes, such as delta-aminolevulinic acid dehydratase, an increase in this enzyme in the urine, as well as zinc protoporphyrin and erythrocyte protoporphyrin, suggests problems of lead toxicity. Another factor favoring examination of these red blood cells enzymes is the fact that 95% of the lead in our bloodstream gets attached to our red blood cells. (This red cell accumulation is also the reason that it is better to measure lead in whole blood instead of just the serum.) A blood level of zinc protoporphyrin (ZPP) is currently the best way to assess lead toxicity.

Sources of contamination. Lead exposure and body lead levels are higher in North America than anywhere else in the world. In the United States alone, it is estimated that approximately 1.3 million tons of lead are used yearly in batteries, solder, pottery, pigments, gasoline, paint, ammunitions, and many other useful substances. Somewhere between 400,000 and 600,000 tons per year go into our atmosphere, onto our Earth, into our food, and into our bodies and tissues. So there is a lot of lead around. The following are some of the common contaminants:

Leaded gasoline. Tetraethyl lead used to be added to all gasoline; it is now used only for older vehicles. After combustion, this lead goes directly into the atmosphere as air pollution and is inhaled by us and other living, breathing entities. It settles into the Earth and its living vegetation; heavily traveled roadways show higher concentrations of lead in the air, soil, and nearby vegetation.

Paint. Although, by law, the amount of lead in paints must be reduced, some still contain lead. Many homes retain lead paints, so this change may not affect us in environmental lead exposure for a couple of decades. Paints found in art supply stores may also contain lead. The most common lead-containing pigments are Chrome Yellow (also called Chrome Lemon and Yellow No. 34), Naples Yellow (Yellow No. 41), and Flake White (also called Cremintz White or White No. 1).

Food. Lead is contained in many foods, especially in those grown near industrial areas or busy cities or roadways. Grains, legumes, commercial and garden fruit, and most meat products pick up some lead. Liver and lunch meats are usually higher. Liverwurst and other sausages may contain more lead than other foods. Roadside vegetation, such as herbs, fruits, and vegetables, has higher concentrations of lead than vegetation growing in more secluded areas. Measurements of lead in trees growing along roads show much more than was present in the 1930s. Bonemeal, a source of calcium and magnesium, is usually made from cattle bones and may contain high amounts of lead. Dolomite, a rock source of calcium and magnesium, is usually lower in lead. Pet foods may also be high. In several industrialized European countries, the lead content of foods like grains and legumes has fallen into a general range of about 2 to 50 ppb. Fruit juices manufactured outside of the United States in leaded cans would merit special concern for lead contamination, because former manufacture of these products in the United States is known to have produced lead levels in the juice of up to 250 ppb.

Water. Drinking water may be contaminated with lead. Lead solder in pipes or lead plumbing in older homes and drinking fountains can leach into the water, especially soft water. A more acid water will pull lead and other toxic and nontoxic minerals from the piping.

Pottery. "Earthenware" in general has potential for lead exposure. Although some potters refrain from using much lead, it is hard to avoid. When the glazing is inefficient, lead containers can contaminate food stored in them. Fruit juices or acidic foods, such as tomatoes, tend to pull out more minerals. Glazed coffee mugs should be avoided. Beginning in 1971, the FDA began to set informal guidelines for levels of lead leaching from ceramic ware products. Current recommended limits are from 7 to 3 ppm for plates, saucers, and other flatware; from 5 to 2 ppm for small holloware, such as cereal bowls, but not cups and mugs; from 5.0 to 0.5 ppm for cups and mugs; from 2.5 to 1.0 ppm for large (greater than 1.1 liters) holloware, such as bowls, but not pitchers; and from 2.5 to 0.5 ppm for pitchers.

Foil capsules. The necks of beer and wine bottles, as well as some liquid herbal products, may be capped with lead-containing foil capsules. With respect to wine, the FDA banned lead capsules in 1996 after a study by the Bureau of Alcohol, Tobacco, and Firearms found that 3% to 4% of wines examined could become contaminated during pouring from lead residues deposited on the mouth of the bottle by the foil capsule. While many U.S. winemakers voluntarily stopped using lead foils about 3 to 4 years before the ban, older bottles with the foils may still be around. Lead capsules on wine have largely been replaced by plastic or aluminum and, in some rarer cases, tin.

Glassware. Leaded crystal glassware can leach lead. In this area, the crystalware industry has itself established some voluntary limits on lead use, and in 1998 the FDA began to develop guidelines for use of lead (and cadmium) in coloration of the lip rim area of glassware.

Cans. Solder in tin cans, usually used to hold the seam together, contains lead; some are nearly 100% lead. Some can manufacturers are changing this, but progress is slow. Avoid lead-lined containers or cans whose seams have a shiny, metallic solder appearance. Many imported cans contain lead. The leaded plugs in evaporated milk cans may contaminate the milk. The FDA has estimated that up to 10% of imported food may be packaged in lead-soldered cans. This percent would translate into about 230 million pounds.

Cosmetics. Many pigments and other substances used for makeup and other cosmetics contain lead. Historically, lead has been part of face paints and other beauty creams.

Cigarettes. Lead is a common contaminant in cigarettes. Lead arsenate may be used as an insecticide in tobacco growing. When lead is found in tobacco and cigarette smoke, it is often present in the 10 to 40 ppb range.

Pesticides. Many pesticides and insecticides contain some lead, mainly as the lead-arsenate base.

Methods of toxicity. Although this is not completely clear, lead most likely interferes with functions performed by such essential minerals as calcium, copper, iron, and zinc. Lead interrupts several red blood cell enzyme systems, including delta-aminolevulinic acid dehydratase and ferrochelatase. Especially in brain chemistry, lead may create abnormal function by inactivating important zinc-, copper-, and iron-dependent enzymes. (When body levels of these 3 minerals are high, there is first less absorption of lead and then more competition with lead for enzyme-binding sites.) Lead affects both the brain and the peripheral nerves. **Lead can interfere with the formation of heme—the iron-binding protein in the middle of the red blood cell—and in this way can cause anemia.**

In the lungs, bloodstream, and retina, lead has been shown to trigger the programmed cell death process called *apoptosis*. Essentially, the cell decides to shut down its function, disassemble itself, and recycle its parts in the face of what appears to be a too-toxic future. If too many cells shut down, of course, the organ system itself becomes weakened and cannot help sustain our health.

Lead can displace calcium in bone, deposit there, and form softer, denser spots that can be seen on X-rays as "lead lines." Because vitamin D is essential in calcium metabolism, the negative impact of lead on calcium is further worsened by the tendency of lead to block vitamin D synthesis. Lead also binds with the sulfhydryl bonds and inactivates the cysteine-containing enzymes, thus allowing more internal toxicity from free radicals, chemicals, and other heavy metals. In addition to cysteine-containing enzymes, lead also depletes our supply of glutathione, a cysteine-containing tripeptide. (Few molecules in the body are as important in detoxification and oxygen metabolism as glutathione, which is discussed in more detail in chapter 3, Proteins.)

Lead is also an immunosuppressant; it lowers host resistance to bacteria and viruses and thus allows an increase in infections. It may also influence our cancer risk. How lead affects the gastrointestinal tract, causing symptoms including a coliclike pain, is still uncertain.

Symptoms of toxicity. An estimated nearly 20% of men and 10% of women have problems with lead toxicity, although it is not clear what levels of chronic lead toxicity, which is most common, will produce symptoms. Lead in the body subtly interferes with optimum function and general health, and other toxicity factors may affect this. Lead accumulation may also cause shifts in important body minerals, such as calcium, manganese, and zinc.

Early signs of lead toxicity may be overlooked, as they are fairly vague: headache, fatigue, muscle pains, anorexia, constipation, vomiting, pallor, and anemia. These can be followed by agitation, irritability, rest-lessness, memory loss, poor coordination and vertigo, and depression. Acute lead toxicity symptoms include abdominal pain similar to colic, nausea and vomiting, anemia, muscle weakness, and encephalopathy. Lead encephalopathy is a brain syndrome that can arise also from advanced chronic toxicity. It is characterized by poor balance, confusion, vertigo, hallucinations, and speech and hearing problems.

A low level of lead intoxication may affect brain function and activity more subtly, influencing intelligence, attention span, language, and memory. Insomnia and nightmares may be experienced. Hyperactivity and even retardation and senility may also result. Moderate levels of lead may reduce immune and kidney function and increase risk of infection and may be another factor in increasing blood pressure. There is some suggestion that lead intoxication may correlate with cancer rates. Further research is needed in this area. With heavy lead intoxication, death may result.

In children, lead is a special cause for concern. Hyperactivity and learning disorders have been correlated with lead intoxication; children with these problems should be checked. Several studies have shown a relationship between lead levels and learning defects, including daydreaming, being easily frustrated or distracted, experiencing a decreased ability to follow instruction or a low persistence in learning, and possessing a general excitability and hyperactivity. There is also a recent correlation between sudden infant death syndrome (SIDS) and increased lead levels. This needs further research to implicate lead intoxication as a cause of death. Fortunately, progress has been made in decreasing some aspects of lead exposure for kids. In 1980, children's average blood lead level was 15 mcg (per deciliter of blood). In 1994, this average had dropped to just under 3 mcg. That is still too high, but the direction is good.

Amounts leading to toxicity. The Centers for Disease Control have set 10 mcg per liter of blood as the maximum safe level for children with 25 micrograms per liter as the maximum safe level for adults. Our daily exposure to lead has dropped substantially since the 1970s and 1980s, and average blood lead levels range between about 10 and 50 mcg per deciliter in adults. Inhaled lead fumes, lead in drinking water, and lead in food all contribute to this daily average. Average absorption is about 10% to 15%, so most of us should be able to eliminate most of what we get. Actually, with proper function, we can excrete many times more lead than that daily.

Nevertheless, lead is still an enormous health and environmental concern, and in some communities and in some occupations, it is the number-one concern. The CDC estimates that nationwide, about 900,000 children have blood levels greater than 10 mcg per deciliter—the jumping off point for major health problems. In 2000, more than 10,000 adults were identified by the CDC as having blood lead levels of at least 25 mcg, and this number is likely to be just the tip of the iceberg, because most adults never bother to have their blood tested for lead.

It is not clear what exposures or body levels of lead actually produce functional difficulties or specific symptoms; this probably varies from person to person. In measurements of any nutrient or chemical in the body, there is an estimated normal, or reference, range, above which some problems or symptoms may appear. For the level of lead in hair, the reference range of the lab that my office uses is about 0 to 30 ppm. Many authorities set lower levels, perhaps below 15 to 20 ppm, as a concern; Doctor's Data in Chicago uses 10 ppm. Even lower amounts, especially in children, may be a body burden and interfere with optimum brain and metabolic functions. For whole blood measurements, below 0.40 ppm is usually considered within the normal range; less than 0.20 ppm is probably ideal. In children, lower levels than that, even 0.10 ppm, may be a concern.

Who is susceptible? There is a long list (hundreds) of industrial and other workers who have a higher than average potential for exposure to lead. Obviously, anyone who works directly with lead has more exposure. Working in zinc or vanadium mining can also increase lead exposure. As stated, children are especially at risk for lead toxicity. For instance, teething children may be exposed to lead; children living in older or low-income housing or who live and play near busy streets may also be especially at risk. Much less exposure than would affect adults can lead to problems in children, because their absorption is better and their bodies are smaller. A small amount of leaded paint can increase body levels enough to create symptoms of toxicity. Children showing signs of hyperactivity or poor learning should be screened for lead levels.

Pregnant women and even the fetus are at risk of lead exposure. Anyone who works around car exhaust or in any of the many industries in which lead is used, from printing to painting to plumbing, should be aware of lead problems and probably get checked for lead levels every few years until we, as a society, are able to lower our lead use and environmental exposure.

Treatment of toxicity. EDTA, a synthetic amino acid, is the standard intravenous medical treatment for lead poisoning. It is a strong chelating agent, as it "claws" or latches onto metals and increases their urinary excretion. This treatment for lead intoxication led to use of the newer "chelation therapy" for other problems as well, as some of the patients treated

Lead-Susceptible Occupations

Battery makers	Garage mechanics	Metal workers and	Soap makers
Bookbinders	Glass makers and	refiners	Solder makers and
Bronzers	polishers	Munitions workers	solderers
Cable makers	Highway workers	Paint makers and	Toll booth collectors
Canners	Ink makers	painters	TV picture tube makers
Crop dusters	Insecticide makers	Plumbers	Vehicle tunnel workers
Dentists and dental	and users	Police and firefighters	Wallpaper makers and
technicians	Lead miners and other	Pottery glaze workers	hangers
Dye makers and dyers	lead workers	Printers	Welders
Enamel workers	Linoleum and tile	Rubber makers	Wood stainers
Farmers	makers	Shellac, varnish, and	
Firing range personnel	Match makers	lacquer makers	

for lead poisoning also experienced improvement of cardiovascular symptoms. This benefit may be a result of pulling out extra calcium and other metals that may be clogging arteries. Although chelation therapy is a controversial treatment that warrants further research, EDTA does much for lead and most heavy metal intoxication. This intravenous treatment is administered by a doctor, often in a hospital setting. Other medical treatments for lead intoxication include dimercaprol (British antilewisite, or BAL), given intramuscularly, and oral D-penicillamine. Treatment by any of these pharmaceutical agents has risks, so the level of lead intoxication should be accurately assessed. An EDTA (or DMSA or DMPS) challenge test is also sometimes used to help diagnose the degree of lead toxicity and help determine the need for chelation therapy. Oral DMSA (dimercaptosuccinic acid) and DMPS (dimercapto propane sulfonate, actually 2,3-dimercapto-1-propane sulfonate) can also be used to help the body clear lead and reduce tissue levels.

To reduce lead toxicity, a high-calcium diet or supplemental calcium inhibits further lead absorption. Injections of calcium chloride and extra vitamin D increases body levels of calcium, which may even displace some lead stored in the tissues, particularly the bones. Vitamin C also helps improve elimination of lead and other metals. The amino acids cysteine and methionine have some effect in detoxifying lead and other toxins, and foods such as eggs and beans, which contain these sulfhydryl-group amino acids, may also help bind and clear additional lead.

Prevention of toxicity (exposure). Obviously, the number-one prevention is to restrict lead exposure. That involves awareness of increased lead contamination potential. **The following are some ways to practice this prevention:**

- Do not exercise along freeways or in heavy traffic.

- Do not allow children to play near busy streets.

- Do not store food in pottery.

- Avoid soldered cans—mostly tin cans.

- Evaluate for lead levels any questionable substances, such as water or bonemeal, that are used regularly.

More positive things we can do to reduce lead problems in our body include eating a wholesome diet with plenty of organic fresh fruits, vegetables, and whole grains to obtain adequate minerals; avoiding refined foods; and possibly taking a mineral supplement to competitively reduce lead absorption. Calcium and magnesium do this well, so a good level of these minerals in our diet, as well as supplements, can reduce lead contamination. Iron, copper, and zinc also do this. With low mineral intake, lead absorption and potential toxicity are increased.

Algin in the diet, as from kelp (seaweed) or the supplement sodium alginate, helps to bind lead and other heavy metals in the gastrointestinal tract and carry them to elimination. Pectin and other fiber foods in the diet also tend to bind the heavier metals and reduce absorption. With this, however, we need to take more of our essential vitamins and minerals, such as the Bs, vitamin C, iron, calcium, zinc, copper, and chromium, to help decrease lead absorption. As mentioned, L-cysteine, 250 mg twice daily, is a sulfur-containing, detoxifying amino acid that helps bind and eliminate lead.

Children can be somewhat protected by getting adequate iron, calcium, and vitamins C and E in their diet and as supplements in appropriate amounts for their age. This program may also help get a little of that lead out and keep them clear thinking, more balanced, and active (but not hyperactive). Our understanding of lead is just beginning. Better prevention and treatments for lead intoxication, along with reduced lead use by industry in fuels, paints, and so on, should enable us to control the problems associated with this widespread contaminant.

Mercury

Mercury, or quicksilver, is a shiny liquid metal that is a widespread environmental contaminant. We are exposed to mercury in three basic forms: (1) the element itself, (2) electrically charged forms of the element (ionic compounds), and (3) organic forms like methylmercury, which are the most highly absorbed. **All forms are toxic, although methylmercury is the worst, followed by some of the ionic compounds.** Dental amalgams are the most common source of elemental mercury; nonfish foods expose us to the most mercury in ionic form; and fish are our greatest concern when it comes to the organic form methylmercury.

Mercury currently ranks as the country's third-most-hazardous substance on the government's CERCLA Priority List of Hazardous Substances, just behind arsenic and lead. Yet many practitioners and patients in California list this as a key concern, maybe because they eat lots of ocean fish and have higher exposures from the mercury-intoxicated waters. Mercury has been used for more than 2,000 years. Modern humans have much higher body levels of mercury than did our ancestors, because of its greater use in recent times. Nowadays, mercury is employed daily by medical and dental practices in thermometers, drugs (more so in the past), and amalgam for fillings; by agriculture in fungicides and pesticides; in solid and hazardous waste incinerators; in cement kilns; in coal combustors; by manufacture of chlorine products; and by the cosmetics industry. Most vaccinations are still preserved with mercury in the form of thimerosal. Certain kinds of fluorescent lights can contain mercury vapor, and for the first time in the United States, lights containing mercury now have to be labeled in at least one state (Vermont). **Mercury in industrial waste has polluted our waters and contaminated our fresh- and saltwater plants and fish.**

In the 1950s, Minamata Bay in Japan was poisoned with industrial mercury; it was measured in the waters at between 5 and 15 ppm, about 20 times the normal level. Many people experienced serious nervous system symptoms, staggering, and even comas and death before the pollution was discovered. In the early 1970s, the "mercury in the fish" scare spread across the United States. Swordfish, tuna, and other large fish were the subjects of concern and, in some areas, were measured with much higher than acceptable levels of mercury. Although the mercury-fish connection may not be as much of a crisis as we originally perceived, it is still high up on the list of toxic concerns. In 2002, mercury-safe seafood bills were introduced in the legislatures of 19 states, as well as in the U.S. Congress. In addition, 8% of all women of childbearing age in the United States are estimated to have unsafe levels of mercury in their blood, stemming in significant part from seafood consumption, especially canned tuna. The blood does not truly show high levels in the body unless there was recent expo-sure, as mercury moves quickly from the blood; tissue levels, the easiest being hair, is a better screen for longer-term exposure.

According to the EPA, our average exposure to elemental mercury is 3 to 17 mcg per day from mercury amalgam fillings in our teeth. For ionic mercury, it is only 0.25 mcg from nonfish foods, including milk, meat, mushrooms, broccoli, cabbage, and other vegetables. For methylmercury, it is 1 to 6 mcg, exclusively from fish. The total for all of these forms adds up to 4 to 23 mcg per day. These numbers do not take into account mercury vapor in the air, workplace exposures, or vaccinations.

Inhaled mercury, regardless of its form, is fairly highly absorbed, in the 40% to 85% range. More important, it more easily reaches the brain and nervous system, where mercury toxicity is of greatest concern. When it comes to eating and drinking, however, the form of the mercury makes a big difference. For elemental mercury, there is virtually no absorption from eating or drinking. For mercury in ionic form, absorption is still very low, at 7% to 15%. For methylmercury, though, absorption is as high as 95%. Clearly, this huge difference in absorption is why we need to be concerned about fish that accumulate mercury primarily as methylmercury. It is also worth mentioning here that we absorb all 3 forms, at a rate of about 2% to 3%, through our skin.

Today, the average person's body contains about 10 to 15 mg of mercury. Some of this mercury is retained in body tissues, mainly in the kidneys, which store about 50% of the body mercury. The blood, bones, liver, spleen, brain, and fat tissue also hold mercury. This potentially toxic metal does get into the brain and nerve tissue, so central nervous system symptoms may develop. **Mercury can also get into a growing fetus as well as into breast milk.** But mercury is eliminated daily through the urine and feces. Hair tissue analysis is the best way to measure body stores of mercury, while urine levels show whether the body is actively working to eliminate it.

Sources of contamination. Mercury is widely used in industry, agriculture, and health care. Even though hatmakers are safer and saner these days since the mercury used for the felt linings of hats was reduced, there are still people walking about "mad as a hatter" from mercury. Common uses of mercury include:

Fungicides and pesticides. These are a large source, used worldwide to treat grains and seeds. Methylmercury is the most common form.

Cosmetics. Mercury is added to decrease bacterial growth.

Dental fillings. Mercury is widely used, although many dentists no longer employ the silver-mercury amalgam, as they feel that it leads to a variety of problems. The American Dental Association, however, still claims that there is no proven mercury toxicity due to dental amalgams.

Medicines. Organic mercurial diuretics have been the most common, although these are less used these days. Mercury-containing cathartics, anthelmintics, and teething powders were also employed in the past. Broken thermometers can increase mercury exposure, and Mercurochrome also contains mercury. **Thimerosal, an ethyl form of mercury, is still used in many vaccinations.**

Coal burning. This releases mercury into the atmosphere.

Fish. Fish may contain varying amounts of mercury. Ocean bacteria, algae, and small fish may all contain some; mercury concentrations usually increase with the size of the fish. An excessive intake of fish foods may lead to increased body levels of mercury. The FDA has set a level of 1 ppm (1,000 ppb) as the maximum safe level for mercury in fish, but that allowance is clearly too high—twice as high as the level allowed in Canada (500 ppb). The Canadian guideline makes more sense, especially considering studies in Japan that have shown neurological damage at levels of 200 ppb.

Water. Mercury is routinely present in drinking water and the U.S. Environmental Protection Agency has established 2 mcg per liter (of inorganic mercury) as the maximum contaminant level for this heavy metal. Because of its relatively low absorption rate, however, inorganic mercury in drinking water is probably not among our highest concerns.

Other sources of mercury are mirrors, latex paints, fabric softeners, felt, floor waxes and polishes, sewage sludge, solid and hazardous waste incineration, cement finishing, copper smelting, laxatives containing calomel, cinnabar jewelry, tattoo dyes, and many others. Most of these are not specifically toxic, as they do not give off high amounts of volatile mercury. Fungicides are the most widely used and probably the most potentially toxic.

Methods of toxicity. Mercury has no known essential functions, although it was once used to treat syphilis, with some success. Mercury probably affects the inherent protein structure that may interfere with functions relating to protein production. Mercury has a strong affinity for sulfhydryl, amine, phosphoryl, and carboxyl groups, and inactivates a wide range of enzyme systems, as well as causing injury to cell membranes. In the case of mercury's affinity for sulfur, there is an especially problematic consequence because the sulfur in glutathione can be bound by mercury, and our glutathione supply can be directly decreased in this way. This special connection may be one of the reasons that mercury can show up so readily in hair analysis, because of the high concentration of sulfur-containing amino acids in hair.

The effects of mercury on the nervous system are well researched and far-reaching. We know that mercury disrupts energy production processes in the mitochondria of nerve cells—effectively poisoning energy production so that the cells no longer have enough resources to function. Mercury can also block the calcium channels that are needed to trigger nerve firing and can interfere with nervous system function in this way. Because mercury depletes our glutathione and disrupts our oxygen-based energy production processes, mercury also increases the likelihood that our nerve cells will be damaged by oxygen. Many types of nerve cells in the brain have been shown to suffer all of the toxic effects of mercury just described.

This heavy metal is also capable of shifting our cells into their programmed death cycles (apoptosis), in which they deliberately shut down and dismantle. We know that mercury can trigger this process in several kinds of immune cells, including T cells, and can there act as an immunosuppressant.

It is possible that mercury interferes with the metabolism of selenium. However, for the most part, the clear connection between these two elements seems to work most strongly in the opposite direction, in which selenium can reduce the toxicity of mercury.

Symptoms of toxicity. The symptoms we get from mercury toxicity depend largely on the form of mercury that we are exposed to. Mercury vapors that we breathe into our lungs can move quickly into our bloodstream, and from there into our nervous system and, if concentrated enough, into our brain. The resulting symptoms can include tremors, changes in vision including narrowing of the visual field, deafness, muscle incoordination, decrease in sensation, and memory problems. Also possible are personality changes, including nervousness, shyness, or irritability. Organic mercury, which I discuss below, can also trigger these symptoms.

Metallic mercury, and all other forms, can damage the kidneys if present in sufficiently high amounts. However, because kidney damage is usually related to accumulation and storage of mercury, the organic forms are a greater worry here. Symptoms here can include reduced urination, discoloration of the urine or change in odor, body swelling, shortness of breath, and, of course, altered lab tests involving kidney function. Metallic mercury vapors can readily damage the lungs, either from short-term high doses, or long-term low-level ones. Burning sensations in the lungs, tightness of the chest, and coughing are common symptoms, as are nausea, diarrhea, vomiting, increase in blood pressure, and increase in heart rate. Skin contact with metallic mercury vapors can also cause allergic reaction, most commonly rashes.

Ionic compounds from mercury, including mercuric chloride, can damage the digestive tract. Accidental swallowing of these compounds by children has shown many problems in this regard. Diarrhea, nausea, vomiting, stomatitis and gastrointestinal inflammation, abdominal pain, and bloody diarrhea are possible symptoms. Rapid heart rate and increased blood pressure are likely symptoms, and if the dose is high enough, severe ulcers can also result.

The organic forms of mercury, including the ethyl forms like thimerosal and the methylmercury forms found in contaminated fish, have the widest range of symptoms. These forms damage not only the kidneys and digestive tract, but also the reproductive organs, immune system, endocrine system, sperm, and, in the case of pregnancy, the developing fetus.

There is still some debate over the cancer-causing properties of mercury. The EPA has classified this heavy metal as a possible human carcinogen, but several well-respected international agencies have yet to do so. It seems clear to me that researchers will eventually reach agreement on the role of mercury as a cancer-causing agent, because too many underlying activities of our cells are fundamentally disrupted in the presence of excess mercury.

Before leaving the topic of toxicity, I want to explain a little more about the relationship between mercury dose, length of exposure, and symptoms. Some symptoms of mercury are truly "acute" and occur from short-term exposure at a high dose. For example, inhaling high levels of metallic mercury (in an industrial setting or a dentist's office) can cause acute symptoms, such as fever, chills, coughing, and chest pain. With low, long-term exposure, more subtle symptoms—such as fatigue, headache, insomnia, nervousness, impaired judgment and coordination, emotional instability and loss of sex drive—may be experienced. Ingested mercury may cause stomatitis and gastrointestinal inflammation, with nausea, vomiting, abdominal pain, and bloody diarrhea, progressing to neurological problems. These symptoms, which are often confused with psychogenic causes, are referred to as *micromercurialism.*

Mild or early symptoms of mercury intoxication include fatigue, insomnia, irritability, anorexia, loss of sex drive, headache, and forgetfulness or poor memory. Nervous system symptoms—such as dizziness, tremors, incoordination, and depression—may often be later-stage symptoms, progressing further over time to numbness and tingling, most commonly of the hands, feet, or lips, and to further weakness, worse memory and coordination, reduced hearing and speech, paralysis, and psychosis. Some of the later-stage neurological symptoms of mercury toxicity suggest a connection with multiple sclerosis. Other problems of severe mercury intoxication are kidney and brain damage as well as birth defects in pregnant women. Luckily, these extreme symptoms are unusual.

Amounts leading to toxicity. The average intake of mercury varies with location and diet. It may range from 10 mcg to more than 500 mcg, mainly depending on air contamination. Industrial cities and heavily sprayed farmland have the highest levels. The average overall daily intake is probably about 30 to 50 mcg. This amount may or may not be toxic to us, depending on our state of health and detox capabilities.

Blood levels of mercury should be below 0.02 ppm, while hair levels may be higher, up to about 3 to 5 ppm. More than 5 ppm becomes a concern. When these

---

Occupations with Potential Mercury Exposure

Barometer and thermometer makers

Cement finishers

Chlorine product makers

Copper smelters

Dental amalgam makers

Dentists and dental workers

Dye makers

Embalmers

Explosives and fireworks makers

Fluorescent (mercury-vapor) light makers

Hazardous waste workers

Ink makers

Insecticide makers

Jewelers

Mirror makers

Neon light makers

Paint makers

Paper makers

Pesticide workers

Photographers

Waste incineration workers

Wood preservative workers

---

levels are exceeded, we should look for the sources of increased exposure and work toward avoiding or eliminating them.

Who is susceptible? Anyone working with mercury, especially methyl or ethyl mercury or mercuric chloride, is more likely to have problems of mercury toxicity. Farmers using mercury products should be careful with them and should be aware of mercury toxicity symptoms or have mercury levels checked every couple of years. All of us, however, are subject to life-long, continuous, low-dose exposure to mercury as a result of the air we breathe and the food we eat. We need to continue reducing our industrial, medical, and agricultural use of this heavy metal to lower its presence in soil and eliminate it as a major factor in fish and other aspects of our food.

Treatment of toxicity. Drinking milk helps reduce the acute effects of mercury, as the mercury acts on the protein in the milk instead of on the stomach and intes-

tinal lining. This may prevent the acute symptoms of gastrointestinal tissue irritation, such as vomiting and bleeding. Penicillamine is a chelating drug that can pull mercury out of the circulation. It works best when given soon after exposure, rather than after tissue storage occurs. Penicillamine itself, however, is potentially toxic. Dimercaprol (BAL) has also been used. EDTA, a stronger chelating agent, can also be used to pull out body mercury. It usually has fewer side effects than penicillamine. Vitamin C, selenium, and the fibers pectin and algin may also reduce mercury levels and toxicity, although usually only in cases of less severity. I currently use DMSA in my patients, prescribing it for 3 days every other weekend, and this helps reduce mercury tissue levels, and thus toxicity, slowly over time. This then allows the mercury gradient to move from the nervous system, the most concerning area for toxicity, out into body. There are no readily available agents that actually go into the brain and spinal system to remove mercury. Other integrated medicine practitioners use DMPS (2,3-dimercapto-1-propane sulfonate) instead of DMSA; however, I find that DMSA is better tolerated and less costly than DMPS.

Prevention of toxicity (exposure). Avoidance of mercury contamination is foremost in preventing mercury toxicity. Staying clear of mercury fungicides and avoiding fungicide-treated foods or eating only organically grown grains and produce may be helpful. Many health-oriented dentists now avoid mercury-containing amalgam to prevent further mercury exposure. Silver-mercury fillings during pregnancy, I believe, should be particularly avoided.

Pectin and algin can decrease absorption of mercury, especially inorganic mercury. Selenium binds both inorganic and methylmercury; mercury selenide is formed and excreted in fecal matter. Selenium is, for many reasons, an important nutrient for all of us, and in an amount of at least 100 mcg, it does seem to help protect against heavy metal toxicity.

Other Metal Concerns

 Antimony is probably only slightly toxic in human beings, although in rats it affects the heart and reduces the life span. We obtain antimony mainly from food and water, with some from the air. Other sources are pottery glazes and cooking utensils. Naples Yellow, also called Yellow No. 41, is a commonly used paint pigment that contains antimony. The approximately 100 mcg consumed daily is poorly absorbed, and most is eliminated in the feces and urine. Our body stores some in the liver, spleen, kidneys, blood, and hair. Antimony is really only of mild concern in humans. Industrial antimony toxicity from gaseous stibine (SbH_3) or ingestion of antimony materials is uncommon. High levels can cause acute symptoms of the gastrointestinal tract and cause damage to the kidneys, liver, and heart.

Ba **Barium** compounds are used in medical testing for X-ray evaluations; in printing, ceramics, plastics, textiles, and dyes; in fuel additives; in the production of glass, paints, paper, soap, and rubber; and in some pesticides and rat poisons. Manganese Violet, also called Permanent Mauve and Violet 16, is a commonly used paint pigment that contains barium. Barium toxicity is relatively low unless there is ingestion of large amounts or aerosol exposure. Inhalation may cause short-term lung irritation. Accidental or intentional ingestion of barium may lead to vomiting, diarrhea, and abdominal pain. As barium becomes absorbed, it can displace potassium intracellularly and cause mild to severe effects in muscle tone, heart function, and the nervous system. Barium can also follow calcium pathways in the body and can be deposited in bone. Treatment with potassium and diuresis may reduce symptoms. Across the country, there appear to be some pockets of barium that affect public drinking water supplies and private wells. The states of Illinois, Kentucky, New Mexico, and Pennsylvania have all experienced some problems in this regard.

Be **Beryllium** is interesting as a metal; it is strong, light, and heat resistant (like aluminum), and has a high melting point. Thus it is a good metal to use in airplanes and rockets. Its use has increased in recent years, and it is found in neon signs and some electrical devices. When it is used in metal alloys, beryllium improves resistance to vibration, shock, and metal fatigue, and thus its use in bicycle wheels, fishing rods, and metal household gadgets.

However, this light metal is toxic in humans. Beryllium can reduce stores of magnesium and decrease organ function, possibly through interference with enzymes. Contamination with beryllium, primarily from its industrial uses, is becoming more widespread. Industrial smoke and rocket exhaust may contain higher than healthful levels of beryllium. Beryllium inhalation can cause shortness of breath, coughing, phlegm, and lung inflammation, which can lead to chronic scarring and disability. There is actually a lung disease named for this metal, called *berylliosis*. One problem with our understanding of beryllium toxicity involves the long latency period—sometimes up to 25 years after exposure—before symptoms may appear. Later-life onset of emphysema, for example, has in some cases been linked to early-life beryllium exposure. There is also some question as to whether airborne beryllium may accumulate in the lungs and create an increased risk of cancer. Although it is not very widely used and its toxicity is fairly minor, more intense use could lead to further problems for people exposed to higher levels of beryllium dust.

Bi **Bismuth** is essentially nontoxic in ordinary amounts, but prolonged exposure or excessive use may lead to toxicity. This could cause mental confusion, memory loss, incoordination, slurred speech, joint pain, or muscle twitching and spasm. The human body contains about 3 mg of bismuth. Many people take in 20 to 30 mcg per day, most of it in water, a minimal amount in food, and some from airborne contamination. Most bismuth is eliminated in the feces and urine. Some drugs, particularly remedies for the stomach, such as Pepto-Bismol, contain bismuth.

Br **Bromine,** like chlorine and fluorine, is a halogen element and poisonous gas. Bromine salts have been used to treat acid indigestion or for sedation. Bromine can displace chlorine in some body functions. Too much can cause toxicity. Mild symptoms may include fatigue, weakness, irritability, disturbed sleep, slow mental processes and poor memory. More severe toxicity can cause confusion and drowsiness, delirium, stupor, depression, hallucinations, and, in the extreme, psychosis. Because it is in the same halogen family as chlorine, and because problems with chlorine toxicity have received widespread attention, manufacturers of chlorine-containing products have sometimes switched to bromine as an alternative component in their products. For example, many home spa products offer a line of bromine-based disinfectants alongside of their traditional chlorine-based ones. Similarly, when PCBs (polychlorinated byphenyls) hit the toxicity spotlight in the 1970s, we saw an upward turn in the manufacture of products using PBBs (polybrominated byphenyls). Fortunately, neither PCBs nor PBBs are still manufactured in the United States, although hazardous residual levels of both toxic substances remain in the air and water. Because PBBs were used as fire retardants in machinery, and especially in plastic-based machinery that was subject to high heat, bromine-containing PBB residues can be found in landfills and hazardous waste sites throughout the United States.

Th **Thallium** has again become a toxicity concern. Discovered in the 1800s by Sir William Crookes, it was used in medical treatments for venereal diseases, gout, and tuberculosis. Its toxicity caused it to fall into disuse, however, although thallium acetate continued to be employed for fungal skin infections for some time.

Industrial use of thallium has increased in recent years. It can form useful alloys with silver or lead and may be a by-product of zinc and lead production. In electronics, thallium is used in power systems, such as batteries or semiconductors. It is also employed in optical lenses, photo film, jewelry, dyes and pigments, and fireworks. In the medical world, the thallium 201 isotope is used in a variety of imaging procedures that assess heart function. A bigger concern was its use in pesticides and rodenticides, which were banned in 1975. Thallium sulfate was used with starch and glycerin to treat grains for poisoning squirrels and rodents. This led to some fatalities when humans mistakenly consumed some of that grain.

Thallium is in low concentration in the Earth's crust. **Humans cannot tolerate much thallium in their bodies.** This mineral and its salts can enter the body through our skin, respiratory tract, or gastrointestinal route. It can be toxic in several ways. First, it can substitute for potassium in certain functions within the red blood cells, such as in the sodium-potassium ATPase. Thallium also has a strong attraction to sulfhydryl groups and thus may interact with these active enzyme sites. Thallium can pass through

the placenta into the fetus. There is some suggestion that thallium has teratogenic effects.

Thallium has significant toxicity effects both with acute exposure to large amounts and lower-level, chronic intake. Acute ingestion can lead to nausea, vomiting, abdominal pain, bloody diarrhea, fatigue, and fever. This can be fatal through its secondary agitation state, which can cause seizures and then coma and respiratory failure. If people survive this exposure, further problems can affect the kidneys, heart, and nervous system. Sensory and motor changes, peripheral neuropathy, loss of reflexes, hair loss, arrhythmias, and renal disease may result. This may progress over several weeks. Most ingested thallium goes to and is excreted by the kidneys; the remainder is stored in many other tissues.

Chronic poisoning may cause polyneuritis with an inability to walk, fatigue, weight loss, and possibly reduced immunity. Thallium acetate has been used as a purposeful poison on several known occasions. Because it has no color or taste, it is well concealed in food and drinks, and it is not commonly looked for. Thallium can be measured in the blood or urine. A 24-hour urine collection may reveal increased levels of this toxic mineral. A treatment with potassium chloride or EDTA may show increased levels of thallium in the urine. Treatment for thallium poisoning is somewhat complex. Agents such as EDTA, dimercaprol, penicillamine, sodium iodide, and thiouracil have all been used with some benefit. Diuresis and potassium chloride are used more standardly to reduce thallium toxicity by increasing excretion levels. Prussian Blue (potassium ferric cyanoferrate) dye has been used to trap thallium in the gut after initial ingestion. Hemoperfusion or dialysis is used to reduce blood concentrations of thallium. Overall, we would be wise to avoid exposure to thallium.

Other Metals of Concern

Cesium, a radioactive element, has been used since the 1940s and 1950s in relationship to nuclear weapons production. One isotope, cesium 137, is currently used in food irradiation as a means of destroying potentially harmful bacteria found in food. **Palladium,** an old treatment for obesity, may be carcinogenic, but this needs further research. **Platinum** may cause allergic pulmonary reactions in platinum workers. **Pluto-nium** is a potent carcinogen, and exposure, even small amounts in workers, is a concern. **Tellurium** may create some mild and infrequent toxicity. **Titanium,** once used to treat skin disorders and now made into beautiful jewelry, is not thought to be very toxic in the body, although there have been a few cases of high exposure causing problems.

Uranium is probably toxic, but there is little direct exposure to it. Recently, several studies have reported on the health and environmental consequences of the use of depleted uranium. Depleted uranium is a heavy metal that is also radioactive. It is commonly used in missiles as a counterweight because of its very high density (1.6 times more than lead). Immediate health risks associated with exposure to depleted uranium include kidney and respiratory problems, with conditions such as kidney stones, chronic cough, and severe dermatitis. Long-term risks include lung and bone cancer. Several published reports implicated exposure to depleted uranium in kidney damage, mutagenicity, cancer, inhibition of bone metabolism, neurological deficits, significant decrease in the pregnancy rate in mice, and adverse effects on the reproductive and central nervous systems. Acute poisoning with depleted uranium elicites renal failure that could lead to death. The environmental consequences of its residue will be felt for thousands of years. It is inhaled and passed through the skin and eyes, transferred through the placenta into the fetus, distributed into tissues, and eliminated in urine. The use of depleted uranium during the Gulf, Kosovo, and Balkan Wars and the crash of a Boeing airplane carrying depleted uranium in Amsterdam in 1992 were implicated in a health concern related to exposure to depleted uranium. The focus here was on the inhalation of uranium-containing dust following weapons explosion, but the poor solubility of uranium has made researchers less worried about transfer to groundwater.

Radon, however, which comes from the radioactive decay of uranium, is a pollution concern in both air and water and is a surprisingly common cause of lung cancer. High concentrations of radon appear to be distributed in different soils throughout the United States, with passage of radon gas up from the soil into homes as the primary source of exposure. Indoor air is therefore the key source of exposure, and the average homeowner in this country has a 1 in 300 chance of developing lung cancer from radon exposure. For about 1 million homes in the country sitting atop concentrated radon deposits, the risk is more like 1 in 40. **Cigarette smokers are at particularly high risk for lung cancer when simultaneously exposed to radon**.

The government has become more concerned about radon exposure, and now there are new devices and organizations that will help us assess the levels of this radioactive element at home or at work. Radon levels are measured in picocuries per liter of air (pCi/L), and the EPA guidelines suggest levels of 4 and below are reasonably safe, 20 and below probably safe, 20 to 200 as requiring reduction, and above 200 often requiring relocation. Some drinking waters, both city and well, also contain radon. It is a radioactive element and, like most others, disintegrates eventually into lead. We have about 90 mcg of uranium in our body. We obtain some in food and water, although it has low absorption and fair elimination. Toxicity, if it occurs, usually affects the kidneys.

For as long as these metals remain in common use by industry, they will continue to accumulate in our bodies. Further research is needed to better understand their effects on human health and well-being.

THE FUTURE OF MINERALS

Remember the word *attachment* when you think about the future minerals, because attachment is going to rule the day when it comes to mineral nourishment. Already, we have a good handle on the idea of chelation (*chela* = "claw"), and in the supplement world we are already producing a variety of mineral chelates by attaching minerals to different amino acids. We're going to see the partnership becoming as important as the mineral itself. "Who" the mineral hangs out with is going to become more and more critical. We're going to see particular amino acids and organic acids as being essential for mineral nourishment, and we're going to start insisting on more and more specialized mineral delivery forms. We will also start treating minerals more like lovers than loners.

Magnesium with calcium, copper with zinc—the relationships are going to captivate more and more of our health energy.

The question of which minerals are essential and which are toxic is going to advance greatly, with new functions identified for some minerals we know little about. Looking at mercury and lead and their body and earthly concerns will become a widespread issue, and learning to detoxify the body of these metals will become more mainstream. Trace minerals in special forms will balance the body and enhance functions, especially of the nervous system, brain, and energy. We'll find out more about natural lithium, vanadium, germanium, and so many more. Scientific studies of minerals' impacts on disease will show new and exciting therapies. Mineral transport and mineral combinations, as just mentioned, will bring new understanding, as will mineral interference and deficiency issues. We will validate the importance of digestion for mineral assimilation and body health and discover better ways to get each mineral into the body and to the places where it functions. Healing and nourishing the Earth's soils will bring higher levels of minerals into our foods, the primary way we receive these vital nutrients.

What to Look For in the Future of Minerals

- Strontium supplementation for bone density will show safety and effectiveness.

- Selenium value in therapy (and the common deficiency of this important mineral) and in many detoxification and metabolic pathways, such as thyroid hormone regulation.

- Vanadium use in glucose metabolism and the possible prevention of diabetes.

- The chemical exposures of modern society as well as the invasiveness of elements such as chlorine and fluoride and the subsequent interference with proper body physiology, and utilization of nutrients such as the mineral iodine for normal thyroid function and vitamins like folic acid, plus many more areas of nutritional concern.

- Low dose lithium, such as lithium orotate or aspartate, for mood stabilization, depression, and anxiety.

- Magnesium taurate for cell and electrical rhythm stabilization, and seizure reduction.

- Magnesium deficiency (the most important macromineral deficiency) in relation to cardiovascular disease, heart arrhythmias, and asthma, as well as magnesium's importance as a nutrient that powers antioxidant activity in the body.

Chapter 7

Special Supplements

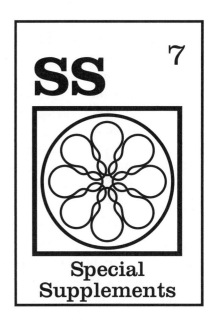

SS 7

Special Supplements

In addition to the nutrients already discussed in chapters 1 through 6, there is a wide variety of products on the dietary supplement shelves that I explore in this chapter. These products, such as enzymes or anti-inflammatory, weight-loss, or anti-depressant supplements, might be prescribed by health practitioners; or they may be sitting on the shelf of your grocery, pharmacy, or natural foods store; or they might be advertised in a magazine or on the Internet. Their claims may pique your interest, and you may wish to know some basics about these supplements.

Literally hundreds of new preparations are marketed each year. The supplement market has greatly improved and expanded since the mid-1980s, but the wide availability, heavy advertising, and variety of opinions about what is best can make it difficult for the individual to know what he or she needs. The literature from the manufacturers backing up their claims for these supplements ranges from common promotional tales to good scientific research. In this chapter I provide the most current, accurate information, based on both science and experience.

This chapter deals with a variety of supplements, and I have grouped them (for the most part) according to the way they are commonly used. The table below details the specific categories of special supplements discussed here. Many of these are new to the marketplace, while others are as old as folklore itself. Often, new methods of production allow a nutrient to be more usable in the body. On the whole, the adventure that lies in deciding what medicinals and nutritional supplements we might take is another part of life's excitement and the quest for better health.

Special Supplement Categories	
Antibiotics	Genetic support and
Anti-inflammatories	RNA/DNA
Antioxidants	Glandulars
Bone and joint	Green foods
strengtheners	Immune support
Circulatory aids	Mental and nervous
Detoxifiers	system support
Digestive support	Metabolic and cellular aids
Energy boosters and	Mood balancers
stress reducers	Plant oils and fatty acids

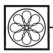

ANTIBIOTICS

Since their discovery in 1928, prescription antibiotics have gone on to become some of the superstars of conventional medicine. Multiple Nobel Prizes in medicine have been awarded for antibiotic research, and about 175 million prescriptions for antibiotics are written each year in the United States. Another 20 million pounds of antibiotics are used each year in connection with animal and plant food production. The reasons for this are simple: antibiotics can have the almost magical quality of killing disease-causing bacteria without killing our own cells or the cells of plants or animals.

At the same time, however, enormous questions have been raised about antibiotic use by many health-care providers, public health officials, and ecologists, many of whom see a huge downside to antibiotic use—antibiotic resistance. All prescription antibiotics lose their effectiveness over time, because bacteria learn to live with these chemicals. The more antibiotics we use, therefore, the quicker the bacteria adjust. *Adjusting* in this case means that the bacteria learn to thrive despite the presence of the antibiotic. The result is that the antibiotics become ineffective and the bacterial world is thrown out of balance. Many bacteria produce the same antibiotics that we use as medicines as a way of protecting themselves from other bacteria. This protective mechanism stops working when too many bacteria become resistant. The downside of prescription antibiotic use has prompted many in the natural health field to look for effective alternatives to these prescription drugs.

In the following section, I discuss some of the best options I have seen personally, recognizing that there are others that may have worked just as well for other practitioners.

Antibiotic Nutrients

You are unlikely to find any nutrients being sold as antibiotics, because the dose of a nutrient it would take to kill bacteria or fungi would be higher than we would want for ourselves. However, you are likely to see nutritional supplements that are recommended when a person is taking antibiotic drugs to help offset the side effects. Folate and other B complex vitamins, flavonoids, and carotenoids are popular in this context. Although not nutrients, probiotic bacterial supplements containing *Lactobacillus* and *Bifidobacterium* species are also commonly used.

Antibiotic Herbs	
Aloe vera	Oregano oil
Garlic	Oregon grape
Ginger	Propolis
Goldenseal	St. John's wort
Grapefruit seed	Tea tree oil
Licorice	Turmeric

Antibiotic Herbs

Aloe vera Although I am including aloe *(Aloe barbadensis)* among the natural antibiotics, it is a plant with a wide range of potential health benefits. You will find these benefits listed in other sections of this chapter. The aloe "cactus," actually a desert succulent, has been touted as a "miracle plant," and its antibiotic activity is definitely a part of its reputation. The gel in the leaves of the aloe plant contains a fairly long list of unique substances that account for many of its healing properties. These substances include aloe resins, anthraquinones, salicylates, and polysaccharide-type compounds.

In this last category is found acemannan, perhaps the best-studied of the aloe's phytonutrients. Acemannan has been successfully used to treat feline leukemia in cats, a sometimes fatal disease that is caused by a retrovirus. For this reason, it has been approved for veterinary use in injectable form. Acemannan has also been successfully used in the form of a topical patch to help prevent infection in patients following oral surgery, and it has gained FDA approval for use as an oral ulcer remedy. Carrington Labs, in Irving, Texas, produces acemannan by extracting juice from the aloe plant, freeze-drying it, and then crushing it into a powder. This freeze-dried powder is then sold under the brand name Carrisyn. Because AIDS is a disease caused by a retrovirus similar to the retrovirus that causes feline leukemia, acemannan from aloe has also been used experimentally to treat AIDS patients and has FDA approval as an investigational drug in this area.

Fighting viruses is not aloe's only antibiotic activity, however. It is also an antibacterial and antifungal. Aloe is a known bactericide against a dozen or so different kinds of bacteria, including the pneumonia-causing bacterium *Klebsiella pneumoniae.* It has also been shown to inhibit the fungus *Candida albicans,* responsible for most yeast infections.

Most of the aloe found in stores comes in the form of topical skin care products like a soap, lotion, or cream. Because the active compounds in aloe kill or halt the growth of bacteria in laboratory studies, it seems highly likely that these products are also bacteriostatic (bacteria controlling) or bactericidal (bacteria killing), even though I have not seen research studies confirming this effect.

The common oral preparation of the aloe plant currently available is aloe vera juice, a partially refined and diluted extract of the active gel. It is important to select a high-quality product that is as much like the inner gel of the plant as possible and that has not been subjected to high heat or unnecessary filtering during its manufacture. Aloe juice is sold in pints, quarts, and even gallons. Mouthwashes and rinses are also commonly formulated with aloe. Once again, I have not seen studies that demonstrate antibiotic activity in the mouth or digestive tract when aloe juice is consumed, but this activity seems likely based on laboratory studies.

Aloe also has a low risk of toxicity, enabling it to be consumed as a drink on a regular basis. Many people start out with 1 ounce twice daily and increase to about 6 ounces per day. Many users describe positive health effects from drinking aloe vera juice on this kind of routine basis. I have taken this nutrient, and it seems at least to be soothing and vitalizing, if you can get past the taste (some preparations taste better than others).

Garlic. This is one of the big shots in herbal lore. Garlic *(Allium sativum)* has been used effectively through the centuries for a variety of concerns and is probably among the best-known herb foods. Many people use garlic regularly in their diets, easily identified by the telltale odor. In recent years, odorless garlic extracts have been used to treat a wide range of conditions without creating the bad breath, although many nat-

uralists and scientists believe that this is not as beneficial as fresh garlic.

Garlic is in the antibiotic herb section because its role as an antimicrobial has been well documented. Studies have even pitted garlic directly against prescription antibiotics to see which was more effective, and garlic has come up looking as good as penicillin, streptomycin, erythromycin, and tetracyclines in some studies. In addition, it has proven effective against some resistant bacteria that no longer respond to these prescription antibiotics. The list of microbes that garlic seems effective in stopping includes the yeast *Candida albicans,* the jock itch fungus *Tinea cruris,* the virus *Herpes simplex,* and several of the rhinoviruses that can cause the common cold. Some of the roundworms and hookworms that can set up shop in our intestine are also killed off by garlic. **In higher amounts, garlic can be irritating to the gastrointestinal tract, and when applied to the skin as raw garlic, it can cause burns.** Some women have used it intravaginally to treat infections; however, this is not recommended as it can cause more irritation if the shell coating of an individual clove is disrupted.

For internal use, fresh garlic is probably best. Researchers in Japan have used a deodorized garlic prepared by an aging-fermentation process. This garlic seems to retain the natural effects, but not all deodorized garlic is prepared in this way, and it may or may not have the same benefits as fresh garlic.

Garlic oil capsules are commonly used as a therapeutic supplement. We can make our own garlic oil from chopped fresh garlic that is soaked a few days in olive oil. It can be used as an external or internal treatment, such as by applying it to the feet or chest during colds or taking it orally as a simple means of obtaining garlic. Garlic oil is good in salad dressings, too.

Ginger. The root of this plant *(Zingiber officinale)* is used effectively with a variety of intestinal disorders, where its antibiotic effects appear to be the key to its success. Protozoal infections, like the amoebic dysentery caused by *Entamoeba histolytica* or the giardiasis caused by *Giardia lamblia,* have some fairly well-researched responsiveness to ginger. Helping to prevent food poisoning from bad fish is another interesting area of research, because *Anisakis* larvae—nematodes in fish that can make us fairly sick—are

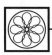

readily killed by the 6-shogaol and 6-gingerol molecules in this marvelous root.

Goldenseal. The roots of goldenseal (*Hydrastis canadensis*) have been a cure-all used by many herbalists as well as a popular herb to the Native Americans. Its range of uses is probably as wide as that of any other herb. **Goldenseal's active alkaloids, hydrastine and berberine, appear to have many body actions, and this bitter, tonifying herb is used as an antibacterial and antiparasitic, especially for giardia and amoebic infections, as well as other infections with yeast, worms, or other germs.** The table below details just how many different types of bacteria, protozoa, and fungi are affected by berberine alone. Many people take goldenseal capsules at the first sign of a flu or other infection and claim good results.

Berberine-Sensitive Organisms

Candida albicans	*Shigella dysenteriae*
Chlamydia species	*Staphylococcus* species
E. coli	*Streptococcus* species
Entamoeba hystolytica	*Trichomonas vaginalis*
Giardia lamblia	*Vibrio cholerae*

Also very interesting with respect to goldenseal is the major jump in effectiveness that occurs as the pH of our body fluids increases. When our gastrointestinal tract is fairly alkaline, with a pH of 7, goldenseal is up to 4 times more effective than when the pH is just 1 notch lower (more acidic), at 6.

Grapefruit seed. Extracts from the seeds and pulp of this widely loved fruit (*Citrus paridisi*) have become especially popular in vegetable washes and countertop disinfectants, and they have a significant history of use in the food industry as germicides and disinfectants. There is evidence for using grapefruit seed extract as a helpful antibiotic in some cases of skin infection (where you would be using it topically) as well as for some cases of parasitic infection in the digestive tract.

Licorice. It is the root of this popular plant (*Glycyrrhiza glabra*) that has been most closely linked with its antibiotic activity. Because I have considered this herb an important option particularly for bacterial problems in the digestive tract, I have been quite excited to see recent research studies showing its effectiveness in blocking the growth of *Helicobacter pylori*, the bacterium that is almost always associated with peptic ulcers. Some unusual isoflavonoid pigments seem to be the compounds most responsible for this ulcer-reducing effect. There are widely available liquid extracts of licorice root, but I also sometimes consider what is called the *solid extract form*, even though it is less widely available. Solid extracts are extremely thick syrups formed by taking plants like licorice root and then distilling and evaporating to obtain the desired consistency. (See page 256 in the "Anti-inflammatory" section of this chapter for more about licorice.)

Oregano. The antibiotic properties of this plant's oils have made it so popular that the marketplace is now dotted with oregano-labeled products that are not even extracted from *Origanum vulgare* but from Spanish thyme or a similar herb. Most genuine oregano oils come from drier, high-mountain climates surrounding the Mediterranean, including Turkey and Syria. **Oregano is used both topically and orally, and when you use it directly on your skin, you need to mix it with a milder oil (like almond, castor, or olive oil) to reduce its harshness.**

Research studies show oil of oregano to be as effective as, or more effective than, some prescription antifungal drugs in treating the yeast *Candida albicans*. Certain intestinal parasites—including *Blastocystis hominis*, *Entamoeba hartmanni*, and *Endolimax nana*—are also killed by some of the principle components in this oil. Oregano oil is also used to treat infection with the protozoa *Giardia lamblia*.

Oregon grape. Although not as well-known as some of the other antibiotic herbs, Oregon grape (*Berberis aquifolium*) is one of the berberine-containing plants that, like goldenseal, can be effective with a wide variety of microbes, including protozoa, fungi, and bacteria. Like goldenseal, Oregon grape has been found to inhibit growth of intestinal parasites, including *Entamoeba histolytica*, *Giardia lamblia*, and *Tricomonas vaginalis*. The form of this herb I most recommend is a liquid extract from the root of the plant. The most common antibiotic use of this extract is for respiratory tract infection.

Propolis. Also called "bee glue," propolis is a unique, sticky fluid that bees make from a diverse mixture of resins found in many different plants. Because of the vast diversity of plants around the world, propolis from different parts of the globe can have widely varying chemical compositions. Although many of the nutrient components in propolis, like minerals and B vitamins, remain relatively constant from country to country, the phytonutrient content of propolis can vary widely. Galangin and pinocembrin were the first antibiotic compounds found in bee propolis, almost 35 years ago. Since then, a growing list of phenolic acids, including caffeic acid and ferulic acid, have emerged as key antibiotic substances in propolis. Studies have compared propolis from many different parts of the world—including Brazil, Bulgaria, the Canary Islands, and Europe—and each different propolis seems to act a little differently in terms of its antibiotic activity.

In general, however, propolis is known to inhibit the growth of *Helicobacter pylori*, the bacterium associated with peptic ulcer, as well as some strains of *E. coli* bacteria. It has been used effectively to treat fungal infections caused by *Candida albicans* and has antiviral activity, although it is not yet clear how propolis works to limit a viral infection. Propolis has been compared with silver sulfadiazine cream in the treatment of minor burns and is definitely helpful when used in this topical way. It is important to purchase propolis that is free of toxic contaminants.

St. John's wort. Although antibiotic use is not the best-known application for this vastly popular herb, this use should definitely be considered, particularly for viral and bacterial infections. St. John's wort *(Hypericum perforatum)* can have beneficial effects in treatment of influenza viruses A and B, *Herpes simplex* I and II viruses (HSV-1 and HSV-2), and also the Epstein-Barr virus. Both staphylococcus and streptococcus infections can be responsive to this herb, along with several other types of bacterial infection. Many of the research studies on St. John's wort have been carried out using fluid extract forms of the herb, which I often recommend.

Turmeric. This long-standing staple spice in Indian and Asian cooking has far-reaching medicinal properties, including well-researched benefits as an antibiotic. Turmeric *(Curcuma longa)* is able to inhibit the growth of certain fungi and bacteria and is also effective against the intestinal parasite *Entamoeba histolytica*. I have also seen particularly good results when using turmeric to treat infections related to the liver, bile duct, and gallbladder. Turmeric is also an excellent anti-inflammatory herb (see page 256).

Tea tree oil. Consumers of tea tree oil can thank New South Wales, Australia, for this wonderful oil, because that is the only place that the tea tree *(Melaleuca alternifolia)* is native. It is an impossible oil to miss because of its almost overpowering aroma. **Tea tree oil is used topically for a wide variety of skin infections. There is convincing research for its use with acne, athlete's foot, and nail fungus infections.** Vaginal yeast infections can also be treated with this oil; studies showing its effectiveness for this condition have typically used a tampon or sponge pad saturated with a 40% tea tree oil solution.

Amino Acids

Lysine. Although it is not very common to see an amino acid like lysine listed as an antibiotic, it should be considered in this context because of its role in treating infections from HSV-1 and HSV-2. There is some controversy in this area about effectiveness, but I believe most of the conflicting research results are explained by too-low doses of supplemental lysine or inadequate shifting of the diet to obtain a strong lysine-to-arginine ratio. Generally, 1 gram of supplemental lysine 3 times a day seems to be the level needed to help with this kind of viral infection. Lysine appears to work better in the prevention and treatment of oral herpes, usually caused by HSV-1, and less so with genital herpes, which is usually HSV-2.

ANTI-INFLAMMATORIES

This category of natural supplements may not be readily familiar, but I encourage people to consider it. Basically, any health problem ending with -*itis* can involve inflammation—for example, arthritis (inflammation of the joints) or pruritis (itchy skin inflammation). All inflammation is a response to injury of some kind, but this injury does not have to be physical. For some people, stress is enough to cause inflammation. Many over-the-counter medicines are popular anti-inflammatories, including aspirin and cortisone-containing skin creams. However, most of these products are formulated on a one-size-fits-all basis and do not take into account the exact type of injury that is responsible for the inflammation. This section details some natural alternatives in this regard.

There is a final distinction to make about the use of anti-inflammatory supplements. We can remain basically healthy and develop an inflammatory condition that has a specific cause and needs healing, and often we will heal more readily with some supplementation. Below I point out which types of supplements are best used in this context. But on the flipside, our general health can also become compromised to the point that our inflammatory response takes over too much of our basic metabolic energy and the body gets caught up in a proinflammatory pattern—even when there is no real cause for the inflammation. In this situation, we need to approach our anti-inflammatory supplementation a little differently. For example, I have found Siberian ginseng (*Eleutherococcus senticosus*) can sometimes be helpful for chronic fatigue, along with whole root licorice.

Anti-inflammatory Nutritionals

Nutrients	Herbs
Bromelain	Aloe vera
Carotenoids	Echinacea
Flavonoids	Garlic
Magnesium salicylate	Ginger
	Licorice
Amino Acids	Turmeric
Glutamine	
Lysine	

Anti-inflammatory Nutrients

Bromelain. This sulfur-containing enzyme from the pineapple has been used by clinicians for almost 50 years in the treatment of inflammatory problems, and there is some solid research backing its effective-

ness. Researchers know, for example, that bromelain can turn down the volume on inflammatory processes by blocking production of molecules that trigger inflammation (like prostaglandin E2). The most impressive applications of bromelain are for respiratory tract problems like chronic bronchitis or sinusitis.

Carotenoids. The carotenoid nutrients—including alpha-carotene, beta-carotene, cryptoxanthin, lycopene, lutein, and zeaxanthin—have been getting a lot of press lately, especially as cancer-protective and heart-protective antioxidant nutrients. They have not yet been proven to prevent inflammation, however, except perhaps in the skin, but they clearly get depleted as a result of inflammation and need to be replaced or supplemented alongside of chronic inflammatory problems. Researchers know that the inflammatory process can be quieted down in this way, because they have tried cartenoid supplementation in rheumatoid arthritis—a classic inflammatory condition—and have had success. Because high levels of beta-carotene, when supplemented alone, can decrease the body's supplies of lutein (an equally important carotenoid), I suggest supplementing the carotenoids as a family and including all of the important family members rather than focusing on an individual type. A common dose range for carotenoids is about 25,000 to 50,000 international units (IU) several times daily.

Flavonoids. Unlike carotenoids, which appear to be highly supportive but not directly anti-inflammatory in their effects, the flavonoids have been shown to directly counter inflammation. Some of the best research in this area involves the flavonoids quercetin, hesperidin, and rutin—all found in citrus fruits and in many other foods. **The flavonoids often reduce inflammation by blocking synthesis of messenger molecules that promote inflammation.** These messenger molecules, called *proinflammatory* molecules, are needed for the body to engage in a full inflammatory response. The proinflammatory prostaglandins are especially important in triggering inflammation, and it is precisely these molecules that the flavonoids can help shut down.

Magnesium salicylate. This nutrient combination is sold over-the-counter; you may have seen it in the drugstore sold as a backache relief medication. It is classified as a nonsteroidal anti-inflammatory drug (NSAID). There is also a prescription form of magnesium salicylate that adds choline to the mix, forming choline magnesium salicylate. Salicylates are found in many over-the-counter products, including aspirin (acetylsalicylic acid). I like the idea of bringing both choline and magnesium into the picture when dealing with inflammation, but I do not see salicylic acid as a supportive nutrient so much as a symptom-suppressing kind of chemical. In addition, some people are sensitive to salicylates in medicines and in foods.

Anti-inflammatory Herbs

The list of herbs with anti-inflammatory properties is a fairly long one. Most of the herbs seem to impact the inflammatory process in the same basic way—by turning down the volume on inflammation. **They accomplish this feat by altering the levels of molecules that stimulate inflammation.** (These molecules include cytokines, eicosanoids, transcription factors, and enzymes.) Included on my list of anti-inflammatory herbs would be aloe, astragalus, boswellia, cohosh, devil's claw, echinacea, feverfew, garlic, horse chestnut, lomatium, maitake mushroom, marigold, Oregon grape, pokeroot, reishi mushroom, shiitake mushroom, stinging nettle, St. John's wort, and willow (such as white willow bark). Some of these herbs also work to reduce the consequences of inflammation, especially damage to the linings of organs or blood vessels. Below I single out a few of these anti-inflammatory herbs because of their special considerations.

Aloe vera. The most common use of aloe vera is the application of its gel (the inside of the leaf) for burns. This is very soothing, and many people experience reduced inflammation and blistering as well as more rapid healing. Aloe is somewhat unique in containing the anti-inflammatory fatty acids gamma-linolenic acid (GLA) and eicosatetraenoic acid (ETA).

Echinacea. Echinacea root, most often as the species *Echinacea angustifolia* (Kansas snakeroot, purple coneflower), has been a popular medicine with American herbalists for more than a century. They have used it in the treatment of various infections, fevers, snake and insect bites, and many skin problems, such as acne, boils, abscesses, and ulcers. More recently, echinacea has become popular with the general public, mostly for cold and flu prevention, treatment of infections, and purification of the blood and lymph. For treating skin problems, most natural practitioners feel that blood purification is important. Michael Tierra, in his popular book *The Way of Herbs,* calls echinacea the "king of blood purifiers." The availability of fine-quality tinctures and powdered root extracts has made the bitter echinacea more easily accessible.

Recent experiments have shown that echinacea root can increase the white blood count and thus the body's ability to handle bacteria and viruses, stimulate the important T lymphocytes' activity, and generally stimulate the lymphatic system to clear wastes. The immune-supporting aspect of this valuable herb makes it effective in the treatment of mild infections, such as vaginitis and prostatitis, poison oak and poison ivy, acne and boils, and respiratory infections. Although more research is needed to verify its effectiveness, many people describe a very good response to taking echinacea root products, either singly or in combination with other purifying, anti-infectious herbs and vitamins. Although echinacea use appears basically nontoxic, until more research can clarify its safety, **I do not advise extended use for more than 3 or 4 weeks due to such possible effects as liver irritation or changes in the normal intestinal flora.**

Garlic. Recent research has demonstrated clear anti-inflammatory properties for garlic. The route of action is complex and involves alteration of immune system messages and quieting of the molecule NF-kappa B. In the future, expect to hear much more about garlic's anti-inflammatory benefits, with likely application to conditions like inflammatory bowel disease.

Ginger. Ginger has been used in studies of osteoarthritis and rheumatism to reduce several aspects of inflammation, including swelling and joint pain. One study comparing ginger to ibuprofen showed no significant results in favor of ginger, but it did show both ibuprofen and ginger to provide benefits. In ayurvedic medicine, ginger has a long history of use as an anti-inflammatory. Ginger may lessen inflammation by lowering the levels of messaging molecules (thromboxanes and leukotrienes) that trigger inflammation in the first place.

Licorice. Licorice likely has the most celebrated herbal past, extending thousands of years, beginning in the Orient and progressing around the world. It has many actions and clearly many uses. **Also known as sweetwood or sweetroot, the "great detoxifier," and the "great peacemaker," this root contains many steroid-like chemicals related to adrenal and ovarian secretions.** Historically, it was used for colds and coughs, and it has become popular as a laxative and for use in children, who tolerate its sweet flavor more readily than bitter herbs, with such problems as fevers, colds, and constipation.

Licorice root has many apparent actions. It is a cough suppressant and an expectorant, an anti-inflammatory and an antiarthritic, an antitoxic (through liver support and protection) and an antibiotic, possibly an anticancer herb (recent research has shown licorice to have an inhibitory effect in some tumor growth), and a laxative. It also acts as a demulcent and emollient, meaning it softens and soothes tissues and mucous membranes. Licorice further offers adrenal support with its mineralocorticoid-like substances, and it contains such estrogenic chemicals as beta-sitosterol and stigmasterol. Its adrenal stimulation allows licorice to be an antistress herb, to be helpful in such inflammatory problems as arthritis, and to be useful to those with hypoglycemia, a problem related to weak adrenals.

The estrogenic support allows its use in women as a sexual and uterine tonic and for problems of infertility. Licorice root has also been used as a stomach and intestinal remedy for such problems as indigestion, nausea, and constipation; for infections of the respiratory tract, including colds and flus, and for hoarseness, sore throat, and wheezing; in patients with hepatitis, ulcers, and hemorrhoids; for skin problems; for muscle spasms and fevers associated with sweating; and for general weakness. Licorice has also been suggested for people with high blood pressure, yet there is concern in this use because excessive intake can elevate blood pressure.

It appears that the whole root or deglycyrrhizinated licorice (DGL) is safe and has the positive attributes of licorice extract without side effects. DGL has been the subject of recent interest and research, and it apparently helps in healing ulcers. Usually, licorice root is used in herbal combinations, not by itself; it balances the flavor of these formulas. In Chinese herbology, licorice is among the most commonly used herbs, along with ginger. It is available in hard roots, soft ground roots, powdered in capsules, in elixirs, and as DGL. The dosage would be as recommended on the product or in an herbal text.

Turmeric. This much-loved spice has come up with glowing reports as an anti-inflammatory. Most of the focus has been centered on curcumin, a curcuminoid polyphenol found in turmeric. Curcumin gets its name from the scientific name for turmeric, *Curcuma longa.* This plant is a member of the ginger family and shares some of its anti-inflammatory properties with that spice as well. Like ginger, turmeric lowers the level of messaging molecules that trigger inflammation. It also lowers levels of nitric oxide and is associated with a more favorable overall balance of immune system messaging molecules (called *cytokines*). In the coming years, I expect to see more research on turmeric in relation to lower bowel problems, including colitis and inflammatory bowel syndrome.

Anti-inflammatory Amino Acids

Glutamine. I have included glutamine as an anti-inflammatory because of its track record in the digestive tract. **Glutamine is the preferred fuel of cells lining the small intestine, and so it is already widely used for intestinal support outside of its anti-inflammatory properties.** Supplementation of this amino acid has also been tried in the lower bowel with colitis and inflammatory bowel syndrome, and there is evidence that glutamine can help lower levels of messaging molecules like IL-8, which stands for interleukin-8, an immune messaging molecule that is generally regarded as increasing inflammation in the lower intestine. Part of the difficulty with oral glutamine supplementation, however, appears to be getting a sufficient amount of glutamine all the way down to the lower intestine; some animal studies have begun to look at delivery of glutamine via enema or suppository as a way of improving its effectiveness.

Lysine. Although lysine has not clearly been shown to be an anti-inflammatory in its own right, researchers know that it can help decrease some aspects of inflammation when added onto other molecules. For example, when added onto aspirin, lysine can improve aspirin's anti-inflammatory effects in heart disease patients. Lysine is often included in anti-inflammatory supplements for this reason.

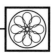

ANTIOXIDANTS

Health-care professionals, researchers, and consumers all need to update their thinking in the absolutely critical area of antioxidant supplements. In the 1980s, when antioxidants made their big-time debut in the marketplace, many professionals and consumers alike characterized these supplements as the good guys that the body desperately needs to do battle with free radicals caused by pollution, bad lifestyle habits, and crummy food, including food with chemical additives and hydrogenated fats. We figured that the most problematic lifestyle habits—like heavy cigarette smoking—would call for the most aggressive antioxidant supplementation, and so we started out the 1990s by launching a series of large-scale research studies involving smokers, heart patients, and other population groups to test out this theory about antioxidants.

Unfortunately, researchers did not get the results they had expected. Since the mid-1990s, several of these major studies have been canceled before completion because of problems caused by antioxidant supplementation. Some individuals receiving high-dose antioxidant supplements actually got worse. These studies included the Alpha-Tocopherol, Beta-Carotene and Cancer (ATBC) Prevention Study, with 29,000 subjects; the Physicians' Health Study (PHS), with 22,000 subjects, and the Carotene and Retinol Efficacy Trial (CARET) study, with 18,000 subjects.

There is still plenty of debate about what happened in these studies. The 1990s sent a message that we need to take heed with antioxidants and the way they work. Antioxidants are not simply the good guys— that is, they do not go off and do battle with anything. In fact, we probably should not even be using the word *antioxidants* in the first place. **What antioxidants do is shuffle energy, or electrons. They keep energy flowing in a way that prevents damage to the cells and tissue.** I like to think of antioxidants as participants in a game of hot potato, where all of the antioxidants are standing around in a circle. In the real game of hot potato, the object of the game is to pass the potato very quickly from person to person so that no one's hands get burned. Everything works just fine as long as the hot potato keeps moving from person to person. Well, it's the same with antioxidants. The circle of antioxidants must be large and unbroken, so that no single antioxidant is called on to touch the potato too often. Of course, the potato must also be kept moving at all times.

During the 1990s, not a single antioxidant food study was canceled or produced negative results. The only canceled studies involved relatively high doses of a single antioxidant (or a few isolated antioxidants)— but never a diverse group of antioxidants or antioxidants supplied through food. One message here seems pretty likely: there were not enough antioxidants standing around in the circle to keep energy flowing smoothly, and researchers may not have understood exactly which antioxidants were needed to help fill in the empty spots in the circle.

Antioxidant Nutrients and Herbs

Nutrients

Vitamin C

Vitamin E

NADH

Selenium

Sulfur

Carotenoids

Lutein

Flavonoids (quercetin, hesperidin, rutin, etc.)

Glutathione and N-acetyl cysteine (NAC)

Lipoic acid

Butylated hydroxytoluene (BHT)

Coenzyme Q_{10} (CoQ_{10})

Carnosine

Catalase

Glutathione peroxidase

Superoxide dismutase

Herbs

Aloe vera

Bilberry

Garlic

Ginkgo

Green tea

Hawthorn

Milk thistle

Wolfberry, Mangosteen, Gac (spiny bitter cucumber), and Goji berries

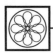

It has been mind-boggling to watch the list of antioxidant nutrients grow. In the 1980s researchers thought that the list of antioxidant nutrients was relatively limited to such well-known substances as vitamin C, vitamin E, or zinc. But now we know that the most active antioxidant in the bloodstream is uric acid, and that there are literally thousands of antioxidant pigments in plants that in some cases do not even exist except in a single type of plant. The world of antioxidants has opened up dramatically, as has the shelf space devoted to them in groceries, pharmacies, and natural food stores.

Antioxidant Nutrients

There is a select group of nutrients that are particularly active participants in the antioxidant game of electron hot potato, headed by five antioxidants: vitamin E, vitamin C, glutathione, lipoic acid, and NAD (a special form of vitamin B3, or niacin). As the game continues, however, each of these antioxidants must also be recycled, and 4 additional nutrients are required for this recycling: carotenoids, flavonoids, selenium, and sulfur. I discuss more about each of these 9 antioxidants in just a moment, but here I want to emphasize the importance of this core group when forming the antioxidant circle that allows energy to flow smoothly in the body's cells.

Vitamins E, C, and NADH. In chapter 5, Vitamins, I discuss these critical antioxidant vitamins, including the tocopherols and tocotrienols (forms of vitamin E), ascorbates and ascorbate esters (forms of vitamin C), and NADH (a bioactive form of vitamin B3). Vitamins E and C actually participate in each other's recycling. NADH plays a direct role in the recycling of lipoid acid. Although more recent attention has been focused on some of the other antioxidant supplements, maintaining an optimal supply of these three vitamins is critical for the body's antioxidant balance. Therapeutic doses of vitamin C range from about 1 to 10 grams daily; for vitamin E, 400 to 1,200 IU daily; and for NADH, 10-mg capsules twice daily.

Selenium and sulfur. Both of these minerals are critical for antioxidant balance. In the case of selenium, it is the recycling of glutathione that researchers are most concerned about. In the case of sulfur, it is the structure of lipoic acid and cysteine that come into play, because both require the presence of sulfur. I discuss these minerals in detail—including their antioxidant function—in chapter 6, Minerals. A common therapeutic dose range for selenium is 150 to 200 mcg daily. We usually obtain our sulfur through the amino acids methionine, cysteine, and taurine, or through organic acids like lipoic acid. Methylsulfonylmethane (MSM), dimethylsulfoxide (DMSO), and mineral chelates containing sulfur (like magnesium sulfate) are other supplemental forms of sulfur. When obtaining supplemental sulfur in the form of amino acids, a typical dose range is 1 to 5 grams of sulfur-containing amino acids daily.

Carotenoids. Carotenoids have already made an appearance in the chapter as helpful anti-inflammatory nutrients. **Although there are more than 600 fully identified carotenoids, the six best-researched are alpha-carotene, beta-carotene, cryptoxanthin, lycopene, lutein, and zeaxanthin.** All of these function as antioxidants as well. One member of this group—beta-carotene—took a pretty good beating in the late 1990s, when several large-scale supplementation trials showed high levels of beta-carotene to be harmful rather than helpful. Such studies as the Carotene and Retinol Efficacy Trial (CARET) are still the subject of much controversy. I include myself among the group of skeptics who are not convinced that it was beta-carotene per se that caused harm, however. From my perspective, it is clear that the carotenoids have important antioxidant functions in the body. It is just as clear that their antioxidant capacity depends on many factors, including how they get incorporated into cell membranes and how they interact with other antioxidants, like vitamins E and C. Because many theories of aging involve a free-radical component, it is not surprising that research studies on aging and carotenoids show benefits of higher carotenoid intake—for example, greater intake of tomatoes that contain the carotenoid lycopene. The antioxidant properties of lycopene undoubtedly account for much of this benefit. The ability of carotenoids to act as antioxidants is also related to decreased risk of certain cancers, like esophageal cancer, associated with the intake of such high-carotenoid foods as tomatoes.

Lutein. Lutein is another carotenoid that deserves special mention because of its antioxidant relationship to our eyesight. **The macular region of the eye is actually yellow in color because three carotenoids—lutein, zeaxanthin, and mesozeaxanthin—are found there in very high amounts.** This carotenoid-filled layer protects the underlying cells from damage by absorbing blue light and preventing free-radical formation. As we age, this macular layer tends to thin in a process called *age-related macular degeneration.* This is the primary cause of blindness in old age. Supplements containing lutein can help rebuild the macular layer, as can foods that are high in lutein and other carotenoids, such as dark green leafy vegetables.

For beta-carotene, a minimum of about 25,000 IU a day is recommended for antioxidant protection. For lycopene, the equivalent dose is about 25 to 30 mg daily. For lutein, a minimum dose would be 20 to 40 mcg, but in the case of macular degeneration, rebuilding of the macular layer may require a much higher level of intake in the range of 5 mg per day.

Flavonoids. You might notice that flavonoids pop up throughout this chapter—they are substances with a wide range of health benefits, and their antioxidant properties are high up on the list. More than 4,000 different flavonoids are known to exist in the plant world, and most of the flavonoids that have been researched to date function as antioxidants. Some also turn out to function as pro-oxidants, however. **This means they can promote oxidation and free-radical formation just as much as they can prevent it.** (Two of the flavonoids found in citrus fruit—naringenin and chalconaringenin—fall into this category.) We don't need to worry about this pro-oxidant potential when it comes to food, but when supplementing, we need to think about getting a balance and a wider variety of flavonoids rather than large doses of 1 or 2 molecules.

A unique feature of flavonoids in comparison with other antioxidants like vitamin C and E is the potential for us to consume high levels in our diet. We might easily get 500 to 1,000 mg of total flavonoids in our food if we consume substantial amounts of fresh fruits and vegetables. It would be difficult for us to get anywhere near this amount for vitamins C or E. When our intake of fruits and vegetables is healthy, we are much less likely to need supplemental forms of these phytonutrients.

Quercetin, hesperidin, and rutin are the most common flavonoid antioxidants not obtained from herbs. They are usually obtained from citrus fruit (mainly from the white, inner rind), but they are also found in many other sources, including blue-green algae, onion, and eucalyptus. Most of the other antioxidant flavonoids are derived from herbs (see the section below on antioxidant herbs).

Glutathione and N-acetyl-cysteine (NAC). Few antioxidants have received as much attention since the mid-1990s as glutathione. This much-heralded substance is a tripeptide, a proteinlike molecule made up of three amino acids—cysteine, glutamic acid, and glycine. Of these three, perhaps the most valued of the group is cysteine, because deficiency of this amino acid tends to have the most negative impact on formation of glutathione. In some studies, supplementation with cysteine is sometimes more effective in boosting the body's glutathione supply than supplementation with glutathione itself. **The NAC form of the amino acid seems most effective in boosting the body's glutathione supply.**

In order to act as an antioxidant, glutathione has to cycle back and forth between two forms. In one form (called the reduced form, sometimes abbreviated GSH), glutathione has its full antioxidant function. Once it has interacted with other molecules, including free radicals, glutathione gets switched over to its oxidized form (sometimes abbreviated GSSG). **It takes selenium to help recycle glutathione back to its reduced form.** This distinction is important, because we want supplements containing glutathione in its reduced (optimal antioxidant) form. My recommendation is to take l-cysteine 250 mg twice daily, NAC 500 mg 2 to 3 times daily, or glutathione 60 to 100 mg twice daily.

Lipoic acid. Also called *alpha-lipoic acid* or *thioctic acid,* lipoic acid is an amazingly underappreciated antioxidant. R-lipoic acid may have even better antioxidant function, and this new product is being researched. This relatively small, sulfur-containing molecule is unique in being able to scavenge free radicals in both fat-soluble and water-soluble environments. It was first shown to help prevent scurvy, just like vitamin C. (It does this by helping to recycle vitamin C.) I think of lipoic acid as working alongside of glutathione, because hydrogen peroxide, a key oxygen compound neutralized by glutathione (through glutathione peroxidase, or GPO), is one of the few reactive oxygen compounds *not* altered by lipoic acid. (Hydroxyl radicals and singlet oxygen are the key free radicals that lipoic acid helps to neutralize.) Minimal dose ranges for lipoic acid fall into the 50 to 75 mg range, although 100 to 600 mg is the dose range in many studies looking at potential benefits for diabetes, cataracts, and glaucoma. Lipoic acid is also used in creams for skin protection.

Additional Antioxidant Supplements

In addition to the core group of antioxidants just described, several others are bound to catch your attention. The information in this section can help you decide when (and when not) to consider these supplements in your own nutritional program.

Butylated hydroxytoluene (BHT). Although not as popular as it once was, BHT as a dietary supplement has been valued for its antioxidant properties and has sometimes been used in the treatment of herpes. Few studies have come out since the mid-1980s on the use of BHT with herpes, but older animal studies showed that this antioxidant could be used topically, or orally, to help reduce infection. In addition, the effectiveness of BHT was linked to its impact on the virus's fat-coated membrane, which could be disrupted by BHT. Some of the reluctance to use this antioxidant, however, may be related to its potential for toxicity. BHT is a widely used food preservative, and it is included on the FDA's Generally Recognized as Safe (GRAS) list of foods. **However, it clearly has toxic potential and needs further study with respect to *Herpes simplex* as well as other health conditions.**

Coenzyme Q10 (CoQ10)—ubiquinone. Coenzyme Q is a greatly underappreciated substance that is both made by our bodies and obtained in the diet, mainly in oily fish (like mackerel, salmon, and sardines), organ meats (like liver, kidney, and heart), and, to a lesser extent, the germs of whole grains. In chemical terms, CoQ10 has a 6-ring structure and a long tail that has 10 pieces. Coenzyme Q7 has 7, and

so on. The conventional wisdom has been to buy this supplement with all 10 pieces and let the body decide whether to chop some off and make CoQ7, and so on. This does not seem like a bad strategy to me, but some day researchers may know more about the exact form needed for specific health problems.

CoQ is a mainstay of the energy production process in the body's cells. Our cells have trouble generating energy without CoQ, particularly when those cells are in organs that are highly active in terms of energy and oxygen processing. The heart is our number-one organ in this regard, and has almost twice the CoQ concentration of any other organ. Therefore, it is not surprising that heart problems are the number-one spot for supplementing with CoQ. **The list of heart problems that have been helped by CoQ supplementation include angina, arrhythmias, cardiomyopathy, congestive heart failure, and mitral valve prolapse.** I strongly recommend taking CoQ when high cholesterol is being treated with lovastatin (Mevacor) or another one of the statin drugs (pravastatin, simvastatin, and so on). While these drugs can be helpful in lowering cholesterol, they also block the body's production of CoQ. There is research on the use of CoQ with other chronic health problems, including cancer (especially breast cancer), diabetes, obesity, AIDS, muscular dystrophy, and infertility. Although some of these areas may hold much promise for the use of CoQ, none are as well established as the heart disease area at this point in time.

Doses for CoQ range widely, from about 30 to 100 mg per day. Although general support calls for a dosage of about 30 mg divided up into three 10 mg doses spread throughout the day, more typical amounts are 30 to 50 mg 2 or 3 times daily. With the more severe cardiovascular problems, the required amount often seems to be substantially greater. People are also supplementing about 100 to 300 mg for cancer concerns.

Carnosine. Researchers are just beginning to get the full picture on this relative newcomer to the antioxidant scene. Carnosine is a dipeptide consisting of the amino acids alanine and histidine. It is found mainly in animal muscle, making beef the number-one dietary source, followed by chicken. Carnosine can neutralize certain free radicals in the body, including peroxyl radicals, and it can help protect cell structures from potential oxygen damage in this way. There is an equally interesting theme related to carnosine involving its antioxidant activities and aging. One problem commonly associated with aging involves the excessive attachment of sugars to cell proteins. (These overly sugared proteins are called *advanced glycation end products,* or AGEs.) We know that they play a role not only in the aging process, but also in development of adult-onset diabetes. Carnosine can help prevent formations of AGEs and may turn out to be preventive in development of chronic conditions like diabetes or Alzheimer's disease in later life.

There is a second form of carnosine, called *anserine,* that is also available in the marketplace. Anserine is a methylated form of carnosine. Researchers do not know enough about anserine yet to decide about its usefulness as a supplement, but I would be surprised if it did not turn out to have useful applications. Dose ranges for carnosine vary widely. In some studies, as little as 50 mg of carnosine daily have been used to help prevent oxidative damage to tissue in adult subjects. At the same time, 800 mg of carnosine have been used to improve function in children diagnosed with autism. I consider the 100 to 500 mg per day range to be an appropriate starting place under most circumstances.

Catalase. Catalase is an iron-containing enzyme that is found throughout the body. It seems designed to prevent hydrogen peroxide from building up inside the cells because it converts hydrogen peroxide into oxygen and water. Although it is not used widely in supplements, it is found in antioxidant formulas, usually together with the enzyme superoxide dismutase (SOD). There is very little research on catalase supplementation. However, there is some evidence of its ability to protect the intestine and the eyes from certain kinds of oxidative damage. A typical dose of catalase would be about 20 mcg per day.

Glutathione peroxidase (GPO). When it comes to reactive oxygen molecules and avoiding oxygen-based damage to the body's cells, GPO is critical. This enzyme takes hydrogen peroxide and converts it into water. The enzyme itself contains four atoms of selenium (a micromineral often found in antioxidant supplements). In order to function, GPO also needs to have a supply of vitamin B3 (in a special form called

NADP) as well as glutathione itself. You seldom see this enzyme itself in antioxidant supplements, but research has clearly shown that supplemental selenium can increase GPO activity in individuals who have selenium deficiency.

Superoxide dismutase (SOD, MnSOD, Cu/ZnSOD). SOD is an interesting enzyme nutrient. In the body, it exists in two forms. Cu/ZnSOD is the form of SOD in cellular fluids. The Cu/Zn refers to the minerals copper and zinc, which are required for this SOD to function. The ratio of copper to zinc allows this form of SOD to work properly, which is among the reasons why many antioxidant formulations include both copper and zinc. The second form of SOD is MnSOD, with Mn referring to manganese, the mineral required for this second type of SOD to work properly. MnSOD is found exclusively in mitochondria, the oxygen-based energy production factories in cells. Both forms of SOD are important for health. **SOD is critical in controlling free-radical levels, because it can take a potent free radical, called a *superoxide anion radical,* and convert it into hydrogen peroxide.** Although hydrogen peroxide can still cause problems, it is far less dangerous than superoxide radicals. Of course, MnSOD needs plenty of available manganese to carry out this conversion, just as Cu/ZnSOD needs ample supplies of copper and zinc.

Like most of the antioxidant enzymes, you won't find SOD being used directly in most supplements. Although orally ingested enzymes are likely to have some activity in the digestive tract, their ability to be absorbed intact and be transported where the body needs them is questionable and has not been documented in research. Some animal-research studies, however, show both oral and intravenously administered SOD being helpful in treatment of radiation-induced fibrosis, stroke, and severe burns from mustard gas. An amount of 350 to 500 mg is a common dose range for most SOD products currently in the marketplace.

Although good research on direct supplementation of the SOD enzymes is lacking, there is evidence that supplementation with copper, zinc, and manganese can improve SOD function in people with these mineral deficiencies.

Antioxidant Herbs

Aloe vera. Only since 2000 have researchers begun to identify antioxidant compounds in aloe, even though we have know for a while that aloe extracts contain SOD enzymes and anthraquinones that can help protect cell membranes from free-radical damage. Expect to hear more about antioxidant uses of this herb in the near future.

Bilberry. As far as we know, it is the flavonoid composition of bilberry that lets it function as an antioxidant herb. **The anthocyanosides in this herb, for example, have been shown to be helpful in supporting eye functions, and it is possible that this support involves antioxidant balance.**

Garlic. The anticancer activities of garlic are not as well defined as its heart supportive ones, yet the research here is promising. Three different cancer-preventive or cancer-treating roles for garlic have been proposed. The first involves its ability to neutralize oxygen radicals in the tissue. Aged garlic extracts are especially interesting here, because the molecules in garlic that have the most powerful radical-neutralizing effects only form as the garlic is aged.

Ginkgo. Ginkgo is one of the better-researched herbs in terms of its antioxidant function. Although known to have benefits for the circulatory system and the eyes (including many eye problems related to aging, such as cataracts and macular degeneration), the application I am most excited about involves the brain and the nervous system. Preventing free-radical damage in these areas seems to be a special talent of ginkgo's, and it may be turn out to be particularly important in the treatment of chronic neurodegenerative problems like Alzheimer's and senile dementia.

Green tea. The green tea polyphenols, including epicatechin and epigallocatechin, have an impressive history of research and use as antioxidants. Green tea extracts can be taken orally or used topically. **There is good evidence that green tea extracts can help prevent oxidative damage from excess exposure of the skin to UVB radiation.** Prevention of skin cancer has also been associated with the intake of green tea. There has also been some suggestion that the use of green tea to improve recovery from alcohol intoxication involves the antioxidant capacity of its polyphenols. Drink 1 to 2 cups daily. Because the antioxidant benefits of green tea do not involve the presence of caffeine, people sensitive to caffeine can buy a decaf form of green tea and still get the antioxidant benefits.

Hawthorn. Hawthorn primarily is a cardiovascular herb and it can be helpful in improving circulation and strengthening the heart. I include it here because it contains an impressive array of antioxidant phytonutrients, including phenols, proanthocyanidins, catechins, and flavonoids. Its support of the cardiovascular system definitely includes the ability of these antioxidants to protect blood vessel linings.

Milk thistle. Milk thistle's well-researched antioxidant properties are largely due to one of its unique flavonoids, silymarin. Amazingly, this flavonoid (undoubtedly along with other phytonutrients in milk thistle) can help increase the glutathione levels in liver cells by as much as 50%. **Thus it is common for people with liver diseases or those taking any drugs that may stress the liver to supplement with milk thistle, typically about 60 to 100 mg twice daily.** I have also seen milk thistle used in clinical studies on animals to help neutralize free radicals that are damaging the bladder (in bladder cancer), the skin (in skin cancer), and the colon (in colon cancer). There is also some evidence that milk thistle might be helpful in preventing diabetes by helping to protect the cells of the pancreas from free-radical damage.

Wolfberry, mangosteen, gac, and goji. There are several other herbal extracts that are new on the market, namely Young Living's wolfberry, Nature's Sunshine's mangosteen (called Thai-Go), and Pharmanex's Gac Superfruit Blend. They are all quite yummy in taste and have touted very good antioxidant and energy-enhancing effects. All of these extracts are used juices. The wolfberry plant has many nutrients and bioflavonoids that support and protect tissues, much as bilberry does for the eyes and hawthorn berry does for the heart. Mangosteen also has purported strong antioxidant effects and the Thai-Go drink has other fruit extracts, including wolfberry. Gac juice is the newest to the market here but has been used by natives of Southeast Asia for centuries. This "fruit from heaven" is used for longevity and vitality. Siberian pineapple and Chinese lycium are also added to Pharmanex's product. Goji berries are also a popular antioxidant fruit.

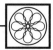

BONE AND JOINT STRENGTHENERS

Thanks to the National Dairy Council, most of us grew up with the impression that calcium, and specifically milk, was the key to strong bones and strong teeth. Unfortunately, it has never been quite that simple. Bones are complicated in their composition and have dozens of components that are every bit as essential as calcium. And when it comes to joints, where bones come together, the situation is even more complex. In this case it is fair to say that calcium plays a minor role in comparison with other nutrients. This section explores the way that bone and joint strengtheners work and covers several widely advertised and readily available substances.

Let's start out with the bones. Most people do not realize how active our bones are. The bone cells continuously exchange minerals and other substances with the rest of the body. This exchange needs to take place for the bones to stay healthy. Mineral exchange is important, because the bones are 70% mineral. But they are also 30% organic and include collagen and noncollagen proteins. **Most of bone's mineral matrix is formed from a substance called *hydroxyapatite*, which consists mostly of calcium and phosphorus.** Excess phosphates in the diet (like the phosphoric acid that is added to many soft drinks) can disrupt this calcium/phosphorus balance and be harmful to bones. Many mineral supplements can help support bone integrity, including calcium, phosphorus, magnesium, boron, silicon, and, to a lesser extent, zinc, copper, and manganese. Among the vitamins, D is most important when it comes to bone strengthening, because calcium is better absorbed into bones when supplemented with vitamin D. Vitamin K also comes into play here, because it is necessary to make the correct form of osteocalcin, which is among the most important noncollagen proteins found in parts of bone. Problems with bone mineral balance can be increased during and after menopause, when cortical bone may begin to be lost at a rate of 2% to 3% per year, so this is a particularly important time to pay attention to possible nutrient supplementation. (See discussions of the various minerals in chapter 6 for how each mineral affects bone health.)

The joints are more complex in terms of nutrient involvement. The synovial cavity—the spot where most bones come together—is filled with a special fluid called *synovial fluid,* the composition of which is important to joint health. **Maintaining optimal intake of high-quality water is absolutely essential in this context.** When we supplement to strengthen our joints, we are often supplementing to increase the stability of the cartilage that lines the joint cavity. Chondroitin sulfate, glucosamine sulfate, galactosamine sulfate, dermatan sulfate, and keratan sulfate are especially important substances found in cartilage (especially the hyaline cartilage at the ends of the bones). All of these substances are chemically classified as glycosaminoglycans (or, in the older terminology, mucopolysaccharides).

Cartilage is not the only type of substance found in the joints, however. The connective tissue also includes many unique proteins, such as the collagen proteins, which are somewhat unusual in their balance of amino acids. About one-third of all the amino acids in collagen are glycine. Collagen is also especially rich in lysine and proline. These two amino acids have to be converted into a special form (hydroxylysine and hydroxyproline), and the enzyme that converts them requires vitamin C to operate. Thus proline, lysine, and vitamin C are often included in joint-strengthening formulas.

Bone and Joint Strengtheners

Mineral and Vitamin Nutrients

Boron	Manganese	Strontium
Calcium	Phosphorus	Vitamin D
Magnesium	Silicon	Vitamin C

Other Nutrients

Amino acids lysine and proline

Chondroitin sulfate

Glucosamine sulfate

Ipriflavone

Glycosaminoglycans (mucopolysaccharides)

Bone and Joint Support Nutrients

Supplemental amounts of vitamins and minerals in support of bone health really depend on a person's diet and other lifestyle factors. However, as a general rule, bone-strengthening supplements should contain a little bit over the DRI (Dietary Reference Intake) level for each nutrient. For calcium, this would mean about 1,200 mg a day; for magnesium, about 400 to 600 mg; for boron, about 3 to 5 mg; and for vitamin D, about 400 IU. I also personally recommend vitamin K supplementation in the case of osteoporosis and other bone problems, because this vitamin is needed to produce the correct form of osteocalcin, among the most plentiful noncollagen proteins found in parts of the bone. As little as 1 mg of K seems to show up as significant in the research on bone health.

Glycosaminoglycans (GAGs). The GAGs are essential for joint health as key components of cartilage, and there is plenty of evidence supporting their use in both osteoarthritis and degenerative joint disease. The doses in these studies involve about 1,500 mg of glucosamine sulfate (or a combination of GAGs) per day, often in three 500 mg capsules or tablets. I have often recommended 2,000 to 3,000 mg daily for acute joint inflammation with some success. Chondroitin sulfate does not appear to be highly absorbed and thus may not be so advantageous; however, some patients experience better results with both chondroitin and glucosamine.

Ipriflavone. Particularly in menopausal and postmenopausal women, this flavonoid has shown promise for preventing or halting bone loss. Ipriflavone is not a naturally occurring flavonoid; rather, it is made in chemistry labs from daidzein, an isoflavone naturally occurring in soy. Ipriflavone helps calcium move back into the bones, and it also helps increase the effectiveness of a woman's existing estrogen supplies. A typical dosage of ipriflavone is about 600 mg per day, usually divided into 2 to 3 portions. Some bone-related uses of ipriflavone that may turn out to be unusually helpful include its possible use with Paget's disease and also with tinnitus (ringing in the ears) when that problem is caused by immobilization of the stapes bone in the ear.

CIRCULATORY AIDS

Supplements that support the circulatory system fall into two broad categories. **First are those products that focus on the integrity of the blood vessels.** These supplements might simply contain substances that help keep the blood vessels vital and functioning. But they might also contain antioxidant nutrients that help protect the blood vessels from damage, as researchers now believe that inflammation may be the primary culprit in the onset of atherosclerosis and cardiovascular disease. In addition to conventional nutrients like vitamin E, there are many phytonutrients (especially the flavonoids) found in plants that have been shown to provide extra protection for blood vessels.

The second kind of supplements targets blood flow itself. These may include substances that actually stimulate blood flow or substances that help the blood stay "clean"—that is, they keep the total amount of fat (in the form of triglycerides) and cholesterol (in the form of LDL cholesterol) in check. Because well over one-third of all deaths in the United States involve heart disease, supplementation in this area may turn out to be even more prevalent in the coming years.

Circulatory Aids	
Nutrients	**Herbs**
CoQ10	Alfalfa
B vitamins	Aloe vera
Vitamin E	Bilberry
Vitamin C	Cayenne
Magnesium	Coleus
	Garlic
	Ginger
	Ginkgo
	Horse chestnut
	Policosanol
	Red yeast rice

Circulatory Support Nutrients

Coenzyme Q (CoQ). Alongside of magnesium, CoQ would definitely qualify as one of my top-level recommendations for circulatory support. CoQ impacts the cardiovascular system in three basic ways. First, the heart is the body's most active aerobic organ, constantly engaging in oxygen-based energy production. **CoQ is essential for the mitochondria in the heart cells to keep producing energy.** Second, a key sub-

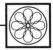

stance we circulate around through blood is oxygen, which brings along with it potential risk of blood vessel damage. CoQ functions as an antioxidant that can help prevent this damage. Third, lower levels of CoQ have been observed in persons with high blood pressure, and normalizing blood pressure is essential for healthy circulation.

There is another heart-related role of CoQ. Many individuals with high cholesterol have been given a statin drug to help reduce their levels. Although lovastatin (Mevacor) is the most common, similar drugs like atorvastatin (Lipitor) and simvastatin (Zocor) are also commonly used. These statin drugs shut down the body's ability to make CoQ, so people taking these prescription drugs should supplement with CoQ as long as they remain on these meds. The amount required here is about 50 to 150 mg per day. For general supplementation, however, the dose range would typically be 30 to 60 mg per day.

B vitamins. It is impossible to talk about circulatory support without mentioning the B vitamins. Vitamin B_6, vitamin B_{12}, and folate are especially important in controlling the level of homocysteine in the bloodstream. (Elevated homocysteine has been closely connected with circulatory problems, particularly atherosclerosis.) For these vitamins, a supplement containing about 200% of the DRI would generally be recommended. Read more about these important B vitamins in chapter 5, on pages 109–138.

Vitamin E. The cells found in the bloodstream and the walls of the blood vessels need continuous protection from free-radical damage. No single nutrient is more involved in their protection than vitamin E, which acts somewhat like a lightning rod on the cells, drawing the energy from the free radicals to itself and preventing it from damaging the other parts of the cell. A customary dose of vitamin E in relationship to circulatory support would be 200 to 800 IU. I recommend a supplement containing vitamin E in its variety of forms, including the mixed tocopherols and tocotrienols, not the synthetic (cheaper) dl-alpha-tocopherol acetate.

Vitamin C. This mainstay of antioxidant support is helpful alongside of vitamin E in protecting both the blood cells and the blood vessel linings. I tend to supplement here on the higher side, with my dose ranges varying from 300 to 1,000 mg per day for circulatory support, up to 2,000 mg day.

Magnesium. Magnesium has an impressive research track record relating to such cardiovascular problems as angina, arrhythmia, heart attack, and high blood pressure. This connection makes a good bit of common sense, because **magnesium is well-known as a muscle relaxant that can reduce the impact of stressors on the cardiovascular system.** Men in particular often have inadequate intake of magnesium, as do people who supplement with calcium alone. The dose range for circulatory support with magnesium is 200 to 400 mg per day, depending on dietary intake. The ratio of magnesium to calcium is also important to keep in mind. In most women, a 2:1 ratio of calcium to magnesium would be appropriate unless there is high blood pressure or menstrual cramps, where higher magnesium levels work better. For these situations and for most men, a 1:1 ratio is typically used. There are also instances where that ratio would be reversed, with a 2:1 ratio of magnesium to calcium. Most everyone's needs would fall somewhere in between these ratios, however.

Circulatory Support Herbs

Alfalfa. These little green tablets come from the very green plants with the prolific and deep root system so loved by rabbits. Alfalfa is actually a legume plant and contains the eight essential amino acids. It is also high in chlorophyll, vitamins A, D, B_6, and E, and some calcium and phosphorus. **Alfalfa is among the few foods with good levels of vitamin K, the blood-clotting vitamin.**

People who use alfalfa take it mainly as a natural supportive supplement for its nutrient content, much as they might take brewer's yeast or kelp. Alfalfa seeds are commonly sprouted, which are also highly nutritious. No grand claims are made for alfalfa, although recent research suggests that both the alfalfa plant and powdered alfalfa seed have a cholesterol-lowering and antiatherosclerotic effect. It is thought that the saponins contained in alfalfa help bind cholesterol and bile salts in the gut. High doses of alfalfa, 50 grams daily, were shown to reduce arterial plaques in monkeys. Some people are sensitive to alfalfa supplementation, and it has produced a lupuslike syndrome in monkeys. Overall, however, alfalfa is a safe and nutritious supplement.

Aloe vera. More full descriptions of aloe are in the "Antibiotic Herbs" and "Anti-inflammatory Herbs" sections of this chapter (on pages 250 and 255, respectively), but I wanted to mention it here because of its beta-sitosterol content. Like its name suggests, beta-sitosterol closely resembles cholesterol, and its presence allows an enzyme called LCAT (lecithin-cholesterol acyltransferase) to process more cholesterol and eliminate it from the bloodstream. Scientists have known about the cholesterol-lowering effects of beta-sitosterol since about the mid-1970s. Campesterol and stigmasterol may have the same cholesterol-lowering ability as beta-sitosterol. As a good source of beta-sitosterol, aloe can be used to help support the circulatory system by keeping the blood cholesterol levels in check. It is also possible to supplement with beta-sitosterol directly, and a typical dose range is 100 to 300 mg. **Until further research is available, however, beta-sitosterol supplementation should be avoided by women who are pregnant or nursing.**

Bilberry. This herb's support specialty is the veins and capillaries. Capillaries are the smallest of our blood vessels, where actual exchange of nutrients takes place with the cells' tissues. The anthocyanosides in bilberry help restore proper capillary function. Included in this category are cyanidin, delphinidin, malvidin, petunidin, and sometimes bilberry extracts are standardized for this anthocyanoside content. Some promising applications of bilberry involve the brain, where ability to support circulation may be able to improve neurological function. Bilberry, also included on page 262 in the "Antioxidants" section of this chapter, supports circulation by providing protection for the blood vessels.

Cayenne. If you like life a little spicy, try some cayenne pepper. It can be taken in capsules or as powder in water or used in cooking. Also called *capsicum* (the Latin name is *Capsicum frutescens*) or African bird pepper, it is the most useful of the red peppers and **among the true natural stimulants for both energy and metabolism.** Cayenne pepper, actually a small red berry from the *Capsicum annum* or *C. frutescens* plants, creates heat when taken into the body, but it is not irritating or burning. Blood flow in the brain and digestive system and skin is known to be stimulated by the capsaicin found in cayenne. In animal studies, cayenne has been shown to lower blood fat levels when a high-fat diet is consumed and also to decrease risk of atherosclerosis. Supplemental doses of cayenne vary widely between 100 and 500 mg. In topical form, capsaicin-containing creams should usually contain about 0.075% capsaicin. In the diet, of course, we are free to include cayenne peppers up to our individual level of heat tolerance!

Coleus. This member of the mint family is getting more attention in the supplement marketplace, and for good reason. One of its main constituents, forskolin, has been studied medicinally for more than thirty years. (Forskolin takes its name from the plant itself, which in the Latin naming system is *Coleus forskohlii*.) The circulatory effects of coleus are by far the best researched. This herb has been proven helpful in treating angina, congestive heart failure, high blood pressure, and general vascular insufficiency. Forskolin is a key part of this herb's circulatory support, because it can help relax the blood vessels by increasing levels of cyclic adenosine monophosphate (cAMP) in many different cell types. **Forskolin also helps prevent platelet cells from clumping together in the blood and increasing the risk of clogged blood vessels.**

Garlic. Garlic seems to be an energy stimulant, helps circulation, and has amassed an impressive list of benefits related to the heart. A 10 mg daily dose of allicin, one of the sulfur-containing compounds in garlic, works over a period of about 4 to 6 weeks to lower total cholesterol, LDL cholesterol, and triglycerides between 10% and 15% and to raise HDL cholesterol by 5% to 10%. Garlic supplements taken over a 1- to 3-month period have been seen to lower blood pressure by about 11 points (systolic pressure) and 5 points (diastolic pressure). Because garlic can inhibit the clumping together of platelet cells in the blood, it can also decrease risk of clogged arteries and stroke. **Some constituents in garlic have antioxidant activities, and there is evidence that garlic can help prevent oxidation of LDL cholesterol—a landmark problem in the development of atherosclerosis.**

Ginger. Ginger root extracts as tea and capsules are very good for enhancing warmth and circulation in the body. Too much can cause profuse sweating (diaphoresis), which happened to me with the first strong cup of ginger tea that I drank. Ginger stimulates blood flow and has been used for nausea and motion sickness problems, supports digestion, and does many other good things. There is some preliminary research evidence that ginger acts as an antioxidant and that it can help lower cholesterol and prevent cardiovascular disease. It also inhibits platelet aggregation, a factor contributing to atherosclerosis and clotting problems. By decreasing the "stickiness" of platelets, ginger can help protect our cardiovascular health.

Ginkgo. One of the oldest living plant species is the ginkgo tree, estimated at more than 100 million years old. The leaves from this tree have a bilobal, brainlike appearance, hence the name. Though fairly new to Western culture, the leaves of the gingko tree have been used for centuries in the Orient for complaints associated with aging.

An extract of ginkgo biloba leaves has been tested and reported to be effective at reducing ischemic symptoms—vascular insufficiency associated with aging and atherosclerosis. **Ginkgo biloba appears to increase cerebral blood flow and thus help oxygenation; it also may inhibit platelet aggregation.** In a study of geriatric patients, ginkgo was shown to reduce symptoms of vertigo, memory loss, tinnitus, and headache. In a study of lower-limb claudication symptoms, ginkgo helped reduce pain and improve walking tolerance over the placebo group. Thus the use of gingko biloba extracts, which have been marketed in Europe for years, appears to help in both cerebral and peripheral arterial insufficiency.

Ginkgo biloba is easily absorbed and has no known toxicity. Either extracts or capsules can be used. Therapeutic amounts range from 40 to 200 mg taken 3 times daily. More research is needed to test the therapeutic value of gingko biloba. Its use in treating symptoms of Alzheimer's disease, other forms of dementia, and neurological and cardiovascular diseases, as well as its potential antioxidant effects, are some possible areas of investigation.

Horse chestnut. Not well studied in the United States but better researched in Europe, horse chestnut has been primarily used to help improve chronic venous insufficiency, in which blood flow back to the heart from the veins is impaired. The saponins in horse chestnut appear to accomplish this task, especially aescin. Horse chestnut creams are also used topically to help improve circulation following physical injury like a sprain. The dose is usually 500 to 1,000 mg per day when taken orally, and horse chestnut creams are usually standardized to contain at least 2% aescin.

Policosanol is the proprietary name for a commercially-developed product that is derived from sugar alcohols in sugarcane wax. The natural alcohols contained in policosanol are primarily 1-octacosa-nol, 1-dotriacontanol, 1-triacontanol, 1-tetracosanol, 1-tetra-triacontanol, 1-hexacosanol, 1-heptacosanol, and 1-nonacosanol. These substances are classified as sugar alcohols, not as polyphenols, and even though they have been shown to have some health-supportive effects, these effects are different than the ones associated with polyphenols. As of 2005, there were about 80 published studies on policosanol, most of them focusing on its cholesterol-lowering effect. This supplemental blend does appear to work effectively in lowering LDL cholesterol, total cholesterol, and triglycerides—in some studies, with the same level of effectiveness or superior effectiveness to popular prescription medications like lovastatin (Mevacor). The typical dosage is about 10 mg twice daily, and it seems to be well tolerated. It also can be used in conjunction with red yeast rice since their mechanisms of cholesterol lowering are slightly different.

Red yeast rice is a dietary supplement consisting of red yeast *(Monascus purpureus)* grown on rice. Red yeast rice contains HMG-CoA reductase inhibiting compounds similar to statin class lipid-lowering medications. Originally described during the Ming dynasty in China as Xuezhikang, some limited but well-conducted research shows red yeast rice significantly decreases LDL cholesterol, triglycerides, and hsCRP (C-reactive protein). There are about 20 mg of the statin-type compounds in a standard supplemental dose of red yeast rice (usually 600 mg of the product). Red yeast rice also contains plant sterols and isoflavones that might act synergistically to lower cholesterol and reduce inflammation. However, there are already some animal studies that question the desirability of red yeast rice, since it appears to lower coenzyme Q levels in a dose-dependent way. For individuals with cardiovascular risk, CoQ is definitely a nutrient that should not be lowered. Therefore, as with people taking statin drugs, supplementing CoQ is essential, at least 50 to 100 mg daily. For red yeast rice, I suggest the amounts of 600 to 1,200 mg twice daily, at breakfast and dinner. At this time, lowering cholesterol appears to still be a focus in reducing cardiovascular risk even though cholesterol is an important body substance. Ultimately, we'll see that maintaining alkalinity and lowering inflammation in the body with consistent good nutrition and regular exercise is going to be our best program for ensuring (and insuring) cardiovascular health.

DETOXIFIERS

In chapter 18, Detoxification and Cleansing Programs, many different programs are covered in great detail, including supplementation protocols for each type of detoxification. I will not duplicate that information here; rather, this section provides an overview of the detox supplements and some tips on what to look for when you are shopping for detox products.

Detoxifying Nutrients

I divide all detox nutrients into two categories. First are those nutrients that provide direct support for steps in the detoxification process. Sulfur would be a good example, because an optimal supply of sulfur is needed to detox many substances we routinely encounter, including drugs, environmental toxins, and even excess hormones produced by our own bodies. This support may come in the form of preventing problems that can occur during detoxification (like the generation of too many free-radical molecules) or supporting specific steps in the detox process. Second are those nutrients that help prevent problems that can occur during detoxification. A good example would be the antioxidant nutrients, because generation of too many free-radical molecules can be a common metabolic problem when people try to detox. There are a couple of nutrient categories that deserve special attention when it comes to detox. Here I cover the methyl-containing molecules and the sulfur-containing ones.

Methyl-containing molecules. These molecules sound complicated, but they are not. Methyl groups are one of the simplest of all chemical compounds—they consist of 1 carbon atom surrounded by 3 hydrogens. Methyl groups are pivotal in metabolism. Our genes often get switched on or off by methyl groups, a process called *methylation.* **And when it comes to detox,**

many substances that would otherwise be poisonous get methylated so they will not cause damage. Arsenic, arsenic-containing pesticides, the heavy metals lead and mercury, and the fumigant carbon tetrachloride are examples of toxins that have to be methylated in order to be made water-soluble and excreted from the body.

It naturally helps to have a good supply of methyl-donating molecules when one is trying to detox, and there has been a huge expansion in the availability of methyl-donating molecules in the natural products marketplace. **These molecules, also called *methyl donors,* include betaine, sarcosine, dimethyl glycine (DMG), trimethyl glycine (TMG), dimethyl sulfoxide (DMSO), choline, and methylsulfonylmethane (MSM).** DMSO is no longer FDA-approved except for use in treatment of interstitial cystitis. Other methyl donors include the amino acid methionine, and possibly vitamin B12 in its methylcobalamin form.

Sulfur-containing molecules. Sulfur-containing molecules stand right alongside of methyl-donors at the center stage of detox. The list of environmental toxins that get neutralized through combination with sulfur is long, encompassing dozens of herbicides and pesticides, including many of the carbamate and organochlorine pesticides. Food additives, including common texturizing agents like ethylene glycol and propylene glycol, also get detoxed using sulfur. So does the over-the-counter drug acetaminophen. Sulfur is used to deactivate many of the body's hormones, including estrogen, testosterone, cortisol, and the thyroid hormones. **Where do we get all of this sulfur needed for detox? Amino acids in the food proteins we eat may be the main source. The sulfur-containing amino acids commonly found in food include methionine, cysteine, and taurine.** The vitamins thiamin (B1) and biotin also contain sulfur. Other important sulfur-containing molecules include acetyl CoA, glutathione, lipoic acid, taurocholic acid (a component of bile), as well as metallothionein and cerulosplasmin (both key mineral transporters).

In this list of sulfur-containing molecules, glutathione deserves special mention. Some toxins can *only* be detoxified with glutathione. These toxins include the packaging materials styrene and polystyrene, the fumigant methyl bromide, and one of the coffee-decaffeinating agents, methylene chloride. For a detailed look at glutathione, please see chapter 3, Proteins.

Detoxifying Herbs

I like to think of the detoxifying herbs as cleansers that act on different organs or body systems to restore vitality. A circulatory cleanser, for example, could relieve congestion in the blood vessels. A liver cleanser could rejuvenate the liver cells and strengthen their ability to process toxins. A colon cleanser could help restore digestive function. Are detoxifiers truly cleansers or maybe tonics in that support function? Overall, I think of detoxifying as cleansing.

Milk thistle. Because the liver is the primary organ for processing toxins, milk thistle is at the top of my list as a detoxifying herb, as it can bring amazing protection to this important organ. Cirrhosis of the liver and hepatitis have both been successfully treated in research studies with milk thistle, and **this herb clearly helps protect the liver cells from toxic damage.** A typical dose of milk thistle is about 150 to 300 mg per day, usually divided into 2 or 3 tablets or capsules.

Licorice should also be considered as a liver-protecting herb. Like milk thistle, it has been used in clinical studies to treat both liver cirrhosis and hepatitis. Licorice is able to act not only as a liver protectant, however. It also acts in the digestive tract like an anti-inflammatory and antibacterial, so it can help us get rid of potential bacterial toxins while simultaneously protecting the intestinal walls during the detoxifying process.

Dandelion, artichoke leaves, and turmeric. Making bile is one of the liver's main ways of eliminating toxins. For this reason, increasing bile flow is often helpful in detoxifying. **The herbs dandelion root, artichoke leaves, and turmeric help increase bile flow.** All three are thus liver cleansers that can be instrumental in detoxifying.

Goldenseal and garlic. When we are detoxifying, we may often need to get rid of potentially toxic bacteria and yeasts in the digestive tract. For this reason, the herbs goldenseal and garlic are digestive cleansers. Goldenseal not only kills potentially harmful bacteria, but it can also help shut down certain enzymes found in these bacteria. This enzyme shutdown can be highly beneficial, because many bacteria are not toxic in and of themselves but because of the substances they produce using their enzyme systems.

Gentian and ginger. Gentian is among the strongest digestive bitters; it has long been popular as a gastric stimulant that can increase digestive function. I think of this herb as a detoxifier because vital flow through the digestive tract is one of the primary means of detoxifying. Ginger can also act as a bitter and can stimulate sluggish digestion. It is a classic digestive tonic that actually has multiple benefits for the digestive tract, including toning of the intestinal muscles, improving bile flow, helping in the digestion of fats, and lessening the risk of inflammation along the lining of the intestines.

Nettle and burdock. I wanted to make special mention of these herbs as urinary cleansers, because both are known to have diuretic effects on the kidneys and can help us eliminate toxins through this route. Although both of these herbs have detoxifying effects throughout the body, their cleansing action on the kidneys makes them somewhat unique. Although the roots of both nettle and burdock have been mostly closely associated with their impact on the urinary tract, other parts of these herbs may also have beneficial effects.

DIGESTIVE SUPPORT

A great many factors contribute to proper digestion, absorption, and utilization of the foods so needed to nourish cells, tissues, and organs. **The stomach, small intestine, liver, gallbladder, pancreas, and large intestine are primarily involved in the digestive process. More subtly, the emotions, stress level, and balance within the endocrine and nervous systems also affect digestive functioning.** A wide range of supplements support the digestive system. A healthy system does not need additional support.

However, research shows that the natural level of hydrochloric acid (HCl) and digestive enzymes decrease as we age or if we abuse our gastrointestinal tracts and whole bodies through food excesses, chemical use, and stress. I have found that the elderly population and many younger people with digestive complaints do

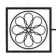

better with digestion-supporting nutrients. (Many of the special programs detailed in part 4 of this book, Nutritional Application: 32 Special Diets and Supplement Programs, suggest digestive enzymes, HCl, and other digestive aids.) Most people older than 50 will have improved breakdown of foods and utilization of nutrients, along with fewer gastrointestinal symptoms, when supportive HCl supplements are taken with meals and additional digestive enzymes (usually pancreas extracts) are taken after eating. Occasionally, people have increased HCl secretion with acute stress, but usually over time, chronic stress causes HCl production to decrease. The level of HCl can be measured easily, although most often an individual's symptoms will reveal if he or she is hyperacid. In that case, inappropriate supplements of HCl would create additional discomfort.

Digestive Support Nutrients

For the most part, when nutrition practitioners mention digestive support nutrients, they are talking about enzymes. In chemistry, the names of nearly all enzymes end in the suffix *-ase*. And for the most part, the first part of the name tells you what the enzyme helps digest. *Lactase,* for example, is the enzyme that helps us digest lactose. A *protease* enzyme helps us digest protein. Many digestive supplements contain a full complement of enzymes that are found in the digestive tract. These enzymes include amylases, cellulases, disaccharidases, invertases, lactase, lipases, maltase, peptidases, proteases, saccharidases, and sucrase. Some digestive enzymes that do *not* end with *-ase* are bromelain, chymotrypsin, papain, trypsin, and pancreatin. The following section provides a little more information about these important digestive aids. **Note that the use of digestive enzymes is not suggested when there is inflammation of the stomach lining.**

A number of digestive enzyme supplements are available. The simple ones are extracted from tropical fruits: **papain** from papayas and **bromelain** from pineapple. Papain has a mild, soothing effect on the stomach and aids in protein digestion. Bromelain is probably more important; it is an anti-inflammatory enzyme useful in post-traumatic responses and swelling and after surgery. It is also part of an antiaging program, as it reduces tissue irritation. This proteolytic

enzyme of pineapple also has several actions that make it helpful in the prevention and treatment of cardiovascular disease. It reduces platelet aggregation, arterial plaquing, and clot formation; 400 to 1,000 mg daily has been shown to reduce the symptoms of angina pectoris. Bromelain's most popular use has been to reduce joint inflammation in rheumatoid arthritis. The ranges for bromelain's anti-inflammatory effects appear to be from 500 to 2,000 mg daily, usually taken in 2 doses. More research is needed to clearly evaluate the potential medical uses of this enzyme as well as those secreted by the pancreas itself.

The pancreas secretes lipases, amylases, and proteases such as trypsin and chymotrypsin. Individual enzymes can be extracted and then added to nutritional formulas, but usually the best support is with the whole (glandular) pancreas, which is discussed on page 279 in the "Glandulars" section of this chapter. Of all enzyme treatments, pancreatic enzyme support has the greatest potential in medicine. Preliminary research on pancreatic enzymes suggests a favorable response to all those problems mentioned as helped by bromelain. Furthermore, cancer may be influenced by high doses of pancreatic enzymes. Many doctors believe that pancreatic insufficiency is at the root of many degenerative diseases, including cancer.

Hydrochloric acid (HCl). Note that people should use discretion in taking HCl, as its intake when there is already normal or excessive stomach acid production or gastritis may increase the risk of gastric irritation or ulcer development. The parietal cells of the stomach produce HCl and secrete it primarily in response to ingested protein or fat. Stress also may stimulate acid output. When we eat more frequently than required by the body or overconsume fats and proteins, acid production begins to decrease. **Decreased HCl production may lead to poor digestion, with such symptoms as gas, bloating, and discomfort after rich meals.** An HCl supplement may improve digestion of meals containing protein and/or fat, although not for such foods as rice and vegetables, which are largely carbohydrate and thus need less HCl for digestion.

Hydrochloric acid is available primarily as betaine hydrochloride. When a 5 to 10 grain (1 grain = 64 mg) tablet is taken before, during, or after meals, it should help proteins break down into peptides and amino acids, and fats into triglycerides. Glutamic acid hydrochloride is used sometimes in formulas, but this amino acid is only mildly acidic and does not work as well as betaine hydrochloride. Betaine may be used alone, in supplements, or along with pepsin or other digestive agents.

The use of HCl support is part of the antiaging process outlined throughout this book, provided of course that HCl production is low. A Heidelberg capsule gastric pH test (which directly measures stomach pH) can be done to verify a low or high acidity; then a supplement can be administered to see what effect it has on stomach pH. One reason that stress can cause more rapid aging is that it diminishes HCl production and weakens digestion. More often, however, the culprit is the low-grade, long-term, emotionally oriented life stress. Stress in intense worriers or high-achieving businesspeople is associated more with HCl hypersecretion and peptic ulcer disease (at least initially).

On the other hand, low HCl production is associated with many problems as well. Iron deficiency anemia (owing to poor iron absorption) and osteoporosis (resulting in part from decreased calcium absorption) are two important problems. General allergies and specifically food allergies are correlated with low HCl. Poor food breakdown and the "leaky gut" syndrome are associated with food allergies (see the allergy program on page 704 in chapter 17, Medical Treatment Programs). More than half the people with gallstones show decreased HCl secretion compared with gallstone-free patients. Diabetics have lower secretion, as do people with eczema, psoriasis, seborrheic dermatitis, vitiligo, and tooth and periodontal disease. With low stomach acid levels, there can be an increase in bacteria, yeasts, and parasites growing in the intestines.

But many patients feel they don't want to take an HCl supplement forever. Fortunately, most people can correct low stomach acid by eating a balanced diet of wholesome foods and by reducing the daily stress level. Niacin (vitamin B3) stimulates HCl production. This can be taken before meals, as can magnesium chloride and pyridoxal-5-phosphate (the active form of vitamin B6) to help stimulate the body's own HCl. With some success, I have suggested drinking the juice of half a lemon squeezed in water or 1 teaspoon of apple cider vinegar in a glass of warm water 20 to 30 minutes before meals. Rosemary, ginger, cumin, or orange peel, used to make tea and ingested before meals, can also be helpful.

I believe that the digestive tract and its function may be the single most important body component determining health and disease. Maintaining normal digestion, assimilation, and elimination is a necessity, and when these functions are faulty, we may not be aware that these dysfunctions are contributing to so many other problems. Another key digestive factor is that HCl is a stimulus to pancreatic secretions, containing the majority of enzymes that actively break down foods. The poor digestion of proteins, fats, and carbohydrates then further contributes to poor assimilation and nutritional problems. Thus, when it is needed, supplemental support of digestive enzymes may be even more important than HCl.

Intestinal Lining Support

When we detoxify, it is especially important for the linings of the digestive tract to be well protected. The detox process means mobilizing toxins, and many of these will need to pass out through the intestines. The last thing we want in this situation is a weakened stomach or intestinal lining that would be at such great risk for damage.

Glutamine and short-chain fatty acids (including butyrate). These are top-level recommendations for support of the intestinal lining. Both are well researched. Glutamine is clearly the preferred fuel for the cells (enterocytes) of the small intestine. These cells would rather use glutamine for energy than any other fuel source, including glucose. In the large intestine, butyrate plays the same role. In hospitals, glutamine is being added more frequently to tube-fed or intravenous formulas because of its amazing benefits to the intestinal lining.

Raw cabbage juice is an excellent source of glutamine, and some practitioners recommend consumption of cabbage juice as a way of supporting the digestive tract linings. Of course, as whole food, cabbage juice has a wide range of supportive nutrients. A 1957 study compared cabbage juice to glutamine in treatment of stomach ulcer (peptic ulcer), and in that study glutamine supplementation appeared to be the more effective approach. Despite this finding, I still see a place for cabbage juice in providing support for the digestive tract.

Probiotics and Prebiotics

Using probiotics for digestive support has really taken off since the mid-1990s, and in addition to the original title of *probiotics,* we now have the second domain of *prebiotics.* Probiotic supplements are simply supplements that contain "friendly" bacteria that we generally want present in the digestive tract in large numbers. Prebiotic supplements contain the nutrients that these bacteria need to grow and thrive. The key probiotic bacteria are bifidobacteria and lactobacilli. The key prebiotic nutrients are fructo-oligosaccharides (FOSs), short-chain fatty acids (SCFAs, including butyrate), and inulin (a fiber). Chicory root and Jerusalem artichoke are common sources from which FOSs can be obtained, so you will also often see them in prebiotic supplements.

Several friendly intestinal bacteria perform many important bodily functions. There are actually a great many lactobacillus and other bacteria that can inhabit the human colon, but the three that seem to be most important are *Lactobacillus acidophilus* (the most famous), *Bifidobacterium bifidum* (more common to the baby colon), and *Streptococcus faecium* (not *S. faecalis,* a possible pathogenic bacteria).

Various cultures of acidophilus are available in many stores, particularly health food stores, as powders, capsules, tablets, and liquids and measured by the amount of viable bacteria per dosage. There are many claims for the use of acidophilus, although it is best known for reimplanting friendly bacteria into the colon to assure return of bodily functions after a course of antibiotic drugs. Actually, acidophilus itself acts as a mild antibiotic—that is, it has antibacterial activity. With regular use, it may even replace harmful bacteria in the colon or vaginal tract, where acidophilus is also commonly used to treat yeast infections. It is further employed as part of the treatment for intestinal yeast overgrowth and the many symptoms that this may generate. These bacteria also help in the production of some B vitamins and vitamin K and in the breakdown of various foods.

Yogurt or acidophilus milk, sometimes with *L. bulgaricus* as well, is often used to provide some stimulus to the colon, although the live bacteria count is not very high in these products. Yogurt can also be used by people with lactose intolerance because of lactase enzyme deficiency, since the bacteria change or ferment the lactose sugar and produce lactic acid. Many people have also described yogurt or, more specifically, acidophilus as helpful for stomach and digestive upset, for intestinal gas, and even for inflammatory problems of the gastrointestinal tract, but these reports are more anecdotal than proved by research. The further suggestions that acidophilus improves immunity, produces its own antibiotics, helps allergies (particularly to foods), improves skin health, is a benefit in herpes infections, reduces cholesterol levels, and lessens cancer risk (especially colon cancer) are also yet unproved, although current research at several universities for one product looks promising.

Bifidobacterium bifidum has become part of intestinal bioculture treatment, often along with acidophilus. The bifidus culture is more prevalent in infants, often as their first organism, but can also be an important part of the adult gastrointestinal tract. Like acidophilus, it helps in the synthesis of B vitamins, in food digestion, and in inhibiting the growth of the coliform bacteria and possibly more pathogenic colon bacteria, such as salmonellae.

Streptococcus faecium is another important colon bacterium that has received recent attention. Its actions are similar to those of acidophilus. It is important in B vitamin biosynthesis, aids the digestion of foods (likely by producing certain enzymes), and inhibits other, more-toxic bacteria; thus supplementation with *S. faecium* may help in some cases of diarrhea. *S. faecalis,* a potentially pathogenic bacterium, has been listed by mistake instead of S. faecium on some bacterial replacement products.

These three bacteria may be taken individually and alternated weekly or every couple of weeks. They can also be taken all together (there are some products that contain all three) on a regular basis when used to balance the effect of a course of antibiotics. There is a possibility that the combination of bacteria works better to rebalance colon health than the individual organisms.

The count of live bacteria in products containing these bacteria is in the millions and billions daily per dose. There has been some question as to whether these bacteria are killed by the acidic stomach juices, but when taken in sufficient quantities, some organisms do make it down to the colon. These bacteria should not be taken regularly, but rather in specific courses to repopulate the colon with these friendly bacteria after antibiotic use or to treat intestinal yeast overgrowth; otherwise, I recommend them for 1 to 2 weeks once or twice a year, or when traveling to underdeveloped countries with higher risks of intestinal contamination from infectious organisms, for which the acidophilus bacteria offer some protection.

Digestive Support Herbs

Aloe vera. Aloe concentrate or dried aloe gel powder is an intestinal purgative that helps stimulate colon activity with less of the cramping that comes with many other herbal preparations. Aloe vera capsules are a useful remedy or preventive for constipation. The dried aloe gel is bitter, so it must be either purified for oral use or dried and capped.

Artichoke. The inulin in artichoke may be responsible for some of its digestive support, but there are also unique flavonoids and caffeoylquinic acids found in artichoke that may have a connection with its ability to aid digestion. Reports indicate that digestive problems—including nausea, bloating, loss of appetite, and even abdominal pain—may be improved with the use of artichoke.

Digestive Bitters

I have already talked about gentian in the "Detoxifying Herbs" section of this chapter (see page 269) as being among the strongest digestive bitters. There are other bitters that are commonly used as gastric stimulants, and these include yellow dock, dandelion root, and blessed thistle. Bitters are not meant to serve as a lifelong replacement for normal digestive tract function, but they can be helpful in the short term for jump-starting digestive flow.

Cinnamon and cayenne. Unlike bitters, which are always taken before a meal, cinnamon often serves as a nice postmeal digestive aid, especially if there is any heartburn or feeling of indigestion following the meal. Cinnamon teas are popular in this regard. As a warming herb, cinnamon is like ginger insofar as it is able to stimulate weak digestion. Cayenne is an interesting component to include in digestive aid formulas because it works in the mouth to stimulate salivary flow and it also increases secretion of digestive fluids by the stomach. Getting digestion off on the right track at the mouth and stomach level can actually carry over into the intestines and provide better nourishment across the board.

Ginger. The ginger used medicinally is from the root of the plant *Zingiber officinale.* Many of its properties and uses are described in the herbal literature. Recently, ginger root has received more medical attention as being useful in treating nausea and motion sickness. Ginger capsules or a cup of ginger root tea seems to allay nausea. Ginger has also been helpful for the nausea of pregnancy.

Ginger root in general seems to be a digestive stimulant and is used to improve weak digestion. Bile flow can be improved with the help of ginger, as can digestion of fat. **A warm cup of tea made by boiling a few slices of root in 1 or 2 cups of water can be ingested about 30 minutes before meals.** Ginger is also a diaphoretic (it causes sweating), and it seems to help in circulation and in warming the body when we feel cold, as can happen in winter. There is some preliminary research evidence that ginger acts as an antioxidant and that it can help lower cholesterol and prevent cardiovascular disease. It also inhibits platelet aggregation, a factor contributing to atherosclerosis and clotting problems. **It has also been shown to help decrease risk of inflammation within the digestive tract.** Ginger is both an energy and circulatory stimulant. Ginger root tea is also used as a compress for sore muscles or congested areas of the body. This is a common macrobiotic therapy.

Ginger root can be used in cooking, too, or as a tea with other herbs. It is a helpful and safe herb. For improving body heat, 1 or 2 capsules of ginger root powder can be taken once or twice a day for about a month. Cayenne pepper can also be used in this way.

Goldenseal. Goldenseal may be helpful for many problems of the stomach and gastrointestinal tract, such as nausea, indigestion, infection, and constipation or diarrhea; it can also reduce bacterial or parasitic proliferation, increase gastrointestinal tone, and stimulate bile secretion and digestion. For most of these situations, goldenseal can usually be taken as 1 large or 2 small capsules (or 10–20 drops of an extract) twice daily for about 2 to 3 weeks. **I do not recommend long continuous intake of this powerful herb because of possible liver irritation.**

Marshmallow. Marshmallow (like mullein, plantain, and slippery elm) is classified as an herbal demulcent that can soothe and protect the digestive tract lining. This protection stems largely from the high mucilage content of these herbs. Inflammations in the mouth and stomach, stomach ulcers, and colitis are digestive problems that may all involve marshmallow in their treatment.

Peppermint. Peppermint is classified as a carminative herb, which means that it can help tone the digestive tract, both by relaxing the surrounding muscles and by promoting elimination of gas. Colic in infants can often be improved with the use of peppermint, as can problems with gas in adults. Because the oil in peppermint can alter nerve function and reduce spasms, peppermint is also sometimes used in irritable bowel syndrome to restore healthy muscle tone and motility.

ENERGY BOOSTERS AND STRESS REDUCERS

Energy-boosting supplements aid in the creation of a steady, stable vitality that we can depend on throughout the day. The energy extremes created artificially, as with caffeine and other stimulants, are not conducive to optimal health and act like stressors. We may get totally hyper at times, just like we might get totally down, but these kinds of energy swings take a toll on our well-being. The stress of these fluctuations can be enormous. In Western medicine, researchers are discovering that blood sugar balance can often swing toward these extremes. Roller-coastering back and forth between hypoglycemia and hyperglycemia may not only leave us feeling unstable and unequipped to get through the day, but it may also lead to chronic health problems. In this section I focus on supplemental nutrients and herbs that can help us avoid the stress of these extremes and instead help us create a stable flow of optimal energy.

Energy-Boosting and Stress-Reducing Nutrients

Carnitine. Carnitine serves as the key shuttle system into our mitochondria, where aerobic (oxygen-based) energy gets produced. Mitochondria are like the cell's batteries. To produce energy, mitochondria need a steady supply of fatty acids and branched-chain amino acids, and carnitine carries these nutrients to them. (Carnitine also carries waste products back out of the mitochondria and keeps them from getting toxic.) A typical dose range for carnitine as an energy-boosting nutrient would range from 1,000 to 4,000 mg per day, taken in 2 to 3 doses.

CoQ. CoQ was described earlier under "Additional Antioxidant Supplements" (on page 260) and "Circulatory Support Nutrients" (on page 264); check those sections for further information about this singular supplement. It is mentioned again here as an energy booster because it is perhaps the most unique nutrient at work in the mitochondria. No other nutrient is capable of replacing it in the mitochondrial machinery, and when we become deficient, we may quickly begin to suffer from an energy deficit.

Creatine. Creatine is a kind of counterbalance to CoQ. In our muscles, we have two basic ways to obtain energy. The first is aerobically, from the mitochondria, using oxygen. The form of energy that gets produced this way is ATP, and CoQ is a key nutrient in the process of making ATP. The second way for our muscles to obtain energy is nonaerobically (without the use of oxygen). In this case, creatine phosphate gets produced. Here we start with creatine, to which the enzyme creatine kinase attaches a phosphorus-containing group. The muscle cells keep a balance between ATP and creatine phosphate.

Energy-Boosting Supplements	
Nutrients	**Herbs**
Carnitine	Ashwaganda
CoQ10	Codonopsis
Creatine	Garlic
Krebs cycle	Ginkgo
organic acids	Ginseng
	Schizandra

Because creatine phosphate helps spare the supply of ATP, it can be extremely helpful to supplement with this nutrient alongside of the antioxidants we might be taking to support the mitochondrial production of ATP. The dose range for creatine varies widely and should take into account body size and level of physical activity. Anywhere between 2 and 50 grams may be used depending on the individual circumstances.

Krebs cycle organic acids. When the mitochondria set out to make energy in the form of ATP, they run a metabolic process called the *Krebs cycle*. There are "Krebs cycle intermediates" out in the marketplace, and these supplements typically contain all of the nutrients found in this first part of the energy production process, including malic acid, succinic acid, oxaloacetic acid, fumaric acid, citric acid, isocitric acid, and alpha-ketoglutaric acid. All of these nutrients can be classified as organic acids, and you might also see that label on a supplement bottle. There is not much research on the supplemental use of Krebs cycle intermediates, but these supplements are currently being used for energy-related problems like chronic fatigue syndrome, fibromyalgia, myofascial pain, and multiple chemical sensitivity.

Energy-Boosting and Stress-Reducing Herbs

Herbs can boost energy in a wide variety of ways, and the herbs described in this section impact different organ systems in the body and often function in vastly different ways. Panax ginseng (also called Asian ginseng), for example, boosts our vitality by supporting the function of the adrenal glands. Schizandra berry, on the other hand, boosts energy by strengthening and quickening reflexes and by stimulating breathing. Ginkgo is more cardiovascular in its focus and sharpens our awareness by increasing blood flow to the brain. Many of the herbs listed in this section would also be classified as *adaptogenic,* meaning that they help regulate our metabolism, improve our handling of stress, and thereby increase our physical energy and vitality.

Ashwaganda. This herb is sometimes referred to as the "ginseng of ayurvedic medicine" because it has long been used in the ayurvedic tradition in India as a key adaptogen. Ashwaganda is typically used to increase stamina and sometimes to increase immunity as well as sexual energy. Some research suggests that compounds in ashwaganda act on the central nervous system, but it is not really known exactly how this herb works. It has one of the longest traditions of use for energy boosting of any herb.

Codonopsis. Sometimes called "poor man's ginseng," codonopsis is both the scientific and common name for a vine native to northeastern China and widely used in traditional Chinese medicine. Codonopsis may work to boost energy by strengthening the immune response, improving the function of the spleen, strengthening digestive function, and perhaps also by increasing the quality of sleep.

Garlic. Researchers are seeing some new uses for garlic regarding energy balance, primarily because of its impact on blood sugar. Some of the substances that can hook up with insulin and deactivate it end up hooking up with compounds in garlic instead, and the result is increasing availability of insulin and better control of blood sugar. Some of garlic's components can also stimulate the pancreas to produce more insulin. For these reasons, garlic is starting to be used in relationship to diabetes, where it seems able to improve blood sugar regulation and energy balance.

Ginkgo. With ginkgo, there is solid research in understanding how this herb can boost energy levels and reduce stress. Ginkgo supports our circulation, especially at the level of the capillaries, where nutrient exchange occurs with our cells. The ginkgolides in ginkgo also help protect our nerve cells and in this way improve cognitive function.

Ginseng. The root of the ginseng plant, usually *Panax ginseng,* is the active and commonly used part. **It comes mainly from Asian cultures, where it is used extensively as a tonic, stimulant, and rejuvenator, especially for men. It is also used by women for fatigue and sexually related symptoms.** It is often part of formulas used to balance the menstrual cycle, reduce premenstrual symptoms or hot flashes of menopause, or to improve the sex drive or enhance fertility. Probably the most common use of ginseng is to increase energy. Research is showing that it also reduces cholesterol and triglyceride levels, raises HDL, and stimulates the immune system. Its rejuvenating qualities may come from its stimulus to protein synthesis.

This herb is called the "man plant" because of the shape of the roots; its species name *panax* refers to "all healing," as in *panacea*. Other active ginsengs are American ginseng (*Panax quinquefolius*) and Siberian ginseng (*Eleutherococcus senticosus*). The ginsengs have a number of active ingredients, such as peptides, glycosides, and the more recently acknowledged trace mineral germanium (discussed as organo-germanium on page 282), which may turn out to be a very helpful and fascinating supplement. Yet researchers still do not know medically or pharmacologically what gives ginseng its powers. **Siberian ginseng may not be as stimulating as panax, but it may be better at stress balancing.**

Ginseng is used most commonly as a tonic and herb for longevity. It seems to contribute to general well-being and improved physical endurance. It is a stimulant but not an excitant like caffeine, and it is particularly useful for men with fatigue or sexual impotency. Ginseng root is imbibed as a tea or taken in capsules, although the brewed liquid seems to have a better effect. It is available in more forms nowadays—in liquid elixirs, as a paste or powder used to make teas, or as the whole root. These beautiful roots, which come mainly from Korea and China, can be expensive. The cost is often based on the age of the root, older ones being more expensive as their power seems to improve with age. On traveling through China, I was impressed by the many displays of ginseng roots throughout stores, airports, and many other places. There is a wild American ginseng that can also be used, and it is thought to be somewhat helpful, although it probably has somewhat different effects from those produced by the Asian plants.

A daily dose of ginseng root is usually about 500 mg. **Larger amounts can cause overstimulation, which may result in increased blood pressure, diarrhea, skin eruptions, or insomnia.** It may interact with the sensitive hormonal system and may also have some estrogenic activity; thus it may aggravate fibrocystic breast disease in women. Any substance that has potential power and benefit obviously can also be misused. If you wish to try ginseng root as a tonic or remedy, obtain guidance from your physician, acupuncturist, or someone with experience in its use. (See my book *Staying Healthy with the Seasons* for a special preparation of ginseng root.) If there are any

cardiac problems, ginseng should be used carefully, and it should not be used by pregnant women.

Schizandra. Another increasingly popular adaptogenic herb, schizandra has a long tradition of use in China, Korea, and Russia as an herb for increasing stamina and longevity. The berry of this plant is typically used to make extracts and encapsulations. Eye fatigue and adrenal exhaustion are among the interesting applications of this energy booster.

GENETIC SUPPORT AND RNA/DNA

Over the next 10 years, I predict a huge flurry of activity in this area of supplementation as researchers continue to learn more about genetic processes and their modification. Right now, in terms of dietary supplements, knowledge in this arena is still in the infancy stage. DNA (deoxyribonucleic acid) is, of course, the main building block of our genes. RNA (ribonucleic acid) is a bridging-type molecule that helps us take the information contained in the DNA and use it as a blueprint for making proteins that are needed throughout the body. Because you can already find many RNA- and DNA-containing supplements in the marketplace, I provide a little more information about these two molecules in this section.

Deoxyribonucleic and Ribonucleic Acids (DNA and RNA)

These nucleic acid polymers act as the genetic code and translators for the proteins, which in turn are the molecular building blocks of body tissues, and actually stipulate which amino acids go together to form body proteins. **DNA is found mainly in the nuclei of cells and carries the genetic message; small amounts of DNA are also found in the mitochondria.** RNA helps transfer this genetic message to guide the manufacture of proteins from all the amino acids, whether created by the body or extracted from foods.

There are supplements containing good levels of nucleic acids, most commonly yeast or such organ meats as calf thymus, which have been recommended to retard aging, improve memory, or improve the immune or other protein functions. However, there is

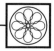

no proof that RNA or DNA, when taken orally, performs any of these fabulous feats. Most of the oral nucleic acid supplement is broken down into purines and pyrimidines, the basic components of RNA and DNA. These purines (such as adenine and guanine) and pyrimidines (such as cytosine, uracil, and thymine) may have some cellular regeneration functions and thus could help slow aging, improve immune functions, and so on. As these components are absorbed, they may aid the production of the body's RNA or DNA, although this has not been proved. Injectable nucleic acids may offer some benefit. These have been used particularly to slow skin aging.

Many foods contain good levels of these primordial nucleic acids. Brewer's yeast is probably the best source. Others include some fish (such as salmon, sardines, and herring), nuts, wheat germ, bran, oats, onions, spinach, and asparagus. Animal meats and eggs are rich in nucleic acids. Most glandular supplements also contain RNA and DNA.

Many nutrients support normal DNA and RNA synthesis. Folic acid is likely the most important. It may become known as a key antiaging nutrient, possibly through its nucleic acid support. One of the theories of aging suggests that distorted genetic messages generated by dysfunctional DNA and RNA allow communication breakdown and decreased cell division and duplication, and thus weakened tissue strength and life force. Other nutrients that contribute to DNA and RNA synthesis and health include the B vitamins pyridoxine, pantothenic acid, riboflavin, biotin, and choline, vitamin C, and the minerals zinc, magnesium, manganese, chromium, and selenium. Keeping all of these at adequate levels in the diet may be the best way to support healthy genes.

GLANDULARS

The use of animal tissues in the treatment of disease and support of health is controversial in medicine, with opinions ranging from useless to miraculous. On the one hand, we have thyroid hormones, insulin, and estrogens, for example, which are commonly used. On the other hand, we have what are called *protomorphogens*, or extracts of tissues from such glands as the adrenal, pancreas, pituitary, thyroid, and ovary, which

can be taken orally to help support those particular tissues in humans.

I used to feel that it was quite simplistic to think that eating an animal's glands would help strengthen my own like glands. Along with many other medical doctors, I also think we should be able to measure the hormone activity of many substances and monitor its effect in the body. The glandulars are usually measured by the amount of the actual glands present, but researchers do not really know what they do. Furthermore, because these glands are broken down into their basic nutrients in the digestive tract, they would not necessarily go directly to improve my own glands. Previously, I was a strict vegetarian, so for that reason alone I did not want to consume animal glands, which might also have a buildup of toxins or chemicals.

Now, however, I feel more open to considering that glandulars have some use in supporting and strengthening specific organ function. On the positive side, it is likely that the basic components of those gland tissues may offer the precursor substances that our own bodies and glands can use to enhance their functions. And there may be hidden factors that may offer some benefit. The glands, like foods, supply basic nutrients, such as amino acids, oils, vitamins, other active ingredients, and a potential "life force," where a drug may not.

In modern medicine, glandular therapy with the use of whole glands began in the late nineteenth century, when doctors suggested that their patients eat the animal parts, usually from cows, that corresponded to the weak areas of their own bodies. So people began eating brains, hearts, kidneys, and so on, as part of their medical treatment. Actually, the ancient Greeks and Egyptians used glandular therapy, following their basic premise that like heals like. Technology and medical endocrinology evolved this therapy by isolating specific hormones at the source of the glands' activities (just as we extract active pharmaceutical drugs from whole plants). These new drugs are more potent, but they also have more potential for dangerous side effects than the whole glands.

For example, desiccated thyroid gland was first used in the late 1800s to help people with goiter and low thyroid function. Then thyroxine (T4) was isolated and used, but many doctors still preferred the whole gland as it was felt to be better absorbed and utilized. Later, the other thyroid hormones, triiodothyronine

(T3) and calcitonin were discovered, but these were always part of the whole gland. Today, both individual synthetic hormones and measured active thyroid tissue are used to support or replace thyroid activity.

In the early 1920s, insulin was isolated by Sir Frederick Banting and Charles H. Best, who received the Nobel Prize for their discovery. Insulin has been a lifesaver for many diabetics, but it is also a dangerous drug because it has such a narrow range of safe use. Overdoses can cause very low blood sugar and shock. Insulin is destroyed in the gut, so it must be injected. It is possible that in the pancreas, as in other glands, certain molecules protect the active hormones from digestive juices, and some of these substances actually get into the body. The whole pancreas gland, which had previously been used, is definitely safer than insulin, but pancreas glandular itself is not strong enough to treat diabetes once it is established.

Currently, opinion is split over the use of animal glands and hormones, separating those in the medical profession from other practitioners, such as naturopaths and chiropractors, who cannot write drug prescriptions. Allopathic medicine usually is not very supportive of the nondrug or natural approaches used by its professional competitors; however, glandular therapy is much more accepted by physicians in other countries, particularly in Europe. Currently in the United States, there is not much definitive research to support those approaches, and the MDs might say those "doctors" are not trained to treat disease. Natural practitioners often feel that what they do is safe and effective for many people who do not have advanced disease; they work preventively to keep a balance and maintain health. But the science and dollars are still behind conventional medicine, even though there is a lot of good experience with the more natural therapies. There does need to be more research to show exactly what effects occur with the use of glandulars so that every practitioner can better apply them to health.

Such glandulars as thyroid, ovary, adrenal, and thymus are not prescription items and can be purchased by anyone in health food stores. Practitioners such as chiropractors, naturopaths, and nutritionists often suggest certain glandular protomorphogens in an attempt to strengthen or balance the internal function and energies of their patients and clients. I, personally, am not sure what to do with glandular

therapy. It does not seem to cause harm, and it may do some good. As I mentioned earlier, I am now more comfortable with this therapy, and I occasionally suggest adrenal, pancreas, thymus, or nonprescription thyroid for people who seem to need that support. I do not use these in medical conditions that I feel need actual hormone therapy, especially in thyroid therapy, where I use prescription glandular (with measured thyroid hormones) medicines. It is clear that more research and understanding are needed in the still-mysterious practice of using glandular substitutes.

Glandular supplements are made in a variety of ways. The best products are prepared from freeze-dried, defatted, fresh glands, as no heat or chemicals that can destroy the enzymes are used. A vacuum process is used to dry the glands after freezing. Because no chemical solvents are used to pull out the fat and potentially toxic chemicals stored in the glands, **it is suggested that the glandular tissue be obtained from range-grazed cattle that have not been given chemicals, hormones, or antibiotics.** Many companies use this type of processing, and the majority of these glandulars are imported from New Zealand. Some practitioners believe that removing the fat from the glands in the least toxic way is important, as the fat can contain any harmful residues of substances contacted by the animal and is subject to oxidizing and going rancid; the remaining protein tissues are stable.

Two methods used for fat removal are the salt precipitation method and the azeotropic method. Salt precipitation means grinding the glandular up in a salt and water solution so that the fat-soluble materials can be separated out. This method avoids the use of a potentially toxic solvent to remove the fat, but it also may result in the loss of certain nutrients because of the high salt level. The azeotropic method begins with quick freezing of the glandular, followed by addition of a solvent (like ethylene dichloride) to get the fat to separate. Like salt precipitation, this method may also result in the loss of certain fat-soluble components of the glandular (like essential fatty acids) and introduce residues of the solvent into the final product. As yet there is no clear answer to which process is best, but these two methods lead the way.

Adrenal. The adrenals are the glands that help us deal with stress, mineral balances, and inflammation. They release adrenaline into the body to increase

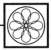

activity and energy. They may be overworked these days in response to stress, caffeine, nicotine, and sugar. **Adrenal glandulars are often suggested for people who experience fatigue, stress, environmental sensitivities or allergies, infections, and hypoglycemia.** The symptoms that come from low blood sugar are probably more related to the adrenal glands than to the pancreas, and supporting the adrenals with freeze-dried adrenal at 50 to 100 mg twice daily, along with other stress-supporting nutrients, such as the B vitamins, vitamins C and A, and zinc, may be helpful.

Pancreas. The pancreas is used mainly to support digestion by providing extra digestive enzymes. Lipases, proteases, and amylases are found in the pancreas gland. Taking digestive enzymes 30 to 60 minutes after meals often helps us to better utilize the meal's nutrition, especially for people whose digestion has been weakened by emotional stress, chemical irritants, or poor eating habits. **Many people, particularly the elderly, need pancreatic enzyme support (and often hydrochloric acid as well) to properly digest and assimilate foods;** this is part of many of the nutritional programs I propose in part 4 of this book, Nutritional Application: 32 Special Diets and Supplement Programs. There are those who suggest that pancreatic insufficiency is at the heart of aging and much disease, including allergies, weight problems, arthritis and other inflammatory problems, gastrointestinal problems, and cancer. Pancreatic support is important in some nutritional cancer programs and the use of pork-derived pancreas for therapy is currently under investigation.

Thymus. The thymus is important to immunological activity. It contains the active hormone thymosin, which stimulates T lymphocyte (T cell) production and activity. T cells help the body defend itself against infection. **The thymus gland tends to weaken with age, and this may affect our defense system.** If we experience fatigue, recurrent infections, or measurable immune deficiency, intake of oral thymus gland may be helpful. This is not well researched, but it most likely will not cause any problems. Injectable thymus has been shown definitely to stimulate immune activity.

Thyroid. Thyroid weakness can be caused by lack of iodine or too little protein in the diet as well as by emotional stress and blocked creativity. In such cases, thyroid glandular may be helpful in supporting the gland to work better. **Nutrients that contain precursors for thyroid tissue and hormones, such as iodine and tyrosine, seem to be helpful. Thyroid glandular has been used for fatigue and to support immune function.** This is different from true hypothyroidism, wherein the thyroid hormone production is low, or relatively low. It is more common practice nowadays to provide some thyroid hormone support for people who demonstrate low thyroid symptoms. Often they feel better. This topic can be reviewed more thoroughly in *Thyroid Power: Ten Steps to Total Health,* written by my friends and associates Richard Shames, MD, and Karilee Shames, RN.

Other glandulars. Many other glandular tissues are available for support of body organs. Brain tissue has been used for ages to stimulate brain function. Likewise, heart or lung extracts have supported those organs. Stomach and duodenum, testicular and ovarian tissue, prostate, pituitary, and hypothalamus have all been employed to enhance body organ functions. Spleen glandular tissue has been popular for immunological support, to help boost lymphocyte activity, and to protect the body from infections. High-nutrient liver tissue is also part of many glandular programs to support this important metabolic organ. As many people describe, liver may help us energetically and functionally, but it should be good liver from healthy, nontoxic animals, as this organ in particular can have high concentrations of many toxins.

GREEN FOODS

The idea of "green foods" may be something of a misnomer, since most of the 350,000 different plants on Earth are green and are eaten for food by some creature. But this label has definitely stuck in the natural products world and refers primarily to algae and freshly sprouted grasses, like wheatgrass or barley grass. On the green food list you will therefore find blue-green algae (including spirulina), green algae (including chlorella), wheatgrass and wheatgrass juice, barley grass and barley grass juice, and dried barley leaf juice. Red algae (including carrageenan, a phycocolloid derived from the red algae *Eucheuma* spp.) and brown algae (including the sea plants commonly referred to as "kelps") are also sometimes referred to as "green foods."

Common to all plants that eat sunlight, of course, is the molecule chlorophyll, which itself can rightly be considered a green food and is a best-selling product in the marketplace. Chlorophyll and the high-chlorophyll grasses are cleansing greens, in contrast with the building greens that are represented by vegetables and other foods. The cleansing greens seem like a good idea for support during detox, because they are highly nutrient dense without saddling the body with a large amount of material to metabolize. I use them routinely in my 10-day fasts or juice cleanses. In the remainder of this section, I provide a little more about some of these green food supplements and their possible use.

Algae. Algae are green, red, brown, or blue-green aqueous, one-celled organisms that can be grown, dried, and safely used by the body. They are now available in the nutritional product arena as supplemental nutrients to enhance body functions only. Spirulina, one of the best-selling green food products, is an example of the blue-green algae. There are about 1,800 species of blue-green algae, but spirulina remains the best known. In the United States, a particular strain of blue-green algae found in Oregon's Klamath Lake has become especially popular. Chlorella is part of the green algae family, which includes about 7,000 total species. This green food, one of those I use in my 10-day fasts, has also been especially popular.

Both spirulina and chlorella have been used as "high-protein" nutrients that contain all of the amino acids. Of course, both also contain a large amount of chlorophyll. They are considered a tonic and rejuvenator of the body and are used commonly during weight-loss programs or fasting. I have spoken with many people who have done a juice–spirulina powder cleanse and felt extremely well, with more energy than usual. Besides the higher protein and low fat levels of these algae, they contain substantial amounts of vitamins and minerals and plant chlorophyll; spirulina has been measured as rich in gamma-linolenic acid (GLA), the oil found in the evening primrose plant. When I say *rich* here, I am using this term on a nutrient density basis—that is, we get a lot

more GLA than we would expect from a small amount of food. Still, if we are looking for 5 to 10 grams of any high-quality fat, we are probably going to have to look elsewhere to get it, because we just do not use large amounts of these green foods when supplementing.

It is possible that the GLA found in spirulina and possibly these other products accounts for some of the positive effects that people experience when using them, including decreased appetite, weight loss, and improved energy levels, especially mental energy. I personally have used all of these products, and I have experienced a subtle increase in mental clarity and alertness (not like a nervous, caffeine-type stimulation). These algae must subtly stimulate our nervous systems or release certain internal neurochemicals that create this "up" feeling.

There has not been much medical research on any of these products, but there should be. When people find interesting substances from the natural world, it is medicine's duty to investigate the activity of these products so we can apply them effectively in our lives. Such analysis with herbs has brought the whole field of pharmacognosy/pharmaceutical medicine, and perhaps continued analysis of Nature's potential remedies will bring useful new substances and help us to better integrate the drug and nondrug therapies.

Kelp. This term is used to loosely refer to many different species of brown algae, a common health-food supplement. **It is taken primarily for its iodine content by people who want to improve thyroid function, although there is no proof that kelp changes this function.** The thyroid gland must have sufficient iodine, however, and if we do not use iodized salt or eat a lot of fish and seaweed, kelp may be a helpful adjunct. It is also high in other vitamins and minerals, such as calcium, magnesium, potassium, niacin, riboflavin, and choline. Algin, which is helpful at pulling out intestinal toxins and heavy metals, is also found in kelp. Several tablets per day will usually supply the needed iodine; kelp powder used on food is a good salt substitute but should not be overused.

Wheatgrass and barley grass. These juice extracts of grain greens seem to offer an energy lift and act as a purifier and rejuvenator, probably because of their chlorophyll and nutrient content. That, at least, is what users state. But these grasses may also help protect against cancer, and chlorophyll, as an antioxidant, can have an antiaging function. Although the research has remained unpublished, barley grass has been studied in Japan, where it has been shown to protect human cells and animal DNA from damage by X-rays and some cancer-causing chemicals. Of course, this effect was seen when the grass juice was given before exposure. This preliminary evidence suggests some possibilities. Along with the other nutrients available in wheatgrass or barley grass, these juices may be useful in healing and disease prevention. There is a lot of enthusiasm about them in certain areas of the health community.

IMMUNE SUPPORT

It is the ongoing job of the immune system to recognize dangers to the body and respond in a way that keeps it safe. Recognizing potential dangers means being able to distinguish between toxic and nontoxic substances; being able to respond to potentially harmful bacteria; and even providing protection against any of our own cells that no longer function properly. As you can imagine, the list of nutrients required to carry out these tasks is a comprehensive one. **Many conventional nutrients are absolutely essential for healthy immune function, and these include vitamins A, C, and E, the minerals selenium and zinc, essential fatty acids, and ample, well-balanced protein intake.** No special supplement can make up for the lack of these basic nutrients, but several deserve special mention for their excellent track record in boosting immune function.

Immune Support Nutrients

Arabinogalactan. This polysaccharide fiber derived from the wood of the larch tree is a relative newcomer to the immune support scene, but one that holds much promise. In research studies, it has already been show to stimulate natural killer cell activity and to inhibit the metastasis of tumor cells to the liver. It has also been shown to boost the immunosupportive properties of echinacea when given together with this herb. A typical dose range for arabinogalactan is 1 to 4 grams per day.

Lactoferrin. Lactoferrin is a glycoprotein and a component of the whey fraction in cow's milk. It has

Immune Support Nutritionals	
Nutrients	**Herbs**
Vitamins A, C, and E	Aloe vera
Zinc	Astragalus
Selenium	Boswellia
Essential fatty acids	Echinacea
Adequate protein	Garlic
intake	Goldenseal
Arabinogalactan	Licorice
Lactoferrin	Lomatium
Lysine	Maitake mushroom
Orango-germanium	Marigold
	Oregon grape
	Pokeroot
	Redroot
	Reishi mushroom
	Shiitake mushroom
	St. John's wort

been clearly shown to modify immune function and can directly alter the production and function of several types of immune cells, including neutrophils and monocytes. Lactoferrin also has antibacterial and antiviral properties, possibly related to its strong capacity for binding iron and other minerals that might be needed by those microorganisms. It has also been used successfully in the case of stomach infections related to the overgrowth of *Helicobacter pylori*. A typical dose range for lactoferrin is 50 to 500 mg per day.

Lysine. This amino acid is an immune support nutrient because of its popularity in treating *Herpes simplex* infections, particularly oral herpes (HSV-1), which causes most of the cold sores or fever blisters. (For some reason, lysine is not as effective in preventing or treating genital herpes, which are usually caused by HSV-2.) High-lysine, low-arginine protocols have become popular in the treatment of *Herpes simplex*, because the virus appears to need high levels of arginine and low levels of lysine to replicate. Presumably, if the balance can be reversed, it can stop replication. The studies on this approach to *Herpes simplex* are mixed, although lack of success in some cases may simply be due to the low levels of lysine used. An amount of 3 grams per day over a 6-month period seems most like the effective dose range, compared to 1 to 2 grams per day used in some of these negative outcome studies. Let's keep in mind that this approach is not a cure for *Herpes simplex*, just a way to temporarily improve the infection while researchers work on long-term immune balance and vitality.

Organo-germanium. Germanium is a trace mineral that has come to the attention of the health world through the work of a medical doctor in Japan. In the 1950s, Dr. Kazuhiko Asai noticed that fairly high amounts of germanium were present in coal, peat, and some of the more powerful and useful Oriental healing herbs. In 1967, Asai and his associates isolated an organo-germanium compound soluble in water and labeled it Ge-132 (bis-carboxyethyl germanium sesquioxide, the 132nd form they had synthesized). In 1968, Asai founded the Asai Germanium Research Institute to study the clinical application of Ge-132 further. **Since that time, researchers have learned, almost exclusively from animal studies, that germanium may be helpful in protecting the liver from toxic damage and may support various aspects of immune function.** More recently, germanium has been shown to help prevent formation of glycated proteins—proteins that get hooked together with sugar molecules in a way that disrupts their function.

Advanced glycation end products (AGEs) are thought to be a major disruptive force in the body that is related to loss of body function in aging and to the progression of cataracts.

There is still debate over the safety of this mineral, which is FDA-approved for sale as a dietary supplement. Most of the problems reported in relationship with germanium have involved the kidneys and have been related to the inorganic form of this mineral, so I recommend its consumption only if used in the organic form.

Immune-Support Herbs

Herbs can support the immune system in two basic ways. First, they can have a direct impact on bacteria and viruses, just like our own immune cells, or like antibiotics do. There are probably hundreds of herbs that have antiviral and antibacterial properties, but in this section I have selected only the best-researched and most popular herbs. A second way for herbs to support the immune system is by enhancing the function of our own immune cells and organs, including the thymus and liver. Herbs can stimulate these organ systems to produce more immune cells, or they can increase the activity level of existing cells, or both.

Immune-Support Herbs				
Herb	Antiviral	Antibacterial	Increased Cell Production	Increased Cell Activity
Aloe vera	x	x	x	x
Astragalus	x			x
Boswellia		x		x
Echinacea	x	x	x	x
Garlic	x	x		x
Goldenseal	x	x	x	x
Licorice	x	x	x	x
Lomatium	x	x		x
Maitake mushroom			x	x
Oregon grape		x		x
Pokeroot	x			
Redroot		x		
Reishi mushroom	x	x	x	x
Shiitake mushroom	x	x	x	x
St. John's wort	x	x		

Based on these criteria, my list of immunosupportive herbs includes aloe, astragalus, boswellia, echinacea, garlic, goldenseal, licorice, lomatium, maitake mushroom, marigold, Oregon grape, pokeroot, redroot, reishi mushroom, shiitake mushroom, and St. John's wort. The table opposite lists some of the basic immune support properties for each of these herbs (see the various discussions of each herb throughout this chapter). Specifically, echinacea and licorice roots are important immune-supporting herbs, as shown in this chart.

MENTAL AND NERVOUS SYSTEM SUPPORT

When it comes to mental and nervous system support, most of the marketplace focus has been on conventional nutrients, especially the B complex vitamins, amino acids, and essential fatty acids. This focus makes sense. **B vitamins are especially important in supporting nerve cell activity and in allowing the nerve cells to produce their chemical messengers (neurotransmitters).** The B vitamin list here includes not only vitamins B_1, B_2, B_3, B_5, B_6, B_{12} and folate, but also biotin, choline, inositol, and PABA. The neurotransmitters that carry messages from nerve to nerve are often amino acids, so it also makes sense for support supplements to focus on these nutrients. Glycine, serine, tryptophan, and tyrosine are particularly important to consider. The myelin sheath that wraps around most nerves and allows them to function properly is also a focus of supplemental support, and its fatty acid composition includes a large amount of the omega-3 fatty acid DHA (docosahexaenoic acid). Supplementing this fatty acid directly, or encouraging its production by supplementing alpha-linolenic acid that the nerve cells can use to make DHA, also makes sense.

Mental and Nervous System Support Nutrients

In addition to the conventional nutrients, there are also some new mental and nerve support supplements on the shelves; this section explores some of these innovative newcomers.

Carnosine. Carnosine is a dipeptide (consisting of the two amino acids alanine and histidine) found in our nerve cells and in several types of brain cells, as well as in our muscle tissue. Our cells can synthesize carnosine, and its metabolism is the subject of much current research. At present, carnosine's overall role in our health is unclear, but some research points in the direction of an antiaging-type substance that is especially effective in regulating blood flow and preventing free-radical damage to our brain cells. Carnosine may turn out to be particularly important in preventing excessive attachment of sugar to brain proteins (to form advanced glycation end products, or AGEs) as well as to prevent cross-linking of DNA strands. Both of these roles would be considered as antiaging, because AGEs and DNA cross-linking are both considered to accelerate the aging process.

Phosphatidylcholine and phosphatidylserine. These two phospholipids are present in nearly all cell membranes, but they have been particularly interesting to look at in relation to the brain and its nerve cells. The ability of nerve cells to function properly seems to depend specifically on their phosphatidylserine content, and there have been a few studies showing improvement in cognitive function in older individuals following supplementation with phosphatidylserine. This supplement also has some successful use regarding the early stages of Alzheimer's disease. Still, the results in human studies with phosphatidylserine have been mixed, and for phosphatidylcholine, the only strongly positive studies have come in animal research. Phosphatidylcholine supplementation has been shown to improve short-term memory in animal studies, but there is not yet the same clear evidence for humans. Both of these supplements appear to have a strong margin of safety, and both are most commonly derived from soy. Short-term doses of these nutrients range from about 250 to 750 mg, with long-term supplementation recommended at a much lower range of about 100 to 200 mg per day.

Vinpocetine. This is a substance that can be made from an alkaloid found in the periwinkle plant (called vincamine). This substance passes rapidly across the blood-brain barrier and acts inside the brain like a neuroprotectant. Some of the nerve protection provided by vinpocetine may be related to its antioxidant activity, as well as to its ability to stop overactivation of the nerves and to prevent depletion of ATP. **Vinpocetine has been successfully used to help improve**

"cerebrovascular deficiencies"—problems related to insufficient blood flow throughout the brain. Vascular dementia, Alzheimer's, and acute ischemic stroke are all conditions in which vinpocetine supplementation has been used successfully.

A dose range of 30 to 120 mg was used in most of these studies, and I am comfortable with that range over a short-term period of several months. Until researchers know a little more about this nutrient, however, I suggest that routine supplementation with vinpocetine be kept under 20 mg per day.

Mental and Nervous System Support Herbs

Feverfew. The leaves of feverfew (*Chrysanthemum parthenium* and *Tanecetum parthenium*) have been more available recently as a supplement, and I have found it to be particularly effective in reducing the incidence and intensity of migraine headaches. Research tends to support this as well. **Reports indicate that feverfew also has a moderate anti-inflammatory effect and inhibits platelet aggregation, suggesting possible use in circulatory disease and other pain problems.**

At the first sign of a headache, 1 capsule is taken, and then another in 30 minutes. If this treatment is effective, another follow-up capsule should be taken in 3 or 4 hours. If the first 2 capsules do not work, a third might be attempted in 1 hour.

If no therapeutic response is seen in 2 separate trials, feverfew herb will not likely be an effective migraine treatment. If it works, however, I then usually suggest one 500 mg capsule once or twice daily for prevention. Although it appears fairly nontoxic, I suggest using it for only 2 to 3 weeks prophylactically and then stopping for 1 week. It can also be effective with no regular use, taking it only when a headache begins.

Ginkgo. Because the bioflavonoids in ginkgo have unique effectiveness in restoring healthy blood flow to the brain, ginkgo deserves special mention as an herb that can support mental health. Improvement of memory, especially in older people, has been demonstrated in studies on ginkgo. The lessening of depression also turns out to be a possible benefit from the use of ginkgo, because poor circulation to the brain can be a major factor in the occurrence of this problem.

St. John's wort. This herb has become a mainstay in treatment of depression because of its ability to inhibit the enzyme monoamine oxidase (MAO). When MAO is overactive, it depletes the brain's supply of norepinephrine (noradrenaline) that is needed to keep the nervous system activated. By lowering the activity level of MAO, St. John's wort boosts norepinephrine levels and increases the activation of the nervous system. When using solid extracts of this herb, a typical dose range is 750 to 2,000 mg per day, usually divided into 250 to 600 mg at a time.

METABOLIC AND CELLULAR AIDS

This category of supplement has become increasing popular with consumers, although it probably has the least research basis at this point in time. It makes sense for us to try and directly support our cells and their metabolism, and nutrition practitioners certainly know many of the nutrients that are essential for their function. However, because there are about 100 trillion cells in the body, including hundreds of different cell types, cellular supplementation can pose a challenge.

Researchers are finding new roles for amino acid and fatty acid supplementation in the cell support area, because both types of conventional nutrients have special roles to play in the cell. There are also two metabolic cycles run by many cells—the Krebs cycle and the SAM cycle (s-adenosylmethionine cycle)—that are becoming popular targets of nutritional support.

Metabolic and Cellular Support Nutrients

Amino acids. Many people take supplemental amino acid powders, capsules, or tablets as insurance for obtaining all the essential and nonessential building blocks for protein. In my practice, I have found amino acid therapy, using both complete formulas and individual L-amino acids, to be helpful for many patients' medical problems and concerns, including vegetarians or people with allergies, stress-related fatigue, or hypoglycemia. In chapter 3, Proteins, I discussed each amino acid and its application to nutritional medicine. Please refer to that chapter for current information on amino acid functions, metabolism, and therapy. However, the research and new findings in regard to amino acid use in medicine are moving rapidly, so watch the medical literature and news for future applications.

The most common amino acids used in treating health conditions have been tryptophan, lysine, and phenylalanine. On the upswing are arginine, carnitine, cysteine, glutamine, and tyrosine. All of these, except phenylalanine, are used in their L-form. (Both D- and DL-phenylalanine also have uses.) Each of the other individual amino acids has some possible uses as well. Their therapeutic amounts may range from 250 mg to 5 to 10 grams daily. **I suggest that single L-amino acids not be used with regularity, as this may affect the balance and functions of the others.** (This is also true when taking higher amounts of single B vitamins or minerals.) I suggest 2 weeks as the limit for taking any single nutrient to the exclusion of the others of its family. After that time, either it should be stopped, or the other amino acids or B vitamins, as the case may be, should be taken at the same time.

Krebs cycle organic acids. See the "Energy-Boosting and Stress-Reducing Nutrients" section of this chapter for a description of the Krebs cycle intermediates (page 274); this metabolic cycle takes place in the cell's energy production facilities (the mitochondria). Included in the Krebs cycle nutrients are malic acid, succinic acid, oxaloacetic acid, fumaric acid, citric acid, isocitric acid, and alpha-ketoglutaric acid. All of these nutrients can be made in the body and are not necessary from diet or supplements. Under many different circumstances, however, the body may not be making enough of them to meet an individual's needs. In principle, supporting the Krebs cycle is a way for us to boost our cells' energy supply (of ATP) while allowing them to continue to run their own metabolic processes.

SAM cycle intermediates. SAM cycle support is a relative newcomer to the consumer marketplace but a long-standing focus in cell science. This cycle is also called the *one-carbon cycle,* and its main job is to keep the cell well supplied with single-carbon molecules (called methyl groups). I also discuss methyl groups on page 747 in chapter 18, Detoxification and Cleansing Programs, because they can be critical to the detox process. You may already recognize many members of the SAM cycle from your trips to the health food store, because they include SAM itself (also abbreviated SAM-e, standing for S-adenosylmethionine), choline, betaine, sarcosine, DMAE (dimethylaminoethanol), serine, and glycine. Vitamins B6, B12, and folate are also necessary to run this metabolic cycle.

There are two related supplements that can also assist the SAM cycle: DMG (dimethylglycine) and TMG (trimethylglycine). DMG, in particular, steps into the marketplace with a long history of controversy and a mixed outcome in terms of research studies. This supplement has not been extensively studied, but it has been studied across a wide range of conditions, including child autism, athletic performance, gastric ulcer, and arthritis. The most consistent results show benefits in the area of tissue oxygenation and increase in stamina, but once again, these results are mixed. Because methyl groups and glycine play such a wide range of important metabolic roles in the body, more research must be done on DMG to refine its use as a supplement. In the meantime, the toxicity of DMG is very low, if any, especially in the usual amounts of 50 to 200 mg daily. DMG is available in oral or sublingual tablets and is taken 2 or 3 times daily. Dissolving these tablets under the tongue is currently the simplest and most efficacious way to utilize DMG.

MOOD BALANCERS

It might sound like I am talking about the nervous system again, but I am not. Mood balancing supplements are not building block–type supplements that are used to supply the organ systems and cells with the nutrients they need. The mood balancers have much more to do with energy and attitude. Balancing our moods is more a question of finding the right blend of activity and quiet, of rough and smooth, than a question of physiological balance. Many things in our lives affect our moods, including sugar, caffeine, alcohol, drugs and chemicals, life stages (adolescence and menopause, as examples), relationships, and expectations. Mood balancing supplements often involve hormones or their precursors, because hormones are the body's key substances for balancing the way we experience everyday life. Below I discuss the more prominent participants in this category of supplements.

Mood-Balancing Nutrients and Hormones

Dehydroepiandrosterone (DHEA). DHEA is a steroid hormone made by our adrenal glands. It is also the jumping-off point for the cells to make other steroid hormones, including estrogen and testosterone (an androgen). Because DHEA levels decrease with aging, there has been a focus on its ability to help prevent diseases related to aging, including cancers, cardiovascular diseases, dementia, and osteoporosis. The balance of our steroid hormone levels, however, is closely associated with our mood. This includes the balance between estrogens and androgens, as well as other steroid hormones. Mood swings related to depression, pregnancy, premenstrual syndrome, and menopause have all been related to fluctuations in steroid hormone levels.

Giving the body optimal flexibility to regulate steroid hormone balance makes a good bit of sense, and that is where DHEA may fit in. This supplement has been used successfully in a mindfulness-based stress-reduction program for older adults, as well as in treatment of depression and anxiety related to aging. **An amount of 5 to 15 mg per day for women and 10 to 30 mg per day for men would be conservative dose ranges for DHEA, but because this is a powerful steroid hormone, I favor lower doses to start treatment and working up as needed.** Many of the supplements in the stores are higher amounts, like 25 to 50 mg; this may be too high for many people.

Melatonin. One of the premier hormones secreted by the pineal gland, melatonin is a substance that helps us stay in sync with the world around us by keeping us attuned to the seasonal balance between day and night, and the daily balance of light and dark. Melatonin is part of the way we keep our sleep-wake cycle matched up with our environment, despite the great changes in daylight and darkness that take place between the winter and summer solstice. It is not surprising that this supplement has been used to help treat insomnia and seasonal affective disorder, and even jet lag, because all of these problems are related to the passage of time and our experience of it. **A range of 1 to 5 mg per day, often taken at bedtime, is a normal dose for melatonin.** When traveling between time zones, the suggestion is to take melatonin at the new bedtime to become in sync with the sleep cycle of your new place. See more on page 620 in the "Executives and Healthy Travel" section in chapter 16, Performance Enhancement Programs.

Pregnenalone. Like DHEA, pregnenalone is a steroid hormone that serves as a jumping-off point for production of other steroid hormones. Pregnenalone may sit in an even more fundamental spot than DHEA, however, because its fate determines whether we make *any* of the estrogenic or androgenic hormones, or instead focus on production of cortisol and other corticosteroids. Research on the use of this supplement is sketchy at this point, but the most common applications have involved age-related health problems, especially bone, joint, and cognitive problems experienced by postmenopausal women. There is not enough evidence quite yet to determine the value of pregnenalone as a dietary supplement, so I recommend its use only in consultation with a health-care practitioner who can help you take a closer look at your specific hormonal balance and needs. Pregnenalone can be measured, as can DHEA and other hormones, and then with these findings, an appropriate rebalance of hormones can be created.

Serotonin, 5-hydroxytryptophan (5-HTP), and L-tryptophan. The neurotransmitter serotonin and amino acid metabolite and serotonin precursor 5-HTP are made by the pineal gland in the same way as melatonin. In fact, the pineal gland starts with the amino acid tryptophan and then converts it into 5-HPT. From there, it takes 5-HTP and converts it into serotonin. From there, it takes two other steps and produces melatonin. All of these supplements are closely related in terms of the pineal cell metabolism.

Although serotonin cannot be sold directly as a dietary supplement, 5-HTP can, and 5-HTP supplementation has been shown to boost serotonin levels. This supplement has proven helpful in treatment of insomnia and also depression. There is minimal risk or side effects when supplementing with 5-HTP or L-tryptophan, and some people respond better to one than the other although either should work effectively. A typical dose range for 5-HTP is 50 to 200 mg, usually taken at bedtime, or it can divided into 2 or 3 daily installments of 100 mg each. Please note that L-tryptophan is available again from practitioners and compounding pharmacies, after being removed from the

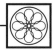

marketplace in 1989 by the FDA following research showing its connection with national outbreak of a disease called eosinophilia-myalgia syndrome (EMS). Before that, it was used safely by millions for several decades without problems. Since the withdrawal, the FDA has reinterpreted this connection between tryptophan and EMS and has stated that the outbreak of 1,500 cases was not caused by the L-tryptophan. Accordingly, in 2001, the FDA allowed reintroduction of L-tryptophan into the marketplace, while still keeping an "important alert" in effect until further research on L-tryptophan becomes available. This amino acid has value in treating sleep disorders and depression. The tryptophan dosage is 500 to 1,000 mg at bedtime.

L-theanine. This amino acid found in green tea is becoming increasingly popular, not in the natural products world, but in the world of cancer treatment. Theanine is currently being used alongside of many prescription anticancer drugs to enhance their effectiveness in fighting tumors and to prevent unwanted side effects. I include theanine here because this substance can alter brain levels of serotonin and change nervous system balance in this way. The shifts in serotonin levels may be related to the possible antiobesity effects that theanine has shown in some animal studies, but the jury is still out in this regard. The standard marketplace dose for theanine is about 100 mg per day. Many users say it has a mild tranquilizing effect.

Mood Balancing Nutritionals

Nutrients	Herbs
Amino acids—L-tryptophan and 5-HTP, L-theanine	Chamomile
	Kava
Hormone-related nutrients— DHEA, melatonin, pregnenolone	Valerian

---

Mood-Balancing Herbs

Chamomile. This gentle and sweet-smelling herb (*Matricaria recutita*) is calming to the body and helpful with irritations of all kinds. I include it here because of its amazing affect on children. For kids who have digestive upset or colic, or who are teething and upset,

chamomile can be an almost miraculous mood balancer. It is not as strong a sleep aid as valerian, but it is a sleep aid nonetheless. And because it is usually consumed as a tea, there is the pleasure of sipping and enjoying its warmth. I have also seen chamomile added to bath water to aid in relaxation.

Kava. Kava (*Piper methysticum*) works through the nervous system to lessen anxiety, reduce pain, and promote relaxation. As a muscle relaxant, it can also work as an anticonvulsant. I like kava's ability to bring about relaxation without causing "brain fog" or any lack of mental clarity. It is also an herb that can improve sleep. It may take 1 or 2 months of regular kava use to realize these benefits, however. A standard dose range for kava is 200 to 300 mg per day, usually divided into 2 or 3 installments. Some people react to kava and it is being used less frequently now. Be sure not to drink kava and then drive, as you may appear to be intoxicated.

Valerian root. Valerian (*Valeriana officinalis*) is a fascinating tonic-type herb that is truly mood balancing. By this I mean that valerian can act as a sedative that calms the nervous system when we are stressed or anxious, but at the same time, if we are feeling low or extremely fatigued, valerian can act as a stimulant and help perk us back up. The most common uses for this herb, however, involve calming the nervous system under conditions of anxiety or stress. The best-studied use of valerian is for insomnia, and it actually compares favorably to prescription drugs like triazolam (a benzodiazepine). A typical dose of valerian would be 300 to 500 mg, and if taken for insomnia, consumed about 1 hour before bedtime.

PLANT OILS, FISH OILS, AND FATTY ACIDS

Most of the information you will need about fats and fatty acids is included in chapter 4, Lipids—Fats and Oils. My focus in this section is on the specialty plant oils one might find in natural food stores and on the Internet. All seeds and nuts are primarily composed of fat and can be pressed to extract their oil. In principle, then, there are literally hundreds of thousands of "specialty oils" available to us from the plant world. I think of oil as a "partitioned" food that lacks the

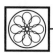

wholeness of the seed or nut. Because all oils lack the nutrient protection that is found in the seed, it is especially important to buy the highest quality and freshest oils, to refrigerate them, to keep them tightly capped when not in use, and to purchase smaller amounts so that one's supply stays fresh. Encapsulated oils are a convenient alternative, although more expensive on an ounce-by-ounce basis.

Common Oil Supplements

Black currant oil. This is usually singled out from the rest of the specialty oils because of its unique fatty acid combination—it contains both GLA (gamma-linolenic acid) and ALA (alpha-linolenic acid). ALA is the essential omega-3 fatty acid the body uses to make all other omega-3s—including EPA (eicosapentaenoic acid) and DHA (decosahexaenoic acid). GLA is the most anti-inflammatory of the omega-6 fatty acids, so the combination of GLA and ALA is considered unique. I have found this oil particularly useful in the case of eczema and allergic dermatitis, and I also consider it a good immune support oil.

Borage seed oil. This oil is known for its high GLA content, and it does appear to contain more GLA than either black currant oil or evening primrose oil. Unlike black currant, however, borage seed oil does not supply an appreciable amount of any omega-3 fatty acid. For this reason, it is often blended together with another oil, like flaxseed, to produce a balanced combination of GLA and omega-3s. Like black currant oil, it is also useful for skin problems, including plain old dry skin.

Cod liver oil. This has perhaps the longest track record of any specialty oil. The first studies on cod liver oil were published more than 50 years ago. It is one of the most concentrated food sources available for omega-3 fatty acids, including both EPA and DHA. The big problem, however, is with making sure you have obtained a high-quality, toxin-free oil. Because cod fish can be contaminated with mercury, cadmium, lead, PCBs, and dozens of other contaminants (and the liver also deals with most toxins), and because the oils themselves can be subjected to chemical processing, it is important to take the extra trouble to find an oil that is certified to be free from these contaminants.

If large amounts of cod liver oil are taken, it is worth calculating the total amount of vitamins A and D consumed for the day from all supplements and foods combined. Above 10,000 IU of preformed vitamin A (retinol) may be reason for concern in some individuals, and for pregnant women, the level of concern would lower down to approximately 5,000 IU. For vitamin D, there may be some concern with daily totals exceeding about 2,000 IU.

Evening primrose oil. The oil that comes from the seeds of the evening primrose plant contains a high amount of its active ingredient, GLA, an oil much like the essential fatty acids (EFA) of the omega-6 variety. In fact, GLA is a precursor of the EFA arachidonic acid, but even more important to its potential therapeutic benefits, GLA leads to the important prostaglandin E1 series (PGE1). **The use of evening primrose oil as a nontoxic source of GLA is a good mix of nutrition and herbal medicine.**

Actually, this night-blooming, bright yellow flowering plant is not a true primrose but is part of the willow-herb family. The name comes from the fact that its flowers resemble those of the primrose plant. This herb has been used medicinally for centuries—externally as a poultice for skin problems and internally to treat a variety of complaints, such as asthma, gastrointestinal problems, gynecological problems, or to enhance wound healing. Native Americans used this plant and its seeds commonly, and in England it was known as "King's cure-all."

There has been a great deal of research with GLA since the mid-1980s, much of it conducted in England, where the majority of evening primrose oil is made. With more than 100 research papers published and many more in progress, the results are mixed. Most of the findings, however, are positive and promising, particularly in regard to clearing or reducing symptoms in arthritis, skin problems, and premenstrual syndrome, as well as for all kinds of inflammatory problems, cardiovascular disease, and immunosuppression.

Our bodies can make some GLA from an essential fatty acid, linoleic acid, and from this GLA, we form PGE1 series. Many symptoms occur from deficiency of linoleic acid, and many of these may be contributed to by low PGE1 levels, which also may arise from reduced or blocked steps in fatty acid metabolism. Many of these aspects are still unknown. When we take additional GLA, we encourage increased formation of PGE1, which produces a variety of effects. The PGE1

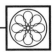

series is probably the most important of the hormone-like prostaglandins. These substances help inhibit or reduce inflammation, platelet aggregation, thrombosis, cholesterol synthesis, blood vessel tone, and the formation of abnormal cells. PGE1 is also thought to help lower blood pressure and protect the liver from the effects of alcohol and other irritating drugs. This prostaglandin also functions in maintaining the salt and water balance, insulin secretion, nerve conduction, and gastrointestinal function.

Studies on the use of evening primrose oil have focused on the skin and the joints. This oil has proven effective in treating atopic dermatitis and atopic eczema (atopy is genetic allergy potential and involves eczema, asthma, and hay fever), and researchers have measured its quieting effects on the immune system. Evening primrose oil is clearly able to reduce antibody levels in these conditions, although not as much as some prescription medications. Given the fact that these prescription medicines have unwanted side effects, however, I would call these results positive. Clear benefits for the use of evening primrose oil have also been shown in the treatment of rheumatoid arthritis. In some studies where the benefits were mild instead of significant, I believe the dose of evening primrose oil used and the duration of the study partly account for the lack of stronger results.

Side effects from the use of evening primrose oil are almost nonexistent. Some nausea may be experienced initially because of the oils, but this can be avoided if it is taken with food. Mild skin rashes or acne can occur occasionally; otherwise, no problems have been noticed. The recommended amount is between 500 and 1,000 mg, taken 2 or 3 times daily, with possibly higher doses (4–6 grams daily) for such problems as arthritis, asthma, or eczema. Most good primrose oils contain about 35 to 40 mg of GLA per 500 mg capsule; I call for a therapeutic amount of 150 to 250 mg GLA daily. Usually I suggest a good-quality vitamin E, particularly for premenstrual and breast soreness and tenderness problems and specifically the natural mixed tocopherols in 1 or 2 doses of 200 to 400 IU each to act with the GLA.

It is likely there will be some interesting new research concerning this nutrient in the upcoming years. Other recently available sources of gamma-linoleic acid include black currant seed and borage seed oils, which can be even more concentrated in GLA than primrose, producing similar effects with less capsules and expense. Although these sources have not been evaluated as extensively as evening primrose oil, they may be good substitutes.

Eicosapentaenoic acid and decosahexaenoic acid (EPA and DHA). EPA and DHA are omega-3 long-chain unsaturated fatty acids found in fish oils. EPA and DHA, which are usually found together, have become very popular recently in the literature and as supplements. Like GLA, EPA and DHA also seem to affect the synthesis of the prostaglandins in series 1, but even more so those in series 3, which may give them additional anti-inflammatory benefits. However, their main effect is to help lower blood fat levels. The intake of dietary EPA and DHA is enhanced by eating cold-water fish regularly, such as salmon, herring, mackerel, or sardines, which feed on certain plankton, or by taking additional oil supplements. Increased intake of EPA and DHA has been shown in numerous studies to lower blood triglyceride and cholesterol levels while raising the level of high-density lipoprotein (HDL), the "good" cholesterol.

I need to add some precautions about consuming cold-water fish and, for that matter, fish in general. Most everything we call "waste" sooner or later ends up in the Earth's waters. The process can take generations, but it eventually happens. **The FDA took action in 2003 by telling pregnant women not to consume more than 12 ounces per week of mercury-containing fish, including canned tuna.** By this time, the FDA had already put swordfish, king mackerel, shark, and tilefish on its list. It is nearly impossible to purchase a contaminant-free fish, but it is possible to minimize the risk. In the case of cold-water fish like salmon, farmed fish are *not* the way to go. These fish have been shown to have higher levels of polychlorinated biphenyls (PCBs), a group of industrial

---

Fish High in EPA and/or DHA

Bluefish	Herring	Salmon
Bonita	Kippers	Sardines
Butterfish	Mackerel	Trout
Eel	Pompano	

chemicals widely used in the 1960s and 1970s, because of their feeding regimen, and synthetic pigments (canthaxanthans) are often added to the fish to improve their pinkish color. Wild-caught salmon are by far the best choice. I would personally avoid the suggested FDA-listed mercury-contaminated fish, pregnant or not, unless I knew their source to be relatively low risk in terms of contamination. There are some specialty canned tunas in the marketplace that are certified mercury-free and that retain significantly greater amounts of the omega-3 fatty acids because they are cooked in the can with their original oils intact. These specialty tunas are more expensive, but they may be worth the price.

The lipid-lowering effects of EPA and DHA, along with some benefits in reducing platelet aggregation and clotting potential, make their use important in the treatment or prevention of cardiovascular disease or in anyone with high blood fats or low HDL. The decreased blood viscosity and lower fat levels help reduce the risk of heart attacks. The mild anti-inflammatory effects, possibly a result of increased PGE1 and PGE3 prostaglandins, may also be helpful and this has suggested the possible use of EPA and DHA in arthritis and other inflammatory conditions. In rheumatoid arthritis, for example, EPA and DHA supplementation has been shown to reduce joint stiffness and soreness and to improve flexibility.

There are no significant side effects from the use of EPA and DHA, except for mild nausea that some people experience from taking these oils. Fish oils contain no vitamin C or E and are more likely to oxidize and go rancid. Therefore many of the commercial preparations have vitamin E added to prevent oxidation. Fish liver oils are not recommended, even though they contain some EPA and DHA, because they are too high in vitamins A and D and because livers tend to concentrate any toxic materials the fish (or any animal) have absorbed.

In general, as a preventive for cardiovascular disease, it is recommended that we eat a portion of the oily fishes 2 or 3 times weekly. If we do have high blood fats, low HDL, or increased risk of cardiovascular disease, we can supplement 500 to 1,000 mg of EPA and DHA twice daily to improve these conditions, although in my experience, it does not work that well to lower cholesterol. Higher amounts may be needed

for this effect. Higher amounts may also be needed for treating asthma and inflammatory disorders. Simple, moderate exercise works better, however, and as for nutritional supplements, it seems that such other agents as niacin or L-carnitine may be better at lowering lipids (see "Cardiovascular Disease Prevention" on page 651 in chapter 16, Performance Enhancement Programs). Also, for supplying the valuable omega-3 fatty acids, cold-pressed flaxseed oil is a less expensive source. EPA and DHA are also discussed in chapter 4, Lipids— Fats and Oils and under "Seafood" in chapter 8, Foods (see page 343).

Flaxseed oil. As the best-selling of the specialty oils, flaxseed oil has drawn increased research attention since the mid-1990s, with some fairly impressive results. One study I particularly liked showed the ALA and EPA content of human milk to increase in nursing mothers who supplemented with this oil. (Interestingly, DHA did not increase in the milk, for reasons that are still not understood.) In obese individuals, flaxseed oil has been determined to improve arterial blood flow, and in young men, to decrease risk of heart problems by decreasing the tendency of platelet cells to clump together inappropriately.

Flax is a nicely balanced oil, containing the essential building blocks for both omega-6 (linoleic acid) and omega-3 (alpha-linolenic acid) fatty acids. I find that problems of dry skin are helped with the use of flaxseed oil, organically grown flax being ideal. The recommended dosage is 2 to 3 capsules or 1/2 to 1 tablespoon taken twice daily at meals. Flaxseed oil can also be used in salad dressings. Although it does not contain high levels of the advanced omega-3s (EPA and DHA), that may be a benefit in long-term supplementation, because we would ideally like our bodies to

---

Possible Uses of EPA and/or DHA

Angina pectoris	Hypertension
Atherosclerosis	Lupus and other
Bronchial asthma	autoimmune diseases
Cardiovascular	Migraine headaches
disease	Rheumatoid arthritis
Cerebrovascular	Tinnitus
disease	

decide when to make EPA and DHA from ALA. Very high doses of EPA and DHA cannot be obtained from flax, making cod liver oil, salmon oil, and other fish oils preferable in some situations.

Wheat germ oil and octacosanol. Wheat germ oil is high in vitamin E and was often used as a source of vitamin E for internal use or for external application to burns, sores, and other skin problems. **The antioxidant properties of vitamin E make wheat germ oil more stable to oxidation or rancidity than many other oils.** Octacosanol is another active ingredient of wheat germ oil. Many users and manufacturers of octacosanol capsules claim that it enhances endurance, reaction time, and general vitality, yet these effects may take several weeks to notice. Although no benefits of this kind have been demonstrated so far in human subjects, animal studies have shown octacosanol to increase the oxidative capacity of the muscles and to help spare muscle glycogen, thus resulting in improved performance in exercise-trained animals.

More research is needed on octacosanol, which may turn out to have potential benefits for a wide range of muscle-related problems. Wheat germ itself is a good source of protein, B vitamins, vitamin E, and many minerals, particularly iron, calcium, copper, magnesium, manganese, zinc, phosphorus, and potassium. Nutritionally, it is more balanced overall than its isolated oil, which is almost exclusively vitamin E plus other oils and is more caloric. We do, however, need some oils for tissue health and to obtain natural vitamin E, so wheat germ oil supplements can be a good addition to a low-fat or low–vitamin E diet.

Part 2

Foods, Diets, Nutritional Habits, and the Environment

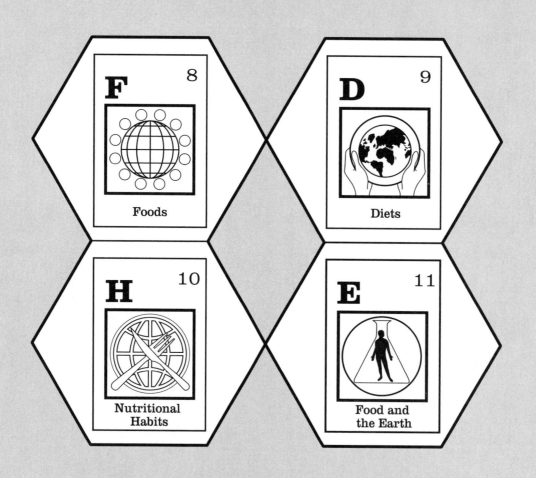

In part 1 of this book, I discussed the building blocks—the nutrients found in foods and other substances on the planet that make up the body's tissues and guide body functions. Part 2 looks at the many foods and diets that contain these important and essential nutrients. If we think of nutrition as a communication system, then the macro- and micronutrients discussed in part 1 are the letters of the alphabet. Individual foods create words, with their special mix of letters (nutrients), and meals are the sentences, combinations of letters and words that bring together multiple components of nutrition.

After reviewing the various food groups and individual foods in chapter 8, Foods, I then discuss in chapter 9, Diets, the various types of diets eaten in Western culture as well as throughout the world. Chapter 10, Nutritional Habits, elaborates on healthy and unhealthy dietary habits, and chapter 11, Food and the Earth, explores concerns about the state of food and the use of chemicals, as well as the effects on the planet's environment. All of these chapters in part 2 provide the hands-on guidelines that will make the technical information earlier in the book work better for you. Enjoy.

Chapter 8

Foods

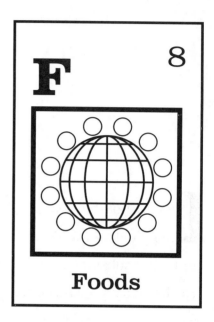

Foods

This chapter provides an evaluation of the various food categories, such as fruits, vegetables, grains, and so on. This is not a discussion of the four food groups classically used to describe a wholesome diet. These aspects of our diet, along with many other nutritional principles, are discussed later in part 2.

Food availability varies around the world. Earth provides different plants according to the climate. People throughout the world have also spread pleasurable and nutritious foods from culture to culture and country to country by carrying seeds or plants to cultivate in a new area. Such foods now present in the United States as potatoes, rice, and even wheat were not originally native to this country.

One of the most natural concepts of eating is that of consuming locally grown and seasonally appropriate fresh foods. Some foods—such as root vegetables, grains, nuts, and seeds—store better than others and may be consumed in winter, when in many areas most foods are not available in their fresh state. It is important to eat a variety of foods. Eating only a single type of food will provide limited nutrition and an imbalanced diet. **I also advocate eating a predominantly natural diet containing fresh fruits and vegetables, whole grains, nuts, seeds, and beans,** with only moderate amounts of the more concentrated proteins such as eggs, milk products, and animal meats. Unfortunately, the opposite diet—consisting mainly of meats, dairy products, and refined foods, and only occasional fresh foods—is all too common in the United States.

Here I discuss the basic foods from the least concentrated to the most, basically from fruits to animal meats. I begin with higher-vibration foods (flowers and pollens) and move through the food chain to animal products, finishing the discussion with seasonings and beverages. With each category, I describe the basic nutrient makeup as well as the vitamin and mineral content, giving specific examples of foods that are part of that group. I also talk about the phytonutrients found in foods, the nutrients that can't be classified as vitamins, minerals, proteins, carbohydrates, or fats but that are diverse and far-reaching in their powers of nourishment and for sustaining good health. For the exact nutrient content of each food, I refer readers to such food sourcebooks as Jean Pennington, Anna Bowes, and Charles Church's *Food Values of Portions Commonly Used.* Using the nutrient content of food, we

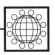

can analyze what we eat in regards to our exact nutrient intake. That is a fairly complex and time-consuming process, however. I often suggest that individuals do a diet survey to see how their diet is balanced and what specific nutrients it contains. A diet survey basically involves recording all food consumed over a 1-week period. This information is transferred into a computer programmed to analyze the daily intake of calories, fiber, cholesterol, and nutrients from vitamin A to zinc. The percentages of fats, carbohydrates, and proteins are also important, as is the percentage of calories from various food groups. Although a nutritionist can be helpful when interpreting the results, these percentages can help any of us see more clearly if the diet is balanced and how to shift to a potentially healthier one. This is a valuable exercise for anyone interested in personal nutrition.

FIBER

Before discussing the particular types of food, I want to say a few words about **two important components of many of the foods from nature—namely, fiber and phytonutrients.** Although a good bit of information about fiber as a nutrient is discussed in chapter 2, Carbohydrates, here I provide a second look at fiber as a health hallmark of food. Fiber is found exclusively in plant foods, and it is among the keys to their health benefits. Exactly how important are fiber-containing plants to our well-being? I answer this question by relating the following surprising set of events.

During the 1990s, several large-scale clinical studies involving more than 75,000 participants were carried out to determine the effects of isolated nutrients (as opposed to whole foods) on health. Most of these studies focused on cancer prevention. The most common nutrient given to subjects in these studies was beta-carotene, the orange-colored pigment found in such plant foods as carrots. At least three of these studies were canceled midstream; letters were sent to the subjects informing them that the beta-carotene supplements they had been taking may in fact have increased their risk of cancer. Researchers were shocked at this outcome, and even today debate continues over the results of these studies. What seems so striking to

me about the cancellation of the studies is the fact that the 1990s also gave rise to several large-scale studies involving whole foods and cancer prevention—and not one of these studies was ever canceled. In fact, the studies found whole foods (particularly fruits and vegetables) to be cancer preventive. Unlike the studies of beta-carotene and other supplements, whole fruit and vegetable studies never failed to reduce the risk of cancer.

Why did whole carrots lower cancer risk 100% of the time when the beta-carotene extracted from carrots did not? I am convinced that the fiber in high-carotene vegetables played a role here. **So much of our nourishment depends on the healthy passage of food through our digestive tract. Without fiber it is impossible for digestion to take place in a balanced way.** With imbalanced digestion comes the risk of poor nutrient absorption, and along with that comes compromised metabolism and inadequate health protection. The risk of most chronic diseases is lowest when whole plant foods, especially vegetables, are plentiful in the diet. Diabetes, heart disease, high blood pressure, obesity, and several types of cancer are least likely to occur when a person's diet is high in vegetables and other high-fiber plant foods.

The connection between fiber and foods is so unique that I consider it the single best principle to follow when selecting grocery products. Particularly if you are purchasing a prepackaged food, looking on the nutrition label for grams of fiber per serving is the best way to go. It is difficult to find a crummy food that has 10 to 15 grams of fiber per serving.

PHYTONUTRIENTS

No greater shift has occurred in nutritional thinking about food since the mid-1990s than the shift related to *phytonutrients*, which simply means "plant nutrients." The term refers to all nontraditional substances in plants that provide specific health benefits. By *nontraditional* here, I mean everything except vitamins, minerals, proteins, carbohydrates, and fats. What is left for phytonutrients?

Surprisingly, phytonutrients outnumber traditional nutrients by about 10,000 to 1. All of the wonderful qualities that we associate with good food —the way it looks, the way it smells, the way it tastes—are the result of a food's phytonutrients. When steamed kale starts to change color, that change is centered around phytonutrients. When a sliced onion releases its smell, phytonutrients are the reason. When we taste the bitterness in beer, that taste is based on phytonutrients. Our *experience* of food is not based on essential nutrients (which, from the scientist's point of view, are also sometimes called *primary metabolites*) but on secondary metabolites that we have come to call *phytonutrients.*

Even if you have not heard about phytonutrients, you may be more familiar with them than you might think. You may not have realized that the way foods look and smell is also connected with their nutritional value. Maybe some people have stopped making this connection because they have gotten too used to eating highly processed foods that smell or taste great but provide little nourishment.

Researchers are finding out more about the way phytonutrients keep us healthy. The phytonutrients beta-carotene and carotenoids give foods like carrots their bright orange color, and at the same time they help protect us from the development of such diseases as cancer or heart disease. Carotenoids are only a single category of phytonutrients, however, and most of the other phytonutrient groups are not as familiar to most people. For example, the color of food comes primarily from carotenoids and flavonoids, but it also comes from porphyrins, alkaloids, and tannins. The taste of food often comes from terpenoids and phenylpropanoids. These phytonutrient groups have not gotten much press, so next I discuss how they relate to the colors, tastes, and smells of food.

Phytonutrients and the Color of Food

The potpourri of colors in the produce section of the grocery store is actually courtesy of a highly organized group of phytonutrients that are found in special locations in all plants. Most of the color-giving substances in food, called pigments, can be grouped together. The cells of plants have small water sacs called *vacuoles,* and inside of these vacuoles are two special types of pigments. Flavonoids—especially a division of flavonoids called *anthocyanins*—are the first type. The reds, blues, purples, and magentas found in food are created by anthocyanin pigments. Other types of flavonoid pigments, called *flavones* and *flavonols,* are also found alongside the anthocyanins and provide foods with some of their vibrant yellow colors. Scientists have identified more than 3,000 different flavonoids in the plant food world. Some of the better known flavonoids include apigenin, butin, catechin, cyanidin, delphinidin, eriodictyol, fustin, hesperidin, leucocyanidin, luteolin, myricetin, naringinen, quercetin, rutin, and taxifolin. Betalains are a second type of pigment found in the plant vacuoles. The betalains are nitrogen-containing pigments, and they come in two basic shades. The betacyanins provide food with varying shades of violet, and the betaxanthins provide food with varying shades of yellow.

In addition to the vacuoles found in plant cells, there are other specialized components called *plastids*. There are two basic types of plastids: chromoplasts and chloroplasts. Inside the chromoplasts are the carotenoid pigments. This well-studied group contains more than 600 different color-providing substances. Carotenoids include such carotenes as alpha-carotene, beta-carotene, gamma-carotene, and lycopene, as well as such xanthophylls as astaxanthin, canthaxanthin, cryptoxanthin, and zeaxanthin. Carotenoids are light-absorbing pigments; they help trap the sun's solar energy and convert it into chemical energy. Many of the oranges and yellows in food, and sometimes even some of the red shades, are provided by carotenoids in the plant's chromoplasts. Chromoplasts are not the star performers, however, when it comes to the absorption of sunlight. That distinction goes to chlorophylls found inside the plant's chloroplasts.

Chlorophylls give plant foods their vital green colors, and they are the plants' primary mechanism for trapping sunlight and transforming it into cell fuel. Sometimes a food contains so much chlorophyll in its chloroplasts that the carotenoid colors become masked to the naked eye. The flavonoid and betalain colors provided in the vacuoles also get masked. While these other pigments are masked, the leaves and other high-chlorophyll parts of the plants appear completely green. It takes a change in season, from summer to fall, for these other pigments to become "unmasked," as the chloroplasts shut down shop for the winter and the greens of summer start dissolving into the reds, oranges, yellows, and browns of autumn.

Phytonutrients and the Taste of Food

Food also depends on phytonutrients for its taste. These categories of phytonutrients, such as terpenoids and phenylpropanoids, are equally important in terms of their health benefits. Terpenoids are responsible for some of the bitter and more astringent tastes. Darjeeling tea, for example, is rich in terpenoids. Carrots are another interesting example, because they depend on just the right balance of sugars and terpenoids for their flavor. Like flavonoids, terpenoids are a major category of phytonutrient, including thousands of unique compounds. The phenylpropanoids are all partly derived from the amino acid phenylalanine, and their flavor-providing qualities are well-known in the food world. In this category are the hydroxycinnamic acids that get released from grapes during a wine pressing. Some of the more subtle and unique differences between wines in terms of bitterness and astringency are created by this phytonutrient mixture.

But most bitterness and astringency is provided by another type of phytonutrient called *tannins*. Tannins are cousins to flavonoids: both are polyphenolic substances and both involve thousands of different compounds that are sometimes unique to a small number of foods, that commonly have antioxidant and cancer-protective properties, and that we should think of as nutritionally essential. The proanthocyanidins that have become so popular as a component of grape seed extract are in fact condensed tannins. Some of the better known cancer-preventive substances like gallic acid, caffeic acid (which can be found in the coffee bean), and their derivatives are also made from tannins.

Phytonutrients and the Smell of Food

Like color and taste, the magnificent aromas of food also stem from phytonutrients. The terpenoid category of phytonutrients is especially important, with many of the distinctive aromas of such essential oils as lavender oil or bergamot oil (the distinctive aroma-producing component in Earl Grey tea) and the rich aroma of a Muscat wine coming directly from its terpenoid content. The phenylpropanoid phytonutrients are also key players when it comes to aroma. Included in this category is the unique smell of cloves provided by its eugenol content as well as the distinct aromas of different coffees, which are closely connected with their phenylpropanoid content (in this case more specifically with the hydroxycinnamic acids content).

In addition, sulfur-containing compounds play a key role in the aroma of food. Unfortunately, the best known example of sulfur's attention-getting odor involves rotten eggs, whose yolks are rich in unique sulfur compounds. The smells of chopped onions or crushed garlic are derived from sulfur metabolism. Hundreds of unique sulfur-containing molecules have already been identified in food, with particular attention paid to the cruciferous vegetables (like broccoli, cabbage, and cauliflower). I predict these sulfur-containing compounds will get more and more attention in the future.

The terms *glucosinolates, thiocyanates,* and *isothiocyanates* each refer to sulfur-containing compounds. In chemistry, the prefix *thio-* and the category *thiol* both refer to substances that contain sulfur. Glucosinolates are actually the precursors for both thiocyanates and isothiocyanates. They are made from amino acids, especially tryptophan, methionine, and cysteine. Glucosinolates are also sometimes called *thioglycosides.* Sulforaphane is perhaps the best known of the isothiocyanates and, like other molecules in this group, is made from a glucosinolate.

How we prepare food makes a difference in the sulfur-containing phytonutrients. When sulfur-containing foods like raw garlic or raw onions are sliced (or chopped, crushed, and simply chewed), enzymes in the food become activated and start converting some sulfur compounds into other forms. In chemical terms, sulfoxides get converted into thiosulfonates. This process also takes place when cruciferous vegetables like cabbage or broccoli get chopped. **The net result is an increase in many of the sulfur-containing phytonutrients that have been linked to cancer prevention and other aspects of improved health.** One group of sulfur-containing compounds you don't want to mess around with are the thiocarbamates. Although this group sounds like it contains phytonutrients, it is actually a group of pesticides, each of which contains sulfur. Dithianon, maneb, mancozeb, and thiobencarb are examples of thiocarbamate pesticides.

Phytonutrients

Type	Description	Examples
Flavonoids (polyphenols)	**GENERAL** Color-providing pigments and related compounds that often have antioxidant, antibiotic, cancer-preventive, anti-inflammatory, and other tissue-supportive and tissue-protective properties. **SUBTYPES** Flavonols, dihydroflavonols, flavones, flavonones, and anthocyanidins	quercetin, rutin, hesperidin, myricetin, fustin, taxifolin, leuco-cyanidin, apigenin, luteolin, naringinen, butin, eriodictyol, eriocitrin, cyanidin, delphinidin, catechin, epicatechin, gallocatechin, myricetin, and rhamnetin
Tannins (polyphenols)	**GENERAL** Polyphenolic substances like flavonoids that often have antioxidant and cancer-preventing properties; some are color-providing pigments; unlike flavonoids, however, tannins can bind tightly to other molecules and are less likely to be absorbed because of their larger size. **SUBTYPES** Condensed tannins (including proanthocyanidins) and hydrolyzable tannins (including gallotannins and ellagitannins)	profisetinidin, punicalagin, punicalin, and gallic and ellagic acid (tannin derivatives)
Terpenoids (isoprenoids)	**GENERAL** Diverse group of molecules originally derived from a vitamin B_5-containing compound and usually containing oxygen; includes all carotenoids; includes substances with antioxidant, immunosupportive, anti-inflammatory, and cancer-preventive properties. **SUBTYPES** Monoterpenoids, diterpenoids (gibberellins), triterpenoids (steroids), tetraterpenoids (carotenoids), and sesquiterpenoids	all carotenoids (including all carotenes like beta-carotene and lycopene and all xanthophylls like zeaxanthin and cryptoxanthin), limonene, terpineol, camphor, thujone, farnesol, abscisic acid, all gibberellic acids, beta-sitosterol, stigmasterol, and squalene

Phytonutrients

Type	Description	Examples
Alkaloids	**GENERAL** Nitrogen-containing compounds derived from amino acids that commonly have antioxidant, immunosupportive, and cancer-preventive properties. **SUBTYPES** Betalains and tetracyclic and pentacyclic alkaloids; many other groups, including oxindole alkaloids, acridone alkaloids, and vinca alkaloids	betacyanin, betaxanthin, piperidine, quinoline, pyrrolidine, berberine, oxyberberine, jatrorrhizine, columbamine, magnoflorine, corytuberine, fumarophycine, vinblastine, vincristine, isopteropodine, pteropodine, and caffeine
Phenylpropanoids (phenols and polyphenols)	**GENERAL** Phenolic and polyphenolic substances that are all initially derived from the amino acid phenylalanine; many of the substances studied have shown antioxidant, anti-inflammatory, and immune stimulating properties. **SUBTYPES** Hydroxycinnamic acids, coumarins, and lignans (derived from cinnamic acid)	hydroxycinnamic acid, coumarin, eugenol, caffeic acid, ferulic acid, chlorogenic acid, and lignans
Glycosides	**GENERAL** Molecules containing carbohydrate and non-carbohydrate portions linked together; includes substances with anti-inflammatory, anticancer, immunosupportive, and antioxidant properties. **SUBTYPES** Saponins, phenylpropanoid glycosides, and cardiac glycosides	glycyrrhizinic acid and isoverbascoside
Sulfur compounds	**GENERAL** Sulfur-containing substances that are often derived from amino acids and that commonly have anti-inflammatory, anticancer, immunosupportive, and antibiotic properties. **SUBTYPES** Glucosinolates, thiocyanates, isothiocyanates, thiosulfinates, and thiols	indole-3-carbinol (not itself sulfur-containing but released from sulfur compounds), sulforaphane, alliin, allicin, ajoene, methiin, and sinigrin

Alkaloids and Glycosides

There are two other types of phytonutrients—alkaloids and glycosides—both of which are important to our health, although they are not as widely involved in the look, smell, and taste of food as some of the other phytonutrients just described. Both alkaloids and glycosides will be much examined in food research in the years to come.

More than 12,000 alkaloids have been identified in food, constituting a major category of phytonutrient like terpenoids or flavonoids (polyphenols). All alkaloids are derived from amino acids and all contain nitrogen. Some of the better known alkaloid substances include piperidine, pyrrolidine, and quinoline. Many of the alkaloids are naturally alkaline (having a high pH). Some food alkaloids are frequently identified as unwanted components of food with potential toxicity. Included here are the Solanaceae alkaloids from the nightshade vegetables—for example, the potentially toxic substances found in green potatoes. But the alkaloid phytonutrients, like all types of phytonutrients, are generally supportive of health and add to the nourishing properties of food.

Glycosides are substances containing a carbohydrate and a noncarbohydrate portion together in the same molecule. There are thousands of unique glycosides already identified in food. Saponins are a particularly important subdivision of glycosides. You might want to think about licorice when you think about the saponin glycosides, because its glycyrrhizinic acid is just such a molecule. It is also responsible for some of the sweetness found in licorice, since on a bite-for-bite basis, it is 50 times sweeter than table sugar (sucrose).

The world of phytonutrients is more diverse and complex than the world of vitamins and minerals, and phytonutrients are absolutely essential to the body's nourishment because they lie at the heart of our food experience, giving food its look, taste, and aromas. Phytonutrients are not "accessory" nutrients or "secondary" nutrients in the sense of being second-class or lower in importance. In fact, they may turn out to be the primary reason why food is nourishing. The table on pages 298–299 summarizes a basic road map to follow when thinking about the phytonutrients in food. Now, as I move through each individual food in

this chapter, I provide a list of its key phytonutrients. Return to this table to understand how a particular food and its unique substances fit into the overall phytonutrient framework.

FLOWERS

 This could be considered an eccentric category but one that is of import to those people interested in beautiful and sensitive eating for the eyes and the body. I am referring here to colorful plant flowers and not to the fruits or vegetables of flowering plants, such as oranges, tomatoes, or zucchini. Those are discussed in upcoming sections later in this chapter. This part actually refers to those colorful flowers from the gardens or meadows.

Many flowers are edible and tasty. Many are not, however, and some could make us sick. Really, there are only a few poisonous flowers. Many flowers have medicinal properties, and eating or using flowers in teas, poultices (compresses), or salves is often more a subject of herbology, the use of plants as medicines. Flowers are the most subtle and often fragrant part of plants. They are not very concentrated in nutrition and are considered more a "food for the spirit," both as a delight to our mouths and in their appeal to our eyes and noses.

Commonly consumed edible flowers include nasturtiums, borage, and marigolds; there are also the many flowering seasoning herbs, such as basil and thyme, although we usually consume only the greenery of these. Mustard, radish, and watercress flowers are spicy additions to salads. Chrysanthemum petals are edible, as are squash blossoms (see recipe in the spring diet in my book *A Cookbook for All Seasons*). Flowers of such common herbs as rosemary, dill, oregano, chives, sage, and marjoram are also edible.

Most of these flowers have a little carbohydrate, no fat, and not much protein. Many contain some vitamin C, and vitamin A is found in others. A few of the minerals, such as calcium, magnesium, and zinc, may also be found in certain flowers. Ten years ago, we probably would not have thought about eating flowers for their nutrient content. Thanks to research on phytonutrients, however, today we probably would. For example, when it comes to the carotenoids lutein and zeaxanthin, marigold flowers are every bit as concentrated a source as collards, kale, or spinach. Similarly, chrysanthemum flowers are now recognized to contain the essential oils camphene, camphor, carvone, and chrysanthenone, as well as the flavonoid chrysanthemin and the carotenoid chrysanthemaxanthin. (Sometimes this collection of phytonutrients in chrysanthemum flowers has been used in herbal smoking-cessation formulas.)

Flowers can also be a welcomed addition to food because of other subtle and lovely qualities they may offer. Borage is said to help us forget our troubles, and marigold or calendula flowers, to fill us with happiness. People should know which flowers are edible and be able to clearly identify them before consuming any to ensure against getting sick or poisoned from eating those delicacies. Many are now available in gourmet markets.

BEE AND FLOWER POLLEN

Although allergists are not overly excited about the use of bee and flower pollens, the general public loves and supports these forms of concentrated energy. Bee pollen is likely the first food supplement ever used. The common claim for bee pollen is that it improves energy and endurance in its users. Many athletes and health enthusiasts use bee pollen. There seems to be some scientific proof, scanty as it may be, that bee pollen does improve physical performance, but its many other claims for helping arthritis, heart disease, or bowel and prostate problems have not been verified. Many use bee pollen to enhance immunity, reduce allergy, lose weight, and relieve stress, but there is no evidence for these claims either.

Bee pollen is collected from bees' legs when special pollen scrapers and collectors are attached to their hive. It is essentially concentrated pollens from flowers, so its nutrient content may vary dramatically. This variation in content applies not only to the nutrients found in bee pollen, but also to potential toxins that could be present as a result of environmental pollution or pesticide use. **Be sure to purchase bee pollen gathered in a pesticide-free environment.**

Although there are usually some amino acids (protein), vitamins, and minerals in most pollens, the most recent research on pollen content points directly toward phytonutrients. Flavonoids found in many samples of bee pollen include tricetin, luteolin, myricetin, and quercetin. From this group, tricetin may turn out to be especially important in some of the potential antibiotic properties of bee pollen.

Because bee pollen is concentrated flower pollen, there is some theoretical concern about its use by people who have pollen allergies, although in practice there seems to be a big difference between the effects of inhaled and ingested pollens. The gastrointestinal action on the pollens, I am sure, changes their allergenicity. Theoretically as well, it would seem that pollens ingested might work to desensitize people who are environmentally allergic, but this has not been proved either.

There are some new flower pollen products on the market as well; these are different from bee pollen in that they are not collected from bees. The companies who promote them and people who use them speak very highly of their positive benefits to energy and health, but again more research is needed to actually show what these products do. Suffice it to say that bee and flower pollens are those extra products used more by personal choice and not because they are a necessary part of the diet. They are more often recommended by friends or health enthusiasts than by medical practitioners. Many people realize some positive benefits from pollens; others may not notice much. Often the amounts used are begun at low levels and built up over days and weeks to a handful at a time to produce the desired effects. **Physical energy and athletic performance probably are the reasons for most pollen use, rather than for disease or symptom treatment.** Bee and flower pollen's effects may range from subtle for many to very strong for others, but most people claim that when they eat bee pollen, which has a slightly sweet and unique taste, they tend to buzz around (pun intended) with more life.

FRUITS

Fruits are considered Nature's perfect foods. They are Nature's only pure offering, as a ripe fruit from the tree may actually drop into our hand. The fruit is the result of a healthy growing cycle for most plants and the bearer or potentiator of life, as it carries the seeds for the next generation of trees and plants. Fruits have many positive qualities. They are natural and healthy (and best from organic sources), and they are juicy, with a high water content, like the human body itself. Fruits are also well stocked in nutrients, particularly such important vitamins as A and C, a little of the Bs, and E in the seeds. Many minerals—such as calcium, copper, a little iron, manganese, magnesium, and other trace minerals—are present in fruits, especially when they are contained in the water and soil that nourishes the plants or trees. **Fruits are low in fat and high in fiber, both healthful attributes in this commonly high-fat, low-fiber culture.**

Fruits are also relatively low in calories and sodium. Most are sweet, colorful, and cooling and can be crunchy too. Fruits' colors are some of the most beautiful in Nature, covering every hue in the rainbow. Fruits are high in natural sugars, thus making them a good substitute for those higher-calorie sugar treats when we feel we want something sweet. The sweet flavor of fruit is the most prevalent flavor in many diets. According to Chinese medical theory, too much sweet food may cause many problems. **But eating whole fruits is the most natural way to obtain this sweet flavor.**

Fruit juices are an important beverage. Ideally consumed fresh, they are higher in vitamins and minerals than many other drinks. They are particularly a good replacement for sugary soda pops. Fruits and fruit juices without added sugars also tend to be purifying and help with the body's elimination. Such juices are often part of a cleansing or detoxification program. Fruits are also easy to digest and utilize, so they usually have low allergenic potential (allergy results mainly from the protein components of food). Occasionally, someone is sensitive to such fruits as oranges or tomatoes, but this is less common than with other regularly used foods like milk, wheat, and other grains. Note: When people do have any reactions to fruit (or to any foods for that matter), it is possible that they are reacting to a chemical in the fruit or even to a combination of the fruit and foods eaten with it. Fruits are simple foods that digest more easily than most others, and they can ferment more easily when having to sit in the stomach juices longer. (See the food combining discussion on page 395 in chapter 10, Nutritional Habits.)

Fruits may have a cooling and calming action for the body and nervous system and may be helpful in reducing body stress. Because of the natural nutrient and antioxidant content, fruit consumption may help strengthen our immune system as well.

It is most natural and economical to eat fruits fresh in season. It is ideal to wash them to clean off any sprays, germs, and environmental contaminants and to eat organic fruits whenever possible. Eating fruit in its ripe state is probably best for the body, as the "green" or unripe fruits may be more irritating to the digestive tract. Fresh is best from a nutritional standpoint as well. Fresh frozen is next, as the fruits lose very little of their nutrients in the freezing process. Drying fruits for storage is probably a little better than canning, although fresh "canned" (really, glass jar–stored fruits in water that produce their own fruit juices) is much better than those with added sugars or syrups. Drying fruit pieces is more economical for storage purposes, and they will keep a long time if protected. Fruit is not usually cooked, although stewed prunes, baked apples, and others are very tasty and can be eaten or used in some recipes; these may be easier to ingest for the elderly, who may not chew well, and this form is good for assisting normal intestinal activity. After cooking fruits, consuming the natural juices in which some of the fruits' nutrients are contained makes them more wholesome.

Fruits fall into such categories as common fruits (like apples and pears), citrus fruits, melons, berries, tropical fruits, and dried fruits. Most fruits grow on trees, but some are found on bushes (berries) or on ground vines (melons). Most fruits follow the flower of the plant and are available during the summer, late summer, and autumn, although there are exceptions. Fruits have also been categorized as sweet, subacid, and acid. The sweet fruits are mainly the dried fruits, such as raisins and figs, and some tropical ones, such as bananas. Most juicy fruits are considered subacid. These include peaches, plums, apples, pears, grapes, cherries, mangoes, papayas, and so on. Citrus fruits, some berries, pineapples, and pomegranates are examples of acid-tasting fruits. They have a higher level of acid, often ascorbic acid (vitamin C), and this may make them helpful in cutting fats or helping fat digestion. **When broken down in the body, however, these fruits become more alkaline.** Cranberries, prunes, plums, and possibly strawberries and pomegranates are the main acid-forming fruits. When fruits are utilized or burned, the minerals and ash that are left, even from lemons and pineapples, are alkaline, supporting the body's acid-alkaline balance. Regarding food combining, fruits are digested easily and therefore are best eaten by themselves, rather than with other, more concentrated foods that take longer to pass through the stomach and digestive tract.

Common Fruits

Apples	Grapes	Pears
Apricots	Peaches	Plums
Cherries		

The common tree fruits (except for grapes) of the United States and much of the world include apples, apricots, cherries, peaches, pears, and plums. Most of these are in the subacid variety of fruits. Apples and pears are similar in their growth and in the climates where they grow, as well as in their multiseeded cores. The single-seeded apricots, cherries, peaches, and plums each have their own unique flavor and avid followers. Grapes are a special vine fruit with many varieties used for eating, seasonal decor, and making wine. All of these fruits are tasty and juicy, and best eaten fresh; however, there is concern over the use of pesticides sprayed on them and the effects of these chemicals on health, especially that of children. If possible, buying and consuming organically grown fruits is ideal.

Apples (*Malus communis, Malus domestica, Malus pumila, Malus sylvestris*). Apple history is rich. From the Garden of Eden to Snow White and the wicked queen, the life of the apple has had a questionable past, yet a better future. As the myth goes, however, Johnny Appleseed spread apples throughout the land and made them one of America's popular fruits. Now they help to keep doctors away and shine up one's schoolteacher. Apples are a very nutritious fruit. They are high in fiber, and apple pectin has a detoxifying quality and is used in many cleansing formulas. Eating apples also helps clean the teeth. Recent concerns over chemicals used in growing and harvesting apples has tainted the image of this "health"

fruit, but organic apples or unsprayed apples are still among our culture's favorite fruits.

One apple has about 100 calories, mainly from carbohydrate; nearly 2 grams of fiber; about 10 mg vitamin C; 150 IU of vitamin A; and some modest amounts of B vitamins—B_1, B_2, B_3, B_6, and biotin. Apples also contain various minerals—lots of potassium; more than 15 mg each of calcium, magnesium, and phosphorus; about 330 mcg of iron; and traces of copper, manganese, selenium, and zinc. Apples even have some vitamin E, mostly in the seeds. Apples are like mini multivitamins—they have a little of everything. The phytonutrients in apples are quercetin and pectin.

Apricots (*Prunus armeniaca*). Apricots have received recent notoriety because of their laetrile-laden kernels. But the fruit itself is nutritious and tasty. It is high in vitamin A, mainly as beta-carotene, the vitamin A precursor. Each little apricot has nearly 1,000 IU of vitamin A. The vitamin C content is fairly good, although lower than in some other fruits, as are the B vitamins. Potassium and other minerals, such as calcium and iron, are also contained in apricots. The trace minerals copper, manganese, and zinc are also present. Dried apricots may have even higher concentrations of vitamin A and minerals. Apricots are considered among the longevity fruits contained in high amounts in the long-living Hunzas' diet. The Hunzas are a group of about 30,000 people living at high altitude in the Himalaya Mountains in the Kashmir region of what is now northern Pakistan. Although no peer-reviewed research on this group is available, many health-care professionals traveling to this region report unusual longevity in the Hunzas ranging from 100 to 120 years; the Hunza diet is often singled out as a main reason for the long-lived nature of this group. The phytonutrients in apricots are lycopene, beta-carotene, and quercetin.

Cherries (*Prunus avium, Prunus cerasus*). Cherries can be sweet or sour, red or black. They are good colon cleansers, as they enhance bowel motility. They are fairly high in vitamin C content, about 15 mg per cup of cherries. Vitamin A content is good, the Bs are modest, and minerals are high. Potassium content is very high, calcium content is good, as is phosphorus content, and there are modest levels of magnesium and manganese as well as fair amounts of copper and iron, thus making this "bloody" fruit good for building the body's blood. The phytonutrients in cherries are anthocyanins, cyanidins, neochlorogenic acid, epicatechin, pelargonidin, and peonidin.

Grapes *(Vitus labrusca, Vitus rotundifolia, Vitus vinifera)*. There are many varieties of this vine fruit. Wines made from grapes are used in most cultures as part of both religious rites and secular celebrations. And many people celebrate daily!

Green Thompson seedless grapes are those most commonly consumed in the United States, although red seedless, larger seeded Ribier grapes, and other kinds are a real treat as well. Grapes have lots of nutrients and also help cleanse the bowels. Grape fasting—consuming only grapes and grape juice for days and weeks at a time—is a fairly popular therapeutic tool in the natural healing fields. Many anecdotal positive experiences have been described by those grape fasters, but, as with any kind of fasting, there is not much research to demonstrate its value. Nor do grapes maintain a balanced diet.

Grapes are fairly high in fruit sugar (fructose) and are mainly carbohydrate foods. They contain no fat and minimum protein but a good amount of fiber. Grapes have about 100 calories per cup. They contain decent amounts of vitamin A; good vitamin C levels; some B vitamins; lots of potassium; some calcium, magnesium, and phosphorus; traces of iron and copper; and a fairly high level of the important mineral manganese. Because bugs are attracted to the sweet grapes, these fruits are often heavily sprayed. In fact, there have been grape boycotts by the United Farm Workers Union to protest the use of dangerous pesticides that jeopardize the workers' health—and the consumers' as well. More organic grapes and wines are currently available. The phytonutrients in grapes include resveratrol, saponins, and quercetin.

Peaches *(Prunus persica)*. Peaches have very good press—they are sweet, fuzzy, and friendly, and when all is going well, life is known to be "peachy." In season, peaches are usually so juicy that they should be eaten outdoors or with bibs. Peaches have good levels of vitamins A and C, potassium, and phosphorus; fair amounts of calcium and magnesium; and traces of the important minerals copper, iron, iodine, manganese, selenium, sulfur, and zinc. The B vitamin content is modest, as in most fruits. The phytonutrients in peaches include hydrocinnamic acids, catechins, procyanidins, kaempferol, and quercetin.

Pears *(Pyrus communis)*. Pears are similar to apples in that they have modest to moderate amounts of many nutrients. There are many varieties, ranging from crunchy to very juicy. They are lower in vitamin A than other fruits but do contain good fiber. They have decent levels of vitamin C and folic acid and have high amounts of potassium and surprisingly good levels of manganese and selenium. Like apples, pears also have good cleansing and detoxification potential, probably related to their high fiber content. The phytonutrients in pears are epicatechin, catechin, isorhamnetin, and quercetin.

Plums *(Prunus americana, Prunus angustifolia, Prunus cerasifera, Prunus domestica, Prunus salicina)*. Plums come in many varieties and are among the few purple foods. They range in flavor from sour to very sweet and are mildly acid-forming when broken down in the body. Plums are low in calories and have good levels of vitamin A and potassium. They contain a bit of calcium and magnesium, some iron and copper, vitamin C and phosphorous, and traces of B vitamins. The phytonutrients in plums include chlorogenic acid, neochlorogenic acid, kaempferol, quercetin, and hydrocinnamic acids.

Citrus Fruits

Grapefruits	Limes
Lemons	Oranges

Citrus fruits are warm-climate fruits containing almost all juice. They seem to be available nearly year-round in such hot states as Florida, Texas, and California, but most citrus fruits are harvested mainly in late spring to early summer, with certain types (such as navel oranges) giving a winter crop.

Citrus fruits are known for their vitamin C content. An average orange, for example, contains about 65 mg (about the recommended daily allowance) of this important vitamin. Citruses are also high in potassium and other minerals. Like most other fruits, they are low in salt (sodium).

Citrus fruits are used commonly for cleansing the body, as during colds and flus, and for cooling it down in the summertime. Citrus juice seems to help cut

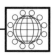

grease on the hands or dishes, and it likely has the same effect on the body, helping fat digestion and utilization. Citrus and vitamin C are thought to help reduce cholesterol. Gallbladder and liver function is thought to be supported by citrus fruits, especially lemons, and lemon water may help stimulate digestive juice secretions. More research is needed to evaluate the actions and effects of citrus juices in the body.

Grapefruits *(Citrus paradisi).* Grapefruits are used in many diets to reduce the appetite and to help digestion and utilization of foods. They are low in calories, and consuming them probably burns as many calories as they contain. Thus, among the citrus fruits, grapefruits are an especially good weight-loss food. One grapefruit contains about 75 mg of vitamin C. Amounts of vitamin A and the Bs are fairly low, although there is some biotin. Potassium content is very good, and there is some calcium, magnesium, and phosphorus as well. Grapefruit juice straight or mixed with orange juice is a high-vitamin C meal. The phytonutrients in grapefruits include glucarates, limonoids, limonene, lycopene, and pectin.

Lemons *(Citrus limon).* Lemons have been a useful food throughout my life. Lemonade fasting has done wonders for me and for thousands of others who have attempted the "master cleanse" described in my books *Staying Healthy with the Seasons* and *The New Detox Diet.* Lemon water, as a half lemon squeezed into a glass of water, drunk 20 to 30 minutes before meals, seems to help stimulate gastric juices and help digestion. In general, liquids drunk a while before meals can reduce our appetite and thus help prevent overeating; lemon water is a good choice for this purpose.

I consider lemons a cleanser, purifier, rejuvenator, and detoxifier, especially for the liver, as they help in fat metabolism. These functions come mainly from their astringent qualities, supported by high vitamin C and potassium levels. Like other citruses, lemons contain calcium, magnesium, and phosphorus, but most of these minerals are present more in the white part of the rind and in the pulp. Lemon juice is used in salads and, more for its biochemical behavior, in cutting fats and oils (even in dishwashing liquid). It is more often used diluted in water as lemon water or lemonade (with sweeteners) than as a separate beverage, because its sour flavor limits its straight use. Lemon peel tea can be drunk after a meal as a diges-

tive aid. The phytonutrients in lemons are eriodictyol, coumarins, kaempferol, eriocitrin, and limonene.

Limes *(Citrus aurantifolia).* Limes are like mini lemons in terms of nutritional content. Limes helped save the British sailors (thereafter known as "limeys") from scurvy by means of their vitamin C content. This little citrus is not as prevalent in U.S. culture as many other citrus fruits; however, it is used in key lime pie and commonly in alcoholic or refreshment drinks, as it is not quite as sour as lemon. The phytonutrients in limes are coumarins, kaempferol, and eriocitrin.

Oranges *(Citrus aurantium, Citrus sinensis, Citrus nobilis).* Oranges are one of the most commonly used fruits in the United States. As orange juice (OJ), they are popular as a breakfast drink. One orange can give us our minimum vitamin C requirement of 65 mg, and one glass of OJ provides about 125 mg. The high potassium and good calcium levels of oranges are also helpful. Actually, oranges contain almost all the vitamins and minerals, at least in modest amounts. Because people can daily consume more oranges, as juice or fruit, than the other citruses, we are able to obtain higher vitamin C levels with OJ, often the drink for the common cold. Oranges also have more vitamin A, as beta-carotene, than other citruses, which may help fight infections and protect us from cancer by supporting the body's immune system. The phytonutrients in oranges include hesperidin, narigenin, hesperetin, eriodictyol, beta-myrcene, limonene, and quercetin.

Melons

Cantaloupes	Honeydews
Casabas	Watermelons

Melons are high-water-content fruits that grow on the ground in the heat of summer. Most are harvested in late summer; casabas and honeydew melons are more of an autumn or winter crop. When we are dry and thirsty in the summer, melons are a good answer. They are also high in calcium, potassium, vitamin C, and vitamin A as beta-carotene, especially cantaloupe and watermelon. Because of the high water and fruit sugar content of most melons, they are more easily digested

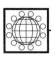

than most any other food. **For this reason, it is suggested that they be eaten by themselves to avoid abdominal gas and bloating, as fermentation may occur more easily when they are eaten with other, harder-to-digest foods.** There are many varieties and colors of melons. Here I discuss a few—one red, one green, and a couple of orange melons.

Cantaloupes *(Cucumis melo* var. *cantalupensis).* Although the terms *cantaloupe* and *musk-melon* are used fairly interchangeably, true cantaloupe corresponds to the cantalupensis variety of melon and muskmelon to the reticulatus variety. Cantaloupes are high in beta-carotene, a precursor of vitamin A. One-quarter of a cantaloupe may give up to 3,000 IU of vitamin A as well as about 30 mg vitamin C; some Bs; potassium (about 250 mg); a little calcium, magnesium, and phosphorus; and traces of iron, copper, manganese, and zinc. The phytonutrients in cantaloupes are beta-carotene, caffeic acid, ferulic acid, and rutin.

Casabas *(Cucumis melo* var. *inodorus).* The casaba is a muskmelon that is higher in the minerals than in vitamins A and C. Potassium, calcium, and phosphorus are all found in good levels. The casaba-type melons are a little higher in sodium than other fruits. The phytonutrients in casabas include beta-cryptoxanthin, caffeic acid, eugenol, and rutin.

Honeydews *(Cucumis melo* var. *inodorus).* Sweet, juicy, green melons, honeydews have a fairly good vitamin C content. The amounts of vitamin A and the Bs are lower, but potassium is high, as are calcium and phosphorus. The phytonutrients of honeydews include anthocyanins, catechins, and ferulic acid.

Watermelons *(Citrullus lanatus).* Eating watermelon can be quite an art. Red and juicy, watermelons are really America's national melon. They are almost all water and nutrients—high in beta-carotene, vitamin C, potassium, and magnesium. Watermelon is a great treat in the hot summer. Most people experience this fruit as a diuretic, stimulating urine flow. The ground seeds have been used as an herbal diuretic and kidney cleanser. I make a tasty organic watermelon juice (from Walt Baptiste's purification diet) in the blender, seeds and all (except the outer dark rind); it is cleansing and nourishing with the additional nutrients (protein and oils) contained in the seeds. The phytonutrients in watermelons are lycopene and lutein.

Berries

Blackberries	Cranberries
Blueberries	Raspberries
Boysenberries	Strawberries

There are many varieties of edible berries found all over the world. Discussed here are some more common berries available in both wild and cultivated forms. Berries usually can be found or harvested in late summer or early autumn, depending on the climate. Depending on ripeness, they may vary in flavor from very sour to very sweet. Most berries have some vitamin C, about 20 to 30 mg per cup. Vitamin A content varies, but at least 150 to 300 IU can be found in 1 cup of berries. B vitamin content is generally low, but minerals are fairly plentiful, with potassium content the best. Amounts of calcium, magnesium, silicon, and iron are actually pretty good. Most of the berries have good fiber content as well.

Berries are a treat for young and old. Berry pie made with fresh-picked berries can be a flavorful and nutritious dessert, ideally consumed at least 1 or 2 hours after dinner. Kids love frozen berry juice popsicles. Berries with cream or a la mode can be a little heavy and harder to digest but definitely a taste treat. Berries with cereals are also fairly popular, but overall berries are best by themselves.

Blackberries *(Rubus plicatus, Rubis* spp., *Rubis vitifolius).* Blackberries are almost exclusively wild and local, even to city folk. Come midsummer, we can stain our hands and get a few stickers picking and eating blackberries. They need to be black and ripe to be sweet; otherwise they can make us pucker. They have pretty good amounts of calcium, magnesium, iron, and other minerals. Both vitamins A and C are found in blackberries. The phytonutrients in blackberries include epicatechin, gallic acid, kaempferol, and quercetin.

Blueberries *(Vaccinium corymbosum).* Blueberries are sweeter and meatier and a little lower in vitamins A and C and minerals than the other berries, although they still have lots of nutrients. The phytonutrients include ellagic acid, anthocyanins, antho-

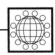

cyanidins, ellagic acid cyanidin, delphinidin, malvidin, peonidin, petunidin, myricetin, and kaempferol.

Boysenberries (Rubus ursinus). A really special treat, boysenberries may come earlier than the other dark bush berries. They are similar to blackberries in their nutrient content. The phytonutrients include cyanidins, anthocyanins, gallic acid, and ellagic acid.

Cranberries (Vaccinium macrocarpon, Vaccinium oxycoccus, Vaccinium vitis-idaea). Cranberries are tart berries used mainly in their cooked and sauced form for celebration. Cranberry juice is commonly used to help acidify the urine to reduce symptoms and clear mild urinary bladder infections. They are lower in minerals and vitamins A and C than the other berries, but cranberries are still nutritious. The phytonutrients include epicatechin, catechin, myricetin, and quercetin.

Raspberries (Rubus idaeus). Both red and black raspberries are another summertime treat. They are fairly high in vitamin C and especially abundant in the minerals calcium, magnesium, and iron. The phytonutrients in raspberries are ellagic acid, tannins, quercetin, kaempferol, cyanidin-3-glucosylrutinoside, and cyanidin-3-rutinoside.

Strawberries (Fragaria virginiana). The most popular American berry, strawberries grow in little ground bushes without prickers. Maybe their friendliness is what gives them top billing. But they are very tasty as well, and they are highest in vitamin C, although a bit lower in vitamin A, and better in iron and potassium than the other berries. Strawberries are unique in that their seeds are on the outside. That trait, along with their red color, makes them the most yang, or activating, fruit from an Asian perspective. I surely liked strawberries in my milk and cereal when I was growing up, especially drinking that pink, sweet milk at the end, with the extra white sugar, of course. Yum! Yet, I have given that up and most of my other bad habits I learned as part of the bad American diet. The phytonutrients are ellagitannins, gallocatechin, quercetin, lutein, ellagic acid, chlorogenic acid, and caffeic acid.

Tropical Fruits

Bananas	Mangoes	Pineapples
Guavas	Papayas	

Tropical fruits are those that grow in a hot or tropical climate, usually one with lots of rain and sun—like Hawaii, Tahiti, the Caribbean, South America, or even Southern California or Florida. The tropical fruits vary in type of plants, fruits, and nutrients, but all are fairly exotic tasting. Each one is known for its unique taste and a particular nutrient in which it is high. **Bananas are great in potassium, for example, and are likely the most popular fruit in the United States (and worldwide), even though they are not grown in this country.** Papayas are high in beta-carotene and the papain enzyme; guavas in vitamin C; pineapples in manganese and the digestive enzyme bromelain; and avocados, a tropical and temperate fruit (discussed on page 308 under "Unusual and Special Fruits"), have some protein and fat (they are really more like nuts in nutrient makeup). Some other, less common varieties of tropical fruits are cherimoya, lychee, and sapote.

Bananas (Musa paradisiaca). Bananas have the number-one vote as Americans' favorite fruit. They are commonly recommended as a potassium source in those patients on potassium-losing diuretic therapy. Bananas are almost completely carbohydrate. They contain many vitamins and minerals, including iron, selenium, and magnesium. They are used in flavoring for desserts, as in banana splits or banana bread, in breakfast cereals, or even in sandwiches. Most commonly, however, they are eaten after peeling the skin as a snack or dessert carried in lunch pails to work or school. As far as treats go, bananas are one of the healthiest. But there is concern, because bananas are not indigenous in the continental United States, over the pesticides that are used to fumigate these fruits when they come from Mexico or Hawaii. Also, some people do not digest bananas well, some are allergic, and others may become constipated from their use. The phytonutrients in bananas are alpha-carotene, gallocatechin, cyanidin, delphinidin, leucocyanidin, leucodelphinidin, lutein, malvidin, peonidin, petunidin, and rutin.

Guavas *(Psidium guajava)*. A common tree fruit in such tropical areas as Hawaii, guavas taste similar to soft pears and have big seeds. They are very high in vitamin C, with a medium-sized fruit having close to 200 mg. They are also good in fiber content, are high in vitamin A and potassium, and have modest amounts of phosphorus, calcium, and magnesium. Although fairly popular in the tropics, guavas are not commonly imported. The phytonutrients of guavas are ellagic acid, gallic acid, leucoanthocyanin, leucocyanidins, limonene, lycopene, myricetin, and quercetin.

Mangoes *(Mangifera indica)*. Mangoes are a tasty and juicy fruit that I first learned to eat in Mexico, peeled and eaten like a Popsicle, using a fork stuck in the pit as a holder. Mangoes are fairly high in vitamin C and have some vitamin E, but they are extremely rich in vitamin A, with a high concentration of beta-carotene. One mango may have nearly 10,000 IU of vitamin A. Mangoes are also fairly rich in many minerals, including zinc, magnesium, and potassium. The phytonutrients are catechin, arabinose, ellagic acid, gallic acid, limonene, leucocyanidins, myricetin, quercetin, and xanthophyll.

Papayas *(Carica papaya)*. Papayas are best known for their digestive support, as they contain the enzyme papain. Their taste is delicious, rather like that of a melon. Papayas also may have a disinfectant property when used to clean wounds and skin or mouth sores. Papayas are rich in beta-carotene (and thus vitamin A activity) and vitamin C as well as potassium and other minerals. This is probably a fruit that can be used as an appetizer or dessert because of its digestive enzyme papain. The phytonutrients in papayas are papain, chymopapain, cotinine, flavonols, gamma-carotene, cryptoxanthin, lycopene, neoxanthin, tannins, and violaxanthin.

Pineapples *(Ananas comosus)*. An interesting bush fruit most commonly grown in Hawaii, pineapples are juicy and mildly acidic, more like a citrus fruit. They contain the digestive enzyme bromelain, allowing for their easy digestion, so pineapples can happily be eaten following a meal. Bromelain may also have an anti-inflammatory action in the body. Pineapples contain some vitamin A and C content as well as potassium, calcium, and the trace minerals manganese and selenium. Manganese levels are in fact quite good; 1 cup of pineapple will supply the body's minimum daily needs, about 2.5 mg.

There is a concern, however, that pineapples more easily accumulate chemicals from the fertilizers and pesticides commonly used in their cultivation, because of their porous skins. For this reason, it is unwise to consume a great deal of pineapple or its juice unless the fruit is organic. It is more difficult to find organic tropical fruits from Hawaii or Mexico, however, than it is the more locally cultivated fruits like apples or oranges, possibly because of the higher amounts of insects and germs that also thrive in those climates. Bromelain is a unique extract from pineapple that contains protein-digesting enzymes and would qualify as one of this fruit's most heralded phytonutrients. Other phytonutrients found in pineapple (and many other foods) include ferulic acid and carotenoids.

Unusual and Special Fruits

Avocados	Persimmons
Kiwis	Pomegranates
Olives	

This section includes uncommon fruits that grow on trees, contain inner seeds, and do not clearly fall into the other categories I have discussed. None of these are eaten commonly, other than olives possibly by some people. But olives are unusual because they cannot be eaten fresh and also contain a high amount of oil, much like avocados. They are really more like a nut than a fruit. Kiwis have recently become more popular because of their unique taste, visual appeal, and modest caloric count. They are probably closest to grapes or the tropical guava; kiwis grow in more temperate climates, including northern California and New Zealand. Persimmons and pomegranates are also unusual in taste and appearance as well as in the adventure of eating these fruits. These festive and seasonal bright orange or red fruits can be seen dangling from near-naked trees in autumn and early winter in the temperate climates in which they grow.

Avocados *(Persea americana)*. Avocados are unique among the fruits in that they are a very con-

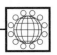

centrated food, more like a nut than a fruit. They are high in calories—1 average avocado has about 300 calories and about 30 grams of fat, as well as 12 grams of carbohydrate and 4 to 5 grams of protein. They are fairly high in most of the B vitamins except B12, being particularly good in folic acid, niacin, and pantothenic acid. They also have some vitamin C, good amounts of vitamin A, and a bit of vitamin E. **Avocados are rich in potassium and are also particularly good in many other minerals, including magnesium, iron, and manganese.**

For vegetarians who do not eat a lot of fatty foods, avocados may be a good source of needed oils, but for those who consume more fat and calories, these fruits may add excess fat and weight. Avocados are commonly used in salads, dips such as guacamole, in sandwiches, or stuffed with seafood. The phytonutrients are alpha-carotene, caffeic acid, cryptoxanthin, isolutein, lutein, coumaric acid, pinene, quercetin, and violaxanthin.

Kiwis *(Actinidia deliciosa).* Little fruits with a tiny name, kiwis reveal a beautiful pattern when the green juicy fruit with furry skin is sliced. Kiwis are another fruit high in vitamin C and potassium and may contain an enzyme that helps reduce cholesterol and improve circulation. The phytonutrients are actinidin, carotenoids, cryptoxanthin, cyanidin, delphinidin, lutein, coumaric acid, quercetin, violaxanthin, and zeaxanthin.

Olives *(Olea europaea).* Horticulturally, olives are considered a fruit, but in their nutritional makeup they are more like nuts, with a high oil content. In the fruit family, they are most like avocados. Olives grow in large quantities on small trees. They are most widely cultivated in the Mediterranean countries of Italy and Spain, although they are now being grown more in the United States, mainly in California.

The best use of olives is in the form of the clear, sweet oil pressed from their pulp. After the olives are harvested and cleaned, the first amounts of the oil are pressed out as virgin olive oil. This can be bright yellow to green-yellow in color and varies subtly in flavor. Fresh olive oil is used classically in salads and can be drunk in small amounts as a nutritive lubricant to the intestinal tract. **Olive oil is one of the best oils for cooking, as it is mainly a monounsaturated fat, which is more stable to heat degradation than the common polyunsaturated oils.** Olive oil also

helps lower LDL (low-density lipoprotein) cholesterol, which is implicated in heart disease.

Olives cannot be consumed just off the tree or even after ripening. They must first be pickled (cooked in vinegar). Green olives stuffed with pimento are familiar to the bartender for drinks. Black olives are more often used in cooking. Most table or dinner olives are much larger than the oil olives. Olives are rich in oil (and calories) and the essential fatty acids and generally have a good variety of vitamins and minerals, along with some protein. They contain vitamin E, vitamin A, and many of the B vitamins. They further contain many minerals, such as zinc, copper, iron, calcium, magnesium, and phosphorus. However, people avoiding salt or vinegar, or those on a low-fat, low-calorie diet, would best minimize their olive intake. The phytonutrients in olives are apigenin, caffeic acid, catechin, cyanidins, kaempferol, luteolin, olivin, quercetin, quinone, rutin, squalene, and tannins.

Persimmons *(Diospyros kaki).* A seasonal fruit (late autumn and winter), persimmons are common in the Orient, where they are associated with celebration. They also grow in the United States in temperate climates and are harvested in the autumn and winter as well. A fully fruited persimmon tree that has lost its leaves and is left with many bright orange fruits is a beautiful sight. Persimmons must be eaten when very ripe. It is the cold weather or frost that aids the ripening process. If you buy them hard, you can freeze them overnight and they will ripen as they thaw. Persimmons have a unique, slightly acidic taste and are messy to eat. They have some beta-carotene, as do most orange fruits and vegetables, as well as some vitamin C, a little potassium, iron, and calcium.

There are more than 200 varieties of persimmon. Many of the varieties are originally native to Japan and Central Asia and were grown there for many centuries before being brought to the United States. Of the varieties native to Asia, there is an especially common astringent variety (Tanenashi, meaning "seedless") and a nonastringent variety (Fuyu). The Fuyu persimmon is ripe when still hard and has a texture more like an apple. The phytonutrients in persimmons are plumbagin, lycopene, tannins, and carotenoids.

Pomegranates *(Punica granatum).* Another autumn celebration fruit in U.S. culture, pomegranates are eaten from around Halloween through the winter holidays. Parents may dread pomegranate season because they are not very easy to eat and the bright red juice contained in the hundreds of little seed fruits stains clothes and skin. Pomegranates have some vitamin C and potassium but overall are not very nutrient rich. However, they are rich with antioxidants. The phytonutrients are various alkaloids, betulinic acid, carotenes, cyanidins, delphinidins, ellagic acid, ellagitannin, gallic acid, granatin, isoquercitin, malvidin, pelargonidin, and punicalin.

Dried Fruits

Apples	Currants	Figs	Raisins
Apricots	Dates	Prunes	

Just about any fruit can be dried, but some are more typically eaten in their dried form. Drying fruits allows them greater longevity and shelf life. However, some of the vitamins, such as C, and minerals may be reduced with time. Also, many dried fruits may be preserved with sulfur dioxide, to which some people, particularly those with asthma or allergies, may be sensitive. Generally, sulfur dioxide in small amounts is not too big a problem and may help maintain higher levels of vitamin C. Because dried fruit has lost its water content, eating too much of it can make the intestinal matter drier, which may cause or worsen constipation. **Rehydrating some of these dried fruits in filtered or spring water will make them juicy and more flavorful and prevent the problem of constipation.**

Apples. Dried apples have only recently become popular commercially. Many of the trace minerals are lost in the drying process, however, but potassium and the apple pectin, which helps intestinal detoxification, are more concentrated in dried apples.

Apricots. Apricots are tasty in their dried form. They usually have sulfur dioxide added to preserve their color, but organic, untreated dried apricots are also available. Dried apricots are rich in vitamin A from beta-carotene and also contain a high concentration of potassium.

Currants. Black currants are tasty raisinlike fruits that contain good amounts of vitamin C and decent levels of vitamin A, niacin, pantothenic acid, and biotin. They also contain good amounts of iron and potassium, as well as some calcium, phosphorus, magnesium, and manganese. Dried currants can be eaten alone or used on cereal or in baking. Recently, the seeds of the black currant have been used for their concentrated oil, gamma-linolenic acid (GLA), also found in evening primrose.

Dates. A sweet, high-carbohydrate fruit harvested from date palm trees, dates are found naturally in the dried state, although fresh dates may have a little more moisture. Date sugar extracted from dates is used as a sweetener. Dates are fairly rich in niacin, pantothenic acid, potassium, calcium, and magnesium. They are surprisingly concentrated in iron; about 10 medium dates contain 3 mg iron.

Figs. Figs can be eaten in the fresh or dried form, although packaged, dried figs are most common. Fresh figs, especially fresh picked, can be an exotic taste treat and great for cleansing the intestines. Dried figs in general are fairly rich in potassium, calcium, phosphorus, magnesium, iron, copper, and manganese. They are good energy foods, support blood formation, and, when soaked and rehydrated, figs are helpful to intestinal function.

Prunes. Prunes are best known for their laxative effect. A few prunes a day, especially soaked, rehydrated prunes, can keep us regular, and the elderly population favors them for this purpose. Prunes are essentially dried plums and are rich in iron, with the highest amount of all the fruits. A cup of prunes may have 4 to 6 mg of iron, and 1 cup of prune juice, the most common way prunes are used medicinally, contains nearly 10 mg of iron. Prunes are also high in vitamin A, niacin, potassium, and phosphorus and have some calcium, magnesium, and copper as well.

Raisins. Dried seedless grapes, raisins are a common snack food or used in cereals, cookies, and puddings. They are fairly high in iron, with 1 cup of raisins containing nearly 6 mg. Raisins are also rich in potassium, calcium, magnesium, and phosphorus and have traces of copper, zinc, and manganese as well. They have fair amounts of the B vitamins and are often helpful in providing quick energy.

VEGETABLES

 Vegetables are likely our most important nutritional topic. I believe they should be the primary part of most everyone's diet. Health and vitality are dependent, I believe, on eating these fresh, nutritious, and vital foods. Fresh vegetables have life force; in fact, the Latin word for vegetables, *vegetare,* means "to enliven or animate."

Most vegetables are high in water and necessary vitamins and minerals and low in fat and protein. Thus they are a perfect complement to animal-protein foods to help supply the needed nutrients that aid the digestion and utilization of those concentrated foods. Most vegetables are predominantly carbohydrate, with important fiber bulk. Vitamins C and A, potassium, calcium, magnesium, and iron are the most commonly rich nutrients, along with some B vitamins and other trace minerals. The dark leafy greens, yellow or orange vegetables (such as squash and carrots), and red ones (such as peppers) are all high in beta-carotene, which produces vitamin A in the body. Many of the nutrients may be partially lost when cooking vegetables. Vitamin C and some minerals may dissolve in the water, and the B vitamins may be destroyed by heat and also lost in the water, but overall the basic nutrition and fiber remains.

The positive flavors, many colors, and variety of textures of vegetables are a distinct advantage to those who enjoy natural tastes and aesthetic eating. The low salt and fat content of vegetables, however, tends to reduce their interest for people who have developed a taste for salt and fat. And many times children refrain, often passionately, from the pleasures of vegetables, as their tastes may tend toward sweet flavors and they may oppose the often slightly bitter flavors of the greenery.

The chlorophyll that is part of most plants, especially high in the green vegetables, has special properties. It is the basic component of the plants' blood, just as hemoglobin is to the human body. Whereas iron is the focal part in the body, magnesium is the center of the chlorophyll molecule. Thus many plants have a good magnesium level. **Chlorophyll is produced as a result of the sun's effects on the plants, and it is known to have revitalizing and refreshing effects when used in humans.** Many studies have been done with chlorophyll extracts. It seems to provide intestinal

nourishment and has a soothing or healing effect on the mucous linings. It also has been used beneficially for skin ulcers and to help detoxify or purify the system, the liver in particular. Chlorophyll may even have antimutagenic potential, although this needs further study. Because of their beta-carotene and selenium levels, vegetables are also thought to help reduce cancer rates. The cruciferous family vegetables (such as broccoli, brussels sprouts, and cauliflower) have a further anticancer effect, although the exact mechanism has not yet been determined.

The most nutritious way to eat vegetables is fresh and raw. But raw vegetables eaten in too much quantity are harder for some people to chew and digest and can produce intestinal gas. **Light steaming of vegetables softens them without depleting much of their nutrients, and hot vegetables with a little seasoning may be more pleasing to the palate.** Baked vegetables are also sound nutritionally. If we boil vegetables, many of the nutrients go into the water, so unless we plan to consume the water, by drinking it or making it into a sauce or soup, boiling is not ideal. Frozen vegetables, when they are frozen fresh, have not suffered much loss of nutrients and may keep for quite a long time, remaining nutritionally rich. Dried vegetables tend to lose vitamins and minerals, however, and canned vegetables often lose the most, but this can vary depending on the additives canned along with them. With water canning, many of the nutrients often dissolve into the liquid out of the vegetables. You can conserve water and gain nutrients by using leftover vegetable water for soup bases, gravies, or watering plants.

Many vegetables are sprayed or absorb some chemicals from the ground, water, or air. These are often most concentrated in the skin or on the surface. Washing or soaking the vegetables in water may help remove some of these chemicals. Some people even soak vegetables suspected to be contaminated in diluted bleach (Clorox, or sodium hypochlorite), then rinse them before preparing them for eating.

Fresh vegetable juices can be an invigorating beverage. Their vitamins and minerals are concentrated in the juices. Many people have fasted on vegetable juices with positive effects, such as enhanced vitality and a diminishment of congestive-type symptoms. Vegetable juices are better the fresher they are. Carrot juice is probably the most common, although other veggies (such as beets, celery, or spinach) can be added for a mixed-vegetable cocktail. Really, almost any vegetable can be made into juice.

Leafy Greens

Cabbage	Collards	Lettuce	Watercress
Chard	Kale	Spinach	

The leafy greens are probably the richest in nutrients of any foods in the vegetable kingdom. And usually the greener they are, the more nutritious they are. They are high in vitamins A and C as well as the minerals magnesium, potassium, and iron. The leafy greens are well-known for their abundance of folic acid (the name is derived from *foliage*). Calcium is also high in the greens, although some of it gets bound up in certain ones (such as chard, spinach, and beet greens) that are high in oxalic acid. During cooking or in the intestines, calcium oxalate, which is not very soluble or absorbable, is formed. But an appreciable amount of calcium can still be obtained from the green leafy vegetables. Kale, collards, and mustard and turnip greens have a lower oxalic acid level and thus more available calcium. Dandelion greens are one of the richest sources of vitamin A.

To give an example of the rich nutrition of the leafy green vegetables, let's analyze 1 cup of cooked kale, which is a fairly large portion, requiring 2 to 3 cups of fresh kale. This has just over 50 calories, nearly 10 grams of carbohydrate, several grams of protein, 2 to 3 grams of fiber, and hardly any fat, less than 1 gram. The vitamin A activity is nearly 8,000 IU, more than the RDA for A. Calcium content is between 150 and 200 mg, magnesium about 30 mg, iron 2 mg, potassium nearly 300 mg, and vitamin C 100 to 150 mg, and there are traces of manganese, copper, and zinc. Sodium is fairly low, less than 50 mg. There are also trace amounts of most of the amino acids. The vitamin B levels are fairly low except for important folic acid, about 40 micrograms (mcg). Also, kale is hearty and relatively easy to grow. There are many edible leafy green vegetables. Following are some of the more common ones.

Cabbage *(Brassica oleracea* var. *capitata, Brassica rapa).* A nutritious anticancer cruciferous veg-

etable, cabbage is low in fat and may even help reduce body fat levels. Although it is not as high in nutrients as some of the other greens, cabbage is still rich in chlorophyll, folic acid, and vitamin C and especially good in that it contains some selenium, another known antioxidant and anticancer nutrient, and the detoxifying minerals sulfur and chlorine. Red cabbage is higher than green cabbage in vitamins A and C but lower in folic acid and chlorophyll. In longevity cultures, such as the Hunzas, cabbage is popular in the diet in both raw and cooked forms and as fermented sauerkraut (mostly in eastern Europe), which adds digestive enzymes. The phytonutrients in cabbage are brassinin, caffeic acid, carvone, cyanidins, ferulic acid, fumaric acid, kaempferol, lutein, quercetin, violaxanthin, indole-3-carbinol, sulforaphane and other isothiocyanates, as well as beta-carotene.

Chard *(Beta vulgaris).* Chard, mainly the Swiss variety, is a rich source of vitamin A; 1 cup of uncooked chard has about 1,200 IU—and fewer than 10 calories. Chard is also about one-third protein and a good fiber food. It is fair in vitamin C content as well as folic acid, calcium, magnesium, sodium, and potassium. Hot cooked chard served with a bit of melted butter or cold-pressed vegetable oil and a pinch of salt is a delicious vegetable. Chard is also sometimes called "red beet" or "silver beet." The phytonutrients in chard are beta-carotene, anthocyans, and lutein, as well as sulforaphane and other isothiocyanates.

Collards *(Brassica oleracea).* Common to the Southern diet, these greens are among the richer sources of vitamin A, with some protein and a good fiber content. Folic acid and vitamin C are also strong. The minerals calcium, potassium, iron, and zinc are plentiful. The phytonutrients in collards are glucosinolates, isothiocyanates, sulforaphane, lutein, beta-carotene, gluconapin, and sinigrin.

Kale *(Brassica oleracea* var. *sabellica).* Kale is a fairly tasty vegetable with a special and rich array of nutrients. It is an especially good source of calcium. Kale is also sometimes called "Scotch cabbage." The phytonutrients in kale include glucosinolates, isothiocyanates, luteins, zeaxanthin, sulforaphane, kaempferol, indole-3-carboxylic acid, quercetin, and sinigrin.

Lettuce *(Lactuca sativa).* This is the common name for a number of related plants that grow in "heads." Head lettuce has been classically identified with the iceberg variety, which is a solid, round ball of lettuce leaves that stores longer than most other types, so that many restaurants and homes prefer it. Iceberg lettuce, however, is less nutritious than some of the other lettuces, such as romaine, red leaf, green leaf, or butter lettuce, which are gaining in popularity. These are generally darker green in color and richer in chlorophyll, vitamin A, and folic acid. Lettuces also contain some calcium, potassium, and iron and are good fiber foods. They are low in sodium and calories as well. The phytonutrients in lettuce are lutein, lactucerol, lactucin, ferulic acid, caffeic acid, luteolin, kaempferol, and pectin.

Spinach (Spinacia oleracea, Basella alba [Malabar spinach], Tetragonia tetragonioides [New Zealand spinach]). "Spinach makes ya strong!" That has been the Popeye tale for most of us, because this dark leafy green food is rich in iron. One cup of uncooked spinach has nearly 2 mg of iron—and for only 15 calories. It is also a good fiber food and has some protein. Vitamin A activity is high, about 4,500 IU for that 1 cup. B vitamins are low except for folic acid; vitamin C content is good, and there is some vitamin E as well. Potassium, magnesium, and calcium are high, and copper, manganese, and zinc are also present. Raw spinach, however, contains oxalic acid, which may bind some of the calcium and other minerals. Spinach is a good substitute for lettuce in salads, and lightly cooked spinach is concentrated in nutrients. Once fresh spinach is cooked or a can is opened, however, it should be consumed within the day and not stored, especially in contact to a metal container, because of the potential oxidation of iron. The phytonutrients in spinach are methylenedioxyflavonol glucuronides, isothiocyanates, sulforaphane, lutein, zeaxanthin, beta-carotene, kaempferol, ferulic acid, coumaric acid, and spinasaponins.

Watercress (Rorippa nasturtium-aquaticum). A special, spicy green from the mustard family, watercress is a nice addition to salads. It grows by or in streambeds in the early spring. Watercress is particularly high in vitamin A and calcium and also contains vitamin C, potassium, iron, magnesium, and traces of nearly all the B vitamins. Many herbalists claim that watercress is a good blood purifier. The phytonutrients in watercress are gluconasturtin, isothiocyanates, and carotenoids.

Stems

Asparagus	Leeks
Celery	Rhubarb

The stem category is basically what is left after the roots, leaves, and flowers. Leeks are probably more similar to the bulb or root group, while asparagus is in a world of its own. Most of these plants are low in calories and good in fiber content.

Asparagus (Asparagus officinalis). This is a spring vegetable, and the edible part is actually the young sprouts or shoots. The asparagus tips are actually little flowers. Asparagus spears are often more expensive than other vegetables because of their short season and the work it takes to harvest them. Asparagus has good amounts of vitamin C, vitamin A, sulfur, folic acid, and potassium. It has some iron, calcium, magnesium, iodine, and zinc as well. As an early sprout, it is relatively high in protein for a vegetable, and it is a good fiber food. Asparagus is also low in calories and sodium. The unusual smell that our urine may acquire after eating asparagus comes from the amino acid asparagine, which actually acquired its name from this springtime plant. The phytonutrients in asparagus are alpha-carotene, asparagine, asparasaponins, cyanidins, inulin, kaempferol, lutein, quercetin, rutin, sarsapogenin, and zeaxanthin.

Celery (Apium graveolens). A popular crunchy stem often used for oral gratification during weight-loss programs, celery is low in calories (fewer than 10 per stalk), although it is higher in sodium than other veggies. Celery is a good fiber and carbohydrate food with a high water content. It is also rich in potassium, with some calcium and folic acid, and it is relatively high in vitamins A and C. This vegetable is thought to have a relaxing effect by calming the nerves. The phytonutrients are apigenin, apigravin, asparagine, caffeic acid, celerin, coumarin, ferulic acid, luteolin, myristicin, quercetin, rutin, scopolin, and thymol.

Leeks (Allium porrum, Allium ampeloprasum). Leeks are a nutrient-rich, high-fiber food related to green onions. They are mainly carbohydrate and fiber, although they are rich in potassium, folic acid, iron, and calcium and fairly high in vitamin C, some Bs, silicon, sulfur, magnesium, and phosphorus. They can be steamed or sautéed with other vegetables or used in soup. The phytonutrients in leeks are kaempferol, alliin, allicin, isothiocyanates, sulforaphane, and chlorophyllins.

Rhubarb (*Rheum rhabarbarum*). This interesting plant comes from Tibet. The only edible part is the stem, which is actually an early sprout of the rhizome (large bulb) of the plant. **The leaves are poisonous, and the stems, when eaten raw, may be toxic as well.** When the stems are cooked or stewed, they can be eaten in a pie or sauce, usually with some sweetener to cover up the bitter taste. Rhubarb is a good fiber food and has some calcium and other minerals. Most of the vitamin C is lost with cooking. The phytonutrients present in rhubarb are catechins, caffeic acid, chrysarone, cyanidins, ferulic acid, fumaric acid, gallic acid, lutein, pectins, quercetin, rhaponticin, rhapontigenin, rutin, and sennosides.

Roots and Tubers

Beets	Parsnips	Sweet Potatoes
Carrots	Potatoes	Turnips
Garlic	Radishes	Yams
Onions	Rutabagas	

The root vegetables, which also include the tubers (potatoes) and bulbs (garlic and onions), are probably the most commonly consumed group of vegetables throughout the world. One of these root vegetables might be cooked along with the main meal or as a dish in itself, as part of a mixed vegetable dish, or as a seasoning for other dishes. Potatoes, carrots, garlic, and onions are the most popular. These vegetables vary in their nutrient content, although they all are "starchy"—that is, they contain a high portion of complex carbohydrates. Both carrots and sweet potatoes are high in beta-carotene, which generates vitamin A. Cooking potatoes are high in vitamin C and lots of other nutrients. Most of these root vegetables, especially yams, are rich in potassium.

Beets (*Beta vulgaris* var. *vulgaris*). Beets are those red-purple roots that stain the other vegetables red when cooked with them. Some people can have a scare after eating beets when they pass bloody-looking stools or see red water in the toilet after elimination. In fact, beets can be used to measure intestinal transit time. Eat a couple of fresh raw beets, usually shredded in a salad, check the time, and watch when the first sign of them appears in the bowel movement. Canned beets will not work for this purpose, as much of the red pigment (and a lot of the nutrients as well) is lost in canning and storage.

Beet greens are particularly high in vitamin A, iron, and calcium, while beet roots are richest in iron, potassium, niacin, copper, and vitamin C. Folic acid, zinc, calcium, manganese, magnesium, and phosphorus are also present. Beet borscht is a classic Russian beet soup, but steamed, raw in salads, or cooked in soups are also simple ways to get these stimulating roots. A mixed carrot, beet, and parsley juice is supportive for women during their menstrual cycle. The phytonutrients caffeic acid, ferulic acid, betanin, kaempferol, neobetanin, and quercetin are present in beets.

Carrots (*Daucus carota*). Carrots are among the more commonly eaten vegetables. Children will often eat raw carrots when they will eat few other vegetables, but cooked carrots are another story. Carrots are amazing in their vitamin A content. One cup of carrots, with only 50 calories, contains more than 20,000 IU of vitamin A, mainly as beta-carotene. Folic acid, vitamin C, potassium, calcium, iron, and magnesium are also present. And carrots usually contain selenium, a hard-to-find and important nutrient. Of course, the freshness and quality of the vegetable determines its content, and accordingly, carrots may range widely in their vitamin A value.

Carrots are most often eaten cleaned and raw, cooked in vegetable dishes (steamed is best for nutrition), or as part of soups or salads. Sliced, diced, shredded, or swirled, they all contain lots of vitamin A. An 8-ounce glass of carrot juice contains almost 5 times (25,000 IU) the RDA for vitamin A and various concentrated minerals; it has the most nourishment when it is drunk within a short time of preparing it. With this vitamin A content, carrots and carrot juice are helpful in supporting skin health and providing immune protection.

The phytonutrients present in carrots are many and include alpha-carotene, alpha-pinene, alpha-terpinene, alpha-thujene, apigenin, beta-carotene, beta-cryptoxanthin, caffeic acid, campesterol, chrysin,

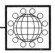

cinnamic acid, coumarins, cyanidins, daucic acid, eugenol, ferulic acid, gamma-carotene, kaempferol, lutein, luteolin, lycopene, malvidin, pipecolic acid, quercetin, and violaxanthin.

Garlic *(Allium sativum)*. A whole book could be devoted to all the tales and remedies of which garlic has been a part for centuries. Its strong odor, from sulfur gas, accounts for the theory that garlic keeps away evil spirits—or any spirits, for that matter, other than other garlic-eating ones. But it is with good reason that garlic has been known as the "king of herbs": it has been used for medicinal purposes including the treatment of high blood pressure, atherosclerosis, worms and other parasites, the common cold and flu, and generally as the "poor person's antibiotic." It seems to help purify the body and may have immune-enhancing properties. The mineral sulfur promotes elimination of toxins from the blood, lymph, and body. Garlic has been shown to help lower fat levels and platelet aggregation, which can lower blood-clotting potential.

Garlic is actually a bulb made up of cloves, each of which is the seed for a future plant. In the low amounts usually used, it is not of high nutritional value. It is used raw in salads or in dressings or cooked with meats, fish, or poultry or with other vegetables. The hot or spicy nature of garlic gives it a stimulating action and aromatherapy effect. The phytonutrients present in garlic are ajoene, alliin, allicin, allyl sulfides, caffeic acid, ferulic acid, kaempferol, coumaric acid, quercetin, and scordinins.

Onions *(Allium cepa)*. The effect of onions is similar to, although more subtle than, that of garlic. There are many varieties of these root bulbs. The standard yellow cooking onion is most common in U.S. culture, although red onions, white onions, green onions, and chives are used frequently also. Onions can be eaten raw in salads or in dips, used as flavorings, or cooked in soups or in just about any kind of food dish. Liver and onions is a fairly popular (and unpopular) high-nutrient entrée. Onion is a universal food and, like garlic, has a characteristic odor from the active sulfur bonds that release its purifying properties. Onions' antiseptic effects also come from its natural oils.

Onions are not high in nutrients, although they have a wide mix. They have some plant protein, calcium, iron, folic acid, and vitamins C, E, and A. They are also a source of selenium and zinc, which they can pick up from the soil. Green onions are higher in vitamins A and C and iron and are used most often fresh as chives in salads or with potatoes and sour cream. The phytonutrients present in onions are allyl sulfides, isofucosterol, allicin, alliin, alpha-sitosterol, caffeic acid, campesterol, catechol, cyanidins, ferulic acid, fumaric acid, quercetin, rutin, and saponins.

Parsnips *(Pastinaca sativa)*, rutabagas *(Brassica napus)*, and turnips *(Brassica rapa)*. These three root vegetables are often among our stranger and less consumed foods, unless they are passed on in a cultural diet. They are mainly starchy vegetables, without a high amount of any single nutrient but with a good mixture. They have some B vitamins, A, and C and are high in potassium, with a blend of other minerals. They are almost exclusively eaten cooked—steamed, baked, or in soups. Turnip greens are rich in vitamins A and C and folic acid. The phytonutrients present in parsnips are alpha-thujene, beta-carotene, beta-pinene, isobergapten, isorhamnetin, kaempferol, limonene, quercetin, and rutin; in rutabagas, allantoin, beta-carotene, and lycopene; and in turnips, allontoin, beta-carotene, campesterol, and lycopene.

Potatoes *(Solanum tuberosum)*. Probably the most universal and highly consumed vegetable, potatoes are actually a tuber, like Jerusalem artichokes or taro root, meaning that they grow underground off the root after the plant has grown and flowered. **I seek organic, nongreen potatoes particularly, as potatoes can concentrate chemicals and produce their own toxicity when they turn color or are exposed to sunlight.** The green color is actually chlorophyll, but it suggests that excessive solanine has been produced in the potato. Solanine in large amounts can produce such symptoms as headache, nausea, diarrhea, or fatigue. Potatoes that have sprouted should also be avoided, yet can be planted to make more potatoes.

Potatoes are rich in nutrients, low in sodium, fairly low in calories (1 potato has between 100 and 150 calories), and negligible in fats. Potatoes are approximately two-thirds starch carbohydrate and about 10% protein. They contain a reasonable portion of vitamin C and B vitamins (especially folic acid, thiamin, niacin, and pantothenic acid) and are high in potassium, with moderate amounts of magnesium, manganese, iron, and zinc.

Potatoes are versatile in the kitchen as well. They can be baked, steamed, boiled, fried, cooked in soups or vegetable dishes, and more. They get costar billing in the standard poorly balanced meat-and-potatoes diet, but they are the least of any dietary problem, unless the diet is high in french fries or the potatoes are slathered in butter, sour cream, or highly chemical bacon bits. The basic potato, however, is really that—a basic nutritious food from the Earth. Boiled potatoes can calm the intestines and reduce bloating. Externally, raw potato can draw out skin boils as well as reduce inflammation. Sliced raw potatoes on sunburns or other mild burns may help their healing. The phytonutrients present in potatoes are allantoin, alpha-solanine, caffeic acid, campesterol, cryptoxanthin, cyanins, delphinidins, ferulic acid, gibberellins, kaempferol, lutein, luteolin, myricetin, petanin, quercetin, rutin, scopoletin, scopolin, solanine, and tuberosin.

Radishes (Raphanus sativus). These spicy, crunchy little roots that grow fast are really low in calories. They are nearly all water, with some vitamin C, folic acid, and most of the trace minerals, including iron, zinc, silicon, and selenium. The chlorine content may actually help in digestion. The spicier radishes can help clear the sinuses and any mucus in the upper airways. Wild radish flowers are also edible and can help spice up a salad. Radish sprouts make a good blend with the common alfalfa sprouts and are nice for those who like a little bite in their salads. The phytonutrients in radishes are beta-carotene, caffeic acid, diallyl sulfide, ferulic acid, glucoraphanin, sulforaphane, methyl mercaptan, and raphanusin.

Sweet potatoes (Ipomoea batatas) and yams (Dioscorea alata, Dioscorea batatas). These potato-related tubers are considered the celebration potatoes in U.S. culture. Usually baked or steamed, they are a real taste treat. Sweet potato pie and candied yams are special holiday favorites. Sweet potatoes are high in beta-carotene and fairly good in the B vitamins, vitamin C, potassium, and iron. Yams are rich in potassium, folic acid, and magnesium but lower in vitamin A and some of the other nutrients. The phytonutrients in sweet potatoes are beta-carotene, other carotenoids, cyanidins, ipomoeanine, isoquercitin, pectin, phytoene, squalene, trans-cinnamic acid, and zeta-carotene; in yams, beta-carotene, dioscorin, and diosgenin.

Vegetable Flowers

Artichokes	Brussels Sprouts
Broccoli	Cauliflower

This group is different from both the flowers and the flowering vegetables, such as tomatoes and squashes, that grow to replace the flower of the plant. Vegetable flowers are actually the early part of the potential flower of the plant, picked and eaten before they progress into a "real" flower. These vegetables tend to be low in calories and high in carbohydrates but also have some protein and good fiber content. They are all good in vitamin C, folic acid, and potassium, and broccoli is rich in vitamin A. Artichokes are actually the flower of a thistle plant that is beautiful when left to fully flower, while cauliflower and broccoli are members of the highly nutritious cruciferous family, thought to help reduce the incidence of cancer.

Artichokes (Cynara scolymus). These are a special treat and a meditation to eat, unless we gobble or add to our salad the oil-marinated artichoke hearts. Eating the fresh, steamed artichoke involves trimming the stickers and then peeling the tender leaves one by one to slide the edible parts through our teeth into our mouths; and then we eventually get down to the hairy heart, which, after a shave, is a real delicacy. Artichokes are good in fiber, low in calories (if not drenched in butter or mayonnaise), and pretty well endowed with folic acid and potassium. Some vitamin A and C as well as calcium, magnesium, phosphorus, and iron are part of the artichoke. The phytonutrients are caffeoylquinic acid, beta-carotene, cyanidols, cyanarin, eugenol, ferulic acid, luteolins, and tannins.

Broccoli (Brassica oleracea). Broccoli is nutritious and low in calories. The protein content is about one-third of its nourishment. **Broccoli is a cruciferous vegetable that is thought to have anti-cancer properties and is rich in vitamins A, C, and folic acid.** Some other B vitamins and most of the minerals are also present, being particularly best in potassium, along with calcium, phosphorus, magnesium, and iron. Broccoli should be eaten raw or lightly steamed, not boiled or overcooked, to maintain its nourishment. The phytonutrients present in

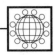

broccoli are glucosinolates, indole-3-carbinol, isothiocyanates, lutein, sulforaphane, and zeaxanthin.

Brussels sprouts (Brassica oleracea var. gemmifera). These are among the cruciferous vegetables known for their ability to reduce cancer potential. Even though they are not many people's favorite vegetable because of their peculiar taste (sulfur) and the fact that they seem to be gas producing, they are definitely loaded with nutrition.

Brussels sprouts are high in vitamins A and C, folic acid, and fiber and fairly high in calcium, sulfur, phosphorus, potassium, magnesium, and iron. These are nearly half protein, although not completely balanced in their amino acid distribution. Getting children to eat brussels sprouts—that is a real victory on several levels. The phytonutrients present are beta-carotene, caffeic acid, ferulic acid, glucosinolates, indole-3-carbinol, coumaric acid, and quercetin.

Cauliflower (Brassica oleracea var. botrytis). A cauliflower is really a little head of thousands of compact flowers. It is white because it contains no carotene pigment and is thus low in vitamin A, but it is rich in potassium, folic acid, and vitamin C. It is also about 25% protein and among the cancer-preventive cruciferous vegetables. Cauliflower can be eaten raw with dips or cooked with other vegetables. Curried in eastern Indian cooking is a tasty way to eat cauliflower. The phytonutrients present are glucobrassicin, glucosinolates, isothiocyanates, alpha-carotene, beta-carotene, beta-sitosterol, caffeic acid, ferulic acid, glucoraphanin, indole-3-carbinol, and quercetin.

Flowering Vegetables

Cucumbers	Pumpkins
Eggplant	Squashes
Peppers	Tomatoes

These plants are many, mainly growing on small bushes and vines. Each one discussed here has many different varieties. The flowering vegetables are botanically like fruits in that they carry the plant's matured seeds for the next generation. These vegetables grow after and in replacement of the flowers, much like a citrus tree.

Tomatoes, the popular "fruit of the vine," were once thought to be poisonous. There was also a question as to whether they were a fruit or a vegetable until the United States Supreme Court ruled in 1893 that they are in fact vegetables. **Actually, tomatoes, eggplants, and peppers are all members of the nightshade family of plants, which are thought to be possible joint irritants in arthritis. Potatoes and tobacco are also in the nightshade family.**

Squashes are multiple and vary from small, soft, high water-content zucchini and summer squash to hard, starchy drier ones, such as acorn and Hubbard squash. Even the pumpkin is in the squash family. Many beans, especially green peas and green beans, are also flowering vegetables (although I discuss these in the legumes section).

Cucumbers (Cucumis sativa). The "coolest" of vegetables, cucumbers are used medicinally for burns or irritated tissues. Laying a slice of cucumber over each eye is a soothing treatment for stressed or inflamed eyes; they're also helpful for hot or burned skin. Cucumbers are eaten in their unripe state, usually raw, although some cultures cook them. The smaller cucumbers may be pickled to make a fermented vinegary fruit known as pickles. Some people find cucumbers difficult to digest, in particular the skins, although they contain the cuke's folic acid. Cucumbers are not really high in any nutrients, but they are almost devoid of calories. They provide the best source of vitamin E (in the seeds) of all the vegetables, however. Cucumbers also have some vitamins A and C as well as potassium and other minerals. The phytonutrients present in cucumbers are beta-carotene, beta-sitosterol, cucurbitacins, cucurbitin, ferulic acid, isoorientin, lupeol, and stigmasterol.

Eggplant (Solanum melongena). This purple vegetable is usually eaten cooked. It is low in calories unless sautéed in oils; we must be careful with eggplant because it is like a sponge and therefore can soak up large amounts of fats. It is best to bake eggplant first before cooking it in other recipes. It is used in many dishes throughout the world. Eggplants are mainly carbohydrate and contain no fat. They are not particularly high in nutrients, except for niacin and potassium. Calcium, magnesium, iron, vitamins A and C, and folic acid are also present. Eggplant is a member of the nightshade family and thus may be avoided by people with concern about arthritis. It includes the phytonutrients aubergenone, beta-carotene, caffeic acid, delphinidin, ferulic acid, lycopene, lycoxanthin, nasunin, pectin, pipecolic acid, scopoletin, and tannin.

Peppers *(Capsicum frutescens, Capsicum annum).* Peppers are grown and eaten throughout the world in a great many varieties, shapes, and flavors, from sweet to very hot. In the United States, we are most familiar with red or green bell peppers and the hotter chile, cayenne, and jalapeño peppers. Bell peppers may be eaten fresh in salads or sliced with dips or stuffed with other foods, such as grains or meats, and baked. Some people have difficulty digesting peppers, however, especially the pepper's skin. The hot peppers are used to spice up salsas, cheeses, and in many dishes of South America, where they originated. **The chiles and cayenne peppers contain capsaicin, with medicinal properties in cleansing the blood and stimulating the circulation and perhaps in reducing cardiovascular disease and cancer.** They also stimulate the gastric secretions and help digestion.

All peppers are high in vitamin C, bioflavonoids, and vitamin A. One sweet pepper might have more than 500 IU of A and nearly 150 mg of vitamin C. A smaller hot chile pepper is more concentrated and so may have similar levels. Folic acid, potassium, and niacin are also present in fairly good levels, as are some other minerals and B vitamins. The seeds surround the inner core of the peppers and often concentrate the hot nature. The phytonutrients present in peppers include cineol, alpha-carotene, alpha-terpineol, antheraxanthin, apiin, beta-carotene, caffeic acid, campesterol, capsaicin, capsanthin, capsiamide, capsolutein, capsorubin, citroxanthin, kaempferol, lutein, quercetin, scopoletin, stigmasterol, and thujone.

Pumpkins *(Curcubita pepo, Curcubita maxima).* Another festive vegetable, pumpkins are used decoratively for Halloween and cooked for the tasty pumpkin pie dessert, eaten mainly around Thanksgiving and Christmas. Pumpkin seeds are also fairly popular. Pumpkins are also high in vitamin A, as beta-carotene, provides the natural orange coloring. They are mainly a starchy carbohydrate with good water content. Pumpkins have some vitamin C, niacin, and pantothenic acid and are high in potassium. Other prevalent minerals include phosphorus, silicon, iron, magnesium,

and calcium. Pumpkin seeds are high in zinc and other minerals (see "Seeds" on page 333 in this chapter). The phytonutrients present in pumpkins are beta-sitosterol, caffeic acid, cryptoxanthin, curcubitin, cucurbitaxanthin, ferulic acid, flavoxanthin, gibberellins, kaempferol, lutein, neoxanthin, quercetin, rutinosides, and zeaxanthin.

Squashes *(Curcubita pepo, Curcubita spp.).* These are mainly autumn harvest vegetables. Many squashes need to be cooked by baking or steaming, although the popular zucchini and yellow crookneck (both summer vegetables) can be sliced and eaten raw in salads or with dips. Most of the squashes are high in carbohydrates, mainly as starch, with a high fiber content. Many are high in vitamin A, especially the orange or yellow squashes. Vitamin C and potassium are also present in varying amounts, as are calcium, magnesium, and iron.

Zucchinis are probably the most commonly used squash in U.S. culture because they are so easy to prepare. They are juicy and flavorful after light steaming. The bigger ones can be stuffed and baked. Zucchinis can also be used raw in salads or for dips, or in soups or dipped in egg and breaded for deep frying. This vegetable seems to have a mild diuretic action and stimulates the intestines, probably because of its mucilage content. The phytonutrients present in squashes are beta-carotene, beta-cryptoxanthin, cucubitacins, pectin, and squalene.

Tomatoes *(Lycopersicon lycopersicum).* The vegetable mainstay of many Americans' diets and the diets of many cultures around the world, tomatoes have a wide variety of uses—as juices and soups, raw in salads, stuffed, in sauces, in ketchups and condiments, in salad dressings, and in pizza, to name just a few. In 1980, it was estimated that nearly 60 pounds of tomatoes per person were consumed in the Unites States, although most of this was probably in ketchups and sauces. The tomato, which is related to the belladonna plant, was thought to be poisonous until a brave soul ate a tomato in public and didn't die. Whether tomatoes are a fruit or vegetable doesn't really matter; they are a delicious, mildly acidic food. **The tomato skins are difficult to digest, and some people can suffer allergic reactions or irritation from too much tomato intake.** Also, as a nightshade plant, they appear to be a joint irritant in some

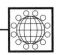

people with arthritis. It is not known whether this is from allergy, acidity, or some other factor.

Tomatoes are not highly nutritious, although they are pretty well spiked with potassium, vitamin C, and vitamin A. They are low in calories and are mostly liquid and carbohydrate. Whole tomatoes contain some vitamin E, folic acid, and other B vitamins (such as biotin and niacin) as well as a bit of iron, sodium, calcium, magnesium, and zinc. Tomato juice and tomato paste are more concentrated in some of the nutrients. Fresh-picked tomatoes are the best and tastiest way to eat those red, ripe jewels of the garden. The phytonutrients present in tomatoes are kaempferol, lycopene, myricetin, phytoene, phytofluene, and quercetin.

Ocean Vegetables—Seaweed

Agar-agar	Hijiki	Nori
Arame	Kelp	Purple Laver
Dulse	Kombu	Wakame

The vegetables that come from the sea are some of the most nutrient-rich foods available, particularly rich in iodine, calcium, potassium, and iron. Some are very high in protein as well. Because these plants are constantly bathed in the mineral-rich ocean waters, they have a regular supply of nutrients. Sodium, however, can also be concentrated in these saltwater vegetables that supply food for many fishes. Most seaweeds contain algin, a fiber molecule that binds minerals. When taken into the body, it can attract various metals within the digestive tract, possibly including such heavy metals as lead and mercury, as well as take them out of the body's system. It is wise to include sea vegetables more regularly in the diet to provide good mineral nutrition and reduce possible absorption and utilization of similar radioactive compounds, such as iodine 131, from environmental or medical sources. Kelp is a good high-mineral salt substitute, relatively low in sodium compared to regular salt, and may be useful for those with hypertension.

Agar-agar (*Eucheuma* spp.). Agar-agar is a gelatin made from various types of seaweed—primarily red algae—that is used as a thickening and stabilizing agent in cooking and for desserts. Agar-agar is usually harvested from a particular type of red algae called *gelidium*. It has no taste and no fishy smell and is healthier than gelatin made from animal by-products. Agar-agar is probably a good place to begin for children or for people who want to bring these sea vegetables into their diet.

Arame (*Eisenia bicyclis*). This is a dark, thin seaweed thread that can be used in soups or salads or mixed with rice. It is fairly rich in protein, iodine, calcium, and iron and is one of the tastier seaweeds. The phytonutrients present in arame are fucoxanthin (the reason for the brown color of these sea plants), diadinoxanthin, diatoxanthin, flavoxanthin, lutein, neoxanthin, and violaxanthin.

Dulse (*Palmaria palmata*). A red-purple leaf that is rich in iodine, iron, and calcium, dulse is a tasty seaweed that can be used fresh in salads or cooked in soups. It is helpful to rinse the dulse before use to wash away some of the salt and the more fishy ocean flavor. Dulse powder, like kelp, is also available as a seasoning. The common name for this sea plant is also sometimes spelled *dulce*. The phytonutrients in dulse are phycobilins (including phycoerythrin).

Hijiki (*Hijiki fusiforme*). This is a mineral-rich, high-fiber seaweed. Its dark, long strands look like thick hairs. Hijiki is about 10% to 20% protein, contains some vitamin A, and is richest in calcium, iron, and phosphorus. Soaked in water, it can be cooked in soup or is good combined and eaten with rice. It is similar to arame. The phytonutrients present in hijiki are fucoxanthin, diadinoxanthin, diatoxanthin, flavoxanthin, lutein, neoxanthin, and violaxanthin.

Kelp (*Fucus vesiculosus*). Kelp is usually used in smaller quantities than the other seaweeds, mostly as a seasoning. It has some protein and is rich in iodine, calcium, and potassium, along with some of the B vitamins. Kelp is a common food supplement, used mainly for its iodine. The phytonutrients present in kelp are fucosterol, phloroglucinol, vanillin, fucoxanthin, diadinoxanthin, diatoxanthin, flavoxanthin, lutein, neoxanthin, and violaxanthin.

Kombu (*Laminaria japonica*). A richer, meatier, higher-protein seaweed, kombu is most often used in soups—it adds minerals and flavor to the stock. Kombu contains vitamin A, some Bs, and lots of calcium and iron, yet it is higher in sodium than most of the other seaweeds. One strip of kombu can also be added to the pot when cooking beans to reduce some of the potential gas-inducing qualities of the beans. The phytonutrients present in kombu include fucoxanthin, diadinoxanthin, diatoxanthin, flavoxanthin, laminarin, lutein, neoxanthin, and violaxanthin.

Nori (*Porphyra tenera*). Nori is probably one of the most commonly used seaweeds. The dark sheets, as it is usually available, are nearly 50% protein. Nori is high in fiber as well. The sheets are used to wrap and hold rice, vegetables, and raw or cooked fish in small rolls that can be eaten with the hands. Nori is also high in vitamin A, calcium, iodine, iron, and phosphorus, and it has one of the sweeter flavors of the seaweeds. Nori is great as a wrap for salad and rice and is commonly used in Japanese restaurants. The phytonutrients present are sulfated galactans, allophycocyanin, and phycobilins (including phycoerythrin).

Purple laver (*Porphyra umbilicalis*). One of the lesser known of the red seaweeds, purple laver is usually purchased in dried sheets and then soaked in water before using. Phytonutrients present in laver include beta-carotene, lutein, and phicobilins, the unique blue- and green-absorbing pigments that give laver its unique purple color.

Wakame (*Undaria pinnatifida*). Another high-protein, flat, and thinner seaweed, wakame is used mainly in soups. It contains some vitamin A, lots of calcium, iron, and sodium, as well as a bit of vitamin C. The phytonutrients present include fucoxanthin, diadinoxanthin, diatoxanthin, flavoxanthin, lutein, neoxanthin, and violaxanthin.

Red Algae	**Brown Algae**
Nori	Arame
Dulse	Hijiki
Purple laver	Kelp
Source for carrageenan	Kombu
compounds	Wakame
Source for agar-agar (gelatin)	
Green Algae	
Sea lettuce	

Fungi

Fungi can make some people a little apprehensive when it comes to eating, but this amazing group of foods is both nutrient-dense and found in cuisines across the globe. Fungi are plantlike organisms, but they do not contain chlorophyll pigments and so they cannot use sunlight to make energy. Since they don't make use of the sun, they are often found in habitats that are both dark and damp. There are over 100,000 species of fungi, and when it comes to food, the best-known are the mushrooms. You should be extremely careful when consuming mushrooms, making sure they are indeed the edible varieties; I recommend buying mushrooms from markets or experienced foragers, and do not recommend that novices do their own foraging.

Mushrooms (*Agaricus bisporus* [button], *Lentinus edodes* [shiitake], *Volvaria volvacea* [straw], *Pleurotus ostreatus* [oyster], *Cantharellus cibarius* [chanterelle], *Grifola frondosa* [maitake], *Ganodema lucidum* [reishi] *Morchella* spp. [morels]). Edible fungi are fascinating. When they are eaten, almost the entire plant is consumed. There are literally thousands of varieties, although probably only about twenty-five are consumed by humans. **Most mushrooms are poisonous in varying degrees, with effects ranging from digestive upset to paralysis and death.** It is important, especially with wild mushrooms, to know the species that are edible and not make any mistakes. I remember a beautiful post-rain walk with herbalist Rob Menzies, where we discovered nearly 100 species of mushrooms in the woods of Point Reyes, California.

White button, or field, mushrooms are found in most grocery stores and are the most commonly consumed. They may be the only variety known to most consumers, yet they have little nutrition. Japanese shiitake mushrooms, boletus mushrooms, chanterelles, oyster mushrooms, and the tiny tree mushrooms are some other fairly common, more nutritious mushroom delicacies. Most mushrooms have a fairly good protein content. I often describe them as the "meat" of the vegetable kingdom, especially some of those exotic forms found in Asian cooking. The average button mushroom is low in calories and about one-third protein, while other varieties may have even more protein. Shiitake mushrooms are noted to have all eight essential amino acids and thus are quite nutritious. Many mushrooms are also high in two other, harder-to-find vegetable nutrients—iron and selenium. The B vitamins biotin, niacin, folic acid, and pantothenic acid are often found in good quantities. Potassium and phosphorus are usually the next most highly concentrated minerals, although other minerals are present in varying amounts, depending on the soil content.

Some people are allergic or sensitive to mushrooms. Also, people with intestinal yeast overgrowth, yeast sensitivities, or mold allergies may have crossover reactions to the fungi family. Many people mistake kombucha as a mushroom, but it is not. Rather, it is actually a combination of different bacteria and fungal yeast cells that can live symbiotically. Although kombucha can be cultured at home by fermenting green and black teas combined with sugar, producing a high-quality tea that can be trusted for content and safety is not easy. The phytonutrients in mushrooms include beta-glucans (including lentinan in shiitake mushrooms), ganoderic acid, and lucidenic acid.

Legumes

Peas and beans *(Pisum sativum* **[green pea]***, Vigna angularis* **[adzuki]***, Cicer arietinum* **[garbanzo]***, Phaseolus limensis* **[lima]***, Vigna radiata* **[mung]***, Phaseolus vulgaris* **[black bean, kidney bean, field bean, navy bean, wax bean, green bean, snap bean]).** The legume vegetables are a special class of the pea and bean plants, which contain edible seeds inside pods that grow after the plant flowers. These include adzuki beans, black beans, black-eyed peas, garbanzo beans, great northerns, green peas, kidney beans, lentils, lima beans, mung beans, navy beans, peanuts, pinto beans, and soybeans. There are also many other types of peas and beans. In fact, peanuts are actually a legume vegetable and not a true nut; but because they are so commonly thought of as nuts, I discuss them in the nut section.

The legumes are an interesting food, mainly a mixture of protein and starch, with many positive qualities as a food. They are low in calories, low in fat, a good complex carbohydrate, and fairly high in fiber, which may help intestinal action and even help to reduce cholesterol levels. **Most importantly, especially for the vegetarian, the legumes are a good**

and inexpensive protein source. They cost on the average about $3 per pound of protein, whereas egg protein may cost about $6 per pound, and meat protein more like $12 per pound. And the extra advantage is that the beans have less than 10% fat content. So, although beans may be considered the poor people's meat, they might better be known as the healthy people's meat.

One concern, however, is that the protein in most of the peas and beans is not as complete as the animal proteins (although the protein present is well utilized). In other words, all the essential amino acids are not contained in near-equal amounts. Tryptophan and methionine are the two amino acids most commonly low in the vegetable proteins. So we must eat more of these vegetable protein foods or mix them with different vegetable protein foods such as grains (which are commonly higher than legumes in methionine but lower in lysine) to get all the essential amino acids at more optimum levels. This mixing of protein foods, called "protein complementarity," is discussed more in on page 57 of chapter 3, Proteins, and in chapter 9, Diets, under "Lacto-ovo Vegetarian" on page 359. Soybeans and peanuts are the most complete proteins of the legumes and, for that matter, of the vegetable kingdom.

Another concern with legumes, especially beans, is that in many people they cause increased intestinal gas, which leads to burping, flatulence, or abdominal discomfort. This is caused mainly by the oligosaccharides in the beans fermenting in the lower intestine. Because these starch-type molecules are contained primarily in the coverings of the beans, we can soak the beans in water, usually overnight, and then discard that water first before cooking them in fresh water to help leach out some of their fermenting properties. This definitely reduces the gas-producing potential for which beans are notorious. Also, combining such beans as mung, adzuki, lentil, or black with such grains as rice or millet in a 1:3 (bean-to-grain) ratio will provide low gas but good fuel as a complete protein. Overall, however, the legumes are an important class of foods. They are especially important to the American diet, where we need to find lower-fat, lower-sodium, and lower-calorie (and lower-cost) protein foods to substitute in the diets that are currently too high in meat, sodium, and fat and contribute so much to disease. The legumes are one of the best substitutes we have.

For this discussion, the legumes are divided into three main categories: *fresh beans, fresh peas, and dried beans.* In terms of nutrient content, fresh peas and beans are more like the basic green vegetables, and dried beans are more similar to the grains as starchier, protein-containing foods higher in B vitamins. Fresh beans, for example, include basic "green" beans and their many varieties, as well as lima beans (also available dried) and yellow wax beans. These beans are usually higher in vitamins A and C than the dried varieties. Green beans are also usually good in folic acid and limas in potassium and iron, while yellow wax beans are lower in the supportive nutrients, although they have some vitamin A. Fresh beans are usually eaten steamed or cooked by themselves or with other vegetables.

The fresh peas include the standard green peas, as well as sweet, snap, snow, and sugar peas. When picked young, the whole pod and baby peas can be eaten fresh in salads or right off the bush, or they may be cooked. When more mature, the peas are bigger and the pods are stringier and less easy to chew and digest. This group is the highest in vitamin C of all the legumes, fairly high in the B vitamins (with some folic acid), high in vitamin A, and fairly well endowed with most of the minerals, including iron, potassium, calcium, and magnesium. Green peas even contain some vitamin E. The phytonutrients present in green peas are alpha-carotene, beta-carotene, jasmonic acid, kaempferol, lutein, and pipecolinic acid; in snap beans, beta-carotene, ferulic acid, genistein, gibberellins, luteolin, phaseolin, pipecolic acid, and trigonelline.

Dried beans are the category in which most of the legumes fall. There are many varieties, and their use tends to vary among cultures. Lentils, often eaten with wheat or peas for complete protein, are common in Middle Eastern diets, as are garbanzo beans, also known as chickpeas. Hummus and falafel are Middle Eastern foods based on this bean. Pintos and black beans, usually eaten with rice or corn, are more common in Latin American countries. Kidney, navy, and great northern beans seem more Western-type beans, although most of the world's beans are consumed in the United States. Flavorful "baked beans" commonly use the red kidney bean. Soybeans have classically come from the Asian cultures in the form of tofu, or soybean curd, but in the past 20 years, soybean use has expanded rapidly worldwide.

Most of these dried and cooked beans contain some basic B vitamins, although the content is not really high. In general, the levels of thiamin, niacin, and pantothenic acid are best. There is a surprisingly high level of iron in most of these beans; calcium, potassium, and phosphorus are also abundant. Black beans, for example, are high in iron, calcium, potassium, and phosphorus; garbanzos are rich in those same minerals and good in vitamins B_1, B_2, and B_3; kidney beans are good in iron and potassium, as are navy beans and lentils. Soybeans are among the better protein sources, although they are a little less well endowed with the supportive vitamins and minerals, so eating them with more vegetables will help provide those nutrients. Soybeans contain some A and C as well as some niacin and are actually fairly high in iron, calcium, potassium, and phosphorus. The phytonutrients present in these legumes are apigenin, ferulic acid, genistein, gibberellins, kaempferol, luteolin, and quercetin.

Soybeans *(Glycine max)* are an important food. They are very versatile and could supply much of the world's hungry population with better protein and improved general nutrition. Growing soybeans for direct human consumption is a much more productive use of the land than raising meat. Raising soybeans can provide nearly 20 times the protein per acre that raising beef can. They contain complete protein as well, although not as concentrated as in beef. The amino acid balance of the soybeans is not perfect, being a little low in tryptophan and methionine, but a good intake of soybeans and soybean products can supply us with a fair amount of protein. Soybeans also contain very little if any saturated fat; most of their fat is the unsaturated variety. Soybean oil, commonly used, is high in linoleic acid and polyunsaturated fat and is more stable to oxidation and rancidification than some other oils because of its high content of lecithin and vitamin E, an important antioxidant. Note: please be aware that genetically modified (GM) soybeans are grown in the U.S., and since we do not really know the human effects from regular consumption of this "food" I encourage use of organically grown soy and soy products as much as possible; at

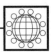

this time, the label "organic" cannot be used on GM foods.

Other soybean products that have hit the American scene in recent years include tempeh, or fermented soybean cakes, and soy burgers made from straight soybeans, tempeh, or tofu. Tofu, the classic soybean product made by fermenting the soybean and concentrating the curd, is now used by many cultures. It has become known as the "food of 10,000 flavors" because it picks up the flavors from the other foods cooked with it. Tofu is a versatile food. It can be used in salads, blended into dressings, eaten in sandwiches, or added to stir-fries or cooked vegetables. Tofu is not as high in protein and other nutrients as the whole soybean, although it retains fairly good levels of calcium, iron, and phosphorus. The sodium level is usually higher, however. Soybean-based ice cream has also become popular as a low-cholesterol, lower-fat dessert treat. Ice Bean, another soybean dessert, contains more soybean and less sweetener than the Tofutti.

Soybean sprouts, like any of the legume sprouts, are also nutritious, vital foods (I discuss sprouts in more detail below). The vitamin C content, chlorophyll level, and protein level are all fairly good in soybean sprouts. The general protein concentration may go down a bit, but protein is still found in good quantity, and the fiber content goes up. Anybody, anywhere can make and use these important sprouts as a healthful adjunct to their diet. The phytonutrients present in soybeans are apigenin, ferulic acid, gibberellins, isoflavones (including genistein and daidzein), kaempferol, luteolin, and quercetin.

Sprouts

Adzuki, alfalfa, buckwheat, clover, fenugreek, garbanzo, lentil, mung, radish, soybean, sunflower, wheat—these are only some of the protein- and vitamin-rich sprouts of many possible seeds, grains, and beans. Barley, corn, oats, green peas, and lima beans are a few others. Really, any "seed" that is endowed with the potential for the next generation of plant life is sproutable. When a seed is sprouted into the first beginnings of the new plant, much of the stored nutrient potential bursts forth into the seedling, and these little sprouts—including the seed, grain, or bean with its shoot and greenery—become wealthy with nutrients. Protein content increases by somewhere between 15% and 30%, depending on the plant, as the carbohydrate food source gets converted.

Chlorophyll and fiber content also increase. The chlorophyll content can be high when the sprout becomes green, as in sprouted wheat berries (wheat grass). Chlorophyll itself is rich in nutrients and has many health-giving properties. **Also, sprouts are living foods that contain active enzymes that help digestion and assimilation. With sprouting, most of the B vitamins are greatly increased, some more than tenfold.** Niacin and riboflavin are in particularly good amounts. The vitamin C level is greatly enhanced in sprouts compared with the dry seeds. Beta-carotene, the vitamin A precursor, increases with sprouting, as do vitamins E and K, calcium, phosphorus, and iron, although mineral content is not as greatly affected as that of the vitamins.

Many sprouts can now be purchased in grocery stores. Alfalfa sprouts, by far the most common, are used in salads or sandwiches. They are tasty but should be eaten fresh so that they do not ferment. Clover sprouts are bigger and have a fuller flavor than alfalfa; they are now more available in stores and can also be used fresh in salads or sandwiches. Mung bean sprouts have been used since ancient China and are still popular in much Asian cooking. Mixed bean sprouts (with lentils, peas, and garbanzo beans, for example) are now more commonly available in little plastic bags. These can be eaten raw in salads or cooked in vegetable, grain, or even meat dishes or in soups. More and more people are realizing that the nutrient value and economical price of sprouts make them an ideal food.

Sprouting at home is simple with a large glass jar or flat tray filled with soil. Most seeds, grains, or beans can be placed in a jar, rinsed, then covered with water for approximately 24 hours, being rinsed once or twice. Then, keep them in the jar and out of direct sunlight and rinse them 2 or 3 times a day, pouring off the water and letting the moist sprouts sit. I suggest using purified, chlorine-free water for soaking and rinsing sprouts. When they have sprouted, they can be placed in more light over the next 1 or 2 days, again being rinsed 2 or 3 times daily to keep them clean and fresh. By this time, the amount of sprouts will have increased

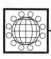
several times over the original volume. The sprouts and greenery are usually edible after 1 or 2 days in the light. Many types of sprouts (such as lentils, garbanzos, or alfalfa) can be eaten earlier than this and are tasty along with being at peak protein levels at day 2 or 3.

Lentils and garbanzos are also easy to sprout, may take only a couple of days, and are rich in protein. Sprouted mung beans, the common bean sprouts used in most Asian cooking, can be used in salads or cooked into vegetable dishes. Fenugreek sprouts have a licorice flavor, while radish sprouts are more spicy. Soybean sprouting takes a little more care, as they must be rinsed more often to prevent fermentation. Sunflower, wheat berry, and buckwheat sprouts all tend to grow better and healthier in a bed of soil. They are placed on top of the soil, watered well, covered with dark plastic or cloth, and left in a dark place for 2 to 3 days. Then they are uncovered and placed in the light, being watered or sprayed as needed. The tall shoots with green tops can be trimmed and eaten fresh in salads, or they may continue to grow even further.

Some practitioners feel that sprouts as a basic part of the diet can be very healthy and can in fact help heal a lot of medical problems. When the Hippocrates Health Institute in West Palm Beach, Florida, and the Optimum Health Institute in San Diego, California, and Austin, Texas, take people in for health care, for example, they feed them mainly sprouts of various kinds, raw foods, and juices. These centers have been inspired by the work of Ann Wigmore, late founder of the Ann Wigmore Natural Health Institute in Rincón, Puerto Rico. Author Viktoras Kulvinskas, best known for his book *Survival into the Twenty-First Century*, has also published an entire book on sprouts, *Sprouts for the Love of Every Body*. In more recent years, Steve Meyerwitz, the "Sproutman" has published several books on consuming sprouts and their benefits, and books on cleansing and detoxification; see www.sproutman.com for more information.

These authors feel, and I agree, that sprouts are likely the most vitally alive and nourishing foods we can eat. They are a great survival food, too. We can sprout these seeds, beans, and grains all year round. Eating high amounts of sprouted foods, along with other vegetables and fruits, promotes health and vitality. Also, for overweight people, sprouts provide low-calorie, high-nutrient foods that also tend to support improved metabolism. Sprouts are a good source of nutrients in the wintertime, when there are less leafy greens and other vegetables available. And the amount of nourishment per dollar surpasses most any other food.

GRAINS

 The grains are the most commonly consumed foods worldwide. Wheat, rice, and corn, in that order, are the three largest crops. They are also some of the oldest foods. Knowledge of their use goes back 10,000 years. **Grains are a key human fuel and are a good source of complex carbohydrates, which are slower burning and provide more sustained energy than the simple sugars.** These rich sources of starch and fiber are also the cheapest caloric supply for the world masses. The whole (unprocessed) grains provide a healthy amount of B vitamins, vitamin E, and many minerals.

The grains, often known as the "cereal" grains, are the seeds of various grasses. There are three primary parts to each kernel, or seed, of the grains—the central core, or endosperm, which is about 80% to 85% of the grain; the germ and future sprout, about 3%; and the bran coverings of the grain, approximately 15% of the entire kernel. The endosperm, the bulk of the grain, is composed mainly of starch (and some protein) for energy to nourish the future seed. It has the nutrients to help the seed, and we humans, to grow. Although it is the major portion of the grain, it has fewer B vitamins and minerals as well as less fiber than the germ and bran coverings. So when a grain is refined, most of these nutrients are lost along with the outer layers. The endosperm of wheat, for example, is what is contained in white flour.

The germ is only a small part of the grain, albeit the most essential part. It is the little embryo at the base of the kernel that is the future life. The rest of the grain is there to serve the germ; the coverings protect it, and the endosperm nourishes it in its new life. The germ actually is the part that grows, sprouting out through the bran covers when moisture and the sun bathe it. It will grow leaves and continue as roots going into the soil to gather more moisture and

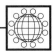

nutrients for continued growth. The germ is also the most nutrient-rich part of the grain. It contains protein, oils, and many vitamins and minerals. The germ is high in the B vitamins, particularly thiamin, riboflavin, niacin, and pyridoxine. Magnesium, zinc, potassium, and iron are some of the minerals contained in this part of the grain. **Wheat germ particularly is high in vitamin E, and wheat germ oil is one of the richest sources.** When the grain is broken apart, as in making flour, the germ content of whole wheat flour is less stable because of potential oxidation of the oils. This is a major reason for the wide use of white flour, which is devoid of the nutrient-rich wheat germ.

The bran of the grain consists of several protective coverings, which add most of the fiber and much of the nutrients. These include the B vitamins and some minerals, especially zinc. The outermost layers of the bran are mainly indigestible cellulose fiber and are not really high in nutrients. These layers also come off most grains more easily than the deeper layers, which contain more of the nutrients. Soft milling or hand milling can clean these outermost coverings and improve the digestibility and utilization of the protein and nutrients from the grain.

Another advantage in removing these outer bran coverings is that they also contain most of the phytic acid present in the grains. In chapter 6, Minerals, I mentioned that phytic acid can bind such minerals as calcium, iron, zinc, and magnesium in the gut and carry them out through the intestines so that they are not assimilated and utilized. This is not helpful for people who are not obtaining sufficient nutrients, such as the elderly or younger people on poor diets. Even though bran, usually wheat or sometimes oat bran, is used by many people to add fiber content to the diet to help reduce or prevent constipation and is known to reduce risks of colon and rectal cancer, I do not recommend its regular, long-term use because of the potential mineral depletion. Rather, I suggest eating more fiber-containing foods, such as the whole grains, vegetables, and most fresh fruits, plus drinking more water. Examples of other high-fiber foods include miller's bran, with about 40% fiber; high-fiber cereals, which may contain up to 30% fiber; and whole wheat bread, with about 10% fiber. This use of high-fiber and whole foods is overall a more healthful approach to bowel care, cancer prevention, and general nutrition.

Grains are the earth's most basic whole foods. The seeds of these grasses, or cereal grains, are a good source of complex carbohydrates, calories, energy, and fiber, as well as being a light source of protein. Vitamins B_1, B_2, and B_3 are the B vitamins most plentifully found in grains. Most grains are relatively low in vitamins A and C; however, these are prevalent in many vegetables, which go well with grains at meals. Vitamin E is found in the germ of the grain. The whole grains are rich in many minerals, especially magnesium, zinc, iron, and potassium, though calcium, phosphorus, and copper are often present. **Rice and wheat are usually good sources of hard-to-find selenium.**

The fiber content of the whole grains is probably the biggest difference between the natural or primitive diet and the industrial or Westernized diet. This is the likely difference between poor health and good health. The diet of the early inhabitants of the United States averaged several times more fiber than the modern, "more refined" way of eating. And lack of fiber may likely be the most significant cause in the advance of chronic, serious, deadly diseases. **Medical research has shown that a low-fiber diet correlates with many diseases, and, conversely, an increase in fiber can reduce the risk of those same diseases.**

The increase in dietary fat and refined flours cannot easily be separated from the lowered dietary fiber, and all of these factors probably contribute to such symptoms and diseases as colon cancer (and possibly other cancers), constipation, hemorrhoids, diverticulitis, gallstones and gallbladder problems, high cholesterol, hypertensive heart disease, ulcers, and varicose veins. As the fiber coverings of the grain are its vital life protection, the fiber content of our diet may protect us from many common problems. Just keeping our bowels moving regularly is an important daily step toward health. Eating more whole grains and vegetables as the mainstay of the diet is the best way to approach the fiber issue.

There are two main aspects regarding protein in the grains. The first is that grains do not contain "complete proteins." This is a relative term because they contain all the essential amino acids, but the proportion of lysine is often low. In the section "Legumes" on page 321, I mentioned that most beans have a good level of lysine but are low in methionine. **So when we eat the grains and legumes together, they complement each**

other and provide us with good levels of all the essential amino acids. Most cultures in the world have learned this important balance. Recent thinking suggests that in the short term, such as for a single meal, combining like this is not absolutely necessary, but over the course of a day we need to get this variety of foods to maintain protein balance.

The second aspect of grain protein is that much of it is as gluten. **Gluten is primarily a protein-carbohydrate mixture that is contained mainly in wheat. Rye and barley, and to a much lesser extent oats, can also trigger gluten-related reactions.** These glutenous grains tend to have a higher protein content than the nonglutenous ones, such as millet, corn, rice, and buckwheat. Some people have a sensitivity to gluten. This is most often intestinal, although a general allergy, most commonly to wheat, may involve the body's interaction with the gluten protein. Celiac disease (a type of malabsorption) may in part be generated by an inability to handle wheat, and for the most sensitive, any of the gluten grains. Many intestinal symptoms, weight loss, and anemia may result. Usually symptoms can be alleviated by avoiding the gluten grains and substituting others. However, certain nutritional deficiencies, psychological factors, and other aspects of diet, such as protein-fat ratios, may contribute as well to these intestinal symptoms of celiac disease.

Grains are consumed without problems by most of the world's population. They are versatile foods and are considered the "staff of life," a phrase often given to breads. Breads, the heated baked paste (flour) made from the grains, are in some form part of the diet of all the world's populations. From hand milling to using large machinery, breaking down the whole grains into fine powder (flour) is the beginning process in making all kinds of edibles, such as breads, crackers, tortillas, cereals, pastas, pastries, and cookies. Wheat, of course, is the most commonly used grain, and most breads, especially in the United States, contain wheat or refined wheat flour as the main ingredient. In 1977, it was estimated that nearly one-third of the world's population obtained at least half of its nutrition from wheat—that is, wheat was the main food in their diets. It is a good overall food, especially whole wheat, but it must be balanced with other nutrients, protein, vitamin A, and vitamin C, for example—all of which may be consumed in amounts insufficient to sustain health. **Another concern, especially in Western cultures, is that many people, children in particular, obtain many of their grains from packaged cereals and refined-flour breads, which provide less nutrition than the whole grain.**

The refinement of grains and its contribution to nutrition and health is a major issue in nutrition circles, and I discuss it briefly here. Refined grains and flours used to make breads, pastas, crackers, cookies, pastries, and so on, have a couple of advantages over whole grains and flours. First, they are more stable in storage; there are no oils in them as there are in the germ, so they do not oxidize and rancidify as easily. Second, the refined grain products may be easier to digest and utilize in the body. They may also have somewhat less allergenic potential than the whole grains. The decrease in gluten in white flour, for example, reduces sensitivity to that protein.

But refining grains and flours also creates a number of problems. The major one is the loss of nutrients that occurs from this processing, particularly the loss of most of the B vitamins, vitamin E, and the many minerals that are found naturally in whole grains. The protein content is only slightly decreased, the level of calories and the amount of starch content, which is found mainly in the inner kernel, remain the same, but just about everything else is greatly reduced. In the United States, by law, thiamin, riboflavin, niacin, and iron must be added back into the grain products,

Potential Grain Allergies in the United States	
Wheat	Most Common
Barley Corn Oats Rye	Less Common
Amaranth Buckwheat Millet Quinoa Rice	Uncommon

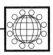

making the "enriched" breads, pastas, cereals, and so on. But other important nutrients are lost and not replaced. These include pyridoxine (B6), pantothenic acid, folic acid, vitamin E, and chromium, zinc, and manganese, plus other trace minerals—all of which are essential to human health. Refined white flour contains about 75% of the whole wheat kernels but fewer than half of their nutrients. Eating too much of refined grain products also increases consumption of the toxic mineral cadmium in relationship to zinc. Zinc is lost in the outer layers, and cadmium, when it is present, is contained in the internal kernel, so this can lead to cadmium toxicity problems (see the discussions of cadmium and zinc on pages 232 and 208, respectively, in chapter 6, Minerals).

Here are a few suggestions for using the grains and their by-products. First, when using whole grain flours, it is best to refrigerate them so they do not rancidify. This will greatly increase their longevity. Also, most people are not allergic to whole grains, so these more wholesome and nourishing foods may be a good source of fuel. Regarding the issue of whole grains and allergies, some allergists and other practitioners theorize that allergies to food may in part be generated by early and excessive intake of processed foods, sugars, refined flours, and pasteurized, homogenized milk. It is wise to eat more whole-grain products, if for no other reason than the increased fiber and nutrients. A taste for the richer and nuttier flavor of whole grains can be reacquired as well. For children, starting them early on whole-grain cereal and such foods as cream of wheat or rice, cooked brown rice or oats, can get them started with a healthy base.

Many natural foods stores carry all kinds of new, wholesome breakfast cereals in place of many of the high-sugar packaged cereals to which kids can easily become addicted. Some of the better big cereal company brands are the puffed grains, Cheerios, the various grains offered as Chex cereals, Kix, Grape Nuts, and many bran cereals. Avoiding sugary foods and refined foods in the early years will help children maintain their taste for natural foods.

In review, the grain foods represent the bulk of the world's food supply, with wheat, rice, and corn being the three top crops. Whole grains are rich in energy-generating starch and complex carbohydrates, fiber, B vitamins, vitamin E, and lots of min-

erals. Each kernel of grain needs to have all of its parts intact to stay alive, or to keep the potential of life, which it can maintain for many years, perhaps hundreds or even thousands. Once the outer shell is disrupted or the grain is refined, it will slowly decay. But if nourished with water, sun, and good soil, it will generate new life and provide much nourishment for our new life for generations.

Specific Grains

Amaranth	Corn	Quinoa	Wheat
Barley	Millet	Rice	
Buckwheat	Oats	Rye	

Amaranth (*Amaranthus caudatus, Amaranthus cruentus, Amaranthus hypochondriacus, Amaranthus tricolor*). Amaranth is a fairly new grain in North American food stores (often pearled or polished), but it is an ancient food native to Central America and used by such cultures as the Aztecs and the Mayan Indians. This high-protein, high-iron grain can be cooked whole as a breakfast cereal or served along with vegetables or other foods for lunch or dinner. It is suggested to rinse first the grain and then dry roast it before cooking. Ideally, it is best used as a flour for baking and can be found in breads, cookies, pastas, or tortillas. It is a substitute for wheat and other grains, although it is still a bit more expensive than the more common cereal grains. Besides iron and protein, amaranth is high in calcium, and it contains most of the B vitamins as well as other minerals. Like most grains, amaranth is a good source of dietary fiber. The phytonutrients present in amaranth include carotenoids, saponins, and ionol-derived glycosides.

Barley (*Hordeum vulgare*). This glutenous grain is much used as cattle feed. It is also used to make beer and whiskey. As eaten by humans, barley is most commonly employed in making soups. Its gluten content gives it a pastalike consistency, and barley is a good heat-generating food. In ancient times, barley bread was popular, especially in Egypt and the Far East. Barley grows well in cold climates, as do buckwheat and rye. Russia cultivates the most barley. Sprouted barley is high in the sugar maltose, which can be extracted, and the remaining malt syrup can be used to make beer and to sweeten other foods. Barley water has been employed for thousands of years for a variety of medicinal purposes.

Pearling is a refining process used to remove the barley's bran covering. The pearled barley is easier to cook but has less nutrient content than the whole barley. This whole grain contains about 10% to 15% protein, with the remainder being carbohydrate. Niacin and folic acid are the best represented of the B vitamins, while magnesium, calcium, iron, phosphorus, and potassium are barley's highest minerals. The phytonutrients present in barley include apigenin, beta-carotene, caffeic acid, calmodulin, catechin, coumarin, cyanidins, ferulic acid, flavone glycosides, gamma-carotene, gibberellins, hordeumin, leucocyanidin, lutein, neoxanthin, oxycinnamic acid, saponarin, and violaxanthin.

Buckwheat (Fagopyrum esculentum, Fagopyrum cymosum). Buckwheat is not really a grass but a thistle plant that produces fragrant flowers, followed by the buckwheat groats, little fruits each covered by their own fibrous shell. Buckwheat does not have the bran and germ that characterize grains, but its flavor, consistency, and nutrient content are so much like those of the grains that it is essentially treated like one. The use of the triangular buckwheat groats originated in China as early as 2600 BC and was not introduced to Europe and Russia until 1300 to 1400 AD. Kasha, a mashed and cooked buckwheat dish, became particularly popular at that time.

Buckwheat can be mixed with other grains, and buckwheat flour can be used to make pancakes and other baked goods. This grain variant is about 15% to 20% protein. It contains a good amount of fiber, an assortment of B vitamins, lots of potassium, and some iron, calcium, manganese, and phosphorus. The phytonutrients caffeic acid, campesterol, cyanidin, rutin, and quercetin are present in buckwheat.

Corn (Zea mays). Though a true grain, corn is different from the other grains in that its kernels are larger and softer, and they can be eaten fresh, like a vegetable. Dried corn can be ground into flour or used to grow the next generation of corn stalks. Corn is a real American grain, possibly the only grain that originated in the United States, and was used as a primary food by the Native Americans. Corn spread easily to Mexico and South America and has also been grown in Europe and, more recently, in the Eastern world. Corn production has increased greatly in the twentieth century and is now approaching that of wheat and rice. Formerly it was grown primarily in the southeastern and northwestern United States, but now its cultivation is fairly widespread. A current concern about corn is that there is a fairly high production in genetically modified corn, and we don't really know its effects on human consumption. If you wish to avoid GM corn, buy products that use organic corn. I also have a concern about the production and high use of high-fructose corn syrup due to its effects on obesity and diabetes.

Corn, or maize, has many uses. Eaten fresh, usually steamed or boiled, corn is a delicious summer and autumn treat. Popcorn is a popular and fairly healthy snack food, as it is low in calories. Its high fiber content helps intestinal activity. Cornmeal or corn flour can be made into cornbread or corn tortillas. Young corn is high in oil, and corn oil is commonly used in cooking, especially in baked goods, and in margarines. The mash left after the oil is pressed is made into a polenta that is much like cornmeal. Polenta can be mixed with beans to increase a meal's total protein content or with leafy greens to improve the vitamin and mineral content.

Corn itself is fairly rich in vitamin B_1. It is about 10% to 15% protein, although mostly carbohydrate. Fresh corn has some vitamin C, folic acid, and other B vitamins, lots of potassium and magnesium, as well as some iron, zinc, and selenium. Actually, much of the manufactured vitamin C in this country is extracted primarily from corn. Cornmeal and corn flour lose the vitamin C and some of the Bs, but the minerals are fairly well retained. Corn oil is usually rich in vitamin E. The niacin in corn is not easily available unless the cornmeal is specially prepared. The American Indians, who used corn as the staple in their diet, were able to prevent pellagra, the vitamin B3 deficiency disease, by pounding, soaking, and boiling the corn into a mineral ash (see the discussion on niacin on page 115 in chapter 5, Vitamins). This sweet yellow grain can provide a lot of nourishment, especially when combined properly with other foods. The phytonutrients present in corn include alpha-carotene, alpha-sitosterol, beta-carotene, caffeic acid, cryptoxanthin, cyanidins, gallic acid, gibberellins, neocryptoxanthin, quercetin, and zeaxanthin.

Millet *(Pennisetum glaucum [pearl or cattail millet], Setaria italica [foxtail millet], Panicum miliaceum [proso millet], Echinochloa frumentacea [barnyard or Japanese millet], Panicum ramosum [browntop millet]).* Previously used in the United States mainly as fodder and as birdfeed, millet has recently become a more commonly eaten grain, although its food use goes back many thousands of years in China. There are many different kinds of millet, and many of them have nutritional profiles, including protein qualities, that compare favorably to other grain foods like corn, wheat, and sorghum. Millet is a nonglutenous grain. It is the most alkaline of the grains and thus potentially the least congesting. It is tasty and a good nutrient grain, with nearly 15% protein, high amounts of fiber, good amounts of niacin, thiamin, and riboflavin, a little vitamin E, and particularly high amounts of iron, magnesium, and potassium. Millet is a warming grain, helping to heat the body in cold or rainy climates. It is a good winter grain and a healthy grain to use more regularly. The phytonutrients carotenoids, catechins, and tannins are present in millet.

Oats *(Avena sativa).* Oats have a growing role in feeding the world's population. Although oats have traditionally been placed right alongside of wheat as "gluten grains" that should be omitted from certain diets, recent research in this area provides good reason for thinking about oats as distinct from wheat and not part of a bigger category called "gluten grains." Its primary use has traditionally been as a breakfast cereal, as in oatmeal, or porridge, and more recently granola. Oats are a soft grain; when rolled and flattened, they cook fairly easily. The nutritional level of the oats is much less affected by this process than is the case with other types of grain refinement. The harder whole oats take longer to cook and are richer in flavor and chewier than rolled or steel-cut oats.

Oats have a great many uses. They have been commonly fed to cattle. **Oatmeal is among the healthier breakfast cereals; its high amount of complex carbohydrate provides sustained energy.** Rolled oats can also be toasted to make a fairly healthy granola. This cereal is often sweetened with honey, maple syrup, brown sugar, or malt syrup and may have raisins, seeds, or nuts added to it. It is a nourishing snack but definitely still a sweet treat and not a staple food. Oat flour can be used to make breads, oatmeal cookies, or biscuits. Oat bran is a good substitute for wheat bran, especially for those sensitive to wheat, and some preliminary research suggests that oat bran used regularly may help lower cholesterol levels. Recent cardiovascular research supports the use of oats and oat bran for heart health. In some ways, oats as an unrefined food are the most accepted whole grain in American society. Oatmeal is the most available whole grain in restaurants across the United States.

Oats are about 10% to 15% protein and provide a source of fiber as well as a mixture of B vitamins. They have a modest level of folic acid, niacin, pyridoxine, and pantothenic acid, as well as decent amounts of iron, magnesium, zinc, potassium, manganese, calcium, and copper. Fortified oat cereals have a higher vitamin A content than natural oats. However, they usually also contain more sodium, as do most processed foods. The phytonutrients present in oats include apigenins, avenin, carotenes, ferulic acid, limonene, luteolin, scopolin, hypoxanthin, vitexin, and isovitexin.

Quinoa *(Chenopodium quinoa).* Quinoa is another new grain on the American scene that, like amaranth, is native to Central America. I am a little reluctant to simply refer to quinoa as a "grain," however, because it is more closely related to beets and to green leafy vegetables like spinach and chard than it is to wheat, oats, barley, or rye. Perhaps we should call it a "vege-grain." It can be cooked in a main or side dish, or in soups and puddings, or used as a flour in baking. Rinse quinoa thoroughly before cooking because it has a saponin (soaplike) coating. Quinoa is a quick-cooking whole grain (20 minutes) and is high in protein, iron, and calcium, with a mix of the B vitamins and other minerals.

The amount of protein as well as the quality of protein in quinoa is worth mentioning. When it comes to the amino acid patterns in grains, lysine is usually the odd man out. Lysine deficiency is a problem when a culture relies too heavily on cereal grains for protein. With quinoa, this lysine deficiency problem is not the case, however, because this grain contains a fairly nice balance of all essential amino acids, including lysine. The phytonutrients present in quinoa include kaempferol, quercetin, and flavonol glycosides.

Rice *(Oryza sativa [common rice]; Zizania palustris [wild rice])*. Rice is the second-most-highly consumed grain in the world; more than 200 million tons are produced each year. Rice is a staple food throughout much of Asia; in China, the same word *(fan)* is used for rice and for food. In the United States, annual rice intake has increased from approximately 11 pounds per person in 1988 to 27 pounds per person in 2002. Some of this market growth involves increasing awareness on the part of consumers about the nature of Asian cuisine and prominent role of this grain. Macrobiotic diets and many natural food diets use whole (brown) rice and its products as a main part of the diet. **Also, concerns over wheat allergy and sensitivity have brought forth many new rice-based products as substitutes.**

The primary place of origin of rice is Southeast Asia, where an average of more than 200 pounds per person a year are eaten. China, India, Japan, and Vietnam are some of the major rice-consuming countries. Warmer climates with abundant water are ideal for rice growth. Larger crops are now being cultivated in California and the southern United States, and a number of varieties of rice are now commonly available. Sweet rice is more gelatinous than other varieties and is used mostly for desserts such as rice pudding. Long- and short-grain brown rice are also commonly available, with many varieties providing different flavors. Besides just being boiled to be eaten with vegetables, tofu, fish, and so on, rice can be popped and used as a breakfast cereal; cream of rice, another breakfast cereal, is made from ground rice.

Rice cakes have become popular and can be found in most stores. They can be a low-calorie, low-sodium, low-cholesterol, high-fiber snack and may be eaten plain, with butter, or with nut butters. **As is the case with all foods, however, quality counts, and it's still worth watching ingredient lists here for added sugar and salt.** Rice flour can be used in breads, cookies, and other baked goods; more of these products are available now for people who have moved away from wheat for various reasons. Several other rice products that are very good include mochi, a hard cake made from sweet rice that can be baked into crunchy and tasty rice balls; rice-based ice creams and crackers; and amazake, a rich and sweet rice drink or nectar that is a tasty and nourishing milk substitute

for diet-restricted people. The almond variety is delicious and high in calcium. Children may love these products.

However, especially in the Asian countries, most rice is refined or polished. Although removing just the outer bran layers would still leave most of the nutrients, further milling takes place. The rice is then bleached, cleaned, pearled (polished with talc), then often oiled and coated. This may make the rice more pleasing because it creates a smoother, less chewy texture, even perhaps more digestible, but it unfortunately removes a great deal of the nutrients. The oils are lost, the protein decreases, and most (80%) of the B_1 is removed, as well as other B vitamins (for example, 50% of the B_6 and B_2, as well as two-thirds of the B_3, and some of the minerals are removed).

Polished or refined rice is easier for most people to digest because of the increased starch level and loss of the outer hulls. Refined rice flour is also more stable because, as with wheat, the oils that can rancidify are lost. But what is the point if we lose the overall nutrition? In parts of Asia, off and on for at least 1,000 years, people following diets high in polished rice would sometimes get into trouble with the disease called beri-beri until it was learned in the late 1800s that this disease was the result of a thiamin deficiency from eating refined rice. (Interestingly, in some parts of Asia, cultures found a partial way around this problem. By parboiling rice before milling and polishing it, some of the thiamin was drawn in toward the center of the grain from the outside layer, so that removal of this outside layer did not remove all the thiamin. Groups that engaged in this parboiling practice escaped the problem of beri-beri.) In China, the white rice was considered a more prestigious food than the whole, "dirty" rice that the peasants commonly ate.

Rice is comparable to wheat in terms of its total protein content (about 5 to 6 grams per cup) and protein quality. (In both cases, the least plentiful amino acid in the protein matrix is lysine, which only shows up in the 150–200 mg per cup range.) However, as I'll discuss in detail in chapter 17, Medical Treatment Programs, when describing allergies, the proteins in wheat are the most likely of all grains to provoke an immune response, and the proteins in rice are the least likely. Brown rice is better in thiamin, biotin, niacin, pyri-

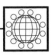

doxine, pantothenic, and folic acids than it is in riboflavin and vitamin B12. It has no vitamin A or C but some vitamin E. Rice, if grown in selenium-rich soil, is rich in selenium, a scarce but important trace mineral. Magnesium, manganese, potassium, zinc, and iron are all found in good amounts. Sodium is low, but phosphorus, copper, and calcium are all available in brown rice. White rice, even when enriched, is lower in all of these minerals; whole-grain rice is one of our more broad-based, nutrient-rich foods.

Wild rice is a special and more expensive type of rice (it is actually not rice but a different grain plant). It has nearly twice as much protein as regular rice as well as more niacin, riboflavin, iron, and phosphorus than brown rice, although it contains less of many other nutrients. The phytonutrients present in rice include campesterol, ceramides, cyanidins, ferulic acid, isoeugenol, lutein, oryzanol, oryzalexin, pelargonic acid, tricin, and violaxanthin.

Rye *(Secale cereale)*. Rye grows best in a cold climate and is much used in Russia, Scandinavia, and northern Europe. Rye is more resistant than wheat and will sustain itself in mountainous northern climates and sandy plains. Rye is often mixed with wheat to make what is called "rye" bread. Pure rye bread (not readily available) is a nourishing black bread with a rich flavor. Light ryes are usually made with a combination of refined rye and wheat flours. Dark rye breads are often made of wheat flour with some rye and dyes to darken the flour. Rye is also used to make whiskey and is not often used as an animal feed. The rye stalks are strong and occasionally used in basket weaving. Rye is also a gluten-containing grain and should be avoided in people with celiac, or gluten, sensitivity.

Rye is nearly 20% protein and a good fiber food, with a mixture of the B vitamins. Iron, magnesium, and potassium are found in the greatest levels, although phosphorus, calcium, and copper are also present. The phytonutrients are pectins, raffinose, beta-glucans, secasterol, typhasterol, hydroxycinnamic acid, ferulic acid, and coumaric acid.

Wheat *(Triticum aestivum, Triticum durum)*. The most important and oldest of the cereal grains, wheat feeds more people in the world than any other food and is now cultivated worldwide, with the exceptions of in the colder climates and tropical areas. Russia, the United States, and China are the top-three wheat-producing nations. Production more than doubled in the twentieth century, and close to 2 billion people worldwide use wheat regularly in their diets. There are two basic varieties of wheat—"hard" (durum) wheat and soft wheat. Hard wheat tends to have a little more protein and is often used to make macaroni and pasta. It also can be ground into flour to make bread, although the soft wheat is more commonly used for bread making.

Wheat is the ideal grain for bread, because of its starch content as well as its gluten content. Gluten is not actually a protein as is commonly thought. Rather, it is a mixture of nutrients that remain after the starches are washed away from a ball of dough made from wheat flour and water. This unique mixture is about 80% protein and 20% carbohydrates, fats, and minerals. Interestingly, this gluten fraction found in wheat is so unique that oats and rye—previously lumped together with wheat and referred to as "gluten grains" are now fairly widely used in diets even when wheat allergy is suspected or diagnosed.

Gluten gives wheat its tenacious elasticity so characteristic of good dough, and it is primarily the gluten that responds and expands with yeast treatment. Refined soft wheat flour is used by most people to make pastries, cookies, and cakes, although whole wheat flour can be used as well. **When buying flours, get them fresh and store them in the freezer or fridge if possible to prevent oxidation and rancidity or infestation with bugs.**

The nutrient content of wheat may vary somewhat depending on the soil availability. The protein content may also vary between 10% and 20% of the wheat kernel. Wheat protein is of good quality and easily usable, but it does not contain high or equal amounts of all the essential amino acids. It is low in lysine and isoleucine. There is a meatlike substitute that can be made from the gluten fraction in wheat. This wheat derivative, called *seitan*, is made by cooking gluten in a broth (usually consisting of shoyu, ginger, and kombu). Seitan has long been used in Asian cooking, although the name itself was coined fairly recently by George Ohsawa, one of the founders of macrobiotics, and the word itself means "simmered in shoyu." Wheat is also relatively high in the B vitamins (except B12). Vitamin E is present in whole wheat, as well as potassium, magnesium, iron, zinc, phosphorus, selenium, calcium, and copper. Vitamins C and A are not available, and wheat contains little sodium and no manganese.

Bulgur wheat is a special preparation of the wheat grain that is commonly used in Middle Eastern countries, although its use has spread throughout the world, especially to Europe and the United States. The wheat kernels are washed, scrubbed, cracked, and then dried. These smaller grains can then be cooked or even just soaked in water, where they swell in size. This grain is most commonly used in tabbouleh salad. Another variety of cracked wheat, smaller than the bulgur, is called couscous. It is used commonly in the Middle Eastern diet, where mutton and couscous is the traditional fare in those countries. Couscous is also good with lentils or chickpeas, and this versatile grain can be used in a main dish, as a salad, or even in desserts. It is easily prepared by pouring boiling water over this soft grain or by light cooking. The phytonutrients present in wheat include apigenin, campesterol, caffeic acid, carotenes, citrin, ferulic acid, gibberellins, lutein, pectin, and quercetin.

SEEDS

Seeds are the potential for new life that are grown as part of a plant and in some way reach the Earth to carry on their species. Long-lived plants, such as trees, may generate seeds of some kind at various intervals. The seeds discussed in this section, however, are from annual plants and are contained within a hard shell that protects this potential for the next generation of life. These seeds are slightly different from the grains, which have softer shells and a different structural makeup, although they are similar in many ways. Beans and peas are actually seeds as well. Most seeds can be stored in their whole form. In fact, some seeds discovered from centuries past are still able to germinate. Seeds were originally used in their ground form as seasonings or herbal flavorings for foods. Celery, cumin, mustard, cardamom, and coriander seeds, as well as many others, are still used in this way. But seeds are also very concentrated food. They are the initial source of the nutrition for the new plant.

The three main seeds discussed here—pumpkin, sesame, and sunflower—are high-protein foods, with more protein than the grains. Pumpkin seeds, for example, are more than 30% protein. High in vitamin E, these seeds are also a good source of fat, containing more than half by weight. Luckily, most of that (more than 80%) is polyunsaturated fats, the essential fatty acids, and oil-soluble vitamins A, D, and E. So seeds can be rather high in calories, which is good for those who are attempting to gain weight. There are some B vitamins in seeds, the levels of which vary depending on the seed. Seeds are rich in minerals, iron and zinc are plentiful. The amount of magnesium is good, especially in pumpkin seeds. Most seeds are a great source of copper. Calcium and potassium levels are also fairly good, yet there is very little sodium. Phosphorus levels are high, especially compared with calcium, thus an excess of seed intake can throw off this important balance. Iodine is usually present in most seeds as well.

Seeds can be eaten raw after shelling and bought fresh, either in shells or unshelled. They are a good protein addition to salads, can be cooked into grain or vegetable dishes, or can be blended to make a low-sodium protein sprinkle for food dishes. Unhulled seeds have a better shelf life than the hulled seeds, which should be kept refrigerated. Unhulled seeds can be stored in a cool, dry place. All seeds can be sprouted to make a highly nutritious seed-vegetable combination. Sunflower and alfalfa are common and can be used in salads or sandwiches.

Most commonly, seeds are used to make oils. Sunflower, safflower, and sesame oils can be used in cooking (sunflower is the most stable for storage and cooking) or to make margarines, but they are best used fresh on such foods as salads and cooked grains or vegetables. Usually, cold-processed oils (not heat-refined) give good nourishment, and using them uncooked is best, as discussed in chapter 4, Lipids— Fats and Oils.

Seeds

| Pumpkin | Sunflower | Sesame |

Pumpkin seeds (*Curcubita pepo, Curcubita maxima*). These are best known for their concentration of zinc and their use in the treatment and prevention of male prostate problems. Pumpkin seeds have also been used in the treatment of intestinal worms. They are a good source of protein and contain a good balance of the amino acids, although tryptophan, methionine, and cysteine are a little lower in concentration than the others. Their fat content, mostly unsaturated, is more than 50% of the seeds.

Pumpkin seeds are very high in iron as well as calcium and phosphorus, with some magnesium and copper; they also contain vitamin E and essential fatty acids. There is a mix of B vitamins, with niacin being the richest. Pumpkin seeds are usually eaten raw, roasted, or blended into a seed meal and used on other foods. Like most squash seeds, pumpkin seeds are found within the hard vegetable and can be toasted and eaten. The phytonutrients in these seeds are beta-carotene, curcubitin, and citrullin.

Sesame seeds (*Sesamum indicum*). These are probably the most commonly used seeds worldwide, especially in the Middle East, where the sesame foods tahini (sesame mash) and halvah (a sesame candy) originated. These foods and other sesame products are used today in many countries. In the United States, sesame seeds are often used in breads or on bread crusts; as tahini or sesame butter to spread on bread or crackers or used in sauces; as halvah candy; and as gomasio, a roasted, blended sesame salt that originated in Japan. Sesame seeds can be eaten raw, dried, or roasted or cooked with all kinds of foods. They are also great to add to other foods, such as grains and legumes, because they provide additional amino acids that may be low in those foods. Sesame seeds can also be used with many seasonings, with other nuts or seeds, such as almonds or sunflower seeds, or blended with such seasoning seeds as caraway, poppy, dill, or anise, and used over various food dishes. Black sesame seeds, also very nourishing, can be used in these seasonings as well. (Note: As do all seeds, sesame seeds need to be chewed well to help them be digested and assimilated; otherwise, many of these tiny seeds may pass through the intestinal tract unused.)

Sesame seeds come from little seed pods of one of the oldest of cultivated plants. In the Middle East, they are still called the "seed of immortality." The seeds are rich in oil, more than 55%. Sesame oil is a useful and common oil, especially in Asian cultures, where toasted and even hot-spiced sesame oil is used in cooking. Sesame seeds are about 20% protein and contain some vitamins A and E and most of the B vitamins (except B12 and folic acid). Minerals are abundant in sesame, as in most seeds. Zinc is high, as are calcium, copper, magnesium, phosphorus, and potassium. Sesame seeds are an excellent source of calcium for those avoiding cow's milk. The phosphorus content is much higher, however, as is true of most seeds, thus making it not quite as good for bone support. The iron content in these seeds is fairly high and the sodium is fairly low, unless, of course, they are salted. The phytonutrients in sesame seeds are beta-carotene, beta-sitosterol, sesamin, sesamol, sesamolin, and sesanol.

Sunflower seeds (*Helianthus annuus*). Sunflowers are native to South and North America. These tall, strong flowers that open bright yellow to the sun are filled tightly with hundreds of seeds to carry on life. Sunflower seeds have been used throughout history as a medicine as well as to enhance energy. The American Indians and other herbalists have used sunflower seeds as a diuretic, to avoid constipation, to alleviate chest pain, to soothe ulcers, to treat worms, and to improve eyesight. Baseball players chew on them in the dugout, likely for salt and energy; eating them one by one, it's difficult to feel very full, so the players can still run and play. Smokers who are quitting smoking also use sunflower seeds as a way to appease the hand-to-mouth energy to which they were accustomed.

Raw sunflower seeds are probably the best, higher in nutrition than roasted and definitely better than salted seeds. **For people with blood pressure problems, unsalted sunflower seeds are very high in potassium and low in sodium, a balance sorely needed by most of us these days with so many salty foods available.** One cup of sunflower seeds contains more than 1,300 mg of potassium and only 4 mg of sodium. This is helpful as a diuretic, or for people who already take diuretics, to help replace some potassium. The high amount of oil in sunflower seeds as polyunsaturated fats, essential linoleic acid, and vitamin E is also helpful in reducing cholesterol levels and improving or preventing cardiovascular disease.

However, sunflower seeds are caloric; ½ cup of hulled seeds is approximately 400 calories. Those wanting to lose weight should go easy on sunflower seeds; otherwise, they are a good food, considering all other aspects of nutrition. For those who need to gain weight or substitute more vegetable oils for saturated fats, sunflower seeds can be a great option. They are about 25% protein, have a good fiber content (the best of the seeds), and are richer in the B vitamins, particularly in thiamin, pyridoxine, niacin, and pantothenic acid. With their high potassium and low sodium, and with zinc, iron, and calcium all at good levels, sunflower seeds are a very mineral-rich food. The vitamin D that gets stored in these sun-filled seeds helps the utilization of calcium. Copper, manganese, and phosphorus levels are also relatively high; they are lower in magnesium than in calcium, which is different from other seeds.

Sunflower seed oil is often used in margarines or cooking oils. It is rich in polyunsaturates and linoleic acid and has a fairly low rancidity level compared with other oils. This may be because of its vitamin E content. **Cold-pressed sunflower oil is the best. It should be refrigerated once opened to avoid spoilage.** Cold storage of most nuts and seeds is generally suggested.

Sunflower seeds have many other uses besides as an oil or a nutritious snack food. They can be sprinkled on salads, are used in baking breads and cookies, and can be baked in vegetable casseroles to add protein, flavor, and crunch. A ground or blended sunflower-sesame sprinkle with a bit of salt or other seasonings can be a nutrient-rich, low-sodium seasoning. Almond-sunflower blend is also good, and a spicy high-mineral protein blend includes ground sunflower and sesame seeds (either white or black), nori seaweed flakes, and cayenne pepper. If sunflower seeds are soaked overnight, it makes them more digestible and alkaline forming. When added to green salads, they supply a tasty crunch, along with some protein and fatty acids. This is also true for nuts. A

great combination is soaked almonds, sunflower seeds, and peanuts. The phytonutrients present in sunflower seeds are beta-carotene, beta-sitosterol, campesterol, cinnamic acid, giberellins, gossypol, jasmonic acid, shikimic acid, and squalene.

NUTS

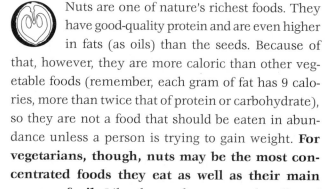 Nuts are one of nature's richest foods. They have good-quality protein and are even higher in fats (as oils) than the seeds. Because of that, however, they are more caloric than other vegetable foods (remember, each gram of fat has 9 calories, more than twice that of protein or carbohydrate), so they are not a food that should be eaten in abundance unless a person is trying to gain weight. **For vegetarians, though, nuts may be the most concentrated foods they eat as well as their main source of oil.** Like the seeds, nuts are bundles of potential—the part of the plant that feeds the future generations. Their calories, proteins, fatty acids, and many vitamins and minerals are what provide the energy for the early growth of the next nut tree.

There are more than 300 types of nuts. Besides those discussed in this section (almonds, Brazil nuts, cashews, chestnuts, coconuts, hazelnuts, peanuts, pecans, pistachios, and walnuts), hickory nuts, macadamias, and pine nuts are also common. Most nuts are the fruit or seed that follows the blossoming of the tree. They are usually contained in a hard shell to protect them from birds, insects, and germs and also to keep them fresh, because the concentrated oils contained in nuts can easily rancidify and spoil in the air. Because of the spoilage problem of these oil-rich nuts, picking or buying the fresh, raw, nuts in their shells is important. They will store longer. **Once the shells are removed, nuts should be kept in closed containers or plastic bags in the refrigerator or even the freezer to prevent rancidity.** If left out in containers or bags, they should be eaten within a month. Nuts will store longer in a cool, dry place in closed containers than if left in the air or in damp areas.

Roasted, salted nuts are best avoided. Most of us do not need the extra salt, and roasting affects the oils and decreases the B vitamin and mineral content. Be aware of places that feed you free salted nuts, such

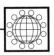

as bars or airplanes, to increase your thirst—and your drink tab! Sadly, most nuts in American society are eaten after they are roasted in even more oil and salted, often with other additives or sugars. Eating raw nuts (especially almonds, walnuts, and hazelnuts) is better for us. Peanuts, particularly in peanut butter, are not easy to digest, and there is concern about potentially toxic molds containing aflatoxin, a potential carcinogen that grows on this leguminous nut/bean.

Many people have trouble digesting nuts because of their high fat content, which is even worse after roasting in oil. This is true especially in people with low stomach acid or gallbladder problems. Overweight individuals with gallstone or gallbladder disease often have difficulty digesting fatty foods in general. To process the nuts in the body, we usually need a good level of hydrochloric acid, fat-digesting enzymes (lipases), and bile secreted by the gallbladder and liver.

Besides raw, fresh nuts and the roasted varieties, nuts can be cooked into such foods as grains and vegetable dishes. This will often add the other needed essential amino acids to a meal to make more complete proteins. A nut-seed blended mix such as almond-sunflower-sesame with a little added sea salt can be kept in a jar in the refrigerator and used as a protein seasoning. Nuts can be blended into a flour, as well as used in baking with other flours. The use of nut butters as snack foods is growing. Peanut butter is, of course, the most common, but many other butters (almond, cashew, and even pistachio and macadamia) are also commercially available, as many people move away from peanut butter. Nut milks are also becoming popular as nourishing milk substitutes and as wholesome drinks, especially for children. Nuts and even a little bit of the nut butters are a much healthier snack than sugary foods, particularly regarding the sustained level of energy that comes from their metabolism.

In terms of nutrient content, nuts are among the best of the vegetable foods. Their fat content is fairly high, of course, but it is mostly unsaturated fats, which are better than the saturated. The inner white meat of the dried coconut, however, is rich in saturated fats and thus more of a concern regarding cardiovascular problems. The essential fatty acids and vitamin E are also part of the nut oils. Almonds, Brazil nuts, hazelnuts, and peanuts are the best in vitamin E content.

Total fat content varies—from peanuts at 50% to pecans (and macadamias), the richest, at 95% fat.

The protein content of nuts is very good, with a fairly balanced amino acid distribution, which may be why the edible part of nuts is termed the "meat." Nuts are the meat of the plant world. But they are somewhat lower in tryptophan and methionine, so the amino acids are more balanced when nuts are combined with a grain food at meals. Most nuts have a general cross section of the B vitamins, but they are not high in any particular one (although peanuts are pretty rich in niacin). They are, however, well endowed with the minerals, particularly calcium, iron, magnesium, potassium, zinc, and other trace minerals. Nuts are low in sodium when unsalted, and some nuts (such as almonds, Brazil nuts, and pecans) even have some selenium.

In general, nuts can be used as a protein- and energy-rich snack food as a midmorning or midafternoon treat. Eaten alone in their raw state, and not much more than a handful, they should be fairly easily digested and assimilated by our bodies.

Nuts

Almonds	Hazelnuts
Brazil nuts	Peanuts
Cashews	Pecans
Chestnuts	Pistachios
Coconuts	Walnuts

Almonds (*Prunus dulcis*). The almond nuts are the fruits of a tree that grows nearly 30 feet tall and is abundant in many areas of the world, including Asia, the Mediterranean, and North America. The soft-shell varieties possess a sweeter nut than those in hard shells, which may be slightly bitter. The presence of 2% to 4% of amygdalin, commonly known as laetrile, has caused almonds to be considered as a cancer-preventing nut. Most of the fats of the almond are polyunsaturated and high in linoleic acid, the body's main essential fatty acid. Almond oil is a stable oil used in pharmaceutical preparations, to hold scents in fragrant oils, or for massage therapy. Almonds are high in vitamin E and contain some B vitamins. Calcium is also found in high amounts, and almonds or home-made almond milk (see recipe on page 538 in chapter 14, Seasonal Menu Plans and Recipes) can be used as a tasty calcium source. Copper, iron, phosphorus, potassium, and zinc are also present in good amounts, as are magnesium and manganese. Sodium content is very low, and some selenium is present. The phytonutrients present in almonds are beta-glucosides, isorhamnetin glucosides, kaempferol, catechin, protocatechuic acid, naringinen, and glucopyraniosides.

Brazil nuts *(Bertholletia excelsa)*. These are the very meaty and high-fat hard-shelled "seeds" of which about 10 to 20 are found in each big fruit of the very large Brazil nut trees (nearly 100 feet high). Brazil nuts are a good-quality protein, yet are also about two-thirds fat, of which more than 20% is saturated. The oil from this nut turns rancid easily and is not used commercially. Brazil nuts are known to be rich in calcium as well as magnesium, manganese, copper, phosphorus, potassium, and selenium. Zinc and iron are also found in good proportions in this high-mineral nut. The phytonutrients included therein are beta-carotene and gadoleic acid.

Cashews *(Anacardium occidentale)*. Cashews are thought by some to be a toxic nut, probably because of the caustic oils found in the hard shell. Lightly roasting cashews may help to clear these oils. These sweet nuts are the real fruit of their 25- to 30-foot trees that grow best in tropical climates. These trees also provide another "fruit," the edible "cashew apple" that grows prior to the nut. Cashews are fairly rich in magnesium, potassium, iron, and zinc. The calcium and manganese content is lower in cashews than in other nuts; cashews also have a lower fat and higher carbohydrate level than most other nuts. Some B vitamins are present, as is vitamin A. Very little vitamin E is found in cashews, however. The phytonutrients present in this nut are alpha-catechin, beta-carotene, beta-sitosterol, cardanol, gallic acid, epicatechin, leucocyanidin, leucopelargonidine, limonene, and naringinen.

Chestnuts *(Castanea alnifolia, Castanea pumila, Castanea floridana, Castanea ozarkensis, Castanea sativa, Castanea dentata, Castanea mollissima)*. These are the classic nut of the winter holidays throughout the world. Hot, roasted chestnuts can be a warming and nourishing snack. Chestnuts are high in starch (carbohydrate) and low in protein and fats and there-fore lower in calories (less than half) than other nuts. Chestnuts have lower levels of most minerals compared with other nuts, but they contain good levels of manganese, potassium, magnesium, and iron. The phytonutrients present in chestnuts are caffeic acid, castalagin, castalin, ellagic acid, gallic acid, kaempferol, and vescalin.

Coconuts *(Cocus nucifera)*. The big nuts (fruits) of the common tropical palm tree, this large fruit has a thick husk covering, a hard shell that surrounds the rich coconut meat. Coconut milk, a nourishing liquid, comes from the soft meat of the fresh green coconut. When the coconut dries or ripens, this meat becomes hard and much of the oils becomes saturated. The dried meat contains about 65% oil, mainly as saturated fat, which is solid or semisolid at room temperature. This oil, however, also has some nourishment and essential fatty acids and has been used in cooking and baking as well as in soaps, shampoos, and cosmetics.

Coconuts are used in cooking much more in the South Pacific and Southeast Asian cultures than in the United States, probably because they have fewer foods with good fat content. The fresh milk can be used as a marinade for fish, as salad dressing, or made into a yogurtlike dish. Coconut has a little protein, about 10%; some carbohydrate and fiber; and traces of the B vitamins, vitamin C, and vitamin E. It has some amounts of many minerals, with potassium, magnesium, manganese, copper, and iron being the best. The phytonutrients galactomannan, pectin, shikimic acid, squalene, and vanillin are present in coconuts.

Hazelnuts *(Corylus avellana)*. These are the fruits or seeds of a small shrub or tree that usually grows between 6 and 12 feet tall. They are also called "filberts" because they ripen about the time of St. Philibert's Day, August 20. The numerous varieties produce either round or elongated nuts. They are usually eaten raw or fried and are often used in confection making or as flavorings in sweet sauces. Hazelnuts have one of the higher vitamin E levels of the nuts. Their protein content is about 15%, and they are nearly 65% fat, mostly unsaturated, being high in essential linoleic acid. Hazelnuts have a fairly good level of the B vitamins and are rich in most minerals (calcium, magnesium, manganese, iron, copper, and potassium) as well as some trace minerals (zinc and selenium). The phytonutrients present in this nut are

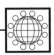

avenasterol, beta-carotene, campesterol, myricitrin, and stigmasterol.

Peanuts *(Arachis hypogaea).* The most peculiar of the nuts, and the most common in U.S. culture, peanuts are not in fact a true nut but a legume or pea (thus "peanuts"). This legume grows on a small bush that yields small, soft, fibrous shells, each containing usually two or three "nuts." Peanuts grow commonly in the southern United States but are now grown largely in China and India, where their oil is used widely in cooking. In poorer, more populated countries, such as Africa, China, and India, peanuts are used in the daily diet in many vegetarian dishes, to which they add more-complete proteins.

Peanuts probably have as good an amino acid balance as any vegetable food. They are about 20% protein and rich in nutrients. Their fat content is about 75% of the nut, three-fourths of that being unsaturated. The B vitamin content of peanuts is better than that of most nuts, probably because they are a legume. Niacin and biotin are best, but all B vitamins except B12 are represented. Potassium, magnesium, and phosphorus are highest of the minerals, while calcium, iron, zinc, copper, and manganese are also found in substantial amounts.

Stored peanuts may easily become moldy, a particular concern for those sensitive to molds. Peanuts have been known to become contaminated with molds containing aflatoxin, a substance that is thought to be carcinogenic. Also of concern is that much of the peanut butter consumed in the United States is the processed variety, with not only the high fat and oil content of peanuts but additional hydrogenated fats, which are more toxic in the body. (See the discussion of hydrogenated oils on page 67 in chapter 4, Lipids—Fats and Oils, as well as in the next section in this chapter, "Oils.") More additives—salt, sugar, dextrose, and others—make this manufactured peanut butter a poor-quality food. Many companies now use only ground peanuts to make their butters; better yet, some stores have nut grinders where customers can make their own peanut butter right on the spot. It is best to refrigerate shelled peanuts and peanut butter to avoid rancidity.

Many people eat roasted and salted peanuts more than the fresh variety. Although a mild roasting of the peanut may make it a little easier to digest and not lower the nutrient value too much, the extra salt is not really needed. Some people do not do well with peanuts at all. Digestive problems, gallbladder irritation, or just plain allergy to these nuts are possible. Despite this, however, they are still the most popular American nut and a good-quality food. The phytonutrients present in peanuts are arachin, beta-carotene, beta-sitosterol, caffeic acid, conarachin, daucosterin, ferulic acid, isoquercitin, luteolin, rutin, sarkosin, and stigmasterol.

Pecans *(Carya illinoensis).* Pecans are nuts for a special treat, such as for holidays or in the traditional pecan pie, usually sweetened with maple syrup. Pecans (and macadamias) contain the lowest protein (5% to 10%) and the highest fat (80% to 95%) of all the nuts. They grow on large trees often taller than 100 feet; the nuts are about four to a pecan fruit, each nut protected by a hard, woodlike shell. In fact, pecan shells can be ground and used as wood sculpture material (I have a pecan shell lion in my personal collection). Pecans contain some vitamins A, E, and C, niacin, and other B vitamins. They are low in sodium and high in most other minerals, including zinc, iron, potassium, selenium, and magnesium. Copper, calcium, and manganese are present in fairly good amounts as well. The phytonutrients in pecans are azaleatin, beta-carotene, caryatin, catechin, and quercetin derivatives.

Pistachios *(Pistacia vera).* Pistachios are those sweet and flavorful nuts of which it is hard to eat just 1. The pistachio nut or fruit grows on a small tree usually about 10 to 15 feet high and is popular in the Mediterranean and Middle Eastern countries. It is most commonly eaten in the shell but is also used in cooking, in making sauces, in baking cakes (as flavoring), and in ice creams. It is best to avoid the less healthy salted and red-dyed pistachio nut, however; go with the natural variety.

Pistachios are about 15% to 20% protein and about 50% to 70% fat. They have good levels of thiamin, niacin, folic acid, and a little vitamin A. The potassium and iron levels are also high; the sodium content is low; phosphorus, magnesium, and calcium are all present in fair amounts; while zinc, copper, and manganese are at modest levels. The phytonutrients are beta-carotene, beta-sitosterol, cyanidin, pectin, and stigmasterol.

Walnuts *(Juglans nigra [black walnut], Juglans regia [English walnut]).* Another of the great nuts, walnuts are real brain food; in fact, when shelled the walnut looks remarkably like the human cerebral cortex. The fatty acids and the 10% to 15% protein level nourish the nervous system. The walnut is about 80% to 90% fat. They can be eaten raw or used in baking, and the pressed walnut oil can be used in cooking or even for oiling wood. It should be used fresh, though, as it is not resistant to spoilage.

Walnuts have a modest mix of vitamin A, the Bs (including biotin), C, and E. Their mix of minerals is similar to that of most of the other nuts, with many at good levels. Probably iron and potassium are the best in this balanced nut, which grows on large trees as high as 40 to 50 feet in many parts of the world, including the United States. The phytonutrients present are beta-carotene, ellagic acid, juglone, myricetin, sakuranin, and tannin.

OILS

The edible oils are all liquid fats extracted from vegetable sources, with the exceptions of coconut, palm, and palm kernel oils. They are virtually 100% lipid, or fat, and most are high in unsaturated fat and low in the saturated component (10% to 20%). Commonly used oils include almond, avocado, corn, olive, peanut, safflower, sesame, soybean, and sunflower. Olive oil, a monounsaturated oil, is the main vegetable oil, along with canola (rapeseed) oil, that should be used for cooking; most of the other oils contain more polyunsaturated fats and should not be heated. (Some companies do manufacture specially conditioned and refined oils, however, that can be of high quality and appropriately used for cooking). *Polyunsaturated* means that the oils have more than 1 unsaturated bond available in their carbon chain to which hydrogen atoms can be attached. These oils should be used on salads and other dishes in their cold-pressed form or consumed with extra vitamin E to prevent oxidation. The polyunsaturated fats can help to reduce blood cholesterol rather than raise it, and more important, they can improve our ratios of LDL to HDL cholesterol to help reduce cardiovascular disease risk. These vegetable oils do not contain cholesterol because they are derived from plants.

All of the vegetable oils are liquid at room temperature except coconut oil, one of the few saturated vegetable oils. When the unsaturated vegetable oils are hydrogenated through a special industrial process, they become partially saturated, as in the solid vegetable margarines. These are usually fortified with vitamin A and have other additives, and they tend to function differently in the body. They may increase blood cholesterol and thus the risk of cardiovascular problems; they have been associated with increased cancer risk as well. The animal fats—lard, butter, and chicken fat—have a much higher percentage of saturated fats and more cholesterol, and these fats are implicated as well in these chronic, serious cardiovascular diseases and cancer. Of particular concern is the presence of more trans fats in hydrogenated oils. These trans fats are created by the hydrogenation process itself and have been shown to increase the risk of several chronic diseases, including the cardiovascular diseases and cancer, as already mentioned.

All of the vegetable oils contain 9 calories per gram of pure fat; 1 tablespoon of vegetable oil contains about 120 calories, so it should be used sparingly by people concerned about weight. These oils are rich in essential fatty acids, particularly linoleic acid, which is also present in the foods from which these oils are extracted. Linoleic and linolenic acids are needed for the growth and maintenance of cells, tissues, and the entire body. Other than vitamin E, these vegetable oils contain negligible amounts, if any, of other nutrients such as the B vitamins and minerals. Some of the oils richer in vitamin E are soybean, safflower, cottonseed, corn, and wheat germ.

Oils can be used in salad dressings, in sauces, in baking, and in cooking. **Heating the polyunsaturated oils is not recommended, as heat may affect their chemical structure making them less usable and more difficult for the body to process (these oils are also possibly carcinogenic).** Overall, it is ideal not to fry foods but to add the uncooked oils after cooking the food. In general, the saturated fats are more stable when used in cooking but are not the healthiest for us. I recommend either canola or olive oil, which are primarily monounsaturated and more stable vegetable oils, or butter when cooking or sautéing foods.

Although usually slightly more expensive, I recommend the cold-pressed oils for two reasons. First,

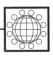

they are subjected to less heat than the solvent-extracted oils, and lower heat means less breakdown of nutrients. Second, they are processed without the use of solvents, eliminating the potentially toxic residues of these solvents in food. Cold-pressed oils can be refined and conditioned or unrefined and unconditioned. I think there is a place for both types when cooking. Unrefined, unconditioned oils are great for salads and low-heat items like soups, sauces, or very lightly sautéed foods. Conditioned oils are best for medium heat dishes like oven-baked or normally sautéed foods. Refined oils are a good choice with high heat dishes like stir-fries.

In chapter 4, Lipids—Fats and Oils, on page 67, I talked about omega-3 and omega-6 types of fat and how imbalanced the ratio of omega-3 to omega-6 is in the modern diet. We need more omega-3s! One of the ways we can get them is through careful selection of cooking oils. We can use cold-pressed, unrefined, and unconditioned walnut oil or pumpkin seed oil, for example, on our salads or in a gently heated soups. By doing so, we would increase our omega-3 intake while enjoying the delicate flavors of these unique oils. Overall, the vegetable oils should contribute a higher percentage of the total fat in our diet than they currently do, as this would increase the proportion of polyunsaturated to saturated fats, which is helpful. But total blood cholesterol is influenced most by total fat intake, so for best health we should reduce our total fat intake. (The topic of fats in the diet is discussed in detail in chapter 4, Lipids—Fats and Oils.)

DAIRY PRODUCTS

With this food category, I enter the animal kingdom. This section explores the foods made from and by animals and their products, such as milk, butter, cheese, and yogurt. These are, in general, denser and higher-protein foods, more concentrated bodybuilding foods, and also higher-fat foods. They are most important in growth years and during pregnancy and lactation, but because of their prevalence in our early years, many people (especially in Western cultures) continue to consume an excess of these protein and fatty foods. This may then contribute to the congestive problems and degenera-

tive diseases that occur in later years. **I believe that these animal-product foods should be consumed moderately in the diet, probably not more than 10% to 20% of total intake. They can even be totally avoided with proper nutritional care to create a balanced strict vegetarian (vegan) diet.**

Milk Products

Milk	Cheeses
Butter	Processed cheeses
Yogurt	Cream cheese
Kefir	Cottage cheese
Buttermilk	Ice cream

Milk. This is a special food—the primary baby food, the first food of most mammals. It is considered the basic food of life, the connection between mother and child. Milk is often associated in early years with survival, with our love from and for Mother, so it is no wonder that many develop a lifelong addiction to this sweet essence of life. Theoretically, the relationship to sweet food, of which milk is our first, may be the basis of so many people's acceptance and use of sugar and sweet foods throughout life. An excess of sweets in the diet creates all kinds of problems, from tooth decay to obesity to diabetes. (See more about sugar on page 30 in chapter 2, Carbohydrates.)

Lactose, a simple sugar, should be easy to digest and use in the body for energy, but some lactose-intolerant children may be unable to utilize this sugar. Even more adults are sensitive to milk sugar; this is a separate issue from milk allergy, and a major one. **Nearly half of the world population is lactose intolerant, which may cause bloating, abdominal pain, and diarrhea after milk is consumed.** Luckily, though, most children can handle at least mother's milk and do all right on milk products, at least in their early years. One of the reasons most infants do fine on their mother's milk is quite fascinating. Although human milk, like cow's milk, contains the simple sugar lactose, it also contains the lactase enzyme that is required for digesting lactose. So the nursing infant gets the potentially problematic sugar but also the enzyme needed to digest it.

When other milks, such as cow's or goat's milk, are substituted for mother's milk in infancy, however, milk allergy is very common. These milks are richer in proteins and have new protein molecules for the baby's system to handle. Lactalbumin and milk casein are among the proteins to which people, especially children, may react. **Milk is the most common food allergen.** Milk allergies may manifest as skin rashes, eczema, chronic otitis media (fluid and infections in the ears), hyperactivity, and other problems. Taking a child off milk products for a 3- to 4-week trial period and seeing how he or she does and then retesting with a meal of milk products is probably the best way to evaluate whether milk is a problem. If there are mild allergies, it is still possible to bring milk products back into the diet later after eliminating them for 1 or 2 months, which reduces the allergic capacity, possibly to a degree that they can be tolerated in moderation. Then a rotating diet whereby these products are consumed only every four days will often be better tolerated. Sometimes substituting goat's milk or, even better, soymilk or nut milks, will make a difference. (See more about this in the allergy program discussion on page 704 in chapter 16, Performance Enhancement Programs.)

In the rest of this section, when discussing milk, I am referring to cow's milk, which is by far the most commonly consumed. Cow's milk and products made from this food are a controversial dietary component, especially for adults. This controversy centers around three issues. The first is lactose intolerance, as discussed above. As many as 50 million U.S. adults (and many more millions throughout the world) may have problems digesting lactose, the primary sugar in cow's milk. Another 10 million may experience allergic reactions to casein and lactalbumin, the primary proteins found in milk products and a second reason for the cow's milk controversy. Dairy foods also seem to be congesting for many consumers. The third primary issue involves treatment of dairy cattle from a physical-health as well as humanitarian standpoint. Feedlot-raised dairy cattle often need prescription medicines to prevent infection and artificial stimulants to increase rate of milk production. They are also often raised under conditions that are unnatural at best. John Robbins, in his powerful book, *Diet for a New America*, discusses this at length, as well as the treatment of chickens and other farm ani-

mals. I have taken the stance throughout my career that our adult population especially would be healthier without the use of dairy products. I know, as an avid milk drinker and cheese eater for my first quarter century of life, my health changed dramatically for the better when I gave up dairy products nearly 30 years ago.

On the more positive side, milk is a very good protein food and an important source of calcium. One glass of milk contains about 300 to 350 mg of calcium, a level hard to find in many other foods. And this calcium is also in balance with phosphorus, so milk may be good for bone health; I say "may be" because the research is confusing on the bioavailability of milk calcium and absorbing it into the body and the bones. It has a better balance than vegetable foods in all the essential amino acids. Milk is considered a complete protein food from which we can build bodily tissue proteins. Milk also contains many of the B vitamins, including B6 and B12; has vitamins A, D, and E; and contains most of the minerals (mainly calcium and phosphorus, along with potassium and some sodium). It has traces of zinc, iron, selenium, manganese, and copper as well as a little vitamin C, but certainly not enough to meet the daily needs for any of these essential nutrients.

Many cheeses made from milk are also concentrated in calcium. Some extra calcium is helpful for elderly individuals or people with high blood pressure, as it helps to relax the vascular tone and some-

Fat and Calorie Content of Milk (one glass = 8 oz)			
	Whole milk	2% milk	Skim milk
Calories	150.0	120.0	86.0
Protein (g)	8.0	8.1	8.4
Carbohydrates (g)	11.4	11.7	11.9
Fiber (g)	0.0	0.0	0.0
Total fat (g)	8.2	4.7	0.4
Saturated fat (g)	5.1	2.9	0.3
Unsaturated fat (g)	3.0	1.5	0.1
Cholesterol (mg)	33.2	18.0	4.0

Source: Food Processor for Windows, Version 7.60, Database Version December 2000, ESHA Research, Salem, Oregon.

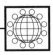

times reduces muscle tension. However, recent research has shown that the actual calcium utilization is not that good from milk or meat, or when consuming a high-protein diet. **More important, though, the higher fat levels of milk may increase cholesterol and blood triglyceride levels, which increases the atherosclerosis risk and may create more long-range problems with hypertension and other cardiovascular diseases.** Thus drinking milk or eating a lot of milk products is not generally recommended in the adult population.

A big concern with milk is its fat content. The regular drinking of whole milk and intake of dairy products leads to excess fat intake and all of its potential problems. Whole milk is described as 3.5% fat, but about half of the 150 calories in an 8-ounce glass are from the 8 to 9 grams of fat (at 9 calories per gram). Skim milk has most of the fat removed and has about half of the calories of whole milk; low-fat, or 2%, milk is in between, with about 50 of the 120 calories coming from fat (two-thirds saturated). Yet whole, low-fat, and skim milks are similar in their vitamin and mineral makeup, as well as their protein and carbohydrate levels. The only difference is the amount of fat.

Another concern is that these milks are processed products. This natural white substance that comes from cows is heated, treated, and diluted to make even the "normal" homogenized, pasteurized milk. It loses some vitamin E, biotin, B_{12}, and other vitamins with pasteurization; often vitamin A and irradiated vitamin D are then added to fortify this food, which some erroneously consider a drink. Homogenization is possibly the biggest concern in milk. It basically involves the conversion of the milk fat into small globules through the use of high pressure so that it does not separate as it normally will do when it sits. It is possible that this process interferes with the body's ability to digest and utilize this fat in homogenized milk. **The increase in cardiovascular disease has been correlated with the rise in the use of homogenized milk;** however, this relationship remains unproven and further epidemiological study is needed.

In general, I do not recommend the drinking of milk for adults. A warm glass before bed can be helpful for sleep, likely because of the tryptophan content. Generally, though, an adult's calcium and protein needs can be met with many other foods. Chamomile flower or valerian root tea may be helpful for sleep in nonmilk drinkers. For adults who seem to tolerate milk products well, are not overweight, and do not have high blood pressure, high blood fats, or a family history of heart disease, I would suggest moderate use of milk products, but not daily because of the possibility of developing milk sensitivities. I think that yogurt and kefir, the cultured milk products that get predigested by friendly bacteria, are probably the best choices in the dairy family. Low-fat milk products and a low-fat diet in general are wise guidelines to follow.

Butter. Butter, made from whole milk through a churning process, is mainly the milk fat. It is a high-fat (two-thirds saturated fats) and high-cholesterol food that is also high in vitamin A and added vitamin D. There is at least 1 advantage to butter's high-fat content: its relatively high concentration of the short-chain saturated fat butyric acid. This type of fat is the fuel of choice for most of the cells in the large intestine and it helps keep the digestive system on track. Butter always reminds me to point out that all saturated fats are not equal. We can apparently handle larger doses of the shorter ones (like butyric acid) much more readily than the longer ones (like palmitic acid). Butter has minimal amounts of some other vitamins and minerals, usually is salted so that it is high in sodium, and is fairly high in calories (100 per tablespoon). Because of its sweet flavor and the fact that it is saturated and so does not break down as easily as the unsaturated fats, it is used commonly in cooking and baking and slathered on potatoes, noodles, vegetables, and other hot foods or poured over popcorn. **A little butter is okay, but it is easy to overuse it.** If you use butter, I suggest investing in organic, since butter is all fat and the most concerning chemicals, like pesticides and herbicides, stay in the fats of foods.

Yogurt. Yogurt is considered the health food of the milk family. One of the foods thought to promote longevity, it is commonly consumed by those who tend to live a long time. Many embrace yogurt as an aid to digestion. Acidophilus yogurt tends to help reimplant normal colon bacteria, which can then act more effectively in the complete digestion and utilization of high-fiber foods. The body's friendly bacteria also aid in the production of many of the needed B vitamins.

Yogurt is the end product of the fermentation process of either whole milk or low-fat or nonfat milk acted upon by bacteria and yeasts. The friendly human intestinal bacteria *Lactobacillus acidophilus* and the one originally used to make yogurt, *Lactobacillus bulgaricus,* are the common ones used to make yogurt, which resembles a milk custard. Yogurt is a form of soured milk that becomes reduced in fat and calories, usually with an increase in the B vitamin levels. Many of the minerals become more concentrated as well. The calcium content of yogurt is good. Like the other cultured or soured milk products, yogurt is more stable and resistant to spoilage than fresh milk, and this can be helpful in many instances.

Yogurt can be eaten alone as a snack or dessert, mixed with cereal, or made into sauces or dips. Lower-fat yogurts are becoming more popular as people watch their fat intake. Frozen yogurt has also increased in use as a slight improvement in fat content over ice cream. Fruited and sugared yogurt is commonly available, but I do not recommend them. Often people who have a lactase deficiency do all right when eating yogurt because much of the lactose has already been acted on by the bacterial process and turned into lactic acid.

It is interesting that, on the one hand, we are trying to get rid of bacteria in milk products through pasteurization, and on the other, we are trying to obtain more bacteria in yogurt and kefir. What we want to do is to keep the friendly colon bacteria *L. acidophilus, Bifidobacterium bifidum* and *Streptococcus faecium. Faecium* working for our benefit, not to obtain pathogenic organisms that can make us sick. **People often eat yogurt (or take healthy bacteria supplements) after antibiotic therapy, which kills off some of their normal bacteria in the intestine or in a woman's vaginal tract**. This may lead to an overgrowth of yeast organisms, such as *Candida albicans,* which may then need treatment to clear. (See the discussion in the section "Yeast Syndrome" on page 698 of chapter 17, Medical Treatment Programs.) Yogurt or acidophilus culture douches or cultures of bacteria taken orally seem to be helpful clinically to prevent these problems, although further research is needed to clarify what is really happening with this interplay of organisms. In some areas of Europe, acidophilus and vitamin B12 are prescribed together with antibiotics.

Kefir. Another soured and fermented milk product, kefir is more of a drink than yogurt. It has simi-

lar properties, although most kefir available is flavored and sweetened with fruit. It is a good nutritious substitute for milk, especially for children.

Buttermilk. Basically soured milk, buttermilk provides good nourishment with a reduced fat content while remaining high in calcium and protein, although its vitamin A content is lower (unless added) than that of whole milk. Buttermilk may be helpful for digestion, as are the other soured products, for those who tolerate its fairly strong taste.

Cheeses. Cheeses have been made for centuries worldwide, directly from milk, by separating the curd, or milk solids, from the whey and then aging the curd. Cheese is a concentrated food; it takes about 1 gallon of milk to make 1 pound of cheese. In general, cheese is a high-protein, high-calcium food with good levels of vitamin A and an assortment of various vitamins and minerals.

Cheese has some of the problems of milk products in general, however. It is high in fats, mainly saturated fats, and high in cholesterol, and too much of it can cause the many problems that come from high-fat diets. Cheese is even more commonly abused in the adult population than milk. The sodium content is also usually higher in cheeses than in milk. There are some lower-fat cheeses available, such as mozzarella, farmer cheese, and cheeses made from skim milk. Recently, goat's milk cheese and fetas made from sheep or goat's milk have become available, which can be particularly helpful for those avoiding cow's milk products.

Most cultures around the world have their own cheeses, for which they may be famous. The French have Brie, blue cheese, and Camembert; the Swiss have Swiss; Italians are known for mozzarella, Parmigiano, and ricotta; Greeks for feta; and Americans for cheddars, Monterey Jacks, and Colbys. The classic "American" sliced cheese is a junk food and not part of the real cheese culture. It is often high in sodium and unnecessary additives. Cheeses are used in a great variety of food dishes, such as sauces, quiche, and omelets.

Processed cheeses. Processed cheeses and cheese spreads are often higher than natural cheeses in fat and sodium, neither of which is needed by most people. They are often fortified with vitamin A, but most of the B vitamins and minerals other than cal-

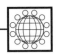
cium and phosphorus are fairly low. Sodium levels are about 400 to 500 mg per ounce. It is a good idea to avoid these cheeses.

Cream cheese. This mildly processed cheese is higher in fat and lower in protein and calcium than other cheeses. Other than vitamin A, its nutrient content is fairly scarce. However, children like it, it is better nutritionally speaking than other cheese spreads, and many people feel they cannot live without their Sunday cream cheese and bagels. But, overall, cream cheese should be used sparingly, if at all.

Cottage cheese. Made from soured milk, cottage cheese is mainly the curd extracted from the whey. This curd is high in protein, and cottage cheese is somewhat lower in calories and fats than other cheeses. The low-fat cottage cheese is even better. Although the sodium content of most cottage cheeses is pretty high and the calcium content low, overall, cottage cheese is fairly good to use as the main part of an occasional meal.

Ice cream. Ice cream is both the greatest joy and the greatest tragedy of our food culture, probably the biggest treat and the biggest threat to health of any food. **The high-fat congesting nature of ice cream, along with the usual high-sugar content, makes it a food that should be eaten only infrequently and sparingly, if at all.** Some high-quality frozen yogurts as well as soy- and rice-based frozen treats are also widely available in the freezer sections of the grocery. Check the sugar and fat content of these desserts before proceeding, however; sometimes (but not always) they can be nutritious alternatives to ice cream.

SEAFOOD

Fish	Mollosks
Shellfish	Crustaceans

 Fish are among the most ideal foods. Seafood offers a good protein balance to a primarily vegetarian diet. **Fish is a good-quality protein, easily usable by the body, and a complete protein as it contains all of the essential amino acids.** It is also low in fats, and the fat that is present in fish is very helpful. In fact, recent evidence suggests that the eicosapentaenoic acid (EPA) and docosahexaenoic acid (DHA) that are contained in many fish help to lower blood cholesterol and protect us from hardening of the arteries, or atherosclerosis. EPA and DHA also seem to reduce platelet stickiness, which then reduces clotting potential and increases clotting time. This effect then decreases the likelihood of arterial thrombosis, heart attacks, and strokes.

This information comes from an investigation of the reason why people in certain fishing villages in Japan and Alaska who eat a high-fat diet, consisting mainly of fish oils and fats from animals who eat fish, had a low incidence of heart disease. This seemed contrary to scientists' knowledge that fat was tied to high cholesterol levels and heart disease. Yet the fish that these villagers eat are high in EPA and DHA and, further, these fatty acids have a different and possibly opposite effect from that of other animal fats. Many of the fish that contain EPA and DHA also contain cholesterol, although shrimp and lobster contain the highest levels, but this cholesterol does not seem to be a problem when accompanied by these helpful fats. With further investigation, researchers are finding that some of those fats in fish that we thought were cholesterol are probably beneficial oils.

Examples of fish that are high in these special lipid-lowering fats are salmon, mackerel, sardines, trout, cod, and haddock. Eating these fish 2 or 3 times a week can help protect us from cardiovascular disease. A popular trend supported by both doctors and the vitamin industry is to supplement the diet with EPA and DHA oils in a dose of about 3 grams of fish oil per day (for example, 3 grams of salmon oil may contain about 350–700 mg EPA and 250–500 mg DHA). This can help to lower blood cholesterol and triglyceride levels, especially if they are elevated, and reduce the risk of coronary artery disease. We can get about 3 grams of omega-3s (including about 1,700 mg of EPA and 1,200 mg of DHA) in 6 ounces of broiled salmon, making this deliciously flavored fish a pretty attractive option.

Outside of the high omega-3 category, fish are fairly low in fat, containing about 5% to 10%, and compare favorably with red meats, which are usually between 30% and 40%. **The types of fat present in fish are more health promoting than disease causing, unlike the saturated fats.** Furthermore, besides being relatively low in calories, seafood is rich in vitamins and minerals. The first few times I ate fish after 5 or 6 years of being a lacto-ovo vegetarian, vegan, and raw fooder, I could feel my body absorb and utilize this concentrated nourishment like a dry sponge soaking up water droplets. It was like the increased efficiency of food utilization after a period of fasting.

Fish liver is especially high in vitamins A and D. Cod liver oil is a common old-time supplement used mainly to obtain these two important fat-soluble vitamins. Most seafood contains some B vitamins, although usually in low amounts, but biotin, niacin, B6, and especially vitamin B12 are often found in higher amounts in such nutritious fish as salmon, halibut, herring, mackerel, crab, and oysters. Vitamin E is found in such oilier fishes as mackerel and herring.

Seafood is a also good source of minerals, especially such harder-to-get trace minerals as iodine, selenium, and zinc. Oysters are especially high in zinc, while crab and lobster also carry fairly high levels; selenium is present in high amounts in most of the shellfish, in mollusks, and in codfish. Most fish are high in potassium and phosphorus. Iron levels are usually very good, and calcium can be high, especially if the fish bones are consumed (as in sardines, salmon, shrimp, and herring). Calcium levels are higher in the seaweeds or sea vegetation, which are ideal foods to eat with fish. This is commonly done in Japan, and it makes good sense.

Shellfish. This refers to a variety of small, meaty, and mineral-rich fish from two families, the mollusks and the crustaceans. The **mollusks** are the sea filterers or "garbage eaters." These include clams, oysters, mussels, and scallops. I suggest that people avoid eating much of these foods. Because these shellfish eat by pumping water through their bodies, they can easily concentrate pollutants from the ocean. Whenever there is water contamination, I suggest that these seafoods specifically be avoided. They can pick up chemicals, such heavy metals as mercury, and germs from sewage, for example. The mollusks can be delicious and high in nutrients, but unless they come from waters known to be clear, they are risky foods to eat and can be toxic. In chapter 11, Food and the Earth, many more details about the relationship between water pollution and fish are addressed. This area is particularly important

regarding potential mercury toxicity and PCBs (polychlorinated biphenyls).

The **crustaceans** are of less concern. They are not sea filterers and live in deeper and usually cleaner waters than the mollusks. The major crustaceans, or soft-shelled sea creatures, are crabs, lobsters, and shrimp. These shellfish had been avoided because they were thought to be too high in cholesterol, but it turns out that what they contain is not all cholesterol but a mixture of lipids. Crustaceans are also fairly low in calories and high in protein and are used commonly by people who are trying to lose or maintain weight. Some religions, such as Judaism, forbid the consumption of crustaceans.

The most nutritious fish overall I think are halibut, swordfish, tuna, flounder, snapper, sea bass, salmon,

Seafood Sources of Vitamins and Minerals

Vitamin or Mineral	Source
Vitamin A	swordfish, whitefish, crab, halibut, salmon
B vitamins	crab, salmon, trout, halibut, mackerel, oysters
Vitamin B12	herring, mackerel, salmon, oysters, trout, crab
Vitamin E	herring, mackerel, haddock
Calcium	salmon, sardines, shrimp, oysters, herring
Copper	oysters, lobster, shrimp, crab, trout
Iodine	most saltwater fish
Iron	oysters, abalone, carp, perch, salmon, scallops, shrimp, trout
Magnesium	mackerel, oysters, salmon, snails, shrimp, crab
Phosphorus	cod, trout, halibut, perch, scallops, snapper, salmon
Potassium	cod, trout, halibut, perch, scallops, snapper, salmon
Selenium	lobster, scallops, shrimp, oysters, cod
Sodium	shrimp, lobster, mackerel, herring
Zinc	oysters, lobster, crab, halibut

mackerel, and cod from the sea, as well as freshwater trout, whitefish, and perch. Most of these fish are high in protein and low in carbohydrates. They vary in calories from about 400 to 800 per pound. The fattier fish—such as salmon, mackerel, eel, herring, and trout—often have twice the calories of the less fatty fish and the shellfish. So even though these are thought to be helpful fats, the calorie count can lead to increased weight.

Many people eat raw fish, known as sashimi or sushi, which is common in the Japanese culture. Typically served with white rice and usually eaten with salty (soy) and spicy (wasabi) sauces, raw fish can be a nutritious and low-calorie meal. The fish must be fresh and clean, of course, as bacterial and parasitic contamination can lead to sickness. More common, however, is baked or broiled fish with seasonings and lemons, often with some oil or butter and garlic and other herbs. This is probably the most healthy choice. Steamed or lightly sautéed fish can be good. Fried fish and especially breaded fried fish should be avoided because of the high content of fat, calories, and salt— none of which are good for us in excess. Besides, the hydrogenated vegetable oils or polyunsaturated oils used for frying are difficult for the body to process, and this can lead to other problems.

For weight loss, fish and vegetable meals are ideal, without extra oils, carbohydrates, or breads, and no dessert, of course. Fish with rice or pasta and vegetables, often cooked with the flavors of garlic or onions, is a good balanced meal. (For weight watching and proper food combining, have just the fish and vegetables.) Shrimp, tuna, or sardines added to a salad with lots of greens and other vegetables can be a wholesome, healthy, and filling meal.

POULTRY AND EGGS

The raising and selling of poultry and eggs is a huge business worldwide. Some types of bird or fowl are consumed in most countries, chickens being far and away the most common. In the United States alone, more than 4 billion chickens are consumed each year; that is more than 50 pounds per person. The next most common bird is turkey, which has been associated with holiday celebrations and

feasts. Like chicken, it is a fairly low-calorie, high-protein, moderate-fat meat. Ducks and geese are also eaten, but these birds have much more fat in their skins and tissues (meat) and are therefore much higher in calories. Pheasant and quail are also eaten, and these birds are high in protein. Yet all of these birds other than chickens make up only a small percentage of the poultry business.

In general, chicken can be a high-protein (complete protein) food that is fairly low in fat. It contains about 11% fat, whereas beef may be more like 30% to 40% fat; and more of the chicken fat, about two-thirds, is polyunsaturated. Also, most of the fat in chickens is in the skin. **Chicken eaten without skin is only about 4% to 5% fat, a better choice for a low-fat diet.** These figures pertain to the entire bird, however; the protein and fat levels vary among the parts. The light meat is lower in fat than the dark by about half. The backs and legs have the highest fat content, followed by the thigh and breast, but the breast also has the most protein. Eating just the meat, not the skin, of the chicken (and especially avoiding any fried chicken) is a way to reduce the fat and calorie content of this billion-seller bird.

Chicken also contains good levels of other nutrients, although they are not as concentrated as in the vegetable foods, because most of the chicken is protein and fat, and much of the vitamins and minerals are contained in the water and carbohydrate portions of foods. The dark meat of chicken is a little higher in the vitamins and minerals. Overall, chickens have some vitamin A and a bit of the B vitamins, with niacin and pantothenic acid being the best. Some pyridoxine (B6) and cobalamin (B12) are present as well. There is some potassium, sodium, phosphorus, zinc, and iron. Levels of other trace minerals and calcium and magnesium are fairly low.

In turkey, the light meat is richer in protein than the dark, with about the same amount of fat. As with chicken, about two-thirds of the turkey's fat is the unsaturated type, and the vitamin and mineral makeup is similar to that of chicken. Turkey has a little more zinc, iron, potassium, and phosphorus, with less vitamin A and some of the B vitamins. Ducks and geese have more than four times the amount of fats and calories than do the leaner turkey and chicken.

Throughout the world there are so many recipes for cooking and eating chicken, and even within each country, we could likely travel a lifetime eating a different preparation daily. Baking, broiling, roasting, boiling, and frying are some methods, each with its special spices or sauces. The Italians like chicken cacciatore, the French are known for coq au vin, and Asians for sautéed chicken and vegetables. Here in fat-fed America, fried chicken is the style. Baked or broiled is probably the healthiest manner of preparation, and without the skin to be very fat conscious.

Many chickens are raised for the purpose of producing eggs. Chicken eggs are consumed in tremendous quantities worldwide, and many nutritional authorities suggest that eggs are among the best proteins available. The egg protein, which is about 50% of its makeup, contains all the essential amino acids to be readily used by the system. Other proteins are compared with eggs on a bioavailability basis (see page 57 in chapter 3, Proteins, for more on this matter). Most of the rest of the egg is fat, about two-thirds of it unsaturated. Eggs also contain a fair amount of cholesterol, which has brought these little chickens under great scrutiny. Two large eggs contain about 10 grams of fat and 425 mg of cholesterol, which is a little higher than the suggested daily intake of cholesterol. **However, research suggests that the regular use of eggs alone when not associated with a high-fat diet does not appreciably raise the serum cholesterol.** Thus occasionally eating some eggs without much fried butter or oils, especially in place of other fatty foods (such as meats, bacon, or sausage), is probably a good choice. If there is a cholesterol problem or cardiovascular disease, however, eggs and all fat-containing foods should be consumed only with a good bit of forethought.

Eggs are also fairly low in calories, each egg having about 75. Besides the fat and protein, eggs also have some vitamins and minerals. The white of the egg contains about half the protein, no fat, no vitamin A, about 20% of the calories, and less of the other nutrients except for sodium and potassium. The yolk is fairly high in vitamin A, has some B vitamins, vitamin D, and vitamin E, all the fat and cholesterol, and most of the calcium, iron, phosphorus, and zinc. Both the yolk and the egg white contain some selenium. Lecithin (phosphatidylcholine) is fairly concentrated in the egg yolk; this substance is vital to the body's cell membranes. Because these membranes include the ones surrounding nerve cells in the brain, memory and other cognitive processes appear related to the lecithin supply.

Eggs are used in a great variety of ways. They are eaten scrambled, boiled, fried, poached, and over-easy. They are used to make omelets that can be filled with vegetables, such as onions or mushrooms, cheese, or herbs. Eggs can also be baked in casseroles or quiches or dropped into soups, such as Chinese egg drop soup. Eggs are occasionally eaten raw or blended into high-power drinks. Too many raw eggs should be avoided, however, as a part of the protein, avidin, can bind biotin (one of the B vitamins) in the intestines and cause a biotin deficiency. Fried eggs are best avoided because of the problem with fried fats.

There is also some concern about the inhumane conditions of the mass production of chickens and their eggs in the United States. Overcrowded housing, the use of antibiotics to prevent infections in those close quarters, lack of exercise, excessive feeding to increase size, and the use of stimulants or hormones such as estrogen (which has been banned since the 1980s) to increase growth have made the poultry business more like a production line of processed food. Researchers do not know the long-range effects of eating chickens and eggs produced in this manner. For this and other reasons, I personally eat eggs and chicken only occasionally and choose organic eggs and poultry raised without antibiotics or hormones, and organic Rosie chicken when possible. Anyone interested further in the economic, ecological, and health aspects of the poultry-egg agribusiness can review John Robbin's book *Diet for a New America*. I talk more about the risk of toxicity related to the mass production of chicken and eggs in chapter 11, Food and the Earth.

One way to reduce the potential dangers from the mass chicken industry is to try to find the more natural or organic chickens and eggs for consumption. These can often be free-range chickens that have more room to roam and are fed nonchemical food with no added stimulants, antibiotics, or hormones. Eating eggs from these chickens or the chickens themselves is probably better for us.

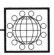

RED MEATS

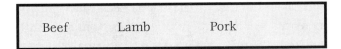

The "red meats" are probably the most controversial of the food categories. It is clear that an excess of meat in the diet can cause all kinds of problems from its high amounts of fat and sodium, and likely from excess protein as well. The saturated fat concentration is probably the worst aspect of meat. But many doctors and other people believe that they have to eat red meats for a balanced diet—that without the protein and iron from meat, they will be undernourished. **Eating meat does make it a little easier to obtain these nutrients, but I believe the negative aspects of beef and other cultivated red meats outweigh the positive, especially when meat is eaten regularly.** I personally have chosen not to eat red meats, and many other health-oriented people have made that same choice.

Red Meats

Beef	Lamb	Pork

Beef. The cow-steer-cattle family is what most people think when we say "meat." I call this "beef," and most of this discussion refers to this flesh of the cattle, because that is the commonly consumed meat, although in some cultures lamb or pork is more common. Meat is basically the muscles of these animals. Such organs as the liver and the heart are usually referred to by their specific name or as "organ meats." There are many parts of the steer that are commonly eaten. These parts all provide a high amount of complete protein, as these muscle meats are close in makeup to human protein. Meats, then, probably supply the best mixture of the amino acids to build human tissues. But the different cuts of meat may vary greatly in their fat content, and this is, again, the greatest concern with meat.

If eating meat, it is wise to eat more of the leaner cuts, which almost always come from the back leg muscles. (Because the cow makes extensive use of these back legs for movement, the tissue around the back leg bones—called the round bones—is relatively high muscle and low fat.) All of the round bone cuts of beef—including top round, bottom round, and eye of round—are relatively low in fat in comparison to other cuts. Beef from the underbelly—including rib, rib eye and rib roast—is typically high in fat, as are the brisket, porterhouse, loin, stew beef, rump roast, filet mignon, and T-bone cuts. The richer and fattier meats also tend to have the richer flavor, as it is the fats, especially the saturated ones, that tend to add flavor to these foods. T-bone and porterhouse steaks, ribs, rib roast, brisket, pork chops, and ham are higher in fats, about 35% to 45%; this may vary somewhat depending on the grade of meat—choice, prime, or good.

The good grades usually contain less fat, which can make these meats a little less tender. The higher-grade meats are usually fattened on special foods just before they are slaughtered to make them more flavorful and tender, as well as higher priced. The highest-fat meats are the processed ones, such as bacon, lunch meat, canned hams, and salami. **These "foods" also usually have high sodium levels and chemical additives, such as nitrates, which may add further dangers.** I explore more about specific toxicity risks in chapter 11, Food and the Earth.

Besides the protein, fat, and calories in the meats, there are many other nutrients. The iron content is good and more usable by the body than iron from any other source. Zinc and selenium are found in some meats, particularly in beef. The B vitamins are there in fairly good levels, especially hard-to-get vitamin B_{12}. Niacin, folic acid, thiamin, and pantothenic acid are also found in most meats. Vitamin A levels are only moderate, although they are very high in liver. Levels of vitamins E and D are minimal. Potassium and phosphorus are the highest of the other minerals. The low amount of calcium makes the calcium-to-phosphorus ratio of meats another concern in terms of the health of our bones and kidneys. Sodium is also found in larger amounts in meats than in other foods, but if the meat is unsalted, it is not very high.

Beef or calf liver is known to be one of the most concentrated sources of nutrition available. The liver, however, may concentrate chemicals and other pollutants as well, because it handles much of the body's detoxification in humans and animals. Liver is fairly low in fat and high in protein. It is high in preformed vitamin A—8 ounces of liver have 100,000 IU, which may cause some side effects, although this is rare with infrequent intake. The vitamin B12 level is also the highest of any food. The content of other B vitamins—such as riboflavin (B2), niacin (B3), pyridoxine (B6), biotin, and folic acid—is also high. Many of the minerals are good, too, such as iron, zinc, copper, chromium, selenium, potassium, phosphorus, and sodium. **Liver is often suggested as a medicinal food for anemia or fatigue because of its high iron and blood-building nutrients.**

Other organs, such as tongue, heart, brains, and kidneys, are occasionally consumed by people with a taste for those things. These organs usually have a higher vitamin and mineral content than do the muscle meats, but they are not nearly as concentrated as in the liver. As with liver, however, high-quality, toxin-free sources are important to look for when purchasing these organ foods.

Lamb. Another red meat consumed fairly commonly, especially in the Middle Eastern countries, lamb is similar to beef in its nutrient makeup and high-protein content, and is said biblically to be the closest to human flesh. Its fat content is about midway between that of the richer and the leaner cuts of beef, although the percentage of fat varies with the specific cut from the young sheep, just like it does with the cow.

Pork. Pork comes from pigs and has been eaten by many cultures. In the first edition of this book, I wrote that pig muscles are similar to beef and lamb in their content of protein, fat, and other nutrients. However, I received comments from pork people that this animal protein is the "other white meat" and has nutrition closer to chicken; in truth, it is a blend of nutrition between the two categories and the health of the pork products are also based on the husbandry practices involved. **Definitely, the cured pork products, such as ham and bacon, have high sodium levels and contain other additives, making them foods to be avoided.** Also, pork may at times become more easily infected with bacteria and parasites. Raw pork should be refrigerated at all times until it is cooked very well before being eaten.

In general, all meats must be refrigerated and cooked. The high amount of fats can rapidly lead to spoilage at room temperature. Steak tartare (raw), as served in some restaurants, should be very fresh or avoided. Uncooked meat should not even sit in the refrigerator for more than 2 days. It is best frozen until

ready for use. The meats can be used in a variety of ways—roasted, baked, fried, broiled, made into stews with vegetables, in soups, and to flavor broth and sauces. There are many kinds of meat dishes, and different cultures use meats differently. In Western countries, for example, large pieces of meat are eaten as the main part of a meal, while in Asian cultures, most meals contain some meat, but in a small portion compared with the vegetables and rice. Meat foods are really not used as a staple in the diet in many cultures.

There are many philosophical and health reasons for not consuming modern meats, at least not large amounts. The main problem with the meat that is cultivated today is that it is not like the wild animals on which our ancestors lived. They used meat for feasts and special occasions, not as a main food. Also, the free-ranging animals (such as deer, moose, bison, and elk) had a much lower fat content than the present-day animals. They lived naturally only on vegetation and were not force-fed grains often containing pesticide sprays and many other chemicals while experiencing less activity. These practices have greatly increased the fat content of animals from about 5% with only 2% to 3% saturated fats (cattle have slightly more) to the modern-day levels of 5 or 6 times that. These extra amounts of fat in cultivated meats may make the difference, especially in a less active culture, between disease and health.

Also, like chicken, cattle nowadays live in close quarters and are fed more food and more stimulants and antibiotics to prevent infection. On page 434 in chapter 11, Food and the Earth, more detail is presented regarding the potentially toxic residues commonly found in nearly all nonorganic and nonnaturally raised chicken and beef. The meat known as veal comes from imprisoned baby cows whose lack of activity keeps their muscles weak, undeveloped, and tender. They are fed an iron-deficient slosh to keep them anemic, which also makes their muscles (meat) white. Wild game, such as venison and rabbit, tend to be lower in fats and possibly more healthy to eat because they tend to graze and eat naturally. If we want these meats, however, we often need, as in olden times, to go out and hunt them.

This is not a serious attempt at building an emotional case against the eating of meat. Rather, I am providing a logical understanding of eating in general

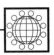

from a sensible and balanced point of view—and to provide information for consumers to make the right choices for them. The medical concerns over beef include increased cholesterol levels, high blood pressure, and atherosclerosis. This may lead to coronary artery disease and heart attacks or strokes. **Vegetarians usually have much lower levels of cholesterol and triglycerides than meat eaters and also have less atherosclerosis and heart disease.** Circulating fats tend to increase arterial plaque formation. Vegetarians also tend to have lower blood pressure. Some epidemiological studies with Seventh-day Adventists, who eat a vegetarian diet, showed a decreased death rate from heart disease and an increased longevity. If they do develop heart disease, it is about 10 years later than the average population. Other factors (such as exercise, stress, sugar, and salt in the diet or the eating of more natural foods) may also affect these statistics.

Cancer rates are increased with the higher amounts of dietary fats, which many studies relate particularly to colon, rectal, and breast cancer, although the risk of other types of cancer is probably increased as well. The American diet averages more than 40% fat, much of this the saturated variety. Dietary changes may reduce cancer risks. High-meat diets may also influence kidney disease and osteoporosis, two other serious diseases of aging. And in recent years, the occurrence of mad cow disease has many people concerned about meat consumption. See page 480 in chapter 11, Food and the Earth, for a more thorough discussion of mad cow disease.)

Overall, the best way to use meat in the diet is to apply the following 10 principles:

1. Eat meat only in moderation. This means less meat than the average American now eats. Try more vegetarian dishes.

2. When eating meats, try the leaner cuts. For most cuts, trim the excess fat.

3. Especially avoid all of the cured meats, such as bacon, ham, lunch meat, sausage, and franks, because of their higher fat content, high amounts of sodium, and cancer-causing chemicals such as nitrates. Chemical-free turkey franks and soy franks are now available as substitutes.

4. When using meats, try them as smaller parts of other dishes, such as casseroles and big salads, or cooked with such vegetables as onions, garlic, carrots, or greens. This helps the meat go a long way in both cost and health.

5. Add more fish to the diet in place of red meat dishes. This will help cut cholesterol and fats and protect us from cardiovascular diseases.

6. Increase intake of some of the anticancer and disease-protecting nutrients, such as zinc, vitamin E, vitamin C, beta-carotene, and selenium.

7. Eat more fiber foods, such as whole grains and vegetables. This also balances our diet and is protective against the degenerating diseases.

8. Exercise regularly.

9. Do not use meat as a dietary staple. If it is consumed, use it as a special treat or celebration.

10. It is not necessary to eat meat at all. Try going without it for a month and see how you feel.

SEASONINGS

A great number of seasonings are used in preparing food, to enhance or add flavor and not usually for their nutritional value, because such small amounts are generally eaten. But many of the herbs and spices (ginger, for example) are used for medicinal purposes, such as stimulating the appetite or aiding digestion. These seasonings vary throughout the world, each culture having its favorites and traditions, but the 5 basic flavors—salty, sweet, spicy, sour, and bitter—seem to cover the common uses.

Seasonings

Salt	Extracts
Peppers	Condiments
Herbs and Spices	Sweeteners

Salt. As common table salt or as soy sauce, salt is definitely the most widely used seasoning. **In fact, in many cultures, especially the Western ones, salt is much overused and may contribute to such problems as hypertension, fluid retention, electrolyte imbalance, and difficult pregnancies.** Most salt is sodium chloride, although potassium chloride is also now common, as are other salt substitutes. Salt is mined from the Earth or taken from the sea. Soy sauce is made through a fermentation process with soybeans. Salt is commonly used in cooking foods, adding flavor after preparation, or in preserving foods. (For more on salt, see "Sodium" on page 171 in chapter 6, Minerals.)

Peppers. Peppers seem to have a marriage to salt in many cultures. Black pepper is most frequently used, especially in U.S. culture, in cooking, freshly ground onto salads, or sprinkled with salt on eggs and other dishes. Even though black pepper has some good minerals, such as chromium, zinc, and selenium, it may be a little irritating to the digestive tract in many people. Hot red pepper or cayenne is a berry that is dried and ground and used on foods for a spicy taste. Cayenne is a much healthier pepper, and it and chile peppers are much better for us, even though they are a bit spicier. **Red peppers help the digestion, warm the body, herbally act as a mild diuretic, and are thought to cleanse the blood.** Cayenne is one of the true natural stimulants and is also high in vitamins C and A.

Herbs and spices. These seasonings come mostly from plants—from seeds (mustard, caraway, poppy), leaves (basil, oregano), tree bark (cinnamon), berries (cayenne, black pepper), roots (ginger, licorice), or bulbs (onion, garlic). These and many other herbs and spices are best used fresh, and some of them can be easily grown at home. Their flavors vary widely, and the more aromatic, the less stable they are—that is, the more easily they lose their potency. Most herbal seasonings should be stored in tightly sealed jars or kept in the refrigerator and certainly out of direct sunlight.

Many herbs can be grown in pots on your deck or windowsill and harvested as needed.

The list of phytonutrients found in spices and seasonings is virtually endless. Many of the unique compounds in these leaves and seeds are actually named for the plants themselves, based on either their common or scientific names. Some examples include cinnzeylanol (cinnamon), dillanoside (dill), fenchone (fennel), gingerols (ginger), isomenthone (mint), and thymol (thyme). Some of the more commonly used spices are listed in the table below.

Commonly Used Herbs and Spices and Their Scientific Names

Spice	Scientific Name
Anise	*Pimpinella anisum*
Basil	*Ocimum basilicum*
Bay	*Laurus nobilis*
Borage	*Borago officinalis*
Chive	*Allium schoenoprasum*
Cinnamon	*Cinnamomum verum*
Coriander	*Coriandrum sativum*
Dandelion	*Taraxacum officinale*
Dill	*Anethum graveolens*
Fennel	*Foeniculum vulgare*
Ginger	*Zingiber officinale*
Lavender	*Lavandula* spp.
Lemon Balm	*Melissa officinalis*
Lemongrass	*Cymbopogon citratus*
Mint	*Mentha piperita* (peppermint)
	Mentha spicata (spearmint)
Mustard	*Brassica nigra* (black mustard)
Oregano	*Origanum* spp.
Parsley	*Petroselinum crispum*
Rosemary	*Rosmarinus officinalis*
Rue	*Ruta graveolens*
Sage	*Salvia officinalis*
Tarragon	*Tagetes lucinda*
	Artemisia dracunculus
Thyme	*Thymus vulgaris*

Extracts. Flavorings come mostly from such foods as lemons, oranges, almonds, or vanilla beans. These concentrated liquid extracts have little nutritional value and are mostly employed in flavoring baked goods, drinks, or candies. These extracts also should be kept out of direct light and in tightly sealed dark glass to prevent spoiling.

Condiments. Typically, in U.S. culture, what is used most often for seasonings are some processed foods that have generally been well accepted as toppings or dressings for many dishes. Besides refined salt (which is used in great excess), common condiments are mustard (which is a more natural blend of the oily mustard seed), ketchup, and mayonnaise (often called "salad dressing"). Ketchup is a tomato-based sauce often made with sweeteners, salt, and additives (although there are now more natural ketchups on the market) that goes with the oft-eaten hamburger and french fries and, for some people, with eggs and other dishes. Mayonnaise is a gelatinous blend of eggs, vegetable oil, sugar, salt, lemon juice, flavorings, and additives. It is high in calories and fats, with some nutritional value. Mayonnaise is commonly used on sandwiches, as the basis of salad dressings and sauces, in salads such as potato salad and coleslaw, and mixed into other dishes for flavoring. Many people overuse this dressing.

Then there are the real salad dressings—the liquid flavoring for salad that is composed of mixes of the vegetable oils, vinegars or lemon, the basic condiments, and various seasonings. **The manufactured varieties are usually high in chemical additives, and I recommend either purchasing natural dressings or making them at home fresh.**

Sweeteners. Sweeteners are a large category of highly used flavorings for foods. The eating of sugary foods is destructive to the tooth enamel because of its support for germ growth. All of these sweeteners, other than the current artificial sweeteners I call "chemical sweets," are simple sugars or carbohydrate foods that provide quick energy. They are easily assimilated and converted into blood sugar, which is potential energy for the cells. **However, a concern is that these sweeteners overstimulate the hormonal glands—particularly the pancreas and adrenals—and cause problems in blood sugar, energy, and emotions.** Most of these sweeteners are low in or devoid of nutrition.

White refined sugar. Extracted from the sugar beet or sugarcane, white refined sugar is the prime exam-

ple and the most used of these destructive sweeteners. Most things are tolerated in sensible quantities but the desire for sweet tastes has generated an excessive use by both the food industry and consumers. There are literally tablespoonfuls of sugar in a can of soda pop. It is present in most of the aforementioned condiments, in baby foods, and in most pastries, candies, cookies, other baked goods, syrups, and jellies. The excessive use of sugar can deplete certain vitamins and minerals that are needed to metabolize it, and its use has been associated with dental caries, pyorrhea, diabetes, hypoglycemia, obesity, nervous system disorders, and mental illness. Obesity and diabetes are associated further with increases in atherosclerosis, heart disease, nerve disease, and cancer. More information on sugar is detailed on pages 31–32 in chapter 2, Carbohydrates, and in many other books, particularly *Sugar Blues* by William Dufty.

Natural fruit sugar. Also known as fructose, this can be used in place of sucrose (white sugar), but it still may overstimulate the hormonal system and irritate the teeth. Eating fruit is the best way to obtain this sweet, along with the bulk, fiber, and nutrients that probably even help digest and utilize the sugar.

Honey. This common sweetener is considered by many to be a more healthful energy food. It may contain some B vitamins, vitamins C, D, and E, and traces of minerals. Honey is essentially a flower pollen extract digested and regurgitated by bees (sounds great), but it is clean, actually sterile. Germs do not really grow well in honey. Even this slightly more wholesome sweetener should be used in moderation, however. Overall, it is best to obtain our sweet flavor from foods. Most fruits, vegetables, and grains are considered sweet foods. This flavor is already overconsumed in the U.S. diet, so further sugar is best avoided.

Date sugar. An extract from dates, this can be substituted for white sugar in baking or candies. Because it is made from whole, ground dates, this sweetener is a major step up nutritionally from white sugar.

Maple syrup is the partially refined sap of the maple tree. It has a unique flavor and is commonly used to top pancakes and waffles but can also be employed in baking, candies, and so on. The best maple syrup to buy is the organic, grade B version. Grade A maple syrups are further refined than grade B and as a result have lost more nutrients. The inexpensive, nonpure maple syrup is high in white sugar water with a little maple flavor and often a few chemicals. It is best avoided.

Chocolate or cocoa (Theobroma cacao). By itself this is more a bitter than a sweet, but it is often used in candy and as flavoring. Along with the added sweetness, chocolate has its own well-loved taste. The cocoa used to make chocolates comes from the cocoa bean, which has some caffeinelike substances, so it is a mild stimulant. Some people are sensitive, even allergic, to chocolate. It is one of the more common food cravings, and chocolate may even have antidepressant properties. Apparently it contains a substance, possibly beta-phenethylamine, a neurotransmitter and mood elevator, that is similar in chemical structure to a hormone secreted by women when sexually aroused. The phytonutrients present are cafesterol, caffetannic acid, stigmasterol, tannins, epicatechin, and avanoids.

Carob (Ceratonia siliqua). Another bean, sometimes referred to as "locust bean," this tastes similar to chocolate; it is more naturally sweet and contains some protein, although it is mainly a carbohydrate food, along with calcium, phosphorus, and some B vitamins. The carob bean is also known as St. John's bread because of its biblical reference as an important food to John the Baptist's survival in the wilderness. Carob is now commonly used to flavor sweets, in baking, and as a drink, mainly as a substitute for chocolate, although some people prefer the carob flavor. The phytonutrients present in carob are concanavalin, gallic acid, leucodelphinidin, pectin, saponin, and tannin.

Stevia (Stevia rebaudiana). Stevia, or "sweetleaf," is an herb that is a fairly strong natural sweetener. It has no calories and can be used by people with diabetes or hypoglycemia. This green leaf can be used straight or in cooking. The phytonutrients present include beta-carotene, dulcosides, steviol, and stevioside.

Artificial sweeteners. These chemical sweets are not recommended. Cyclamate was popular for a while but has since been taken off the market because of cancer-producing tendencies. Saccharin has been around for a while and is still used, although there are long-range health concerns associated with its use. Aspartame, a more recently developed sweetener made from amino acids (aspartic acid and phenylalanine) is also under scrutiny. It is still not a natural substance and many people have problems with aspartame; it appears to agitate people and affect their

moods and nervous system, and it may have effects similar to those of MSG (monosodium glutamate), another amino acid derivative. Splenda (sucralose, a chlorinated sugar) is another new sweetener that may be tolerated better, yet it still poses some concerns. (See "Common Food Additives" on page 455 in Chapter 11, Food and the Earth, for more about these sweeteners.) Ideally, it is best to bring our cultural sweet tooth into balance and focus it on naturally sweet foods, such as apples and carrots.

BEVERAGES

Beverages are those fluid substances that we drink for the primary reasons of satisfying thirst and maintaining the body's 65% water content. There are other reasons for consuming different liquids, including body detoxification, energy stimulation, relaxation, and nourishment, as well as merriment and celebration.

Different people and cultures have their favorite beverages. Many of the substances we drink have the potential for addiction and may produce certain problems when consumed in excess. Alcohol and caffeine, in the United States mainly as coffee, are 2 commonly abused ones. Milk use can create difficulties for many adults and children because of lactose intolerance or allergy, or because of its calorie and fat levels. Sugared soda pops, many of them containing caffeine, have become a common addictive problem, especially in

Common Beverages of Various Countries	
Country	**Beverage**
Australia	beer, milk
China	tea
France	wine, coffee, mineral water
Germany	beer, schnapps, fruit juices
Great Britain	tea, beer
Italy	wine, coffee, mineral water
Japan	tea, wine (sake)
Russia	kvas, tea, vodka
United States	coffee, beer, sodas, milk

young people. We all need to consume liquids to maintain life. It is best for as much as possible of our liquid intake to be water and for the other beverages to be used only as special treats. In this way, along with a diet containing the essential nutrients, we will more easily provide the body and cells with what they need, rather than make it harder for the digestive and other systems to obtain the replenishment they require.

Beverages

Water	Teas
Fruit juices	Coffee
Vegetable juices	Sodas
Milk	Alcohol

Water. Water has been discussed rather thoroughly in the beginning of this book (see chapter 1). Ideally, we should consume about 6 to 8 glasses of water a day with average activity and a fairly balanced diet, consuming a fair portion of high-water-content fruits and vegetables. If we are more active and sweat, or if we consume a higher proportion of richer or fattier foods, we usually need more water. I believe the water that is best for us is not city-processed tap water but well water, springwater, or home-purified water. Any water can be checked for basic minerals, toxic minerals, or chemical contamination. This is suggested when there is any concern about the water that we use for regular consumption. Solid carbon block water filtration, reverse osmosis, and distillation are the predominant water purification processes. Each has its advantages and disadvantages, but all are effective and helpful systems for home water use (see pages 20–24 in chapter 1, Water). All living things need water to thrive and survive. Animals, both domestic and wild, the plants of Nature, our gardens, trees, and the grass on our front lawns—all require water to stay alive and grow. All of the other substances discussed in this section are basically water with some other nutrients or chemicals added, for which the water is the vehicle that carries them to the appropriate areas of the body.

Fruit juices. The extracted liquids from fruits are particularly high in fructose (fruit sugar), so they provide calories and energy. They also contain some vitamins and minerals, most commonly vitamin C and potassium. Other B vitamins, some vitamin A, and other minerals (such as calcium and magnesium) may be found in various fruit juices. Orange juice and apple juice are the most consumed of the fruit juices. Grape juice, grapefruit juice, and prune juice are also used, most often as breakfast drinks. The nectars of pears, peaches, or apricots may be special treats as well. Some juices are used therapeutically, such as papaya or pineapple for digestion or cranberry juice for soothing urinary tract irritations.

Children may drink a lot of fruit juice, more than adults, who are more given to coffee, tea, or alcoholic beverages, although soda pops have replaced some of the more natural fruit juices among young people as well. Fruit juices are still useful, nourishing, and often a good way to obtain the concentrated juice of several pieces of fruit at one sitting.

Vegetable juices. These are similar to fruit juices except that they are, of course, the extracted liquids of various vegetables. These are also liquids with concentrated nourishment, even more than the fruit juices. Levels of vitamins A and C may be high, with some B vitamins also. The mineral content is usually fairly rich in potassium, calcium, magnesium, and phosphorus. Tomato juice is the most commonly consumed vegetable juice, although other juices from carrots, beets, celery, and greens are also used. Fresh vegetable juices are available in health food stores more frequently now. Making vegetable juices at home requires special equipment, although there are some simple, relatively inexpensive juicers to accomplish this.

More and more people are going back to juice fasting or cleansing for brief or extended periods of time as part of their yearly dietary program. Juice or liquid fasting is a traditional part of many cultures, both human and animal, and may be a beneficial process to clear the body of maladies and to revitalize the life force. (See chapter 18, Detoxification and Cleansing Programs, of this book and *The New Detox Diet* for more information on healthy detoxification.)

Milk. Milk is more of a food than a beverage. Its high-fat, protein, calorie, and vitamin and mineral content, in fact, makes it a nourishing food. And at mealtime, it should be considered a food—not something to be drunk along with meals. Even though it is such a nourishing food, milk can pose problems. As discussed more thoroughly in the section "Dairy" in this chapter (see page 339), milk can provide excessive fat and lead to cardiovascular problems in those who consume it in excess. And many people are allergic to milk or lactose intolerant, not possessing the enzyme lactase to metabolize the milk sugar.

Teas. Teas are classified as the basic commercial tea, or black tea, the herbal teas, and green tea. Tea is essentially a drink, usually hot, made from soaking various plants in boiling water. Teas should be considered more as drugs, like coffee, or medicinals than just as liquid beverages. **The commercial teas contain theobromine, a central nervous system stimulant like caffeine, and tannin, or tannic acid, which can be an irritant to the intestinal mucous linings and kidneys.** Other than fairly high amounts of fluoride, common tea provides little nutrition. It is used commonly in the United States, in the Orient, and in the United Kingdom as a social beverage. Teatime is an afternoon relaxation period often involving caffeine restimulation.

Herbal teas are better overall than the caffeine-tannic acid teas and are becoming more popular. The berries, barks, flowers, leaves, stems, and roots of all kinds of plants have specific therapeutic actions when consumed in sufficient dosages. The knowledge of these medicinal properties has been passed down through the ages and can be found in a variety of texts. Green tea has become popular for its antioxidant effects and health benefits; more important health research on green and herbal teas is being conducted. (The science of the use of herbs is termed *herbology*.) The phytonutrients present in teas include catechins, epicatechins, gallocatechins, epigallocatechins, apigenin, beta-carotene, beta-sitosterol, caffeic acid, campesterol, cinnamic acid, cryptoxanthin, eugenol, gallic acid, geraniol, and theaflavins.

Coffee (*Coffea arabica*). Coffee is probably the most commonly used and abused drug (caffeine) in the United States—and in many other cultures, for that matter. The caffeine-containing coffee bean is roasted and ground and then brewed by passing boiling water through the coffee grounds. Caffeine has a number of metabolic effects as a central nervous system stimulant. It increases the heart rate, blood pressure, respiration, gastrointestinal activity, stomach acid output, kidney function, and mental activity.

Some people use it to relieve fatigue, although many develop a taste and love for the unusual, slightly bitter flavor.

Coffee abuse is common, with regular drinking of it throughout the day, especially in the 9-to-5 workforce. This may create cardiac sensitivity, with abnormal heartbeats, anxiety and irritability, stomach and intestinal irritation, insomnia, and such withdrawal symptoms as fatigue or headaches. **Coffee can also interfere with the absorption of many vitamins and minerals, such as calcium and iron.**

Caffeine addiction can be a problem, although usually not too major, and withdrawal from coffee may be difficult. Many coffee substitutes are available, and decaffeinated coffee is used much more commonly by those who like the flavor and social scene of coffee drinking yet do not like the caffeine stimulation. **There are some concerns over the chemicals used to decaffeinate coffee and about coffee in general.** It is wise to reduce and minimize the regular intake of coffee. (See more about coffee in "Caffeine" on page 761 in chapter 18, Detoxification and Cleansing Programs and my book *The New Detox Diet*.) The phytonutrients present in coffee are caffesterol, caffeic acid, caffeol, eugenol, glucogalactomannan, stigmasterol, and tannins.

Sodas. Sodas are beverages carbonated with carbon dioxide gas; their use has increased greatly since the mid-1970s. **I believe that these beverages have a fairly destructive nutritional pattern and are greatly abused.** They have no nutritional value, contain high amounts of phosphates, which can influence calcium and bone metabolism, and often contain tremendous amounts of white sugar or chemicals that may rot the teeth—and the body too, for that matter. The cola drinks often contain high amounts of caffeine as well, which prepare the children who often drink them for later coffee abuse. I have seen people completely addicted to colas, drinking 10 to 12 bottles or cans a day.

These drinks can deplete the body of nutrients as well as overstimulate the body. Most of the noncola drinks are also high in sugar or chemicals. If these beverages are used regularly or in excess, it is wise to replace them with good, clean water or other more nutritious drinks, and use these soda pops only as an occasional treat. Although the huge industry that pro-

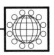

motes the use of these drinks and their availability in all stores and restaurants make this more difficult, as with other tantalizing treats of our society, having the willpower and discipline to avoid or replace these sugars or drugs that can hurt us with more healthful habits or substances is one of the challenges of life.

Alcohol. This is another commonly used and abused drug, even more so by the younger population in recent years. Alcoholic beverages come in many varieties, such as beer, wine, and more alcohol-concentrated liquors. These are produced by means of fermentation (usually by yeasts) or distillation. They have little nutritive value but a fair amount of calories. The gut or beer belly is characteristic of the regular beer drinker who must consume higher amounts of liquid and calories to obtain the drug effect of alcohol.

Alcohol is different from caffeine; it is a central nervous system depressant, or sedative. Even though it seems to loosen people up, it does so by sedating the usual inhibitory mechanisms. **Alcohol slows the brain actions and affects physical coordination and reaction time. It is also irritating to the gastrointestinal tract and liver, which handles the detoxification of this drug.** Furthermore, the chemicals used in alcoholic beverage production are a big concern. Often grapes and grains are heavily sprayed with pesticides, and sulfites and heavy metals may also be contaminants.

Many people drink too much and too often; some become addicted to alcohol and are then known as alcoholics. This disease can be devastating to the individuals and their families. Usually there is an underlying emotional problem (possibly a genetic predisposition as well) or inability to make contact with and express the emotions. Drinking alcohol in excess is also greatly influenced by social and peer pressure. In general, alcohol is not something that is particularly beneficial to health. Although some medical articles suggest that moderate alcohol consumption (1 or 2 drinks a day) may be helpful to cardiovascular health, this is most likely through its action as a mild stress reducer. Other forms of stress management, such as exercise and a variety of relaxation techniques, are much healthier, although they may take more work. Occasional drinking for celebration may be beneficial in some ways. However, if we are drinking daily or in excess regularly, it is wise to reduce or even eliminate this potentially addicting drug. If it is not possible by oneself, it is wise to seek help. (A complete discussion of alcohol and its problems can be found on page 758 of chapter 18, Detoxification and Cleansing Programs, and in my book *The New Detox Diet.*) **Drink good water and nourish yourself with real foods from Nature.**

Chapter 9

Diets

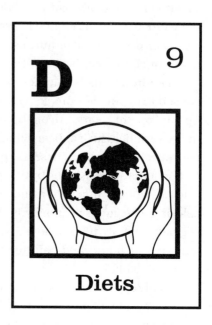

Diets

A diet is whatever we eat, and there are literally millions of them. What each of us eats is our individualized diet. When we say the word *diet,* many of us may think of a particular time when we tried to lose or gain weight before going back to what we usually eat. Who we are, how we feel, and how we look in size and shape are the results of what we eat, our eating habits, and all that we do and think. So, if we wish to change in any way, we probably need to *change our diet*—that is, what and how we eat—rather than *go on a diet.*

In this chapter, I discuss the variations in diets, their different classifications (such as vegetarian or omnivorous diets), and the common cultural diets throughout the world. I define each and then discuss its strengths and weaknesses, along with ways to modify it or additional supplements needed to make the diet healthier. In chapter 10, Nutritional Habits, I review the various eating habits—both health supporting and not—on my way to part 3, Building a Healthy Diet, where I put all of these basics of nutrition together.

Diets are influenced by a number of factors. First, the classification of the diet is based on its content. This used to be based on availability of foods indigenous to locale—what could be grown or hunted, gathered or caught. Nowadays, however, it is even wiser to eat locally and minimize imported foods, which often are heavily treated per government regulations to protect them from decay and germ and insect infestation. Eating locally obviously has its limitations, however, as foods are subject to seasonal and climatic influences.

Each culture has its own dietary patterns regarding what is eaten and how it is prepared. These patterns are strong, as are our individual tastes and food conditioning. Even stronger are family influences. Thus both our culture and our environment affect our eating patterns. Specifically, diets and habits seem to run in families, as do many of the problems that come from these diets and habits. In many cases, such diseases as hypertension, heart disease, adult diabetes, obesity, and even cancer are related more to familial influences, both psychological and nutritional, than to a genetic predisposition. Genetics do play a factor in our diet, however. Over generations, our bodies adapt to the foods we eat, and our physical well-being is influenced by our ability to digest, assimilate, and utilize any food. Although the human species is adaptable, genetic mutation is a slow process. When we shift cultures or markedly change diets, we may consume foods that the body will react to rather than receive easily. Digestive problems, other sensitivities, and allergies may occur from this. We should pay close attention to how the body handles new foods and new recipes.

As I mentioned, our general eating patterns and habits are greatly influenced by our upbringing. Such preferences as when we eat, whether we snack rather than eating meals, or whether we like to eat on our own or socially may have their origins in childhood. The emotional ties between love and food or between love and cleaning our plate are deep-seated and influence our whole life. Sweets such as ice cream or milk and cookies after dinner or before bed or sweets and treats as rewards may create lifelong problems with our relationship to food. These eating patterns, likes, and dislikes develop early and are difficult to change. (I discuss these aspects in more detail in chapter 10, Nutritional Habits.) Our individual constitution determines how we respond to these influences and how we grow on the diet we are fed as children. As we age, our individuality usually creates a new diet that fills our own needs, and that, occasionally, varies a fair amount from our family's diet.

The increased availability of foods due to society's industrialization has influenced dietary changes more than any other factor since the 1950s. Technology has led to food refinement, increased storage, and flavor control. Salt, sugar, and fried foods have never been so prevalent. Diets have shifted from more natural ones to fast foods and snack foods. The working class has always looked for ways to save time and effort in food preparation. Even since the 1980s, we have seen a shift from TV dinners and other frozen foods to the huge fast food restaurant business and microwave meals. As journalist Eric Schlosser has pointed out in his 2001 best seller *Fast Food Nation,* Americans spent $6 billion on fast food in 1970 and more than $110 billion in 2000. During this time, McDonald's also became the world's biggest owner of retail property; this company has also been challenged for its contribution to obesity, and has changed their menu somewhat due to public health concerns.

The influence of technology on the food chain, although it has helped somewhat in extending the shelf life of food, has had a bad overall effect on general nutrition. The Western or American diet has been the most affected by these industrial changes, which are spreading rapidly to other nations.

These technological influences have also played a major role in the field of nutritional medicine. The main concern in the past was deficiency disease, caused by not getting enough of certain important nutrients. Although this still occurs in some people, and unfortunately in some nations, there is now the added concern about problems that arise from excesses found in the new world diet. There is no longer any doubt about the important relationship between diet and disease. The federal government began to acknowledge this relationship with the publication of the 1988 *Surgeon General's Report on Nutrition and Health.* In that report, the most common diseases that plague U.S. society—including high blood pressure, coronary artery disease, cancers, diabetes, and obesity—were all linked to unhealthy dietary habits. More recently, in March 2003, an independent expert report commissioned by the World Health Organization (WHO) reaffirmed diet as a "key factor" contributing to the increased burden of chronic disease, including all of the diseases mentioned by the surgeon general years earlier.

Probably the most significant aspects of diet are the fat and fiber content. Protein sources are a concern, and vitamin and mineral levels are also important. But overall, the high amount of fat, specifically saturated fat, is associated with the major diseases like cancer, cardiovascular disease, and hypertension and their secondary problems. Although the high-fat (and high-protein) diet has contributed to making Americans and others consuming this diet larger (in both height and weight) than most of the more vegetarian cultures, it is not necessarily healthier. Cancer and cardiovascular disease, both nutritionally related, are the two biggest killers of the adult population in the United States and the two greatest costs to society, in terms of direct medical costs and lost work. But much of the incidence of these diseases can be avoided. The incidence is changing, as more doctors as well as the general public and food stores respond to the suggestions contained in this book and many other good nutrition texts.

There are usually big differences between the diets of rural and urban families. The availability of restaurants, fast food outlets, and giant supermarkets has become an obstacle to good nutrition for many people. Growing our food, either as a means of making a living or in our own gardens, brings us back into contact with the Earth and provides us with the freshest, most vital nutrition on the planet. This influence often will affect the rest of our diet for the better. Words such as *natural* (as nature provides), *organic* (chemical free), and *fresh* (just picked) are becoming popular again in societies that have moved far from these qualities.

Each of us needs eventually to find our own balance in diet. Through knowledge and experimentation, we can learn what works best for us. Each culture must find this balance as well. Each has its basic natural diet as well as extremes or abuses that may undermine health. For example, the typical Asian diet is high in fiber and complex carbohydrate, with a good balance of fat and protein. But it uses a lot of salted or pickled preserved foods, which influence the incidence of stomach cancer. Those Western cultures that consume more fat and less fiber have a much higher incidence of colon cancer. Balancing the diet requires developing new tastes. Sometimes it involves taking some supplements to assure that we consume some hard-to-get nutrients or those that may be deficient in our soil or foods. Supplements can also provide more of those nutrients that help protect against cancer and atherosclerosis, such as the fish oils and the antioxidant nutrients vitamin C, vitamin E, beta-carotene, zinc, and selenium.

Historically, the evolution of the human diet began with the nomadic tribes who moved with the seasons, eating those foods available through hunting and gathering. With more stable village life, however, humans had to learn anew to feed themselves—to cultivate, to store, and to prepare foods to feed the growing numbers of people. Both farming and hunting were necessary for survival, and these were believed to be influenced by both the climate and the spirits. Droughts or floods affected feasts or famines as well as health, disease, and war. Different areas of the world had different foods available, and this led to culture-specific diets. Knowledge and recipes to nourish the family were passed from generation to generation, and each generation usually added something new. The increase in food cultivation and industrial-

ization went hand in hand with the rise in the population and urban living. More food was needed to feed the masses.

Survival was dependent on the food supply. People had to become more adaptable and learn to eat new foods and even change their diets. Adaptability is still key to survival. Even if we have eaten a certain type of diet for 40 years, we can still change if we feel that shifts may be helpful. Such change is often important for continued health or to reduce the level or incidence of many diseases. Adaptability is even more important as we age. **Changing our diet or lifestyle is not necessarily easy, but it can be done, and it may influence many other aspects of our life for the better.**

TYPES OF DIETS

Most diets can be placed within one of several different categories. I've found these various categories to be quite helpful in thinking about food and would like to describe them for you here.

Omnivorous

An omnivorous diet is one in which both animal and vegetable foods are consumed. Most people of the world are omnivorous, and this type of diet is the easiest to balance, as there are no limitations. Of course, the knowledge of how much and what specific foods to eat is needed. These types of diets are discussed in more detail in the sections below on the specific cultural diets. In the animal kingdom, however, many species are either vegetarian or carnivorous; some animals, such as bears and crows, are omnivorous.

Carnivorous

A carnivorous diet is one that contains animal flesh—that is, meat. From a vegetarian viewpoint, anyone who eats meat is a carnivore, but truly most people who eat meat are omnivores. True carnivores who eat only meat are hard to find; in the animal kingdom, they include the canine and feline families, which naturally subsist on the flesh of other animals. These animals are naturally adapted to hunt and to consume flesh. Their speed, power, pointed teeth, and sharp claws help them a great deal in this quest. They have no molars and cannot really chew; they rip the flesh from their prey and swallow it. Their digestive tracts are specifically designed to process the high-protein, sometimes fatty meals. They only eat vegetables, local greens, when they are sick.

The human, though, has different characteristics: a longer digestive tract makes us more adapted to eating as vegetarians and processing the vegetable foods. Our long and convoluted intestinal tubing is different from the carnivore's short system, where the meats can move through rapidly before they putrefy. Our digestive tracts are more like those of the herbivores, where the length allows increased absorption area to help break down the plant fibers and utilize their nutrients. We are adaptable and most likely can function as omnivores, although there are varying opinions on this question. Meats are a concentrated food, high in protein, with varying degrees of fat, only certain vitamins and minerals, and almost no fiber. The protein helps in growth and many other functions, such as tissue repair, and the iron content is very good. Without the proper balance of fiber, however, a high-meat diet will increase the risk of disease of the colon and other organs. The high-fat types of meat increase the risk of cancer, atherosclerosis, heart disease, and other problems. To balance the meat in our diet, we need supplementary fiber and more of the B vitamins, vitamins C and E, and the many minerals found in the vegetable foods.

Lacto-ovo Vegetarian

This is the most common of the vegetarian diets. It does not include animal flesh but does use the byproducts of the chicken and cow—eggs and milk products (vegans, or strict vegetarians, do not eat these foods). Some vegetarians are lacto only (not ovo); they may espouse many reasons for not eating eggs and may have a moral aversion to eating unborn chickens. Other vegetarians may be sensitive to milk but find eggs okay. Whatever the nuances, however, vegetable foods are usually the largest part of the lacto-ovo vegetarian diet, which consists mainly of fruits, vegetables, grains, legumes, nuts, and seeds. Throughout history, most people's diets have been primarily vegetarian, with meats eaten only occasionally. This is still true today throughout much of the world. Only in the twentieth century have the meat foods been so heavily consumed in the Westernized cultures, such as North and South America, Australia, and the European countries. This is due mainly to the commercial herding, slaughtering, and packaging of flesh foods to make them readily available at the corner store.

I myself lean strongly toward a more natural and vegetarian-type diet as the choice that is more healthful, especially when compared with the typical

---

Food Complements for a Vegetarian Diet

To combine daily proteins, eat

Grains + legumes (main combination)—
    rice and lentils, wheat and peas, bean burritos

Seeds or nuts + legumes—garbanzo and
    sesame (hummus), tofu and sesame

Grains + milk or eggs*— quiche, rice and eggs,
    French toast, lasagna

Vegetables + milk or eggs—cream soups,
    vegetables with eggs or cheese sauce, salad
    with sliced eggs, omelet, eggplant parmesan

---

* Not if following food combining.

Food Complementarity

Complete Proteins	Incomplete Proteins
Milk	Grains (low in lysine, isoleucine)
Eggs	Legumes (low in tryptophan, methionine)
Fish	Seeds and nuts (low in lysine, isoleucine)
Poultry	Vegetables (vary—most low in methionine, isoleucine)
Red meats	

American diet. My suggestion is not that people become vegetarians, which is a scary proposition to many—What? Give up my meat?!—but that people become *more* vegetarian, eating less meat and animal fats. Moving toward meatless meals is a beginning step. **A more vegetarian diet clearly reduces the risk of many common chronic diseases, and as long as we consume adequate protein, we are safe from deficiency problems.**

The most common reason for not giving up meat, besides being used to the taste, is the fear of not getting enough protein. I believe the protein concepts perpetrated by American nutritionists to be among the biggest fallacies about our diet. We do not really need as much protein as we might think, and it is likely that excess protein is a bigger concern than protein deficiency, at least in Westernized cultures. Having said that, however, vegetarians need to be aware of obtaining adequate protein and maintaining efficient digestion and assimilation; I have seen many vegetarians with problems in these areas.

A mixed vegetarian diet with or without eggs or dairy products can theoretically supply adequate protein, although it may take more effort than with the omnivorous diet. As long as the diet is not filled with a lot of sugars and other empty calories, the protein content is usually adequate. Protein combination, or complementarity, suggests that we mix two or more plant protein foods at a meal to provide sufficient levels of all the essential amino acids. Usually one or two of these amino acids may be low in each food, and mixing them at the same meal means that the body has what it needs to make new proteins. Recent research in this area has made it clear that protein combining within a single meal is unnecessary. In other words, we do not have to mix rice with beans to make sure that the lysine missing in the rice gets supplied by the beans, and the tryptophan missing in the beans gets supplied by the rice. As long as both rice and beans are eaten sometime during the day, the body will do fine at making new proteins. Some researchers believe that the time frame for protein combining is even longer than 1 day, but I think we should err on the conservative side and get the combinations we need over a 24-hour period.

Carbohydrates and fats are more readily used for fuel, and it is they, not protein, that actually nourish the active muscles. Protein (amino acids) builds the tissue during growth, though, and this may come from dietary protein of either animal or vegetable origin. Another fallacy in many people's concepts about protein is that animal proteins are needed for strength and endurance or athletic prowess. Although the percentage of vegetarians in U.S. culture is generally low compared with omnivores, there have been some outstanding athletes and record setters through the years who were vegetarians.

The strengths of the lacto-ovo vegetarian diet are many and the weaknesses few. Both are more pronounced for the strict vegan diet, but here I focus on the lacto-ovo diet, which usually provides sufficient protein, calcium, iron, and vitamin B_{12}—all of which are concerns for any vegetarian. If eggs or milk products are eaten once a day along with other wholesome foods, the diet should be fairly balanced in all respects. Vegetarians in general have lower blood pressure and weight than their meat-eating companions. Their incidence of hypertension, obesity, high cholesterol, atherosclerosis, heart disease, osteoporosis, and cancer are all reduced. Studies of the Seventh-day Adventists, for example, a large vegetarian population, shows their incidence of coronary artery disease about half that of the average population. Throughout the world, the incidence of coronary artery and heart disease correlates with each country's intake of meat.

The high amount of fiber and the lower amount of fat in the vegetarian diet are also helpful in keeping cholesterol down and digestive tract diseases at a minimum. The high amounts of vitamins and minerals present in vegetables, especially, are also an advantage. Many vegetarians find that they have a higher level of energy. I certainly did when I changed to vegetarianism, and this has continued through the years. My diet has been re-created numerous times to suit my lifestyle and the changing seasons. It is still primarily vegetarian, with occasional fresh fish or organic poultry.

Potential problems for vegetarians include a reduced iron and vitamin B_{12} intake and thus a higher incidence of anemia. As stated earlier, this is less a concern for the lacto-ovo vegetarian than for the strict vegan, but it is still something of which to be aware. Oral iron and vitamin B_{12}, or even B_{12} injections, could be needed to fulfill the body's needs (more likely with poor digestion and low hydrochloric acid output) and maintain the tissue stores of these important nutrients.

There is some concern among health-care practitioners that infants, growing children, and women who are pregnant or lactating should avoid vegetarianism. This is unfounded, particularly for the lacto-ovo diet. Pure veganism in these cases should be avoided. If children can eat a wholesome diet with a good protein balance, they can grow well and be healthy on a lacto-ovo vegetarian diet, as can pregnant women. Sometimes they may be even healthier, perhaps because vegetarians tend to have better food habits and less tendencies to abuse foods and other substances, in general, than the average population.

Vegan

This is the strict, pure form of vegetarianism. No animal products are consumed (and many choose not to wear leather goods from animals as well), only fruits, vegetables, legumes, grains, nuts, and seeds. No eggs, cheese, yogurt, ice cream, butter, or other milk products are eaten. This diet is not advisable for children unless the parents can painstakingly oversee it and select the right foods. It is difficult with this diet to obtain a balanced intake of all the nutrients that are needed during growth; however, it can be done. This is true also in pregnancy and lactation, where higher intakes of most nutrients are needed. I am not suggesting that this cannot be done; it just is more dangerous in its risk of creating deficiencies and subsequent health problems.

Overall, the vegan is often of a lower than average weight, even underweight for his or her size, and usually has a low cholesterol level. Many of the advantages of the lacto-ovo vegetarian diet are even truer of the vegan diet. There is a much lower incidence of hypertension, obesity, heart disease, and some cancers, most notably of the colon, breast, uterus, and prostate. The fiber content of the diet is usually very good. However, the potential nutrient deficiencies are a concern. Vitamin B12 is the main one. Iron and calcium may also be low. Protein levels may be all right if the person is conscious of protein intake and complementing food. Vitamin A may be low unless a high amount of the orange, yellow, and green vegetables is consumed. Vitamin D is often low; some sunshine

will help. Zinc may also be low unless seeds and nuts are consumed regularly.

In general, I suggest a good supplement program for vegans. A vitamin B12 level and general biochemical profile every few years will help reassure us that the diet is providing adequately for bodily functions. As with any type of diet, if health is faltering or sickness is recurring, an investigation should be made. Overall, however, with the right intention and knowledge, the vegan diet can be a healthy one.

Macrobiotic

Macrobiotics is a philosophy of life centered around a diet originally brought to this country from Japan by George Ohsawa. Although Ohsawa began writing and teaching about macrobiotics in Japan in the early 1930s, he did not begin his work in the United States until 1959. Over the next 10 years, his work in macrobiotics helped it gain popularity, particularly in New York and California, where he focused his involvement. Ohsawa's efforts have been expanded upon and shared with many by teachers and authors Michio and Aveline Kushi, a Japanese couple living in the Boston area, and by the magazine *East West Journal.* Macrobiotic diets, either very strict or more liberal, have been adopted by a great many people in this country and throughout the world. The diet consists almost exclusively of cooked foods, as raw foods are felt to be difficult to digest and too cooling for the system. A minimum of fruits is consumed, less than 5% of the diet, and most of those should be cooked. Dairy foods and eggs are usually avoided; the only animal products recommended are such whitefish as halibut, trout, and sole, and these are also kept to less than 5% of the diet. Thus it is primarily a vegetarian, almost vegan, diet, but it seems to contain more protein (from soy products and other types of beans) and nutrients than the standard vegetarian cuisine.

The macrobiotic meal includes between 50% and 60% whole cereal grains, such as brown rice, whole oats, millet, barley, corn, wheat berries, rye, and buckwheat. Flour products and baked goodies are avoided, and pastas and breads are eaten only occasionally. Vegetables make up about 20% to 25% of the meal; members of the nightshade family, such as potatoes, peppers, tomatoes, and eggplant, as well as avocados,

Macrobiotic Diet	
Includes	**Avoids**
Cooked whole grains	Meats
Cooked vegetables	Poultry
Legumes	Eggs
Soybean products	Dairy foods
Cooked beans	Sugar
Tofu	Nightshade
Tempeh	vegetables
Pickled vegetables	Yams and sweet
Sea vegetables	potatoes
Soups	Spinach
Bancha twig tea	Avocado
Whitefish (less than 5%)	Fruit juices
Cooked fruit (less than 5%)	Baked goods

spinach, yams, and sweet potatoes, are all avoided. Beans and sea vegetables (seaweeds) are suggested to complement the meal, making up 5% to 10% of its quantity. The primary beans eaten are adzukis, lentils, and garbanzos, along with such fermented soybean products as tofu, tempeh, and miso. Most other beans can be eaten occasionally in this diet. Some seeds, nuts, and vegetable oils may be used. Soups and "wilted" (slightly steamed) salads can also be eaten, constituting about 5% of the meal. Such other exotic foods as umeboshi plums (and other pickled foods, such as daikon radish and ginger, usually eaten at the end of a meal to aid digestion), tamari soy sauce, sesame salt (gomasio), and bancha twig tea are also included.

Overall, these are basic and wholesome foods, but the diet is somewhat controversial. There is limited research on macrobiotic eating, but the few studies available point to possible problems with vitamin D and vitamin B12 deficiency, particularly in infancy, childhood, and adolescence. I am in favor of nutritional supplementation to help avoid these possible problems. On the positive side, though, this diet is considered to have a nice overall balance. It provides a lot of vitamins and minerals and is good in complex carbohydrates and fiber. The protein content is usually adequate, and the fat content is low. By "balanced," I also mean that a majority of the foods are from the

center of the food spectrum, such as vegetables and whole grains, with a minimum of foods from the extremes, such as fruits and sugars (which are more cooling) and the meat and dairy foods (which are more stimulating). Also, herbs and spices, such as garlic, onions, and cayenne are considered too stimulating. From the viewpoint of Eastern philosophy, this diet is felt to be a good balance of yin and yang and to be stabilizing, nourishing, and healing. With the avoidance of chemicals, sugars, refined foods, and high-fat foods, it is a good step toward a more balanced and healthful diet for many Americans.

Many readers of my first book, *Staying Healthy with the Seasons,* felt it recommended a macrobiotic diet, but it was liberal macrobiotics at most. Whole grains and vegetables are the mainstay of a healthy diet. They provide wholesome fuel without being too rich and clogging for the finely tuned body machine. But I believe that fruits, salads, and more raw foods can be tolerated well, especially in warmer climates or in late spring and summer. These are often richer in many nutrients that might be lost during cooking and other preparations. Also, many of the special foods recommended in the strict macrobiotic diet are not readily available locally, making it difficult for macrobiotic practitioners everywhere to eat a similar diet. Furthermore, I am an advocate of juice fasting, a process that macrobiotics does not support; fasting may be an extreme practice, but I feel it is a useful therapeutic tool in many situations.

Another drawback to macrobiotics, especially for Americans, is that it is sometimes served with a whole philosophy—almost a religion, if you will—a way of life that goes along with the diet. Given this book's scope on nutrition, I cannot get into a discussion of this philosophy here, but for many people it can become a psychological barrier against acceptance of the dietary principles. With some of its proponents and in much of its literature, there is almost a fanaticism that this system will solve many problems and difficulties in the world. Although much has been written about the theory that a macrobiotic diet can help cure many diseases, including cancer, there is limited evidence in this area. A review by researchers at Columbia University published in 2001 in *The Journal of Nutrition* suggested that higher phytoestrogen intake and slightly lower circulating estrogen levels in women who follow a macrobiotic diet might be associated with a lower risk of breast cancer. This suggestion makes sense to me, and in fact many of the dietary factors recommended by a macrobiotic diet seem consistent to me with prevention of cancer and other chronic diseases.

Overall, I am much more supportive than otherwise of a macrobiotic-type diet. Except for my period as a raw-fooder, my own diet through the years has been closer to macrobiotic than to any other type, although I usually eat more raw vegetables and fruits than that diet allows. I feel that it has a lot to offer, including some sound, wholesome information, that may provide many Westerners with an improved sense of health, peace, and well-being, as well as health-care savings from reduced disease.

Noodletarian Diet: 21ST-Century Update by Bethany Argisle

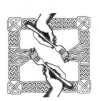

Noodletarian is a term coined by Bethany Argisle for people who love noodles as a main part of the diet.

For me, eating is an adventure, a joy. In my lifetime, I have investigated many styles of appetite fulfillment, from pablum to school cafeteria food, from steak tartare to caviar, from McDonald's to Julia Child's—to now, a healthy, low-fat diet of natural and organic foods.

As a young child my mother served me elbow marcaroni with melted butter, salt and pepper, and a little sprinkle of Parmesean cheese. This lacto-ovo cuisine led me to realize that well-informed, sincere, earnest food combining techniques coupled with soul satisfaction were the keys to my now evolved noodletarian diet.

The noodle, through history and myriad cultures, has become a universal means of food communication and is included in all types of diets, even wheat-free diets, since there are now many products available for people with reactions to wheat. Fresh-made noodles are delightful, yet in the cupboard, well-sealed packages seem to have a shelf life that future archaeologists may find themselves researching and cataloging.

Some say noodles themselves aren't so healthy, too much starch in our low-carb craze. Yet, they can be the basis of a healthy dish with fresh tomato sauce and vegetables added. And there are many healthier versions, such as oat bran noodles, rice sticks, black squid noodles, beet red noodles, and my all time favorite, chocolate noodles (well, maybe they're not as healthy). There are many, many shapes and textures. Noodles are high-performance food and in many cultures have been the very survival of the people. Noodles can be eaten as leftovers, served in the best restaurants, as a side dish, or for a quality, high-performance, athletic endurance meal. In fact, I have hardly met a person who didn't like noodles in one form or another.

The elements for noodletarians are basic. First, the choice is made of the type of noodles and this in itself can be quite an adventure. Then, good water—with a bit of sea salt in the water. Next, the water is boiled and then the noodles are added, or in some cultures, grain, cornmeal, or gruel is used.

When the noodle is al dente, the flame is turned off, the noodle is drained and rinsed, when appropriate, and other ingredients can be added for flavor, for perfect food combining, and for ultimate digestion. If you are very, very aware, you'll note that it doesn't mess up your kitchen much to make a one-dish meal.

There are as many methods of eating noodles as there are shapes and types of noodles; some swear by the fork, some use a wedge of bread, and others delve deftly with chopsticks. Noodles seem to be available for all types of budgets and can be eaten at any meal of the day; I have even had noodle pancakes.

Noodles are an emotional food with savorability enhanced by many other ingredients. Whoever invented noodles hit upon another food language. Noodles are the glue (the paste, quite literally) that holds the bones of the soul together, while chocolate, another food language component, is the putty (often quite nutty) which seeps into the breaks of the heart and seals them.

Whereas lamb, beef, or chicken, or even tofu, used to be in the center of my plate, now noodles sit in an Argisle pile in front of me—with salad or a vegetable on the side. As history changes, it appears our diets do, too. We have come a long way from food gathering in the forests and fields, to pushing our carts down the aisle, or have we?

KELP NOODLES

I recently discovered kelp noodles from the Sea Tangle Noodle Company. These noodles have low carbohydrates and are wheat free. The ingredients used in these noodles are kelp, water, and sodium alginate from sea kelp. They look like plastic, require refrigeration, and need no cooking. These noodles are clear in appearance and have no flavor of their own; they are very similar in form to a mung bean thread or rice noodle, yet with minimal carbohydrates.

From crunchy to tender, they can be added to a soup, a stir-fry, or placed in a divine noodle salad. Include your favorite ingredient combinations; my godson Orion added tamari, sesame oil, cucumber, ginger, and lemon juice with seasoned tofu that was thinly sliced—very satisfying. Kelp noodles are also wonderful heated and served with spaghetti sauce. Sea tangle, also called gonpo, is another name for certain varieties of sea vegetables, such as kombu and kelp. There are dishes prepared from oceanic plants under the name of "sea tangles"; however, these are not the same as kelp noodles, which are derived from, not solely, kelp.

For the sake of nutritionists and students everywhere, here are the noodle's nutritional values:

Based on a 2,000 calorie diet
Serving size: 4 ounces
Servings per container: 3
Cholesterol: 0
Calories: 6
Total Carbohydrates: 1 gram
Dietary Fiber: 1 gram
Calcium: 15% DV
Sodium: 35 mg
Iron: 4% DV

If you wish to enjoy these cleansing and palate-pleasing kelp noodles, look for them, or request them, at your local health food market; they can also be found in some Korean markets. Alternately, you can order them from the Sea Tangle Noodle Company (530 Quarry Road, San Marcos, CA 92069; 760-744-3066) in 12-ounce bags.

PURE LENTIL BEAN PASTA

Another one of my favorite noodles products is Papadini Hi-Protein Pure Lentil Bean Pasta from Adrienne's Gourmet Foods. This is a revolutionary new source of nutrition that is so unique it has been awarded a U.S. patent. This pasta has a rich flavor and provides significant amounts of protein, complex carbohydrates, and soluble fiber; it cooks quicker than semolina and is terrific tossed warm into a salad, dressed, or by itself with one or two veggies. You can find this pasta on the web at at Adrienne's Gourmet Foods' website, www.adriennes.com/pasta.htm.

100% SOBA

Clearspring's 100% Soba is wheat-free noodles made from whole buckwheat flour and sea salt. Buckwheat is tolerated well by most people who have reactions to wheat. The soba noodle is originally from Japan. These soba noodles are a product of the United Kingdom, and not only are they tasty, they are organic as well. Suggested preparation: Cook noodles with miso or soy sauce broth, and add tempura, vegetables, or tofu. Garnish with green onions. To learn more about these noodles, visit Clearspring's website, www.clearspring.co.uk.

Raw Foods

A raw food diet is an interesting concept and potentially very healthy or healing for those who have congestive maladies. It basically consists of uncooked whole foods. Foods are eaten in their uncooked, most potentially nutritious state, with the vital elements of Nature still contained in them. The sun's energy, water, and nutrients from the Earth invigorate fruits, vegetables, legumes, nuts, and seeds. Sprouted beans and seeds are often a nutritious component of the diet. Sprouted grains can be made into breads and wafers. Raw (unpasteurized) milk products may be used. Water, fresh juices, and sun teas are the main drinks in this diet. All stimulants, chemicals, and alcoholic beverages are avoided.

Although this diet can be healthy and adventurous, unless it is astutely balanced, it is not good for long periods of time. It can provide good vitality and nutrient content, but it is usually low in protein, calcium, and iron—all of which could lead to problems in the long run. Also, with no heat added to the foods and an avoidance of the more concentrated and heat-producing foods, the body could become cold. People in warmer climates, those who are overweight, or those with good body heat are more likely to do well on this diet. Many people lose weight on a raw foods diet. Proper chewing and good digestion help with this diet; some people experience more difficulty in their digestive tract than on a more cooked diet, however.

For one spring and summer, I ate a completely raw food diet—lots of fresh fruit and vegetable juices, blended fruit shakes, sprouts and vegetable salads, nuts and seeds, and a special treat I used to call "nice cream," made solely from frozen fruit, such as bananas or berries, put through a Champion juicer. The neighborhood kids used to come running to see me when they heard Dr. Elson was making "nice cream." During that particular dietary experience, I felt great, very light and more open spiritually. I weighed the least I have in my adult life, although I definitely felt less grounded—more spacey you might say—than when on a more cooked diet, and my intestines were very active and somewhat gassy. In lecturing about nutrition and fasting, I have talked to many people who eat a raw food diet, often for a period of from 1 to 3 years. They speak highly of their experiences and especially how healthy and alive they feel. The raw foods diet is really the "living food" diet. It definitely goes against the flow of Western (and most) dietary traditions, but for those with an adventurous spirit who want to lighten up and cleanse themselves on deeper levels, it is something to try. Many of the same concerns must be watched for as on the vegan diet.

Natural Hygiene

The so-called natural hygiene diet is not the latest fad but an ancient system of a raw foods diet supported by cleansing the colon and occasional fasting. This program and philosophy began with the Essenes, an ancient tribe of Jewish scholars. They believed in preparation for the Messiah via detoxification of their bodies, minds, and spirits through clean living and keeping the body free of waste. This pure diet and evolved lifestyle is written about in the *Essene Gospel of Peace,* by Edmond Bordeaux Szekely, and in other texts. The natural hygiene diet was repopularized in

the 1930s in Germany and has had its followers in Europe and America since that time. I review more of the Essenes' concepts and practices of natural hygiene in chapter 18, Detoxification and Cleansing Programs, in the sections "General Detoxification and Cleansing" and "Fasting and Juice Cleansing," on pages 741 and 769, respectively, and in the Futureword under "Immortality and Beyond."

Fruitarian

There are some people who attempt to subsist solely on Nature's true gift of nourishment—fruits. But fruits do not contain all the nutrients that human beings need to live, at least not on a long-term basis. Their protein content is very low, and many of the B vitamins, iron, calcium, magnesium, and other minerals are scarce in fruits. They are also deficient in fats, although if the seeds of the fruits are eaten, the essential fatty acids, the only fats that are truly needed, can be obtained. Overall, a fruitarian diet is limited, and it is generally considered poor nutrition. It can be invigorating and purifying on a short-term basis, about a week or so at the most; staying on such a diet any longer than that could be dangerous.

Fasting

True fasting is consuming only water—and air, of course. This provides a strong inner experience, but I believe that it should be done only under certain circumstances and ideally with the guidance and supervision of a physician or experienced nutritionist. However, a surprising number of people have done water fasting successfully for short periods of time on their own. It is undertaken basically as a detoxification-cleansing-purifying process. It is not really a diet, because it does not provide any nutrients.

Juice fasting is more common, provides more nutrients, and can be undertaken for a much longer period than water fasting, but it is still deficient in total nutrition. Drinking only fruit and vegetable juices can be done for several days, 1 or 2 weeks, or even longer; the longer fasting is done, the more problems (called "cleansing reactions" by those experiencing them) and deficiencies may be experienced. I have known people who have fasted for longer than

2 months and have personally monitored some patients through 30-day fasts, most often on the Master Cleanser, or lemonade, diet. This fast and others, as well as the how-tos of fasting, are discussed in many books on the subject, including my first book, *Staying Healthy with the Seasons,* and my book *The New Detox Diet.*

The fasting process is best used as a means of transformation to enhance the potential for change in habits and lifestyle during the reevaluation and detoxification period. Weight is usually lost during the process, although I do not suggest fasting as a weight-loss diet. I feel that it is among the best natural therapeutic tools available to the healing arts, given the right situation. Resting from foods and letting the body process what is already stored is the perfect balance to the typical excessive and congestive way of eating. Body-organ-cell congestion comes from eating more fat and protein foods than we need. I have called fasting, or the cleansing process, the "missing link" in the American diet.

Weight Reduction

Weight-loss diets come and go by the hundreds. Every year at least half a dozen new diets become popular with Americans, who are always looking for the latest, greatest, shortest route to that trim figure. There is usually at least one diet book on the best-seller list, and publishers are always on the lookout for a hot new book that can make a few million dollars creating wallet weight loss.

There is no single specific type of reducing diet but a whole collection of diets that either reduce calories, restructure eating habits, or add a special food that cuts fat. I will not discuss all of them here; several are described in some of the therapeutic diets in part 4 of this book, and most specifically in the weight loss section on page 684 in chapter 17, Medical Treatment Programs. Overall, those who are overweight or who easily put on extra pounds need to think of "diet" as a basic wholesome daily food intake, rather than a special project to be struggled through on occasion until returning to the enjoyable habitual way of eating that created the body that necessitated the original struggle.

Very simply, for the average overweight person, the best diet to reduce weight will provide fewer calories and burn more with exercise: less intake plus more output equals decreased mass, or "sweat equity." Eating small meals and drinking lots of water helps. Avoiding breads, sweets, dairy foods, and excess fats and oils will greatly reduce calories. Low-calorie fruit or vegetable snacks are best. Importantly, though, simple meals of lean proteins and lots of vegetables provide a good level of nutrients, enhance digestion and metabolism, and, if not overdone, will cause us to burn more calories and stored fat and thus reduce weight. Developing good shopping and eating habits to change the basic diet is the only way to create the body we want in the long run.

Warrior's

The *warrior's diet* is a term that I have used to describe the way I often eat, especially on the days when I am busy and want to be productive. This diet consists of small meals or snacks eaten every 2 to 3 hours throughout the day. These are simple meals and often only simple foods (or "mono" meals), such as a handful of almonds or sunflower seeds, 1 or 2 apples, carrots or celery sticks, crackers with avocado, or a bowl of rice with sprouts or cooked beans. Consuming the contents of 1 small to medium bowl should generate sufficient fuel to continue energetically along the day's path.

A warrior is always ready for action, with energy available whenever he or she is called. Big meals or lots of different foods can act as a mental and physical sedative, as they cause a lot of energy and blood to be shunted to the abdomen (liver, stomach, intestines) to digest and assimilate food. The warrior eats large meals only in celebration or ritual, or given modern society, at the end of a workday to relax at home alone or with friends or family. At this time, we can let go more of physical concerns and tensions, be more aware of inner levels, and digest a meal and the day's experiences.

The warrior's concept is that food is our fuel; we give our body what it needs for continued combustion of energy. When referring to being a warrior, I am talking about embracing the challenges of life with some feeling or passion. Food nourishment should support this and not devitalize us or generate excess aggressiveness or moodiness. Because I am a strong supporter of peace and positive action, I think of the warrior as one who does battle not with others but rather with life, the main struggle being to conquer our own weaknesses. Illness is, in a sense, succumbing to that battle; from a nutritional standpoint, when we take in too much, we may block the energy that is needed to cope with stress, and then we get stuck in the specifics of the battle, such as conflict with a person or job. Keeping ourselves clear through light and simple eating allows our full energy to be available to us so that we can be the true "spiritual warriors" or "spiritual athletes" we were intended to be.

Natural Foods

The natural or whole foods diet is the original native or tribal diet intrinsic to all cultures prior to the industrial age. What was available from Nature varied according to the area of the world, but all people cultivated their own food or gathered or captured wild vegetable and animal foods. Whatever the culture—North or South American Indian, Mexican, African, Mediterranean, European, or Asian—the diets consisted of similar food components. The foods that Nature provided were used directly and in a multitude of ways to feed all the people. And Nature still provides all the world's people with the best possible diet when we use our land harmoniously and productively, as caretakers cultivating respect for Earth's resources.

The whole-grain cereals, such as wheat, rice, and corn, have been and still are the predominant cultivated foods on Earth. Fruits and nuts can be cultivated and gathered from the trees. Fruits were often a special treat, eaten freshly picked, ripe, and juicy. Vegetables could be grown in abundance—the greens, legumes, and root vegetables alike. Most native cultures knew to mix their grains and legumes or seeds together for complete protein nourishment, likely through instincts and experience. Most of these cultures, however, were not vegetarian, although their diets consisted largely of vegetable nutrition. Fish was a good source of protein for the tribes who lived near big lakes or streams or by the ocean. The wild birds or animals, when found, provided an important source of food for some people, according to the skills of their hunters. Water or brews from their foods were drunk freely. And there was occasional fasting from foods, either voluntarily or because availability was low. This may have helped keep the people in balance—and

most definitely sustained their reverence and appreciation of food.

Nowadays, a "natural foods" diet is followed by many people. The health food industry and local farmers' markets have grown greatly, and many stores provide the wholesome or basic foods as Nature provides them; we may find bags, boxes, or bins containing a variety of grains, beans, nuts, seeds, and so on, at most markets. Fruits and vegetables are usually widely available, and some natural food stores attempt to find or specialize in organic produce, as the natural foods diet is as low as possible in chemical sprays. It also avoids food additives and prefabricated and refined foods with extra sugars, salts, flavorings, and chemicals added to increase shelf life and to appeal to the addicted taste buds of the industrial-age consumer. The natural food diet is rich in natural flavors, colors, and aromas. Foods are prepared so that the flavor of each food can be tasted, and that usually means with the least amount of tampering. Herbs and spices may be used to enhance flavor when desired.

I am particularly enthusiastic about this topic, because these are the dietary principles that I follow and advocate—*eating foods as wholesome, as chemical free, and as much from the local environment as possible.* Foods are chosen for their quality, even though the more wholesome foods may be slightly more expensive. When we prepare our own foods and eat a more vegetarian diet, the average cost is usually lower than that of the typical American diet, high in fats and sugar, and our health-care costs are typically less as well. If a minimum of animal foods is eaten, we should take special care to get sufficient protein, calcium, iron, zinc, and vitamin B12. A natural foods diet can be omnivorous or vegetarian; if properly balanced, it provides a good level of all the nutrients we need for the body to function optimally.

Paleolithic (Hunter-Gatherer)

This is among the more fascinating of the diet plans of recent years. And yet, it is based on some of the most ancient, evolutionary eating patterns—the "caveman" or "caveperson" diet. (This is not to be confused with the dinosaur era, which was some 70 million years ago.) Actually, these peoples belonged to nomadic tribes and mainly used caves for winter shelter. This hunter-gatherer diet of the Paleolithic humans, our ancestors who inhabited Earth from 2.5 million to 10,000 years ago, has been carried on in many tribal cultures. Nowadays, however, it is essentially only a few of that ancient species of humankind that continues to hunt wild game and gather their foods (fruits, vegetables, nuts, and seeds) as available on a seasonal basis.

Recent archeological findings suggest that these ancient ancestors were a healthy bunch—tall, with strong bones and body structures like modern-day athletes—they appear to be most similar to us regarding stature, and as long as they survived accidents, infections, and childbirth, their longevity was similar to ours, but with much less chronic degenerative disease. Further anthropological studies suggest some of the food and life habits of these early human beings: They had regular vigorous exercise through hunting and gathering their food for survival. Flesh foods provided their proteins, seeds and nuts their oils. Fruits and berries were available for quick energy, and some starchy vegetable tubers provided more complex carbohydrate fuel.

Boyd Eaton, MD, on faculty at the Department of Anthropology at Emory University in Atlanta, Georgia, has been studying Paleolithic eating patterns since the late 1970s. His publications in this area have also become the springboard for involvement of several other researchers, including Loren Cordain, PhD, on faculty at the Department of Health and Exercise Science at Colorado State University, to get involved in Paleolithic research. What these investigators have discovered about the Paleolithic diet is fascinating.

First, in terms of the macronutrients, protein intake was fairly high, at 19% to 35% of total calories. Moreover, protein foods always included meat. There was a catch, however. Hunter-gatherer meat was wild game, and its total fat content was much lower than our domestically raised meat is today. Cordain and Eaton have compared Paleolithic meats to the wild caribou that still roam across Alaska and parts of Canada. Their percent body fat varies from a high of 16.6% in late fall (storing up energy for the winter) to a low of 2.9% in April. Nine months out of the year, it stays under 10%. By contrast, today's feedlot-raised cattle average about 30% fat. The saturated-fat content of wild game was also dramatically lower than the amount provided by today's domesticated animals.

The average for Alaskan wild caribou, about 11% of total calories, is believed to be comparable to the amount consumed by our ancestors.

Equally interesting in the fat category was 4 times greater intake of omega-3 fatty acids, and 1.5 times greater intake of monounsaturated fat in Paleolithic times. Nuts and seeds were eaten much more plentifully, and in their raw form, which maximized retention of these delicate fats. Except for honey, there were no refined grains or sugars in Paleolithic days. Berries and vegetables were eaten in much greater proportion and helped bump the daily fiber intake to about 3 times our present level of 10 to 15 grams.

As an overall approach to eating, this Paleolithic strategy has a lot to recommend it. Although it is higher in fat than many present-day health authorities recommend, the fat is of consistently high quality. The trend in today's research is to point the finger less and less at total fat, and more and more at problematic qualities in the fat we eat, including saturated fat, trans fat, and hydrogenated oils. These types of fat were either nonexistent or in more scarce supply in Paleolithic times. It is also impressive that fiber intake was kept fairly high (at 30–50 grams), despite high fat and protein levels. Fiber appears to be critically important for the health of the digestive tract and the regulation of blood sugar. But what about the specific foods that were hunted and gathered?

The average tribe's food consisted of about one-third hunted food to two-thirds gathered, so it was a primarily vegetarian diet that varied seasonally and had added high-protein, low-fat meats based on hunting success. Besides the various wild game available at that time, the majority of the food consumed consisted of the following uncultivated vegetable foods: beans, berries, bulbs, flowers, fruits, fungi, gums, leaves, melons, nuts, roots, seeds, stalks, and tubers. For most tribes, 10 to 20 common foods made up the diet staples, with possibly up to 50 other foods eaten less frequently. Herbs were also used, more as medicinals, often with different parts of the same plant gathered or used at different times of the year.

Interestingly, the evolution of our current diet began with the Neolithic revolution some 10,000 years ago. In the following 2,000 years, the population became more settled and rapidly began to increase. Organized agriculture began then, along with the increase in whole-grain foods, especially wheat. Animals were domesticated and sheep, goats, pigs, and cattle provided various meats and milks that have since been used throughout the centuries. Chickens and their eggs were also eaten. These new, richer, fattier foods are thought to be at the source of many of our chronic degenerative diseases. The whole-grain foods are also the more common allergenic foods, as are cow's milk and chicken eggs. This suggests that in an evolutionary sense, many of us have not yet genetically adapted to these foods.

The Industrial Revolution, only 200 years old, added another dimension to the modern diet—that of refined foods and the use of chemicals in foods. This big problem is discussed in greater detail in the following section, as well as in chapter 11, Food and the Earth. In the book *The Paleolithic Prescription,* Eaton and his coauthors suggest that "modern disease is a result of a mismatch of our genetic makeup and our lifestyle." Eaton calls the twentieth-century diseases "afflictions of affluence" or "diseases of civilization," including atherosclerosis, hypertension and heart disease, heart attacks and strokes, adult-onset diabetes, and cancer.

Following a hunter-gatherer diet is not an easy task in this day and age. Grains, both whole and refined, and milk products are readily available, and wheat and cow's milk are found in a great variety of commercial foods. The wild game and uncultivated vegetable foods are typically not found in supermarkets. Meats are domesticated as well as being high in fats and potential chemicals. Most grains and vegetables are cultivated and sprayed with pesticides and other chemicals. Although more organic foods and meats with lower concentrations of chemicals are now available in the marketplace, they are not always easy to find, and they are still not as devoid of chemicals and heavy metals as the foods of the preindustrial times. Thus it is a chore to adapt the diet and eat in a way that is close to our Paleolithic, Stone Age, Cro-Magnon ancestors, who had no real stoves or refrigerators, shopping carts for stores, or online orders—just the cool stream waters and their own industriousness.

Some suggestions for eating this more natural diet blend together Paleolithic nutrition with more modern foods. This clearly reduces fat intake and the incidences of many of the "diseases of civilization." We

should bake, roast, and steam foods instead of frying or sautéing them, and eating more raw, organic foods is helpful. We need to reduce the fatty meats and all processed meats as well as most of the whole milk products. We can eat a good breakfast of whole grains, fruit and juice, or skim milk. Lunch should be a healthful meal prepared and eaten at home or carried to work or school. It may include a protein like fish or poultry with vegetables or a sandwich and soup. Dinner is a lighter meal of raw salad and soup. Late eating is minimal and the main beverage is water. Many of these suggestions are incorporated into my ideal diet described in chapter 13, The Ideal Diet.

Exercise is as key an issue for good health as is diet. Our Paleolithic ancestors had a good level of physical activity incorporated into their daily lives. If we are tilling, planting, growing, and harvesting our own foods full-time, we all experience that similar benefit, especially if we do a little distance running as the ancient hunters did. Construction workers probably have that level of physical labor, although they are possibly not as aerobically active and are exposed to more noise, dust, and chemical pollution.

Most of us need to develop and maintain a lifelong exercise plan that blends with our more sedentary work lifestyles. This should include a natural seasonal variance that ideally coincides with the cycles of light and darkness in our area. The activity should be outdoors and energy expending during the warmer, lighter months; energy-gathering exercise, such as yoga, done indoors is best in the colder, darker times. The exercise program should provide a balance that leads us to our optimum weight, good strength, and adequate endurance—and should be an integral part of our life, as it was for most of our ancestors.

Industrialized

The industrialized diet is quite different from the natural foods and Paleolithic diets. By *industrialized,* I am referring not to the foods eaten by people who work in industry but to the trend of our times toward mass production and factory processing. The industrialized diet contains a large proportion of refined foods. Many of the basic grains and sugar-containing plants are stripped of their fiber and nutrients, leaving the concentrated sweet or starch powder that can be used to make or flavor other foods. Refined white flour and white sugar are the two basic components. In fact, it has been estimated that about 19% of our total caloric intake—about 380 calories—comes from white flour (bleached and stripped of its more nutritious parts, the germ and the bran). For processed sugars dumped into the daily diet, this number averages about 320 more calories (20 teaspoons!), bringing the grand total for these two nutritionally bankrupt foods to about 700 out of 2,000 calories a day or 30% of everything we eat. These new foods often have additives and preservatives to allow for packaging, shipping, and shelf life. They fit in with the mass production ideology and fast-paced lifestyles of not only the American culture but many other technological and urban cultures of the world. Rural farming peoples in the United States still tend to eat more basically and naturally, yet nowadays many poor people all over the world eat more inexpensive and refined foods.

An interesting fact is that when the industrial or refined foods diet was introduced to different tribal cultures throughout the world, a general degradation of their health followed, usually within a single generation. Tooth decay and diseases such as diabetes, cardiovascular disease, and cancer increased to levels that correlated with those in industrialized societies. Even recently, the breast cancer incidence in China, which was once much lower than in the United States, has risen quickly with their adoption of a more Westernized way of life. Dr. Weston Price, a dentist, studied native cultures eating such diets during the 1940s and compared them with like tribes who were still eating their classical diet. He reported on his own observations as well as the descriptions of the tribal people themselves regarding the changes they had experienced. This whole story is contained in his book *Nutrition and Physical Degeneration: A Comparison of Primitive and Modern Diets and Their Effects.*

Modern medicine and technology have made some fantastic advances that have affected the lives of almost every being on Earth, but the greatest dilemma now is how to balance these industrial changes with a healthier diet. The refined and fast food diet has been one of the greatest economic supporters of our currently expensive health-care system and has made the medical profession (and the pharmaceutical companies) wealthy, profiting from an increasingly diseased population. The dilemma, I believe, lies in the fact that the Western economic structure is dependent on mass production, corporations, fast food restaurant chains, and refined, packaged foods. The American consumer is pushed to consume these products in even greater quantities, as more are being produced all the time. It is possible that if more people cultivate foods and go back (or ahead) to eating more natural, chemical-free foods, it will either bankrupt or totally transform the current big business economy, and health-care systems

---

Problems Associated with the Standard American Diet

Nutritional Problems	Other Problems and Diseases
High calorie	Obesity
Low nutrient	Anemia, immune problems, tooth decay
Low fiber	Atherosclerosis, digestive problems, colon cancer
High fat	Obesity, coronary artery disease
Excess saturated fat	High blood pressure, atherosclerosis, coronary artery disease
Excess hydrogenated oils	Heart attacks, atherosclerosis
High protein	Kidney problems, strokes
Excess salt	Vascular insufficiency
Excess sugar	Diabetes, insulin resistance
Excess alcohol	Breast cancer, cardiovascular disease, liver disease
Excess meats	Prostate cancer, colon cancer, breast cancer
High vitamin D	Hypercalcemia
Excess phosphorus	Bone disease

would have to change in order to survive; plus, there would be room for the small farmers who are now going bankrupt.

But there is a lot of resistance and dollars preventing that from happening. Billions are poured into advertising to brainwash people into buying and eating these nonfoods. Also, sweet and salty flavors are addicting, making it harder for the people eating all those prefabricated snack foods to eat more naturally and to enjoy it. I do not have the answer to this dilemma (maybe more advertising for apples and sunflower seeds) other than exposing these issues in writing this book. Time will tell. Change is usually slow, and adaptability and survival are timeless. It is ultimately an individual choice. As more of us choose to eat more healthfully, more new and natural products will be developed and made available. Good luck to all of us.

CULTURAL DIETS

In my quest for books that deal with the different types of diets and dietary patterns of the many and varying cultures around the globe, I have found little contemporary information. I would like to see more research into cultural diets, especially their relationship to diseases within a culture so that we can attain a more global knowledge of diet and health. Here I share my knowledge of these diets and some theories as to their strengths and weaknesses, related deficiency problems, and supportive nutrients that might make them more complete. Obviously I cannot discuss each and every culture around the world; that would require a whole book in itself (which I hope someone will write). Rather, I discuss some commonly encountered and intriguing ethnic diets. My nutritional portrayals are rather broad and generalized, however, because even within each country the diet may vary greatly from north to south or from province to province based on the climate, local populations living within that region, and available foods. For example, in China, the northern provinces tend toward a diet containing spicier foods, more meat products, and more wheat than in the southern provinces, where a milder diet is consumed, with more rice, greens and other vegetables, special fruits, and generally less meat.

Also, within each nation, the diet of poorer people is usually healthier than that of the middle or wealthier classes. Rather than the richer diet of affluence, which may include more meat, dairy foods, coffee, and sugar, the poorer rural populations (the city poor, more often consume a highly refined and malnourished diet as in the U.S.) still consume the more traditional and natural foods—local grains, vegetables, and fruits—in a generally healthy balance. This factor is less apparent in the United States, however, where the poor-quality and refined foods so readily available in local stores and supermarkets are accessible to nearly the entire population. Happily though, in most cultures there is an improved nutritional awareness with a return, even in the affluent population, to a more wholesome, balanced, and natural diet. Let us make sure that this continues and grows.

In reviewing this section on international dietary issues, Eleonora Manzolini, a traveling cuisine artist who contributed to this original section, offers a different observation as follows. It used to be true that more affluent people throughout the world had access to richer foods and in general more food, but the food was of good quality and natural. Today, globalization of the multinational corporations has created a situation in Western and Westernized countries that is increasingly similar to that of the United States. Advertising for fast foods, prepackaged, microwavable meals, and all kinds of snacks and sugary sodas is rampant, and the more affluent and educated people are the ones who have the tools to resist all that, and the time to prepare wholesome meals or the means to pay someone to do it for them, or to go to expensive restaurants that use higher quality ingredients. The rural population has it better, because natural wholesome foods are available to them, although the young people in most Western countries do not want to work on the farm anymore, and they watch television that tells them that it is cool to go to MacDonald's. The European community has resisted genetically modified (GM) foods and other blatantly unhealthy practices that the globalized "food" manufacturing corporations want to impose, but still the trend is not a healthy one.

You may want to check out the slow food movement. It is a movement that started in Italy with the purpose to oppose the fast food industry. It has now grown into an international organization, Slow Food, that is very well-known in the United States, and Slow Foods USA is based in New York. They have cookbooks, a magazine, and member restaurants, and they advocate growing our own food organically and processing it according to ancient traditions. You may want to check out www.slowfood.com.

I really don't think that we can keep saying that the poor eat better. The poor eat less, that's for sure, because they don't have the money to buy as much, but the quality of what they eat is also poor, and if we are talking nations, the poor nations, such as most of Africa, are literally starving from deficiency diseases while we are overconsuming junk and dying from diseases of affluence.

WESTERN DIETS

The so-called Western diet is that of the Westernized cultures, including Australia, Canada, many European countries, New Zealand, and the United States. Although the diets of these cultures are similar, let's first look at the modern North American diet. Many concerns about this diet and the problems that arise from its consumption also plague other Westernized countries. Many European populations eat a diet similar to the North American diet, although it is somewhat shaped around each country's basic cultural practices. For example, people in Australia and New Zealand probably consume even more meat and milk products than we do in the United States; however, their meats and animals are not raised with added hormones, which New Zealand in particular has laws against, as well as strict rules on the use of chemicals in foods. Most have a high intake of red meat, fat, sodium as well as regular alcohol use. (Most Anglo-Saxon populations consume a lot of alcohol and process it badly.) The meat consumption rates in New Zealand, Australia, and the Scandinavian countries, as well as in some South American countries (such as Argentina, Brazil, and Venezuela) are among the highest in the world. The incidence of the diseases generated by this food component correlates with its intake. Many Europeans consume less meat and fats (maybe other than the French and Germans), often as much sugar and alcohol, and definitely more tobacco, which all generate their own diseases.

The Western dietary influence affects many cultures. Technological advances can bring benefits to everyone, but sometimes the time-saving, mass-processing chemical preservation of food is not in the best interest of nutrition. The health of people of all cultures can be affected by sweeter or saltier foods, or new and different foods altogether. We all like change, especially if it appears to be a step up. But often it is not (see the previous discussion of the industrialized diet on page 369 of this chapter). Eating refined flour or sugar products may be all right occasionally, but the natural, wholesome, and homemade foods are better. Although these refined foods might be tastier, easier to chew, or a status symbol, the trouble begins when they replace the basic staples of the diet.

North American

Although the North American diet varies regionally and culturally, I focus here on the common trends that cross over and influence so much of the population. The Canadian diet, in my understanding, is similar to that of the United States. Diet-linked diseases that are common in both countries similarly affect immigrants, even though those diseases may be rare in their native lands. This has been demonstrated in studies of the incidence of breast cancer among Japanese women living in the United States, of colon cancer among Asians, and of diabetes among Japanese men living in the Pacific Northwest, to give a few examples.

All the factors I mentioned earlier under the industrialized diet apply particularly to the North American diet, which has been most affected by technology in the food industry. The evolution in the tastes of the average food consumer has involved a significant desensitization to the natural flavors in food. Many modern consumers are attracted to the rich taste and smells of fatty meats and fried oily foods, salty and sugary snacks, artificial flavorings and additives, and coffee, colas, and other stimulating beverages. To speak of the refined food diet is actually a contradiction in terms, as this does not represent a "refined" taste at all, but taste buds that need to be knocked with a sledgehammer to wake up. Many nutritionists consider such refined flour products as breads, pastries, and doughnuts as well as the refined sugary goodies like cereals and sodas as hardly foods at all. It is difficult for people used to these processed foods to experience much enjoyment or psychological satisfaction from a simple meal of rice and vegetables, with or without some animal protein. The diet of our culture has become an "anticultural" diet—one that our ancestors would definitely not have approved.

How processed the diet is varies according to the quantities of fast foods, junk foods, sweets, sodas, and other "dead" foods consumed. Teenagers are often the worst offenders, eating too much of these foods and little of anything else. Some refined breads and pastas or occasional sodas, sweets, or fatty meats will not hurt most people, but when they become the predominant foods in the diet, it is poor nutrition. It is among the greatest sins of the U.S. health-care system that doctors so readily accept and support (often simply by not condemning) the industrialized American diet. With awareness of and attention to these problem areas, we can make our nation's diet healthier.

There are also some positive aspects of the American diet. There are many wonderful foods available to nourish us. We grow all types of grains, vegetables, legumes, nuts, and fruits and raise cattle and other animals for milk, eggs, and meats. (The main concern with all of these foods is the chemicals used in growing and raising them, however, and the impact on sustainability of the Earth and our future.) **We can certainly choose most of our foods in their more nourishing, untreated and unprocessed state.** Another positive aspect is the growth patterns that our children develop from eating the typical protein- and calcium-rich diet. North Americans are growing bigger and stronger with each generation, and the average height of the population continues to rise as well.

With the change in our taste for foods that has occurred throughout the twentieth century, there has been a decrease in the consumption of fresh fruits and vegetables and the complex carbohydrates, with an accompanying decrease in fiber intake and an increase in the consumption of salt, sugars, and fat. This eating pattern, with its overall increase in calories and decrease in nutrition, is associated with many chronic diseases, such as obesity, diabetes, atherosclerosis, cardiac disease, and a variety of cancers, as well as liver disease and nervous system problems from alcohol abuse.

Each of these potentially negative dietary choices contributes to specific pathogenic processes. First, the standard North American diet provides less nutrition per calorie consumed than does a diet of natural foods. The body needs a certain amount of nourishment to function. The high amounts of white sugar and refined flour in the current American diet provide useless calories with few nutrients. Therefore we require more food on this diet to obtain all the needed nutrients. This is a crucial aspect underlying one of America's biggest problems: obesity. Refer to the weight-loss program on page 684 in chapter 17, Medical Treatment Programs, where you will see the many diseases associated with obesity. It is often the psychological impact that both causes and worsens this problem, influencing our diet, self-esteem, and inability to change, and the subsequent effects on our health and the costs of dealing with chronic diseases. It is clear that improving the diet both lessens the diseases and the costs of aging.

The decreased consumption of vegetable and complex carbohydrates foods means a lower intake of vitamins, minerals, and fiber. This lack of fiber has significant adverse effects on digestive function, which may lead to such colon diseases as diverticulitis and colon cancer. The decrease in nutrient intake resulting from an unbalanced diet with a lot of empty-calorie foods may lead to a wide variety of depletion and deficiency symptoms and diseases. This may occur in the diets of both the poor and the rich of the U.S. population.

Higher protein levels, especially from the protein-concentrated meat foods, may contribute to kidney problems, hypertension, and an increased risk for certain cancers, although this has not been well documented. The dairy foods may also cause digestive problems because of many adults' inability to properly utilize them (due to lactose intolerance), as well as common allergy or hypersensitivity reactions to milk. Another concern is with the chemicals fed to dairy cows that may then end up in the milk supply. At about 6 months of age, cattle are commonly injected with slow-release pellets of estrogen, which can speed up growth and add 40 to 50 pounds by the time of slaughter. About 0.25 pound of antibiotics is also commonly added to their daily feed to help prevent infection related to their unnatural and unhealthy feedlot environment. Thus, many of us are exposed to drugs and hormones, which can cause side effects and allergic reactions.

Dairy foods add more saturated fats to the diet unless only nonfat products are used. The higher calcium content of milk can be helpful, but the extra vitamin D intake can cause problems when combined with even higher phosphorus ingestion from more meats and carbonated beverages. This mixture of nutrients affects bone metabolism and may be a major factor in osteoporosis. Maintaining adequate calcium intake while keeping it in balance with phosphorus is probably important in this regard.

The three aspects of the American diet that have received the most attention are salt, red meats, and fats. Salt restriction is often suggested for people only after they are diagnosed with high blood pressure, but there should be attention to avoiding high-salt foods and reducing total sodium intake (and raising potassium, calcium, and magnesium intake) before this problem arises. Salt can contribute not only to high blood pressure but also to kidney and heart disease. Salt is contained in so many foods, often hidden, that we may need to read labels and avoid certain restaurant foods to really reduce the intake of sodium.

Eating red meat—the cooked muscles (and organs) of cattle, sheep, or pigs—is both a nutritional and a philosophical issue. Nutritionally, these meats (especially the domesticated, overfed animals) contain a high amount of fat, and regular consumption of meats may add to an already fatty diet. Meats are high in protein, phosphorus, and usually sodium, and are low in fiber—all of which may contribute to other difficulties. Meats, of course, do provide nourishment; we just need to moderate their intake and, for most people, increase the consumption of water and vegetables.

Some thinkers have postulated the interesting idea of an association between meat eating and war. Throughout history, meat eating has been correlated with hunting, fighting, conquering, and a desire for power. Eating meats seems to stimulate aggressiveness, hostility, and competitive feelings. Now that most people do not hunt for food, meat consumption may stimulate these same feelings of aggressiveness,

which they may take to the streets, to jobs, or to the home and their families. In contrast, the vegetarian diet has typically been associated with peace and nonresistance and a general respect for life, as manifested in a spiritual sense of a connection to all living beings. This is seen in the peoples of India and exemplified by the life of Mahatma Gandhi. Maybe we'll need to watch the next 50 years to assess whether a reduction in animal meat consumption will be met with less war and greater planetary harmony, an interesting postulate to which many would agree. As for fat, meats and milk products contribute to our total fat intake. Vegetable oils are all fat, but of greater concern are the hydrogenated fats, which may contribute more specifically to disease. The use of fats in cooked or fried foods, in baked goods, and in margarine has greatly increased since the mid- twentieth century; the trend should be in the other direction, however. Fats in the diet contribute specifically to increased cholesterol levels, atherosclerosis, cardiovascular disease, and many types of cancer, particularly cancer of the breast, colon, prostate, and uterus. Atherosclerosis, or clogging of the arteries with fatty plaque, is the basic process that contributes to all kinds of cardiovascular diseases. **Reducing total fat intake is probably the most important step to creating a healthier diet.**

Overall, how can the American diet be improved so that it will nourish a healthy and long-lived people? What can we do with this diet based on quick eating, fast preparation, microwave meals, stop-and-go diets; the diet we can fit between two pieces of white bread; the diet we can eat with one hand while driving our car or working at our desk; this processed, refined, junk food, high-sodium, high-fat diet; this diet that generates death more than life? I suggest going back to the basics, back to Nature, back to the garden.

Getting back to the basics means learning to take the time to shop for (or grow) and prepare, as well as to sit down and eat, wholesome nourishing meals— to generally be more conscious and conscientious with the diet. This is a tough request for a busy population that seems to always be trying to catch up with their bills and credit cards. Believe me, it is worth the price, though, because we will feel better longer and be more productive, and not spend our life savings on disease care.

22 Suggestions for Making the American Diet Healthier

1. Consume less low-quality fat.
2. Consume less red meat, lunch meat, bacon, ham, and so on.
3. Consume less milk and milk products.
4. Consume less fried foods.
5. Consume less hydrogenated oils.
6. Eat fewer refined flour products,
7. Eat less white sugar and simple sugars.
8. Eat less salt and salty foods, such as crackers, pretzels, chips, and pickled foods.
9. Consume fewer calories.
10. Consume less coffee and alcohol.
11. Smoke less or not at all.
12. Eat more fresh fruit (especially berries).
13. Eat more fresh vegetables (especially green leafies).
14. Eat more legumes and keep grain products 100% whole, including wheat breads, oatmeal, rice, and noodles.
15. Eat more fiber foods—fruits, vegetables, legumes, nuts, and grains.
16. Eat more fresh fish and poultry to replace red meats.
17. Eat more vegetable protein, such as nuts, seeds, and beans, as well as the sprouts of these foods to replace animal proteins.
18. Drink more filtered water or springwater.
19. Drink more dilute fruit juices and vegetable juices as well as herbal teas to replace coffee, black teas, soda pops, and other stimulating beverages.
20. Get more regular exercise (preferably daily) with some aerobics—that is, more-vigorous exercise.
21. Take better care of our air.
22. Keep our waters free of pollution.

New Healthy American

The new healthy American diet is basically what I assert throughout this book. Many of us have turned to this diet as we have realized the consequences of the refined, processed, and chemicalized American diet.

The new health food industry and health or natural food stores are providing us with the ingredients needed to create a new diet. And the bounty from our own gardens can also help. More supermarkets and chain stores are supplying many of the new, more natural, less processed health foods. This just proves that the dollar can stimulate more positive results. Furthermore, the use of chemical farming (see chapter 11, Food and the Earth, for more on this issue) has brought the term *organic,* grown without chemicals, to national attention. Animals are now considered "chemical" when they are factory farmed, treated with antibiotics or hormones, and fed chemically treated foods. They are considered "natural" when they are fed well, without chemicals and drugs, and given space to live.

This new American diet is thus more natural and really the traditional diet, but with the advantage of industrialization. The basis requires a return to whole, unprocessed foods—fruits, vegetables, nuts, seeds, legumes, and whole grains. There is an avoidance of refined flour products and sugar, red meats, lunch meats and sausages, high-fat and high-salt foods, and the regular use of dairy products and alcohol. More people are turning to a vegan or lacto-ovo vegetarian diet.

At times, I have also followed a "pesca-vegan" diet, which is fish added to the vegan diet. In this diet, milk and egg products are avoided, as are poultry and meats. All the foods eaten are high in nutrients, and fish protein and oils are chosen over milk and eggs, which many people do not handle well. (And yes, I am concerned with mercury toxicity in seafood and the pollution of our planet Earth, and yet, I still think occasional fish consumption, varying the types, has greater nutritional and health value than concern. A few times a week is good if fish is among your key protein foods. See chapter 11, Foods and the Earth, and "88 Survival Suggestions" on page 785 in the Futureword.) More recently, I have added occasional eggs and some free-range and organic poultry as I focus a bit more on fewer grains and better proteins. I also add some sprouted beans and nuts and seeds to my diet. Because my weight rises so easily with my usual love for foods, I focus my diet on vegetables. I also occasionally consume only fruits and juices (even fasting) when my body feels the need to lighten up and clean out.

At the beginning of each spring, I organize a 10-day fast for myself and my patients. It always feels so good, so right for me, that I often continue longer. I typically feel light and productive with lots of energy on this lemonade diet known as the Master Cleanser. (See "Fasting and Juice Cleansing" on page 768 in chapter 18, Detoxification and Cleansing Programs, as well as my book *Staying Healthy with the Seasons,* for the formula and further discussion.) Although cleansing like this is not for everyone, it certainly works for me. Now my diet is moving slowly back into a vegan diet, with more raw foods during spring and summer; I maintain a high-alkaline diet, consisting of green salads, fruits, sprouts, millet, soybean products, and some soaked nuts and seeds. Meals are protein and vegetable or starch and vegetable, as described in chapter 13, The Ideal Diet. I avoid refined foods and wheat and other gluten grains (oats, barley, and rye). And I minimize rice and corn, which I so love. This is stricter than I have been in years, but my body and energy are already experiencing the benefits.

Australian and New Zealand

Since the mid-1990s, health consciousness in Australia and New Zealand has increased significantly and made this region increasingly interesting in terms of diet and health-care practices. For example, Australia (unlike the United States) requires labeling of genetically modified food. Currently, only buying organically grown foods protects Americans from GM foods. The country has also established stricter standards for food irradiation. Australia and New Zealand are similar in terms of dietary fat intake and obesity rate, with about 62% of men and 47% of women in both countries showing up as overweight or obese.

As in the United States and other industrialized countries, the intake of milk, cheese, and other dairy products in this region is fairly high. Alcohol consumption, especially beer intake, is quite different, however. In the United States, we average 1.2 gallons per person per year, while in Australia, this average is slightly more than 18 gallons. Mutton and beef are staple foods in this region, although the annual intake is decreasing somewhat. A healthy aspect of food intake in this region is the willingness of many people to grow their own vegetables, which continue to be eaten in good quantities along with other foods.

British Isles

The diet in Great Britain is notorious in Europe as among the worst, both in quality and taste. It is actually quite similar to the typical U.S. diet, however, both in terms of total fat intake and total calories consumed. In both countries, men average 2,300 to 2,400 calories of food a day, and about 34% come from fat. (Women average about the same percentage fat but eat about 700 fewer calories.) The diets of surrounding Scotland and Ireland, which make up the British Isles, are similar. Overall, there is a high amount of industrialized, processed foods consumed, along with the classic meat-and-potatoes diet. At the same time, however, there are some good signs pointing to more awareness of food and diet. The British government's Department for Environment, Food, and Rural Affairs, its Rural Development Programme (focused on organic farming), and new organizations like the Wholesome Food Association are sparking increased interest in food change.

In general, this northern, cold-climate island does not have much agriculture and therefore does not produce many fresh foods throughout the year. Most of the fresh fruits, vegetables, grains, and nuts must be imported, which is usually expensive and seasonal. Often visitors from Europe will carry fresh food with them. Although fresh fruit consumption in England is almost identical to that of the United States (with an average of 1.5 servings per day), vegetable intake is significantly lower. Less than $1/4$ cup of salad and less than $1/4$ cup of fresh or cooked vegetables is the British average, as compared with 3 servings in the United States. And both countries are far below the high-nutrient, whole foods focus that is so important to health.

The consumption of red meat in the British Isles is also high, with pork and mutton eaten as much as beef. Raising sheep for food is common in the countryside. Fish is readily available for those who live near the sea, but most often it is eaten fried, with fried potatoes, a meal known as fish-and-chips. Butter is the main cooking fat, and milk, cheese, and butter are regularly consumed. All of these animal foods provide a high-fat diet, and because this is generally not an exercise-oriented culture but does have a lot of smokers, cardiovascular diseases are a prevalent process of aging. With its industry-oriented culture, chemical carcinogenesis is another big concern in Great Britain.

Other aspects of the diet include refined flour products, with a lot of bread, pies, cakes, and pudding. Whole-grain products are seldom consumed, save a bit o' porridge for some in the morning. Sugar is eaten regularly in desserts, along with sugar in tea. The British drink a lot of black tea, with its caffeinelike agents and tannic acid, contributing to teeth stains and stomach ulcers. Also, beer and ales are drunk throughout the British Isles, with local brews abounding.

Overall, the health and nutrition wave is just starting in the British Isles. It would be wise for them, as for all of us, to push ahead with reduced intake of animal foods, refined flour and sugar products, alcohol, and nicotine. Obtaining more fresh foods via agriculture and importation, as well as storage for the colder, wetter months, would help. Dehydrating vegetables and making sprouts are a couple of ways to obtain these important foods, and eating more whole grains and the products made from them will improve this diet.

WESTERN AND EASTERN EUROPEAN DIETS

The Germanic diet (including Austria, Germany, and Switzerland) is a little spicier and even sweeter than the British diet, with more breads, cakes and other sweets, potatoes, and meats (beef, venison, and pork, especially the sausage-type meats). Each region of Germany has its own type of sausage. Butter and lard are used as the main cooking fats. Baked goods are a staple of the German diet. In Switzerland, chocolate and cheese are popular. Austria is known for its sweets and cakes. Hot chocolate and pastries are a favorite late-afternoon tradition, followed by a light dinner. Fermented foods, such as sauerkraut and sour cream, may help the intestinal tract handle this higher-fat, low-fiber diet. Fresh fruits are less available, and the colder-climate vegetables, such as cabbage, cauliflower, and potatoes, are used more than others. Beer consumption is high, leading to more weight problems than in many other cultures.

The eastern European countries (including the Czech Republic, Hungary, and Poland) are basically poor and consume a less industrialized diet with less sugar and fewer desserts. They still use more natural food preparation and preservation, such as pickling foods for the colder winters. The diet is changing fast in those nations that are now part of the EU, and they are now experiencing an economic boom with all the related health issues. Western Europeans definitely ate a healthier, more natural diet before industrialization. The people of Hungary and Poland consume more rye bread, cabbage, potatoes and other root vegetables, buckwheat, paprika, onions, peppers, pork, pickled fish, and cottage cheese. Food is expensive and not always readily available. More fresh vegetables, fruits, and whole grains could be added, but overall, this is a poorer yet healthier diet than that of many of the more Westernized nations.

Russian

The Russian diet is usually higher in complex carbohydrates and lower in protein, especially animal protein, than most other European diets—and the Russian people have better longevity than most other cultures. There are more centenarians there than anywhere in the world, particularly in a colder region where they are physically active in the more mountainous air. The Russian diet includes dark bread, buckwheat (kasha), wheat, goat's milk and yogurt, potatoes and other root vegetables, cabbage, beet borscht, and some meats. The grain and vegetable basis of the diet, with less consumption of refined flours and sugars, makes it among the healthier diets in Europe. Concerns may include the high consumption of vodka and the animal fats used for cooking. Also, because there is less variety of available foods, vitamin and mineral deficiencies may pose a problem.

Scandinavian

The Nordic diet of Sweden, Norway, and Finland has many healthy aspects for such a low agricultural area, and certainly produces people of strong constitution; however, there are several types of food that are overconsumed in this region, thus increasing the potential for and incidence of a number of chronic degenerative diseases. Because of the cold climate, a higher-fat diet is the common fare and is probably handled better than in most other areas of the world. This would be more beneficial if they ate less animal foods and more coldwater fish (freshly cooked) from the surrounding seas. Cod and herring are popular, but these are often pickled or smoked. Fish is widely consumed, as are other meats and milk products. Finland's high animal food consumption has given it the distinction of having the highest average blood cholesterol level of any place on Earth. The high-salt Scandinavian diet also increases incidence of hypertension and other cardiovascular problems. Alcohol use, particularly beer and schnapps consumption, adds another health concern; black teas are also popular.

Some wholesome traits of the Scandinavian diet include the regular use of rye as crackers and whole-grain breads, which adds fiber and important nutrients. This emphasis on rye is especially interesting, because it seems to be connected with the relatively low rates of bowel cancers in Scandinavia as compared with other parts of Europe. The apparently protective effect of rye against bowel and other cancers appears related to its unique lignan content. Expect to hear more accolades about this aspect of the Scandinavian diet in the years ahead. In these northern European countries, sweets are not common and pastries tend to be light. Fresh fruits and vegetables are available during the three to four warmer months of the year. Nordic peoples would be wise to dry and store more wholesome fruits, vegetables, nuts, seeds, and legumes to use through their long winters. Sprouted foods are ideal for cold climates or areas of low agriculture. Scandinavians would benefit by foregoing their "smorgasbord" style of eating (with too many choices and poor food combining) in favor of simpler meals.

MEDITERRANEAN DIETS

Several dozen diet books and cookbooks have recently been published that trumpet the virtues of the so-called Mediterranean diet. Although all of these popularized versions focus on some specific nutritional components, here I provide a broader context. The area referred to in these popularized diets usually includes a cross section of Greece, Italy, Portugal, Southern France, and Spain. Not usually included, but also part of the Mediterranean region, are the North African countries (like Morocco), which offer a mix of Mediterranean and Middle Eastern

cuisine. Also nearby are the Turkish and Middle Eastern diets, with wheat, rice, lamb (and goat), cheeses, yogurt, olives, and olive oil as major components. All along the Mediterranean, there is an emphasis on whole grains, including couscous (North Africa), polenta (Southern Europe), and bulgur (Eastern Mediterranean), as well as on legumes (including chickpeas and the tasty hummus spread that can be made from them). Also interesting in this part of the world is the tendency to eat breads without butter or margarine.

No single food is more central to the popularized Mediterranean diet books than olives (and their oil). Inhabitants of this area have been singing the virtues of this fruit for centuries, and now the research world is catching up. Unlike most of the other plant oils, olive oil is highly monounsaturated, less likely to be damaged by oxygen and heat, and much more amenable to low cholesterol levels. But the big news about the olive involves its phytonutrient content. Here the people of Greece, Italy, and Spain are in luck! The olive and its oil contain cancer-protective, blood-sugar stabilizing, and atherosclerosis-preventing compounds are becoming legendary. These compounds include olive oil's key polyphenol, oleuropein, as well as its key terpenoids—squalene, beta-sitosterol and tyrosol. Moderate (although sometimes excessively high) consumption of red wine in this region is another positive factor when it comes to dietary health. I explore more on this red wine phenomenon on page 379 under discussion of the French diet.

When you add greater fish intake and lower saturated fat from land animals together to these olive oil and red wine benefits, you get a regional cuisine that is associated with a much lower rate of heart disease than would otherwise be expected. Contributing to this healthy outcome is the fact that fresh fruits and vegetables are more plentiful in these warm coastal areas than anywhere else in Europe. Daily shopping in outdoor markets is a Mediterranean tradition. Tomatoes, peppers, citrus fruits, nuts, and fresh and dried herbs give this diet even greater variety. Such fruits as apples, pears, cherries, and apricots may be eaten fresh or cooked. Negative aspects of the Mediterranean diets include excessive use of coffee and cigarettes. Another negative aspect of the Mediterranean diet is eating late at night. In Italy and France dinner is around 9 p.m.; in Spain it is never before 10 to 10:30 p.m.

Italian

The Italian diet contains more breads, pastas, and cheeses than that of other European countries. Italians drink more wine than beer. In many regions of this coastal country, they produce local wines, cheeses, and prosciutto (cured ham). In general, though, dairy product consumption is low, primarily as such cheeses as mozzarella and Parmigiano. Italy has a great variety of cheeses, and they are very regional, but you can safely say that mozzarella and parmesan are ubiquitous. Spaghetti is classically Italian, as is a thin-crusted pizza (nothing like heavy American pizza). Meats (such as prosciutto, veal, and chicken) as well as the fatty, processed spicy meats (such as salami and pepperoni) are popular. Vegetables are usually consumed in decent amounts, especially tomatoes, as are fresh herbs like basil, oregano, thyme, and marjoram. Minestrone is the common soup. Olive oil is used regularly as the main cooking fat and on salads and other foods; even though it is better than other fats, it is high in calories when used in quantity. Other foods prominent in the Italian diet include garlic, hot peppers, wild local greens, white breads and breadsticks, and fresh figs and melons in the summer.

A typical Italian meal is served in several courses, as is true in much of Europe. Breakfast is light if at all, consisting of coffee, juice, and croissants. Lunch is the main meal, with most businesses closed between 1 and 4 p.m. The first course is pasta, followed by meat or fish with vegetables and a green salad. Dessert is often fruit, followed by an espresso, which has a stronger taste but less caffeine than a typical American cup of coffee. After a rest, people go back to work. Dinner is generally light or just a social time, with some soup, bread, and wine. Luckily, the portions in Italian meals are modest; thus there is less overeating than is typically stereotyped in Italian Americans. Some concerns about the Italian diet include recent increases in refined and processed foods. As elsewhere in Europe, the heavy consumption of alcoholic beverages, cigarettes, caffeine, and sweets may lead to health problems. Furthermore, globalization is changing the good aspects of cultural diets in the Mediterranean, yet even more so in many other parts of the world.

French

Since the highly publicized report on *60 Minutes* in 1991, the "French paradox" has been become a popular buzzword in discussions of regional cuisine. This paradox refers to the fact that death from heart disease in France is much lower than one would expect, given the high-fat nature of the French diet. Although the French paradox has yet to be fully explained, researchers are beginning to put their fingers on more of the factors involved. But first I'll paint a broader picture of the French and their cuisine.

In this large European country (as is true in many larger countries), the diet may vary widely from north to south, in response to climate, cultural differences, and available foods. The mid-Europe northern area consumes more meat and a generally heavier diet, while the southern, Mediterranean regions eat more fish, local vegetables, and a lighter diet overall. In most countries of the world, especially the European ones, the native, rural, or peasant-type diet contains a higher amount of natural foods than the urban diet. For example, a typical meal served in American "French" restaurants is rich in creamy sauces, gravies, pastries, sweets, fats, cheeses, bread, pâtés, and, of course, wine. This type of food is also consumed by the wealthier classes and in the fancier restaurants in France, yet in very small portions and using very good quality ingredients. The French culture is about pleasure, don't forget.

In general, the French are very involved with food and often consume multiple-course meals, as is true in much of Europe. There are local street markets that provide fresh seasonal foods and special cheeses and sausages. The French tend to shop often, preparing their meals to suit the locally available foods. This emphasis on locally grown and seasonal foods may be an important component of the French paradox, because many of the heart-protective phytonutrients can only be found in fresh fruits and vegetables. The more rural or peasant diet in France consists of potatoes, some meats and charcuterie (sausages and cold cuts), poultry, breads and cheeses, and vegetables. Meals often include a small green salad and finish with cheese as "dessert." Breads, croissants, and pastries are often consumed daily. Wine and strong coffee are the national beverages.

The daily consumption of red wine may also be part of France's high-fat, low-heart disease paradox. Like fresh fruits and vegetables, red wine has its own unique phytonutrients. Its heart-protective substances include polyphenols like resveratrol and tannins as well as several kinds of saponin glycosides. A glass of red wine each day appears to have reduced the risk of heart disease in this country by helping to raise HDL levels, lower total cholesterol levels, and prevent clumping of red blood cells. Despite these heart health benefits, however, the overall French diet remains richer and higher in fats and refined flours than many other European countries.

Spanish and Portuguese

The Spanish diet is similar to the Italian, at least along the coastal regions. Having more inland terrain, Spain's beef production and consumption is higher than in other Mediterranean countries. The Spanish enjoy a wide variety of foods, including fish and meats, olive oil, tomatoes, greens, wine, white breads, and figs, as well as citrus and other fruits. Paella is a common dish that combines rice and seasonings, especially saffron, with seafood, shellfish, chicken, and sausage. Wine is consumed regularly with meals. Problems with refined foods and animal fats are beginning to appear in Spain, however. Coffee consumption and cigarette smoking are also high. The Portuguese consume a similar diet to the Spaniards, but being a poorer nation, the people tend to eat simpler, more natural meals of locally available foods. Wine is also consumed regularly.

Greek

This southern, coastal mecca provides a relatively simple diet, mostly cultivated from its own land. Goats and sheep are raised for milk and meats. Goat's milk cheeses, such as feta, and yogurt are eaten regularly, as is lamb meat. Fish is popular. Moussaka is a common local dish—a layered, baked casserole with lamb, eggplant, feta, tomatoes, and onions. Salads are eaten almost daily, made of tomatoes, black olives, red onions, cucumber, feta cheese, and dressed with olive oil and herbs. A yogurt and cucumber appetizer dip for pita bread is also common. Greece is less industrially developed than the other Mediterranean coun-

tries and thus has probably one of the healthier diets in Europe.

ASIAN DIETS

In most Asian countries, people are poor and must cultivate their own food from the land around them; these hardworking people do a good job of it. These cultures are basically noncarnivorous, although not strictly vegetarian either. However, their diets are vegetarian based, focusing on grains and fresh vegetables, usually with some meat, poultry, or fish cooked into one of the dishes. Eggs and milk products, mainly as yogurt, are occasionally consumed by adults.

Because of this generally healthy (more natural, local, and seasonal) diet, there is a reduced incidence of many of the chronic degenerative diseases that are nutritionally related. Thus the elderly population is typically healthier and more active in these cultures and is less plagued by atherosclerosis, high blood pressure, heart disease and their consequences (heart attacks and strokes). However, with the increasing use of refined sugar products, especially in China and Japan, combined with other factors (possibly food and environmental chemicals), adult diabetes and cancer are on the rise. In general, China and Japan are now definitely much closer to Westernized diets than before; only in remote rural areas do you still find traditional natural fare. As times change and there is more industrialization and Americanization of these countries, unfortunately the general diet, nutritional adequacy, basic health, and longevity of their populations will be affected.

Chinese

When we consider that China contains more than 1 billion people, about a fifth of the Earth's population, what the Chinese people eat is the major diet of the world. That diet is primarily vegetarian, with usually only small amounts of animal foods consumed. When I visited China in late 1984, I was most impressed with the agriculture—the incredible use of the land and the masses of people working it. Crops were planted in huge fields, on hillsides, along riverbanks, around houses, literally everywhere. It appeared a green and fruitful country. China has changed a lot since 1984;

the cities have grown and there is more industrialization. I look forward to going back to see the growth. Rice is the main crop, although more wheat is used in the north. The northerners also eat more meat and spicier foods to keep them in balance with the colder climate, although people throughout China make spicy dishes using tiny, hot red peppers; and chile oil, vinegar, and soy sauce are on most tables.

The basic Chinese diet is fairly consistent, containing polished white rice, cooked vegetables, mushrooms, tofu, and small amounts of meat, pork, or fish, with occasional poultry and eggs (often a luxury). Large amounts of meat are rarely consumed at a single meal. Fruits are eaten, as they are available. Soybeans are used in a variety of ways—as tofu (soybean curd) or as soy sauce, a favorite flavoring. Milk products are consumed infrequently, mostly as yogurt, which spoils less easily. Pickled, smoked, and salted foods, usually fish or meats, are also common. There is some concern that these pickled and smoked foods may irritate the gastrointestinal mucosa and, when consumed excessively, may increase the risk of stomach cancer.

Perhaps the most famous expedition to China with the goal of studying the Chinese diet was that of T. Colin Campbell, chair of nutritional biochemistry at Cornell University's medical school and lead researcher for the Cornell-Oxford-China Diet and Health Project. This project, begun in 1983, resulted in the publication of the much-heralded 912-page book *Diet, Lifestyle, and Mortality in China: A Study of the Characteristics of Sixty-Five Chinese Counties*. What Campbell and his colleagues found was an average calorie intake about 30% *higher* in China than in the United States, but drastically less obesity and an average body mass index (a measure of obesity) about 25% *lower* than in the United States. Along with this diet's higher calories but lesser risks of obesity was a high fiber intake (33 grams per day) and 90% of total protein coming from plant (versus animal) foods. What explained the lower rate of obesity despite the higher calorie intake? Better exercise. The people of China are hardworking, especially on the land, and being outdoors cultivating food also contributes to good health. The elderly population seem healthier and more capable because, I believe, they have eaten well and been more connected to the Earth. They are usually more involved in family care,

including the raising and teaching of children, than in Westernized countries, which gives them a sense of purpose and a positive self-image.

Rice is the staple of the diet. In Chinese, the word for rice (*fan*, pronounced "fahn") means "food." White, polished rice does lose some of its nutrients, but in China, it represents status and success. It is considered a little easier to digest and utilize in the body. Peasants still consume a less refined rice with more nutrition. Most Chinese live in rural areas and work the land. In the larger cities, where people have access to refined foods such as sugars and flour products, sugar abuse and poor nutrition from consumption of candy, sodas, and other junk foods are causing concern. But the basic diet is fairly sound and healthy, the product of a culture thousands of years old.

Japanese

The Japanese diet is similar to that of the Chinese, with the basic rice, cooked vegetables, pickled vegetables and fish, and a modest amount of animal products. Because Japan is actually a group of islands, seafood is consumed in much higher quantities than in other Asian countries. Raw fish (sashimi) is characteristic of the Japanese cuisine. Soybeans in the form of tofu and other beans, such as adzuki, are also used. Miso (a fermented soybean paste) is a common salty soup base. Milk products are eaten minimally, and fruits are consumed as available. Raw, fresh vegetables are consumed rarely, as is true throughout the Asian countries. Most everything is cooked (or pickled or smoked), except for raw fish. This practice may have evolved because of concern over spoilage and contamination. Japan is more Westernized than other Asian countries, so concerns over an industrialized diet are present there as well. Also, the higher use of condiments and pickled and fermented foods may offer some concerns in terms of health.

Indian

The Indian diet is similar to the other Asian diets with its basic cooked rice and vegetables. However, in India, the major legume is lentils, rather than the soybean. Dahl is the main Indian lentil dish. Wheat is used to make various flat and pocket breads. Curry flavoring, a hot mixed spice, is used throughout India, and fermented milk products, mainly yogurt, are also consumed regularly, often to cool down the spicy foods. Lassi is a yogurt drink taken with meals. A more common beverage is chai, a spiced black tea served hot or cold with added milk and sugar. White sugar is used all too commonly in India, unfortunately. Fried dishes are fairly popular. Because of heat, hygiene, and concern over food poisoning, few raw foods other than peeled fruits are eaten; most are cooked. The main cooking fat is ghee, a clarified butter. Coconut oil and coconut meat are also used in cooking in some East Indian recipes.

The cow is considered the sacred animal of India, and vegetarianism is much more common there than anywhere else in the world. However, the Hindu people tend to maintain their lactase enzyme function and thus can handle eating cow's milk products, such as milk, yogurt, and paneer, a fermented cheese curd made from milk. The main concern in this quite populated country is basic shortages of food and subsequent malnourishment.

Here I would like to add a few words about ayurveda and the diet that goes along with it. Ayurveda (which means "the science of life") is the oldest system of healing on the planet and is quite complex. The Ayurvedic approach to eating has been practiced for more than 5,000 years in India and throughout the Far East. According to ayurveda, the forces that make a diet healthy or unhealthy are the same forces that govern the entire universe, and the challenge is to understand how those universal forces work through us individually and through our food. Eating in a way that can balance these forces is the crux of an ayurvedic diet. For example, pungent-tasting foods like chile peppers, garlic, and ginger are important when the universal force called *kapha* (the slow, wet, heavy, cold, oily, soft, sweet, and smooth qualities of water and earth) is too strong within us. Conversely, if the *pitta* force (sharp, penetrating, light, and hot) is excessive, these exact same foods should be avoided in favor of raw or lightly cooked and lightly spiced foods like cucumber, cilantro, fennel, and sunflower seeds.

Although this greatly oversimplifies the elegance of the ayurvedic approach, I hope you can see how ingenious this tradition is in taking all of the unique spices and seasonings of the Far East—including cumin, cardamom, clove, turmeric, fenugreek, fennel, cayenne, asafetida, and at least a dozen others—and creating an approach to health that brings diversity and balance to a fairly simple group of staple foods.

Thai

Thai cuisine is becoming increasingly popular in the United States. This diet is close to that of southern China, which Thailand borders. This food can range from mild to spicy, and the Thai people are quite artful in their use of special spices and flavors. In the Thai tradition, there are five basic flavors: sweet, sour, salty, bitter, and pungent. (Ayurveda follows this same list but adds a sixth: astringent.) Thai cuisine uses all five flavors and seeks to blend them in a variety of ways, because the right balance in food is said to correspond to the right balance in one's health. Spicy, curried dishes are some of my personal favorites.

Some of the essential and unique foods in Thai cooking include jasmine rice, fish sauce, tamarind, coconut milk, shrimp paste, oyster sauce, salted plum, kaffir lime leaf, holy basil, palm sugar, lemongrass, galanga root, and Thai chiles. Because Thailand is so fertile, fresh foods especially green vegetables, are readily available much of the year.

DIETS IN OTHER COUNTRIES

Even though there's been less dietary research conducted in other parts of the world, some rich culinary traditions have developed in various countries that now influence more universal eating in the United States. Before concluding the chapter, I'd like to introduce you to several of these food approaches.

Middle Eastern (Morocco, North Africa, and the Arabian Countries)

The Middle Eastern nations consume a variant of the Indian diet, although wheat is used more than rice, eaten both as breads and crackers and as cooked wheat grain (couscous), often with peas or lentils. More types of legumes are used, including lentils, peas, and garbanzo beans. Meat, mainly lamb, is eaten regularly; yogurt and some cheeses are an important part of the diet as well. Vegetables are usually cooked with meats. Olives are also eaten. Few fruit trees (other than date and occasionally fig) grow in these desert climates. Alcohol is forbidden by Muslim law, as is pork. Sweets are popular, such as halvah, a sweetened sesame seed candy, as well as sugared fruits.

African

The diet of the white population of South Africa is similar to that of Australia and England, with the same high consumption of meat and dairy products that leads to an increase in disease. There is also an acceptance of many of the refined foods. The traditional diet of the native black Africans is closer to the natural (cultural) food diet. Cultivated and gathered grains and vegetables with some hunted meats (for rural tribes) and fish (for coastal tribes) make up the basic diet that has supported this culture for many generations. But the acceptance of more refined foods and sugars has been to the detriment of these already malnourished people. It is very difficult to talk about native Africa, I think, because the situation in most native African countries is really dismal and I don't see how we can address the issue without getting into a political arena that is beyond the scope of this book. Leave it to say that there is insufficient food, especially good quality food, and there is a great deal of deficiency and starvation. The excesses from much of the world that is overfed could be used to balance this nourishment problem. And that will take some major work.

Mexican

The staples of this North American country are rice, beans, and corn, with a bit of shredded beef or chicken. Tomatoes and chile peppers are particularly common, as Mexican people like their food spicy. The spicy chiles stimulate the digestive function, clean the blood, and may help prevent certain degenerative diseases.

Corn is used in a variety of ways, mainly ground for tortillas or corn bread. Red beans are the most commonly used legumes. The rice used varies in its degree of refinement. *Burritos, tostadas, tamales,* and *enchiladas* are Mexican names for a variety of dishes, rather like sandwiches, made of meat, beans, cheese, or vegetables and corn or flour tortillas.

Refined foods have become more common in the Mexican diet. Breads, sugars, cookies, and candies are eaten more and more by young children. Hydrogenated oils and lard for cooking may be a problem too, related to obesity and atherosclerosis. The Mexican people would do better with less refined foods and more whole grains and vegetables for fiber. Fruits are plentiful and should be eaten more. Excessive alcohol intake should, of course, be avoided. Because water and food contamination are common, most foods are well cooked before eating, although eating more fresh fruits and vegetables for their cooling effect would probably be healthier for the hot climate.

South American

The South American diet varies a bit from country to country. Most are similar to the Mexican diet, with a fair amount of the staples corn, rice, and beans. In the wealthier countries such as Argentina and Venezuela, where cattle are raised on a large scale, beef consumption is high. Fresh vegetables are not consumed often, although fruits are available. More dairy foods are eaten than in Mexico, but the basic diet is meat, grains, beans, and fruit. A more natural diet with less beef consumption, both in South America and elsewhere internationally, would reduce the necessity to convert rain forests into cattle grazing areas and save these beautiful environments.

TROPICAL DIETS

The diet of such tropical locales as Hawaii, the Caribbean, and other ocean islands seems to be potentially healthful. Fruit and fish are both plentiful, although they are not usually eaten together. Some vegetables are grown and eaten, especially the sweet potato, taro root, the banana-like plantain, and breadfruit. The coconut is also popular; its inner water is drunk for nourishment by many natives before eating its meat. Both the milk and meat of coconuts are used in many tropical dishes. The island diet is generally light, often with more raw foods than cooked ones, appropriate for keeping energy up in these humid climates. However, problems of malnourishment, obesity, loss of teeth, diabetes, and other diseases have increased since the islanders have adopted a more Westernized diet, consuming more refined, canned, and fried foods, sodas, and other sugar products. **This trend, occurring within native cultures around the world, must be addressed and changed for the peoples of this Earth to be healthier.**

KOSHER DIETS

Although the laws of kashruth (kosher dietary laws) have been important to people practicing Judaism for literally thousands of years, in the United States, only about 1 in 6 people who practice Judaism keep kosher. In fact, only 20% of kosher products sold in the United States are sold to persons who identify themselves as practicing Jews. The other 80% are sold to members of the Muslim faith, to vegetarians, to lactose-intolerant individuals, and to those who just want a healthier diet.

Because the kosher dietary laws bring with them a long and rich cultural heritage, different aspects of these laws have naturally been woven into a way of eating that I here I refer to as "Jewish," even though there are Jews living around the world who eat differently than I describe. In addition, some aspects of the Jewish diet are really based on eastern European cuisine, because many Jews living within the United States have ancestors who grew up in that region of the world. So there is a clear mixture here, and there are many people practicing Judaism to whom this mixture does not apply.

Jewish traditions may include a rich involvement with food, including associations of food with love and safety. Such associations are common to many cultures in which people have known poverty or starvation, for whom eating to satiation represents security, contentment, and even wealth.

Most of the food eaten is cooked, often involving complex preparations. More flour products than whole grains are eaten, although buckwheat may be more common than in other cultural diets. Vegetables are eaten either in soups or with meats. Tomato soup, beet borscht, and the famous chicken noodle soup are common. Fruits are often eaten cooked, such as baked apples, stewed prunes, compotes (mixed stewed fruit), or fruit soups.

The kosher diet usually includes only a single animal protein at a meal, and for religious reasons, the tra-

ditional menu does not include meat and milk foods at the same meal. This aspect of the tradition points straight back to the kosher dietary laws described in the Book of Leviticus. Of the red meats, only those of cud-chewing animals, such as cattle, goats, or lambs, are eaten; pork is avoided. Roasts and beef brisket are popular cuts of beef. Chicken is eaten regularly, most often baked, broiled, or boiled for soup. Fish, usually whitefish, is consumed fairly often. In the laws of kashruth, fish with scales are viewed as healthy, but ocean creatures lacking in scales (like shellfish) are something to avoid. Gefilte fish—balls of grain meal and whitefish—are a Kosher classic. Other common foods are potato pancakes (latkes), matzo balls, kreplach, blintzes, and flour pastries, such as apple strudel.

The Jewish diet may cause weight problems. Including more natural foods, such as fresh fruit, vegetables, and whole-grain products, would increase fiber, decrease calories and sweet cravings, and help to prevent some chronic disease problems. **Learning not to overeat and avoiding too many sweets are important habits to develop, not just for this diet but for any diet.**

ENOUGH FOOD?

Many cultures of the Western world have plenty of available food and have a tendency to excesses and the many congestive and degenerative problems that this creates. But others, such as the African countries, India, and China, do not have advanced agricultural technology and thus still count on manual labor. Many countries do not have enough resources or enough usable agricultural land to feed their ever-growing populations. Even if they can grow enough food, slow or nonexistent transportation may not be available to distribute the food, and thus many people are underfed. Often, they do not get enough nutritious food to support normal growth and development in young people or maintenance for adults. Malnourishment and starvation are among the greatest diseases humans confront on a global basis. The high consumption of animals, who eat half of the world's grain before they themselves are eaten, is considered a poor use of energy, poor economics, and poor sense. We need to change this focus from the excessive amounts of meat we eat to move toward a more healthy, vegetarian-based diet; this will help reduce the destruction of the Earth, the only home we have.

Further complicating this set of problems are international trade agreements and global economic alliances that force countries to export food that is actually needed at home. There are numerous examples of countries suffering from food shortages or outright famine and at the same time shipping staple crops off to other countries, or investing precious agricultural energies in specialty crops designed exclusively for export. These kinds of problems are clearly not problems of food sufficiency. They are problems of social justice and food fairness. As global citizens, we need to work hard on both fronts—ensuring the plentiful resources by moving in a more vegetarian and sustainable direction and also envisioning a "just food" that is fairly distributed and accessible to all.

Keeping people healthy enough to recultivate the Earth, and teaching and inspiring them to do so will go a long way toward solving one of humanity's greatest challenges: malnourishment and starvation. Feeding the world's hungry babies, adults, and elderly is a growing and vital concern for everyone.

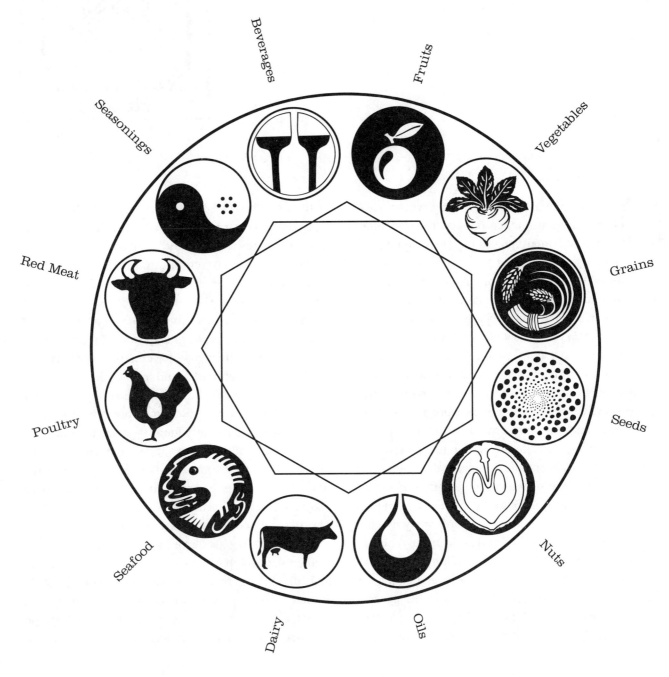

Chapter 10

Nutritional Habits

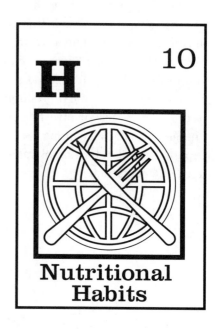

H 10
Nutritional Habits

Our nutritional habits—that is, the way we eat—probably influence our health even more than our food choices do. Developing good dietary habits should begin as early as possible, because these lifestyle habits will help or hinder us for life. Once they are "under our belt," so to speak, they are a challenge to change. For example, obesity is as much a result of *how* and *when* we eat as it is of *what* we eat. Overeating, eating late at night, or eating too many different foods at a meal may weaken digestive functions and make it much easier to gain weight (which may lower self-respect, whereby our discipline worsens). Overeating at meals and snacking between meals are common eating problems, and often these habits are picked up from other family members during our developmental years, as is substituting television and other media for simple ongoing healthier parenting. The focus on food and the socialization around eating are family dynamics that become deep-seated early on. Our psychological and emotional states are often tied into these habits. Equating food with love or prosperity and eating for emotional satisfaction or security are powerful psychological factors that are influenced by eating patterns and problems, and further influence social interactions of all sorts. Thus weight reduction is a significant challenge that encompasses major shifts in our psyche, attitudes, emotions, and, hopefully, physique.

Specific food attractions are also part of our personal eating pattern. These likes and dislikes often develop when we are children and are usually difficult to change. They also influence personal health and weight as well as attitude and aptitude. Breads, pastas, meats, peanut butter, chips, ice cream, fried foods, sugars, hot dogs, hamburgers, and french fries are not our most healthful foods, but these are surely in greater demand than carrots, celery, and apples. The Western family's attraction to fatty foods (and sugar) continues to influence children, teenagers, and young adults toward the trend of obesity and cardiovascular disease. And what we are served at holidays, birthday, schools, and so on, influences the association of junk food and rewards and poor choices later in life.

Tastes for specific flavors, such as for salty or sweet foods, also develop when we are young and are accordingly difficult to change. Occasionally, people become attracted to sour or spicy foods, to bitter foods such as leafy greens, or to other, less common, flavors. In the U.S. food culture, abuse of or addiction to sugar and salt is widespread and influences health significantly. From sugar added to baby food, cereal, coffee, or tea and salt added to almost everything else, to further hidden salt and sugar in most restaurant or fast foods, we are constantly bombarded with these two flavors. The Chinese consider that there are five flavors—sweet, salty, sour, spicy, and bitter—all of which must be balanced to create a healthy diet (see "Balance—Flavors and Colors" on page 503 in chapter 12, The Components of a Healthy Diet, for further discussion of this topic).

The abuse of sugar and salt in the United States and even worldwide is significantly influencing the types of diseases we see (and create with our choices). Too much sugar affects the teeth, contributes to obesity, and may be an important factor in the development of adult diabetes and immune problems. The connections are becoming more and more obvious. In the United States, for example, we are averaging 20 teaspoons of added sugar each day—20 teaspoons in addition to the sugar naturally found in our food. We are also getting nearly 20% of all our calories from bleached, highly processed wheat flour. Extra salt (sodium and chloride) and too few of the other minerals are affecting the body's water balance, thereby affecting kidneys, blood pressure, and, eventually, the entire cardiovascular system. Most of these problems could be greatly reduced with a more balanced diet.

In addition, there has been a dramatic increase in fast foods, snack foods, artificial foods, and foods containing excessive amounts of sugar, salt, or fats beginning in the early 1970s. Although these foods may be less expensive for the consumer, the overall costs are more than just what it takes to pay for big factories, expensive equipment, and many employees; this industry affects the health of our internal and external environment, and that is a high price to pay! Nowadays, nearly 40% of the food dollar is spent in restaurants. In fact, in 1993, for the first time in U.S. history, surveys showed Americans spending more money on food in restaurants than on food prepared in the home, and the amount has only increased since then. **Fat intake is more than 40% of the average American's diet.** A large portion of this diet consists of those poor-nutrition foods with their empty calories and excess fat, salt, and sugar—hamburgers, french fries, soft drinks, pizza, hot dogs, fried chicken, bacon, potato chips, candy, pastries, and so on. The attraction

to and the regular intake of these foods because of their flavors, consistency, availability, or social acceptance easily become habits—we seek them out without thinking, and they become a regular part of the diet, often taking the place of more nutritious foods. They become so ingrained (and inbrained) that we cannot even fathom going without them.

Luckily, however, we can change these habits and become healthier in the process. We can change (choose) what we eat, how we eat, and when we eat. We can shed addictions to sugar, salt, or other specific foods. We can gain new attractions to more wholesome foods, and lose weight and improve other conditions, allowing the body to find its more optimal shape and metabolism. Any change, though, requires motivation and time to allow for physiological readjustments and even withdrawal to take place; this usually takes at least a few weeks. Now more and more people are choosing natural foods and losing their taste for unnatural, oversweetened, salty, greasy, meaty foods. Preparing simpler meals with simpler foods in modest quantities spread throughout the day is a healthful way of eating that has come back into vogue.

In preparation for this next section, learn be a food and digestion detective. Throughout my career, I have believed it important for me to motivate people to think about—and to be more aware of—what they eat and how that makes them feel. When you are hungry or are searching for food, ask yourself, "What do I want to eat? What do I need to eat? What's best for my body? Am I even hungry? What will nurture me the best?" and so on.

THE FOOD HABIT INTERVIEW

There are many factors involved in eating to achieve a balance of physical nourishment, mental relaxation, and emotional harmony. These goals are easily undermined when we let certain patterns develop and lose our sense of eating as a way of nourishing the body, mind, and spirit. When we do not take the time to prepare wholesome food, or if we hurry our meal or eat in unpeaceful settings, we risk creating difficulties in digestion and assimilation and losing our food's basic nurturing potential. Below I have outlined a brief look at a healthful way to approach food and our relationship to it.

Who, What, When, Where, Why, and How?

Who is eating? Each of us is ultimately responsible for our own nutrition, except when we are babies or young children. However, many of us never grow up when it comes to being responsible for what we consume and learning about healthful nutrition—how to shop, how to store food, and especially how to prepare it. It is not the responsibility of our spouse or the cook at the local restaurant; we all need to experience the art of food preparation so that we can ultimately nourish ourselves and others. Anyone who feels that his or her only role is to go out into the world and make money is selling himself or herself short as a complete human being. I am not suggesting that we all become gourmet chefs, but I urge everyone to learn the basics of meal preparation so that when left to our own devices we will not just survive but thrive.

As we grow, we need to develop our sense of what is the best diet for each of us and not live by the needs of our housemates, spouse, parents, or children. And we should all review and maybe challenge the diet on which we were raised (especially if we are experiencing health problems) to see if it is still right for us. This individual process is an essential part of good nutrition throughout life, and this may also be in a state of ongoing adjustment, definitely shifting with the seasons as well as changing over the years with new insights of health issues. For example, I grew up eating the average and then-new American diet, and lots of it—meats mainly as burgers, fries, sodas, cookies, ice cream, and other junk with a few fresh fruits and vegetables thrown in for good measure. Of course, I was overweight and congested/allergic all the time until I awakened to eating better and then feeling better. The results and awareness are what you are reading in this book. I truly believe that if I had continued eating the industrialized, modern diet I would be in much poorer health, on several medicines to control diseases, and without the vitality and healthy appearance that I currently have.

With whom we eat is also important. Creating a peaceful setting around food preparation and food consumption is a vital part of the nutrition process. "What goes in is what comes out" is a wise saying regarding the transformative powers of energy—and if love and a nourishing spirit go into food while it is being prepared, it is likely that the person eating the food will experience and exude those qualities as well. When a meal is prepared by someone who is frustrated or angry, it may take on a whole different nature. That is why loving mothers and grandmas (as well as loving fathers and husbands) are often the best cooks—they put their love into everything they make.

This leads to another important aspect of eating: the social setting in which we eat. The family meal, with everyone sitting around the table sharing the day's experiences, is potentially wholesome and relaxing. But if there is more stress than peace, more argument than discussion, or too much coming and going, digestion and nourishment can be negatively affected. If we are particularly sensitive to others or easily upset, it might be best to eat in peace by ourselves or with another who likes to eat quietly. But many families and cultures use mealtimes to socialize, and I believe that we can adapt to this with the right attitudes.

Everyone could take the time to relax and breathe before eating—before receiving new energy. To receive nourishment, be receptive. Eating on the run or while doing other things, even having an intense conversation during a meal, does not really allow us to pay attention to the whole process of eating—chewing, tasting, and swallowing food. Overeating is common in these situations. I believe that when individuals, couples, or families have their main or primary contact around the dinner table, inappropriate attitudes toward food can be created. Some resulting problems are associating being social or close to others while eating or even using food as a barrier against social interactions and closeness. It is a good idea to ask ourselves with whom and in what kind of setting we like to eat—quietly alone, with a certain friend over an intimate dinner, or in a quick, move-'em-through meal. When we tune into our own preferences, we can nourish ourselves to the fullest potential.

What we eat is probably the most important factor. (However, even the healthiest diet will not be utilized properly if we are stressed, upset, or eat on the run.) A balanced diet is, of course, what we all need. What this actually is may vary from person to person. Our diet is ultimately based on our individual needs, our cultural background, our current knowledge and tastes, and food availability and expense. At best, we should eat moderately and eat a variety of foods. A balanced diet contains seasonal fresh foods—fruits, vegetables, whole grains, seeds, and nuts. More concentrated foods such as eggs, milk products, and animal meats can be added as desired and tolerated, although they should make up a much smaller percentage of the diet than the vegetable-source foods. An even smaller amount of manufactured, processed, or baked goods should be included; these are really not needed at all and should be considered treats.

Food combining and rotating our foods to avoid eating the same things every day may help alleviate or prevent such problems as poor digestion or allergies. We may find that certain foods feel good in the body both short- and long-term, while other foods do not resonate very well. A good part of this book is really about what to eat. Also, see part 3, Building a Healthy Diet.

When we eat is a fairly controversial concept in nutrition. Although most cultures have regular mealtimes, this is ultimately an individual choice based on body cycles, work, energy levels, and sleep patterns. The first rule of eating is to eat only when we are hungry. The message of hunger tells us that the body has digested and used the last food we consumed and is now ready for more. Many people, especially those who are overweight, experience more emotional or psychological hunger than the physical feeling I am discussing here.

To balance this hunger response with regular eating patterns, it is also important to plan meals and have food available when we are hungry. If your schedule is such that you have specific times for breakfast, lunch, and dinner, eat sufficiently but not excessively so that you are feeling some hunger at the time of the next meal. There are many people in the world, especially in Western cultures, who rarely experience hunger. There are also millions of impoverished people on this Earth who rarely experience nutritional satisfaction.

When to eat what kinds of foods and how much food to eat are nutritional issues about which there have been a variety of theories. That we should not eat too much too late in the day is a pretty unanimous viewpoint. Eating a wholesome, well-balanced dinner in the late afternoon or early evening is a fairly well-accepted activity. Dinner tends to be the most social meal, a time to relax after a hard day at work, school, or home. In many parts of the world, particularly Europe, people tend to eat lightly in the morning and then eat their main meal in the early

afternoon. Dinner is usually light, with soup and bread or salad, and often a social time with friends or family. See the Italian diet, discussed on page 379 of chapter 9, Diets, as an example.

Breakfast is a more open question. The word *breakfast* means to "break the fast" after not eating overnight, often for nearly 12 hours. Some traditional schools of thought feel that breakfast is the most important meal of the day—that a big breakfast consisting of fruit, starch, protein, fats, muffins, and so on is what gets us going. Clearly, if we finish eating for the day by 6 or 7 p.m. (with the light), the next morning we should be hungry again and need a wholesome, nourishing breakfast. However, many adults eat later in the evening. Thus many nutrition specialists, myself included, think that the fast should be broken in the morning very lightly, with fruit, for example, and that we should progress throughout the day with more concentrated foods.

The principle of "eat the most before you do the most" seems to apply to the best daily meal patterns. When I talk about "doing the most" here, I am talking about physical activity. We cannot eat "backward"—that is, food that we eat at night cannot go backward after we have eaten it and help give us energy for events that happened earlier in the day. Food works forward. It takes time to digest and absorb what we eat. It also takes energy to turn food into energy for the body. Some of us face a heavy physical workload in the early morning, not all that long after we get up. A construction worker, for example, tapping deep into his or her nutrient reserves on the morning job, is probably going to need a substantial, warming, and fuel-oriented breakfast. For this individual a light start probably would not work. For a writer, however, wanting to feel cleansed and focused and not bogged down with digesting food, a substantial, fuel-oriented breakfast probably makes a lot less sense. In this situation, fruit alone may be the perfect fit, with a gradual tapering into the more substantial-type meals as the day progresses. What does your lifestyle require? How long has it been since you looked at your eating habits? In many traditions, including the tradition of Oriental medicine, fruits are typically eaten by themselves anyway because they are fairly quickly metabolized and viewed as monopolizing some of the digestive function needed for other types of foods.

Often we do not know our own needs unless we experiment. By eating different amounts at different times of the day, we can see what will work best for our work and energy schedules. If we get fatigued in the afternoon after lunch, we may need to shift things around. A big dinner and light breakfast may be best for us, or it may be the other way around. We will not know unless we try it. Just because we have been doing things a certain way for a long time does not mean that it is the best way to reach nutritional health.

Where we eat can be particularly important for people who are overweight because of poor eating habits. With our concerns about time, convenience, and comfort, it is easy to find places to eat or snack away from our usual ones, such as the dinner table. Eating in front of the television, in the car, or while walking around leads to an increased intake of food, especially of the more highly caloric snack foods. This can become an extra assault on our digestive tract, which gets no chance to rest. While eating, avoid "techno-traps," such as telephones, television, and computers. This will reduce electrical interference in our digestive, assimilative, and mental abilities (see "Electricity and Electropollution" on page 483 in chapter 11, Food and the Earth).

I suggest to people on weight-loss programs or to those who have developed poor eating habits that they pick one or two places to consume their food, usually one indoors and the other out. Eating outdoors, especially in a natural setting, can contribute to the relaxation and enjoyment of the meal. The dining room table is usually the best indoor spot, so that eating is mainly centered around meals instead of snacks. Restaurant eating involves another place we may need to include, but for a variety of reasons restaurant eating is best done only occasionally.

People who are overweight tend to snack or eat while watching television, or they become prowlers in their own homes, checking the refrigerator and cupboards for treats even after a good-sized meal. Retraining ourselves to eat in a limited number of places (and at certain times) may be difficult, but it is a good habit to develop. Where do you usually eat? Do you like quiet meals, with nice music, or social meals?

Why we eat is definitely an interesting question. We should basically eat to nourish our being— our organs, our tissues, every cell in the body. Food is the main human fuel for life; it provides heat and all of the specific nutrients that have been discussed so far in this book. It helps the body function. For a period of time when we rest or fast, the body can use stored nutrients to run itself, but eventually we need to refuel. Think of bringing nourishment into our bodies rather than just feeding ourselves. And nourishment can come on many levels and from all of the senses. As my associate Bethany Argisle has suggested, we have many more mouths to feed other than just our oral cavity. Our eyes need to be nourished with color and beauty, our ears with music and the sounds of Nature, our nose with the natural aromas of the world, our hands and body with the touch of another, and, of course, our heart and spirit with the love and friendship of other living beings (in other words, using vitamin L, love for self and others, the activator of all healthy choices). Many people feed their bellies but not their souls; this will not lead us where we are meant to go in health and in life if we are not healthy or have less energy.

There are, of course, many other reasons why we eat—loneliness, frustration, reward, and punishment, to name a few. Some people use food like a drug to sedate or numb themselves. Everyone's awareness of this aspect of eating is critical. Most of us at some times eat for social reasons. Sharing food is a custom of friendship. When we are asked to join someone in their creative cuisine or for a drink or snack, it is often taken as a rejection or even an insult if we decline. Because my diet throughout the years has usually been so different from those around me, I have learned to share what I was or was not doing and why as a means to educate or inspire friends or relatives to other possibilities. But it is often difficult not to succumb to the temptations of others. If we are planning to go to a social gathering for eating, it would be wise to eat lightly in the hours before our arrival; the extra hunger will allow us to really enjoy the meal, although we must be careful not to overeat. We all, on some level, want our friends or family to be like us. Still, individuality is the beauty of the species and among the most important aspects of nutrition.

Many of these different motivational aspects of eating point to a single conclusion: there is always some component of desire when we eat—the desire to nourish ourselves, to be alive, to live life, both privately and with others. Losing this element of desire can mean losing the ability to eat; thus it is possible for us to become anorexic, which in Greek literally means "without desire." In some respects, eating should always involve a little celebration, recognizing the desire in our lives and embracing the goal of nourishing our whole selves.

How we eat can also make a big difference in our nutrition. Eating slowly and chewing our food well are important. Starting the digestive process in the mouth saves a lot of wear and tear on the stomach (which does not have teeth) and digestive tract. We can then more easily break down the food and utilize the nutrients contained in it. When we rush through meals, we are doing the body and digestion a disservice. Our emotions influence our digestive functions as much as any system in the body, so getting into a peaceful and receptive state is important to healthy food consumption. Allotting enough time to nourish ourselves is also helpful.

How we get the food from the plate or bowl to our mouth—what utensils we use—is also an interesting topic. The choice of the Western world is silverware (or other metalware). Personally I do not like to eat with metals. Forks are sharp and hard, and if the metal hits the metal fillings in the mouth, well, that is no fun. Those of us who enjoy Eastern influences prefer chopsticks, especially the wooden (not plastic) variety. My favorite utensils, though, are my god-given chopsticks called "fingers." My mother and my more "proper" friends have never been very supportive of this habit. Whether with fingers or chopsticks, eating can be a primal and personal experience. Many foods, such as fruits, vegetables, nuts, and seeds, adapt easily to hand- or finger-eating. Soup may be drunk, and soft foods such as mashed potatoes or oatmeal may need a little creativity and practice. If we adapt to the individual characteristics of the food and the individual dietary needs of the body, we should do well and enjoy good foods and greater health.

HABITS TO CHANGE

Healthy eating habits are a mainstay of good nutrition. A patient recently told me, "Dr. Haas, make a note about this because it's so important. All of my digestive problems have cleared up because I am chewing my food more thoroughly and I am not drinking two large glasses of water or soda with my meals. Thank you for that." Too much fluid with meals dilutes digestive juices and causes inefficient digestion and assimilation of the nutrients contained in the foods. This patient has also changed her food choices, which is helping her begin to lose the nearly 100 extra pounds she carried around. The challenge for her now is to be prepared and have her new food choices available at work to nourish her; or if she needs to work late, she has an early dinner and is not starved when she arrives home later (when she would typically overeat, sleep poorly, and feel bad the next day). We can make a huge difference in our overall health, weight, and energy levels by incorporating some of the healthy eating habits discussed in this chapter.

Overeating

Overeating is among the most common and dangerous dietary habits. It is natural, on festive occasions such as holidays or parties, to eat more than usual, but many of us have turned up the level of our satiation state so that we need to eat a large amount of food to feel satisfied all the time. A great many emotional and psychological factors that may have started in our early years contribute to overeating. It is often influenced by our parents and family members as well as by our own insecurities and self-image.

Overeating often leads to obesity, which is a factor in many other diseases. The overconsumption of food also causes stress to the digestive tract and other organs and can lead to the overworking and weakening of those areas. Congestion or stagnation also occurs more easily with overeating. These problems need to be dealt with at the level from which they arise. If they stem from a nutritional deficiency, so that the body is craving missing nutrients, this issue should be discovered and corrected. If they are of recent onset, stress may be the source. More often, though, overeating is a long-term and deep-seated problem that needs to be dealt with on both the psycho-emotional and nutritional levels. Moderation in eating is an important habit to develop. Eating small meals several times a day instead of 1 or 2 large meals is probably better for most people. Balancing flavors as well as types of food will help satisfy us and may lessen the desire to eat more.

Undereating

In recent years, there has been growing concern over problems associated with undereating, such as the medical conditions known as *anorexia nervosa* and *bulimia.* Undereating usually has a strong stress or psychological component, which can range from being too nervous or concerned about an upcoming event or relationship to part of a full-blown psychosis. All forms of undereating—skipping meals or eating only limited foods—will lead to poor nutrition and eventually to problems from protein, calorie, vitamin, or mineral deficiencies that occur over time. Other symptoms include lack of energy and subsequent weakness, malnourishment of internal organs, skin problems, hair loss, and lack of sexual desire. Severe weight loss despite regular eating may indicate an underlying medical condition and warrants an evaluation by a doctor, especially one who is knowledgeable about nutrition.

People who undereat are often overly concerned about obesity or have a distorted self-image. This is more common in women and in teenage girls who become overly body conscious or are concerned about becoming too shapely. Often, being thin is similar to being fat in that it makes us less attractive and is a protection against intimacy with others. These issues may come up during adolescent sexual development.

As mentioned earlier, *anorexia* literally translates as "lack of desire," but in the everyday medical work, anorexia simply means "loss of appetite." Anorexia nervosa means not eating because of "nervous" or psychological problems. Although many people with this condition are young females who want to be trim, or to be models or ballerinas, which requires a long and lean body, there are a growing number of cases involving women of all ages as well as men. A long and lean body may not be the natural body shape of many people, who literally need to starve themselves to maintain that weight or shape. To be diagnosed with anorexia, a person has to be no more than 85% of their normal body weight.

Bulimia involves binge eating followed by inappropriate methods to prevent weight gain. A person diagnosed with bulimia may in fact be a perfectly normal weight and in many respects appear perfectly healthy. Contrary to common belief, it is not necessary to voluntarily vomit or purge in order to be diagnosed

as bulimic. All that is necessary is a feeling of loss of control following eating and attempts to make up for the eating through extreme steps, usually through pushing the food out unnaturally by vomiting or creating diarrhea. Use of laxatives, diuretics, and enemas could fall into this category but so would excessive exercise.

All of these problems have strong psychological bases and usually require counseling as well as generous support from loved ones. Occasionally, these situations become extreme and, as with overeating, can be fatal. Fortunately, these conditions are often short-lived, and those troubled by them see their way clear to begin a new balanced diet and create a newly shaped body and self-image.

On the other hand, systematic undereating has been studied and is being practiced by more people as a way to improve aging and longevity. A lower-calorie diet, especially with good quality and nutrient-rich foods along with supplements to prevent deficiencies, is the primary approach that has been shown to help animals live longer in many studies. And thus, more elders are adopting this practice with a new focus on the old adage "Eat to live (long), and not live to eat." Many people who derive their primary pleasure from foods also suffer the consequences of excess, which is the common imbalance leading to many chronic diseases in Westernized countries. Finding a balance is the key to health and longevity.

Eating Late

This is a common problem among people with busy daily schedules. Food often acts as a sedative and helps us to physically relax. After a meal, more blood goes to the digestive organs and away from the areas of physical and mental activity. So eating lightly during the day, getting hungry at night after work, and then eating the main meal in the evening is a convenient pattern for many people's schedules. However, going to bed on a full stomach is not necessarily helpful for digestion or sleep. The food may just sit there, undigested through the night, so that we wake up full and sluggish. Eating late can become a habit that robs us of our vitality. It also may contribute to overweight (from overlate) problems.

It is best to try to eat earlier in the evening, ideally before dark, and not too heavily; to engage in some activity, both mental and physical, after dinner; and to eat little in the 2 or 3 hours before bedtime. When we have not eaten enough throughout the day, it is wise to eat lightly in the evening also and sleep well to awaken energized for some exercise and a good, hearty breakfast. And remember to breathe fully too: oxygen is a primary food as well.

Rigid Diet

Many people develop rigid eating patterns and consume only a limited selection of foods. This inflexibility is often based on a preference for certain tastes or just a discriminating personality. Teenagers and elderly people are subject to this lack of flexibility (as are some health food fanatics) more often than other areas of the population. Sometimes this is based on fear, rebellion, lack of adventure, or just being stuck in an attitude or rigid physical environment that will not allow them to be open to other ideas. They just maintain themselves on a few foods, such as hamburgers, hot dogs, french fries, and sodas for the younger crowd, or eggs, toast, potatoes, and meat in the older group. All of these items lack the freshness and vitality found in natural foods, however.

There are people who develop what I would call positive restrictions in their diet. We all have certain foods we do not like because of their flavor or past experience with them. Specific allergenic or reactive foods are clearly best avoided. Restricting such foods as meats, milk, wheat, and sugar- or chemical-containing foods may be based on certain philosophical or health choices. But being too rigid in the diet is usually not in our best interest. It is difficult to get people to change when they do not wish to, especially regarding what they eat. They already know that they will not like it before they even try it. Sometimes consulting with a nutritionist and doing a diet analysis by evaluation or computer can show people the excess or lack of nutrients in their diet, and this may educate and influence them to make some changes.

Ideally, choosing to eat a variety of foods, from all the groups that I have discussed in earlier chapters, unless there is a particular sensitivity to certain ones, is the most balanced approach. This gives us the opportunity to absorb the nutrients that Nature and the larger world provide. Eating them in moderation while introducing new ones daily is a healthful path to follow.

Emotional Eating

I have already discussed overeating and undereating, but there are other issues surrounding the use of food in dealing with stress and psychological troubles. Some people eat when upset or depressed; others cannot eat at all in this condition. Our emotions strongly influence our eating behavior, so if we want to maintain a more balanced diet, and thus a more balanced life, we need to learn to deal with our emotional states in ways other than with foods' moods.

Using hunger as a guide, integrated with a regular eating plan, we create a basic diet. If we are overweight, we may need to plan meals that include less food and calories; if underweight, we include more food and calories and then maintain a balanced diet when we are at a better weight. We can learn to deal with stress, sadness, frustration, depression, and so on, through self-development techniques, counseling, or mental affirmations and visualization—all good ways to clear these problems—or at least not let them take hold of us and run our lives. There are very few issues that are important enough to take precedence over our health. **And not using food to cover up these important feelings, thoughts, and issues is crucial to maintaining optimum health.**

Liquids and Eating

Many of us drink liquids with our meals. This is not really a good practice, because extra fluids can dilute the digestive juices, making it more difficult to break down food. Drinking water before or after meals is much better. A small amount (less than 1 cup) of water with meals may help dissolve the food and stimulate digestive juices.

Good drinking water is generally the best beverage, and consuming about 8 to 10 glasses a day (though we need less than this as if consume a higher amount of fruits and vegetables) is helpful for weight loss and keeping the body functioning. It is best to drink two or three glasses first thing in the morning, several glasses between meals, and then a couple of glasses about 30 to 60 minutes before dinner to reduce the appetite a bit. Sweetened soda pops should be avoided. Milk is a food (to be used sparingly by adults), not a beverage to be drunk with meals. Many people feel that a bit of alcohol before a meal stimulates the appetite and the digestion of food. There is actually some fascinating research in this area, where wine and beer before a meal have been shown to stimulate secretion of gastrin (a peptide in the stomach that helps regulate digestion). Coffee or tea following a meal is enjoyed by many people and is probably not too detrimental when done occasionally. Overall, it is wise to be aware of needs and drink when thirsty, and it is best to drink only between meals, giving the digestive tract the best shot at getting those nutrients ready for our cells. How about a spot of peppermint tea or warm lemon water? They are nice for digestion.

Additional Habits to Cultivate

Preparation of both ourselves and our food is helpful. Food made with awareness and love adds that little extra, and when we take the time to prepare ourselves to receive nourishment, such as with a little prayer of thanks or some quiet time, we also give ourselves the chance to get the most out of a meal.

Relaxation around eating is a good habit to develop. This is part of preparation and digestion. After a fair-sized meal, it is important to take some time to let digestion begin. After about an hour, we can begin some light activity. A walk is ideal. However, most of us cannot afford the luxury of taking this time around meals. When I cannot, I try to follow the "Warrior's" diet (discussed on page 366 in chapter 9, Diets) of frequent small snacks throughout the day until I can take more time to prepare and eat a proper meal.

Exercise is important to keeping the body healthy and to utilizing the nutrients that we consume. I do not recommend exercising for at least an hour, or longer, after eating. It is usually several hours after a meal before my body feels right doing any vigorous activity. Often I exercise first and use eating as a reward for doing the physical activity. Early in the day before breakfast and after work before dinner are the two best times for exercising.

COMBINING FOODS

Three important factors help us choose what foods to eat in combination and when to eat them. These are acid-alkaline balance, food combining, and food rotation. These are discussed briefly in this section, as they are useful in developing ways to improve general health or digestion or to reduce food allergies. Each factor is discussed more fully in part 3, Building a Healthy Diet.

Acid-Alkaline Balance

Because the body tissues and blood are slightly alkaline, we need to eat more foods that break down into alkaline elements. The ash or residue that remains when a food is metabolized influences the body's pH, or acidity/alkalinity. (Actually, pH stands for "pressure of hydrogen," as the amount of hydrogen ions affect the acid-alkaline state.) The foods that generate an alkaline ash are the fruits and vegetables (even the acid fruits, such as lemons), except for cranberries and most dried fruits. The whole grains, nuts, and seeds are slightly acid in the body, although millet, buckwheat, corn, almonds, and all sprouted seeds tend more toward the alkaline side. The cereal grains tend to be more acid-alkaline balanced than the more acidic nuts, milk products, meats, and refined flour and sugar products.

The way foods break down is not the same as their pH, however. Every food has its own degree of acidity, which is measured on the pH scale. The low-pH foods, like limes, are extremely acidic (limes have a pH around 1.9). The high-pH foods, like cow's milk, are much more alkaline (cow's milk has a pH around 6.5). But pH does not tell us how a food breaks down in the body, and when I talk about acid-alkaline balance, I am talking about the body's response to the food, not the food in isolation.

For a system that does not get too acidic, congested, or mucousy, the diet should contain about 70% alkaline foods. This means the type of diet that I advocate throughout this book—a diet that focuses on fruits and vegetables, with some whole grains, more sprouts, and smaller amounts of animal foods and refined treats. This will keep the system functioning optimally, provided we get the balance of vitamins and minerals we need, as well as the essential fatty acids and amino acids to perform the required fat and protein functions.

Food Combining

Food combining is a somewhat complex issue—and a revolutionary idea in terms of the standard diet. If called on to pinpoint the origins of this idea, I would cite the 2,000-year-old ayurvedic texts written by doctors in India. Here we get fascinating descriptions of specific physiological problems that can occur from improper combination of foods. These ancient writings also seem consistent with present-day ideas about food combining. The basic theory is that for best digestion and utilization of food, we need to observe certain rules for the way we combine foods within a meal. Unfortunately, there is surprisingly little research in this area, so many of the principles described below have yet to be backed up by scientific studies.

Fruits are often thought to be best eaten alone, as they are more easily digested than other foods. This idea means that we would want to consume fruit between meals or perhaps as a cleansing way to start the morning. In the same way that fruits may best be eaten alone, high-protein foods may also require special consideration. Meats in particular require an acid digestive medium, and the same degree of acidity needed for the digestion of meat may be too far from the alkaline environment needed for starches or vegetables. **Thus, food combining principles suggest not mixing proteins and starches.** Eaten together, starches, vegetables, and meats may engage the digestive system in a suboptimal way, such that digestion takes longer and is less efficient.

In some systems of food combining, fruits and simple sugars are not eaten along with or after other foods, because doing so is believed to delay their passage from the stomach and to subject them to an unwanted process of fermentation, allowing gas to go through the intestines. Some food combining advocates recommend that milk not be drunk as a beverage but used as a food, and some proponents also argue that the fruits of the melon family be eaten alone, not even with other fruits.

In most food-combining plans, fruit is usually eaten in the morning or several hours after other foods.

Sources and Choices

To be Earth and body conscious, it makes sense to ask our consumer self, "Where do things come from, and where do they go?" What is the source of what we buy and consume? How was it made and did that production cause air or water pollution, for example? After we use or consume the product, what happens to its packaging and how is the food processed in the body? Is there personal and planetary toxicity in what our choices are? We can really make a difference if many of us, ideally if everyone, becomes more conscientious about health and the products in which we invest. By making better choices, we can change the world and support the products that are better for us and our environment, or as Bethany Argisle has wisely suggested, "Our dollar is our vote."

From this point, it helps for us to learn about the toxins in our food chain and the chemicals used in foods (food additives). Consumers' responsibility is to know the basics about additives and their risks to be able to make the wisest choices in selecting safe and healthy foods. Chapter 11, Food and the Earth, details 100 or so specific food additives; in this chapter, however, I provide the basic information on reading food labels. My book *The Staying Healthy Shopper's Guide*, also goes into detail about food chemicals, safe shopping, and label reading.

Meals are simpler than is usual in the American culture, consisting of lots of vegetables with either a protein food (such as dairy products, eggs, or meats) or a starch food (such as grains, pasta, or potatoes). This type of diet, I believe, may be capable of generating less stress on the intestinal tract and creating overall better health, both immediately and on a long-range basis.

READING FOOD LABELS

Reading a food label takes a little know-how (and very good eyesight or a magnifying glass). Given the more than 3,000 additives used in processed foods, it can be challenging to fully understanding the risks and benefits of all the ingredients that appear on a food's label. However, unless you are going to avoid every fancy packaged or processed product (the healthiest approach), you need to have some basic information on the how-tos of label reading. Below I detail these basics.

Before 1994, food labels provided only an ingredient list. The labels we take for granted today have greatly expanded information that can be quite important to your health, especially to those with specific needs, such as a low-fat or low-salt diet, or even more common today, a low carbohydrate/sugar diet. See the sample label for a common brand of crackers. Knowing how to read a food label enables you to decide if the product is nutritious, if it is best used as an occasional treat, or if it should be avoided altogether.

The Basic Food Label Guidelines

Serving size. This is the calculation upon which all the other numbers on the food label are based. The food manufacturer often tries to limit the serving size so that the amount of calories or fat will appear smaller, especially in foods such as chips or cookies. For example, they might declare a serving as 1 or 2 cookies or 1 ounce of chips when, in reality, the consumer is likely to consume much more at once. So, if you are considering eating "the whole thing," check out the label. You may want to bring your calculator—because you will need to multiply the serving size by the number of servings in the package to determine the actual amount of calories, fat, and carbohydrate you might consume.

Servings per container. This lets you know your multiplication factor, should you consume several servings or the entire container or package. For example, an 8-ounce bag of chips that lists 150 calories (and 40% fat, about 60 fat calories) per 1-ounce serving actually contains a whopping 1,200 calories if you eat the whole bag. And that includes about 500 calories of fat! And we wonder sometimes why it is so easy to be overweight!

Calories. This represents the number of calories in 1 serving. A calorie is a unit of energy or heat that your body generates from the food you eat—from the macronutrients, which include proteins, fats, and carbohydrates. Remember that proteins and carbohy-

drates (sugars and starches) offer about 4 calories of energy per gram; the richer fats give more than double the calories at 9 per gram; and alcohol (a carbohydrate variant) is metabolized at about 7 calories per gram. The body requires calories to run—converting carbohydrates, proteins, and fats into glucose, the essential fuel for the system. If we take in an excess of calories, especially sugars and starches, they are stored in the body as fat, and this can lead to weight gain and obesity. Being continually overweight can be a primary cause of illness and chronic disease.

A key to good nutrition is to consume primarily wholesome foods high in nutrients. **The objective is to eat mostly foods with a high nutrient-to-calorie ratio,** such as vegetables, which are low in calories but have a variety of vitamins and minerals. Seafood also has many quality nutrients and proteins, without excessive calories or much fat; in fact, the fats

---

Food Label Categories

Serving size
Servings per
  container
Calories
Calories from fat
Total fat
  Saturated fat
  Trans fat
  Polyunsaturated fat
  Monosaturated fat
Cholesterol
Sodium
Total Carbohydrate
  Dietary fiber
  Sugars
Protein
Other nutrients
  Vitamin A
  Vitamin C
  Calcium
  Iron
  Others

Nutrition Facts
Serving Size 1 Can (325 mL)
Servings Per Container 6 Cans

Amount Per Serving		
Calories 220 Calories from Fat 25		
		% Daily Value*
Total Fat 3g		5%
Saturated Fat 1g		5%
Trans Fat 0g		
Polyunsaturated Fat 0.5g		
Monounsaturated Fat 1.5g		
Cholesterol 5mg		2%
Sodium 220mg		9%
Potassium 600mg		17%
Total Carbohydrate 40g		13%
Dietary Fiber 5g		20%
Sugars 34g		
Protein 10g		20%

Vitamin A	35%	• Vitamin C	100%
Calcium	40%	• Iron	15%

*Percent Daily Values are based on a 2,000 calorie diet. Your daily values may be higher or lower depending on your calorie needs.

		Calories:	2,000	2,500
Total Fat	Less than		65g	80g
Sat Fat	Less than		20g	25g
Cholesterol	Less than		300mg	300mg
Sodium	Less than		2,400mg	2,400mg
Potassium			3,500mg	3,500mg
Total Carbohydrate			300g	375g
Dietary Fiber			25g	30g
Protein			50g	65g

INGREDIENTS: FAT FREE MILK, WATER, SUGAR, COCOA (PROCESSED WITH ALKALI), GUM ARABIC, GUM ARABIC, CALCIUM CASEINATE, CELLULOSE GEL, CANOLA OIL, POTASSIUM PHOSPHATE, CELLULOSE GUM, SOYBEAN LECITHIN, MONO AND DIGLYCERIDES (EMULSIFIER), ARTIFICIAL FLAVOR, CARRAGEENAN, MALTODEXTRIN AND DEXTROSE.
VITAMINS & MINERALS: MAGNESIUM PHOSPHATE, CALCIUM PHOSPHATE, SODIUM ASCORBATE, VITAMIN E ACETATE, ZINC GLUCONATE, FERRIC ORTHOPHOSPHATE, NIACINAMIDE, CALCIUM PANTOTHENATE, MANGANESE SULFATE, VITAMIN A PALMITATE, PYRIDOXINE HYDROCHLORIDE, RIBOFLAVIN, THIAMIN MONONITRATE, FOLIC ACID, CHROMIUM CHLORIDE, BIOTIN, SODIUM MOLYBDATE, POTASSIUM IODIDE, PHYLLOQUINONE (VITAMIN K1), SODIUM SELENITE, CYANOCOBALAMIN (VITAMIN B12) AND CHOLECALCIFEROL (VITAMIN D3).

Source: Nutrition Facts Label, U.S. Food and Drug Administration, November, 2004.

in fish are known to be healthful. In contrast, processed and packaged foods are lower in nutrients and have too many calories and fats. Even the fat-free foods designed for low-fat diets contain higher levels of sugar and carbohydrate and thus more calories—not ideal for long-term health, high-functioning brains, and trim bodies.

> **For a better diet plan, consume the majority of your calories from natural and whole foods— fresh fruits and vegetables, whole grains, beans, nuts and seeds, fish and poultry, and low-fat or nonfat dairy products.**

Calories from carbohydrates. These are not listed on the label, but you can get this total by multiplying the total grams of carbohydrates by 4 calories. Many people are now following a lower-carb diet, and thus lower calories, to reduce weight, so this is an important area for them. Because food manufacturers do not list total carb calories, it may give us a false sense of security—the sense that if we eat only low-fat products, we are limiting all the foods that might cause excessive weight gain and health problems. Yet eating too many refined carbohydrates (sugars and starches) can cause weight gain and subsequent health degenerative diseases, just as fats do.

Calories from fat. This signifies the number of fat calories per serving. This is an important item for people who are watching their fat intake and calories. The kinds of fat you eat also matters. Much of the fat we consume from processed foods is mainly the unhealthy saturated and hydrogenated fats, which lack the essential fatty acids that the body needs. And typically, eating foods with higher amounts of these "junky" fats is linked to heart disease, stroke, and cancer. These unhealthy hydrogenated and saturated fats are found in many commonly eaten foods, such as potato or corn chips and other fried foods, in baked goods from cookies to crackers to doughnuts and croissants, and in such fatty meats as salami or bologna. These higher-fat foods are often high-calorie foods, with more than half of the calories coming from fat. **Also, remember that the fats in foods, especially animal-based foods, store more of the pesticides and chemicals. So higher-fat foods should be in the "occasional treat" category.**

"Calories from Fat" on the label also lets you know the percentage of fat in the product. In a bag of chips, for example, there may be 150 calories per 1-ounce serving and 60 calories of fat; that is 40% fat. Because the government suggests that the diet contain no more than 30% fat (and 20% to 25% is probably more ideal, and that is of primarily healthy fatty acids from vegetable oils), you may want to avoid foods that have a higher fat content. Obviously, such foods as good-quality, cold-pressed oils or healthy salad dressings are exceptions.

Total fat. This signifies the total grams of fat *in each serving* in the food. The label also tells what percent of the day's total ideal fat intake, termed *% daily value,* is fulfilled by a single serving of the labeled food. Government guidelines suggest that our total fat intake be about 60 grams, or 540 calories; that is 30% of an estimated 1,800-calorie diet. This may be too high, however realistic, for the optimum health of many people, especially those attempting to restrict fat in their diet.

Saturated fat. This describes the total amount of saturated fats per serving. Multiply this figure by 9 to get the saturated fat calories. Limit this type of fat, which is primarily found in animal foods and has been implicated in atherosclerosis and cardiovascular diseases as well as many types of cancer. Hydrogenated fats (found in margarines and many chips and crackers) are also saturated (artificially) and can contribute to these diseases as well. The % daily value allows for 25 grams of saturated fats—this is estimated at 10% to 15% of the average food intake.

Polyunsaturated fat. This signifies the number of grams of polyunsaturated fats per serving. Polyunsaturates are contained primarily in vegetable oils. Ingredients that come from vegetable shortening or oils other than canola and olive are primarily polyunsaturated fatty acids (PUFAs). (The term *unsaturated* is a biochemical term meaning there are unstable bonds on the fat molecule—more than one in this category is thus polyunsaturated.) Because these fats are less stable biochemically, they tend to oxidize and become rancid more easily than other oils. As a result, foods containing these oils need preservatives and antioxidants to protect their stability. Such is the case in most salad dressings, crackers, chips, and many other baked and packaged goods. **Polyunsaturated**

fats are not required to be listed on the label; their listing is voluntary.

Hydrogenated fats and oils, which should generally be avoided, are not described on the label either, other than being listed in the ingredient section. The instability of PUFAs is primarily why the food industry substitutes hydrogenated fats in processed foods—hydrogenation makes fats more stable. Unfortunately, the hydrogenated fats can act as irritants, generating free radicals, which have been implicated in cancer and cardiovascular disease.

Monounsaturated fat. This signifies the number of grams of monounsaturated fats in each serving. These are healthy fats found in such vegetable oils as olive, canola, or peanut oil. They are more stable, with less of a tendency to become rancid. Their listing is also voluntary, and no % daily value is indicated. **We should consume more of the healthier monounsaturates and fewer saturated and polyunsaturated ones.**

Cholesterol. This indicates the number of milligrams of cholesterol per serving. This figure reflects the presence of a particular animal fat (sterol) in the product. Food cholesterol is different from body cholesterols. There are helpful and problematic fractions of cholesterol, namely HDL (the so-called good high-density lipoprotein) and LDL (the so-called bad low-density lipoprotein). **There is clear consensus in the medical and nutrition community that it is important to limit the amount of cholesterol we ingest.** Saturated and hydrogenated fats seem to increase harmful blood cholesterol levels, whereas more healthful monounsaturated fats and fish oils improve cholesterol and protect against cardiovascular disease. The % daily value is accepted at 300 mg per day.

Sodium. This represents the amount of sodium in each serving. (Sodium is one of the minerals in salt, or sodium chloride.) Such processed foods as crackers, canned soups, packaged meats, and potato or other chips have fairly high amounts of sodium. The total daily value acceptable for sodium is 2,500 mg; this amount can be quite easy to surpass, especially if you have a taste for salty foods or add salt to your meals. Restaurant foods and fast foods are often high is this most common flavor enhancer. **People on low-sodium diets should watch this category carefully,** especially those with high blood pressure, heart disease, or problems with fluid retention.

On a food package, the phrase "reduced sodium" indicates 25% or less sodium content than the "normal" version of that food; "light in sodium" means sodium has been reduced by at least 50%; "low-sodium" means the food has 140 mg or less of sodium; "very low sodium" means 35 mg or less; and "sodium-free" means the food has less than 5 mg per serving.

Total carbohydrate. This signifies the number of grams of carbohydrate in each serving. Carbohydrates include starches, sugars, and dietary fibers and contribute 4 calories of energy per gram. Simple carbohydrates include primarily dextrose, glucose, and fructose (from fruits), while complex ones are starches in wheat and rice as well as dietary fiber. The total daily value for carbohydrate appears to about 300 grams (about 1,200 calories and nearly 60% of the average diet), and the label may provide a percentage of that amount. Read the serving size carefully to be sure of how much carbohydrate you are getting in what you eat. For example, a loaf of whole-grain bread I checked recently listed a serving size as one piece, but typically most people eat two or more slices in a single serving. Knowing your total carbohydrate content means multiplying the number of servings consumed by the number of carbs per serving.

Eating too many carbohydrates (fruits, juices, sweets, and starches) in the diet is one of the greatest risk factors for obesity and can cause rapid mood swings. The main concern is with refined carbohydrates—products made with refined flour and sugar. These include white breads, white rice, and most pastas; most baked goods, such as cookies, cakes, doughnuts, and crackers; as well as foods high in sweeteners, such as sodas, candy, and ice cream. Too many sweets or simple sugars can overtax the body's insulin activity. A diet high in refined carbohydrates has been associated with hypoglycemia problems, diabetes, or atherosclerosis, and subsequent cardiovascular problems. Thus focusing as early in life as possible on more wholesome complex carbohydrate foods—whole grains (such as brown rice, oats, and whole wheat), whole-grain pastas, and root vegetables—supports better carbohydrate function and more nutrients per calorie from these healthier foods.

Dietary fiber. This indicates the number of grams of fiber per serving. Because fiber is important for preventing diseases and supporting proper colon health, it is specifically listed. However, this entry applies primarily to fiber added back into processed foods, which typically contain only small amounts of fiber compared with whole foods. Fresh fruits and vegetables, whole grains, and beans are commonly high in natural fiber, but these foods are not usually labeled. The minimal suggested intake for daily dietary fiber is 25 to 30 grams.

Sugars. On the label, "sugars" refers to the number of grams of simple sugar per serving. Multiplying by 4 calories per gram provides the total calories from sugars. Sugar content refers not only to sweeteners added to the product, but also to sugars that occur naturally, such as fructose in fruits and lactose in milk. This is a key area to monitor in order to maintain good health. Limiting refined sugar intake and lowering all simple sugars is important. Also, remember to limit even sugars from juices and natural sweeteners, while increasing the complex carbohydrate intake. Try to moderate both man-made sweeteners (refined cane and beet sugars, corn syrup, corn sweeteners, fructose, and the artificial aspartame and saccharin) as well as natural sugars (honey, maple syrup, malt, molasses, rice syrup, fruit juice concentrates, and dried fruits). **The majority of simple sugars in the diet should come from fresh fruits.**

Protein. This indicates the number of grams of protein per serving. Protein is an essential nutrient that comes primarily from animal tissues, legumes (beans and tofu), nuts and seeds, and dairy products. We can also obtain complete proteins by combining plants, such as rice or corn with beans. Almost all foods, even fruits and vegetables, actually contain some amino acids. We require a certain amount of protein foods, based on our individual body needs, activity level, and state of health.

Protein deficiency can also cause problems, such as fatigue, hypoglycemia, and less resistance to disease. Excess protein, on the other hand, can create problems of long-term toxicity from overconsumption of these more concentrated foods. They make the body more acidic, which may promote osteoporosis and other metabolic disorders. We need at least 40 to 50 grams of dietary protein a day, or roughly 1 ounce of protein per 50 pounds of body weight. We may need additional protein with pregnancy, before and after surgery, when doing more exercise or bodybuilding, or when recovering from an illness. The % daily value may not be mentioned on the label, but it is typically about 60 grams a day.

Other nutrients. This indicates some of the essential vitamins and minerals. Most food labels include four items: vitamin A, vitamin C, calcium, and iron. **It is important to remember that your requirements for nutrients are individual and unique to your body, and that optimum levels of intake are often higher than government standards for the minimal requirements to prevent deficiency.** Like protein and all nutrients, the requirements for vitamins A and C increase when we are ill and under other special circumstances. The needs for calcium and iron are also unique depending on gender (women usually need more) and stage of development, for example adolescence, pregnancy, or menopause. Therefore, if these values are going to be useful for you, you need to understand these issues more completely.

Vitamin A. This is an important nutrient for healthy tissue and skin, for immune function, as well as for helping to fight infections. Both vitamin A and beta-carotene, a precursor for vitamin A, are included in this category; these specific nutrients tend to be interactive. (Specifically, beta-carotene is a double molecule of vitamin A, which must be split by an enzyme found in the liver and small intestine into vitamin A; therefore, beta-carotene represents only potential vitamin A activity.) The basic requirement for vitamin A is 5,000 IU, and there is no specific requirement for beta-carotene, even though it is an important antioxidant nutrient found in fresh fruits and vegetables. Nutritionists are looking at all the carotenoid pigments found in foods, termed *mixed carotenoids,* as important for overall health—not just beta-carotene.

Vitamin C. This is among the most important nutrients for staying healthy. This water-soluble vitamin is an essential antioxidant protecting against many toxins. It also helps fight disease and is used in nutritional medicine for a variety of therapies. The package information suggests a minimum daily intake of 30 to 60 mg, but my experience indicates that many people do best with 1,000 to 3,000 mg daily, which would require the use of an additional supplement.

Calcium. This is an important nutrient to support bones and other functions relating to cell metabolism and electrical conductivity. The daily requirement for calcium is 850 mg, but this may vary depending on gender, menopause status, and other factors.

Iron. This is another required nutrient for the production of hemoglobin in the red blood cells, which carries oxygen around the body to support life. The iron requirement is different for men and women; men need about 10 mg a day, while menstruating women need 18 mg. Pregnant women need more, while postmenopausal women need less. Iron needs depends on the blood count and iron status in the body.

Other nutrients. These may be listed on food labels and include vitamins D and E, niacin (vitamin B3), phosphorus, or zinc.

Ingredients

Another important part of the food label is the list of ingredients. The contents are listed in order by quantity—the predominant ingredient in the product is listed first, the smallest last. This is an important point. Recently, my family found an all-organic treat that sounded pretty healthy, but it contained more sugar than anything else (it was the first ingredient). The ingredient list on the label is also where the *direct additives* are listed (along with the food components, of course)—that is, the additives allowed by the FDA as part of the product.

Indirect Additives and Unlabeled Foods

Sometimes the label does not contain all the information consumers need. Foods frequently also contain *indirect additives.* These are substances that enter the food in any phase of production from the farm to the factory, the grower to the green grocer. In other cases, labeling information may not be available, as in the case of meats, which are currently sold unlabeled, so we have no way of knowing the fat content, particularly the amount of saturated fat, in each ounce.

Using the Label to Avoid Disease

Thousands of research studies have found that there is a real link between what we eat and our health. **Public health authorities report that at least one-third to one-half of all cases of cancer and heart disease in the United States are caused by diets high in fat and salt and low in fiber.** And they have not even made a statement of chemical exposure. Food labels provide the information that can help us choose foods wisely and thereby reduce the risk of heart disease and cancer and help cope with specific health conditions. Below I examine a few common concerns and how each is affected by various dietary factors.

> **On the Label or Not?** Not everything, every chemical, that is in our food is listed on the label. Obviously, during growing, many chemicals are typically used and they are not identified, measured, or listed on the label. Food manufacturers also use a wide variety of chemicals that are not officially added to the food. During processing, for example, the fruits, vegetables, whole grains, and other foods are ground, mashed, boiled, and otherwise manipulated to create the multitude of boxed, canned, packaged, and plastic wrapped "foods" found in the stores.

Allergies. Not all additives are safe for everyone, so be sure to read the ingredients carefully if you or a family member suffer from allergies, reactive digestive problems, or lactose intolerance. Some people with a tendency toward asthma have strong reactions to sulfites, even problems as serious as anaphylactic shock; others react to MSG, experiencing a sense of faintness or chest pains; and many people are allergic to citrus fruits, dairy, eggs, or wheat. Clear labeling information helps you to avoid any allergens you know about.

High blood pressure. Nearly 50 million Americans suffer from high blood pressure (hypertension) and many others are at risk. Food labels can be especially helpful with this concern, because the label states the amount of salt (sodium) per serving. **Keeping sodium at reasonable intake levels is an**

Food Label Terms

FATS

Fat-free: fewer than 0.5 g of fat per serving

Low-fat: 3 g or fewer per serving

Reduced-fat: at least 25% less fat than a correlating food

Cholesterol-free: fewer than 2 mg, and 2 g or fewer of saturated fat per serving

Low-cholesterol: 20 mg or fewer, and 2 g or fewer of saturated fat per serving

Reduced or less cholesterol: at least 25% less than a reference food and 2 g or fewer of saturated fat per serving

MEATS

Lean: fewer than 10 g of total fat, 4.5 g of saturated fat, and 95 mg of cholesterol per serving

Extra lean: fewer than 5 g of total fat, fewer than 2 g of saturated fat, and fewer than 95 mg of cholesterol per 100 g

HEALTHY

Low-fat: less than 3 g per serving

Light (there are 2 meanings):

One-third fewer calories or half the fat of the reference food, but if the food derives 50% or more of its calories from fat, the reduction must be at least 50% of the fat.

A low-calorie or low-fat food whose sodium has been reduced by at least 50% compared to the reference food. "Light in sodium" may also be used when the food has 50% or less sodium than the reference food but does not meet the restrictions for calories and fat.

CALORIES

Calorie-free: fewer than 5 calories per serving

Low-calorie: 40 or fewer calories per serving

Reduced or fewer calories: at least 25% fewer calories than the reference food

FIBER*

High-fiber: 5 g or more per serving

Good source of fiber: 2.5–4.9 g of fiber per serving

More or added fiber: at least 2.5 g more per serving than the reference food.

SUGAR

Sugar-free: fewer than 0.5 g per serving

No added sugar, without added sugar, or no sugar added: no sugar or sugar substitutes (for example, corn syrup or fruit juice) added during processing or packing; or, no ingredients made with added sugars, such as jams, jellies, or concentrated fruit juice

SODIUM OR SALT

Sodium-free or salt-free: fewer than 5 mg per serving

Very low sodium or salt: 35 mg or fewer per serving

Low-sodium: 140 mg or fewer per serving

Light in sodium: at least 50% or less sodium per serving than the reference amount

Lightly salted: at least 50% less sodium per serving than the reference food

Reduced or less sodium: at least 25% less per serving than the reference food

POTASSIUM

High-potassium: 700 mg or more per serving

Good source of potassium: 350–665 mg per serving

More or added potassium: at least 350 mg more per serving than the reference food

CALCIUM

High-calcium: 200 mg or more per serving

Good source of calcium: 100–190 mg per serving

More or added calcium: at least 100 mg more per serving than the reference food

Source: A Food Labeling Guide, U.S. Food and Drug Administration, Center for Food Safety & Applied Nutrition, Revised Version June 1999.

* Foods making claims about increased fiber content also must meet the requirements for "low-fat" or the amount of fat per serving must appear next to the claim.

important key to controlling high blood pressure. Sodium in a number of forms may be added during food processing or occur naturally in such foods as milk, cheese, meat, fish, and certain vegetables. High blood pressure is also more common in overweight people, those with high cholesterol, and those who consume excessive fats in their diet. Anyone with a tendency to hypertension should watch their sodium level as well as calorie and fat intake. **The food label can also be used to monitor fat, calories, and carbohydrate intake to limit weight gain—important because obesity is a causative factor in hypertension.**

Heart disease. If the label has a claim about the relationship of diet to heart disease, the food must be low in total fats, saturated fat, and cholesterol, because high intake of any of these categories is linked to elevated blood cholesterol and increased risk of coronary artery disease, the most common degenerative disease. The current general recommendation is to limit fats to 30% or less of the day's nutritional intake, with saturated fat limited to 10% of total calories. (Thus, for a 2,000 calorie diet, that amounts to about 65 grams of fat a day and only 20 grams of saturated fat.) People with extremely high blood cholesterol or with existing heart disease may need to limit fat intake even further, based on their doctor's recommendation. For example, the diet recommended by Dr. Dean Ornish for reversing and preventing heart disease allows only 10% fat, all from unsaturated sources. You would also want to monitor other nutrients, such as sodium and fiber, to support a low-salt, high-fiber diet.

Diabetes. Labeling information can also be vital to people with diabetes, because diet is very important in managing this condition. Poorly managed diabetes can greatly increase the risk of cardiovascular disease, so diabetics need to monitor fat intake, especially saturated fat and cholesterol. **In addition, of course, diabetics should limit their intake of sweets and refined starches to stabilize their blood sugar.**

STAYING HEALTHY IN THE KITCHEN: HOW TO KEEP CLEAN AND NOT GET FOOD POISONING

Most of us spend a significant part of our daily lives shopping for food, preparing meals, and consuming the by-products of our efforts. For many of us, mealtime is still an important ritual, but we consider the shopping, food preparation, and cleanup aspects to be mundane and tedious tasks. Being lax in these important chores, however, can pose serious risks to our health. This section encourages readers to regard their work in the kitchen as a meaningful contribution to the family's good health. How we handle foods and the cleanliness of our kitchens are vital topics, as important as the way we eat and what we choose to consume.

Food Preparation and Hygiene: Avoiding Contamination

What kinds of problems come up during food preparation and storage? All food in cans, boxes, plastic bags, containers, jars, and bottles have a particular shelf life that may vary from a few hours to several

---

A New Outlook in Food Preparation

- **The mindfulness of cooking.** Food preparation and hygiene are a reflection of our awareness and attentiveness to other aspects of our lives.
- **The elegance of cleanliness.** Even a simple meal can be quite beautiful if it is composed of wholesome ingredients and attractively arranged. However, it is difficult to create elegance when the kitchen or dining areas are cluttered or unclean.
- **The rituals of handling food.** There are certain rituals associated with kitchen hygiene and food preparation that have kept people from harm for ages.
- **Creating order in our lives.** The more organized we are, the less likely we will be to have contamination. An orderly kitchen allows greater efficiency in all aspects of cooking and cleanup.

years. Foods can spoil. Most of the fresh fruits and vegetables, depending on their ripeness and refrigeration, must be used within a few days to 1 or 2 weeks. Fresh-cut meats, poultry, and fish, which are most easily contaminated by microbes or insect larvae, must be refrigerated. Wrapping may give some protection, but these foods should be eaten as soon as possible, within a few days, or frozen and labeled with date and content.

Whole grains and beans store well because of their protective coverings, although bug infestation can be a problem, especially with organic foods. Storing grains and flours in the refrigerator will often help prevent this. Nuts and seeds are definitely best refrigerated, even stored in the freezer, to prevent these oily foods from going rancid. Most foods that are prepackaged in boxes, cans, and jars contain some kind of spoilage retardants and do well when stored in cupboards. Often, open packages of cereals, crackers, and other grain products must be used rapidly or be refrigerated to protect them from insect infestation, especially in the warmer months.

Food preparation presents several other possible problems besides food spoilage. **The main concern is food contamination by microorganisms such as bacteria, viruses, or molds.** Other concerns are the use of chemicals in cooking or seasoning and the hazards involved in the various cooking processes. Food contamination may occur at any step, from the time the food is grown to the time it reaches the plate and palate of the consumer. Molds are the most common microbes that contaminate foods; they may grow on cheeses, nuts, breads, meats, herbs, and grains. In general, most molds are fairly well tolerated when consumed in small amounts. Some people, however, are allergic or sensitive to molds. If one is not overly sensitive, typically the mold can be removed from the cheese, for example, and then the remainder can still be used.

Certain molds and foods may produce specific toxins that can be dangerous. Aflatoxin, produced by the molds *Aspergillus flavus* and *A. parasiticus,* is such a substance that is potentially harmful, especially to the liver, where it can cause a type of hepatitis or even cancer. It has been associated most commonly with peanuts but may also contaminate other nuts as well as corn, wheat, and barley. The fresh peanut butter grinder in the grocery store is a

place where we should take caution in this regard. If the grocery has outstanding sanitation techniques and cleans their peanut-grinding machine regularly, we are on safe ground. But if it is left unclean, the heat from grinding combined with the moisture from the peanuts make a perfect environment for growth of unwanted microorganisms and potential production of aflatoxin. Many bacteria produce toxins, while most mushrooms contain toxic substances that could cause problems ranging from intestinal upset to fatal neurotoxicity. Examples of these bacterial toxins are found with the chemical cycasin, produced by certain nuts grown in Japan, as well as the bracken fern and chewed betel nut leaf (India), which can cause stomach cancer or mouth cancer, respectively.

Another source of food contamination is produced by the widespread use of antibiotics in animals. At least 70% of all large cattle feedlots incorporate antibiotics into the animals' daily food supply. The ratio is approximately .25 pound of antibiotic per 15 to 20 pounds of feed. At least a quarter of all small feedlots also use antibiotics in this way. In the pork industry, for example, 90% of all starter feeds and 75% of all grower feeds contain antibiotics. In this industry, the cost of the antibiotics has been estimated at 3.75% of the total feed cost. But this practice has also been estimated to increase the total revenue to the pork producer by about 7% to 8%.

The Union of Concerned Scientists (www.ucsusa .org) has estimated that a total of 24.6 million total pounds of antibiotics were used for nonmedical purposes in U.S. meat production in 2001, including 10.3 million pounds in hogs, 10.5 millions pounds in chickens, and 3.7 million pounds in cattle. These estimates do not include antibiotics used to treat diseases in these animals. Antibiotic use may lead to the development of resistant, harder-to-treat organisms and toxic residues or antibiotic breakdown products, often stored in the animals' livers and fatty tissues. Most ranchers and farmers allow a drug-withdrawal period before they slaughter their livestock in order to reduce the drug levels in the edible tissues. However, this is not always done, and even after a 2-week withdrawal period, antibiotic levels in tissues may still be high enough that a penicillin or sulfa-sensitive person may have an allergic reaction to the drug residue in the meats.

Potential Sources of Contamination during Production

PHASE	SOURCES
Production and harvest Growing, picking, bundling	Irrigation water, manure, lack of field sanitation
Initial processing Washing, waxing, sorting, boxing	Wash water, handling, inadequate hygiene of environment, pests
Distribution Transport by truck, rail, or sea	Ice, dirty trucks or tankers
Final processing Slicing, squeezing, shredding, peeling, mechanical extraction, mixing of batches	Wash water, handling, poor hygiene of equipment, cross contamination
Display in the supermarket Handling, moisturizing, displaying	Inadequate hygiene of employees, cross contamination in displays, infested produce sprays, airborne microbes

---

Weight-promoting drugs are also used, especially in beef. Various hormones have been and are still used to increase weight and reduce the estrous cycle in animals. Some cancer-producing steroids, such as diethylstilbestrol (DES), an estrogen hormone, have been used. In 1979 DES was banned from use in livestock to be consumed by the public, but that does not mean that it is no longer used. For example, in 2000, DES residues showed up in shipments of beef from the United States to Switzerland. Most of the estrogenic hormones are potentially carcinogenic in humans, particularly in women. A slow-release estrogen pellet is usually injected in the back of the cow's ear at about 6 or 7 months of age to provide this hormonal growth boost. In 1989, the European Union (EU) banned the sales of hormone-treated U.S. meat in member countries because potential for adverse health risk.

A word about organic meat products: Antibiotic use is currently allowed in the production of organically grown beef, chicken, and pork, but only when the antibiotic is necessary to treat an existing disease. Whether this standard is sufficient to protect consumers of organically grown meats remains a matter of debate. Because there are many concerns, besides infection from animal foods, it looks that being more vegetarian—even following a strict vegetarian (vegan) diet that also avoids milk and egg products—is safer. Fewer worries is always helpful. There may also be some concern with microbial contamination of organic foods, because they do not possess the toxic chemicals that keep parasites and their eggs from thriving on them. Because of this, it is helpful in the kitchen to clean even fresh organic fruits and vegetables with water, perhaps also using a food-oriented disinfectant, and to grow them ourselves wherever and whenever we can.

Food poisoning refers mainly to illness caused by bacterial or viral contamination of food that occurs during food shipping, as a result of improper refrigeration, or during preparation. Some foods, such as meats, may be infectious even before the animals are slaughtered. The issues of meat quality and mad cow disease are discussed in more detail on page 480 of chapter 11, Food and the Earth. Most of the problems of food-borne infections come from animal foods. Parasites can also be contracted from these

Food Contamination by Microbes

Disease or Agent	Estimated Total Cases	Reported Cases by Surveillance Type			% Foodborne Transmission	Hospitalization Rate	Case Fatality Rate
		ACTIVE	PASSIVE	OUTBREAK			
BACTERIAL							
Bacillus cereus	*27,360*		720	72	*100*	*0.006*	*0.0000*
Botulism, foodborne	58		29		*100*	*0.800*	*0.0769*
Brucella spp.	*1,554*		111		*50*	*0.550*	*0.0500*
Campylobacter spp.	*2,453,926*	64,577	37,496	146	*80*	*0.201*	*0.0010*
Clostridium perfringens	*248,520*		6,540	654	*100*	*0.003*	*0.0005*
Escherichia coli O157-H7	*73,480*	*3,674*	2,725	500	*85*	*0.295*	*0.0083*
E. coli non-0157 STEC	*36,740*	*1,837*			*85*	*0.295*	*0.0083*
E. coli enterotoxigenic	*79,420*		2,090	209	*70*	*0.005*	*0.0001*
E. coli other diarrheogenic	*79,420*		2,090		*30*	*0.005*	*0.0001*
Listeria monocytogenes	*2,518*	*1,259*	373		*99*	*0.922*	*0.2000*
Salmonella typhi[b]	*824*		412		*80*	*0.750*	*0.0040*
Salmonella nontyphoidal	*1,412,498*	*37,171*	37,842	3,640	*95*	*0.221*	*0.0078*
Shigella spp.	*448,240*	*22,412*	17,324	1,476	*20*	*0.139*	*0.0016*
Staphylococcus food poisoning	*185,060*		4,870	487	*100*	*0.180*	*0.0002*
Streptococcus, foodborne	*50,920*		*1,340*	134	*100*	*0.133*	*0.000*
Vibrio cholerae, toxigenic	*54*		27		*90*	*0.340*	*0.0060*
V. vulnificus	*94*		47		*50*	*0.910*	*0.3900*
Vibrio, other	*7,880*	*393*	112		*65*	*0.126*	*0.0250*
Yersinia enterocolitica	*96,368*	*2,536*			*90*	*0.242*	*0.0005*
SUBTOTAL	*5,204,934*						
PARASITIC							
Cryptosporidium parvum	*300,000*	*6,630*	2,788		*10*	*0.150*	*0.005*
Cyclospora cayetanensis	*16,264*	*428*	98		*90*	*0.020*	*0.0005*
Giardia lamblia	*2,000,000*	*107,000*	22,907		*10*	*n/a*	*n/a*
Toxoplasma gondii	*225,000*		15,000		*50*	*n/a*	*n/a*
Trichinella spiralis	*52*		26		*100*	*0.081*	*0.003*
SUBTOTAL	*2,541,316*						
VIRAL							
Norwalk-like viruses	*23,000,000*				*40*	*n/a*	*n/a*
Rotavirus	*3,900,000*				*1*	*n/a*	*n/a*
Astrovirus	*3,900,000*				*1*	*n/a*	*n/a*
Hepatitus A	*83,391*		27,797		*5*	*0.130*	*0.0030*
SUBTOTAL	*30,883,391*						
GRAND TOTAL	*38,629,641*						

Source of information: P.S. Mead, L. Slutsker, V. Dietz, et al. (1999). "Food-Related Illness and Death in the United States." *Emerging Infectious Diseases* 5(5), 840-842. Table 2. Reported and estimated[a] illnesses, frequency of foodborne transmission, and hospitalization and case-fatality rates for known foodborne pathogens, United States
a) Numbers in italics are estimates, others are measured. b) Greater than 70% of cases acquired abroad.

foods as well as through water. Contamination of the human intestinal tract with pathogenic bacteria and viruses is the cause for most cases of acute diarrhea. The FDA has estimated that somewhere between 100 million and 300 million cases of diarrhea occur yearly, and nearly one-third of those are caused by contaminated foods. Other causes include food allergy, absorption problems, emotional stress, and intestinal diseases.

The U.S. Centers for Disease Control has estimated that food-borne diseases result in 76 million instances of illness, 325,000 hospitalizations, and 5,000 deaths each year. About one-third of these deaths have been directly traced to three organisms—salmonella, listeria, and toxoplasma—and another third can be directly traced to a variety of other specific bacteria or parasites. Many other organisms cause intestinal infections—such bacteria as shigella, campylobacter, and certain E. coli strains (most are normal); such viruses as hepatitis A; and such parasites as cryptosporidium, blastocystis, and various amoebas. Giardia can be a problem from contaminated waters, especially local rivers.

Food can be contaminated in several ways. Contamination can occur before a food is packaged if the cans, jars, or packages already contain microorganisms, or from hands of people touching them. The occurrence of this seems to be decreasing as packaging conditions become safer and more sanitary. Food can also be contaminated by the environment; microorganisms are everywhere, and if food is not properly protected or stored, these germs may multiply and cause disease.

People contaminate food as well, either those working in factories helping to process or package it or, more commonly, those who prepare foods at home or in restaurants. And what about shopping carts and the others who use them? Some viruses, such as those that cause hepatitis A, may be transmitted in this way, but luckily, this is not common. Most intestinal viruses are not thought to be contagious by respiratory transfer. However, staphylococcal germs may get into foods from either the skin or the respiratory tract of the food preparer, and this occasionally causes food poisoning. The symptoms are similar to salmonella poisoning, occurring within several hours of exposure and usually lasting 1 or 2 days. Common experiences with food poisoning include abdominal pain and cramps, dehydration and fatigue, achiness, and of

Avoiding Food Contamination		
FOOD	**PREVENTION OF INFECTION**	**RISK**
Milk, raw salmonella	Purchase only pasteurized milk	Campylobacter, E. coli, Listeria,
Raw cheeses: brie, blue-veined, Camembert, feta	To be avoided by infants, children, elders, and those with chronic illness	Listeria
Water	Filter to "1 micron absolute" or boil for 15 minutes	Campylobacter, Cryptosporidium E. Coli, Giardia
Honey	Do not feed to infants or those who are immunocompromised	Botulism
Fruit juices, cider	Buy pasteurized or bring to a boil	E. coli
Fruits: cantaloupe, raspberries, strawberries, frozen	Wash thoroughly; soak in Organo-Clean or other natural disinfectant	Salmonella, Cyclospora, Hepatitis A
Vegetables and tomatoes	Soak in OrganoClean	Cyclospora, E. coli, Listeria, Salmonella, Shigella
Home canning—avoiding spoilage from storage	Boil for 10 minutes at above 165 degrees F	Botulism
Spices: paprika	Store in refrigerator	Salmonella

Source: National Food Safety Information Network, Center for Food Safety and Applied Nutrition, Food and Drug Administration (www.foodsafety.gov).

course vomiting sometimes and diarrhea often. In general, if the diarrhea is not too severe or does not last very long, food poisoning can be a good means of purging and cleaning out the intestines. People often feel better than ever, and a little lighter, after experiencing it; still I do not recommend this as a new weight-loss program. Contaminated food is a real health issue.

How can we avoid the spread of infections through food? First, it is important that the food preparer, whether at home or in a restaurant, be responsible for keeping his or her hands clean and avoid handling foods when he or she is sick. If there are any cuts or open sores on the hands, rubber gloves will reduce the spread of any bacteria. Make sure to wash

your hands before handling food, especially after handling money or animals, or each other, phones, doorknobs, and the like. It is important to wash while caring for children, particularly after wiping noses or changing diapers. Food-preparation surfaces, such as countertops and cutting boards, should be cleaned after each use so that organisms do not grow. Cutting utensils should also be kept clean.

Foods can also be contaminated before they are purchased. Avoid buying overripe produce; do not buy or use bulging cans, outdated foods, or packaged foods with broken seals. If a food smells or tastes funny or spoiled, take it back or throw it out. Meats and poultry should always be kept refrigerated and used within 1 or 2 days, or else they should be frozen for use later.

Nontoxic Household Cleaners

PRODUCTS	CONCERNS	BEST OPTION
Dishwashing liquid	May have dye, ammonia, artificial fragrance	Green, or environmentally safe, products
Dishwasher detergent	Chlorine	Green products now in health food stores; Seventh Generation products available through mail order
Cleanser	Chlorine; Possible asbestos	Nonchlorinated scouring powder; available in supermarkets and health food stores; baking soda, borax, salt
Germ-killing disinfectants	Cresol, phenol, ethanol, formaldehyde	1/2 cup borax in 1 gallon hot water; hydrogen peroxide; solution of ammonia, chlorine, and benzalkonium chloride
Drain cleaners	Lye (poisonous)	1 handful baking soda and 1/2 cup white vinegar or 1/2 cup each salt and baking soda followed by hot water; follow by using a plunger
Ammonia and all-purpose cleaners	Ammonia (skin irritant, chemical burns); aerosol sprays	1 quart hot water in a spray bottle or bucket with either liquid soap or borax; or green products
Chlorine bleach	Chlorine by-products	Nonchlorine bleach (Seventh Generation)
General cleaner		1/2 tsp washing soda, 2 tsp liquid soap and 2 cups hot water
Oven cleaner	Lye, ammonia, aerosols	Use chemicals carefully for really dirty ovens; or in a spray bottle, add 2 tbsp liquid soap, 2 tsp borax, and warm water; or make a paste of liquid soap and borax
Glass cleaners	Ammonia, blue dye	Solution of half water and half vinegar in spray bottle or bucket
Mold and mildew cleaners	Kerosene, formaldehyde, phenol, pentachlorophenol	Borax or vinegar and water; heat and/or dehumidifier

Courtesy of Debra Lynn Dadd, *The Nontoxic Home and Office* and *Home Safe Home*.

Frozen foods should be kept frozen or used soon after thawing, and usually shouldn't be refrozen.

Care must also be taken to avoid contamination after food is cooked. Bacteria grow rapidly at room temperature but slowly when the food is cold. Cooked foods should not be left sitting out overnight; if they are, they should be thoroughly recooked to kill any bacteria they may have grown. (This is a relatively wise use of microwave ovens.) Home canning or jarring should be done carefully in sterile conditions; if done improperly, this is probably the most common cause of botulism (meats and green beans being the worst culprits). There is also a slight risk of botulism in feeding infants honey.

You can find a lot more details about keeping a safe and healthy kitchen in chapter 9 of my book *The Staying Healthy Shopper's Guide*. If we are not careful and conscientious, we can be exposed to chemicals in our kitchen and other areas of our home. The cleaners we use are a common source of chemical exposure. I encourage people to use more natural cleaners for all purposes in their homes. Many companies now focus on nontoxic dish soaps, counter and glass cleaners, detergents, and so on. I provide a list of some of these companies in the back of my book *The New Detox Diet*. See the table on page 407 on "Nontoxic Household Cleaners" for some options.

Food Storage and Recycling

Another aspect of food safety and protection involves how we store our foods. This starts with proper refrigeration. When I worked with my folks as a teenager in our grocery store, my dad taught me to "rotate and rejuvenate," one of his many one-liners. This means to keep everything fresh, or at least, let the minimum spoil. The newer products go toward the back and the earlier foods move to the front so that they get used first. It is a challenge, but I apply this principle to my refrigerator. First, it helps to organize our shelves so we know what goes where—that is, have a system. Then when I shop and bring home groceries, I look and see what is there and pull out older foods and leftovers, storing the new items further back and in their appropriate area. I have gotten used to this process so that I even cook this way quite often. When I am preparing a meal, rather than finding foods to fit

an exact recipe, I typically begin by looking through my fridge to see what needs to be used most immediately. I then create my meal/menu from these foods.

Cleanliness is not only about keeping clean, but also about not letting things get old and spoil. Even so, foods will spoil; it is wise to just let them go and discard them rather than take the risk of getting sick. Your compost or garbage will handle them better. In storing foods, we need to be aware of foods that mold, like breads and cheeses, and use them before they go bad. If we are using whole-grain breads without many preservatives, we may wish to refrigerate or freeze them to give them a longer life. I use little bread and cheese in my kitchen any more, so this is a small concern for me. To avoid pests like moths and mice, our grains and goodies need to be closed in storage containers to be kept fresh and protected. Leaving breads and baked goods or cereals in open packages in our cupboards can attract these pests. Not keeping counters clean will put out food smells to neighborhood insects, such as ants and flies, to come visit and crawl around our counters.

Regarding recycling, I encourage all of us to recycle as much as we possibly can—newspapers and magazines, glass, aluminum and tin cans, cardboard, and plastic—as well as kitchen scraps for your compost pile and garden. Hopefully this continues to be a worthy business and the technology is efficient, meaning it saves money or creates less toxicity to recycle materials. There is some further discussion about recycling and ideas for conserving materials in chapter 11, Food and the Earth, and in chapter 10 of *The Staying Healthy Shopper's Guide*.

Eating Away from Home and Staying Healthy

With any healthy diet plan, think preparation, ahead of time. I suggest to my patients and groups that when following any special eating program (and I have many) that they focus on what they are eating rather than what they are avoiding. Then make a list of those good foods, shop for them, and have them available in the home (and the car even); then prepare these good foods and have what you need to eat when you are hungry and when they are scheduled for consumption. Sometimes we just need to write out our plan and follow it. Having the foods and meals we plan ready for us at work or school or on the road allows us to implement our individualized program and thus get the expected results.

When we need or wish to eat away from home, our first thought might be a healthy deli and especially the health food store delis, such as those in the many wonderful Whole Foods markets and many other natural food stores. Foods are made fresh with wholesome and often organic choices, and there is usually a selection of soups and a great salad bar to create your own vital green salad. After that, we might learn to make the best choices in the wide variety of local and international restaurants that use the least amount of chemicals and toxins.

When eating out, make sure that the restaurant is clean and the foods used are fresh, if that is possible. If you can see the chef, make sure that he or she looks healthy. When the food is served, smell it and taste it first before gobbling it down so you can more easily tell whether it is of good quality. Watch for heavily salty tastes or extra additives in the food; perhaps even ask whether such additives as MSG or sulfites are used. Nowadays, more Chinese restaurants advertise that they use no MSG, or they will at least avoid using it in your food if you ask.

From chapter 9, Diets, use the concepts of natural foods in your restaurants as much as you can. For example, in my Chinese and Thai restaurant visits, I let my waitperson know that I am nutritionally sensitive, have a strict diet, and experience food reactions (at times I may say I am a nutritional doctor or nutty doc). I ask for no MSG, minimal or no cornstarch (often used to thicken sauces), and, please, only fresh vegetables—not canned. I will add my own soy sauce to taste (and chile paste), so they do not need to add a lot. The typical restaurant wants to serve flavorful and appealing food, and thus they may add fats and oils as well as salts and seasonings to achieve this, which makes those foods higher in hidden calories and sodium. That is why I tell my patients who consume a high amount of restaurant food that it is difficult to lose weight and detoxify their bodies while eating often at restaurants, even supposedly healthy ones.

Another example is my burrito at Mexican restaurants, which I commonly make at home with organic corn tortillas instead of the bigger whole wheat ones

Five Basic Guidelines for Eating Out and Staying Healthy

1. Preparing and eating the majority of your meals at home gives you and your family the greatest control over your diet. This is better for your budget and your health, with less exposure to viruses and other germs.
2. Save dining out as a treat, and when you do, make healthy choices.
3. If you work long hours, develop a repertoire of wholesome, tasty bagged lunches or dinners to bring with you.
4. Try to assess the cleanliness and quality of the restaurant before you decide to dine there. Ask friends or just go in and look around. Your intuition and observations may protect you from discomfort and unnecessary medical bills. Don't be afraid to ask questions; you have a right to know what you are investing in and putting into your body.
5. Carry nutritional supplements with you to aid digestion and protect your health.

that I do not digest as well. If possible, I order grilled vegetables, rice, and beans, as well as guacamole and salsa, and I avoid the cheese and sour cream. So, what is right for you? As you learn more about your body and what foods work best in it, you can guide your favorite restaurant to support you. Thai food, with its spicy curries, is currently my favorite cuisine, and my local Thai restaurant makes my Dr. Sun's Savory Seasonal Soup with a coconut milk base and fresh seasonal vegetables, such as carrots, onion, zucchini, and peppers. To make it a bit spicy, they use hot peppers. Yum!

Chapter 9, Diets, reviews different diets, both types of diets and cultural ones, and points out the strengths and weaknesses for health. In my book *The Staying Healthy Shopper's Guide,* chapter 11 is about eating away from home. This gets into more specifics on how to make healthier choices in each type of restaurant. There are further suggestions about eating better while traveling, which is always a challenge, especially with airplane and hotel food. I also have articles and tips about these topics on my website, www.elsonhaas.com. Also, see the "Executives and Healthy Travel" section on page 620 in chapter 16, Performance Enhancement Programs. Learn to enjoy your food and ideally the simpler, natural flavors of real foods, wherever you are.

Nourishing Our Children

Because most parents feel a duty to keep their kids healthy, yet often succumb to treats and poor food choices and habits to get by, here I include a few guidelines for nourishing children healthfully. I have a fuller discussion of this in chapter 12 of my *Staying Healthy Shopper's Guide* as well as in the health tips and articles on my website (www.elsonhaas.com). I know that it is difficult to change your habits for the benefit of others; this needs to be something you do for yourself. If anyone should make positive changes, however, it is parents for the sake of their children, and ultimately themselves.

Here are my top 10 guidelines for parents who want to teach their children good nutritional habits:

1. **The most effective way to get kids to eat healthfully is to set a good example.** Young people are most influenced by what they see and experience, not by what they are told. Therefore, what you do—how you live—has the greatest effect on shaping your kids' behavior and their diets. Remember that the habits your children form while they are young will probably be with them for life.

2. **Feed your children a balanced diet.** Natural tastes for food develop early. If kids eat real food and develop a taste for fruits, vegetables, and other delicious flavors from Nature, they will not depend on the "enhanced" flavor of processed food. Continue to cultivate their tastes for natural foods, even after they have experienced the intensely sweet flavor of chocolate cake, sodas, and ice cream, or the highly salty flavor of chips and pretzels. Make sure your kids eat a nutritional meal first before allowing treats or desserts. Limit treats and watch out for excess sugar, caffeine in sodas and chocolates, and heavily processed foods laced with chemicals like colored dyes and preservatives.

3. **An important part of a balanced diet also involves getting plenty of fluids—good drinking water should be a basic right for everyone.** Children may need to be encouraged to drink water before having other liquids, especially sugary drinks. Consider getting a filter or buying bottled water so that you can make good-tasting and healthy drinking water available for the entire family.

4. **Do not bribe your kids with sugar and other treats; encourage them with healthy foods and snacks.** It is easy to forget to take the time to deal with children's true needs—love and attention. When you are busy, it is tempting to give them sodas, sweets, or whatever, even TV, instead of you. This can create the habit of trying to satisfy emotional needs with the distraction of food or material things.

5. **Have healthy snacks around the house** for your kids—organic sliced apples, oranges, grapes, or bananas; raisins or dates; almonds or other nuts; yogurt; pieces of cheese with healthy crackers; good chips and guacamole or salsa; and more. Offer your children healthy snacks at least a couple of times a day, such as mid-morning or in their school lunch, and then after school, around 3 to 4 p.m. (a time some parents call the "witching hour," recognizing that their kids are becoming cranky and irritable, but not realizing that they may simply be fatigued or have low blood sugar).

6. **Get your children (over age 5) involved in shopping for and preparing the foods that they like.** When you go to the grocery store, allow them to choose a few appropriate treats. You could give them a budget, maybe $10, to spend on good choices when they help you shop for family groceries. Most children will appreciate learning to prepare food that they like. Typically, kids enjoy making smoothies and shakes, preparing pasta and sauce, or arranging fruit or veggies on a platter in a pretty design. Fruit

salads are often a big hit. Be creative; together you may find some new treats.

7. **Plant a garden with your kids if you have the space, or if not, join with neighbors in a community garden.** If you have only a patio or small deck, you can use planter boxes or hydroponic equipment to cultivate organic, quick-growing produce. Even if you only have a window sill, many food-producing plants will fit in a small space—tomatoes, strawberries, herbs, and lettuce, for example. It is magical for kids to watch things grow and eat foods fresh off the vine. Or get your kids to help you make tasty, nourishing, and vital sprouts from seeds or beans, such as alfalfa, sunflower, lentils, garbanzo, or mung beans.

8. **Organize your refrigerator and pantry in a way that allows the young ones to get the items that you want them to have.** This makes it harder for them to get to the treats that you want to control. Even if they eat too much junk when they are with their friends or at school, encourage them to eat well when they are home and keep setting a good example. It will be worth it for you, too, in the long run!

9. **Help your children to avoid or to limit their intake of foods with unhealthy additives.** The basic additives to watch out for regarding children are artificial food colors, excess refined sugar, MSG (monosodium glutamate), aspartame (an artificial sweetener), sodium nitrite in treated meats, excess sulfites in dried fruits and other preserved foods, hydrogenated fats, and Olestra. It is wise also to limit children's intake of foods containing artificial flavorings, the preservatives BHT and BHA, and excess salt.

10. **Look out for food allergies and reactions, which are so common in children.** You will notice that when children limit foods causing their reactions, they will usually become clearer, more alert, and healthier. A delayed food reaction can cause a hidden problem that may not appear until later that day or the next. For example, chronic ear fluid congestion (otitis media) is quite common in young children. This is often not an infection but is usually treated as though it were, with strong antibiotics. When children who have chronic ear infections are taken off cow's milk products, those with a dairy allergy or sensitivity will stop getting ear problems.

In conclusion, healthy eating and cooking habits are best instilled in our early years, as correcting them later is definitely more challenging, yet still crucial to healthy aging. If we do a good job with our children, perhaps their children will be able to skip over a big chunk of this chapter because they will instinctively welcome food in the way it was meant to be. Eat healthy to stay healthy.

Chapter 11

Food and the Earth

If we want to provide our children with the same opportunities for dignity and enrichment as those our parents gave us, we've got to start by protecting the air, water, wildlife, and landscapes that connect us to our national values and character. It's that simple.

—Robert F. Kennedy Jr., *Crimes Against Nature*

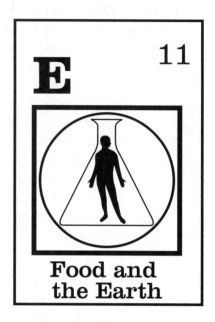

Food and the Earth

We live in a world plagued by pollution from agricultural spraying, industrial chemicals, toxic metals, and war technologies. Pollution of the earth, air, water, and our life-giving foods is really a by-product of our current industrial progress. War is also toxic to the food supply. There are now so many new substances, some highly toxic in nature, that are proving difficult for both the Earth and our bodies to handle. We do not have enzymes to metabolize them. What can we do? Is it too late?

The growth of technology has no doubt increased chemical pollution, but a greater difficulty has been generated by the capitalistic viewpoint: concern for profits often outweighs concern for people, personal health, and the state of the Earth. Those creating or allowing the pollution are often not willing to clean up their own messes. On a more individual level, each of us can easily get caught up in our own misuses of the Earth's resources and our desire for consumption (fitting in with society) and buying the latest new products. This approach is both shortsighted and irresponsible, however. It shall take many years to heal the damage caused by these continuing problems—if that is indeed even possible. And what about stems cells and

genetically modified organisms (GMOs), nuclear power, cancer, global warming, war, and so on? It's amazing that we still have our Earth and some semblance of health. We only can do our best and be aware of what the main concerns are for each of us. We need a greater effort and awareness to care for our planet.

There is also a state of consciousness, a belief or approach to life, that is responsible for our environmental pollution. This attitude is aligned with the "magic bullet" and "attack and conquer" approach of Western medicine—kill the germs, spray the bugs, add more chemicals to the soil to stimulate growth. If things get worse or side effects develop, we will use a different or stronger chemical. There is no end to this cycle because this approach is continually creating a new series of effects rather than addressing the causes. The condition that was originally identified as the problem will never be corrected this way. (This is also a great concern in conventional medicine today.) There have always been germs and insects; they also inhabit the Earth. In the 1960s and 1970s, farmers found that if they sprayed the whole field to kill the insects and those pesky weeds, they would often have a better crop yield and more profits that year. Everything still looked the same, with no apparent side effects. Later, food manufacturers found that if they preserved foods or added new chemicals or colors, the foods would last longer or look better, even if they used cheaper ingredients.

This shortsightedness of just looking at this year's crop or a particular germ lacks the vision to see what might happen to the "host"—Earth or our own bodies. When the concentration of chemicals used in the food chain, at home, or in industry rises to a certain level, there *are* side effects, everything from mild irritations to disorders of the blood and immune system. The body may be stressed by chemical insults, whether we breathe them, drink them, or eat them, and this stress may increase the potential for disease. Indeed, radiation and many airborne chemicals are well-known causes of many specific diseases and cancers. Often, however, we do not find out that these chemicals are dangerous to humans until they have been in use for many years. For instance, chemically induced cancers often take many years, even decades, to develop.

This topic could easily fill many volumes; with chemical testing, reported experiences, new drugs put on the market, and old ones taken off, new knowledge comes to light every day. I provide here some basic information on the subject and look at ways to survive our "new age of industrial chemistry," with a focus on chemicals in foods. I first explore the research about how chemicals are endangering our health and then look at how we can avoid or at least balance out their effects and survive through the twenty-first century.

GENERAL CONCERNS: WHAT IS THE DANGER?

The health of Earth and the health of our bodies are aligned—if Earth is sick, we cannot be entirely healthy. Pollution in many forms pervades everything on the planet and is in everyone's body. Industrial chemicals have surrounded and invaded the entire world. Building a rocket ship to get out of here takes more resources and more pollution. Of course, these chemicals also have a beneficial role in our current consumer-oriented society. The human species has worked diligently to develop ways to make life easier

(although it has really become more complex while Nature itself is simple!), to make new products, to improve worldwide communications systems, and theoretically to improve agriculture and crop yields as well as to develop new foods. New discoveries in the field of chemistry and the use of chemicals have their price, however. I am well aware of and concerned about the impact of industrial chemicals on our personal health and the health of our children, as well as the impact on our local and global environments. This crucial problem in the early twenty-first century must change *now!*

Many U.S. leaders and developers would like us to believe that exposure to tiny amounts of toxic materials presents little or no risk. But this is not true! (The real leaders, individuals like John Robbins, founder of EarthSave International, or Theo Colborn, coauthor of *Our Stolen Planet,* are the ones concerned about the actions we take and what their long-term and ultimate effects will be. Previous leaders were Rachel Carson, author of *Silent Spring,* and David Brower, environmentalist and founder of Friends of the Earth.) Chemicals are tested for their effects on laboratory animals in both small doses and larger than "safe" or usual doses. We must believe that a chemical or drug may be dangerous to humans if it causes problems for rats or mice, but we must also consider that a substance could cause serious problems in humans even if it seems "safe" for these laboratory animals. **The hidden danger is in the repeated small exposures over time with regular use, and in the additive, combined effect of all toxic substances to which we are exposed in this bit-by-bit way.** Partly because many chemicals do not break down (and therefore accumulate), their presence in the body can cause repeated insults or lead to chronic diseases. Nature does not provide the enzymes necessary to break down all of these synthetic chemicals, nor can the body readily metabolize and excrete them.

As Earth becomes more and more polluted, so do our bodies. For example, mercury dumped in the ocean is now at higher levels in the fish we eat and thus in our tissues. Today, most of the common diseases are environmental in nature, involving our interaction with our surroundings—contact with viruses, bacteria, fungi, and other parasites; food intake; and exposure to chemicals and wastes in the air and water.

These exposures can occur at home, at work, and while traveling or shopping. Some of this we can do something about, but in most cases of chemical exposure, we are at the mercy and conscience (and unconsciousness) of others.

There are several factors that influence the potential dangers of chemicals. **First are the repeated insults from the same or similar chemicals;** the more exposures to a potentially toxic synthetic chemical, the greater the danger to our health. **Second, the condition of the host is also important.** Are you in generally good health, or is your body already stressed or dealing with other chemical insults, such as smoking cigarettes, drinking alcohol or caffeine, or eating highly processed or fatty foods? The process is similar to that with germs: some microorganisms are strong enough to cause problems even in the healthiest person, but most germs and parasites need a weakened host or weakened immune system to take hold and multiply in the body.

The third factor is that chemicals can interact with each other. Various industrial chemicals may combine in Nature, in products, or in the body to make new chemicals that may be more toxic than the original. A good example of this is the formation of trihalomethanes (THMs), many of which are carcinogenic. These chemicals are formed when a halogen, such as chlorine or fluorine, combines with an organic hydrocarbon. For example, when we add chlorine to the water supply to disinfect it, this chlorine can interact with

---

Reasons to Be a Proactive Shopper: Chemicals and Toxins in Our Food

How Many of These Are on Your Shopping List?

DIRECT ADDITIVES TO FOODS

- **Labeled additives** such as sugars, salt, sulfites, preservatives, and so on.
- **Additives listed by general category,** not required to be identified by name, include artificial food colors and artificial food flavorings.

POLLUTANTS (unintentional—these are typically not labeled)

- **Pollutants, chemicals, and pesticide residues** from the air, water, or soil.
- **Toxic industrial wastes** in fertilizer that contaminate groundwater, surface water, and soil (270 million pounds from 1990 to 1995—all unlisted, not on fertilizer labels).
- **Toxic concentrations of minerals** in the soil or water (selenium, sodium chloride, and nitrates).
- **Toxic heavy metals** in the water that accumulate in soil, water, and in the tissues of fish and shellfish (lead, mercury, arsenic, cadmium, and chromium).

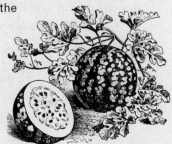

UNLISTED CHEMICALS (used in farming and processing, but not on the label)

- **Pesticides** sprayed on soil, plants, trees, and crops.
- **Equipment cleaners,** such as bleaches, detergents, rinses, and so on.
- **Food sprays,** such as mold inhibitors on fruits, pesticides, and gases applied before shipping.
- **Chemicals** contained in other ingredients, used in the preparation of processed foods (such as MSG), and toxins in lard, as well as pesticide residues in food waxes.
- **Chemicals given to animals,** such as antibiotics, insecticide sprays, pesticides in feed, and steroids and hormones to stimulate growth, as well as sedatives and other drugs used for slaughter.

MICROBES

- In the fields and orchards.
- In shipping from the farm or factory.
- In mass processing and preparation.
- In the slaughter and packing houses.
- In shipping from the factory to families.
- From improper storage in the store or at home.
- Kitchen counters and sponges, refrigerator bins.
- In restaurant preparation or from food handlers.
- In the grocery store, at deli counters and salad bars, in free sampling and open-air displays.

naturally occurring organic compounds in the water to form chloroform. Chloroform is the THM found in the highest concentration in our waters (both drinking water and outdoor lakes and streams), and several studies suggest that exposure to chloroform through daily showering alone may be increasing our risk of certain cancers. Shower dechlorinators may provide some protection.

Another example is the nitrosamines, which are also carcinogenic. These are formed when nitrites and nitrates in foods or in the soil react with other organic compounds in the soil, in the body, or in the foods we eat. Researchers do not fully understand how this process works in the environment, but we suspect that use of manures and fertilizers may be involved. In foods, certain preparation methods—such

as the curing of meats—can produce problematic amounts of nitrosamines. Within our bodies, imbalances in the digestive tract coupled with synthetic food additives or food contaminants introduced through application of fertilizers or pesticides can trigger this same result. For example, the constant trickle of nitrogen-containing fertilizers into our groundwater can increase nitrates in our drinking water. The bacteria in the mouth gets much more access to this nitrate, converts it into nitrite, and on it goes to the stomach for possible conversion—under the right circumstances—into nitrosamines. There are potentially many chemical interactions occurring within the body, although much of this is beyond the scope of scientists' current knowledge.

Reasons to Be a Proactive Shopper: Chemicals and Toxins in Our Food

FOOD PROCESSES RESULTING IN LOSS OF NUTRITIVE VALUE

- **Milling of grains** such as wheat, rice, oats, and barley to create "instant" foods, which removes such essential nutrients as the bran (an important source of fiber) and the germ (a source of essential vitamins, minerals, and oils).
- **Refining,** for example, when the sugarcane is processed to make white sugar, the nutritious portion is discarded.
- **Overprocessing of food,** such as the prolonged and high-temperature heating of foods, chemical cleaning, and automated meat processing.
- **Synthesizing** is a process by which artificial foods are created, such as Olestra and sweeteners. These are low in nutrients and potentially toxic.
- **Artificial processes,** for example, making honey by feeding bees sugar water does not create the same nutrient-rich honey as that derived from free-roaming bees that collect flower pollen and nectar.
- **Storage methods,** such as canning, freezing, and packaging, can decrease the vitamin content of foods.

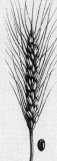

ADDITIONAL UNLISTED FOOD PROCESSES AND ADDITIVES

- **Genetically engineered foods** include vegetables with built-in pesticides; coffee beans with altered caffeine content; and produce manipulated to extend shelf life, such as corn, wheat, peppers, and fruits. Note that these foods do not yet require labeling. Legislation may change this aspect; however, the risk of this process is that it may also contaminate other plants.
- **Genetically engineered hormones,** such as the engineered growth hormones (like BGH) that increase the milk production of dairy cows (no labeling requirement exists).
- **Unlisted additives from processing,** for example, meat products can contain bone, bone marrow, and even spinal cord and lower nutrient levels.
- **Food irradiation** is frequently unlisted and may be more commonplace than is known; its risks to our health are still an unknown. It is used on produce, spices, and animal meats.

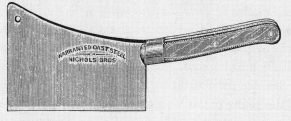

One of our greatest concerns individually and as a species regarding environmental chemical contamination is cancer—the feared, growing "twenty-first-century disease." The carcinogenicity of many chemicals is well documented; there are many other chemicals that may cause cancer but have not yet been sufficiently researched. Cancer is the worst possible outcome, but chemical exposure may also result in weakened immune function with increased susceptibility to germs and allergens, disruption of cell integrity and possible changes in DNA, loss of the body's energy production capacity, and ultimately, increased sensitivity to other chemicals in the environment. Cancer itself is, in part, the inability of the body to process chemical agents that have carcinogenic potential to cells and tissues, causing them to misbehave and grow aggressively.

HOW CHEMICALS CAUSE DAMAGE: A BRIEF REVIEW

Industrial chemicals contaminate as well as interact with life. Some chemicals can even destroy life when they become concentrated enough. Many pesticides, fungicides, herbicides, and preservative chemicals can cause liver disease, cancer, and death. Radioactive fallout and air pollution also affects us. But the focus in this book is on food, both processing additives and the contaminants that get into our food.

Food, water, and air are the main vehicles whereby we receive the chemicals that get into our bodies. Of course, they are interrelated. Crop dusting with pesticides spews toxins into the air and onto plants. These toxins settle down onto the ground and can be incorporated up into the cells of the plants. Rain carries the toxins all the way down through the soil, down into the underlying groundwater. Once diffused into the environment, toxins circulate according to geography, ecological cycles, and regional conditions. Local areas may have an emphasis on a particular type of pollution, such as Los Angeles or Gary, Indiana, with air pollution; the Mississippi River with water contamination; or such active agricultural areas as California's Central Valley with chemical sprays. Ironically, the government agencies charged with ensuring the health of the nation and the safety of our air, food, and water refer to these unsafe industrial and agricultural chemicals as "economic poisons."

The direct irritation by chemicals is known to cause disease, particularly cancer. This causes change at the cellular and DNA level. A chemical that is a potential carcinogen may actually bind to the DNA in the cell nucleus or in the mitochondria, thereby altering its structure and potential for normal duplication. It may also make the DNA more vulnerable to the same or other carcinogens. Further generations of the cell with damaged or transmuted DNA may become malignant. Our bodies have remarkable capabilities when it comes to the repair and even elimination of any abnormal DNA and malignant cells; however, when the immune system is weakened or there are just too many chemical insults for the body to handle, chronic inflammation and cancer may develop. Cancer, or malignancy, is a mass of rapidly dividing, undifferentiated cells that take the body's energy without using it creatively.

The condition of the host's immune system is another important aspect regarding potential carcinogenesis, and indeed this is a contributing factor in a wide variety of diseases. Chemical damage is largely due to the generation of free radicals, unstable molecules that can cause irritation and breakdown of tissues unless they are countered by antioxidants in the body. This oxidation of natural biochemical molecules in the cells and tissues may be a process of degeneration of the body leading to inflammatory problems, allergies, and cardiovascular disease. Stress of all kinds, including aerobic exercise, increases free-radical formation in the body. Environmental chemicals and food additives can also cause increased free-radical generation. Potentially, these are the same kinds of problems caused by radiation, including tissue damage, abnormal effects on cell division (most noticeable in the rapidly dividing cells of the skin, mucous membranes, and gastrointestinal tract), and the production of mutated cells. The antioxidant system is a series of enzymes and essential nutrients within the body that protects us from these chemically induced free radicals, just as a fine-mesh screen protects us and our homes from the shooting sparks generated by burning wood in the fireplace.

Free radicals are a normal product of metabolism; in the body, they are generated by both enzymatic and chemical reactions, including the metabolism of fats.

Peroxides, epoxides, and superoxides are examples of free radicals. The glutathione peroxidase and superoxide dismutase enzyme systems can help neutralize some of these potentially damaging free-radical molecules. Vitamin A and beta-carotene, vitamins C and E, glutathione, and selenium are all important antioxidants that help protect us from disease. This core list has expanded since the mid-1990s to include literally hundreds of phytonutrients naturally found in the foods we eat. In addition, during this same time period, more than 100 clinical trials have looked at the relationship between antioxidants, free radicals, and cancer, with the overwhelming majority of these trials suggesting a need for better food-based antioxidant protection.

Cigarette smoke is a complex mixture including chemical carcinogens. Although exposure to cigarette smoke does not invariably cause cancer, it is irritating to everyone. Smoking is a good example of the factors mentioned earlier: repeated chemical insults over time that make a mild carcinogen progressively stronger. The condition of the smoker and his or her nutrient status and lifestyle are important. Nicotine and tars in cigarettes may interact with other environmental or body

---

Specific Health Issues Regarding Chemicals in Our Food

- **Lack of research data.** The hidden danger is in repeated small exposures over time, about which scientists still have very little real data.
- **Not enough information.** Insufficient information exists about potentially toxic interactions of the many chemicals in the environment and in our bodies.
- **Chemicals that interact and form new toxins.** Chemicals interact with each other. Various industrial chemicals may combine in Nature, in products, or within the body as new chemicals, which can be even more toxic than the original.
- **Our body's inability to cope.** Because our ancestors did not live in a chemical environment, we do not have the enzymes necessary to break down or metabolize and eliminate these synthetic chemicals.
- **Chemicals remain in the body.** Chemicals can accumulate in body tissues and become a source of ongoing toxicity. Chemicals stored in body fat and other tissues may be released regularly and continually into the system over time, thus generating an ongoing toxic effect.
- **Repeated exposures.** When repeated insults occur from the same or similar chemicals, they can damage cells and tissues, endangering our health. Multiple chemical exposures can lead to chronic disease, such as cancer. Harmful effects to the nervous system and to reproductive health may be a more common threat than we realize.

- **Undisclosed exposure.** The majority of the chemicals in our foods are not disclosed on the label, which makes informed choices difficult.
- **Testing falls short.** Because testing looks primarily at very high exposures, researchers lack information on the toxic threshold level of many chemicals in humans—the level at which damage begins to occur. *Scientists do not really know how much is too much.*
- **Exposure and the individual.** Dose and response are highly individual, based on many factors, such as age, size, and metabolism. Legally allowable exposure levels for both food additives and pesticides are based on the tolerance of a healthy adult male. Women, children, the elderly, and people who are already ill are not taken into consideration.
- **Delayed effects.** Researchers found that when infant animals were given neurotoxic doses of food additives they failed to show overt signs of distress. Damage to the nervous system and vision was not evident until the animal approached adulthood.
- **Interplay of chemicals and immune function.** The condition of our health and immunity is important. When we are stressed or overly fatigued, we become more vulnerable to chemical insults.

chemicals to increase the risk of cancer. Researchers do not know much about this area; indeed, there is a lot more to discover regarding the world of chemicals in general, their effect on the human species, and how best to protect ourselves when necessary. Until then, common sense is our most important ally; we must avoid chemical exposure as much as we possibly can.

Chemicals with highly toxic potential are categorized by the Environmental Protection Agency (EPA) and researchers according to their harmful effects on the body as cancer-promoting toxins (carcinogens), mutagenic toxins, reproductive toxins, developmental toxins, endocrine disrupters, and nerve toxins.

Cancer-Promoting Toxins (Carcinogens)

Carcinogens are substances known to increase the incidence of cancer. The EPA labeling actually identifies some agricultural chemicals in current use as "probable human carcinogens." At least 107 different active ingredients in pesticides have been found to cause cancer in animals or humans; of these, 71 are still in use on food crops, according to the National Campaign for Pesticide Policy Reform. Food additives documented to cause cancer in animal studies include artificial food coloring, BHA (butylated hydroxyanisole) and BHT (butylated hydroxytoluene), nitrates, and saccharin.

Mutagenic Toxins

Mutagenic toxins are chemicals in our food that can alter genetic makeup and can have an adverse effect on human development when the exposure occurs during pregnancy. **Many of the toxins that damage our nervous or immune system also damage our genetic processes. Or they may damage our nervous and immune systems by means of genetic damage.** When man-made chemicals that are consumed in food or water appear at the wrong times and in the wrong amounts, unpredictable outcomes can occur.

Reproductive Toxins

A number of adverse effects on the reproductive system have been linked to the influence of toxic chemicals, particularly pesticides. These effects were first noticed in birds: male birds became sterile, eggs devel-oped with damaged shells, and birth defects occurred more frequently. Researchers have linked reproductive damage specifically to pesticides, heavy metal pollutants, and a number of chemicals, including dioxin.

Developmental Toxins

Developmental toxins can cause a number of different toxic effects on both unborn and young children. The potential effects of chemicals are also a concern with growing children. Their ability to fight infections and detoxify chemicals is less well developed than that of adults.

Endocrine Disrupters

Certain pesticides lengthen the estrogen cycle, prolonging the body's exposure to estrogen and significantly increasing the possibility of cancer. DDT is the most well-known of this class of pesticides that has been linked to increased cancer incidence. Although DDT was outlawed in the United States in 1972, its residues persist in the environment and in our bodies.

Other pesticides with extensive use have been linked to hormone disruption. Atrazine, the most frequently used pesticide in the world, is a known endocrine disrupter and has been associated with increased numbers of mammary tumors, uterine cancer, and other cancers in animal studies, according to the National Institute of Cancer at the National Institutes of Health. Between 1998 and 2003, the Environmental Working Group in Washington, DC anazlyzed drinking water supplies throughout the country and found that 19.1 million people in 702 communities were drinking water contaminated with atrazine. In over half of these communities, the level of atrazine was higher than the health-based threshold. The largest amount of atrazine in our diet comes from milk, corn, sugar, and meat.

Nerve Toxins

Since the mid-1970s, pesticide exposure has been linked to neurotoxic effects in both insects and humans. High accident rates among pesticide workers and crop dusters first suggested that these chemicals might have effects on the human nervous system, as they do on those of insects. Information on the Gulf War syndrome, also linked to frequent and intense pesticide and chemical exposure, is providing additional insight into neurotoxic effects, which have included chronic fatigue, headaches, memory loss, and sleep disturbances.

Many researchers consider a number of food additives and artificial food colorings found in prepared foods to be nerve toxins. The molecules of these chemicals can interfere with the chemical and electrical functioning of our brains, and it takes little of the offending chemical to produce a toxic effect. In lab studies, the artificial sweetener aspartame has been linked to seizures, hydrolyzed vegetable protein to demonstrated brain-damaging properties, and MSG (monosodium glutamate) to brain tumors and brain lesions in lab animals. **Such additives as MSG and aspartame are termed** *excitotoxins,* **so even if they do not cause nervous system damage, their chemical effect can overstimulate mental activity.**

Exposure to chemicals, free-radical damage, and immunological changes probably affect us in other ways as well. Chemical sensitivity and food allergy often go hand in hand. Allergies and body immune reactions in general are becoming more common with increased environmental chemical exposure. With the effects of the environment and our emotional stress on our immune system, we can become weaker and more environmentally sensitive overall. Concerns over these interactions have generated a whole new field in medicine, known as *clinical ecology.*

The two main components of environmental disease—food allergy/reactivity and chemical susceptibility—come together in the chemical pollution of foods. Many chemicals are present in food as both additives and contaminants. Contaminants accidentally get into food as residues of fertilizers, pesticides, or pollutants in the water or air. Additives are deliberately added to food, both in processing and as ingredients to improve flavor, color, or shelf life. Only those additives mixed into foods need be listed on the label; neither those used in the various steps of processing (or packaging) nor any contaminants are required to be identified on the label. Until relatively recently, for example, it was common for cereal manufacturers to put preservatives like BHT directly into their cereal. By shifting this practice and injecting BHT into the wax bag containing the cereal (instead of adding

it to the cereal itself), manufacturers could continue to extend the shelf life of their highly processed, nutrient depleted food without having to list the potentially toxic BHT additive on the label, even though it still gets into the food. Chemical contamination is a big problem in the food industry and of great concern to the chemically conscious consumer. Most foods have some additives and contaminants, and the problem is getting worse, not better. Even organic produce has some extraneous chemical contamination from the soil, water, and air; however, certified organic foods should have little or no added chemicals.

In U.S. capitalist culture, there are many instances where profits speak louder than people. This has often seemed true in agriculture as well. The sale of chemicals to farmers is a huge business, based on profits, not on the knowledge of what these chemicals ultimately might do to humans. Forests are sprayed with herbicides such as 2,4-D and 2,4,5-T, which can cause miscarriages and birth defects. Farmers spray their fields with hundreds of different herbicides, insecticides, and fungicides. Many of these chemicals kill natural pests and their predators, throwing off the ecological balance of Nature. The result is that even more potent chemicals are needed to eradicate the pests, which usually develop a resistance to the earlier chemicals used.

INDOOR POLLUTANTS: THE HOME AND THE OFFICE

Despite the dangers of outdoor chemical pollution, it is possible that indoor chemical pollution is a bigger concern. Some estimates suggest that pollution is 5 to 10 times more damaging indoors than outdoors because there are so many sources of it. To name a few, some sources include gas heaters and ranges; insulation; carpets and carpet padding; adhesives; such aerosols as hair sprays and deodorants; insect sprays, pesticide powders, and pest strips; synthetic drapes and clothes; cleaning compounds, detergents, deodorizers, and disinfectants; and cosmetics, perfumes, and colognes. It is difficult to know or evaluate what effects various combinations of specific chemicals will have on us. If we want to reduce chemical exposure, the home is a good place to begin.

Indoor Pollutants: What Are They?

- **Hydrocarbon fuel combustion.** The burning of coal, gasoline, natural gas, and wax candles.
- **Pesticide sprays.** As used on insects and rodents.
- **Cleaning fluids.** Such as cleansers, soaps, bleach, detergents, ammonia, and window cleaners.
- **Paints, adhesives, glues, and solvents.** Used in housework and for hobbies, for example.
- **Plastics.** Used in many areas.
- **Heating systems.** Used in households as well as in other buildings and schools, these can spread toxins.
- **Smoke.** Secondary, or sidestream, smoke is now clearly a big problem; fireplace smoke or barbecue chemicals can also be hazardous.
- **Aerosol sprays.** Such as air sprays, antiperspirants, disinfectants, and cleaners—mostly propellants, which may be fluorocarbons or hydrocarbons, neither of which are good.
- **Dust.** In households and elsewhere, this can carry sensitizing or toxic materials, including mites, molds, bacteria, pollens, cat and dog dander, carbon monoxide, asbestos, pesticides, solvents, sulfur dioxide, lead, smoke, and vinyl chloride.

Indoor air pollution is a large and important topic; however, because it is not directly related to nutrition (unless we consider everything we see, breathe, hear, and contact to be part of our nutrition), I will just summarize the general concerns and give examples of specific risks in this chapter. See the bibliography at the end of this book for useful references that treat the subject more fully. **It is time to save the planet, and now is the time to do it!**

We are exposed to chemical toxins through three main routes—ingestants, inhalants, and contactants. (A fourth route, injectants, is minor in occurrence compared with the others; however, this very direct form of body contamination by chemicals occurs in medical practice or by insect bites and stings and can create problems ranging from minor itching to death.)

The **ingestants** include food, drink, and drugs. Food may contain both intentional (food additives) and unintentional (contaminant) chemicals, as well as the individual protein allergens within the food. Water may, and often does, contain some chemicals, even dangerous ones. Such beverages as alcoholic and caffeinated drinks can cause toxic reactions. Ingested drugs, both prescription and over-the-counter, take effort for the body to metabolize and eliminate.

The **inhalants** are transported by the air, through which toxic substances can be carried both indoors and outdoors. Dust can carry all kinds of things, from mites to molds, as well as many chemicals. These can create allergies, sinus congestion, and lung irritation. **Contactants,** another large class, include cosmetics and cleaning supplies. Skin rashes are the most common problem caused by contactants. Pesticides can be spread by all three methods. When sprayed, they are carried by the air; they get into water; and they contaminate food. Dr. Buck Levin, PhD, RD, who has collaborated with me on this revised version of *Staying Healthy with Nutrition,* has himself written a book that looks comprehensively at toxins found in the food supply. In his *Environmental Nutrition: Understanding the Link between Environment, Food Quality, and Disease,* he explains the exact mechanisms by which these toxins impact our health.

There are many symptoms of chemical toxicity, affecting nearly every system of the body. Some of these symptoms are headache, fatigue, behavior changes, mood swings, nervousness, confusion, depression, loss of sex drive, skin rashes, coughing, wheezing, anorexia, nausea, and edema. A careful personal history may help isolate and correlate specific chemical exposures or environments that precipitate the symptoms. Then the solution often involves avoiding the chemicals, changing jobs or making changes within the work environment, and learning less toxic ways to work, clean, and live, and, of course, detoxification of the body.

Chemicals are ubiquitous and invade our lives more and more. Some are needed and helpful, but many are now created to support the huge chemical and home products industry, with the manufacture and marketing of faster and more powerful cleansers, stronger and lighter plastics, denser insulation, and stronger pesticides. We do not need this. Of course, it is beneficial if the new products are safer and less toxic than what was previously used, but often they are not. Rather, we need to allocate more effort and money toward cleaning up our contaminated environment, homes, workplaces, and bodies.

Pollutants in the Workplace

Although some environmental problems can affect us anywhere, in the work environment there is a much wider range of potential pollutants, depending on the type of job. Pollution in the work environment is caused by the manufacture of specific goods as well as by chemicals in the furniture, carpeting, insulation, and chemical cleaners found in the workplace. Industrial chemical pollution is a major side effect of technology. This affects us individually and as a species,

as we must breathe the air, drink the water, and eat the food. People work in a great variety of situations—indoor and out; cities, suburbs, farms, and industrial locations; small and large offices; big factories; and so on. The types and degree of chemical exposure vary with the situation; see the "High-Risk Occupations for Work Pollution" table below for a list of jobs where people are at particularly high risk.

Tobacco, asbestos, and alcohol also affect health and cancer rates. People who drink alcohol and smoke cigarettes have a higher incidence of cancer—specifically, cancer of the esophagus—than those who have just one of those habits. **People with certain nutrient deficiencies—such as beta-carotene, folic acid, or selenium—usually from poor nutrition, are also predisposed to higher incidences of cancer.**

Some Occupational and Chemical Hazards

Acrylonitrile	Cigarette smoke	Inks	Tin
Aerosols	Detergents	Lead	Toluene
Anesthetic gases	Dry cleaning solvents	Mercury	Trichloroethane
Antimony	Dyes	Methylene chloride	Trichloroethylene
Asbestos	Ethanol (alcohol)	Microwaves	Vinyl chloride
Benzene	Fibers/dust	Noise	X-rays
Bromides	Flame retardants	Photocopier gases	Xylene
Carbon monoxide	Formaldehyde	Silver nitrate	
Carbon tetrachloride	Hair spray resins	Soaps	
Caustics	Industrial chemicals	Solvents	

High-Risk Occupations for Work Pollution*

Airline flight crews	Dental hygienists	Insulation workers	Printers
Anesthesiologists	Dentists	Janitors	Radiologists
Auto mechanics	Dry cleaners	Leather workers	Radiology technicians
Chemical researchers	Electronics assemblers	Manicurists	Soldiers
	Explosives workers	Miners	Steelworkers
Chemical workers	Farmers	Painters	Tanners
Clerical workers	Firefighters	Pharmacists	Textile workers
Computer chip factory workers	Grape harvesters	Photocopy workers	Welders
	Hairdressers	Plastic workers	

* Many of these occupations have above-average risks of cancer, and all of them have more chemical exposure than the average population. **Women of childbearing ages (usually defined as 15 to 44) who work in these jobs are especially at risk.** They should familiarize themselves with particular dangers in their workplace and do their best to minimize their exposures. If this is not possible, it may be worth considering a change in job or occupation. Many of these lead to exposure to substances on the list above, which could be harmful to a fetus.

Although cancer is the most serious outcome of chemical exposure, it is probably not the most frequent; general chemical sensitivity, which can create a great number of symptoms and illnesses, is most prevalent. We might suspect we are sensitive to chemicals if our contact with them causes any of these symptoms: headaches, dizziness, burning eyes or nose, stuffy nose, confusion, light-headedness, inability to concentrate, sore throat or cough, wheezing, slurred speech, blurry vision, itching, or rashes. Some of these symptoms may result from irritations caused by the chemical inhalants.

In addition to chemicals, today's average office setting may pose dangers from fluorescent lights, computer screen radiation (and other electrical equipment), and even noise in some jobs. Of course, people who work directly with chemicals, especially in closed settings, are at greatest risk, but there is a wide variety of dangerous exposure in the typical work environment. In fact, since the mid-1990s, the names *sick building syndrome* (SBS) and *tight building syndrome* (TBS) have been created specifically to identify these indoor exposure problems. In SBS and TBS, acute health problems are associated with time spent in a building, even though no specific illness or cause can be identified. (There is another term, *building-related illness* (BRI), in which a person shows symptoms of a diagnosable disease and the symptoms can be attributed to toxins inside the building.) A World Health Organization committee report has suggested that as many as 30% of all newly remodeled buildings may contribute—for at least a temporary period of time—to SBS.

Adequate ventilation may be among the key remedies for many of these indoor air problems, and the increasing cost of energy has made builders waffle back and forth on minimum ventilation requirements. I am glad to see that the American Society of Heating, Refrigerating, and Air-Conditioning Engineers (ASHRAE) has revised its ventilation standard to provide a minimum of 20 cubic feet per minute per person in indoor office spaces. Many buildings provide much less ventilation than this and simply do not give occupants enough relief from possible air contaminants.

Lighting is much more a cause for concern than most people, especially employers, would believe, not so much by posing a grave danger as by affecting how we feel from day to day. Fluorescent lighting has been shown to increase illness and absenteeism, to reduce

Products Containing Common Chemical Irritants

Art supplies	Paint removers
Car exhaust	Paints
Carpets	Perfumes
Deodorants	Photographic supplies
Gasoline	Room deodorizers
Glues	Scented detergents
Nail polish	Smog
Nail polish remover	Synthetic clothes
Natural gas	Toilet paper
Newspapers	Typewriter correction fluids
Oven cleaners	

productivity, and to diminish morale. Using natural lighting or full-spectrum lights to replace fluorescent ones at work has been shown to reduce illness and improve attitude and productivity. The use of full-spectrum bulbs is increasing, and their price has been reduced in recent years, now making them a wise business and health investment. However, some very sensitive individuals may not even tolerate full-spectrum bulbs and must use the incandescent bulbs.

With the use of computers so widespread in this technological age, I am concerned about the effects of sitting at a video display terminal (VDT) for 8 hours in a stretch. People I see in my practice who spend much of their time working at VDTs often have a variety of symptoms. Fortunately, nowadays technology has improved and LCD (liquid crystal display) monitors, flat panel technology, glare filters, and plasma displays may help to minimize the kind of exposures I saw in my patients with cathode-ray tube (CRT) computer screens.

Noise, even inaudible sounds, can also affect mental and physical health. Both office and factory jobs with high levels of noise definitely affect not only our hearing but our general disposition as well. Printers, tabulating machines, computers, and conversation all combine to increase the decibels in the office. Insulation is not always effective; and in large, open offices with many workers, it is difficult to concentrate and hear ourselves think. Outdoor work in construction or with jackhammers or near a busy airport can be the noisiest. In this type of job, it is wise to protect the ears, but the sound vibrations also penetrate the body and influence organs, tissues, and cells. We need peace and quiet to balance us.

Everyone has the right to work in a safe space. Noise reduction and protection, good lighting, and especially clean air are part of a healthy work environment. Let us educate industry and employers toward the realization that a safe, healthy work environment provides greater health, success, productivity, and prosperity for all concerned.

Pollutants in the Home

Most of us are exposed to more chemicals in the home than anywhere else, mainly because there are so many possible uses for chemicals and also because we spend more of our time in our own or in friends' homes. The use of chemicals in the home affects everyone there, and this is a particular cause for concern when there are small children in the household. It is wise to minimize chemical use at home as much as possible. Besides irritation from contact and inhaling them, generalized chemical sensitivity and allergy can result from recurrent chemical aggravation. In her book *The Nontoxic Home*, consumer advocate Debra Dadd does a wonderful job of outlining the types of toxic products that are available and, in many cases, the possible exposure by using them. I referred to her work and other sources to create the general list of home chemical dangers on page 424. All of those listed are, of course, a greater danger to those who are chemically sensitive. Children, the elderly, and invalids may also experience more serious reactions. All of these products are much worse when ingested, so childproof your chemicals by putting them out of reach.

Most cleaning supplies, cosmetics, and toiletries have a dual route to irritation and toxicity—by contact and by inhalation of the fumes. Of course, if ingested, most of these products may be dangerous, even deadly. In recent years, more and more new products that are less toxic or nontoxic have been created or old ones have been rediscovered. Safe cleaners, for example, include lemon, baking soda, vinegar, salt, and trisodium phosphate, along with good old elbow grease. Check at local health food or environmentally conscious stores for the safer products or see the list compiled in the appendix of my book *The New Detox Diet*.

Plastics have become extremely pervasive in U.S. society, with a great many uses. They are a variety of synthetic materials made from coal or petroleum. Some of them, such as nylon and polyester, are relatively safe; others, such as polyethylene, acrylics, and polyurethane are unsafe for many people; and some, such as polyvinyl chloride (PVC) and formaldehyde, are out-and-out toxic to all of us. These last chemicals should be avoided. I think it best not to microwave food in any kind of plastic container, to avoid the plastic chemicals getting into the food and air. I do not keep water or juices in polyethylene unless they are refrigerated because these thermoplastics tend to soften with heat and release more chemicals. Even when refrigerated, storing in glass would be an even safer practice, but at least cooling helps keep these plastics more stable.

There are many alternatives to the chemical-based home pesticides and other toxic products. Often, they are not as strong or fast acting, just as natural remedies may take more time and effort than strong pharmaceuticals in the treatment of illness. Check health food stores, bookstores, online, and in suppliers' catalogues for less-toxic products to use in place of more harmful chemicals.

In general, our challenge as consumers is to be much more selective in our purchases, and at the same time, to ask more questions of retailers and manufacturers and insist on answers. **Here are some general guidelines to follow:**

- Avoid chlorofluorocarbon (CFC) products, such as polystyrene (Styrofoam) containers and packaging protectors, whose production and breakdown are polluting the atmosphere and destroying the ozone layer.

- Avoid aerosol sprays, such as deodorants, hairsprays, and cleaners.

- Avoid plastic containers or use products with comparably minimal waste; for example, bulk cheese instead of individually wrapped slices.

- Use biodegradable products, such as paper, not plastic; water-based soaps; eggs packed in cardboard products; and waxed paper rather than plastic wrap.

(continued on page 426)

Common Chemical Exposures: Home and Office

HOME CLEANING SUPPLIES

Detergents and fabric softeners. These may cause eye irritation and allergies.

Spray starch. Containing phenol, formaldehyde (aerosol), these are airborne irritants.

Dry cleaning spot removers. The toxic solvent perchloroethylene can irritate the liver and nervous system. Wash and dry your own clothes when possible.

Chlorine bleach. This should not be mixed with ammonia or vinegar, as the resulting chloramines can be toxic fumes.

Ammonia. This may cause a rash or irritate the eyes and skin, especially in aerosols.

Drain cleaners. The caustic lye (sodium hydroxide) is very toxic to skin and when ingested.

Furniture and floor polish. Containing nitrobenzene, naphthalene, and phenols, this group of toxins can disrupt the activity of our red blood cells and increase our risk of certain cancers.

Air fresheners. Containing phenol, cresol, ethanol, and xylene, this group of toxins can disrupt our liver metabolism, lung capacity, and genetic processes.

Germ-killing disinfectants. Containing cresol, phenol, ethanol, and formaldehyde, these can be very irritating to our respiratory and nervous systems.

Mold cleaners. Containing phenol, kerosene, and formaldehyde, these can be especially irritating to the eyes.

Carpet shampoo and upholstery cleaner. Containing perchloroethylene, ethanol, ammonia, and other detergents, this group of toxins can disrupt activity in our nervous and endocrine systems.

Dishwasher detergents. Containing chlorine and other detergents, these should not be mixed with ammonia or ingested **because chlorine gas and ammonia can mix to form chloramine gas that can cause respiratory and immune system problems.**

TOILETRIES

Toothpaste. Containing phenol, cresol, ethanol, artificial color and flavor, this group of toxins can damage our liver metabolism, nervous and immune systems.

Mouthwash. Often containing hydrogen peroxide, phenol, cresol, ethanol, ammonia, formaldehyde, artificial color, and flavor, this group of toxins can damage our nervous and immune systems and disrupt our liver metabolism.

Hairspray. Polyvinyl pyrrolidone (PVP) is not currently used in cosmetics, only in hairspray, and the acronym does not include the words "plastic", artificial colors, plastic resins, alcohol, and formaldehyde; this group of toxins can disrupt our liver metabolism and immune system.

Talcum powder. This may contain asbestos.

Perfume and aftershave. These may contain alcohol, phenol, cresol, trichloroethylene, formaldehyde, and artificial color and fragrance.

Aerosol hairspray. This may contain PVP (polyvinylpyrrolidone), formaldehyde, and artificial color and fragrance.

Antiperspirants and deodorants. These may contain aluminum chlorohydrate, ammonia, alcohol, formaldehyde, and artificial fragrance.

Dandruff shampoo. This may contain PVP, formaldehyde, detergents, and artificial colors and fragrance.

Hair color. This may contain coal tar dyes, ammonia, and other detergents.

Bubble bath. This may contain detergent as well as artificial color and fragrance.

Nail polish and remover. This contains acetone, phenol, toluene, and xylene.

Denture cleaners. Many contain salts, artificial colors and fragrance, and preservatives.

Disposable diapers. These are made with synthetic fibers and various deodorizing chemicals.

CLOTHES

Permanent press. This fabric uses resins and formaldehyde.

Fabric dyes. These can include dichlorobenzene and benzidine.

Flame-resistant fabrics. These are now banned in children's sleepwear because of carcinogenicity.

Synthetic fibers. Nylon, polyester, and acrylic are all plastics.

Common Chemical Exposures: Home and Office

ART AND HOME OFFICE SUPPLIES

Glues. Epoxy contains vinyl chloride, formaldehyde, and ethanol; "super glue" has acrylonitrile, phenol, and naphthalene—all are toxic.

Permanent ink markers. These contain acetone, toluene, xylene, ethanol, and cresol.

Liquid correction fluid. This contains cresol, trichloroethylene, naphthalene, and ethanol.

Computer terminals. Staring at these for long periods may cause eye irritation, headache, and fatigue, as well as neck, shoulder, and back pains.

Television. This may cause eye irritation, headache, and fatigue.

PLASTICS

Polyurethane foam. This is in beds, cushions, and pillows and may be a lung, skin, and eye irritant.

Polyester. In clothing, bedding, diapers, tampons, and upholstery, this may cause irritation, allergy, and skin rash.

Nylon. In clothing, toothbrushes, other brushes, upholstery, carpets, and so on, this is probably safe.

Acrylics. These are made from acrylonitriles and are in acrylic fiber, waxes, paint, and Plexiglas.

Polyethylene. High-density polyethylene (HDPE) and low-density polyethylene (LDPE) are found in containers, wrappers, kitchenware, plastic bags, and squeeze bottles. They are possibly carcinogenic.

Vinyl chloride. This is the worst of the plastics and is carcinogenic.

Polyvinyl chloride. Found in adhesives, containers, records, tapes, toys, beach balls, pacifiers, raincoats, and boots, all of which can release vinyl chloride and cause cancer, liver disease, birth defects, and more.

Urea-formaldehyde plastic resins. Found in particleboard, plywood, insulation, tissues, and towels as outgas formaldehyde, a suspected carcinogen.

Fluorocarbon plastic. Known as tetrafluoroethylene or Teflon, the nonstick coating, this is also found in ironing board covers and can be an irritant to the skin, the eyes, and the respiratory tract.

Plasticizers. Known as MEHP (mono[2-ethylhexyl]phthalate), DEHP (di[2-ethylhexyl]phthalate), and PET (polyethylene terephthalate), these are found in most plastic packaging containing printed labels or logos.

Styrene. This is found in Styrofoam egg cartons, fast food burger packaging, and restaurant take-out meals.

OTHER HOME TOXINS

Smoke. About 96% of cigarette smoke pollutes the air and increases carbon monoxide levels. It is also an irritant and secondary smoking is a legitimate concern.

Garbage. This can bring insects and rodents. Keep the house clean and recycle wastes.

Gas appliances. These emit gas fumes and create carbon monoxide.

Kerosene lamps and heaters. These emit kerosene fumes and create carbon monoxide.

Fireplaces and woodstoves. These emit chemicals in wood and create carbon monoxide.

Particleboard. This is created with urea-formaldehyde, which is possibly carcinogenic.

Foam insulation. This is urea-formaldehyde foam insulator (UFFI), a carcinogenic that was banned in 1982 but then reapproved for use.

HOME PESTICIDES

Rodent killers. Used in mousetraps, these contain arsenic, strychnine, and phosphorus, which are deadly if eaten.

Insecticides. Used for various bugs, many contain chemicals, even as "inert ingredients," that may be dangerous. Pyrethrum, a plant extract derived from white chrysanthemum, can be useful.

Lice shampoos. These contain lindane (as in the brand G-Well), which are available in the United States by prescription but banned in many countries due to risk of nervous system and reproductive system damage as well as possible carcinogenicity. They are used for lice and crabs and also as an insecticide. Pyrethrin powders and sprays may be helpful and useful for animals but not for humans.

- Purchase reusable products, such as cloth napkins and towels, returnable bottles, and rechargeable batteries.

- Support legislation for deposits on bottles, cans, and plastic containers.

- Recycle everything possible, such as glass, cans, paper, cardboard, and plastics.

- Reuse as much as possible, such as paper bags, plastic bags, cardboard boxes, bottles, and Styrofoam packing pellets.

- Buy more-durable products.

- Buy less whenever possible.

- Shop at co-ops and farmers' markets where products are available in bulk, there is less fancy and costly packaging, and they support using recycled plastic and paper bags.

- Join a community supported agriculture (CSA) food subscription program.

- Buy in bulk, for example, larger bottles in place of 6-packs, or large containers of regularly used products, such as soaps, detergents, shampoos, and cleansers.

- Voice your objections to stores and manufacturers when you first see new throwaway, nonrecyclable products; the plastic can and the throwaway camera are two recent examples.

- Ask for more biodegradable products.

- Borrow or rent items that you only need infrequently, and keep other items in good repair; loan them to neighbors also. (Make responsible agreements for shared maintenance and repairs if you do.)

TOXIC PROBLEMS IN OUR FOOD CHAIN: HOW DO CHEMICALS GET INTO OUR FOODS?

In this section, I discuss the contaminants and chemical additives that may enter our food—from the elements that help it through its growing cycle, harvest, and processing until it reaches our tables and mouths.

This involves air, water, soil and food cultivation (growing), and the manufacturing, processing, storage, and preparation of food.

Air

In regard to food, air pollution is probably the least of our concerns. It likely contributes minimal contamination, unless certain chemicals, gases, or metal molecules are present where the food is grown. Some airborne contamination may get into water, which may in turn pass into food. Food grown in fields near industrial plants or along heavily traveled roads may pick up more chemicals, lead, or other auto and truck pollutants. The term *air pollution* does not refer to the flight path of a crop duster as it flies over the crop acreage spraying pesticides down onto the plants, even though that may be the most intense pollution locally.

Some Facts on Waste

- **Twenty-five million tons** of acid rain is generated each year from sulfur dioxide and nitrogen oxides spewed from factories.
- **Packaging** costs about 10% of total product cost.
- **The average American** produces about 4 pounds of garbage daily.
- **Americans** go through 2.5 million plastic bottles every hour.
- **We throw away enough glass bottles** and jars to fill up two 100-story buildings every 2 weeks.
- **We throw away enough iron and steel** every day to supply all the nation's automakers' daily needs.
- **Consumers and industry** in the United States throw away enough aluminum to rebuild the entire commercial air fleet every 3 months.
- **Recycled paper** takes 60% less energy and 15% less water. One ton of recycled paper saves 17 trees, 7,000 gallons of water, 4,200 kilowatts of energy, and 3 cubic yards of landfill. (For more information about the benefits and statistics on recycling, visit the website of the Worldwatch Institute in Washington, D.C., at www.worldwatch.org).

Common Air Pollutants

Acetylene	Formaldehyde
Ammonia	Hydrogen sulfide
Benzene	Methane
Benzopyrenes	Methyl chloride
Beryllium	Nitrogen dioxide
Butane	Nitrogen oxides
Cadmium	Ozone
Carbon monoxide	Propane
Cigarette smoke	Sulfur dioxide
Cis-2-butane	Tetraethyl lead
Ethane	Trans-2-butane
Ethylene	Vinyl chloride
Fluoromethanes	

Air pollution is of greater concern in regard to general health. There are higher levels of chemical irritants in the air in smoggy, heavily populated, or industrial areas. There are numerous studies documenting the relationship between air pollution, weakened immunity, increased infection, and increased risk of cancer (see the bibliography at the end of the book for a sample of these research references). Indoor air pollution at work, at home, in stores, or at the hair salon may be much worse than outdoor air pollution because there is more contamination with less dilution. More chemicals are used in everyday work and home life than most of us imagine. This means that a great deal of pollution occurs virtually unnoticed.

Many air pollutants are released directly into the atmosphere by industry or by the discharge of industrial waste. See the "Common Air Pollutants" table above for a list. It would be best to reduce air pollution as much as possible by enforcing stricter industrial controls and reducing the manufacture of unnecessary products, such as Styrofoam, that may generate more severe pollution. For those of us who are sensitive to indoor air pollution (and we all are, some of us just notice it more), such as people with allergies and asthma, an air filtering device may be a wise investment. **Portable units are relatively inexpensive, and I suggest one with a HEPA (High Efficiency Particulate Air) filter, as these are government tested for their capacity to remove dust particles,** **air chemicals, and molds.** Some air filters include an activated carbon component, which can help trap fumes that might be otherwise be irritating and may leave air smelling cleaner. A newer addition to air filters is ultraviolet (UV) bulbs. Because ultraviolet light may help kill certain types of molds, bacteria, fungi, and airborne spores, UV bulbs may be added to air filters to help remove these types of microorganisms.

Water

Chapter 1, Water, reviews the subject of water in relationship to many topics, especially bodily requirements, types of water to drink, and home purification. It also touches on the major problem of water pollution. This section goes a bit deeper and looks at pollution's effects on us and Earth as well as some ideas for cleaning it up. **Water is probably our biggest area of concern regarding chemical pollution.**

At one time, undrinkable water was thought to be a problem only in so-called Third World countries, but in fact it is a major problem in the United States as well as in the rest of the Western world. When our farmers dump 850 million pounds of pesticides on our food crops, a good bit of this pesticide ends up in our groundwater. Thus it should not be surprising when 95% of municipal water supplies contain traces of pesticides like atrazine. Fortunately, in the United States we do not have the problem of bacterial contamination of our water supplies, a problem in poor nations without proper water treatment plants and sewage systems. For most Americans traveling in these countries, the water can cause illness with immediate gastrointestinal symptoms, such as diarrhea and abdominal cramps; a severe case can even be fatal. The problem in the United States is more subtle, invisible, and long-range—it may even be more dangerous.

The industrial productivity of Western societies has been accompanied by the accumulation of vast quantities of waste, especially chemical waste. In terms of total chemical waste (not just pesticides dumped on food crops), billions of pounds a year are dumped into waters, soil, hundreds of thousands of landfills, and city dumps. This chemical waste is continuously polluting our groundwater. The country relies heavily on groundwater, not only for individual use but also for agricultural production. Seventy-seven billion gallons of groundwater are withdrawn every day in the United States, about two-thirds for agricultural irrigation and one-third for other uses. There is current concern that the world's population is depleting these groundwater sources. Current industrial practices are directly contaminating all of this water. In addition, surface waters (such as our lakes, streams, and rivers) often connect with groundwater sources, allowing chemicals to cross contaminate.

Groundwater and surface water chemical pollution have become serious problems. This is both a political and an economic issue, involving industry, agriculture, and, of course, the water drinkers. This is another example of Western shortsightedness—kill the immediate problem (such as bacteria or bugs) or make the quick buck without a serious thought of the consequences to Earth or its inhabitants in years to come. We all must deal with the consequences of drinking water contaminated by pathogenic microorganisms. The less visible problems of organic, industrial, and agricultural chemical contamination and their potential toxicity and carcinogenesis have been overlooked until recently, but clearly they are a serious concern. Some particularly toxic chemicals found in groundwater include vinyl chloride, methylene chloride, carbon tetrachloride, trichloroethylene (TCE), benzene, xylenes, and petroleum by-products.

Groundwater contamination is currently irreversible; it is estimated that it would take billions of dollars to even begin to clean up our groundwater, rivers, and lakes, and we do not yet really have the technology to do this, even if the money were allocated. The EPA is responsible for keeping our water clean, an almost impossible task, especially given the fact that other political agencies and lobbyists currently support the interests of big business. During the early 1970s, the EPA was quite productive. The Clean Water Act, passed in 1972, helped regulate industrial dumping of chemicals into the environment. However, the problem was so prevalent and the potential fines were so much less than the costs of changing business practices or the profits to be made, that controlling industrial pollution was never accomplished. In 1974, the Safe Drinking Water Act (SDWA) was passed, which set a standard for any water system serving more than 15 homes. Water treatment plants were required to test periodically for certain bacteria, as well as specified organic and inor-

ganic substances. The EPA currently requires that water be tested for approximately 100 potential toxins, including heavy metals like cadmium, lead, and mercury; pesticides like endrin and lindane; and volatile organics like trihalomethanes (THMs). But there are literally thousands of other possible chemical contaminants; this is a tough job to oversee, so this law has not been well enforced.

Since 1972 and the passage of the Clean Water Act, important progress has been made in many areas. About 55% of lakes and streams are now safe for swimming and fishing, as compared with 30% to 40% in 1972. **But 3 of every 4 persons in the United States still lives within 10 miles of a polluted waterway, and recent changes to the Clean Water Act that allow more mining waste to be dumped into streams and wetlands are further increasing our toxic risk.** Wetlands destruction, sewage overflows, and delayed cleanup of existing waters continue to be enormous problems where much remains to be done.

Water can be polluted in a variety of ways and by a wide range of substances. In *The Nontoxic Home and Office*, a very helpful book on reducing chemical exposure in our homes and environment, author Debra Lynn Dadd groups these water-contaminating substances into four categories. **Microorganisms,** such as bacteria and viruses, are the first form of contamination. (Chlorine is usually added to water to reduce these organisms.) **Dissolved solids** are the second group. These are materials that dissolve in the water, many of which come from the soil. Included in this group are the nitrates, the sulfates, fluoride, and various mineral salts. These are relatively safe. The third group contains the **particulates,** undissolved materials such as dirt, rust, asbestos, or heavy metals—lead, mercury, cadmium, silver, aluminum, cobalt, and so on. These are relatively safe unless they are found in high concentrations. The fourth group, **volatile chemicals,** is the biggest concern, because many of these are unsafe even in small amounts. These include pesticides (such as DDT and lindane), chlorinated hydrocarbons, chloroform and other THMs, trichloroethylene, and many more. Chemical water pollutants include both inorganic and organic substances.

There are many chemical contamination problem areas in the United States, often in areas with large industrial facilities. Some examples include New Orleans, which is surrounded by the Mississippi River on one side and Lake Pontchartrain on the other, both

---

Possible Sources of Water Contamination

- **Agricultural activities.** Pesticides, herbicides, selenium, and the nitrates in fertilizers are some examples of substances used as sprays. These accumulate in runoff waters and end up in underground aquifers or in lakes and rivers.
- **Industrial wastes.** These are very common as production by-products dumped into local rivers or lakes, or buried underground if toxic.
- **Chemical dumping and waste sites.** Common outlets for industrial waste, these include the multitude of municipal landfills, many of which may be contaminated, while other chemicals, radioactive wastes, or sewage are injected directly into the Earth. Some chemicals affecting water found near waste dumps include DDT, vinyl chloride, benzene, carbon tetrachloride, TCE, PCBs, and such metals as lead and mercury. Land disposal of wastes is an inefficient way of storing pollutants, but it is less expensive than other, more responsible solutions, and changing established ways of doing things is always difficult. Business and bureaucratic rationalization are often used to sweep major problems under the rug.
- **Underground storage tanks.** Gasoline, probably the most common substance stored in this way, may leak into groundwater.
- **Mining of metals and radioactive materials.**
- **Leaking septic tanks.** According to the National Institute of Environmental Health Sciences, about one-fourth of all U.S. households use a septic tank as part of their wastewater disposal system. Leakage from septic holding tanks is known to be associated with outbreaks of acute infectious diarrhea. In at least 1 state (Wisconsin), public officials have estimated inappropriate leakage to occur in up to 40% of all systems.

---

of which are extremely polluted primarily from chemical dumping by industry. California's Santa Clara Valley, also known as Silicon Valley because it is a major center of the computer industry, is troubled by toxic wastes contaminating the groundwater. Ethylene dibromide (EDB), a pesticide commonly sprayed on citrus trees and other crops, has been found as a water contaminant in Florida and many other states. It has been shown to cause male sterility and cancer.

The military is likely the biggest polluter in the United States. An estimated 1 billion pounds of hazardous wastes are disposed of yearly, much of this as a result of nuclear weapons development and manufacture. California, Colorado, and New Mexico are among the affected areas. The beautiful Snake River in Idaho has been found to have a low level of some radioactive compounds. **Texas, Vermont, Maine, and Nevada are states equally affected by issues involving radioactive waste. According to the EPA, approximately 140,000 cubic feet of "mixed waste" containing low levels of radioactivity or radioactive material were produced in the U.S. in 1990 alone.**

If you live in a dense city or industrial area, you should be wary of your tap water. If your water has a funny taste or odor or stains your tub or sink, have it checked. It is fairly inexpensive to have the bacteria count verified. With all the chlorine added to the city waters, most microorganisms will not grow very well. Analyzing the water for chemicals can be much more difficult and costly. There are a few companies that perform this service, and it can cost hundreds of dollars just to check for the more toxic chemical contaminants, such as the organic halides—trihalomethanes, vinyl chloride, trichloroethylene, ethylene dibromide, and dibromochloropropane. There are many others.

Well water is not necessarily safe, either. It usually comes from groundwater, the underground reservoirs also known as aquifers, which may be contaminated. In recent years, many thousands of wells have been closed in more than half of the states throughout the country because of contamination, and those are only the ones that have been discovered—there may be many more. Even living in the country does not totally protect us if there is much local agriculture. If you are going to use a particular well for a number of years, it is now necessary to check the water for chemicals every few years; your life could depend on it.

It is also worthwhile and fairly inexpensive to use a home filter system. Most are reasonably priced and can remove much or even all of the chemical contamination. Solid carbon block filtration is a good basic system; avoid granulated carbon filters, however. Reverse osmosis filters are also a good choice, but these systems usually have three different filters and are usually more expensive. Reverse osmosis also needs good water pressure and can waste water. (Water filters are discussed in more detail in chapter 1, Water.) Bottled water is usually free of toxic chemicals, but it

---

Can We Really Heal Earth?

Humankind has not yet reached the evolutionary state whereby we can move from our focus on fear and our desire for money and power (which clearly have led to technological progress along with pollution and warfare) toward love and trust and a desire to heal and purify the planet. **Our ingenuity and technology, I believe, can be applied to discover ways to clean up our water and air.** There must be some process, such as using solid carbon and volcanic ash systems, through which we can run our polluted rivers, lakes, and ocean waters, allowing these filtering factories to remove heavy metals and toxic chemicals and to turn out mineral-rich, clean water. Large air-filtering factories could be set up around cities to purify the air. If we would use only a tenth of the monies that we put into nuclear power and weapons, we could do it. These new high-tech buildings and underground sites can replace our nuclear power plants and chemical-producing and smoke-spewing factories that now hasten Earth's demise. Cleaning the air will allow the sun to function for us, as it once did, and not become a danger. We can also harness solar, wind, and water power to further supply our living needs, so that Earth can continue to survive for many millenia. **I believe that the real answer to disease, and specifically to the increasing cancer problems, will not be chemical warfare on the body, but learning to reharmonize and support the body's natural healing forces.** So will the healing of Earth result from our reattunement to its ecosystem.

---

too can come from contaminated groundwater. Polyethylene, a soft plastic commonly used for water containers, can also contaminate water.

For various reasons, I recommend that people not drink city or tap waters. Public water treatment leaves much to be desired. Chlorine has become a panacea to treat and prevent microbial contamination. Although such treatment has helped clean up our water, chlorine can interact with organic wastes, such as dead leaves, and form the carcinogenic trihalomethane (THM) chemicals. Chloroform is commonly found in city waters. In 1979, the EPA set the limit for THMs to be 100 parts per billion (ppb) in water. This regulation applies to any water system serving at least 10,000 people. They estimated that this level would add only 200 cancer deaths a year. Several studies have shown an increased incidence of cancer, especially of the gastrointestinal tract, bladder, and rectum, in people who drink chlorinated water.

There are other problems with tap water. Plastic pipes more easily leak or interact with industrial solvents, pesticides, or gasoline. Polyvinyl chloride (PVC), polybutylene (PB), and polyethylene (PE) are three common pipe plastics; the first two are mild carcinogens. Lead leaks occur in certain pipes. Old asbestos cement (AC) pipes, of which some 200,000 miles were laid after World War II, can leak asbestos and may be associated with an increase in gastrointestinal cancer. Copper pipes may add excess copper to our bodies and often have lead solder lines, which adds to lead contamination. Fluoridation of water is also of concern to many people. Although research in this area is definitely divided, some studies have shown a relationship between risk of oral and bone cancers and lifelong intake of fluoridated water. Most inorganic pollutants are relatively safe at very low concentrations, because our livers and kidneys are usually up to the detox task. However, relatively small amounts of lead and mercury can be neurotoxic, and small amounts of nitrosamines can be carcinogenic. The health impact here depends on many factors, so we should all err on the safe side and limit our exposure to these pollutants as much as possible.

Controlling chemical pollution and polluters at the state level is a problem because most states do not have the financial resources to clean up contaminated waters.

In most cases, this pollution is often not detected, or detected only when it is too late. Low-level contamination creates long-range problems, nothing that we notice immediately unless widespread and expensive testing is done routinely. Cancer, birth defects, reproductive problems, miscarriages, and liver and kidney disease are some of the health problems researchers should look for. Immune weakness that could allow more infection and cancer may be an earlier sign of pollution. We must prevent further

---

Water Chemicals

Common Drinking Water Pollutants

Lead

Mercury

Dichloro-trichloroethane (DDT)

Polychlorinated biphenyls (PCBs)

Polycyclic aromatic
   hydrocarbons (PAHs)

Chloroform

Vinyl chloride

Trans-dichloroethylene

Ethylene dibromide (EDB)

Organophosphate pesticides
   such as aldicarb

Gasoline

Xylene

Toluene

Benzene

Dibromochloropropane (DBCP)

Herbicides like 2,4-D

Chemicals Found in Groundwater

Petroleum by-products

TCE

Vinyl chloride

Methylene chloride

Carbon tetrachloride

Tetrachloroethylene

Cis-dichloroethylene

Mercury

1,1 dichloroethylene

1,1,1 trichloroethylene

Chemicals Found in Waste Dumps That Affect Water

Carbon tetrachloride

DDT

Vinyl chloride

TCE

Benzene

PCBs

Lead

Inorganic Water Pollutants

Lead

Nitrates

Mercury

Cadmium

Cyanide

Arsenic

Silver

Asbestos

Chromium

Selenium

Organic Chemical Water Pollutants

Chloroform	Toluene
TCE	Xylene
Trichloroethane (TCA)	DDT
PCBs	2,4-D
Carbon tetrachloride	2,4,5-T
Tetrachloroethylene	Benzene
Vinyl chloride	Toxaphene
Methoxychlor	Endrin
Dichlorobenzene	Lindane
1,2 dichloroethane	Dioxin
DBCP	Aldicarb
EDB	Gasoline
PAHs	Nitrosamines

Almost all of the organic chemical water pollutants in this table have been shown to cause cancer or to be toxic to the nervous system. This table was compiled with the help of Mike Samuels and Hal Zina Bennett, *Well Body, Well Earth*, and other, more current book sources.

pollution! California, Florida, and New Jersey have recently enacted legislation giving individuals greater power to pursue and legally stop industrial polluters. It remains to be seen what effect such laws will have, however. **In the meantime, here are 10 things that can be done to reduce water pollution:**

1. Do not use toxic agricultural or industrial chemicals.

2. Recycle wastes safely. Find ways to deactivate or recycle dangerous chemicals.

3. Foster awareness of local problems, including water status, common pesticide use, and industrial waste dumping.

4. Find better ways than the use of chlorine to disinfect water. Ozone and UV radiation can be used to disinfect water, although there are still limitations to the use of these methods. Ozonation, like chlorination, can result in the creation of harmful by-products, and either method may yield purified water that is sufficiently stable over time. But if we cannot refine these methods, we need to keep looking until we come up with a pollution-free answer.

5. Enact, support, and enforce better standards and limits for industrial and agricultural contamination.

6. Make examples of polluters (or officials who allow pollution) with more lawsuits, stiffer fines, and even threat of plant closure or jail sentences. **It is not acceptable that the negligence of so few can affect the health of so many.**

7. Support the EPA in doing its job of monitoring industry, agriculture, and water treatment facilities.

8. Test water to make sure of its safety.

9. Use water filters for drinking and cooking water.

10. Foster heightened concern about ecological issues and their future impacts and take action to further natural harmony on Earth.

Soil and Food Cultivation (Growing)

Almost anything in the soil can get into food while it is growing. Plants absorb chemicals and minerals from the soil. Water is a route by which some of the chemicals keep recycling back into the soil and food. Because Earth and our bodies do not break down most of the new chemicals used, they accumulate and last a long time. Nitrogen-based fertilizers are commonly used to stimulate plant growth and create bigger crop yields. These fertilizers can create some imbalances in the soil and produce depletion of other important minerals, such as chromium, selenium, and iodine. Such heavy metals as lead and mercury can also contaminate soil.

Such herbicides as 2,4,5-T and 2,4-D are used on the soil in the preplanting period and in the early stages of plant growth to kill weeds so that there will be less growth competition and easier harvesting. Most of these herbicides are fairly toxic and potentially carcinogenic. These are also sprayed over forests and along highways to reduce foliage and allow easier clearing of timber. Pesticides are applied primarily during food cultivation. Of course, pesticides from previous applications to crops may linger in the soil for years. For example, DDT, which has not been used (legally) since 1972 in the United States, still contaminates most soil, plants, animals, and humans.

Since the passage of the Organic Foods Production Act (which was Title 11 of the 1990 Farm Bill) and full

---

3 Common Misconceptions about Pesticides

- **Pesticides** are considered safe for use as long as they are not actually used during the growth phase of the plant. *Not true!* These chemicals can still contaminate the parts that we consume.
- **"Natural" pesticides** are better than manufactured ones. *Not true!* There are still dangerous plant-based pesticides, such as strychnine and some of the pyrethrum derivatives.
- **Nerve toxins** (most chemicals) that are deadly to insects are not that harmful to humans. *Not true!* They are also toxic to the nervous system of humans.

implementation of this program in 2002, we finally have uniform standards across the country for production of organic foods. Several states, including California, have stricter rules than the national standards. But in every instance, certified organic foods cannot be raised or produced with the use of pesticides or other toxic additives. Of course, organically grown foods cannot be totally screened from ecological drift of pollutants, but the quality of these foods is outstanding in comparison with nonorganic alternatives, and drift pollutants are found in exceedingly low amounts much of the time.

Much of the chemical contamination that gets into our foods comes from pesticide sprays used during cultivation. One way to better understand these chemicals is to look at their subclassifications. The three main classes of chemical pesticides are organochlorines, organophosphates, and carbamates.

Organochlorines. This toxic class of chemicals includes aldrin, endrin, lindane, and 2,4-D. Although they are most known for their pesticide application, they are commonly used disinfectants as well. Organochlorines kill pests by attacking their central nervous system. Most of them have been shown to cause cancer, birth defects, and genetic changes in animals. They are also stored in the body fat when absorbed and accumulate there. Organochlorines were commonly used as pesticides in the 1940s, 1950s, and 1960s. They are used less commonly in the United States now but are still shipped to other countries, so they may return to us in such imported foods as bananas, coffee, sugar, tea, rice, cocoa, and chocolate.

Three of these common organochlorines were banned—DDT in 1972, aldrin in 1974, and endrin in 1979. **These poisons and their relatives still remain in the soil after many years of spraying, but they no longer kill the pests, just the people and the wildlife.** U.S. hazardous waste burners release about 22 million pounds of organochlorine compounds into the air each year, and most of these chemicals have a half-life of about 50 to 100 years.

Organophosphates. These are the most common pesticides used today, with chlorpyrifos and malathion leading the group. Also found in this category are diazinon, disulfoton, fenthion, methyl parathion, phorate, phosmet, and terbufos. They are less dangerous than the organochlorines, because they break down

---

Types of Pesticides Currently in Use

Pesticides can be grouped into several categories.

By use

- **Herbicides.** These are used to kill weeds, usually before growing.
- **Insecticides.** These are used to kill insects and pests during the growing period.
- **Fungicides.** These are applied to retard molds and fungi.
- **Fumigants.** These are used for controlling insects and damage during shipping and storage.

By chemical structure

- **Heavy and toxic metals.** These can include mercury, cadmium, arsenic, and copper.
- **Organochlorides.** These typically strong chlorinated hydrocarbons persist in the soil and our bodies.
- **Organophosphates and carbamates.** Essentially nerve gases, these are shorter-lived and include malathion, parathion, and carbaryl.
- **Triazines and other herbicides.** These toxins designed to kill plants must be stronger than those used for insects; they include Agent Orange, paraquat, and the triazine family, such as atrazine.

---

into less harmful chemicals within weeks of their use. In pests, organophosphates interfere with nerve conduction and can lead to convulsions and death. The human concern is that the organophosphate pesticides may have a genetic effect that could generate cancer or birth defects, or that they may directly cause allergic reactions or neurochemical aberrations in the brains of those exposed. Approximately 60 million pounds of organophosphates are applied to U.S. crops each year.

Carbamates. This variety of chemical pesticides is in fairly wide use today. Included in this category are aldicarb, carbaryl, the ethylenebisdithiocarbonate (EBDC) pesticides (including mancozeb, maneb, metiram, and zineb), naphthol, and carbofuran phenol. Like the other types of pesticides, carbamates disrupt the activity of certain enzymes and alter genetic and energy-production processes. However, unlike these other categories, they appear to be more rapidly excreted by most animals and so they do not become as bioconcentrated. This rule does not apply to fish, though, where the concentration of carbamates is just as problematic as that of the other pesticides.

Pesticides and their residues in food are a growing problem. Each year in California alone, more than 200 million tons of pesticides are dumped on fields and crops, and most of it never reaches the pests. These pesticide products contain more than 1,000 active ingredients. **Nationwide, about three-quarters of all produce has been found to contain detectable residues of pesticides. Pesticides are used because they are toxic to pest life; unfortunately, they are also toxic to wildlife and people.** Many of these chemicals become more concentrated as they move up the food chain. Eagles and other large birds that eat insects and rodents contaminated with DDT, for example, acquire huge and sometimes fatal levels of that chemical. High concentrations of certain chemicals can have serious consequences for humans as well.

The industrial, chemical and agriculture businesses work together. Agribusiness is highly oriented toward the use of chemical fertilizers and pesticides. Often salespeople are out on the farms selling new chemicals before there have been thorough studies to prove their safety. The EPA was created in 1970 partly to control the use and abuse of these pesticides; unfortunately, they often find out that a pesticide is unsafe after it has been used for many years. For example, dibromo-chloropropane (DBCP), which was sprayed on Hawaiian pineapples for years and contaminated the waters there, was banned in 1979 because of its toxicity, but it has remained in the environment for decades after.

Many imported foods, particularly tropical fruits, are sprayed or fumigated to keep bugs away during shipping. Spraying with pesticides is not uncommon for such fruits as papayas, mangoes, and pineapples. Bananas are less likely to be sprayed but may be gassed or fumigated before they are shipped. Spraying after harvesting is of concern because of the high concentrations of the chemicals on the foods when they get to the consumer. Dieldrin, a toxic organochloride pesticide that was banned in 1974 (except for

use on nonfood seeds and termites), used to be sprayed on produce after harvesting to prevent insect infestation. Now other chemicals and sulfurs are used, many of which may turn out to have the same toxicity problems as dieldrin. Many people become sensitive to one or more of these chemicals and may experience symptoms after consuming chemically treated produce; some very sensitive people may get sick just from being around the fruits or vegetables or their boxes. People who become chemically sensitive must often avoid a great number of foods and products that are sprayed or grown with chemicals. Even soaking the fruits in bleach, for example, or washing them with soap may not remove enough spray residues for the fruit to be tolerated. Pesticide spray residues in foods are not only a problem for the chemically sensitive person but are of long-range concern to the general public because of their potential for promoting cancer.

Many chemical sprays are used on cultivated vegetables. In some ways the cruciferous vegetables may be the biggest problem in this regard, because they absorb the chemicals so well. **Cabbage, broccoli, cauliflower, and brussels sprouts may be eaten more these days because of their reduction of cancer potential, but if they are sprayed with subtle carcinogens, the possibility of causing cancer may potentially be increased.** Certified organic produce may be extremely helpful in this regard, especially with vegetables without any skin to protect them. See "Which Foods Are Most Important to Buy Organically Grown?" on page 439 in this chapter.

Sprays can also contaminate meats and poultry. Much of the feed for these animals has been sprayed or may have pesticide residues. The animals themselves may be sprayed on occasion. The fat of animals is where the chemicals become most concentrated, so for that reason and to avoid increased saturated fats. **I recommend that nearly everyone minimize consumption of animal fats.**

Fruits, especially such dried fruits as dates and figs, as well as many grains and legumes, may be fumigated with chemicals like methyl bromide to protect them from insects and molds. Bananas are gassed with ethylene to help them ripen. Sulfuring foods by treating them with sulfur dioxide helps keep them looking fresher and may keep dried fruits brighter and moister.

Corn, for example, may be soaked in sulfur dioxide, and wine may have excess residues of sulfur dioxide. The most common practice when it comes to sulfur, of course, is the use of sulfites as preservatives. The spraying of sulfites on salad bar vegetables was probably the best-known example of sulfite use until this practice was banned by the U.S. Food and Drug Administration (FDA) in 1986. Today, red wines are probably the most well-known of foods/drinks that have added sulfites, but they may also be found in grape juice, sauerkraut juice, molasses, bottled lemon juice, dried potato flakes, pickles, some cookies and crackers, and pie dough. In the case of dried fruits, even if these foods are labeled sulfite-free, they may be fumigated with chemicals that can cause irritations or allergic symptoms.

Food Manufacturing, Processing, Storage, and Preparation

The food industry routinely uses about 2,000 different food additives in a wide variety of packaged and preserved foods. The total number of additives available worldwide has been estimated at about 6,000 to 8,000. These range from added vitamins and minerals to emulsifiers, buffers, natural and artificial flavoring and coloring, and large amounts of salt and sugar. **The average American consumes nearly 150 pounds of food additives a year, supporting a multibillion-dollar food-processing industry.** This includes about 130 pounds of sugar and sweeteners, along with 10 to 15 pounds of salt and 5 to 10 pounds of "enriched" vitamins, flavors, preservatives, and colored dyes. Some people in this world do not consume that much food in 1 year.

Besides the acknowledged additives, there are about 12,000 other chemicals that contaminate food during the various stages of propagation, growth, harvesting, packing, shipping, and preparation. These chemicals include sprays and pesticides, many of which are more dangerous than most food additives. About 400 different pesticides are currently registered for use on food in the United States, and about 850 million pounds of these pesticides are used on food crops each year. These chemicals show up not only in our food, of course, but also in our water supply. In one national survey, for example, the pesticide atrazine

showed up in the municipal drinking water of 718 out of 748 towns studied.

Plastics are another example of contamination. Even though manufacturers in the industry have switched from using PVC-based plastic wraps in favor of plasticizer-free polyethylene versions, every plastic used in the food industry—including low-density polyethylene (LDPE), high-density polyethylene (HDPE), polypropylene (PP), polystyrene (PS), polyethylene terephthalate (PET), and polyvinyl chloride (PVC)—is known to migrate from packaging to food (especially in boil-in-a-bag and microwave-type heating), thus posing a health risk. This risk could involve something relatively mild, like depletion of our nutrient supplies, cellular irritation, increased allergies, or weakened immune function. But it could also involve lifelong chronic disease, as would occur with the development of a cancer.

Why, then, are chemicals used in foods? Originally, foods were grown and eaten directly from relatively unpolluted soil. Wild foods were sought and gathered. The oceans and other waters fed us nutritious fish. Animals in the wild provided food for the hunters and their tribes. As the human population multiplied, however, the world expanded, farming progressed, trade specialties developed, and town markets shared a variety of goods among a diversity of people. Techniques for preparation and preservation (such as pickling, salting, and smoking) were developed to deal with the new problems of storage, waste, and food-borne illnesses.

As technology developed, we learned to create new chemicals to manipulate, preserve, and transform foods—and life changed. The subtle balance of Nature shifted with each new assault on the body's unique biochemical balance. Foods and food processing also changed. Scientists were able to mimic natural flavors, to color foods to make them look more "natural," and to aid in the creation and preservation of breads, crackers, and many more commonly used foods. Now there are even "foods" that are made entirely from chemicals—for example, coffee creamers, sugar substitutes, and candies are made of completely processed ingredients.

But there is a method to this madness. The food industry puts forth reasons (or rationalizations) for using these chemicals besides the fact that processed foods are usually more profitable. **Here are six "reasons" why we have processed foods:**

1. **To improve shelf life or storage time.** This was, I believe, the original reason for using additives. It allowed more food to get to more people and prevented waste and spoilage. Most canned foods are heat treated and vacuum packed so that they can be preserved and stored for years. Many fruits, especially dried fruits, are treated with sulfur dioxide or sprayed with chemicals to prevent their destruction by the air or bugs. Many breads and baked goods are treated or "embalmed" with chemicals to improve shelf life. This may be helpful to the manufacturer but not necessarily beneficial to the health and longevity of the consumer.

2. **To make food more available.** This is achieved not only by improving shelf life, but also through the use of specific types of packaging: separate dishes or entire meals boxed or frozen, such as TV dinners, cake mixes, and microwave meals. This technique of food processing has brought thousands of new products to grocery stores and demonstrates the convenience of modern food technology. Just walk down any grocery aisle; these products are everywhere!

3. **To increase the nutritional value.** Many foods have synthetic vitamins added to them. This can be of moderate benefit to people who consume these enriched foods. Often these added vitamins are the same ones that were removed during processing. The great flaw here, though, is that many important vitamins and minerals are processed out of whole foods and not added back into them. Vitamin B_6, chromium, and zinc are a few examples of important nutrients that are lost during the processing of grains and flours and not replaced. For that reason, it is better to eat whole grains. Occasionally foods are fortified, which means that they have an added nutrient that is not normally found in the original food. Cow's milk fortified with vitamin D is the most common example. A second flaw with this "increase nutritional value" approach is the fact that

Nature does not just plop vitamins and minerals into food. Rather, vitamins and minerals are woven into food, into the organic structure of the food. For example, minerals are often chelated to amino acids on proteins. Food is whole, and its wholeness is matched to our digestive system. Synthetically added nutrients are just that: synthetic additions that are not matched up with our needs in the same way.

4. **To improve the flavor of foods.** Many flavorings, both natural and artificial, are used in an attempt to create greater consumer appeal. Making foods sweeter, saltier, or spicier often tantalizes the taste buds and creates a certain identity and desire for repeated use of those foods. The unique flavor of many processed and packaged foods is created through much time and expense on the part of the manufacturer. Salt and sugar are the 2 most common flavorings. Monosodium glutamate is another common "flavor enhancer."

5. **To make foods easier to prepare.** These days, people take less time with food preparation. Family orientation has changed through the years, and many wives and mothers no longer spend their days at the supermarket, in the kitchen, or in the garden. So the manufacturers prepare the foods for us and package them in boxes or cans, freeze them, or make them "instant" so that we can add water, heat, microwaves, or otherwise take little effort to get them ready to eat. Mashed potatoes, breakfast cereals, instant oatmeal, cookies, cake mixes, hot dogs, lunch meats, and thousands of other products fit into this category.

6. **To improve consumer acceptance.** This is a scary one, because the chemicals used to maintain a food's color or prevent it from being discolored are often the more potentially toxic substances. Even our natural produce, the fruits and vegetables, are exposed to these chemicals. It is still legal in the United States for orange growers to inject Citrus Red No. 2 into orange rinds at 2 ppm to achieve a uniform orange color. Chickens may be treated with yellow dyes to keep their skin looking healthy. Sprays are

used on produce to prevent insects and microorganisms from moving in or consuming them before the consumer. Bananas are gassed, many fruits and vegetables are sprayed with fungicides, and breads have added mold inhibitors. What increases the selling power of many items, in the eyes of the consumer, may not benefit other parts of the body.

I am not a big supporter of food processing, chemical sprays, and food additives. I know there is definite value in these processes to both manufacturers and consumers of "modern foods." Luckily, though, many of them are safe, and more research has been allocated to food additives than to any other areas of industrial chemical use. Our ignorance regarding both food and environmental chemical interactions is an important issue. Individual chemicals that are nontoxic on their own may be combined to form new chemicals. There are literally millions of possibilities that could cause serious problems before they are discovered. I make a concerted effort to avoid or minimize the use of chemicals and processed foods, and I prescribe the same to those who choose to stay healthy and support the planet. Cultivating and consuming wholesome, natural, and organic foods, ideally grown locally and eaten fresh, has long-range benefits for our environment, our bodies, and our health.

People using chemical foods take a risk. The chemical companies and the food processors make a lot of money, most assuredly at our expense, in terms of both our health-care costs and the money spent on their products. The health of the planet is also at stake. It is in our personal health interest to avoid chemical additives and processed foods, and to eat naturally. Even in natural foods such as fruits, vegetables, and grains, however, there is a great deal of potential contamination when these foods and the land on which they are grown are chemically treated. For this reason, we can try to eat organic, but this is not easy, especially in some areas of the country and at certain times of the year. Even organic foods can have small amounts of unavoidable environmental contamination, such as from acid rain, contaminated water, chemical residues in soil, and nuclear fallout. An otherwise healthy lifestyle of exercise, stress management, good dietary habits, and some protective nutritional supplementation will reduce the risks that chemical food additives pose to our health.

WHO IS RESPONSIBLE FOR FOOD SAFETY?

Three government agencies are primarily responsible for regulation of food in the United States. These agencies are the EPA, the U.S. Department of Agriculture (USDA), and the FDA. Responsibilities of the EPA include enforcement of the 1974 Safe Drinking Water Act (SWDA) and the 1996 Food Quality Protection Act (FQPA). It is up to this agency to monitor more than 100 potential toxins routinely present in this country's drinking water and to set levels for the amount a city or town is allowed to pipe out to its residents. It is also up to the EPA to decide what amount of a known carcinogen should be allowed in our food.

The USDA's responsibility is focused on a wide variety of inspection services, including the Animal and Plant Health Inspection Service (APHIS), the Federal Grain and Inspection Service (FGIS), and the Food Safety and Inspection Service (FSIS). This agency polices problems like fruit flies and salmonella in food and samples about 500,000 animal products from production plants across the country for potential contamination.

Regulation of food additives, nutritional labeling, dietary supplements, and food irradiation all fall under the jurisdiction of the FDA, which itself is housed within the Department of Health and Human Services (DHHS). Although much recent attention has been focused on the FDA's role in the regulation of dietary supplements, I believe that its involvement with food is also extremely important. One key area of FDA involvement is food irradiation. Since its approval of irradiation for wheat and wheat powder in 1963, the FDA has now expanded its approval of irradiation to most categories of food. By placing foods on a conveyor belt and passing them briefly under a radioactive element that emits gamma rays (like cesium 137), insects, parasites, bacteria, and other microbes can be killed. In addition, in the case of foods like fruits, ripening can be delayed. (See more under "Food

Irradiation" on page 478 in this chapter.) Thus, irradiation of our food can definitely help reduce risk of bacterial contamination, but it can also serve as a means for industries to increase their profit margin by salvaging foods that are essentially low-quality and past their prime. Irradiation of food is also a risk reducer that avoids asking the basic question, "What is making our food so much more susceptible to bacterial contamination in the first place?"

Like irradiation, food labeling is a key area of FDA involvement. Food labeling is important to the conscientious consumer. The FDA is responsible for overseeing proper labeling, standards of quality and quantity, enriched product standards, and nutritional misinformation, as well as enforcing compliance, researching and accepting new foods, and educating consumers. For certain food creations, such as ketchup, mayonnaise, and jam, there are "standards of identity" required—they must contain certain ingredients to be called by those names.

Everyone who touches food is responsible for consumer safety—the farmer, picker, shipper, manufacturer, grocery store, and cook. Chemical additive manufacturers have a vested interest in new products appearing to be safe. How safe they actually are is an issue of legitimate debate, particularly following the passage of the Food Quality Protection Act by the U.S. Congress in 1996. Although it was intended to reduce our risk of toxic exposure from the foods we eat, a provision of this act may have turned the tables in the opposite direction. The provision involved what was tantamount to a repeal of the Delaney Clause that kept carcinogens out of our food for nearly 40 years.

From 1958 until 1996, we were fortunate to have a zero-tolerance policy with respect to allowing cancer-causing agents in our food—they were not allowed in our food in any amount. During these same years, however, researchers developed the ability to detect smaller and smaller amounts of cancer-causing toxins. By 1996, for example, laboratories were detecting small amounts of cancer-causing pesticides on most all of the fruits and vegetables in our food supply. Short of removing all nonorganic fruits and vegetables from the food supply, Congress decided to allow small amounts of cancer-causing toxins back into the food supply at levels where there was "a reasonable certainty that no harm will result." So our responsibility

as consumers is greater than ever. We need to work toward less use of pesticides and additives in the general (nonorganic) food supply and, at the same time, support organically grown foods as much as possible because they are produced without the use of these carcinogens.

Reading Food Labels

Packaging information laws are slowly changing to help consumers learn more about what they are buying. This chapter provides information to help us make conscientious, healthy, and environmentally sound choices, if we choose to purchase packaged foods.

- Minimize the purchase of food packaged in plastics, Styrofoam, and other nonbiodegradable products. "Precycle" means not buying products you cannot recycle. This will create a demand for the production of environmentally sound packaging.

- Additives to avoid include the artificial colors, excess sugars and salt, BHA and BHT, as well as nitrites and sulfites.

- A shopping guideline to follow is, "If you can't pronounce it, don't buy it."

For a more thorough discussion on food labels, see page 396 in chapter 10, Nutritional Habits. You can also review my book *The Staying Healthy Shopper's Guide,* in which an entire chapter is devoted to reading food labels. There is lots to learn and wisdom to be gained, along with healthier eating by making wiser choices.

ORGANIC FOODS: ANOTHER SOLUTION

Consuming organic foods is a good way to avoid agriculture chemicals. Consuming whole foods from Nature—the fruits and vegetables, whole grains and beans, nuts and seeds, and so on—is a further plan to avoid processed foods that are mixed with chemicals. In *The Staying Healthy Shopper's Guide,* which is all about how chemicals get into our foods and how to avoid them, I have an entire chapter on this topic:

"Organic Foods: Why, When, and What to Buy." Below I include information from that chapter on 25 foods to buy organic. I chose these foods based on three primary criteria. First, foods that are highly treated with chemicals, such as strawberries, are best avoided unless they are organically grown. Second, foods that we consume regularly, like bananas, wheat, or milk products, are best used organic to minimize our overall exposure. And third, those foods where any chemical sprays are absorbed directly into the parts we consume, such as leafy greens, should be organic, ideally grown ourselves. Also, when we are feeding babies, who are more sensitive to chemical exposure, or for people with severe illness or who are very sensitive to chemicals, focusing on organically grown foods is suggested.

Which Foods Are Most Important to Buy Organically Grown?

There are certain key foods that are more important to buy organically grown, because some crops are more heavily treated than others. As much as 70% of produce grown in the United States has been found by the FDA to have some pesticide residues. More than half of everything we usually eat introduces some pesticides into the body. However, no existing research has looked into the long-term effects of small doses of thousands of different chemicals over a lifetime. Having reviewed the most relevant research on pesticides and additives in food, I have come up with **the following list of 25 important foods to buy organically grown.**

   1. Baby foods. Since infants are more sensitive to pesticides because of their more vulnerable nervous and immune systems, organic baby foods are much safer. Unless we specifically buy organic, studies show that babies may be getting toxic chemicals in such common foods as green beans and applesauce. Fortunately, there are several companies marketing organic baby foods in mainstream grocery stores. Even better, make your own fresh baby food in the blender from organic fruits and vegetables.

   2. Strawberries. This is the most heavily contaminated produce item in the United States today, according to data from a number of environmental groups, including a 1993 study by the Environmental Working Group and an analysis by the Pesticide

Action Network North America. Strawberries in California are treated with more than 300 pounds of pesticides per acre, and some areas of the country use up to 500 pounds per acre. As a comparison, conventional farming currently uses about 25 pounds of pesticides per acre on the average crop. Also, some growers may be spraying the harvested strawberries for shipping. This adds to the amount of chemical concentration in the fruit. Strawberries were also found to have the highest level of hormone-affecting pesticides, including benomyl, vinclozolin, and endosulfan. Methyl bromide is another common spray used on strawberries. Note that out-of-season strawberries may be most heavily treated because they come from other countries and are sprayed even more before shipping.

   3. Milk and butter. Because pesticides are pervasive and stored in higher amounts in fat, dairy products tend to retain higher levels of residues and chemicals from feeds and other sources. This is not well researched yet; however, my family has been buying organic milk products for years. Milk is a common source of the herbicide atrazine (a known endocrine disrupter) and the growth hormone BGH, which has been genetically engineered to boost milk production. Almost 80% of the cows treated with BGH get udder infections, so there is also increased risk of antibiotics in the milk. These concerns have motivated shoppers to consider organic milk products more seriously, and the sale of organic milk is now averaging $50 million to $60 million each year. It is becoming more available in mainstream supermarkets.

   4. Bananas. If you are mashing bananas for babies or feeding them frequently to kids, buy them organic whenever possible. Because they are shipped from southern and tropical countries and are exposed to some chemicals at all phases of growth and production, they may be receiving heavier pesticide exposure. Bananas are commonly gassed with ethylene (even some organics) to ripen them and prepare them for shipping, and this seems to be relatively nontoxic to the banana consumer. They are also being fumigated with ethyl bromide to prevent pests from coming in with the fruit. I am most concerned about this exposure, and so I buy organic bananas, which are more available these days. Although the studies suggest that much of the contamination can

Wise Choices to Buy Organic

Product	Concern
Baby foods	Possible effects of neurotoxins on developing infant.
Milk and butter	Pesticides are stored in fats and can be passed on to us.

FRUITS

Strawberries	70% of those tested had residues; the highest content of endocrine disrupters; on average, 300 pounds of pesticides are used per acre.
Bananas	Often baby's first food; banana sprays are highly toxic; many people eat bananas daily (America's favorite fruit).
Peaches, cherries, nectarine, apricots	About 70% of each of these stone fruits have residues.
Apples	Contain a large number of different pesticides.
Grapes	79% of grapes tested from Chile had residues.
Melons	Mexican cantaloupe: 76% residues; honeydew: 69% residues.
Red raspberries	56% had residues; 31% had 5 different residues.
Imported produce	Sprays used that are banned in the United States; always buy U.S. produce in season.

VEGETABLES

Bell peppers	64% had residues; the highest level of neurotoxins.
Leafy greens	Treated with systemic pesticides that cannot be washed off.
Spinach	Systemic pesticides, carcinogens, and most endocrine disrupters.
Green beans	Heavily treated, most sprays are systemic, endocrine disrupters.
Tomatoes	On some samples, 30 different pesticides were found.
Cucumbers	Second-highest level of carcinogenic pesticides used.

be peeled off, organic bananas are the safest option for children.

5. Stone fruits (peaches, cherries, apricots, plums, and nectarines). Stone fruits are often sprayed to protect them because their sweetness attracts many insects. They are often sprayed after they are packed into boxes for shipping. Because their skins are absorptive, they tend to retain more of the chemicals. In FDA spot checks, 71% of the peach crops had pesticide residues, and peach farms also tended to have some of the highest rates of pesticide violations. Cherries are another heavily sprayed crop; the FDA found more pesticide residues on U.S. cherries than they did on the imported ones. Apricots frequently had residues (64% of those tested), and 35% had the carcinogenic pesticide captan present.

6. Leafy greens (lettuces, spinach, kale, and chard). Sprayed chemicals tend to remain on the leaves of these vegetables, which is potentially more harmful because we eat the leafy parts. In FDA studies, spinach was the leafy green most frequently found to contain the more potent pesticides, especially the organophosphates (neurotoxins) and permethrin (noted as mildly carcinogenic). In addition, 10% of the spinach samples had residues of DDT, which was phased out of use in the United States more than 30 years ago.

7. Grapes. Unless they are organically grown, grapes may receive multiple applications of a variety of chemical agents during their growing period. Some fruits and vegetables are more highly sensitive to the environment, particularly those that ripen quickly or attract insects and molds. These crops, including grapes,

Wise Choices to Buy Organic

Product	Concern
GRAINS	
Rice	Conventional fields are heavily treated.
Corn	Corn receives an excessive amount of U.S. pesticides.
Oats	Also may be overtreated.
Whole wheat	More than 90% of all wheat samples had pesticides (according to the FDA).
PROTEIN FOODS	
Eggs	Factory farming increases bacteria and decreases quality.
Seafood	Many rivers and estuaries are polluted; it is important to know the source.
Meats	Animals are often raised with hormones, antibiotics, and other drugs.
BEVERAGES	
Coffee	Sprays are not always burned off in roasting.
Wine	Grapes and wines are frequently treated with chemicals and sulfites (which can be allergenic).

Source: Information compiled from U.S. Food and Drug Administration Pesticide Monitoring Program, 2003, and Report Card: Pesticides in Produce, Environmental Working Group, Washington, D.C., 2006.

tend to be more heavily treated in order to get them to the market (and to protect the financial interest of the grower). FDA research indicates that imported grapes are even more heavily treated than the U.S. samples. During winter and early spring, almost all grapes available in the United States are from Chile, and these are found to have an exceptionally high percentage of pesticide residues (79%). They also have a higher percentage of the carcinogenic pesticides captan and iprodione. However, U.S. grape growers use high amounts of sulfites and the fumigant methyl bromide, so these are all good reasons to buy organic grapes and grape juices.

8. Green beans. Consider buying your green beans organically grown because the EPA has registered more than 60 pesticides in use on green beans, and the FDA found 23 different chemicals on green beans in its 1992–1993 studies. In addition, almost 10% of the imported green beans contained illegal pesticide residues.

9. Apples. A staple in many diets, apples have been found to be nearly as contaminated as strawberries. Forty-eight different pesticides were detected by FDA testing in nearly 2,500 samples from 1984 to 1991, while 36 different chemicals were found in their 1992–1993 evaluations. Nearly half of these chemicals were either neurotoxic or carcinogenic. In the FDA analyses, apples and peaches had seven different pesticides per crop. Fortunately, a shift away from spraying the orchards is occurring in some areas. If you buy nonorganic and/or waxed apples, be sure to peel them and discard the skin before you eat them since most of the chemical residues are on the apple skins. It is time to change the saying to "An *organic* apple a day keeps the doctor away."

10. Rice. This is the most frequently consumed food on the planet. Consider buying organically grown rice and rice products, especially if it is one of your staple foods. The dangerous herbicide 2,4,5-T was sprayed on rice before it was banned in 1984, and many persistent water-soluble herbicides and insecticides have been found to contaminate the groundwater near major rice fields, such as in California's Sacramento River Valley. I suggest buying organic rice in bulk. That way it is as economical as nonorganic prepackaged rice and much safer.

11. Corn products. A primary staple in the American diet, corn is typically heavily treated; nearly 50% of all pesticides are sprayed on corn. Locally grown fresh corn tends to be treated less, so sweet corn on the cob is likely safer than corn by-products, which may have more contamination. Corn is still heavily treated with the herbicide atrazine, however, and it is also typically sprayed after harvesting. Also, nonorganic corn may be genetically modified, as may be soybean products.

12. Bell peppers. Both red and green bell peppers were found to have many chemical residues from the most neurotoxic of the pesticides. In the FDA's measurement of both U.S. and Mexican crops, 64% of peppers contained at least one pesticide, while 36% contained two or more. These vegetables also may be waxed, which makes it difficult to remove the residues and other chemicals within the waxes.

13. Tomatoes. One study found that as many as 30 different pesticides are used to spray tomatoes. Because the skins of tomatoes are thin and absorbent, and since this is a staple in many salads, soups, and sauces, tomatoes are worth buying organically grown. At certain times of year, the price of organic plum tomatoes is competitive with nonorganic varieties. Farmers' markets may be the best source for fresh unsprayed tomatoes. Or they can be easily grown on a deck or in planter boxes at home.

14. Tropical fruits. Pineapples, papayas, and mangoes are attractive to tropical pests and may be more heavily treated during cultivation, preparation, and shipping. Because of their skins, they tend to absorb the sprays, creating higher levels of chemical contamination. These are called "systemic pesticides," and they cannot be washed away as they are contained within the fruit and seeds.

15. Celery. Although most people do not eat a lot of celery all at once, it can be an ideal, low-calorie snack food. This absorptive, watery vegetable understandably retains residues, so it is not surprising that on EPA analyses, 81% of samples contained residues, more pesticides than any other crop. Furthermore, many of the pesticides found were the stronger neurotoxic and carcinogenic ones. After reading the EPA report, I added celery to my list of important foods to buy organically grown.

16. Berries (raspberries, blueberries, blackberries). As with strawberries, these berries have high pesticide exposure during cultivation, and most of these are systemic. More than 50% of EPA-tested raspberries had pesticide residues, and nearly a third had

two or more. It is best to find your own untreated patch to pick from or buy them organically grown.

17. Imported produce. This usually out-of-season produce is often heavily treated for easier growing and shipping to the United States. There is also risk of higher toxicity from the use of chemicals that have been banned in the United States. Cantaloupes and other imported melons were found to have a high concentration of pesticides in two-thirds of tested samples. In Mexican cantaloupes, 48% had two or more residues.

18. Cruciferous vegetables (broccoli, cabbage, brussels sprouts, and cauliflower). Because of their healthy, anticancer nutrient content, high fiber, and low calories, these are excellent foods to eat regularly. But because we eat the parts that may have been sprayed with carcinogenic chemicals, it is best to eat the organically grown versions of these vegetables.

19. Cucumbers. These appear on the Environmental Working Group's buy-organic list because of the potent pesticide dieldrin found in nonorganic cucumber crops. Dieldrin increases cancer risk. Also, the waxes commonly used to make cucumbers shiny should be avoided because they may contain other chemical residues.

20. Wheat. Many grains and legumes, particularly wheat, rice, and corn, are treated with pesticides as crops and then fumigated periodically during storage. In a recent review of pesticide residues, 91% of the wheat sampled by the FDA contained pesticide residues! Wheat can be among the most heavily treated grains, because it is stockpiled as a basic commodity and fumigated periodically to keep down pests. When it is milled, the outer coating—the bran included in whole wheat bread and cereals—is the portion that receives the most chemical treatment. The bran and germ portion of the wheat also retains the most residues. It has been suggested that some forms of so-called wheat allergy, which has been associated with learning problems and difficulty in concentrating, may actually be a neurotoxic reaction to the pesticide residues in the grain. These pesticides are, by definition, neurotoxins— that is how they affect the insects they are intended to destroy. Wheat is on this organic list because it is so heavily consumed by most people in this country and elsewhere throughout the world.

21. Eggs. These are typically produced in factory farms where the hens often live in unhygienic conditions. This may be one of the reasons that salmonella bacteria are found in eggs so frequently. More than 2 million eggs each year are contaminated, resulting in more than 500,000 cases of food poisoning. Factory farm eggs also may be lower in nutrients than organic ones, and they usually do not taste as good as farm-fresh eggs from free-ranging chickens that are not fed antibiotics. Our best egg option is organic eggs, which are becoming more available in mainstream supermarkets.

22. Seafood. Depending on where it is caught or harvested, seafood can be contaminated by polluted water. Because some chemicals persist in water (as well as in the soil), fish taken from pesticide-polluted water contain concentrations of the fat-soluble chemicals, including those that mimic estrogen. Rivers and lakes also contain other contaminants and heavy metals, including arsenic, cadmium, chromium, mercury, and lead. Sadly, more than 1,600 waterways are documented to be polluted with mercury. If you are eating seafood regularly, be sure to consume a variety to avoid overexposure to specific chemicals or contaminants. Seafood will not be labeled as organic because we do not have control over it. Also, farm-raised fish may have even more chemicals in them.

23. Meat. This is reported by researchers to be among the most contaminated products in our food supply. Like poultry, cattle and pigs no longer roam free but are frequently raised under unsanitary feedlot conditions. Their health, productivity, and muscle mass are maintained by an array of drugs that include antibiotics, hormones, and steroids. They also receive antibacterials on their coats; additives and pesticides in their feed; and sedatives and other drugs for slaughter. If available, desirable, and affordable, choose less chemically treated and cured meats and, ideally, organically raised meat. Be sure to store and cook it properly.

24. Coffee. As I write in *The New Detox Diet*, I do not support the regular intake of caffeine and alcohol, but since so many do partake regularly of these psychoactive substances, I feel that it is important to address them in this list. The magic bean is often heavily treated with chemicals. Since people who drink coffee tend to do so regularly and often in quantity, there may be a significant risk of exposure to toxins. Coffee drinking is a questionable health habit, but if you are a regular coffee drinker, make that java organic and use good water.

25. Wine. Grapes and wine may contain a variety of accumulated pesticides and other chemicals. Both grapes and wine—even organic wines—typically contain sulfites, so asthmatics and others sensitive to sulfites should consume only organic, sulfite-free wines if they choose to drink any alcohol. Many people who consume wine tend to be regular drinkers. Because it is thought that some of the adverse and hangover effects from wine drinking may be from the chemicals, try some organic wine, made from organically grown grapes and manufactured without chemicals or contaminated bottles and corks.

FOOD PROCESSING

This section discusses many of the chemicals that are used by food manufacturers. Fruits, vegetables, whole grains, and other plants, as well as animals and fish are ground, mashed, boiled, and taken through many

---

Some Ways to Minimize Pesticides in Your Food

- **Limit** use of out-of-season, imported produce.
- **Wash,** soak, and peel conventionally grown fruits and vegetables.
- **Limit** your intake of red meats and factory-farmed poultry.
- **Limit** your intake of fish known to be caught from polluted waters.
- **Replace** some meat meals with such complementary proteins as corn, beans, whole-grain rice, or soybeans and their products, like tofu and tempeh.
- **Buy** some new bulk foods, such as beans, oats, and some time-honored grains that may be less treated, including millet, quinoa, barley, couscous, amaranth, and spelt.
- **Try** emphasizing fruits and vegetables that can be peeled or those that have been recently found to have low residues.
- **Substitute** one good fresh food for another. The Environmental Working Group has found that just 12 fruits and vegetables contain half the pesticide load in the average diet.

processes to create the multitude of boxed, canned, packaged, and plastic-wrapped "foods" that we find in stores. Chemicals are added to foods in three ways. First, there are the **intentional additives** that become ingredients in the foods. These chemicals are the only ones listed on the packages, but sadly, there are many hidden additives that never appear on our "truth-in-packaging" labels; these are classified as "contaminants." Next are the **chemicals that are used during processing,** which may contaminate the foods without being direct additives. Chemicals used in packaging may get into foods as well. Plastics, cans, and boxes may all pose a danger, because various chemicals and metals are used in their production. Finally, there are the **silent additives,** which are of most concern—the pesticides; chemicals in water and air; antibiotics, hormones, and other medicines given to animals; and ubiquitous industrial chemical pollutants. The best way to prevent harm from these "economic poisons" is to prohibit their use in the first place or avoid all manufactured products.

It sometimes seems that there is more concern about chemical exposures in the home or at work, where little regulation protects us from toxic substances, than about chemical dangers in food. Food additives, in particular, are more closely regulated by the FDA, so that these chemicals pose less short-term risk. However, researchers do not really know the risks posed by the long-term use of most chemicals, especially because we are exposed to so many that if we do develop some health problems, it would be difficult to isolate which specific chemical(s) or other factors may have generated these problems.

Just because certain food additives are used today and deemed "safe," that does not mean that they are, in fact, safe. The FDA must be constantly aware of possible long-range effects. It is currently conducting or overseeing a great deal of research regarding both chemicals in use and potential new ones. The FDA can change the status of any chemical used in food, removing old ones from use or approving new ones. Some additives that were found to be unsafe and removed after years of use include Red No. 2, cyclamates, and cobalt sulfate. There is also a category for "interim approval" additives whose safety has been questioned. The FDA has used this category in recent years to handle a variety of suspicious food additives, including acrylonitrile copolymers, saccharin, and brominated vegetable oil (BVO).

There are currently about 3,000 food additives approved for use in the foods we eat or the beverages we drink. As mentioned earlier, the average American consumes 150 to 160 pounds of additives each year, including 130 pounds of added sweeteners, nearly 90% of it sugar. In 1990, almost 30 billion pounds of sweeteners were consumed by the U.S. public, and that number has only grown since then. Salt intake is about 15 pounds per person per year, while various other food additives account for another 5 to 10 pounds. Additives have really helped the success of both the junk food and fast food markets, where a great deal of that 150 to 160 pounds of additives is consumed. In 1958, the U.S. Congress approved the FDA's Generally Recognized as Safe (GRAS) list when it enacted the Food Additives Amendment. Some several thousand additives that were already in use were reviewed by a number of scientists, and those that were felt to be safe were placed on the GRAS list. This meant that they were accepted without further testing. The accepted list originally included about 700 substances, many of which were salt, sugar, spices, vitamins, minerals, flavorings, preservatives, emulsifiers, and so on. With some of these, levels or application to certain foods are restricted; they are classified as "for intended use based on standard manufacturing processes." Other additives can be used freely.

One of the problems with the GRAS list, however, is lack of knowledge regarding many of the additives. With better testing, some of them have been shown to be unsafe, particularly when increased consumption causes intake to exceed "intended exposure" levels. In the 1970s, a fairly extensive review of the GRAS list (including about 450 additives) was undertaken; many of the additives are still being investigated.

As noted in *A Consumer's Dictionary of Food Additives,* author Ruth Winter clarified a 1980 report of the FDA's 10-year evaluation of 415 common additives (some evaluated as groups). Only 305 were considered safe, a class I rating, for their current and projected uses. Another 68 were given class II ratings—that is, they were deemed safe as currently used, but it was felt that more research was needed to evaluate their effects at higher levels. These included some of the basic vitamins and minerals, such as vitamins A and

D, iron, and zinc salts. Class III included 19 substances, such as BHA, BHT, and caffeine, where further research brought up more questions; their use was approved until further testing might show them to be unsafe. Could the FDA's motto be "better sorry than safe"? Class IV–rated items included five additives that were generally considered safe but that required some use restrictions due to sensitivities in certain individuals. These included salt, modified starches used as thickening agents, and lactic acid and calcium lactate used in infant formulas. Another 18 items, rated as class V, were taken off the list until sufficient data could be gathered to prove them safe. These include some glycerides and specific iron salts.

There is a final piece of information of concern regarding the FDA and its GRAS list. Beginning in the 1970s, the FDA began to contract out some of its scientific research reviews on additives with the primary trade organization for food extracts and flavorings in the United States, called the Flavor and Extract Manufacturers Association (FEMA). Under congressional jurisdiction, and with FDA approval, FEMA began publishing its own GRAS list in 1965. With its most recent, twenty-first version of this FEMA-GRAS list in 2003, FEMA has currently sanctioned approval of about 1,200 flavoring agents.

Types of Additives

Sweeteners. There are many sweeteners used in processed foods in addition to all of the natural sweet flavors from fructose in fruits, lactose in milk, and maltose in breads. Sweeteners are the most common additive, and they are consumed in the largest volume. Natural or nutritional sweeteners are extracts of real food. These sweeteners, as pure carbohydrate and simple sugar, contain 4 calories per gram. For example, 1 tablespoon of cane sugar contains 50 calories but no other nutrition. Honey has about 64 calories, maple syrup about 50, and raw sugar about 15 per tablespoon. Other nutritional sweeteners include beet sugar, brown sugar, molasses, fructose, corn syrup, barley malt, and rice syrup. Stevia, or sweetleaf, is a well-tolerated herbal sweetener with basically no calories.

The nonnutritional, or chemical, sweeteners are also popular, especially in this country's overweight culture. Saccharin and aspartame are both well-known and commonly used artificial sweeteners. Cyclamate was banned in 1969 but is still legal in some countries that feel that the results of cancer studies in rats are not a cause of concern for humans. The FDA has been trying to ban saccharin, but the public continues to demand it. Aspartame has remained controversial since its adoption as a GRAS-listed additive in 1982. As NutraSweet or Equal, it is now the most common artificial sweetener, and there is concern that this chemical (two amino acids bound into a new compound that does not act like amino acids or offer any nutrition) is a nerve system irritant and affects some people adversely, much like monosodium glutamate (MSG) does.

Much more recent entries into the artificial sweetener market include acesulfame-k or ace-K (Sunette), sucralose (Splenda), and neotame (first approved for use in baked goods in 2002). Neotame is actually aspartame that has been hydrogenated and linked up with another chemical to make it 30 to 60 times sweeter. On the fake sugar front, note that a fair number of chemicals have some form of approval (not GRAS approval) for addition to our food as sweeteners. These other sweeteners include the dihydrochalcones (especially neohesperidine dihydrochalcone, which is approved through FEMA and their GRAS list), thaumatin, maltol and ethyl maltol, glycyrrhizin (obtained from licorice), and stevioside (obtained from stevia).

These chemicals are supposedly used to minimize obesity or help regulate blood sugar, but many people use them merely as an opportunity to eat other, more caloric foods and desserts. Studies show that artificial sweeteners do not really help weight loss in the majority of people unless they are already eating a low-calorie diet. It is better to eat the naturally sweet foods, such as the whole grains, fruits, and vegetables, to obtain an adequate level of fiber, vitamins, and minerals along with that sweet flavor, and to reduce intake of the processed, more heavily sweetened foods.

An alternative is the aforementioned stevia, derived from the plant *Stevia rebaudiana*. This plant has the common name sweet leaf of Paraguay because of its naturally sweet taste and native habitat. It is available in granular, powdered, and liquid forms, and may have some unique health-supportive properties in addition to its effect on our taste buds. There continues to be debate about the proper use of this sweetener, however, and it has yet to be granted approval by any regulatory organization in the United States (even though it has not been banned by any organization).

Flavorings. Flavorings constitute the largest number of all the additives, with sweeteners being the biggest portion. There are more than 2,000 different flavorings, 500 natural and more than 1,500 synthetic. Flavor additives are used to attain a certain taste in foods, and this taste needs to be consistent, persistent (last with time), and uniform throughout the food item. Because many ingredients used in preparing foods may vary in flavor, these additives are used to ensure that the consumer's expectations are met.

The natural flavors, which are basically concentrated extracts, include the essential oils, various spices, and oleoresins. Most of these are considered safe and in my opinion are more acceptable for use in foods than are the synthetic versions. A few natural flavors, such as nutmeg and safrole (the oil from saffron) may be toxic under certain circumstances. The synthetic versions of natural flavors are made from a great number of chemicals. Current FDA regulations state that any of these chemicals need be listed on packaging only as "artificial flavor" or "imitation flavor." If there is only 1 such chemical used, it might be listed, but to simulate a particular flavor, a chemist must often use a mixture of a number of chemicals.

Most of the artificial flavors are on the GRAS list. Although they may not be as dangerous as the food col-

Natural Flavorings		
Anise	Garlic	Mustard
Cassia	Ginger	Orange oil
Clove	Kola nut	Other fruit oils
Cocoa	Lemon oil	Peppermint
Fennel	Licorice	Vanilla
Fenugreek		

ors (with the exception of artificial smoke flavorings, which appear to be clearly mutagenic), they are much more widely used. Some of them can be toxic to the nervous system, kidneys, or liver, but still, in comparison to the colorings, they appear less risky when consumed in small amounts.

Flavorings are used in a wide variety of foods. Soft drinks, chewing gum, confections, ice creams, baked goods, puddings, gelatins, and other desserts are some examples. Most of these flavorings are considered fairly safe in modest amounts. There are also "flavor enhancers," substances that seem to bring out or improve the flavors of the foods in which they are used. Salt is probably the most common, although MSG is also used frequently. Maltol is another example of a flavoring agent.

Most labeling on packages does not name specific flavorings, whether artificial or natural; rather, it usually just states "natural" or "artificial flavoring." Also, a single artificial flavor—for example, "artificial

Some Chemicals Used to Provide Artificial Flavor

Amyl alcohol	Ethyl formate	Octyl alcohol and salts
Amyl salts	Formic acid	Phenethyl alcohol and salts
Benzaldehyde	Geraniol	Pinenes
Benzyl acetate	Geranyl acids	Propyl alcohol and salts
Benzyl alcohol	Isoamyl alcohol and acid	Propylene glycol
Butyl acetate and salts	Linalol	Rhodinol
Diacetyl	Linalyl salts	Salicylaldehyde
Ethyl acetate	Nonyl alcohol and salts	
Ethyl butyrate		

Many of these chemicals can be found naturally in some foods, such as fruits or nuts, but most chemicals used to flavor foods are prepared synthetically.

Common Foods That Often Contain Artificial Flavors				
Alcoholic beverages	Gelatins	Jams	Meats	Soda pop
Baked goods	Gum	Jellies	Puddings	Soups
Candy	Ice cream	Liquors	Sauces	Spices
Cereals	Ices	Maple syrup	Seasonings	Syrups
Cordials	Icings	Margarine	Shortening	Yogurts
Desserts				

strawberry flavoring"—may actually be comprised of 50 or more different chemicals, all combined. If we want to avoid the 1,500 or so chemicals used as artificial flavors, we had better start learning some of their names. The table on the opposite page provides the names of some of the more commonly used artificial flavoring agents.

Coloring agents. As a general category, this is probably of most concern. We need to be careful with the artificial colors, not the natural ones. My list of natural food colors includes carotene, annatto, beet red (powdered beets), saffron, turmeric, paprika, and grapes, as well as vegetable and fruit juices. All of these are considered safe in the usual amounts used to color foods. In very high doses—much higher than would be found in a typical meal—there has been some concern about toxicity involving such extracts as safrole and turmeric. Particularly in the case of turmeric, however, there is some pretty solid evidence about the health-supportive properties of this spice and coloring agent, including its value as an anti-inflammatory. Most coloring agents are synthetic and potentially toxic, however. These synthetics are a fake substitute for the natural, fresh color of foods. Artificial colors are chemicals synthesized from petroleum and coal-tar products. Many of these chemicals have been incorporated into foods with insufficient research as to safety, and some have been withdrawn because of studies showing toxicity or carcinogenicity.

Colors derived for food, drugs, and cosmetics (labeled FD&C colors) by the FDA) have been used for many years. Many of the same dyes and pigments are used to color clothing. In 1938, about 15 dyes were certified for use in foods. Through the years, many have been eliminated from food use, however. Over the course of the 1950s, FD&C Orange No. 1 and Orange No. 2 as well as FD&C Red No. 32 were withdrawn after the U.S. Congress initiated hearings on possible carcinogenicity and the FDA conducted a systematic review of all certified food additives. More dyes were removed in 1973 for various reasons (hyperactivity, allergy, general toxicity, carcinogenicity); these included Red No. 1 and No. 4, Yellow No. 1, No. 2, No. 3, and No. 4, as well as Violet No. 1. In 1976, Red No. 2 was removed (except for use in coloring orange skins) because of its carcinogenicity in rats. More recently, Orange B (used in casings for frankfurters and sausage) was withdrawn because of cancer links.

FDA-approved dyes in current use include these:

- **Citrus Red No. 2.** This dye was withdrawn in 1976, except for use in coloring oranges to establish a brighter and more uniform color, because it was shown to cause cancer in animals. It had been widely used in desserts, cereal, and maraschino cherries. To avoid this, use organic oranges when adding grated orange peel in a recipe or eating oranges unpeeled.

- **Red No. 3 (erythrosin).** This dye is used in cherries, cherry pie, gelatins, ice cream, fruit cocktail, candy, sherbet, pudding, cereals, and baked goods. It is on the safe list, but research has suggested that this coal-tar derivative is harmful, possibly causing gene mutations, cancers, or changes in brain chemistry. Clear evidence is lacking, so this dye stays on the safe list and does not have to be listed on labels except as "artificial color."

- **Red No. 40 (Allura Red AC).** This dye took the place of banned Red No. 2 and is used in foods, drugs, and cosmetics. Specific food uses include gelatins, puddings, soft drinks, condiments, dairy products, and candy. It may cause cancer in animals.

- **Blue No. 1.** This coal-tar derivative is used in soft drinks and replenishment fluids, candy, ice cream, icings, syrups, jellies, cereals, and puddings. It is on the permanent safe list. It is a possible allergen, and it can cause tumors in animals at the site of injection.

- **Blue No. 2.** This is used the same way as Blue No. 1 and is on the permanent FDA list. The World Health Organization rates it in category B—questionable for use in food.

- **Green No. 3.** This color is used in such foods as mint jelly, gelatins, candy, frozen desserts, and cereals. It is classified as safe but is a potential allergen and is tumorigenic upon injection.

- **Yellow No. 5 (tartrazine).** This is the most notable color agent, partly because it causes the most immediate allergic reactions in people sensitive to salicylates, such as aspirins (to which it is related), and because, by law, it is the only artificial color that must be listed by name on packaging. Tartrazine is used in such foods as spaghetti, puddings, gelatin, soft drinks, sherbets, ice cream, custards, cereals, and candy. Attempts to ban it have not succeeded. Most people can tolerate some Yellow No. 5 in foods, but those with sensitivity may develop skin reactions or asthma symptoms (problems are worst in sensitive asthmatics).

- **Yellow No. 6.** Another coal-tar color, this dye is used in many foods, such as candies, baked goods, cereals, desserts, carbonated beverages, and gelatins. It is considered safe, although there is some concern about allergy. Another name for this color is Sunset Yellow.

There are several major concerns with colored foods. The first is potential toxicity (including allergic reactions) liver stress from metabolizing these chemicals, and potential carcinogenicity. Another problem is that they may cause behavior problems in children. Benjamin Feingold, MD, a forward-thinking physician, has shown that hyperactivity in children is related to

food colorings. Many kids with short attention spans and learning disabilities improved on a diet without food coloring. Still another concern is that the FDA does not even require food manufacturers to list the specific agents used in their foods; they need only be designated as "artificial colors," so we cannot differentiate between those that are classified as safe and those in question. As stated, Yellow No. 5 is the only one that must be listed, because of possible allergic reactions.

On the basis of all the currently available information, my advice is to avoid all foods that have artificial colors listed on their labels. Many children's (and adult's) drugs and vitamins have added food coloring, and we must be careful with these as well. (It almost seems like a cruel joke that the number one prescription drug used to treat attention-deficit/hyperactivity disorder—Ritalin—is artificially colored using Yellow No. 10, among the most problematic additives on the hyposensitivity list.) If it is necessary to take medications, I advise taking the pure pharmaceutical preparations as white tablets or clear fluids if available. In that way, we are most likely to get the effect we want and avoid other undesired ones. It is possible that some side effects from drugs are caused by ingredients other than the active ones, such as these coloring agents.

Preservatives. This group of about 100 different chemicals is used to prevent spoilage. Each of these is specifically mentioned on the label when added to food. There are three main types of preservatives: antioxidants, mold inhibitors, and sequestrants.

- *Antioxidants.* Antioxidants (such as BHA, BHT, THBQ, and benzoic acid, or sodium benzoate) are used to prevent oxidation of the fats within foods. Oxidation leads to a change in the flavor and odor of certain ingredients, which essentially spoils the whole food. These additives are used commonly in many packaged and bottled foods that contain fats, such as shortening and vegetable oils. Cereals and crackers commonly contain BHA or BHT. Propyl gallate is an antioxidant used in fats and oils.

- *Mold inhibitors.* Also termed *antimycotics,* these are used commonly in breads and baked goods to prevent or retard the growth of yeasts and molds. Cheeses, syrups, and other foods might also contain mold inhibitors. Some common ones are sodium or calcium proprionate, sodium diacetate, sorbic acid, acetic acid, lactic acid, and various sodium and potassium salts. When these are used, they are specifically listed on the label. Most of these are fairly safe.

- *Sequestrants.* These are substances that prevent physical or chemical changes to the color, odor, flavor, or appearance of a food. These are commonly used in dairy foods as sodium, potassium, or calcium salts of citric, tartaric, or pyrophosphoric acids—for example, sodium citrate. EDTA (ethylenediaminetetraacetic acid), a sequestrant that binds metals, is used mainly in such liquids as soda pops and salad dressings. It is also commonly used in commercial beers to chelate out metal particles that wind up in the beer as a result of processing.

Salt, vinegar, and sugar are other common preservatives. Sulfur dioxide is used often to preserve dried fruits.

Acids, alkalis, buffers, and neutralizers. Many of these are common mineral acids or salts that help adjust or balance the pH (acid-alkaline condition) of foods. These items may or may not be listed on the package label. Acids are used in baking to help make the dough rise and in soft drinks (as phosphoric acid or phosphates) for a tangy taste. Citric acid (from citrus fruits), malic acid (from apples), and tartaric acid (from grapes) are other mild acids used in foods. Alkalis, or bases, are substances that reduce the acidity of foods. Some examples are baking powder, baking soda, aluminum hydroxide in cocoa, and aluminum carbonate in various crackers, cookies, and candy. Buffers and neutralizers help to adjust or maintain the acid-base balance of foods. Calcium carbonate, sodium aluminum phosphate, potassium tartrate, and ammonium bicarbonate are some examples.

Bleaching and maturing agents. Most of these are used in flour products and sometimes in cheeses. Such bleaching agents as benzoyl peroxide and chlorine dioxide are used to help oxidation and speed the whitening of fresh-ground flour. These chemicals also act as maturing agents and are sometimes called "bread improvers." Chlorine, nitrosyl chloride, and oxide of nitrogen are some other food bleaches. Milder

ones that are used to aid in yeast and dough conditioning include mineral salts, potassium bromate or iodate, and ammonium sulfate or phosphate. A newer entry into the world of white is titanium dioxide. This inorganic compound has dozens of industrial uses, and it is also the agent that makes many chewing gum coatings and toothpastes white. It is associated with increased risk of lung tumors when inhaled by workers in industrial settings, although risks associated with food use have yet to be clearly documented.

Moisture controls. These chemicals help prevent foods from drying out or from getting too moist. Calcium silicate is used in salt to prevent caking; it attracts the moisture instead of the salt. Moisture controllers are also termed *humectants.* Other examples include propylene glycol, glycerine, and sorbitol. These additives are not always listed on the label.

Activity controls. These agents either slow down or speed up the ripening or aging of foods. They are most often used on fruits or vegetables and so would not be listed on any labels. Ethylene gas is sprayed on bananas to speed ripening. Potatoes and onions may be prevented from sprouting by application of maleic hydrazide. This is a potentially toxic chemical that is also sprayed on most tobacco crops in the United States. Some enzymes such as amylase may be used to stimulate food reactions like the digestion of starch or the fermentation of sugar. This is helpful in brewing alcoholic beverages and making bread, candy, or certain milk concentrates.

Emulsifiers. Emulsifiers help to blend water and oils together to maintain the consistency and homogeneity of such products as mayonnaise and salad dressings. These additives are in part stabilizers and thickeners. They help keep the fineness of the grain and uniformity of the material, which allows cake mixes, for example, to work so well. Lecithin, mono- and diglycerides, and propylene glycol alginate are some examples. These are fairly safe and are listed on labels. Sorbitan and the polysorbates are also useful emulsifiers.

Texturizers. Texturizers are stabilizers and processing aids that give body and texture to food. These additives are mostly safe, natural ones that are usually listed on the label. Agar-agar, gelatin, cellulose, and other gums are some texturizers. They may be used in ice cream for consistency and to maintain the size of the ice crystals. Some gums or carrageenans are used in chocolate milk to thicken it and prevent the cocoa from settling out. Pectin, starch, and gelatin are used in confections, and thickeners such as the alginates might be used in soft drinks. To keep canned tomatoes and potatoes from breaking apart in the fluid, calcium chloride or other calcium salts are used to maintain texture. Nitrites and nitrates are used in curing meats to maintain pink color and texture. These nitrogenous additives and the foods that they are used in are best avoided for a variety of health reasons, including their ability to potentially interfere with the oxygen-carrying capacity of the blood, and their ability to increase long-term risk of cancer development.

Other processing aids and clarifying agents. Sanitizing agents help to clear bacteria and debris from foods. Gelatin and albumin help to remove small particles of copper or iron from such liquids as beer and vinegar. Tannin from teas can be used to clarify such liquids as beer and wine. These agents may or may not be listed on food labels.

Nutritional supplements (for enriched and fortified foods). This category includes a long list of both natural and synthetic vitamins and minerals used to enrich foods (adding what was depleted during processing) or fortify them (adding more than what was there or adding something totally new). The B vitamins are commonly added back into grain and cereal products, as is iron. Vitamin A is used in margarine, D in milk, and C in fruit drinks, while iodine is added to table salt. Some of these additions are helpful, but eating the whole food is a better way to get the nourishment. The supplements most commonly added to foods are thiamin (B1), riboflavin (B2), and iron. Next in use are niacin (B3), calcium salts, and vitamins D and A. According to what is lost during food processing, more pyridoxine (B6), magnesium, chromium, manganese, and many others should be added back to foods.

Since the mid-1990s or so, the sugary breakfast cereal companies have begun adding up to a dozen vitamins and minerals to their cereals, in small amounts sprayed onto the cereals before they are packaged. Most of these nutrients are water-soluble and may end up in the milk. So, to get these extra nutrients, finish your cereal and drink the milk before you head off to school or work. There are, of course, other, healthier ways to obtain a nutritious breakfast.

Potassium iodide was added to salt beginning in 1924 to help relieve the epidemic of goiter, a thyroid enlargement from iodine deficiency. This was the first case of fortification of our food supply. Vitamin D was added to milk in the early 1930s to prevent rickets, a common bone deformity problem at that time caused by vitamin D deficiency, particularly in children. Thiamin (vitamin B1) deficiency causes beri-beri, leading to skin and neurological problems. Most B vitamins are lost in the flour refinement process. In the 1940s and 1950s, vitamins B1, B2 (riboflavin), and B3 (niacin), along with iron, were added to flour.

Vitamin C was first added to foods in the 1950s, specifically to Tang and a variety of fruit juices. The popular sugar drink Hi-C contains added vitamin C. Starting in 1998, folic acid, another B vitamin, is now routinely added to such grain-based foods as breads, cereals, and pastas. Folate deficiency has finally been documented to cause birth defects. The USDA may soon require than candy bars and other snack foods be fortified with a variety of nutrients, because many Americans consume these caloric foods in significant amounts, as much as 10% to 30% or more of their daily diet.

What Is the Best Approach Concerning Food Additives?

First, we must try to reorient ourselves to the natural diet of our ancestors and eat more wholesome foods, such as fresh fruits and vegetables, whole grains, nuts, seeds, beans, and range-fed animals. Find and purchase organic produce (local if possible) and organically fed poultry and beef, thus supporting those farmers and ranchers who raise them. Our support will help make these foods more available and at a better price. And whenever possible, we should grow our own foods, plant more fruit and nut trees, and share or barter our harvest with our friends and neighbors.

It is also important to buy less and eat less of the packaged foods that contain additives. Definitely avoid the nitrates and nitrites, as they can form carcinogenic nitrosamines in the food and in the body. The sulfites—such as sulfur dioxide, sodium sulfite, bisulfites, and metabisulfites, which are commonly used to prevent or reduce spoilage or discoloration—are best avoided, particularly by people with allergies.

BHA and BHT, as well as EDTA, should be consumed minimally, as should the flavor enhancer MSG. Artificial colors should definitely be left out of the diet; artificial flavors should also be minimized. See the chart on page 455 for a list of common additives that are best avoided, those that should be used with caution, and those that are relatively safe.

Food Additives to Avoid

Avoiding toxins in your diet is an initial step toward enhancing your health and lowering your risk of disease. There are several key additives that may undermine health. Those with immediate effects may cause headaches or alter your energy level, or they may affect your mental concentration, behavior, or immune response. Those with long-term effects could increase your risk of cancer, cardiovascular disease, and other degenerative conditions. Make a decision to either cut down on or cut out altogether those food additives that may be hazardous to your health. It may seem difficult to change habits and find substitutes for the foods you enjoy, but remind yourself that you will be adding wholesome new flavors and foods to your diet that you may come to like just as much or even more. Avoidance and discrimination are crucial proactive steps in most natural health-care programs, and are more likely to lead to health rather than disease.

12 Key Additives to Avoid (or Eat Only Occasionally)

1. Hydrogenated fats. These "junky" fats are my number-one no-no. Hydrogenation infuses polyunsaturated fats with hydrogen, changing their biochemical structure and thus "saturating" them. They act like saturated fats in the body and increase the risk of cardiovascular disease and cancer. For a while in the past, researchers thought these artificial fats, such as margarine, were supposedly better than butter, but they were wrong. That does not mean we should consume large amounts of butter either. Reduce any regular use of foods containing significant amounts of hydrogenated fats. These include margarine, most chips, and many manufactured baked goods, such as crackers, cookies, and the like. The natural food brands that avoid hydrogenated fats are a better choice.

2. Artificial food colors. These are coloring agents, many of which have carcinogenic properties; many are allergenic and are also believed to contribute to hyperactivity, learning problems, and concentration difficulties in children and in some adults. I strongly recommend avoiding the regular intake of foods that contain artificial colors. This is especially important for children, who seem to gravitate to the brightly colored artificial foods that pervade the food industry. Foods to avoid include colored drinks, color-coated candies, gummy and chewy candies, most colored cereals, and cookies and cakes with colorful toppings. Most of these "foods" are also heavily sweetened and not particularly nutritious. Be aware of these additives when shopping at candy counters or vending machines. Be especially mindful of food choices on holidays, such as Christmas, Halloween, and birthdays.

3. Nitrites and nitrates. These preservatives can be converted to nitrosamines in the body, and research indicates that these compounds can be highly carcinogenic. Vitamin C seems to be protective against this process, so it is suggested that any time you eat nitrated and nitrited foods, take at least 500 to 1,000 mg of vitamin C. (Little packets of vitamin C powder are available to carry in your pocket or purse.) Nitrites and nitrates are found most often in preserved meats and lunch meats, such as hot dogs, bologna, bacon, and salami. It is wisest to avoid these smoked and preserved meats altogether because they are also sources of saturated fats, meat contaminants, and added chemicals.

4. Sulfites. These include sulfur dioxide in fruits, sulfites in grapes and wines, and metabisulfites in other foods. These agents are now limited to preserving dried fruits and freshly cut potatoes, and in fruit juice concentrates; they are also sprayed on grapes and commonly used in making wine. Sulfites are known to trigger allergic reactions in sensitive individuals. Anyone suffering from allergies or asthma should avoid sulfited foods, while others should keep exposures to a minimum. Sulfites can cause headaches, nausea, diarrhea, irritated membranes, and allergic reactions, particularly in people with asthma. In people prone to certain forms of asthma, sulfites have, on occasion, triggered anaphylactic shock. The FDA receives hundreds of reports yearly regarding sulfite reactions.

5. Sugar and natural sweeteners. These show up in a staggering variety of food products. Common problems from overuse include dental caries, obesity and its associated consequences, diabetes and the secondary effects of elevated blood sugar, hypoglycemia, behavioral changes (such as hyperactivity or difficulty concentrating), yeast problems, excessive food cravings, and more. (Refer to chapter 7, Sugar Detoxification, in *The New Detox Diet* for further information on the sugar problem.) Even natural sweeteners should be limited to no more than 10% of the diet. These include honey, maple syrup, date sugar, brown rice syrup, barley malt, fruit juice and fruit juice concentrates, fructose, Sucanat (dehydrated sugarcane juice), and molasses. Notice the effects on your body and mood during the hours following your consumption of sweeteners. Do your mood and energy levels rapidly improve and then suddenly drop? At that point, do you experience irritability, depression, or both? Or sleepiness or

anxiety? Wouldn't you like to avoid the inevitable lows that follow the initial high of sugar consumption?

6. Artificial sweeteners. Aspartame, saccharin, and acesulfame-K are synthetic sweeteners. Avoid using them regularly or in large quantities. Saccharin is the greatest concern, but it is less available these days, so high exposures are not likely. Research studies have linked saccharin with cancer in laboratory animals as both a cancer initiator and promoter. It has also caused fatal genetic mutations in animal studies. Aspartame is widely used throughout the diet industry—in soft drinks, chewing gum, candies, and other products. Two research studies found it caused brain tumors in lab animals. It does have some calories, however, and some people may be hypersensitive or show reactions after its use. Aspartame is contraindicated in individuals with phenylketonuria (PKU),

12 Key Additives to Avoid and Their Health Risks

1. **Hydrogenated fats.** These may lead to cardiovascular disease and obesity.

2. **Artificial food colors.** These have been shown to lead to allergies, asthma, and hyperactivity; they are possible carcinogens.

3. **Nitrites and nitrates.** These substances can develop into nitrosamines in the body, which can be carcinogenic.

4. **Sulfites (sulfur dioxide, metabisulfites, and others).** These can cause allergic and asthmatic reactions.

5. **Sugar and sweeteners.** These may lead to obesity, dental cavities, diabetes, and hypoglycemia as well as to increased triglycerides (blood fats) or candida (yeast).

6. **Artificial sweeteners (aspartame, acesulfame-K, and saccharin).** These have been linked to behavioral problems, hyperactivity, and allergies, and they are possibly carcinogenic. The government cautions against the use of any artificial sweetener by children and pregnant women. Anyone with PKU (phenylketonuria—problems with metabolizing phenylalanine, an amino acid) should not use aspartame (NutraSweet).

7. **MSG.** Common allergic and behavioral reactions include headaches, dizziness, chest pains, depression, and mood swings; it is also a possible neurotoxin.

8. **Preservatives (BHA, BHT, EDTA, THBQ, and others).** These may cause allergic reactions, hyperactivity, and possibly cancer; BHT may be toxic to the nervous system and the liver.

9. **Artificial flavors.** These may cause allergic or behavioral reactions.

10. **Refined flour.** Low-nutrient calories may lead to obesity, carbohydrate imbalances, and altered insulin production.

11. **Salt (excessive).** Excess salt may lead to fluid retention and blood pressure increases.

12. **Olestra (an artificial fat).** This may cause diarrhea and digestive disturbances.

OTHER CONCERNS

Food waxes. The protective coatings applied to produce, as in cucumbers, peppers, and apples, may trigger allergies and can contain pesticides, fungicide sprays, or animal by-products.

Plastic packaging. Polyvinyl chloride is carcinogenic and may cause immune reactions and lung irritation.

pregnant women, and children under 7. Acesulfame-K (ace-K) is a more recently developed sweetener marketed as the brands Sunette and Sweet One. It is 200 times sweeter than sugar and is utilized as a sweetener and as an additive in chewing gum, beverage mixes, instant tea and coffee, nondairy creamers, and desserts. It has been found to cause brain tumors in animals. One of the newer sweeteners—sucralose, being sold under the brand name Splenda since 1998—has very little long-term research. This sweetener is produced by the chlorination of sugar, and for this reason alone deserves more scrutiny, since many chlorine-containing additives and pesticides have been found to pose health risks.

7. MSG. This flavor enhancer is linked to the common reactions referred to as "Chinese restaurant syndrome," including headaches, agitation, increased heart rate, tightness in the chest, and tingling muscles or skin. Some restaurants avoid using MSG and even advertise that they do so. Avoid the regular intake of the many products that contain this flavor enhancer, from soups and crackers to candies and a variety of other processed foods. You must read the labels to avoid MSG.

8. Preservatives. Preservatives like BHA, BHT, and EDTA are used only in small quantities in grain products (cereals and crackers), soup bases, and other food products containing oils to prevent rancidity and to preserve freshness. Preservatives are chemicals that must be processed by the body and are potentially toxic to the liver and kidneys. They are known to cause allergic reactions and neurotoxic effects. In research studies, BHA and BHT have caused cancer. (BHT is prohibited as a food additive in England.) EDTA does not seem to be quite as harmful as BHT and BHA. Children can be sensitive to preservatives, may demonstrate hyperactivity and behavioral changes, and should therefore avoid regular use of them. In general, it is best to limit preserved foods because the freshest foods tend to be the most nutritious.

9. Artificial flavors. These represent the largest number of additives, the majority of which we do not really need. Most of the products that contain artificial flavoring are industrially processed, highly refined, and best limited to an occasional treat. Adults and children may exhibit a variety of behavioral and allergic reactions to these chemical flavorings.

10. Refined flour. Although not officially a food additive, refined flour can encourage weight gain and is a main cause of obesity when overused. It is an unnecessary "additive" to the diet. Refined flours (processed grains) are typically used in such products as breads, cereals, cakes, cookies, doughnuts, crackers, and croissants in place of more complete and nutritious whole-grain products. The lower fiber content of refined flour can lead to a variety of digestive problems, from constipation to diverticulitis. Eating some refined flour products as an occasional treat is less of a problem within a high-fiber, natural foods diet. There are many delicious whole-grain products now available; these include breads, cereals, pastas, crackers, and cookies, as well as wheat-free corn- and rice-based products. Whatever the source, be sure to check the carbohydrate content on the label to avoid taking in excessive calories and carbohydrates.

11. Salt. Sodium chloride is needed by our bodies for strength and the proper electrical conductivity within cells. Eating too much salt can lead to fluid retention and increased blood pressure. Emotional irritability also may be associated with high salt intake. Too much salt can also influence a woman's menstrual cycle. From the perspective of Chinese medicine, excess use or desire for salty foods may represent an imbalance in the body, signifying potential problems in the kidneys and bladder.

12. Olestra. This is a newly synthesized fat substitute intended to meet the public's desire to stay trim or lose weight while still eating rich-tasting foods. Olestra has been marketed in selected products, including potato chips that have only half the calories (75 versus 150 calories per ounce) of the regular high-calorie, high-fat chips. If you must eat potato chips, these are an improvement in terms of calories, or you could just eat half the chips you usually eat. Either way, potato chips should only be eaten as a special treat. Because Olestra is a nonabsorbable oil polymer, it is not really metabolized by the body. Consumer reports indicate that it causes mainly digestive problems, including abdominal cramping, diarrhea, and fecal incontinence. I do not plan on trying this product myself.

Other Food Additive Problems

Food waxes. These are usually oil- or hydrocarbon-based and are not digestible or usable by the body. They are used on produce as a protective covering and to hold in moisture, most commonly on cucumbers and apples. Although they are not terribly toxic in and of themselves, they may contain other chemical toxins, such as pesticides, mold inhibitors, and other additives, and are thus best avoided.

Food packaging. This comes in many forms. Plastic packaging, such as polyvinyl chloride (PVC, a potentially carcinogenic chemical) and polyethylene, and painted boxes and papers all introduce additional toxins directly into our food, many of which are carcinogenic. In addition, food wraps may outgas (discharge) plastic toxins into the foods. Many grocery stores seal meats, poultry, fish, and other foods in PVC plastic wrap using heat, which releases the PVC as a gas. Limit your exposure to these chemicals by eating fewer packaged and plastic-wrapped foods.

On the Label or Not?

Let's take a closer look at how chemicals are used by food manufacturers. During processing, fruits, vegetables, whole grains, and other foods are ground, mashed, boiled, and otherwise manipulated to create the multitude of boxed, canned, packaged, and plastic wrapped "foods" that we find in our stores. Chemicals are added to foods in a number of ways. First, there are the intentional additives that become ingredients in our foods. These chemicals are the only ones that are listed on the packages. **Sadly, however, there are also many additives that never appear on the "truth-in-packaging" labels; these are classified as** *indirect additives.* The packaging itself can also pose a danger of contamination, because various chemicals and metals are used in their production.

Such secondary contaminants (really hidden ingredients) as chemicals used during processing, additives already in preprepared ingredients, and chemicals used in packaging may all wind up in our foods. The hidden additives that may be contained in other ingredients include possible toxins in lard or MSG, both of which are routinely added to already prepared foods but their contaminants are rarely dis-

closed on the label. There are also the "silent additives," which can be a serious concern: pesticides, pollutants, antibiotics, hormones, and other drugs given to animals or found in animal feed; chemicals in the water and air; and other ever-present industrial chemical pollutants. The best way to prevent harm from these "economic poisons" is to prohibit their use in the first place.

Although the chemicals used as food additives are closely regulated by the FDA and seem to pose less short-term risk, we do not really know the risks posed by their long-term use. We are routinely exposed to so many different subtle toxins that when we develop certain health problems, it can be difficult to isolate a specific chemical or other factors that may have been responsible.

Healthy Diet Tips for Minimizing Additives in Your Diet

At least 50% of your diet should be fresh fruit and vegetables.

1. **Buy or grow** as much organic produce as possible—and start today!
2. **Eat more whole grains,** beans, nuts, and seeds as the other main components of your diet.
3. **Eat seasonally** because this will bring your daily life into harmony with the Earth and its cycles.
4. **Eat primarily locally** available foods. This minimizes the chemicals used in shipping, and these foods are usually less costly. Shop at farmers' markets if they are available.
5. **Limit your consumption** of animal products.
6. **Minimize** processed foods—especially fatty and sugary snacks, sodas, and chips; consider them treats and eat them only occasionally. Notice how you feel when you do eat them.
7. **Drink plenty** of clean, uncontaminated water.
8. **Make a list** of what to buy, what to eat, what to grow, and what *not* to buy or eat. A simple shopping guideline to follow is "If you cannot pronounce it, do not buy it."

FOOD SHOPPING

The "Food Additives" table below summarizes my understanding of the safety of food additives. You may wish to copy this list and take it with you as a shopping guide for choosing more healthful packaged products. Add any of your own concerns to the list, in case you have any allergies, digestive problems, or follow a low-salt, low-sugar, or low-fat diet. The Center for Science in the Public Interest (CSPI) produces a helpful large and colorful chart on this topic titled "Chemical Cuisine." CSPI can be contacted at 1501 16th St. NW, Washington, DC, 20036. See www.cspinet.org for more information.

COMMON FOOD ADDITIVES

This section provides more specific information about individual food additives—what each is used for, in what common foods, and whether it is safe (or its safety is unknown). Of the more than 3,000 different chemicals that are used in preparing foods for sale to consumers, only some are true "food additives"— agents actually added to the foods and listed on the ingredient label, such as the emulsifiers, sweeteners, or preservatives I described earlier in this chapter. Many other additives are not listed but are used in various stages of processing. Some of these are GRAS list additives, while others are not meant to be consumed

---

Guide to Food Additives

Additives to Avoid or to Consume Only Rarely

Artificial colors (FD&C colors)

Aspartame

BHT (butylated hydroxytoluene)

BVO (brominated vegetable oil)

Olestra

Saccharin

Sodium nitrite and nitrate

Sulfites (especially sodium bisulfite)

Sulfur dioxide

Additives to Limit (Use with Caution)

Acesulfame-K

Aluminum salts

Artificial Flavorings

BHA (butylated hydroxyanisole)

Caffeine

EDTA

Gums

Hydrogenated vegetable oils

MSG (monosodium glutamate)

Propyl gallate

Propylene glycol

Salt

Sugars (sucrose, dextrose, corn syrup)

TBHQ (tertiary butylhydroquinone)

Xylitol

Relatively Safe Additives

Acids—citric, sorbic, lactic

Alginates

Annatto

Beta-carotene or carotene

Calcium proprionate

Carrageenan

Casein and lactose

Gelatin

Glycerin

Lecithin

Minerals—iron, zinc, and others

Monoglycerides and diglycerides

Natural Flavorings

Pectin

Polysorbate 60, 65, and 80

Potassium sorbate

Sodium benzoate

Sorbitol

Vanillin

Vitamins A, C, and E

at all (such as solvents like formaldehyde, benzene, and carbon tetrachloride—all carcinogens—used to extract "salad oils," for example). Some of these oils may also be heated up to 400 degrees Fahrenheit, which may change their molecular structure. Lye may even be used to extract the fatty acids. Many people use cold-pressed oils because they are not made with solvents and are subjected to minimal heating. Different detergents and bleaching agents may also be used in processing without being listed on the label.

Although I am mainly talking about food additives in this section, many of these synthetic chemicals are used in the preparation of pharmaceutical drugs, both prescription and over-the-counter. None appear on the labels. Large amounts of FD&C colors are used in drugs, and these are often potentially as toxic as the active ingredients. An analysis of a common female hormone product, Premarin, shows that it contains a conjugated estrogen drug made from pregnant mare's urine (sounds great!) used most commonly in menopausal women. Estrogens are, of course, helpful in relieving menopausal symptoms, but they can also cause other symptoms and may play a role in carcinogenesis. (There are safer, bioidentical estrogens from plants that can include the least carcinogenic estrogen known, estriol.) An analysis of Premarin also shows more than 25 other chemicals, including talc, polyethylene glycol, shellac, edible black ink, carnauba wax, sucrose, corn starch, propyl paraben, Yellow No. 5 (tartrazine), sodium benzoate, and more. Most pharmaceutical drugs, especially children's flavorful liquid preparations, contain many chemicals besides those we think we are getting; and many of these additives can cause problems.

There is also a long list of contaminants that we will never see on food labels. All the pesticides, herbicides, and toxic environmental chemicals from dumps or from the water can get into our food. Closest to the consumer are the fungicides that are often sprayed on crops after they are harvested. These may still be concentrated on crops, in the produce boxes, or in the papers wrapping the foods. Some people may be sensitive to these substances; in addition, the effects of long-term intake of small amounts of these toxic chemicals are not yet known. The best we can do is to be aware of what is known and demand that the government and food growers give us complete

information. Then we can either push for change or find alternatives that meet our needs.

Individual Food Additives

Acacia (gum arabic). This is a vegetable gum, a thick excretion that comes from many species of acacia tree found in Africa and the southern United States. It has been used for many thousands of years, especially in the Middle East. Acacia gum is a complex polysaccharide that is soluble in water and in foods; it tends to blend mixtures together, retards sugar crystallization, and acts as a thickener. For these reasons, it is used in the confection industry for candies, jellies and glazes, and chewing gum. It is also used as a stabilizer in soft drinks and beer. Gum arabic has been on the GRAS list since 1976 and is actually pretty safe, according to most studies. The acacia tree is a fairly common allergen, however, and there are some people who also have allergic responses to oral ingestion of acacia, with possible skin, sinus, or asthmatic reactions. Anyone who is allergic, especially to acacia, should avoid gum arabic. Although most of the foods that contain this additive are overly processed or sweet, acacia gum itself seems safe in modest amounts.

Ace-K (acesulfame potassium). This is a synthetic chemical created by Hoechst AG, a German pharmaceutical company now owned by the French pharmaceutical Aventis. Beginning in 1988, the FDA approved its use in select foods as an artificial sweetener, and then expanded this use for the general food supply in 2003. In the United States, ace-K is sold under the brand name Sunette. Because of its somewhat metallic and bitter taste, it is often used together with other sweeteners like aspartame. The safety of Sunette has been challenged on the grounds of carcinogenicity by organizations like the Center for Science in the Public Interest. Because testing on this additive seems inadequate, I recommend avoiding it.

Agar-agar (seaweed extract). This is a polysaccharide that comes from several varieties of red algae. In liquid, it has the ability to swell and gel. Agar is used in making ice creams, jellies, icings, and preserves, and for thickening milk and cream. It can be used as a substitute for gelatin, which is an extract of animal proteins. Agar also acts as a mild bulk laxative. It is used by the food industry and is also sold in stores for home use. Agar-agar is a safe, even beneficial food additive that is on the GRAS list. Although in rare situations it can be a mild allergen, it is otherwise completely safe.

Alginates (alginic acid; algin gum; ammonium, calcium, potassium, and sodium alginate; propylene glycol alginate). These are all (except for propylene glycol alginate) natural extracts of various seaweeds. They are used in the food industry primarily as thickening and stabilizing agents. Alginates are also water retainers, prevent ice crystal formation, and help uniform distribution of flavors through foods. As a clarifying agent, they add smoothness to mixtures. The alginates are used in ice creams, custards, ices, chocolate milk, cheeses, cheese spreads, salad dressings, jams, jellies, confections, baked goods, toppings, and beverages. All of these alginates are on the GRAS list and were reapproved in 1980. Propylene glycol, an antifreeze and a fairly safe solvent, does pose a little more cause for concern; the propylene glycol alginate salt is used fairly often in food processing.

Aluminum salts—alum (aluminum potassium sulfate), sodium aluminum phosphate, aluminum ammonium sulfate, aluminum calcium silicate, aluminum hydroxide, and others. Although aluminum is found abundantly in the Earth's crust, it remained largely tucked away in the ores bauxite and cryolite until engineers and politicians decided it could be mined and transformed into a lightweight, durable, corrosion-resistant material that could be used for just about everything. Outside of the food world, of course, it is found everywhere, from roofing and aircraft to electrical equipment and over-the-counter stomach antacids. In recent years, there have been increasing concerns about accumulation of aluminum in the body and its effect on brain chemistry and health. (See the discussion on aluminum on page 229 in chapter 6, Minerals.) Problems with cognitive function, osteomalacia, chronic neurodegenerative diseases like Alzheimer's, pregnancy complications, lung cancers, and asthma have all been associated with aluminum exposure. Exposure in these studies was not restricted to food, of course, but in many cases food was factored in as a contributing source.

The burgeoning use of aluminum in cookware (including anodized aluminum and nonstick applications), together with increased use of aluminum in foil liners for aseptic packaging and other containers,

makes me more concerned than ever about our reliance on aluminum-containing additives. Coupled with this concern are the environmental impact of increased bauxite mining and the emission of hydrogen fluorides and polycyclic aromatic hydrocarbons (PAHs) during the smelting of aluminum. All in all, aluminum-containing additives are compounds I would like to see us phasing out of our meal plans. Aluminum compounds are currently used to adjust acidity (that is, as a buffer), as an astringent, to keep canned produce firm, to lighten food texture, and as anticaking agents. Sodium aluminum phosphate, the most commonly used, is found in baking powder and self-rising flours. Alum is used as a clarifier for sugar and as a hardening agent; aluminum calcium silicate is used as an anticaking agent in salt and other powders. Aluminum hydroxide is a strong alkali agent that can be toxic but is safe in small amounts, as a leavening agent in baked goods, for example. It is also used in antiperspirants and antacids. Aluminum ammonium sulfate is used as an astringent, buffer, and neutralizing agent by the cereal industry; it is also used in baking powder.

Ammonium salts (ammonium bicarbonate, ammonium chloride, ammonium phosphate, ammonium sulfate). Ammonium salts occur naturally in foods when ammonia (as in proteins) combines with acids. Ammonium ions are important in the body for acid-base balance, in amino acid metabolism, and in the urinary tract. Ammonium salts are used in foods as leavening agents, dough conditioners, and buffers to lighten texture; to create uniformity within a food mixture; and occasionally as flavor enhancers. Ammonium bicarbonate is most often used as a leavening agent for baked goods and confections. Ammonium chloride is used as a dough conditioner and a nutrient for yeast in breads and baked goods. It is also used in making batteries and dyes. Ammonium phosphate is used in baking powder, as a buffer and leavening agent in breads, rolls, and other baked goods, and in the brewing industry. Ammonium sulfate is also used, mainly as a buffer and dough conditioner. All of these ammonium salts are on the GRAS list. Ammonia by itself can be toxic in large amounts, as it affects basic biochemistry and kidney function, but as salts in small amounts, it seems to be okay.

Annatto. This is a natural coloring agent extracted from the seeds of a tropical tree, *Bixa orellano*. It is a yellow to light orange vegetable dye that is used commonly in such dairy products as butter, buttermilk, cottage cheese, and other cheeses. Annatto is also used to color margarine, ice cream, cake mixes, baked goods, and the casings of hot dogs. Annatto is on the GRAS list and really has no known toxicity. Research, which is still going on, has not yet shown any ill effects.

Ascorbic acid (vitamin C)—ascorbate salts: sodium ascorbate, ascorbyl palmitate. Ascorbic acid, either natural or synthetic, is a popular vitamin supplement. (Esterified forms, such as Ester-C, of this vitamin have also gained a good bit of popularity.) It is found naturally in many fruits and vegetables, such as citrus fruits and green and red peppers. It is also used in food processing as an antioxidant and preservative; vitamin C, as ascorbyl palmitate, prevents oxidation and rancidity, especially in fats, and can help preserve the flavor, color, and aroma foods. Vitamin C is also used as a nutritive additive for artificial fruit drinks and has recently been added to cured meats to prevent the formation of carcinogenic nitrosamines from their added nitrites. Ascorbic acids or ascorbates are also used in soft drinks, alcoholic beverages such as beer and ale, juices, candies, dry milk, and dips. Ascorbic acid is basically nontoxic, even in high doses. Its use in food is often beneficial, as vitamin C is a required nutrient, and a deficiency can cause serious problems. Vitamin C is the most commonly used vitamin supplement in U.S. culture.

Aspartame (NutraSweet, Equal). Aspartame is the most widely used of the artificial sweeteners and is found in approximately 5,000 different food products. In fact, this additive is so pervasive that "Nutra-Sweet sludge"—a by-product of aspartame production—is actually sold as a nitrogen-containing fertilizer for use on food crops. Despite its FDA approval and inclusion on the GRAS list in 1982, many members of the health-care profession continue to question its use. Foremost in raising questions has been Dr. John Olney, a physician on faculty in the Department of Psychiatry at the Washington University School of Medicine in St. Louis, Missouri. Olney's studies—along with several others—have found intake of aspartame to be associated with migraine headache, worsening of seizures in children with epilepsy, and increased risk of brain tumors in animals. Olney classifies NutraSweet as an excitotoxin, because one

of its two key components is an amino acid—aspartic acid.

Aspartic acid and glutamic acid (as found, for example, in MSG) are two primary nerve stimulators in the nervous system. The other key amino acid in aspartame is phenylalanine. People who have a problem metabolizing this amino acid often develop a condition called phenylketonuria (PKU). The use of NutraSweet by these individuals would be so problematic that the FDA requires a warning label on all aspartame products that states "Phenylketonurics: Contains Phenylalanine." Aspartame is about 200 times sweeter than sugar; because of this, very little is needed, so it is much less caloric. This same principle applies to most of the artificial sweeteners, banned or still marketed. Cyclamates, currently banned, are about 30 times sweeter than sugar. Saccharin, which is still sanctioned but under ongoing study, is about 300 times sweeter. Sucralose (Splenda), a newer sweetener, has pushed the envelope even further and is about 500 times as sweet as sugar. Unfortunately, this enormous gain in sweetening power may come at a high price, because sucralose is made by chlorinating sugar. Its cumulative, long-term health effects are almost completely unknown. The name of this chemical, by the way, which is promoted as being "made from sugar so it tastes like sugar," is 1,6-dichloro-1,6-dideoxy-beta-D-fructofuranosyl-4-chloro-4-deoxy-alpha-D-galactopyranoside. Now that is a mouthful we should keep out of our mouths.

In sum, I am not convinced that any of the artificial sweeteners (aspartame, saccharin, or sucralose) are safe to use on a regular basis. I have seen many patients who do not tolerate aspartame, having mood and energy reactions most commonly. A low-calorie diet including foods that are naturally sweet would be my first and foremost recommendation. After that, I would recommend limited use of natural food-based sweeteners like stevia, evaporated cane juice, molasses, maple syrup, and so forth, rather than synthetic "super sweeteners" that have questionable long-term health impact.

Benzoic acid—sodium benzoate (benzoate of sodium). Benzoic acid or its sodium salt is commonly used as a preservative in food processing. Benzoic acid is found naturally in many berries, cherry bark, prunes, anise, cloves, cassia bark or cinnamon, and tea. It was first found in gum benzoin in the 1600s. It is used as a flavoring agent in chocolate, orange, lemon, nut, and other flavors in candies, beverages, baked goods, ice cream, and chewing gums. As a preservative, it is used in a wide variety of processed foods, including margarine, soft drinks, juices, pickles, condiments, jellies, and jams. In perfumes and cosmetics, it prevents spoilage by microorganisms. Benzoic acid is also a mild artifungal agent. In medicine, sodium benzoate is occasionally used in testing liver function, as it is metabolized by the liver.

Benzoic acid and sodium benzoate are probably the safest of the chemical preservatives, certainly much safer than BHA and BHT. Tests have not shown the benzoin derivatives to be carcinogenic. Occasionally, larger amounts can cause intestinal upset, especially with weakened liver function. Benzoic acid can also be slightly irritating to the skin, eyes, and mucous membranes, and both it and sodium benzoate can cause allergic reactions, including urticaria (hives), although these appear to be relatively rare. Overall, small amounts of these additives seem to be relatively safe.

BHA (butylated hydroxyanisole). BHA and BHT are interesting chemicals. They are both petroleum by-products used in preserving foods. BHA (like BHT) acts as a preservative and an antioxidant to prevent the rancidity of fats and fat-containing foods and thus prevent spoilage that causes a change in taste, odor, or appearance. Both of these chemicals were originally developed in the 1970s as preservatives for rubber products, and to this day, only 5% of the total BHA and BHT produced go to food. Production of these two preservatives started out in favor of BHT, with about three times as much BHT being synthesized. Since the mid-1970s, however, production of the two has evened out somewhat, with about 750,000 pounds of each being manufactured each year. The health impact of BHA is controversial. On the one hand, BHA has been shown to disrupt some of the metabolic processes inside of cells. For example, our oxygen-based energy production can be damaged by BHA. On the other hand, however, in animal studies, BHA added into the diets of animals at a low dose has been associated with less occurrence of cancer, especially stomach cancer. At higher doses, though, BHA appears to lose this protective effect and to even promote cancer occurrence. So although the antioxidant

properties of this additive may have certain benefits under certain circumstances, I am reluctant to recommend BHA-containing products based on the overall research evidence.

BHA is used in such foods as dry cereals, crackers, instant potatoes or potato flakes, soup bases, seasonings, dry mixes for desserts or beverages, canned or bottled beverages, lard, shortening, baked goods, ice cream, candy, and more. It is almost always listed on the label, but it may not be when it has been added to lard or shortening that is an ingredient of the food product. BHA is still on the GRAS list; during a 1980 review, additional studies were recommended, although previous studies had revealed no major hazards to public health. The FDA has set limits on the amount of BHA that particular foods may contain, such as 50 parts per million (ppm) in dry cereals or 200 ppm in shortenings. Allergies to BHA and BHT have been known. Liver toxicity is possible but unlikely from the small amounts used in food. There is some suggestion that both these antioxidants may be helpful in preventing disease and aging, as they reduce oxidative and free-radical irritation of the tissues. This has not been scientifically proven, and my advice is to avoid any regular use of the chemical BHA.

BHT (butylated hydroxytoluene). BHT is another common antioxidant that is used to extend shelf life and preserve a variety of foods. Like BHA, it is not permitted for use with fresh foods, so exposure to it comes exclusively through the prepackaged food route. Common foods that contain BHT are enriched rice, breakfast cereals, shortenings, animal fats, dog and cat foods, potato flakes, chewing gum, cake mixes, and vegetable oils At lower doses, BHT (like BHA) may be a cancer preventive. It has recently been used by some people in the treatment of herpes viral infections. If it is helpful in such cases, it is probably because of its antioxidant properties, but there is no good evidence that it works, and the doses that are needed for such treatment have not been established.

BHT can be irritating to the liver and kidneys, especially when there is decreased function of these organs. Allergic reactions have been known. There is also some concern that BHT may convert to other substances in the human body that may be carcinogenic. For example, 1 conversion product of BHT (the hydroperoxide form) has been shown to disrupt the chemical signals that are sent from cell to cell. Some of the research here has been focused on the underpinnings of cancer, where the breakup of cell signals is part of the framework that leads to cancer. The use of BHT is prohibited in England. In the United States, it is on the GRAS list, with further research pending. I suggest avoiding foods with BHT, partly because most of them are prefabricated food-industry creations and also because researchers do not really know whether it is safe.

Bromines (calcium bromate, potassium bromate, brominated vegetable oil [BVO]). The bromates are used in flours and breads as dough conditioners and maturing agents. Because they are used during processing, these ingredients may not be listed on the label. Bromination makes oils heavier so that they can evenly distribute flavoring in soft drinks, especially citrus and fruit-flavored beverages, as well as in ices, ice cream, and some baked goods. BVO also gives drinks a cloudy appearance, so it may make those artificial fruit drinks resemble natural fruit juice.

Bromine, like chlorine, is one of the halogen elements, and its use in food (or manufacturing) merits the same type of concern as chlorine. Some of the upsurge in bromine-containing products has been motivated by increasing consumer awareness of chlorination and its potential risk. PCBs (polychlorinated biphenyls), for example, may get replaced by PBBs (polybrominated biphenyls), and pools and spas may switch from chlorination to bromination. The bromines and BVO are not considered safe, however, and the FDA limits their use. They have been known to cause allergic reactions, with high amounts causing intestinal irritation and food-poisoning symptoms as well as kidney or central nervous system problems. High doses may even be fatal. Small amounts of most of these chemicals can be tolerated, but the FDA currently has them, especially BVO, on the "suspect" list.

Caffeine. This is found naturally in coffee, tea, mate leaves, guarana root, cocoa (chocolate), and kola nuts. As part of coffee, tea, and cola, it is one of the world's big drugs. Caffeine is a stimulant to the heart, central nervous system, and respiratory system. Many people feel it gives them energy. It is currently used as a flavoring in cola and root beer; by regulation, this chemical must be present in any beverage termed "cola," For any food in which it is naturally found (coffee, tea, or cocoa), caffeine need not be listed on the label. Much of the caffeine added to other foods is extracted in making decaffeinated coffee (which has often been done by chemically treating with such solvents as methylene chloride, although I hear this usage is declining). Decaf has become more popular in recent years among those who do not want the caffeine effect, and water-decaffeinated coffees are widely available. I recommend these versions and urge purchase of organic because so many chemicals of concern are used in coffee growing and shipping. But there are also many people who still like their caffeine fix. On a trip to the supermarket to research food additives, for example, I found Jolt cola, for those who want "all the sugar, and twice the caffeine"—fine if you like drinking caffeinated syrup.

Caffeine use is banned in certain types of competitive sports events (like track-and-field events) because it can shift an athlete's metabolism. In sports lingo, it is classified as an *ergogenic aid,* which allows athletes to tap into their fat stores earlier in a competition, before they have depleted their muscle glycogen (starch) stores. It is not clear what this means for us everyday folk, but it indicates the potential whole-body effects of this chemical. Caffeine use is only questionably safe. It is on the GRAS list, but a 1980 review suggested further testing. Caffeine passes the placental barrier, so it can affect the growing fetus. It is therefore not recommended during pregnancy—or during nursing, because it also gets into mother's milk. **Young children or anyone with cardiovascular disease (and especially high blood pressure) or ulcer problems should avoid caffeine.** In general, caffeine should be considered a psychoactive, potentially addictive drug and used intermittently and with caution. Regular or excessive use should clearly be avoided. (See "Caffeine" on page 761 in chapter 18, Detoxification and Cleansing Programs, and *The New Detox Diet* for a more complete discussion of caffeine.)

Calcium proprionate (proprionic acid, sodium proprionate). The proprionates are naturally found in such dairy products as butter and cheese. They are used to inhibit the growth of most fungi and some bacteria. Proprionic acid and its salts are used as mold inhibitors in baked goods, breads, rolls, cakes, and cupcakes and as preservatives in natural and processed cheeses, chocolate products, jelly, and preserves. Calcium proprionate, proprionic acid, and sodium proprionate are all safe. Studies in animals revealed no problems even with levels higher than are usually consumed. They have all been reapproved by the FDA and remain on the GRAS list.

Calcium salts (calcium carbonate, chloride, citrate, gluconate, hydroxide, lactate, oxide, phosphate, and sulfate). The various calcium salts are helpful in providing the important mineral calcium, which the body needs in significant quantity for many functions, especially healthy bones. Various calcium formulas, such as calcium carbonate and calcium gluconate, are taken commonly as dietary supplements to attain adequate calcium levels. Many calcium salts are used as nutrient additives in infant formulas and other enriched foods, especially grain products—cereals, flours, cornmeal, farina, noodles, and breads.

Calcium salts are also used as emulsifiers in evaporated milk, frozen desserts, and breads; as dough conditioners in baked goods; and as clarifying agents in sweets. Some calcium salts (such as calcium carbonate, oxide, and hydroxide) are used as antacids and as buffering agents in milk products, for example, to help control acidity. Calcium lactate is used as a buffer in baking powder. Some salts (such as calcium chloride, gluconate, and hydroxide) act as firming agents. These may be used in jellies or in canned fruits, especially tomatoes or potatoes. Calcium sulfate can act as a carrier for bleaches and is used in the brewing industry. Problems from the use of the many calcium salts are unlikely. High amounts of any of them could cause shifting of the body's acid-base balance, though. Their basic use in foods is considered safe.

Caramel. This is made by heating sugar, giving it a burnt, slightly bittersweet taste. It is used both as a coloring for soft drinks such as colas and root beer, candies, ice cream, and baked goods, and as a flavoring in such products as butterscotch, chocolate, cola, ginger ale, brandy, vanilla, and cream soda. Caramel is used mostly in beverages but also in ice cream, candy, and baked goods. There is some question about the safety of caramel. The heating process uses ammonia, which may be toxic, and the nitrogen going into the caramelized sugar produces compounds that may be harmful. Studies regarding possible carcinogenesis have been negative so far; caramel in modest doses is still considered safe.

Caramel, by the way, is not the same as caramel color. This second chemical is completely synthetic and goes by the chemical shorthand of THI because of its impossibly complicated chemical name (2-acetyl-4(5)-tetrahydroxybutylimidazole). Many non-transparent soft drinks contain THI to darken their color. In animal studies, fairly small amounts of caramel color have been shown to depress the immune system and to alter the shape and function of the thymus gland. For this reason, caramel color is well worth avoiding.

Carob (St. John's bread)—locust bean gum. This is a natural flavoring that has seen increased use since the mid-1980s as a healthier substitute for chocolate and sugar. Carob powder is an extract from the bean pods of the carob tree. It is more nutritious than other flavorings; it is termed "St. John's bread" because it is said in the Bible, in the Book of Mark, that it sustained John the Baptist in the wilderness. As a flavoring, it is sometimes used as a part of caramel, butterscotch, chocolate, cherry, maple, and root beer flavors in beverages, ice cream, candies, baked goods, gelatin desserts, and toppings. Carob gum extract is used as a thickener and stabilizer added to such foods as chocolate milk, syrups, gassed whipped cream, cheeses, ice cream, and sherbet. As a gum, carob is extremely high in water-soluble fiber, which has been shown to help lower cholesterol levels. Carob has also been shown to have some mild antibiotic properties, so that when carob is blended in with other foods, the bacterial growth on those foods is inhibited. This effect of carob may or may not mean anything about health benefits for us humans. Overall, I consider carob to be a safe additive that may turn out to have special benefits.

Carotenes (beta-carotene, provitamin A). Carotenes are found naturally in many vegetables and fruits; for example, carrots, sweet potatoes, spinach, apricots, papaya, and cantaloupe. In the body it can be converted to vitamin A. (For detailed information about carotene as an essential nutrient, see page 92 in chapter 5, Vitamins.) Carotene is a yellow-orange pigment that is used primarily as a natural coloring agent in food manufacturing. It is employed to color butter, buttermilk, margarine, and cottage cheese. Carotene, mostly as beta-carotene, is a useful additive. It is known to be a helpful antioxidant and a cancer-preventing nutrient. It is a safe additive or supplement even in high dosages, where its only side effect is yellowish pigmentation of the skin.

Carrageenan (Irish moss extract)—ammonium, calcium, potassium, and sodium carrageenan. Carrageenan is a useful seaweed extract. This gluey and salty substance is used as a natural stabilizer and emulsifier in food processing, in such foods as French dressings, ice cream, cheese spreads, chocolate milk, evaporated milk, puddings, sherbet, candies, and jellies. As an herb, Irish moss is used as a demulcent and emollient to soothe and soften such irritated tissues as the skin and mucous membranes. It has also been known to be helpful in lung conditions. Carrageenan has passed most of the health safety tests for humans when it comes to small amounts found in food. For this reason, it remains on the GRAS list and is an additive. I do not think we have to be overly concerned about it, although some animal studies have associated carrageenan intake with increased risk of digestive system cancers, and it does bother some people with irritable bowel syndrome. For this reason, researchers need to keep testing and evaluating this additive. Concerns about the health safety of carrageenan also apply to its use as a pharmaceutical drug, which is also under investigation.

Caseinates (sodium, potassium, calcium, and ammonium). Casein is one of two major proteins in cow's milk (lactalbumin is the other). It is used as a texturizer in ice cream, ice milk, sherbet, and frozen custard. Casein is a nutritive protein source in many protein powders. Calcium caseinate is probably the most useful here. Caseinates are also used as binders or extenders in some lunch meats and soups and as a clarifying agent in wine. Casein is essentially nontoxic and is on the GRAS list. However, many people are allergic to the casein molecule present in milk. Those people should avoid foods with added caseinates. In addition to the terms *casein* and *caseinate*, the term *milk protein* will be shown on the ingredient list of foods containing this additive. There continues to be some debate about the whey portion of milk and how it fits into the allergy picture. Caseins are the proteins that form the curd when milk is left to sour. Whey proteins are part of the watery portion that is left over once the curd has been removed. It is possible to have an allergic reaction to whey proteins, casein proteins, or both. However, in practice, I believe there are more problematic reactions to the caseins than to the whey. In addition, the whey fraction of milk has been shown to contain some globulin proteins that support the immune function in the digestive tract, and this desirable effect does not seem to hold for the caseins.

Cellulose derivatives (carboxymethylcellulose, cellulose gum, methyl cellulose, and others). Cellulose is a fiber that forms the basic structure of plant tissues. The cellulose used in food processing as a thickener or stabilizer and emulsifier is extracted from plants, cotton, or even wood. It can help in the blending of ingredients, aiding gel formation and preventing ingredient caking. Cellulose products are used both in foods (such as ice cream, icings, fillings, candies, and jellies) and in toiletries and cosmetics (such as hair gels, shaving creams, shampoos, beauty masks, and dentifrices). They are also used in some medicines (such as laxatives and antacids), as stabilizers. There is some concern about many of the products that contain cellulose, more from the chemical extraction process than the cellulose itself, which is inert. Carcinogenicity of some of the cellulose derivatives is being studied, but they are still accepted as safe and remain on the GRAS list.

Citric acid and its salts (calcium, potassium, and sodium citrate). Citric acid is an old and versatile food additive. It and its salts are found naturally in citrus fruits, tomatoes, coffee, apricots, peaches, pineapples, and some berries. Commercially, citric acid has traditionally been extracted from citrus fruit or made by fermenting crude sugar. Many new techniques for producing citric acid have been investigated in recent years, however, including production from soy whey and cheese whey. Because yeasts and fungi are sometimes used in the citric acid production process, some yeast-free diets recommend avoidance of processed foods containing this additive.

In food processing, citric acid or, occasionally, its salts are used as a flavoring agent or enhancer to impart a tangy, tart, or sour taste to foods, including beverages, candy, ice cream, baked goods, and chewing gum. Citric acid is also used as a buffer, being a mild acid, to maintain acidity in such foods as fruit juices, carbonated beverages, wines, jellies, and sherbet. As a sequestrant, it removes metal contaminants from food and allows preservatives to work better, maintaining food flavor. Calcium citrate is used as a firming agent in canned tomatoes, and the citrate salts, like calcium, are a vehicle for adding various mineral nutrients. Citric acid and its salts are safe food additives, secure on the GRAS list. They are normal constituents of foods and are easily metabolized in the body at levels much higher than those used in foods. These are useful and safe additives, with the possible exception I just mentioned about yeast-free diets and the possible use of yeast to commercially produce this additive.

Cornstarch. This is mainly used to coat foods or containers to prevent sticking. It is also used in home cooking and as a medicinal for irritated mucous membranes or colons. It is basically a safe additive, not always listed on the label, but it may cause mild allergic symptoms of the skin, eyes, or nose in people sensitive to corn.

Corn sweeteners (corn syrup, corn sugar). (Note that sugar, in the form of dextrose, may also be extracted from corn. Corn products in this country may be made from gentically modified (GM) corn, and so you should avoid regular use.) Corn syrup, the most commonly used corn sweetener, is made by chemically splitting cornstarch with a weak acid. This additive is also labeled high fructose corn syrup (HFCS), although that is somewhat misleading, because corn syrup and table sugar actually contain about the same amount of fructose (about 50%). The popularity of HFCS among food manufacturers does not have much to do with the percentage fructose content, but the relatively inexpensive cost of this additive and its unusual resilience as a liquid that is viscous, retains moisture, and blends quite easily. Corn sweeteners are fairly prevalent in the food industry, used for flavoring in various beverages, candies, baked products, and ice cream. Corn syrup is used in a wide variety of products, including the adhesive on postage stamps, envelopes, and various tapes. It is also eaten commonly in ketchup, dressings, Chinese foods, cereals, carbonated beverages, candies, jellies, peanut butter, and processed meats.

Corn sweeteners are on the GRAS list with no limitations, and they seem to be safe overall, although they are caloric sugars that may help create tooth decay and obesity if overused, as well as mood swings. Occasional allergic reactions may occur, although this is much less likely with corn sweeteners than with corn itself or cornstarch, both of which contain some of the corn protein, which is the actual allergen. Just

how much of the pesticides commonly sprayed on cornfields ends up in the corn syrup is currently unknown. The majority of the population tolerates corn syrup, however, and other sweeteners fairly well in moderation.

Cyclamate (Sucaryl). The cyclamates, sodium and calcium, were the diet sweeteners of the 1960s. More than 30 times sweeter than sugar, they were used freely. When research showed that high amounts of cyclamates caused bladder cancer in lab animals, they were removed from the food market by the FDA in 1969. There is some evidence that cyclamate is converted in the body to cyclohexylamine (CHA), which may cause chromosomal changes and damage. More work is needed to fully document these events, however. Cyclamates were used mainly in soft drinks, chewing gums, and diet candies. In fact, these artificial or nonnutritional sweeteners are still used in Canada and other countries. In 1984, the FDA reviewed the research and considered reinstating cyclamates for food use, but the results and long-term effects are still unclear. More investigation is being done. The cyclamates were once a popular noncaloric sweetener, and with saccharin possibly going out again, the diet-conscious population wants other choices besides aspartame, sucralose, and acesulfame-K.

DES (diethylstilbestrol, stilbestrol). This synthetic estrogen has been used commercially to fatten cattle and poultry. It has been found to be carcinogenic, specifically in the daughters of women who have used the drug medically. Its use in animals was recently banned in the United States, but it is still used in other countries. It is wise to purchase meats and poultry that have not been treated with this or other hormones or antibiotics.

Dextrin (starch gum). Dextrins are carbohydrate chains of glucose molecules prepared by heating such starches as cornstarch, potato starch, or tapioca. Dextrin has a variety of uses in food processing. It holds water and is used as a thickener in many sauces and gravies and as an expander in bakery goods. Dextrin is also used in pill coatings, as a diluting agent, and as a foam stabilizer in brewing. It can also be used as a mildly sweet sugar substitute. Nonfood uses include thickening industrial solutions and in such flammables as matches and firecrackers. Dextrin is considered safe, is on the GRAS list, and is basically metabolized easily as starch is in the body. Studies have shown no problems with dextrin. Dextrose is the dextrorotary form of glucose and is used as a sweetener in many beverages and packaged foods. It can be extracted from corn, sugar cane, or sugar beets, and like all sugars, its use should be limited or avoided.

Diacetyl. This ingredient, with a flavor and odor like butter, is found naturally in some cheeses, cocoa, coffee, berries, and pears. It can be made chemically or by fermenting glucose. Diacetyl is the primary component of starter distillates used to culture flours and milk products. It is used predominately, however, as a flavoring agent in margarines, candies, and chewing gum and to help carry a buttery or coffee taste in foods. Many flavors might contain diacetyl, including strawberry and other berries, chocolate, coffee, butterscotch, caramel, rum, nut, and butter. These flavorings may be used in making baked goods, gelatin desserts, ice cream, beverages, gum, and candy. Diacetyl may be listed on the label as such or merely as "artificial flavor." Diacetyl is considered a safe ingredient. Studies have shown no significant problem, and it remains on the GRAS list.

Dihydrochalcone (DHC). This is possibly an upcoming chemical sweetener, but at the moment, it has only been granted low-level approval by the Food and Extract Manufacturers Association (FEMA). It is made by a chemical modification of naturally occurring bioflavonoids. It is about 1,500 times sweeter than sugar, but the sweet flavor takes longer to be released and tasted than other sugars, so use might be limited. DHC is thought to be safe, but further testing is being done before it will be available for use.

Ethyl alcohol (ethanol). Also known as grain (drinking) alcohol, this is used as a solvent in a variety of foods, such as candy, beverages, ice cream, baked goods, pizza crusts, liquors, gelatin desserts, and many medicinals (tinctures and elixirs). Because it is used mostly during processing, ethyl alcohol is not always listed on the packaging label. It is basically a safe additive in small amounts, although higher dosages can be toxic or even fatal.

Ethylenediaminetetraacetic acid (EDTA), calcium disodium EDTA). EDTA is a mineral chelator that binds metals and takes them out of a solution. In medicine it is used (mainly as calcium disodium EDTA) to treat lead poisoning and in chelation therapy. In food processing, EDTA and its acetate salts are used as chelating agents to decrease metals in food mixtures. EDTA is used even more commonly as a preservative in salad dressings, mayonnaise, sandwich spreads, condiments, margarines, juices, and drinks. The sequestering action is a result of its chelating effect, which allows EDTA to prevent changes in the color or flavor of foods, particularly from metals. EDTA is on the safe list even though it is under further study. Results of research for any harmful effects or tumorigenic properties have not been conclusive. It is possible that EDTA has some modest positive effects when metal toxicity is a problem. It is also possible that some of the potential adverse effects of EDTA may involve depletion of our zinc and copper supplies or disruption of our zinc-to-copper ratio simply because of the strong binding ability of EDTA for these minerals.

Fructose. This is a natural sugar found in many fruits and in honey. It is twice as sweet as sucrose, or cane sugar, and is now being used more frequently as a sweetener. It is available in bulk as well as being used in candies, preserves, ice cream, and "natural" beverage drinks and ices. The health food industry often uses fructose instead of sucrose. It seems to stimulate blood sugar and pancreatic insulin less rapidly than glucose (part of sucrose) and is absorbed more slowly. Still, too much fructose can be just as hard on our blood sugar level as too much table sugar or corn syrup. Fructose is basically safe in small amounts, as are most of the simple sugars. When used in excess, however, all sugars seem to affect the emotional, mental, and physical states of the user. It is best to use fructose and other sugars moderately and to consume more natural fruits and vegetables to obtain the simple carbohydrates.

Gelatin. This is a protein made from the skin and connective tissue (collagen) of animals. It can be extracted from hooves, skin, snouts, tendons, or ligaments and is used commonly in the food industry. A series of chemical baths are typically used for this extraction. In the vitamin supplement and pharmaceutical industries, gelatin is an important ingredient for making capsules and pill coverings. In foods, it functions as a thickener or stabilizer by absorbing as much as 5 to 10 times its weight in water. Gelatin itself is tasteless and colorless. It is employed as a base in gelatin desserts, pudding, chocolate milk, whipped cream, and marshmallows and is also used in ice cream, sherbet, custard, cheeses, and cheese spreads. It has also been used as a medicinal to treat weak fingernails.

Gelatin is basically safe, and according to research, the primary problems with it involve allergic reactions. Some strict vegetarians avoid gelatin because of its animal origin. Somewhat incomprehensibly, many brands of gelatin desserts (like Jell-O) have been given the "parve" label by their manufacturers. This is a category of food in kosher dietary laws that is neither meat nor dairy and designates a food that is not animal-derived. The position of the manufacturers is that the origin of the gelatin in animal skin and connective tissue is no longer present in the final product because of the multiple chemical baths and processing steps. Because connective tissue and skin contain protein, gelatin does provide most amino acids but is somewhat low in tryptophan.

Glycerides (monoglycerides, diglycerides). The glycerides are used commonly as emulsifiers to maintain softness and consistency in dressings, gum, milk, ice milk, ice cream, toppings, shortening, chocolates, lard, margarines, confections, and baked goods. The basic monoglycerides and diglycerides are naturally occurring fats (more specifically, alcohol fats) and are easily metabolized in the body. Triglycerides are among the more predominate body fats. These are all basically safe. However, there are a number of chemically synthesized glycerides currently being used, oxystearin being of the highest concern. Fats in general should not be used in high amounts; they seem to correlate with increased incidence of cancer and cardiovascular disease, although clearly some glycerides in foods would add little to this risk.

Glycerin (glycerol, glycerine). This is an alcohol that is part of all fats, about 10% by weight of both animal and vegetable fats. Most of the glycerin used in food processing is made from animal oils and fats. It is a mildly sweet agent that has many functions. Glycerin is a solvent that helps carry food colors and flavors. It absorbs water and so is used as a humectant. It is also used as a thickener in gelatin desserts and chewing gums. Glycerin is also a plasticizer used in the coverings for meats and cheeses, providing a waxy protection when mixed with other ingredients. It is also added to some baked goods, fillings, beverages, and gelatinous

meats. In medicines and cosmetics, it is used in suppositories and a wide range of skin products. Glycerin is on the GRAS list and is basically safe. It causes occasional irritation to mucous membranes in some people, but it can also be a soothing emollient (softener).

Guar gum. This complex carbohydrate, soluble fiber extracted from the guar plant grown in the Middle East acts as a stabilizer, thickener, and binder of foods, as it easily absorbs cold water, forming a thick, pastelike substance. It helps to stabilize and add texture to such foods as ice cream, ices, cheese spreads, dressings, and some meat products. Guar gum is also used in baked goods, fruit drinks, frozen fruits, and bakery glazes. It is on the GRAS list, although there is some concern about its use by pregnant women. Research to date has not shown any specific problems with guar gum, especially in the amounts commonly used. In fact, there are a few studies showing improved control of blood sugar with regular, low-dose supplementation of guar gum.

Gum arabic. See **Acacia.**

Honey. This is being used more commonly as a sweetener by food manufacturers. Many new natural, preservative-free beverages, cereals, ice creams, and candies contain honey instead of cane sugar. Honey contains both glucose and fructose and has less dramatic effects on blood sugar levels than cane sugar. It can be used directly from Nature instead of being chemically extracted and processed. However, consumers should be careful about the quality of honey they buy, because residues from pesticides or other toxins in the flowers and plants forming the bees' habitat can be passed on through the honey. Organic is definitely the safest bet here. Provided it has been obtained from a toxin-free environment, honey is a safe food additive and actually has some preservative action. Of course, it is caloric and, if used in excess, can cause dental cavities and weight gain. It is best used in moderation, as are all sugars.

Hydrogen peroxide. Hydrogen peroxide is a commonly used antiseptic that works by releasing oxygen, thus its bubbling action. It is also used in food processing, although it is not directly added to food, and therefore it is usually not listed on the labels. The peroxides are mild preservative and antibacterial agents used in processing milk and making cheese. They are even more commonly employed as bleaching and oxidizing agents in butter, cheese, and powdered eggs. The Japanese have used hydrogen peroxide to disinfect fish and noodles before they are eaten. Hydrogen peroxide is safe when used in food processing but not when added to food. Studies for carcinogenicity did not reveal any positive findings. The peroxides can be an irritant to the skin and eyes and have a mild allergenic potential. Some people use oral food grade hydrogen peroxide (H_2O_2) for treatment of a variety of ailments.

Related to hydrogen peroxide in terms of their chemical activity are two other peroxides—benzoyl peroxide and calcium peroxide. Calcium peroxide has been primarily used agriculturally as a way of bringing oxygen into the soil. It has also been used in aquaculture, both to oxygenate and to disinfect water. Benzoyl peroxide is the better-known peroxide when it comes to food, because this peroxide has been used to bleach flours, cheeses, and whey powders. (If you are buying a container of protein powder that is based on whey, it is worth finding a product that is free of benzoyl peroxide.) This GRAS-listed additive has been shown to cause breaks in DNA strands as well as cross-linking. Both types of damage to DNA are problematic, require repair, and can lead to increased risk of cancer.

Hydrolyzed vegetable protein (HVP). HVP is used occasionally as a flavor enhancer in soups, gravies, and meats. It is also used in baby foods, although there is some concern about this, as HVP may affect certain growth-related proteins. Certain types of HVP are produced by extraction with petroleum distillates; these petroleum residues are a cause for concern, although studies have been inconclusive regarding specific hazard. On the allergy front, persons allergic to wheat, corn, or soy should avoid products containing this additive, because all of those foods can serve as sources for HVP. With these reservations, however, HVP is considered safe.

Iodine salts (calcium iodate, cuprous iodide, potassium iodate, potassium iodide). Iodine is a mineral that occurs naturally in the soil and sea and is needed by the body for proper thyroid function. It is sometimes found in foods grown in iodine-rich soil and foods harvested from the ocean, such as fish and sea vegetation. Because iodine deficiency is common, potassium iodide is added to table salt to ensure that we receive our daily requirement. Calcium or potassium iodate is added to breads as a nutrient and as a

dough conditioner to improve texture. Potassium iodide is also used in drinking water. Iodine is basically safe and is essential for life. Pregnant or lactating women usually require extra dietary iodine. Occasionally, susceptible people may have mild allergic skin reactions to iodine, but this is not very likely with the small amounts used in foods.

Lactic acid (calcium lactate, butyl lactate, ethyl lactate). Lactic acid is produced naturally in the body as a result of metabolism and exercise as well as by bacterial fermentation of milk. Some lactic acid is found in tomatoes, apples, molasses, beer, and wine. It can also be made by fermenting molasses, whey, cornstarch, and potato starch. Lactic acid is used to give flavor and tartness to carbonated juices and other beverages and to some desserts. Its acidity reduces spoilage in such foods as cheeses, olives, breads, butter, and candy. Lactic acid helps condition dough and stabilize wine as well. Calcium lactate helps to firm some processed foods, to inhibit discoloration in processed fruits and vegetables, and to stabilize powdered milk and some baked goods. Lactic acid is safe and on the GRAS list. Research shows no deleterious effects, although it is not used in infant formulas.

Lactose (milk sugar). This occurs naturally in milk and can be extracted from whey or during cheese making. Lactose represents about 7% of human milk and 5% of cow's milk. It is made up of 1 molecule each of galactose and glucose. Lactose is much less sweet than sucrose (about one-sixth as sweet). In the food industry, it is used in powdered formulas, such as infant formulas and protein powders for weight loss, weight gain, or bodybuilding. Lactose also helps carry flavors and aromas in foods and can improve the texture and flavor of baked goods.

Lactose is quite safe except for people who are sensitive to milk or who are lactose intolerant—that is, they do not have sufficient amounts of the enzyme lactase needed to metabolize lactose. Gastrointestinal symptoms—such as nausea, diarrhea, and bloating—or a variety of other symptoms may occur in the lactose-intolerant person. Lactose may help absorption of some nutrients, most notably calcium. There are several lactase enzyme products out in the marketplace that provide tablet and liquid forms of this enzyme. These tablets and liquids can be swallowed, or the liquid drops can be added to lactose-containing products (like cow's milk or puddings) to assist with breakdown of the milk sugar. When used properly, these products are fairly effective and can be helpful.

Lard and animal fats—pork fat, beef fat (tallow), cheese fat. Fats extracted from animals are commonly used in preparing soups. Saturated fats are also used in various ointments, salves, and lubricants. In food, their main purpose is flavoring, giving a richer taste. These fats, especially lard, may be treated with such preservatives as BHT, which may not be listed on the package label. If lard or shortening is listed, it probably contains other additives as well. Because the vast majority of these fats are obtained from animals that were not raised organically, they routinely bring along with them toxic residues found in these animals, including pesticides, growth hormones, and antibiotics. These toxins may not be as much cause for concern as the saturated animal fat itself, but they are another reason on my list to avoid most lard products.

Lecithin (soy lecithin, phosphatidylcholine). This nutrient is part of the fatty matrix in our cell membranes and is important to many body functions, particularly healthy nerves and cell membranes. Commercially, it is extracted from eggs, soybeans, or corn, and can be produced in the form of an oil or a powder. In food processing, lecithin is used mainly as an emulsifier and stabilizer in oil-containing foods, such as salad dressings, mayonnaise, margarine, chocolate, frozen desserts, cereals, and baked goods. Lecithin also acts as a mild antioxidant, preventing changes in flavor and fragrance of oil-containing products. It is also used in paints. Lecithin is safe and may even have some beneficial effects. Certain chemically prepared lecithins, such as hydroxylated lecithin synthesized with hydrogen or benzoyl peroxide, may be a little more risky, but these too have been found to be basically safe.

Locust bean gum. See **Carob.**

Maleic hydrazide. This dangerous chemical is not listed on food labels, even though it is sprayed on most tobacco leaves, making tobacco smoke even more dangerous. Maleic hydrazide is sometimes sprayed on potatoes and onions to prevent sprouting, but it may cause the sprouting to occur inside the vegetables, which is probably worse. The most common source of exposure to this toxin, by the way, is not sprayed food but automobile exhaust. It is also released into the environment following manufacture of resins and polymers. **Maleic hydrazide is toxic to humans.** Animal studies have shown carcinogenicity and damage to the liver and central nervous system. Some studies have denied this cancer-causing potential. Until the use of maleic hydrazide as a pesticide is discontinued, we should avoid it, if possible, by buying organic produce or by making sure it is not used on the products we buy. Also, by not smoking, we will avoid it and the other toxins in cigarettes.

Malic acid. This occurs naturally in many fruits and vegetables, including apples, cherries, peaches, tomatoes, rhubarb, pears, plums, and berries. It is used to provide a tart taste to various sweets. Malic acid is used in wines, jellies, jams, sherbet, candies, beverages, and frozen milk products. It is basically safe, and studies show no potential hazards.

Malt (malt syrup, malt extract, maltol). Malt is basically an extract from barley. It is a mildly sweet substance that is used commonly in the brewing industry. It is also used as a sweetener in such foods as ice cream, flavored milk, candy, cereals, and dressings and is occasionally used to flavor meat and poultry products. Malt is safe, with no known toxicity, and is on the GRAS list. Although not related to its safety as a food additive, I would like to mention here that malt is often among the first substances to eliminate on a yeast-free diet, because its sugars are especially good growth promoters for yeast. Maltol, which is not malt but an extract from larch trees and pine needles, is also used to flavor foods and give them a fresh-baked smell. Ethyl maltol is the synthetic maltol. Both of these are used in flavorings for frozen desserts, gelatins, soft drinks, ice creams, candy, baked goods, and gums. Maltol is also known to be safe.

Maple syrup. This natural extract from maple trees is a flavorful sweetener. It is now commonly used in place of sugar in many "health" foods, such as baked goods and cereals. Pure maple syrup is also used commonly on pancakes and waffles. Many maple syrup manufacturers in the United States use formaldehyde, a toxic chemical, on their trees to improve the syrup production, which also contaminates them. Canada does not allow formaldehyde use on its maples, however. In addition to formaldehyde, nonorganic versions of maple syrup can contain pesticides and other toxic residues. Many maple syrups are imitations and not pure. They contain a high amount of corn syrup and artificial flavors and maybe a small percentage of actual maple syrup. These types of syrup are best avoided. Genuine maple syrup is a safe food, although excessive use should be avoided, as with all sweeteners. A final note on maple syrup involves its grade. Most maple syrups sold in the marketplace are rated grade A. This version of the syrup is maximally filtered and substantially lower in nutrients that the grade B version. From my point of view, the optimal version is a grade B organic maple syrup.

Monosodium glutamate (MSG). This fairly controversial food additive is used both in food processing and in restaurant and home cooking. It is basically a flavor enhancer that is commercially produced through fermentation of corn, sugar beets, or sugarcane. MSG is the monosodium salt of glutamic acid, an essential amino acid. It is used commonly in seasoning salts, soups, spices, condiments, meats, some baked goods, and candies. Other fermented and Asian food preparations contain MSG, as do most food dishes served in Chinese restaurants. Like other additives, it is a somewhat "hidden" type of ingredient and would not be recognizable without label reading or a question to the restaurant chef.

It might appear that MSG should not be a problem. After all, it is found naturally in such foods as soybeans, beets, and seaweeds. However, glutamic acid is one of two excitatory neurotransmitters in the brain. Along with aspartic acid, glutamic acid is among the body's key chemicals for activating the nerves, and for some people, an MSG-flavored meal is enough to alter their nervous system activity and trigger headaches, tingling, or other symptoms. Asthmatics seem to be particularly susceptible to MSG reactions, as do people who are low in vitamin B6. There was more concern in the past about the use of MSG with infants, as it was added to many baby foods for flavor, but that practice was voluntarily stopped by manufacturers beginning in 1969.

"Chinese restaurant syndrome" is definitely associated with the use of MSG. Symptoms occurring after eating foods high in MSG include headaches, tingling, numbness, and chest pains. These effects have been confirmed by some studies but not by others, although it seems that many people are sensitive to MSG and experience some untoward reactions when using it, especially at the high levels often added to Chinese food. Some researchers theorize that it may be the various mushrooms, sprouts, teas, soy, mustards, fish, or sauces used in Asian cooking; either these foods themselves or their interactions with MSG may cause such symptoms. More research on MSG is needed, and studies are being undertaken. In 1980, the FDA evaluated available research findings and decided that MSG could be left on the GRAS list. I avoid foods with MSG or restaurants that use it, however, because I experience unpleasant reactions to it. I suggest that, until further research clears it as being safe, foods containing MSG should not be eaten.

Neotame. This derivative of aspartame is produced by the processing of aspartame together with another chemical (3,3-dimethylbutyraldehyde). It is 30 to 60 times sweeter than aspartame and more heat stable. The FDA approved it for use in food in 2002 as an artificial sweetener, but there are no widely available commercial products containing neotame yet. The further processing of aspartame would make this sweetener at least as suspect, if not more suspect, than aspartame itself when it comes to safety. I recommend avoiding it for this reason.

Nitrates (sodium nitrate, potassium nitrate [saltpeter]). Nitrates, in relatively low amounts, are found naturally in many vegetables and in most water supplies. The prolonged use of nitrate fertilizers has increased these levels in food and water. Vegetables that are high in nitrates include spinach, beets, celery, radishes, lettuce, and other greens. Nitrates, particularly potassium nitrate, have long been used in curing meats (hams, bacon, sausage, hot dogs, corned beef, lunch meats, and some fish products), acting as a color fixative. The nitrates are not as stable as the nitrites (see the next entry), and therefore sodium nitrite is the main meat-curing chemical used. In fact, nitrate converts easily to nitrite and can interact with amines in the digestive juices or tissues to form nitrosamines, which are highly carcinogenic chemicals.

Nitrates were thought to be safe until recent years, but research has shown otherwise. They are safer when used with vitamin C, which can help prevent nitrosamine production. But nitrates and nitrites have not been banned, and they are still in use in the $100-billion-dollar processed-meat industry. Manufacturers claim that there is no good substitute for these nitrates and nitrites. I suggest avoiding all foods, especially bacon and cured meats, containing these substances for obvious health reasons.

Nitrites (sodium nitrite, potassium nitrite). Sodium nitrite is used primarily to cure meats in that megabusiness. This chemical is a color fixative that works by reacting with the muscle myoglobin to create a red color like that of blood. Sodium nitrite also protects against the growth of the bacterium *Clostridium botulinum,* which causes botulism. It adds a tangy taste to the meats treated with it. These meats include hams, bacon, lunch meats, bologna, frankfurters, meat spreads, some smoke-cured fishes, and corned beef. Sodium nitrite and salt are often added to foods to fix their color, prolong their shelf life, and trigger our taste buds.

There are many problems associated with eating these processed meats. First, they are usually high in both sodium and fats, which endanger the cardiovascular system. The chemicals used in raising animals and found in their meat are also a cause for concern. The biggest health hazard, however, is the direct carcinogenic effect of nitrosamines, which are formed when nitrite interacts with amines (parts of proteins) in the digestive fluids or in the foods eaten. Nitrosamines have been shown to be potent carcinogens in animals, producing increased amounts of cancer in the liver, lungs, and pancreas—all usually fatal. Also, the nitrites can form amyl and butyl nitrites, which have been shown to be carcinogenic as well.

It has been demonstrated that vitamin C reduces the production of nitrosamines. More recently, vitamin E has been shown to help as well. In lieu of banning the use of nitrites, for which the cured-meat industry claims there is no effective substitute, the FDA has asked processors to at least add vitamin C and, more recently, vitamin E to the brines used to cure meats. If you do happen to indulge in any of these fatty, chemical meats, take additional vitamin C and vitamin E when you do. Further research needs to be done to substantiate the clear dangers of nitrite use in human foods. For the many reasons mentioned, it is wise to eliminate all nitrite-containing foods from the diet and substitute more healthful foods.

Olestra. This sucrose polyester, an artificial combination of sucrose and fatty acids, was first developed by Proctor & Gamble in 1968 for use as an artificial, noncaloric fat. The company filed with the FDA for approval of olestra as a drug in 1975 but regrouped and decided to seek approval for its use as a food additive. It was not until 1996, however, that olestra was finally approved for use in savory snacks under the brand name Olean. Amazingly, after research showed olestra to increase loss of the fat-soluble vitamins A, D, E, and K from the body, the FDA announced that it would continue to allow the use of olestra in products but that manufacturers would be required to fortify those products with these four vitamins. Olestra remains in potato chips and some other food products, but I recommend avoiding its use. If nothing else, the vitamin-loss issue suggests that olestra is an unnatural presence inside the digestive tract, and it causes digestive upset and loose bowels in some people.

Palmitic acid. This is a saturated fat found naturally in many animal and vegetable sources, such as butter, celery seed, palm oil, coffee and tea, anise seed, and other herb seeds. Palmitic acid is used occasionally to create butter or cheese flavorings to season foods. It is basically nontoxic and is on the GRAS list. As a long-chain saturated fat, we do not want too much palmitic acid in our diet. But the contribution of palmitic acid to the diet on a food additive basis is relatively small.

Parabens (methyl, butyl, and propyl paraben). Paraben, or parahydroxybenzoic acid, is closely related to benzoic acid and sodium benzoate, both common food preservatives. Methyl and propyl paraben are synthetic compounds that are esters of paraben and also act as preservatives, preventing the growth of molds and yeasts as well as other microbes. They are used commonly in the cosmetics industry and are useful in both liquids and solids. They are also protective in alkaline products. In the food industry, the parabens are used in baked goods, some milk products, frozen desserts, and sugar substitutes as well as the artificially sweetened foods that contain them, such as jellies, jams, and dietic foods and beverages.

Because the paraben esters have been so widely used in the cosmetics industry, and because studies so far have not clearly documented health problems associated with their use, parabens are considered to be basically nontoxic. In fact, their desirability for use in cosmetics is partly because they are nonirritating and nonallergenic. Although some birth defects were noted in rats and hamsters fed high amounts of propyl paraben, the current level of use does not warrant concern. Some people wish to avoid synthetic chemicals with unknown effects, however, and I would put the parabens in that class.

Pectins. These binding agents are found in the cell walls of all land plants, particularly in fruits and vegetables, such as apples and citrus fruits. They are polysaccharides consisting of many simple sugars (especially glucuronic acid) and are extracted for food use from the rinds and pressings of apples, oranges, and lemons after they have been squeezed for their juice. Pectins are used in foods as stabilizers and thickeners; they help food to blend and gel. They are common ingredients in jams, jellies, preserves, ice cream, chocolate milk, sherbet, beverages and juices, and French dressing. Pectins can also be used as antidiarrheal agents. They are safe and even helpful as food additives. I should also note that there are three basic types of plant pectins—homogalacturonan, rhamnogalacturonan I, and rhamnogalacturonan II.

Polysorbate 60 and 80 — polyoxyethylene (20), sorbitan monostearate; sorbitan monooleate. Polysorbate 60 and 80 are sorbitan derivatives made from sorbitol (see entry below), a sugar alcohol that is sweet and that is produced by converting glucose. Polysorbate 60 is made by chemically combining palmitate and stearic acids with sorbitol and sterilizing it with 20 parts of ethylene oxide, a toxic gas. Polysorbate 60 is an emulsifier that helps blend oil and water together and also aids in spreading flavor through the various mixtures to which it is added. Polysorbate 60 is used in many processed foods, including salad dressings, bakery products, dairy products, gelatin desserts, shortenings, cake mixes, whipped vegetable toppings, candy and sugar toppings, and vitamin supplements.

Although there are other polyoxyethylene derivatives besides polysorbate 60 and polysorbate 80 (such as sorbitan monostearate, tristearate, and palmitate), polysorbate 60 is used most commonly. It has been classified as safe, but the FDA wants further study. The effects of the ethylene gas are unknown. I would recommend avoiding it when possible until further information is available. Polysorbate 80 (also sometimes called glycol) is similar to polysorbate 60 except that it contains oleic acid instead of stearic acid. It can be used as an emulsifier and flavor carrier in the same foods and dietary products as polysorbate 60. It is also

employed as a defoaming agent in brewing and yeast production and in chewing gum. It also appears to be basically nontoxic and is on the GRAS list. Studies with it and polysorbate 60 have not revealed specific problems, but further studies are being done. I recommend avoiding polysorbate 80 whenever possible.

Polyvinyl chloride (PVC). This is a potentially toxic plastic (a polymer of vinyl chloride) when it releases vinyl chloride on exposure to heat, light, or chemical solvents. It is more a food contaminant than an additive. Plastic wrap contains polyvinyl chloride and other chemicals that leach into foods, especially meat, when they come in contact with them. Heat increases the release of vinyl chloride into the food which then fixes with the tissues. PVC, which is derived from vinyl chloride, is a stable material, resistant to environmental breakdown. That is why it is used so widely in industry, as in pipes, records, containers, linings, film, toys, and so on. Research linking PVC to the increased risk of cancer has been limited to industrial and manufacturing situations in which workers are exposed to large amounts of PVC through inhalation, and no studies to date show increased cancer risk from food-based applications alone. Still, the toxic potential of this substance makes it worth avoiding. If possible, we should steer clear of prepackaged plastic-wrapped animal foods or other deli take-out-type foods. PVC is not listed on food labels.

Propyl gallate. This synthetic chemical is added to foods for its antioxidant effect. It reduces rancidity and prevents changes in color, taste, and odor in foods containing fats and oils. Propyl gallate is often combined with other antioxidants, such as BHA and BHT, to reduce the level of each used. It might be added to such foods as meats, shortenings, vegetable oils, candy, snack foods, nuts, baked goods, and frozen dairy foods. It has also been used as part of fruit or spice flavorings in beverages, ice cream, candy, and bottled goods. Propyl gallate is on the GRAS list. It has been studied fairly thoroughly, and no research has revealed any carcinogenic or toxic effects. There are some reports of contact dermatitis with bakers and other workers who handle large amounts of this additive, but this problem involves large amounts and is unrelated to ingestion. Propyl gallate is therefore considered a safe additive; however, it is still a synthetic chemical.

Propylene glycol (propylene glycol monostearate and alginate). Propylene glycol is a blending agent used in food processing. It is made from propylene gas (a by-product of petroleum refining) and glycerol. It is a solvent that attracts water and improves the flexibility and spreadability of the products in which it is used. These include confections, ice cream, beverages, toppings, icings, chocolate, shredded coconut, and baked goods. In meats, it helps prevent discoloring. Propylene glycol is also used in a variety of cosmetics, as it promotes absorption through the skin. Propylene glycol alginate is extracted from seaweed with propylene gas. It is a defoamer and stabilizer used in some salad dressings, ice creams, and sherbets. Propylene glycol monostearate acts as an emulsifier, texturizer, and dough conditioner in baked goods, puddings, and toppings. Butylene glycol and polyethylene glycol are related compounds produced with different gases.

These products, especially propylene glycol, have been studied fairly well and have been shown to have very low toxicity. The 1980 review by the FDA substantiated their safety and they remain on the GRAS list. I would still be wary of using these products, however, because of their chemical nature and because the foods in which they are used are not always the healthiest; however, there are apparently worse additives than these.

Quinine (quinine hydrochloride, quinine sulfate). Quinine is a bitter extract from the bark of the cinchona tree. It is used as a flavoring to impart a refreshing bitter taste to such carbonated beverages as tonic water, bitter lemon, and quinine water. It is also used in some over-the-counter medicines and in the treatment of malaria. Quinine hydrochloride and sulfate are synthetic variations used as flavoring agents in various bitters and citrus beverages. Quinine can cause some problems. Although it is generally safe, it is not recommended for use by pregnant women. Some people are allergic to quinine and can have skin reactions or a syndrome named *cinchonism,* consisting of flushing, nausea, vomiting, visual disturbance, and hearing changes. This is usually a result of an overdose of quinine, although sensitive people may experience some symptoms with low intake.

Rennet (rennin). This enzyme extracted from the linings of cow's stomachs is used to make cheese,

as it helps to curdle milk. It has been found to be safe in the small amounts. However, many vegetarians and health-conscious people prefer rennetless cheeses, which are made with various vegetable enzymes.

Saccharin (sodium saccharin). This popular artificial sweetener has been in use for over 100 years. It contains no calories and is several hundred times sweeter than sugar, although it has a slightly bitter aftertaste. After initially sanctioning its use, the FDA turned around and proposed a ban on saccharin in 1977, but the public resisted the ban. The U.S. Congress placed a moratorium on the ban, and the FDA officially withdrew its proposal 14 years later, in 1991. More recently, Congress passed a law removing the required warning label on products containing saccharin. The health research on saccharin has remained controversial. According to the EPA, saccharin is a possible carcinogen. This opinion is based on animal studies showing increased risk of urinary tract and bladder cancers for animals given relatively high doses of saccharin.

In the early 1990s, nearly 5 million pounds of saccharin were used yearly—about 75% in diet drinks, 15% in other diet foods, such as canned fruits and ice cream, and about 10% as a table sweetener. One advantage of saccharin is that it does not convert to glucose in the body, so it is popular among diabetics. However, it is a chemical that must be metabolized and eliminated from the body, and I do not consider saccharin a safe additive for regular use. It may be mildly to moderately carcinogenic, depending on the level of use and the health of the consumer. There is special risk to children, teenagers, and pregnant women. More studies are needed, but my current suggestion is not to use saccharin. It might be helpful in certain medical conditions, such as diabetes or for low-calorie or weight-loss diets, and it probably would be best to make saccharin available only by prescription.

Salicylic acid and salicylates (amyl, phenyl, benzyl, and methyl salicylate). A number of foods— including apples, almonds, apricots, berries, plums, prunes, raisins, cucumbers, cloves, wintergreen, and tomatoes—naturally contain salicylates. Salicylic acid, made synthetically by heating phenol with carbon dioxide, is the basis of aspirin, acetylsalicylic acid. Aspirin is a commonly used anti-inflammatory and pain reliever. White willow bark contains a natural salicylate that has similar effects. Tartrazine, FD&C Yellow No. 5, is a salicylate-type compound used as a food dye. Salicylate-related substances are also used in a variety of flavorings, such as strawberry, root beer, sarsaparilla, spice, walnut, peach, and mint, as well as in some beverages, candies, baking goods, chewing gum, and ice cream.

The salicylates are known to cause symptoms when consumed in higher doses. Ringing of the ears (tinnitus), gastrointestinal irritation, nausea, vomiting, increased respiration, acidosis, and skin rash may occur with salicylate intoxication. Only a small amount is used in foods, so except for those with allergic sensitivity to the salicylate products, they are basically safe. Because of the phenol derivation and possible side effects, however, salicylic acid and aspirin are substances of which to be wary.

Silicates (silicon dioxide, sodium aluminosilicate, calcium and magnesium silicate, sodium calcium aluminosilicate, talc). The silicates are salts of silica oxides, which are found in rocks and sand, in such gems as quartz, amethyst, and agate, and in flint. Silica is related to silicon, an important element in the Earth and probably essential to humans for bone calcification and connective tissue strength. The various silicates are used infrequently in food processing as defoaming agents in beer production or as anticaking agents in such powders as salt, dry mixes, and baking powder. These silica salts absorb water and prevent the powders from sticking together. Silicon dioxide may also be used in vitamin tablets, BHT, sodium proprionate, and other food additives.

There are some concerns about health hazards from the aluminum-containing silicates, and talc may contain asbestos (see "Talc" on page 476); otherwise, the silicates are safe in the usually small amounts used. Environmental aspects of silica production are another matter, and silicates continue to be studied for their impact on ecosystems, especially lakes, where many plants and small organisms at the bottom of the food chain depend on a delicate balance between silicon, phosphorus, and other minerals.

Simplesse (microparticulated whey protein). This artificial fat approved by the FDA for use in frozen deserts in 1990 is produced by taking whey protein concentrates and forcing them at a high pressure through a small tube (1 micron wide) to produce unusual microparticles that provide fatlike qualities to food without providing calories. Although I would place this artificial fat in a better category than its rival olestra when it comes to health safety, I still recommend that it be avoided it in products. It is unlikely that the value of whey proteins are maintained during the highly damaging process used to produce this artificial fat.

Smoke flavoring (liquid smoke, char smoke flavor). Liquid smoke flavorings are manufactured by burning various types of hardwoods, maple and hickory most commonly. They are used for flavoring foods, particularly meats and cheeses. They are also mild antioxidants, protecting against fatty changes and helping to reduce bacterial contamination. Smoked yeast can be made by exposing yeast to the smoke. It may be used in cheese, pizza, soups, crackers, and dips. These flavorings have been studied fairly extensively and have been found to contain a variety of potentially toxic substances. First in this category are the polycyclic aromatic hydrocarbons (PAHs). Present in liquid smoke are at least six different PAHs, all of which are classified as probable or outright carcinogens. There has been some suggestion that smoke flavoring helps prevent bacterial growth in meats, but this would hardly be a reason to expose ourselves to the cancer-causing agents. And it is not only this smoke flavoring additive that should be avoided, but also the charcoaling of meats in general. Charcoal grilling meats has been shown to create these same PAHs and to cause changes in cells that foreshadow the development of cancers.

Sodium acid pyrophosphate (SAP) and tetrasodium pyrophosphate (TSPP). SAP is a diphosphoric acid (pyrophosphate) of sodium used in processing, so it is not usually listed on the label. It is a mild buffer and acid constituent of self-rising leavening mixtures for cakes, pancakes, doughnuts, waffles, and other baked goods, flours, and mixes. SAP and sodium pyrophosphate are added to lunch meats, hot dogs, and sausages to accelerate the development of their red color and to reduce the amount of nitrites needed. They also help hold in the juices of cooked pork. In 1991, the American Conference of Governmental Industrial Hygienists rated SAP as moderately toxic and cited excess acidity in the body and disruption of calcium balance as the 2 toxic consequences of SAP.

Sodium benzoate. See **Benzoic acid.**

Sodium bicarbonate (baking soda, bicarbonate of soda). This alkaline powder is used to balance acid products and as a leavening agent to lighten and help raise dough. It is found in many biscuit, muffin, and pancake mixes; in baking powders; in many crackers; in self-rising flours; and in other foods. Baking soda is also used as an antacid for stomach acidity, topically for insect bites or poison oak, and to absorb odors and freshen refrigerators. This useful substance can be further used to clean our teeth as well as remove the acid-chemical residue found on the surface of foods (see "88 Survival Suggestions" on page 785 of the Futureword). Sodium bicarbonate is a safe product. Bicarbonate is used by the body as a buffer to help maintain acid-base balance. Excess baking soda could affect this balance, but the amount used in foods poses no real problem.

Sodium bisulfite. See **Sulfites.**

Sodium caseinate. See **Caseinates.**

Sodium chloride (common table salt). One of the most widely employed food additives in both processing and preparation as well as at the dining room table, sodium chloride has a number of valuable uses. It is found naturally in small amounts in many foods but is much more concentrated in processed and restaurant foods. It can be used as a pickling and curing agent by soaking foods in a salty brine. It acts as a mild preservative in such foods as vegetables, meats, and butter. It is also used as a dough conditioner and occasionally as a nutritional supplement, although most people acquire plenty of salt without even trying. Sodium chloride can be commercially extracted from salt mines or seawater, or through brine evaporation.

Salt is basically safe when used in modest amounts. Some people with salt-sensitive high blood pressure must avoid it. As a factor in causing high blood pressure, it is implicated in heart and kidney disease. Although salt is safe, it is unwise to consume high-salt-content foods. (See "Sodium" on page 171 in chapter 6, Minerals.) I also believe that relying on salt as a primary source of flavor cheats our taste buds and prevents us from experiencing the rich variety of flavors found in traditional foods and cuisine.

Sodium hydroxide (lye, caustic soda). Sodium hydroxide, a strong alkali, is used in food processing, so it does not usually appear on labels. By itself, it is caustic and dangerous. It is used in the refining of vegetable oils and animal fats, in modifying food starch, and in glazes, cocoa products, and some curdled milk products; it's also used as an acid neutralizer in some canned vegetables. Sodium hydroxide has also been used in liquid drain cleaners, but that use has been limited. When ingested, lye causes internal burns, nausea, and vomiting; it can irritate the lungs when inhaled. In food use, with the small amounts ingested, which are usually balanced by other acid products, sodium hydroxide is basically safe and innocuous.

Sodium nitrate and nitrite. See **Nitrates** and **Nitrites.**

Sorbic acid (potassium sorbate). Sorbic acid is found naturally in the berries of the mountain ash. For use in food processing, it and its salt, potassium sorbate, are made synthetically. Sorbic acid is a mild preservative and is used to inhibit yeast and mold growth, especially in beverages and cheeses. It also reduces bacterial growth and works best in acidic foods. It is used in wine, many cheeses, cheesecakes, chocolates, syrups, fruit juices, baked goods, margarine, premade salads, pie fillings, and artificially sweetened preserves and jellies. Sorbic acid is basically safe and nontoxic. It can cause some skin irritation with contact, but it is one of the safer food preservatives.

Sorbitan derivatives. See **Polysorbate 60 and 80.**

Sorbitol. This natural sugar (technically called a sugar alcohol) is found in berries and other fruits, including pears, plums, apples, and cherries, as well as in sea vegetation. It can also be made chemically by modifying corn sugar (dextrose). In food processing, sorbitol helps control crystallization and viscosity of such foods as candy, frozen desserts, and dietetic fruits and soft drinks. Sorbitol has many functions. It is a thickener, humectant, texturizer, sequestrant, stabilizer, and sweetener and can be used as a sugar substitute by diabetics. It does not act as a sugar metabolically and has minimum potential for causing tooth decay or diabetic problems. Sorbitol is commonly used in chewing gums. It is also the basis of the emulsifiers polysorbate 60 and 80 and other sorbitan derivatives.

Sorbitol is thought to be safe, although it can be irritating to the intestinal tract when taken in larger quantities. Further studies are being done on sorbitol to prove its safety. Although its use in moderation is probably safe, I believe that it should be limited. Thanks to extensive studies involving diabetes, researchers now know that cataract formation involves the excessive depositing of sorbitol in the lens of the eye. Although there is no research to suggest that too much sorbitol in the diet can lead to the accumulation of this sugar in the eye, scientists are at least tipped off here to potential problems involving this sugar alcohol.

Soy protein isolate (texturized vegetable protein [TVP]). Soybeans have become a major commercial crop. When soybean oil is extracted, what is left is a high-protein residue that can be processed to make soy protein isolate. This protein powder can be used in milk-free formulas for infants and in protein-powder formulas for weight loss, weight gain, or bodybuilding. Soy isolate may also be used in soups, sauces, gravies, flavorings, seasonings, artificial bacon bits, cereals, frozen desserts, and meat substitutes. Other soy products are used in soy sauce, salad dressings, Worcestershire sauce, lunch meats, and candies.

Soy proteins are basically safe, especially if they are prepared with minimal chemical processing and without such dangerous chemicals as formaldehyde. In people who are allergic to soy products, however, their use could cause intestinal upset, bloating, headache, or skin rashes. Heat treatment of the powders reduces but does not eliminate allergenic potential. Soy protein may contain a small level of nitrites formed in processing, and these could generate carcinogenic nitrosamines. Soy protein is not a complete food and should not be consumed exclusively. Diet powders usually have added amino acids and vitamins and minerals. Consult a doctor or nutritionist for weight-loss programs with soy protein. In general, moderate amounts of the soy protein isolates are safe.

Soy sauce (hydrolyzed and fermented soybeans, tamari, shoyu). This is a salty food flavoring that can be prepared in two different ways. The traditional way, which I prefer, usually starts with soybeans, wheat, and a special starter mixture containing an aspergillus fungus to help the fermentation process. The traditional fermenting and aging process for soy sauce may take up to 2 years. A modern method speeds up this process by skipping the fermentation.

In this method, the soybeans may be cooked with hydrochloric acid, then neutralized and filtered, and then frequently combined with caramel color, corn syrup, and salt. There are organic, wheat-free versions of soy sauce available, usually labeled as wheat-free tamari. (*Tamari* in Japanese means "little puddle" and is sometimes used to refer to the liquid that collects in the bottom of a barrel used to age miso or soy.) You might also see the word *shoyu* in place of soy sauce. In Japanese, *shoyu* means "soy."

Soy sauce is used in some food preparations, such as soups or crackers, but is also added in cooking, especially in Asian restaurants, or as a tabletop seasoning. Soy sauce is safe and on the GRAS list. Its salt content may be a disadvantage to those with high blood pressure, and some people are sensitive to mold-fermented products or to soy itself. Also, people who are sensitive to wheat may want to purchase the wheat-free versions of this sauce. Soy sauce, like all salt products, should be used sparingly.

Starches (acid-modified, modified, unmodified, and gelatinized). Starch is a complex carbohydrate found in such whole grains as rice, wheat, and corn as well as in such vegetables as squashes, potatoes, and cassava. It can be chemically separated from the proteins and other nutrients in these foods so that the pure starch can be used in food processing as a thickening or gelling agent. After extraction, it can be further chemically modified to make it "easier to digest." To modify starch, it is bleached, oxidized, and treated with such chemicals as aluminum sulfate, sodium hydroxide, and propylene oxide. When the starch molecules are left to swell and burst, they form a gel—gelatinized starch. Starches are used to thicken such foods as baby foods, gelatins, and cake mixes, and sometimes to prevent caking or to dust baked goods to prevent sticking. Often, neither the type of starch used nor the chemicals employed to make the starches are listed on labels. These starches are on the GRAS list. Some of them have been studied and shown to pose no hazards, but there is concern about the chemical modification, extraction, and treatment processes. Starch is basically easy for the body to digest and metabolize. It is best to get our starches from whole foods and avoid starch-added foods as much as possible.

Stearic acid (calcium stearate). This is a saturated fatty acid that occurs naturally in animal fats and some vegetable oils. It is prepared synthetically through hydrogenating such vegetable oils as cottonseed oil and is used in foods to lubricate or help blend them. Synthetic stearic acid is also used in some flavorings, such as butter and vanilla, which may be used in candies, chewing gum, beverages, or bakery products. Calcium stearate is often the form of stearic acid used. It is also employed in cosmetics and medicinals, such as ointments and suppositories. Stearic acid is basically safe and is a by-product of fat-containing foods. Some people are slightly allergic to it, however. I think we should avoid much use of foods containing added stearic acid or calcium stearate. Further research is pending regarding possible dangers from the use of these additives.

Succinic acid. This is found naturally in meats, cheese, fungi, and many vegetables with its distinct tart, acid taste, such as asparagus, broccoli, beets, and rhubarb. Succinic acid is involved in carbohydrate metabolism and can be made synthetically for food processing by chemically changing acetic acid or maleic acid. Succinic acid can be used as a buffering or neutralizing agent. It is added to some foods to give an acid taste. It is also used by the perfume industry. Succinic acid has been rated as safe. Studies have shown that in amounts thousands of times higher than the quantities used in food, succinic acid creates no problems. It is, however, only infrequently used in food processing.

Sucralose. This chlorinated sugar, another new artificial sweetener, is produced by replacing three chemical groups in sugar with three atoms of chlorine. The FDA approved it as a tabletop sweetener in 1998 under the brand name Splenda. Because it is 600 times sweeter than table sugar, sucralose is added in fairly small amounts to a variety of candies and beverages. However, I do not think nearly enough research has been done on this artificial sweetener, and I recommend it be avoided in your diet.

Sucrose (cane or beet sugar)—white sugar, refined sugar, dextrose. Sucrose, or "sugar," is the primary food sweetener and the common table sugar. Sucrose (a disaccharide) is a carbohydrate, each molecule being composed of glucose and fructose. It is obtained mainly from sugarcane and sugar beets. These crops are now grown plentifully throughout the world as the sources of refined sugar. Sugarcane has been engineered to yield more sucrose (see page 482 for a discussion on the genetic modification of food). Sugar is used throughout the food manufacturing industry and is found in a great variety of foods. Condiments, dressings, candy, cereals, baby food, and beverages are some common examples. It can also be the starting substance in the fermentation process and is used widely in pharmaceuticals as a preservative, coating for tablets, or sweetener in syrups and children's formulas. Table sugar is used freely by many adults and children to sweeten coffee or tea, cereals, and fruit dishes and is liberally added in cooking and canning. Bakery products may contain high amounts of sucrose, and the soft drink industry uses millions of pounds each year.

Sucrose is probably the most commonly abused substance on Earth and the number-one food additive, both before and after processing. The average American consumes more than 125 pounds a year—that equates to billions of pounds in the United States alone. On a daily basis, this translates into 20 teaspoons. Sucrose is on the GRAS list, and studies show that it is generally safe—unless, of course, it is overused or there is individual sensitivity. It is not safe for diabetics, however, and sugar use is implicated in causing adult-onset diabetes. In large amounts, it is highly caloric and can contribute greatly to obesity, which increases the risk of diabetes and many other diseases. Tooth decay is much higher in people, especially children, who consume lots of sugar and practice poor oral hygiene. In addition, the pesticides and chemicals sprayed on cane and beet sugar and the chemical bleaching process used to make "white" sugar are potentially hazardous; consumers are not advised about this on sugar packages or food labels. Many people become hypersensitive to sugar, either because of repeated insults to the body or weakened body condition. Sucrose use may affect activity levels, physical energy, and emotional and mental states. It is a substance that should be avoided or used in moderation. It is better to get our natural sugars from the many wholesome foods that contain them.

Sulfites (sodium sulfite, sodium and potassium bisulfite, sodium and potassium metabisulfite). These sulfiting agents, which can release sulfur dioxide (see entry below), are used in food processing as preservatives and sanitizing agents. They prevent bacterial growth and the browning of exposed foods.

475

They are antispoilants and actually prevent undesirable microorganisms from growing during fermentation and food processing, thus preventing food discoloration. They have been used for this purpose in many processed foods, such as syrups and condiments, as well as in preserving fruits and vegetables, in wine making, and as a spray on restaurant salad bars. This latter use, fortunately, has recently been banned. Now sulfites must be listed on packaging labels, including alcoholic beverages.

These sulfites are on the GRAS list and thus considered safe, although they are under review because there are some indications that sulfites can enhance the cancer-causing potential of other substances, even though they may not be cancer-causing themselves. In the body, sulfites are frequently oxygenated and changed to sulfates, which are generally considered harmless. But many people seem to react to sulfites, especially those sprayed on foods or added in restaurants. Allergic reactions are worse in asthmatics, whose condition (wheezing and shortness of breath) can be exacerbated by sulfites. Sulfite reactions, including diarrhea, nausea, and headaches, also occur in nonasthmatic people as well. All of the sulfites are on my personal "avoid" list.

Sulfur dioxide. This gas is formed when sulfur is burned and is used in food processing for a variety of purposes. It is sprayed on many fruits and vegetables to preserve their color and to protect against attacks from microorganisms. Many grapes are so treated, and thus much wine contains this gas or other chemical by-products. Raisins, particularly golden raisins, and many other dried fruits are treated with sulfur dioxide. It is used as a disinfectant in food manufacturing, a bleaching agent, and an antioxidant and preservative, as well as an antibrowning agent. Other foods that may contain sulfur dioxide include beet sugar, corn syrup, jellies, soups, fresh and dehydrated potatoes, condiments, fruits, and beverages.

Sulfur dioxide gas is highly irritating and a strong oxidant. It destroys vitamin A and some B vitamins, such as thiamin. Its use is not allowed in treatment of meats. It is on the GRAS list, however, and reviews have found no apparent hazard. The healthy body can metabolize the reaction products of sulfur dioxide contained in foods. Even so, I recommend avoiding sulfur dioxide as much as possible.

Talc (magnesium silicate)—talcum powder. Talc is a silica chalk (see "Silicates" on page 472) that is used in coating and polishing rice and as an anticaking agent. It is also used externally to help dry the skin and genital areas. Talc appears to be carcinogenic in and of itself; in addition, it may contain asbestos fibers, increasing its potential for toxicity. The substance itself is chemically very similar to asbestos. Americans have so trustingly used it on babies' bottoms for decades, but is it really safe? The FDA has asked that only talc free of asbestos be used in food processing, but at this time, there is no good way to determine the presence of asbestos, and talc appears to be a problem with or without it. I recommend avoiding talc in food, talcum powder, and white rice that is polished and coated with it.

Tannic acid. This is found naturally in coffee and tea, wine, and the barks of some trees, including oak, cherry, and sumac. Commercial tannic acid is derived from the seed pods of palms, from ferns, or from oak nutgalls, little growths on the twigs. Tannic acid is used as a clarifier in brewing, for filtering out proteins, and as a refining agent for fats. Its main use is in flavorings, where it provides its enjoyable astringent taste. Some of these are caramel, nut, maple, butter, brandy, and fruit, which may be used in beverages, candy, bakery goods, ice cream, and liquors. Tannic acid is on the GRAS list, and studies show it to be safe. In fact, several studies have shown tannic acid to prevent growth of certain kinds of tumors to help prevent the formation of cancers in the first place. Tannic acid can stain the skin or irritate the stomach with higher doses, as with high intake of coffee or tea. In food use, where it is probably safe, it is not usually listed on the label.

Tartaric acid. Found in grapes, wine, and a few other fruits, as well as in coffee, it is also formed as a product of grape fermentation. In food processing, tartaric acid is used to augment flavoring and to adjust acidity in beverages, candy, jelly, baked goods, and frozen dairy products. It also acts as a stabilizing agent to prevent color or flavor changes because of rancidity. It is sometimes the acid component of baking powder. Tartaric acid may be a bit irritating to the gastrointestinal tract in large doses; in food use, however, it is safe. Studies show no toxicity, and it is on the GRAS list.

Tertiary butylhydroquinone, or T-butylhydroquinone (TBHQ). This butane gas derivative of petroleum is fairly new in food processing, where it is used as an antioxidant. It is often used along with BHA or BHT, but it may work alone to prevent rancidity of fatty foods, oils, and even low-fat products. It works best on unsaturated fats, particularly the vegetable oils, such as soy and safflower. TBHQ is the most recent antioxidant to be approved by the FDA. It is toxic in even modest amounts if ingested, but it is limited in foods to 0.02% of the fat and oil content (0.02% is the maximum content for antioxidant combinations as well). Because this chemical has been shown to be neurotoxic and to alter red blood cell activity, I suggest avoiding it, even at its currently restricted level.

Trichloroethylene (TCE). This chlorinated hydrocarbon related to vinyl chloride is a strong carcinogen. TCE is also a degreasing solvent. It is used in the process for decaffeinating coffee and in some spice preparations. It is not directly added to food, but it might be a contaminant; it is not be listed on the label. TCE has also been used in medicine as an analgesic and anesthetic. Like other chlorinated hydrocarbons, TCE is dangerous in any concentration when taken into the body. Because it and other solvents are used to make decaffeinated coffees and teas, it is wise to avoid these products. Water-processed decaf, even made from organic coffee beans, is now available.

Vanilla (vanillin, ethyl vanillin). This aromatic and flavorful substance is naturally found in the vanilla bean as well as in some other foods, such as potatoes. Vanillin and ethyl vanillin are stronger, synthetic analogues of vanilla, made from eugenol (an oil from cinnamon or clove). When natural vanilla is used as a food flavoring, it is listed as such. When the synthetic vanillas are used, they are probably listed only as artificial or imitation flavors. Vanilla and its analogs may be used in caramel, chocolate, root beer, butterscotch, butter, and some fruit flavorings for such foods as candy, ice cream, beverages, puddings, gelatin desserts, toppings, frostings, and even margarine. Vanilla, vanillin, and ethyl vanillin seem to be safe flavorings. Even when used in much higher amounts than they would be in foods, studies have shown no adverse effects. All are on the GRAS list.

Whey (whey protein concentrate, milk serum). Whey is the liquid part of milk left after the casein is removed, such as in cheese making. As I mentioned earlier, whey powders are sometimes bleached using benzoyl peroxide, however, so it is worth shopping for a powder that is benzoyl peroxide–free. Whey contains the lactalbumin protein and lactose or milk sugar. Whey can be dried to yield a mildly sweet, high-lactose powder containing such minerals as calcium, phosphorus, and potassium. Whey can be used complete, demineralized, or delactosed for certain purposes. It is used in a variety of foods, such as ice cream, candies, breakfast cereals, baked goods, and eggnog. Whey solids have been used as an extender and binder for meats, meat loaf, and sausage products. Whey protein may be used in powdered formulas for breakfast beverages, weight-control programs, or bodybuilding. All of these products are basically safe. People allergic to milk or with a lactose intolerance may have reactions to whey, however. In addition, when whey is obtained from nonorganic milk, it may retain some of the contaminants that were present in the milk—a good reason for going organic. Otherwise, whey products are well tolerated and may even be extremely helpful as nutritional supplements.

Xanthan gum. This complex carbohydrate is made commercially by fermenting corn sugar with *Xanthomonas campestris* bacteria. The gum formed is used commonly in food processing as an emulsifier and thickener, particularly in salad dressings to create a viscous, thick-pouring substance and to keep oil and water together in suspension. Xanthan gum is also used in dairy products and in low-calorie foods like puddings as a starch replacement. Xanthan gum in itself is safe. Tests show no hazards at very high levels. Often, however, the foods in which it is used are artificial and contain unnecessary chemicals, so I recommend avoiding them for that reason.

Xylitol. This simple carbohydrate alcohol, similar to sorbitol, is found naturally in some berries, fruits, and wood. Wood sugar, or xylose, is used to produce xylitol, a waste product of the wood-pulp industry. Birch is the most common type of tree for obtaining xylose, but other woods, like eucalyptus, can also be used. Once the xylose is obtained from the tree, it is usually fed to a yeast for conversion into xylitol. Finland is the main producer of this sugar. In chemical terms, xylitol is a sugar alcohol made from a pentose sugar (xylose) instead of from a hexose sugar like glucose. As a pentose-derived alcohol, xylitol is metabolized differently and therefore may be easier on the blood sugar and useful for diabetics. It is caloric like sugar, however, although it does not seem to promote dental decay (and may even help reduce cavities), so it is popular for use in chewing gums. It is found in many dietetic foods and beverages. Xylitol does not have as extensive use or research as some of the other sugar alcohols but seems relatively safe from studies so far. In fact, some fairly recent studies show a possible use for xylitol in the prevention of ear infections. Still, until more evidence is in, I suggest using the additive in moderation.

Yeast (baker's, brewer's, dried, nutritional, torula). Yeasts are unicellular fungi that are grown by fermentation of carbohydrates. Yeasts have a wide variety of uses in food processing and preparation and have been used for centuries. Enzymes in yeast help convert simple sugars to alcohol and carbon dioxide. Baker's yeast is used for making breads and baked goods. This type of yeast is different from most of the others available in the marketplace; baker's yeast is a raising yeast that is still active because it has been made from cream yeast at lower temperatures. For nutritional purposes, pick an inactive yeast that has been processed at a higher temperature. Although brewer's yeast is sometimes called "nutritional yeast," these two types are not usually the same. While both may involve the same genus and species of yeast *(Saccharomyces cerevisiae),* brewer's yeast is recovered after the beer brewing process, and its nutritional composition reflects the ingredients used in the beer making (like hops for example). Nutritional yeast is usually grown on a molasses solution specifically for use as a nutritional supplement. Both are safe (unless you are allergic to yeast or have yeast overgrowth) and both are rich in nutrients. These yeasts are particularly good sources of B vitamins, including folate, and at 4 grams of protein per tablespoon, they are a pretty good source of this nutrient as well.

Torula yeast can vary in quality depending on its production method. Sometimes torula is composed of the fungus *Pichia jadinii,* which may be grown on wood sugars from paper mill waste. But torula is also sometimes composed of *Candida utilis* and grown on higher-quality sugar sources like molasses. For this reason, it is best to ask about the source of the torula before purchasing. In addition to their use as nutritional supplements, yeasts are used to enrich refined flour products. Some foods that contain yeast are breads and other baked goods (as leavening and dough conditioners), including crackers, bread crumbs, and pretzels; alcoholic beverages; soup mixes and gravies; vinegars, ketchup, barbecue sauce, and other condiments; mushrooms; many vitamin preparations; and some dried fruits and herbs (as a contaminant).

Smoked yeast used as seasoning should be avoided because of the smoking process. And, as I mentioned earlier, some people are allergic to yeast or may experience intestinal gas, bloating, or indigestion with its use. People with overgrowth of intestinal yeast *(Candida albicans* or *Rhodotorula* spp.) should avoid all yeast-containing foods. Otherwise, yeast can be a nutritious, safe, and useful food additive.

OTHER FOOD AND HEALTH CONCERNS

In this section, I discuss a few of today's crucial food and environmental issues as well as their effects on our health and that of the precious planet. These areas of concern are discussed in the following sections:

1. Food irradiation

2. Microwaves

3. Meat quality and mad cow disease

4. Genetic modification of food

5. Electricity and electropollution

Food Irradiation

This involves short-term exposure of food, often in packaged form on ready-to-send shipping pallets, to electromagnetic radiation in the rage of 10^{-10} to 10^{-14} meters wavelength (million trillionths of a meter) and 1019 to 1022 Hz (one trillion trillion cycles per second). These extremely high-frequency and short-wavelength forces are called *gamma rays,* and the type of radiation is called *gamma radiation.* Irradiation of food has been legal in the United States for more than 35 years, and it is regulated by the FDA, which sets policy, and the USDA, which can order irradiation as a quarantine treatment for food being imported into this country or as an on-the-spot treatment following inspection of meat or poultry. Authorized use of irradiation is surprisingly broad. This sterilization technique is not only available for control of insects, parasites, and bacteria that can contaminate foods; it can also be used as a means of altering the natural life cycles of plants. For example, delaying the ripening of fruit and delaying sprouting of potatoes are approved uses of food irradiation. See the table below for the FDA-approved uses of irradiation.

When you look at the table, among the first things to notice is that the doses of radiation are extremely high in comparison to the doses received by living organisms. An average chest X-ray exposes the human body to approximately 10 millirads of radiation. This level is the same as 0.01 rad, or 300 million times smaller than the allowable dose applied to spices in the marketplace. Supporters of food irradiation have downplayed the difference in magnitude between medical and food irradiation by telling us that food irradiation is used on plants that are already dead, so the danger is nothing like that posed to a living human being. However, research suggests that this difference may not be quite so large. For example, just as radiation therapy has been shown to deplete vitamin B12 and vitamin D in cancer subjects, so has food irradiation been shown to deplete B vitamins as well as fat-soluble vitamins like A and E in irradiated food. Similarly, both human radiation therapy and food irradiation have been shown to alter cell structures and intracellular activity.

The jury is still out, however, on the exact health risks we face from consumption of irradiated food. Perhaps the highest-risk consequence that remains the subject of an unresolved debate is a genetic problem called *polyploidy*. Polyploidy refers to a condition in which 2 or more sets of chromosomes are created within the cells of an organism. Human cells, for example, ordinarily contain a single set of 46 chromosomes. A polyploid human cell might contain 2 sets (92 chromosomes), 3 sets (138 chromosomes), or even more sets of chromosomes. In humans, this type of cell change happens very rarely.

In the early 1970s, about 10 years after irradiation had been approved for use on wheat, a series of studies showed increased polyploidy in the cells of both animals and humans fed irradiated wheat. The nature of these studies, however, left them open to many different interpretations, and follow-up studies have not really clarified the issues involved. So, we are still left with an enormous amount of irradiated food in the food supply, and no clear research understanding of its safety. **For this reason, I think irradiated food should be avoided as much as possible.** I encourage manufacturers and government regulators to look at the real issues underlying food irradiation, which are further discussed in the next section on microwaves.

FDA-Approved Uses of Food Irradiation

Food	Date of Approval	Dose Permitted (rads)	Approved Purpose
Wheat/wheat powder	1963	20,000–50,000	insect decontamination
White potatoes	1965	5,000–15,000	prevention of sprouting
Spices/seasonings	1983	3,000,000	insect decontamination
Dehydrated enzymes	1985	1,000,000	insect decontamination
Pork	1985	30,000–100,000	parasite decontamination
Fresh fruit	1986	100,000	delayed ripening
Dry vegetables	1986	3,000,000	microbe decontamination
Poultry	1990	300,000	microbe decontamination
Beef, lamb	1997	450,000 (fresh)	microbe decontamination
		700,000 (frozen)	microbe decontamination

U.S. Food and Drug Administration, *FDA Consumer*, May-June 1998, Publication No. (FDA) 98-232

Microwaves

Many people confuse the idea of irradiation with the idea of microwaving, but these technologies are very different. Irradiation uses gamma rays—a type of ionizing radiation with extremely high frequencies that are powerful and penetrating. Microwaves, though, are a type of nonionizing radiation occurring at vastly lower frequencies with much less ability to penetrate. Microwaves are fully absorbed by the water found in foods, and heat is produced in this process, cooking the food by heating up the water molecules. Gamma rays, in contrast to microwaves, are so deeply penetrating that they are difficult to fully absorb, so they not only impact the water found in food but the cell structures as well. It is this ability to alter cell structures that make gamma rays effective against bacteria.

Numerous studies have been conducted about the effects of microwave radiation on humans, particularly following the Korean War, where many members of the military were exposed for the first time to microwave radiation in the form of radar signals. (Radar waves are the same as microwaves.) No adverse health effects—including altered risk of cancer—have been found in these studies involving nonionizing radiation. There are plenty of studies showing enzyme deactivation in microwaved foods, and changes in food color or taste that correspond to this enzyme deactivation. But these consequences occur with any type of cooking and are a result of heat rather than wave source. A recent study has suggested that microwave cooking may deplete nutrients in food much more than researchers originally expected. However, even this study is open to interpretation, because the loss of nutrients in the food corresponded to the use of more water and longer cooking times in the microwave oven. So the overcooking may explain the results of this study better than the nature of the microwave oven. All of this is not to say that microwave cooking is absolutely safe, however. There is not enough evidence to arrive at that conclusion. But researchers also do not have evidence of chronic health risk from the use of this energy source.

Microwave packaging is a clear exception in this health risk area. **No one should microwave in plastic!** In fact, most everything we put in the microwave should be removed from its original container and placed in glass, Pyrex, or nonleaded microwavable ceramic. Plastic chemicals leech into microwaved foods from plastic packaging, and these chemicals (like DEHA, DEHP, MEHP, or PET) increase the risk of cancer. They also disrupt the energy production processes in our cells and the chemical messaging from cell to cell. Even brief reheating in the microwave should not be done in plastic. Unfortunately, this even includes the more durable plastic containers that are specifically sold for microwave use.

The first microwave oven to be sold in the marketplace cost $1,300 in 1952. Today 9 out of 10 U.S. households have a microwave oven, and total retail sales for microwavable frozen meals is about $28 billion every year. Most microwaves cost under $100 nowadays. Until there is better evidence about the long-term impact of microwaving on our health, I suggest the following approach: **First, limit use of the microwave to reheating.** This approach will decrease the amount of time foods are exposed to microwave radiation, because actual cooking in the microwave takes longer. **Second, reheat foods in the microwave to a slightly hotter temperature than required.** Microwave heating is fast, but the heat distribution is uneven and follows moisture pockets in the food. For dishes that can be stirred or rotated, both of these steps help to promote even heat distribution. **Third, do not stand in front of the oven door when microwaving,** and if the microwave is old and may possibly have developed a leak, consider purchase of a replacement. **Fourth, take precautions to avoid steam burns** when handling microwave foods by using an oven mitt or potholder and by paying close attention. **Finally, stop microwaving in plastic.**

Meat Quality and Mad Cow Disease

The story of mad cow disease is one of the most remarkable of all stories about food quality, although it is a saga that has yet to receive an ending. The story starts in the 1980s in western Europe, when many cattle began showing symptoms of a nervous system disease in which they lost their ability to do many normal things, including walk. In 1993, the occurrence of this disease reached its peak with more than 100,000 cattle affected. Yet even at the time of this writing, despite a downturn in the number of cattle affected, researchers still do not understand exactly what took place or what is currently taking place. The first case of this disease in the United States occurred in December 2003, with cases in Japan (2001) and Israel (2002) occurring in between.

At first, scientists assumed that this disease must involve some kind of virus, but that assumption turned out to be incorrect (or so we think). The carriers of this disease are simply proteins, although they are not identical to the kind of proteins that we are accustomed to talking about in nutrition. The new type of proteins that appeared responsible for this nervous system disease in cows were named *prions*—a shorthand for "proteinaceous infectious particles." Prions seem capable of reproducing themselves, and they probably do a variety of good things for cows and for humans. In the case of this disease, however, they seem to be excessively produced and to disrupt the activity of the nerve cells. The prion-based disease affecting the cows was given the scientific name *bovine spongiform encephalopathy* (BSE) and the common name became mad cow disease. Scientists are now convinced that a similar disease in humans, variant Creutzfeldt-Jakob disease (CJD), can occur following consumption of meat from cattle with BSE.

But what caused the problems with the prion proteins in cattle? Researchers still are not sure. Many researchers believe that the prion proteins were transmitted to the cattle through incorporation of sheep parts into the cattle feed (for example, incorporation of sheep brain into meat and bonemeal protein supplements for the cattle). The reason for this belief is that sheep also get a prion-related disease, called *scrapie,* and many of the cattle with BSE had been given feed containing sheep parts. However, other facts surrounding BSE are not at all consistent with this assumption. Mark Purdey, a farmer and researcher in Somerset, England, has published several medical hypotheses linking the prion problems in BSE to a unique combination of events that includes exposure to organophosphate pesticides, manganese toxicity, and copper deficiency. His research looks at agricultural practices, mining practices, and other ecologically disruptive events as the key underlying factors in development of prion-related disease.

Regardless of the relationship between prions and mad cow disease, there are steps that anyone eating

beef can take to reduce the risk of consuming BSE-infected meat. The first would be to purchase organically grown beef, because these cattle should not have been exposed to any animal products in their feed. Organic cattle are also, of course, fed only organic feeds. Second would be to choose cuts of beef that are likely to be free of nervous system tissue. Boneless cuts would be the best bet, including boneless steaks, chops, and roasts. Bone-in cuts would probably carry the next lowest risk, including T-bone, porterhouse, and prime rib with the bone. Beef extracts, beef jerky, and some beef hot dogs in which AMR (advanced meat recovery) machines are used to get meat off the carcass would probably be the most risky in terms of contamination. **And overall, for a healthier planet, consume less red meat: the land currently used to raise cattle could feed so many more people if farmers could use some of that land to raise other foods.**

The phenomenon of mad cow disease is not the only time the United States has seen some potentially scary health problems regarding meat. On August 21, 1997, 25 million pounds of beef processed at a meat-packing plant in Columbus, Nebraska, were recalled for fear of contamination with the bacterium E. coli O157:H7. This recall was the largest in U.S. history, and although it was voluntarily carried out by Hudson Foods, the recall actually came at the insistence of the U.S. Department of Agriculture and political pressure following the announcement by Burger King that it would no longer buy beef from Hudson Foods. Fortunately, no deaths were attributed to this batch of contaminated meat, but reports of E. coli poisoning were received as close by as the Colorado Department of Public Health and as far away as Gainesville, Florida.

In response to the E. coli threat in beef and a petition from the Hudson Foods Company, the FDA announced its decision in December 1997 to allow irradiation of beef. This decision was applauded for its responsiveness to a major public health threat but also heavily criticized by environmental groups for failing to address the real reasons for beef contamination. Food researchers have a pretty good idea how E. coli got into the beef in the first place, and the relevant factors have been nicely summarized by Least Cost Formulations, a food consulting company based in Virginia Beach, Virginia. These factors include the failure of ranchers to wash manure off cattle before sending them to market; the failure of ranchers to stop feeding animals at least half a day before slaughter, thus reducing their intestinal contents and lessening the chance of bursting at slaughter; the practice of packagers like Hudson to reuse "reworked" (broken or poorly formed) meat patties 2 and 3 days after initial processing, thus extending the risk of contamination; the failure of workers at fast food restaurants to cook ground beef to 160 degrees Fahrenheit; the lack of E. coli testing at multiple points along the beef production process; and the failure of governmental agencies like the USDA and the FDA to set and enforce regulations preventing all of these failures.

I have concluded from this series of events that from a health standpoint, we have no business trying to salvage millions of pounds of potentially infected beef through irradiation. We need to find other ways to lower the risk of contamination, and the best place to start is in the cow's immediate environment, which is all too often unnatural, unhealthy, and nonsustainable. The threat of mad cow disease has pointed us in the exact same direction as the E. coli O157:H7 scare: toward a closer look at remedying imbalances in the environment as a way of increasing long-term food safety.

The Genetic Modification of Food

One place we are not going to find any long-term answers is in the realm of genetically modified food. The introduction of genetically modified (GM) foods into the U.S. marketplace has been swift and far-reaching. About 70% of all products currently sitting on grocery store shelves are estimated to contain some genetically modified component. The two most likely components are soy and corn, because half of the world's soybeans and a third of the country's corn are genetically engineered. So are most of our tomatoes and potatoes, as well as dozens of other foods. More than 50 GM crops are approved for sale in the United States, and GM acreage has grown from 0 acres in 1994 to about 75 million today. So you see, it is not a lightweight problem even though many people in this country and the world have fears about these so-called Frankenfoods. About 1,000 patents have already been granted for GM foods, and almost none of these patents have been granted for nutritional purposes.

Foods are being genetically engineered to facilitate mechanical harvesting, to allow for planting before the end of the frost-free period, to resist insects, or to resist pesticide sprays, but almost never to improve their nutritional contents. Companies are seeking to control the licensing of seeds and controlling crops, which provides more money and power, but less freedom for farmers and growers.

Much of the above activity has happened unbeknownst to the consumer, because there are no labeling requirements with respect to genetically modified food in the United States, and because the FDA decided in 1992 that GM foods should be handled on a basis of "substantial equivalence." This principle stated that a genetically engineered food was really no different than a naturally occurring one so long as it resembled its natural counterpart in terms of aesthetics, nutrition, and "anti-nutrition." In other words, as long as the modified food was the same color and shape, had most of the same vitamins and minerals, and contained the same kind of nutrient binding agents or other modifying factors as the nonmodified food, it does not matter whether it was genetically engineered or not.

Unfortunately, however, it does matter. For millions of years, plants have evolved alongside of each other and other organisms. They have also evolved within the context of the seasons, regional weather patterns, and local soil conditions, despite dealing with chemical pesticides and herbicides. Scientists now manipulate the "sp" gene in tomato plants to control how far out on the stem tomatoes are formed. By controlling this distance, we can make it easier for the machine that cuts the tomatoes off the plant to do its job. Until recently, however, the decision about where to form a tomato has been left to the tomato plant, which in turn has looked to the arc of the sun, the structure of the soil, the placement of surrounding plants, and many other factors to make its decision. The dance between plants and insects, between plants and soil bacteria, between plants and the position of the sun— all of these delicately coordinated movements are discarded when a plant is genetically engineered.

As with the consumption of irradiated food, very little research exists on the health effects of GM food. One research scientist at the Rowett Research Institute in Scotland, Arpad Pusztai, lost his job at the institute after

36 years of research for publishing articles that raised questions about the health impact of GM food. Pusztai fed GM potatoes to rats and found unexpected changes in their digestive tracts, including thickening of their stomach lining and scattered thinning of their intestinal lining. There was also some excessive stimulation of cell growth in certain areas of the small intestine. Researchers and the public at large do not know how to interpret these results, except to say that they clearly indicate a need for more research until the health consequences of consumption of GM foods become clearer. To me, it makes sense to believe until proven otherwise that GM foods may cause allergic-type reactions and immune dysregulation and possibly contribute to cancer. Until scientists are sure of long-term safety, **I recommend avoiding GM foods as much as possible. One of the best strategies for doing so is by purchasing organic foods, because genetic engineering of food is not allowed under the Organic Foods Production Act that serves as the basis for all nationally certified organics.**

Electricity and Electropollution

It may be hard to accept that something we cannot sense, something that all of us depend on daily at home and work, might be an actual problem in our modern lives—yet electricity may fit into this category. **I have concern that excessive exposure to environmental electricity, electromagnetic radiation (EMR), can be a danger to our health and may even be a factor in carcinogenesis.**

After all, the body is an electromagnetic generator; its electrical potential can be measured in the cells and nerves as well as in the heart and all of the muscles. In fact, many vital functions in the body depend on the electrical energy generated by ionic movement of minerals across cell membranes. An electromagnetic force field can also be measured around the body, and our life force or vitality influences the strength of this field. In fact, we vibrate with direct, not alternating, current, and at very specific frequencies (or hertz, Hz). Why then, wouldn't it make sense that certain machines, wires, homes, and businesses could vibrate or contain EMR at levels that are either harmonious or discordant with the body's own vibration levels? Machines and power lines all have

fields of electricity surrounding them that could be hazardous to our biological force. Overhead power lines, especially high-voltage ones, have been among the main aspects of EMR that may be negatively affecting those who live close to them. The higher frequency radiations, from X-rays to nuclear radiation, are clearly dangerous.

EMR can be divided into two categories. The first is **ionizing radiation** and includes X-rays, gamma rays, and nuclear radiation. Exposing the body to these highly reactive ions at certain levels can dramatically affect the atomic structure. Ionizing radiation can actually rip electrons from atoms and molecules and directly affect cell division and cell structure. It causes problems initially in areas of our bodies that have a rapid cellular turnover, such as the skin, the gastrointestinal tract, and blood.

Nonionizing radiation includes the forms of EMR below 300 Hz, or cycles per second (cps), and notably the 60 Hz alternating currents that power our homes and offices. This form of energy does not clearly destroy the cellular function, but it can "shake" the micro matter, and at higher frequencies, this shaking generates both vibrational changes and heat. This is how microwaves work, by increasing the vibration of the water molecules in the food, which then generates heat. At the lower end of the nonionizing radiation frequencies, ranging from 30 Hz to 100 Hz, this effect is less, and the consequences are not known. The supposition here and in current research, however, is that exaggerated or regular exposure to this extremely low frequency (ELF) level of electricity, such as many hours per day surrounded by or working with electrical objects or wires, is hazardous to our health. Studies have shown 50 Hz exposures to impair sleep and to disrupt some of the chemical communication between cells. Other studies have shown little connection, however, between exposure to 50 Hz energy and some of the chemical benchmarks of sleep—for example, increased melatonin production. I suspect the research will eventually establish a clear connection between these lower frequency energies and a wide variety of health problems.

Electropollution is generated by the constant use and wide variety of electronic instruments and lines. Electricity and other forms of radio waves are how we connect and communicate with each other. Common electropollution components include computers, underground radio transmitter grids, medical imaging, and high-voltage power lines. Home devices that may affect us include hair dryers and electric blankets. Some common avenues of electrical exposure are seen in the table above.

Earth's vibration is approximately 10 Hz, which is in the alpha, or resting, range of the brain. The ELF common range of 45 Hz to 70 Hz of most machinery and power lines is close enough to the vibrations of the body and that of Earth that it influences us, mainly in the sense of agitation or stimulation. These vibrations most assuredly influence our biocycles and, clearly, changes in magnetic energy must alter us as well. I am sure that it also may affect the ability to sleep and rest deeply, as well as increase levels of stress and fatigue. **Research has shown that the pineal gland, which produces serotonin and melatonin and may be at the core of the entire endocrine system, is affected not only by light but also by magnetic fields.** The seasonal light and dark cycles of each day appear to regulate our psycho-emotional being through the pineal gland.

Many birds, insects, and reptiles daily use Earth's natural magnetic influence of 10 Hz (this is the primary frequency of the brain in most animals) for their movement and in structural sense of direction. Subtle changes in magnetism alter their behavior. Research with homing pigeons has clearly shown this. Even the growing patterns and movements of bacteria are influenced by magnetic fields. Atmospheric ionic gases, solar and lunar influences, and the metallic core of Earth all affect its electromagnetic vibration. Electromagnetic energy changes in Earth's field seem to affect responses in animals, as observed in their behavior before earthquakes and dramatic weather shifts; clearly, many species can sense these changes.

Electromagnetic fields (EMFs) also affect the most vital body systems, particularly the central nervous system (CNS) as well as the cardiovascular, endocrine, and immune systems. Similar effects and changes occur with microwaves, radio waves, and electrical and magnetic fields. In the CNS, brain chemistry may be altered, particularly in the hypothalamus and cerebral cortex. Microwave exposure clearly affects stress levels and mood shifts. Possible changes in electron transfer in cellular mitochondria may also occur and thus reduce general energy levels. Research into depression and suicide shows a relationship to EMR exposure. In the cardiovascular system, heart efficiency, oxygen capacity, and hemoglobin and red blood cell levels are all reduced, as is the sodium-potassium response, which is at the base of body electricity (membrane electrical potentials). Immunologically, there is a decreased response. This "electrical" system leaves a large area open for exploration, and some researchers theorize that the current increase in such infectious diseases as herpes, AIDS, and Lyme disease is correlated with changes in EMFs. Cancer and leukemias may also be associated with more specific exposures. The endocrine system is probably influenced by EMR, although research is needed to verify this; thyroid and pituitary functions are additional concerns.

Magnetic fields are measured in gauss. The level found near high-voltage power lines and many high-current appliances is 1 gauss. Government research has revealed that humans in the presence of a 1 gauss field demonstrate reduced performance in adding sets of numbers and in short-term memory than when not surrounded by this type of electromagnetic field. High-voltage power lines, which generate a constant irritating hum, have been studied more than other EMF effects regarding their influence on human behavior and disease. In the 1980s some concerned residents in England living near power lines complained of an increase in headaches, lethargy, memory loss, and the recurrence of illness. Local farmers observed that their vegetable growth and crop production were reduced. Cattle that grazed by the power lines showed lower milk production and more birth defects.

In 1979, researchers Edward Leeper and Nancy Wertheimer reported increased cancer and leukemia rates in children who lived near high-voltage power lines. Other researchers in the United States and Sweden have had similar findings. Researchers working out of the Institute of Environmental Medicine at the Karolinska Institute in Stockholm, Sweden, published findings in 1993 showing a connection between risk of childhood leukemia and residence near high-voltage power lines. An increase in the incidence of brain tumors in electricians, electronic technicians, and utility line workers has also been shown. Pregnant women who sleep under electric blankets have a higher incidence of miscarriages than other pregnant women. EMFs appear to stimulate microbial growth and cell division; this is possibly related to an increased incidence of infections in people who have high exposure. Since the mid-1970s, there has been a higher incidence of birth defects, infertility, and cancer; this may be related to higher levels of electrical exposure, although studies have yet to prove this.

Other than some specific electrical concerns, I believe we are dealing with a total body electrical load, or exposure, regarding these health effects. Making a drink in a blender, cooking on an electric stove, or even using a microwave on occasion are probably minimal risks unless we are particularly sensitive. I see a lot of businesspeople, office workers, airline staff, and medical workers in my practice who receive regular exposure, such as 10 to 12 hours daily, to electrical machinery, computers, and hospital equipment. Most of these people seem to get sick or burned-out more easily, are less able to handle stress, and generally do not appear as vital as those people who work in more natural environments. In my practice as well as in the nutrition courses I teach, I have become aware of the high level of stress and burnout among nurses; fatigue and recurrent infectious illnesses were most common.

Most people who work around electrical machinery, such as nurses, wear rubber-soled shoes. This may reduce the risk of electrocution, but it does not allow them to clear (ground) the electromagnetism they pick up from their surroundings. When I do some form of massage on my patients, I feel uncomfortable whenever I wear my rubber-soled shoes, because I cannot easily clear the energy I pick up from them. Some bodyworkers are adversely affected because they get congested or weakened when they work on others. If we remove our shoes, however, the body is then a conduit for electromagnetic energy, and we can clear ourselves of electricity or another's magnetic energy more easily.

To help balance electromagnetism and electropollution after working around electrical devices, the Earth itself as well as water can be quite helpful. Showering, bathing, or swimming are good ideas. Instead of or in addition to bathing, we can go outdoors and put our bare feet on Mother Earth (grass or dirt) for a few minutes to help ground ourselves and clear body electricity.

In *The Body Electric* and in his companion work, *Cross Currents: The Promise of Electromedicine, the Perils of Electropollution*, Robert O. Becker, MD, has discussed many of the current theories and research about EMR as well as our internal electrical vibration, external electricity and electropollution, and the use of electricity in medicine and healing. The right vibration of electrical energy used correctly may increase the body's own healing forces. Electricity can also be used to stimulate regrowth and regeneration. The body's ability to regenerate and heal may be even more profound than scientists have thought, especially with the right bioelectrical support. Becker describes many cases of this in animal studies and, most spectacularly, in children under 12, who have the ability to grow back a normal fingertip if it is severed above the first crease. In these cases, when surgeons attempted to repair the wound or to sew the finger back, it did not heal as well as when left alone to regenerate anew with bioelectrical support.

Clearly, electropollution is a controversial topic. It has wide political and economic concerns, and it is unlikely that either the government or electric companies would admit to much danger after more than 50 years of use. Yet research may show that certain frequencies may be disruptive to cellular resonance. It is possible that the rates of extremely low electrical frequencies (30–100 Hz) that are in common use interfere more with biochemical impulses or the cell rate for release and absorption of calcium, for example, than might a higher frequency (400 Hz). More research is clearly needed. Burying the big power lines may help reduce some electropollution but could cause other problems as well.

Researchers do not really know the safe level of EMR exposure. With the increased use of EMR and subsequent electropollution ranging from hair dryers to power lines to nuclear radiation, our concerns should grow; continuous or regular high exposure of any type of EMR seems to create problems. From stress activation to impaired cellular growth processes and immune response to increased cancer rates and reproductive problems, there is also a wide range of potential effects. **The combined concerns of EMR and toxic chemical exposure may be an even greater dilemma in upcoming decades as the magnitude of exposures and accumulation of exposures increase.** The U.S. government as well as those of the global community at large have their work ahead of them. We need more regulation regarding pollution of all sorts, perhaps even electropollution in particular.

The art and science of geomancy, carried on throughout the centuries, studies Earth's forces and energy lines and may provide insight for those people who want to live in areas of lower geopathic stress and to avoid areas of electropollution and negative influences from the Earth. Home planning and building

with this in mind as well as clearing negative forces from existing homes and workplaces are part of the future. Learning to live in harmony with the Earth's electromagnetic fields is a part of living in harmony with Nature and its laws.

We all need to address the concerns in this chapter—for ourselves and our families as well as for better health. We must deal with electrical exposure and GM foods. Chemical use is part of all aspects of life; chemistry is here to stay. The question is, "Do we have better living through chemistry?" Learning to live with chemicals and to use them appropriately so that they do not destroy us or the planet is my fervent hope. **On an individual level, this involves maintaining a healthy immune system, a positive attitude, and a high purpose in which there is care for everything found in the natural world.** Protecting ourselves by reducing chemical usage and exposure greatly reduces our chances of disease, cancer, and early death. This is important for everyone, but especially for the chemically sensitive, our infants and young children, the elderly, and invalids, all of whom are more susceptible to chemical toxicity. Making changes and a commitment to living as chemically free as possible is a strong investment in one's personal and collective life insurance plan.

For more specific practical information on how to survive healthfully in these modern times, see "Personal and Planetary Survival in the 21st Century," on page 783 in the Futureword. You will also find my "88 Survival Suggestions" on page 785 in the Futureword. Stay Healthy by making wise and conscientious choices in all you do.

Due to changing weather patterns, chemical use, and genetic modification of food, our beautiful monarch butterfly population as well as other migratory beings, plus all other insects and animals, are suffering and are challenged to extinction. This is not the way to go. What can we do?

Be the Guardian

Protect what we have left

Do not lose

Please choose Life.

You're next!

—Bethany Argisle

Part 3

Building a Healthy Diet

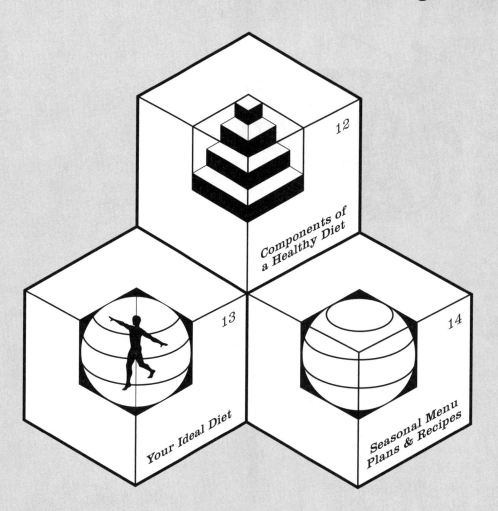

Components of
a Healthy Diet

12

Your Ideal Diet

13

Seasonal Menu
Plans & Recipes

14

In the previous chapters of this book, many aspects of a healthy diet are discussed—the macronutrients (proteins, fats, carbohydrates), the micronutrients (vitamins and minerals), as well as various food groups, possible diets, and nutritional habits, including drinking uncontaminated water and breathing clean air. Now, in these next three chapters, let's put all of this positive information and philosophy together into a healthy diet.

Chapter 12, The Components of a Healthy Diet, further explores food groups and discusses proper dietary balance. Chapter 13 defines the Ideal Diet. Based on diets of the world in people who live close to Nature and eat a natural diet, the Ideal Diet is oriented to the highest good of the individual, the world population, and the Earth itself. Nowadays, there is often a great difference between a culture's rural and urban diets, especially in highly industrialized societies. One of the biggest needs in the technological age is to learn to shift the focus from processed food, the supermarket, fast foods and quick meals to a diet made primarily from the garden with family-oriented, home-cooked meals. Really, God and Nature have already provided us with the means to create and sustain this ideal diet.

The diet also needs to be individual and intuitive. Our cultural upbringing and individual needs are important influences, and learning to listen to our bodies from day to day and season to season is a crucial aspect of creating and maintaining a healthy diet. This ideal diet is based on current knowledge on the part of researchers, clinicians, educators, and all health-conscious individuals about foods and their positive and negative effects on humans, beyond a moral judgment about eating animals or being vegetarian. The ideal diet is an integration of many current ideas and is primarily vegetarian, with some low-fat, good-quality protein foods such as fish and consciously raised poultry for those interested as well as a low intake of milk products for adults.

Currently, less than 1% of the United States population is vegetarian (although this percentage is growing), so we must be realistic to find the proper balance and use of all foods.

This book is not another among the multitude of fad diet books. What we really need to create is a long-term, even lifelong diet that will keep our bodies in their optimum state. Throughout chapters 12 through 14, I provide you with the knowledge to be able to make proper choices and create a healthy diet and way of life, forever. The idea is to transform our diet and eating habits so they work, not just to go on a diet to improve health or lose a few pounds and then return to our old habits. Scientists, practitioners, and dieters know that does not work; rather, we want a diet that nourishes us optimally for life. So the main question is, "What are the basic components that provide the needed nutrients, and how can these foods be prepared and combined to make the best possible diet for us?"

Building a healthy diet is like creating a meal. As we might choose a number of particular foods to make a meal, so too might we mix many foods and food groups together over days, weeks, and months to create our diet. No single diet is perfect for everyone. Each of us has likes and dislikes, often based on the body's chemistry and needs. We have genetic and family backgrounds, our basic foods, and our special feast or celebration foods. We have

our own particular eating patterns and habits regarding foods and even chemicals and substances such as caffeine and sugar. These are what we begin with. Then we must sort out what works and what we need to change to improve our diet and our lifelong health.

Sometimes we must totally change our diet. I know many people who have completely transformed their ways of eating and have made big improvements in their health. I for one used to eat the basic American diet—lots of hamburgers, french fries, and sodas; milk, ice cream, and cookies; peanut butter and jelly on white bread; more meats and chicken; and a sparse amount of fresh fruits and vegetables. I was overweight and congested in a lot of ways as a result of this rich, unbalanced diet. I decided to use fasting as a means to clear old patterns, and then I began eating a more natural and vegetarian diet, continuing this process of slow detoxification, much of which I discussed in my first book, *Staying Healthy with the Seasons.* Since the early 1980s, I have continued to adapt my diet to the seasons and my personal needs, maintaining a natural, primarily vegetarian diet. See chapter 14, Seasonal Menu Plans and Recipes, for some healthy ideas in this regard. And for more recipes to go along with the diet guidelines discussed in these next three chapters, see my companion recipe book, *A Cookbook for All Seasons.*

Chapter 12

The Components of a Healthy Diet

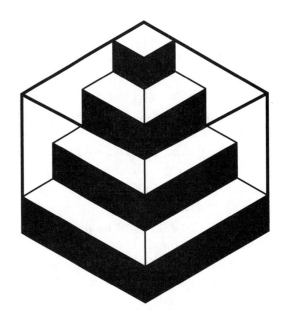

There are many components involved in a healthful diet that can be made quite simple. Nutrition has gotten very complex, and there is a continual flood of new information, both insightful truth as well as propaganda, surfacing daily in the news and various publications. Even though this book provides an immense amount of information, I have attempted to make it simple and easily accessible—easy to digest, assimilate, and use. Basically, though, we need to return to our own instincts of proper nutrition.

Our natural locale provides the best and most wholesome foods available to us. Local stores, however, have a continuing fancy array of new packages, boxes, and cans hyped by equally flashy advertising to entice us to buy these products. Profitability is the key motivation in the food industry, and much of what consumers buy is the packaging and advertising, which often costs more than the actual food in the product. If we take some of this big business money and pay all the mothers and fathers and sisters and brothers to grow food and prepare wholesome, natural meals, we would take a big step in the health and well being of ourselves as well as our planet. This may sound revolutionary when done on

a mass level, but it is exactly what we need to do individually—go back to the basics and redevelop our own nutrition. To do this, we need to transform our thinking and the conditioning of an entire century of misguided advertising that has so strongly influenced and molded the diets of many generations of Americans as well as nutrition worldwide. To begin with, I look at one of the earlier misconceptions that is still taught in most of our nation's schools—four food group nutrition.

FOOD GROUPS: OLD AND NEW

This complex, important concept regarding the basics of our diet is a challenging area of nutrition. For nearly a century, mainstream nutritional thought was centered on the "basic four" food groups—meats, dairy products, cereal grains, and fruits and vegetables. But there are many health-care practitioners and health advocates who feel that this approach, the result of a large advertising campaign that was perpetrated and perpetuated through the highly industrialized twentieth century, is archaic, unhealthy, and part of the reason for the large increase in the chronic degenerative diseases in the United States.

The "basic four" approach has been difficult to change. The main reason is that Americans have been conditioned to believe that these are equally important categories of foods, and that animal, bird, or fish meats, as well as milk, butter, and eggs, are crucial parts of a good meal (and they are yummy for the moment, just as sweets are). This belief is exemplified in the public school cafeteria diet. All of these foods, of course, can be used and are nutritionally helpful, but only in modest amounts—not as 2 out of 4 of the main food groups and not at the level currently consumed by the average person (clearly not at 50% of the diet). Actually, if these meats and dairy foods were all removed from the diets of anyone older than 18 (as well as from the diets of pregnant or nursing mothers), United States society would be much healthier. Even though these foods stimulate growth, younger children need far fewer of these high-protein, high-fat foods than you might think. For goodness sake, I ate plenty of salami and fried bologna sandwiches with mayo on white bread. Protein deficiency is highly unlikely in a balanced diet, as are most mineral and vitamin deficits, and we need less protein to maintain health than most people assume.

Another area of resistance to changing the "basic four" has been the food industry. Billions of dollars have been spent in creating and advertising products that are less healthy for us than the basic foods that Nature provides. And many of the high-fat, high-salt, and high-sugar foods are so intensely promoted that the profit-oriented industry often has more influence on diet and health than do informed parents and nutritionists. (And, of course, it has also worked the other way around. The glitzy array of low-fat, low-sugar, and low-sodium foods has not proven any better for health. Since the introduction of these "about face" products, for example, there has been an increase in the incidence of obesity and diabetes.) We are convinced by distorted advertising to try these new boxes, cans, and frozen treats that imitate natural wholesome foods and create refuse for the Earth as well as for our bodies. Thus this concept of the "basic four," created by the power and advertising of the food industry giants—the dairy, meat, and breakfast cereal industries—and supported by the medical establishment and educational

system, left the farmer with only one category to cover all the nourishing fruits and vegetables.

Of course, in 1992 the U.S. Department of Agriculture (USDA) debuted its now famous (and infamous) Food Guide Pyramid. Many observers looked at this event as marking a positive change in the American approach to eating. I was not one of them. Although the shape of the Food Guide Pyramid may have suggested less meat, milk, and sweets in comparison to fruits, vegetables, and other whole natural plant foods, the politics and the numbers suggested otherwise. Thanks to Marion Nestle, professor and Nutrition Department chair at New York University, and her impeccably well-researched book *Food Politics,* we know exactly what happened with the Food Pyramid. In April 1991, a matter of weeks after preliminarily introducing it to the general public, the USDA withdrew the Food Pyramid following demands from the National Milk Producers Federation and the National Cattlemen's Association. These organizations believed the pyramid would cause Americans to eat less beef and drink less milk. The pyramid was then renegotiated. In the new pyramid, the meat allowance stayed at 2 servings per day, but the recommended amount was changed from 4 to 6 ounces to 5 to 7 ounces. In addition, the actual graphic look of the pyramid was changed to make servings of meats and dairy look like minimum required amounts. In short, milk and meat retained a place of prominence.

Some people have argued that fruit and vegetable intake, fiber intake, and low-fat foods gained a prominence in the pyramid that was missing in the traditional four food groups arrangement. I disagree, however. The *combined* fruit and vegetable recommendations in the pyramid add up to 5 to 9 servings per day. But processed fruit juices containing no pulp and no fiber, as well as potatoes—including french fries!—are counted as fruits and vegetables in this scheme. On top of that, we are asked to have *more* servings from the bread, cereal, rice, and pasta group (6 to 11 servings), with qualifying foods from the group including fiber-free white bread, fiber-free salted pretzels, doughnuts, and cookies! Not much of a time-out from the high-fat, high-salt, high-sugar routine that is prevalent in U.S. culture. And as a major uneducated consumer, my body learned the hard way with extra weight, allergies and congestion, and sluggishness.

In 2005, the U.S. government unleashed a new food pyramid with rainbow colors and all. I am sure we will continue to fine-tune this pyramid over the coming years, and it does continue to improve to reflect a healthier eating program, definitely a vast improvement over the original "four food group" plan.

Finding the proper balance and mix of these foods is the first important step in creating a healthy diet. A starch-centered diet—that is, a diet based on complex-carbohydrates—has been the native or traditional diet throughout the world for the past 1,000 years. This allows the main foods to be high in nutrients and low in calories, with a substantial fiber intake. The food sources for these carbohydrates, however, are not exactly what you might think. Although the traditional cereal grains like wheat play an important role in overall food balance, 17 cereal grains are found on a global scale, including such grains as sorghum and millet. The overall complex-carbohydrate balance includes substantial amounts of the pulses (dry beans, dry peas, chickpeas, and lentils) as well as root crops (cassava, taro, and yam). So when I talk about "starch-centered" here, I am not talking about platefuls of pasta or rice but about many foods that are rarely represented in the typical U.S. diet. The high fiber content of the vegetables and whole grains allows them to be less caloric, as the vegetable fiber material is not used as energy.

Which carbohydrate is used, however, may vary with the culture. Traditional Asian cultures used mainly rice, for example, with some wheat; the Indian diet was similar, with more wheat; in the Middle East, the staple was wheat; and in Africa, sorghum was the second-most-important cereal, and cassava (manioc) was the most important root crop in terms of food security. Europeans ate wheat and potatoes, and the Native Americans used a large amount of corn (also called maize). These cultures also used some peas or beans to balance the grains and make complete proteins, and then many local vegetables were added. This primary diet was usually supplemented with smaller amounts of seasonal fruits, milk products, and animal foods.

As technology developed over the centuries, however, richer living meant richer foods. Meats, eggs, cheeses, and milk became associated with success, as did eating out in "rich food" restaurants, and then high-fat, high-calorie fast food places. No longer did we need to hunt and move with the seasons. We could pen animals and milk or slaughter them for food. **With more technology, shelf life replaced health life.** A rejection of the "peasants'" diet went hand in hand with this high-fat diet. The refinement of foods was also part of this move up. None of these factors has improved nutrition. In fact, many of them have been steps backward in terms of nutritional health.

A NEW BASIC FOUR

What we need is a new basic four food group arrangement. The new basics start with 10 basic food groups, the foods Nature provides, the whole-food ingredients of the diet: fruits, vegetables, whole grains, legumes (beans and peas), nuts, seeds, dairy products and eggs, fish, fowl, and meats. The new basic four consists of fruits, vegetables, whole grains and legumes, as well as proteins and fats/oils (nuts and seeds for the vegetarian, and milk, eggs, and meats for the omnivore).

This is really not very different from the old basic four, but it is the first step in a transition to a healthier diet. The main thrust is the de-emphasis on the meats and dairy products, which need to be combined into 1 category. The vegetables and the whole grains and legumes are the most significant groups and should be the largest part of the diet. The protein and fat foods are really secondary groups and combined, though they also are important to balance out the diet. The specific individual proportions of these groups vary somewhat from person to person and season to season, as I discuss more fully later in this chapter.

A New Basic Four Food Groups

Fruits

Vegetables

Whole grains and legumes (beans and peas)

Proteins and fats/oils:

    Vegetarian—nuts and seeds

    Omnivore—milk, eggs, and meats

COMPONENTS OF A HEALTHY DIET

Next I look at the different components that we should bring together to make up the new, healthy diet. These components are not necessarily listed in order of importance. A balanced diet and moderate consumption of foods, without regular overeating, are likely the most important components of a healthy diet, especially on a long-term basis. Other aspects, such as food combining or rotating foods, may be more important in the fine-tuning of the diet or in treatment of special problems, such as poor digestion or food allergies. However, following these 10 guidelines preventively will assure us of keeping our digestion, immune system, and entire body functioning at its optimum capacity.

Some of these components may also overlap. Freshness and nutritiousness or seasonality and variety may often include the same characteristics and choices in foods. Which foods are tasty and appealing is a more personal thing—to some this may mean a beautiful, colorful salad and to others a burger and fries. This has a lot to do with the conditioning of our taste buds and minds, which may be the most difficult aspects to change to create a healthier diet.

Natural Foods

Natural foods are the best choices. The closer the foods are to the garden, fields, and orchards, the more energy, vitality, and nutrients we will obtain per calorie of food consumed. I do not believe that the human species has improved on our food other than in the artistry of the culinary chef who makes appealing and tasty cuisine with fresh, natural foods. Although the food processing and manufacturing industries have improved somewhat on shelf life and the ease of shipping foods, processed foods in cans, boxes, and various packages are a distant second to the foods that Nature has provided. And many packages themselves contain chemicals or metals that pose toxicity concerns; in addition, the packaging is often a costly waste product that may not be recyclable and thus creates digestive problems for Earth. Many of the earlier chapters of this book and especially chapter 11, Food and the Earth, provide more lengthy discussions of chemical versus natural foods.

10 Key Components of a Healthy Diet	
Natural foods	Tasty and appealing foods
Seasonal foods	Variety and rotation
Fresh foods	Food combining
Nutritious foods	Moderation
Clean foods	Balance

Fruits, nuts, seeds, vegetables, whole grains, and legumes should constitute the majority of the diet, at least 80% to 90%. People eating much more than 10% to 15% of their diet in the form of animal foods should reevaluate their choices, as the high-fat and low-fiber content of these foods can be detrimental to health in the long run. The only times I might suggest a diet higher than this amount in animal products (mainly fish or poultry with vegetables) would be for weight loss or in the treatment of intestinal yeast overgrowth, where it is important to temporarily reduce the foods high in natural sugars and starches. In these two situations, the main foods are vegetables and fish and poultry, with a modest amount of whole grains.

Seasonal Foods: Indigenous Diet

Eating seasonally—eating foods that are available and grown locally—keeps us attuned to Earth, its elements, and the cycles of Nature. This supports eating naturally of Nature's bounty of fresh foods. It gets us thinking about gardens and being able to pick our own food. Eating seasonally is a most economical dietary pattern and gives us potentially the cleanest foods, as fewer chemicals are needed to store or ship them. My first book, *Staying Healthy with the Seasons* (revised in 2003), focuses on nutrition through the seasons, with many concepts and practical suggestions about seasonal awareness and diet. Eating seasonally is important first for providing the right type of fuel to protect us from the climate as our environment provides the best foods to support our health and keep us in balance. For example, in summer's hottest months, the juiciest of fruits are available. Fruits and fruit juices help to cool the body. In contrast, in cold and wet winter, the foods that require most cooking are the most prevalent. Before

494

the advent of twentieth-century technology, these were foods that stored well and were protected by shells or hard skins. These are the grains, nuts, seeds, hard squashes, tubers, and root vegetables—foods that are either higher in protein and fats or that need to be cooked well to make them ready to eat. The fresh, juicier foods are not available then. We often eat somewhat heavier or richer foods when it is colder and may easily gain a few pounds to better protect the body from the cold. Be aware that food availability may vary somewhat, even by a couple of months, around the normal harvest time, because of weather differences, crop timing, and refrigeration.

Being aware of locally grown foods and eating them when they are available helps re-attune us to Nature and, most important, to our own body cycles. This is an essential step in attaining and maintaining health. It is difficult to stay healthy year-round without being sensitive to our inner needs and taking extra measures and time to care for ourselves during times of stress and change. Our personal challenges may be emphasized around the 2 to 3 weeks of seasonal changes that occur at the equinoxes and solstices, the demarcation days of change. Below I summarize some seasonal nutritional advice.

Spring is a time of purification, healing, and rejuvenation. It is the time I most often suggest for a period of cleansing or fasting. In Nature, the greens are growing freely, and these chlorophyll-rich foods are the body's best cleansers. In many climates, citrus fruits also help in the purification process. I usually do 10 days of the Master Cleanser, or lemonade diet (see "Fasting and Juice Cleansing" on page 769 of chapter 18, Detoxification and Cleansing Programs), and invite many to join me in my annual detox programs at the beginning of spring. As spring progresses, the amount of fresh fruits and vegetables in the diet usually increases as the weather warms and in proportion to the other foods, such as whole grains and legumes. The heavier protein and fat foods, which were likely at their peak intake in winter, are now eaten less often. Sprouted seeds and beans are a helpful, nutritious addition to meals. **Spring is a great season to do a whole reevaluation of our health program and create a new one, incorporating whatever changes seem necessary.** Spring is the most creative and fertile time in Nature. That is why we should ready the body by cleaning out the

unnecessary past (our home closets and pantries), that which no longer serves us, and planting new seeds and nourishing them to fruition at a later time.

Summer is a time of growth and activity, when things are expanding. The warmth of summer requires both a lighter diet and fresher, higher water-content foods. It is amazing that those are exactly the foods that Nature provides during this season. After the greens of spring blossom into fruit, many more succulent fruits and vegetables can be harvested to feed us in summer. More raw salads of these available foods can be used, with a reduction of cooked foods in hotter times. The juicy fruits and especially the melons can be eaten, although usually not mixed with other foods (see the section "Food Combining" on page 498). Summer is also a time of more activity, so it is an easier time to slim ourselves, although we may need a fair amount of good foods to support the increased energy output. Our protein and heavier cooked fats are best reduced to allow the simpler fuels to run the body at this time. If a heavier meal is eaten, it is best done in the cooler parts of the day. Drinking more water, juices, and herbal teas will keep us hydrated, especially when we are active in hot weather.

In autumn there is a big shift in energy, climate, and diet. It is the official harvest time of Nature, and we are provided with an abundance of nourishing foods. First the remaining fruits and watery vegetables are harvested, and then the harder root vegetables and squashes come in, most of which require more heat to prepare. Whole grains, legumes, seeds, and nuts also are harvested in this season. The diet thus shifts to more cooked foods, whole grains, and the richer protein and fat foods as the weather cools and the days shorten. Fewer raw fruits and vegetables and more complex carbohydrates are now the mainstay of the diet, especially from later autumn into spring. More indoor-focused activity and exercise need to be developed as well to be in harmony with autumn.

Winter has us craving richer, more warming foods. Foods requiring more preparation are part of our cuisine, and hopefully we can be at home more, resting and recharging, cooking, and of course eating. We often need more fuel to feed our furnace to generate more energy to keep us warm. We do not want to overeat, however, especially the sweets and fatty foods, as the usually decreased activity level can cause us to gain too much weight during this season. As in autumn, the mainstay of the diet is the complex carbohydrates found in the whole grains, squashes, and root vegetables, such as carrots, beets, potatoes, onions, and garlic. Dairy foods and meats might be consumed more during winter but should never be a large proportion of the diet. More fish and the high-mineral seaweeds are good in the winter, and poultry may be eaten more if it is desired.

Seasonal eating really involves a number of the other components of a healthy diet. The Earth-grown foods are natural, usually fresh and appealing, definitely nutritious, and often clean, especially if grown organically; they give us a wide variety of foods throughout the year. I emphasize the seasonal diet throughout this chapter, as it is an essential part of the ideal diet. Also, for more specifics on seasonally available foods, see my *Seasonal Food Guide*—a beautiful and informative poster and booklet.

Fresh Foods

Eating fresh foods is among the healthiest aspects of a diet. This applies obviously to the foods from Nature—the fruits, vegetables, grains, nuts, beans, and seeds. It also applies to most milk and animal products, which can cause more problems if they are old. Spoilage or rancidity of the animal foods can more easily cause microbial diseases, because bacteria, viruses, and parasites, for example, grow very well in these substances. Fruits and vegetables are best eaten as fresh as possible, but most of these foods store well for several weeks. Many of the whole grains and legumes keep for years after harvesting. The nuts and seeds must be more carefully stored (in a closed container in a cool, dark place, or refrigerated), as they may easily go rancid because of their oil content.

Mostly, we just need to be aware of the different foods, how they store, and how to use them appropriately (see chapter 13, The Ideal Diet). Eating seasonally allows us to get the freshest produce. When we say *fresh,* we usually think of fruits or vegetables, not a fresh can of spinach or a fresh box of breakfast cereal. But even though prepackaged foods often have a long

shelf life, they are often better when eaten soon after packaging. What I mean by "fresh eating," however, is eating as close to the garden, field, or orchard as possible, such as eating an apple or apricot off a tree, gathering a salad from the garden, or cooking some just-picked sweet corn.

Nutritious Foods

Eating a nutritious diet primarily means acquiring all the vitamins, minerals, amino acids, fatty acids, and phytonutrients that the body needs to function optimally and to protect health. It also means eating specific foods that contain good levels of many nutrients. These, once again, include such natural, fresh foods as fruits, vegetables, whole grains, legumes, nuts, and seeds. The animal foods, although not as balanced, can be high in certain important nutrients, such as protein, iron, calcium, or vitamin B_{12}, but they are often high in fats as well. The fresher the foods are, the higher in potential nutrients they are, because they lose certain vitamins, minerals, and especially enzymes when they sit around or when cooked, which usually reduces some of the nutrient content. **Several studies show that organically grown foods have higher nutrient levels than the same produce grown commercially.** The industrial processing of foods greatly diminishes the level of nourishment. When speaking of a nutritious diet, I am referring to the consumption of a high percentage of whole foods, as fresh as possible. Eating a variety of foods allows a greater balance of nutrients. Many processed and refined foods are enriched or fortified to make them more "nutritious." This does help some but is a distant second to the nourishment received from natural, fresh foods.

Clean Foods

Eating a clean diet refers to two important areas. The first level regards consuming chemical-free (and not genetically engineered) foods as much as possible. The chemical-free part of this equation means avoiding chemical additives and chemically treated foods, as well as refined-sugar and refined-flour foods. **Finding organically grown produce as well as organic (untreated) milk products, poultry, beef, and**

eggs is becoming even more important as pollution worsens around the world. Buying organic foods from farmers who grow fruits, vegetables, and nuts and from ranchers who raise cattle, chicken, and other animals lets the organic farming industry know there is a market that supports them as opposed to food producers who use many chemicals.

Clean also refers to washing and storing food properly to avoid spoilage and contamination. Washing fresh produce with water or a natural veggie wash before eating or cooking can be helpful to clean off the dirt, bugs, or chemicals. Packing food properly for storage in reusable containers (glass, Pyrex, stainless steel, or nonleaded ceramic) will protect it longer. Keeping ourselves and our homes, kitchen counters, and utensils clean also protects us and others from spreading disease. Drinking clean, filtered, chemical-free water is important as well.

Tasty and Appealing Foods

Eating a diet that is tasty and appealing satisfies the senses, which is important, too. The more we make each meal a feast for our eyes and mouths, the more it nourishes the deeper levels of our being. The diet must be gratifying; a diet of foods we enjoy will satisfy us while a diet of foods we do not enjoy is not fulfilling. Food that is visually appealing and colorful is as important to many people as the taste, because this improves the appetite and the enjoyment of the foods. Often the food tastes especially good when someone has taken the time to prepare a beautiful meal.

All foods have their characteristic flavors. Our attraction to some of these flavors, and thus to certain foods, is inherent in our natures, while other tastes are learned or conditioned. Often, to change the diet more positively, we need to work at changing our tastes or developing new tastes. (This was discussed more thoroughly in chapter 10, Nutritional Habits.) A lot of unnatural or concentrated sweet and salty flavors in foods, as well as chemical tastes, have taken people away from simple, natural eating. To return to or support the many components of the healthy diet discussed throughout this book, we may need to recondition ourselves to enjoy the true natural flavors of Earth's real foods.

Variety and Rotation

Eating a variety of foods provides a variety of nutrients, thus preventing any marked deficiencies. That is, of course, if the variety of foods we choose are mainly nutritious. If we vary among pizza, franks, and hamburgers from day to day, the diet is not going to be balanced. Eating and varying many of the whole foods will assure a proper amount of nutrients without excesses of potentially harmful levels of sugars, fats, or even protein. Rotating the diet means eating different foods from day to day and not repeating the same foods every day. This reduces the potential to become allergic or sensitive to particular foods, which can result from repeatedly stimulating the body's immune and cellular systems with the same nutritional biochemistry.

The molecular protein parts of a food are usually what we become sensitive to; we build up antibodies against these antigens, and then whenever we eat the food, we may get a reactive immune response. Common foods that may generate allergies include cow's milk, wheat, eggs, soybeans, corn, beef, coffee, chocolate, tomatoes, yeast, shellfish, and mushrooms. We may also be intolerant of the sugars found in foods. The most common example, of course, is lactose intolerance, when we do not have a strong capacity (because of small amounts of the enzyme lactase) for breaking down the primary sugar found in cow's milk (lactose). But there can be similar problems with many of the other sugars, including the monosaccharide sugars fructose, fucose, xylose, and sorbose as well as the disaccharide sugars sucrose and maltose.

We may also be genetically sensitive or allergic to foods or have developed allergies and reactions through other stresses or illnesses we have experienced. If we are very reactive to foods—that is, if we do not feel well after we eat, with fatigue, irritability, or such specific symptoms as nasal congestion, itching, or skin rashes—we might want to find out what foods may be causing this. We may then wish to eliminate those foods for a while and go on a specific 4-day rotation diet, with any specific food consumed on 1 day not again consumed in the next 3 following days, thereby allowing the body to deal with it and clear it completely. This reduces the constant stimulation to the immune system that can occur when we consume a food daily. (This topic is discussed in more detail under "Allergies" on page 704 of chapter 17, Medical Treatment Programs, and is the basis of my book *The False Fat Diet*.)

We reduce the potential for food reactions by avoiding repetitive consumption of the same foods, especially the commonly allergenic ones. For this reason, and to obtain all of the important food nutrients, it is wise not to limit food choices or eat the same foods consistently but to consume a wide range of foods from all the various groups on a daily as well as a seasonal basis. Food allergy and sensitivity is a subject of increasing concern with respect to genetically modified foods. Because these foods are rapidly increasing within the marketplace, we need to try to understand possible food reactions.

Food Combining

Food combining (also discussed in chapter 10, Nutritional Habits) is a basic component to good nutrition. It allows us to digest and utilize the foods and their inherent nutrients optimally. Many people overstress their digestive tracts by eating a large number of foods at each meal. Western culture has been conditioned more to the balanced meal than to the balanced diet, and people may eat foods from all the different groups at each sitting. This, as I have stated, is very taxing on the body and may in part be why there is so much digestive disease from stomach to colon in the United States. Simple meals of a few ingredients each, using a variety of foods over time, with concern about balancing the diet over the day or week, is a more overall healthful approach to eating.

Four basic principles and new concepts of food combining are as follows:

1. Meals should be balanced according to our individual needs, not according some preset standard. How many of us have that picture in our mind of the perfectly balanced dinner, where the meat entrée (a piece of chicken, beef, or fish) takes up half of the plate, leaving a quarter plate's worth of a starch (like mashed potato or rice) and a final quarter's worth of a vegetable (like green beans)? Or a perfectly balanced breakfast where we have a token dairy and grain (a bowl of cereal with cow's milk), a token fruit (a glass

of OJ), and a token meat (two slices of bacon)? These visions of balanced meals are not based on reality, however. There is no scientific research to support them. In fact, not only are we not required to balance meals in this way to stay healthy, we may actually be doing harm to ourselves in the process.

I am fully convinced by nutrition research since the mid-1990s that we do not need all nutrients at every meal, even when it comes to the delicate issue of amino acids and protein. Our bodies, when we are healthy, give us plenty of flexibility. If we want to only eat a few kinds of root vegetables for lunch, that is perfectly fine. If we only want fruits in the morning, so be it. As long as we pay attention to the overall intake for the day, and how the combinations make us feel, our bodies can do the rest. (We are not free to eat junk as a food group, of course. The resilience of the body does not apply to processed food.) As long as we are sticking primarily with whole, natural foods, what we need to do most is experiment, spend time finding out what works for our particular metabolism and needs. How long does a food or meal give us energy, or do we feel tired? We can never give up the living and learning aspect of life.

2. Large amounts of a food that is particularly concentrated in a single nutrient area do not work well when combined with other foods. The two most obvious examples here are fruits and meats. Fruits can be an especially concentrated source of sugar. A large banana, or 1 cup of grape juice, for example, can contain about 30 grams of sugar—*more* than 8 ounces of soda pop. A 16-ounce steak has about 140 to 150 grams of protein—the same as 7 to 8 cans of baked beans! When we try to bring these kinds of foods into our meal plan, things become too lopsided, and our digestion is taxed too heavily. We are not *meant* to digest 30 grams of sugar alongside of 100 grams of protein. Indigestion, gas, bloating, and abdominal discomfort are all too possible given this combination. In addition, there is a potential conflict of interest between the more acidic secretions that can be helpful for digesting large amounts of protein and the less concentrated acidity that normally accompanies high-carb intake. The same can be said about large platefuls of processed carbs—and here I mean fiber-free white rice, fiber-free white noodles, and enormous baked potatoes where we scoop out the insides and leave behind the fiber-rich skins.

These kinds of foods do not work well anyway; but combined with other foods, their impact on the digestive tract is even worse.

3. It is fine to eat some foods alone. This principle is particularly relevant when it comes to fruits, which seem to go best either with other fruits or simply as stand-alones in the meal plan. The scientific research does not bear this out, but my personal experience and that of many patients absolutely does. What can be more pleasurable when it comes to food than a cluster of fresh organic red grapes, or a crisp Gravenstein apple, or a handful of freshly picked blackberries, with no napkin and no utensils and no other foods to interrupt the sheer delight of these foods? I also want to mention water in this context of foods eaten alone. Although we all need to keep up fluid intake to remain healthy and well hydrated, drinking large amounts of water along with meals does not seem to work well for most people. It dilutes the strength of digestive juices and makes it more difficult to thoroughly break down foods. This issue may also involve stomach acid levels, or stomach volume, or both, but I have encountered problems enough times to recommend that we treat major water consumption as a between-meal activity.

4. Food combining is something we need to take seriously, despite the position of many health-care practitioners and the current status of nutritional research. I have seen physicians and dietitians all too often reject the importance of food combining, by claiming that we have all of the enzymes and other digestive machinery to eat anything we want anytime we want. We are omnivores, they point out, and thus can eat anything. I strongly disagree, however. When I look at cultural eating practices worldwide, the healthiest cultures do not eat anything anytime they feel like it. They eat seasonally, and locally, and with sacred food restrictions. They may only mix two foods, like plantain and cassava combined into a delightful mixture known as *fufu*, seasoned with local herbs (as is done in many villages in Ghana). The wisdom of world cuisines is always channeled and discriminating. Foods are always combined carefully and never eaten indiscriminately. Only in cultures like the United States, where chronic diseases are most widespread, do we toss all the foods we want onto the plate, without seasonal or regional or religious constraints. As a culture, we need to move in the opposite direction, I believe, and explore combinations that leave us feeling our best. Below are 4 new, science-based guidelines for food combining.

Guidelines for Food Combining

1. Fruits are eaten by themselves or with other fruits.
2. Proteins and starches are not eaten together.
3. Combine protein and vegetables or starches and vegetables.
4. Do not eat more than one protein per meal.

Moderation

Eating moderately, not overeating (or undereating), is probably the basic first habit of good nutrition. Many nutritionists feel that overeating, especially on a regular basis, is the worst thing we can do to the body. Overeating applies to not only the total amount of food consumed, but also, as I explore in the next section, to the overconsumption of specific foods that can lead to improper dietary balance. Overconsumption or abuse of sugars, fats, protein, salt, and chemicals can lead to the most disastrous results. We must be careful to control the intake of foods that contain large amounts of these ingredients.

Eating too much food at any time, as most of us have experienced, causes great stress on the body. After a meal, much more blood is sent to the digestive organs, and we are often sedated and unable to move well until digestion is completed many hours later. Regular overeating also tends to reduce exercise potential, and this, along with the increased calorie intake, contributes to weight increase. Almost all obesity, other than from hormonal imbalance, is caused by overconsumption of calories along with physical underactivity. Obesity leads to an increase in most of the serious and chronic diseases, such as hypertension, heart disease, diabetes, and cancer.

When we follow the other components of a healthy diet, we nourish the body in the best way. This reduces the nutritional reasons for overeating, where the body craves more and more food to satisfy its malnourishment. This happens most often when foods low in nourishment, such as processed foods, or foods high in fat, protein, or sugar are eaten as a major part of the diet. The craving for food will not be diminished until the cells and tissues are nourished.

There are also many common psychological factors that cause overeating. These can be specific short-term stresses or more long-range problems. Early conditioning can cause patterns of overeating to cover up emotional pain or insecurity. These issues must be dealt with also. (See page 391 in chapter 10, Nutritional Habits, for more on overeating.) Whatever the reason, it is wise to do what is needed, even counseling and hypnosis, to learn to eat moderately and to focus on the most nourishing foods. This will contribute to health, both daily and lifelong.

Balance

Eating a balanced diet is probably the most important aspect of nutrition in regard to long-term health. However, the concept of a balanced diet is among the most controversial topics in the nutritional field. Few authorities agree on the specifics of this balance, although there seems to be general agreement on the basic trends. **In this section, I discuss the following five aspects of balance:**

1. **Macronutrients.** Proteins, fats, and carbohydrates.

2. **Micronutrients.** Vitamins, minerals, amino acids, fatty acids, and phytonutrients.

3. **Food groups.** Fruits, vegetables, grains, legumes, nuts, seeds, dairy products, eggs, fish, poultry, and meats.

4. **Flavors and colors.** Sour, bitter, sweet, spicy, and salty; red, orange, yellow, green, blue, and purple.

5. **Acid-alkaline.** Acid-forming and alkalizing foods.

BALANCE—MACRONUTRIENTS

How much of the carbohydrates, fats, and proteins we need is discussed further in several places through chapter 13; also, chapters 2, 3, and 4 discuss the three macronutrients in detail. Here I review specifically the basics of these important nutrients and give my suggestions for the right balance. Carbohydrates, which include simple sugars and starches, provide the body and cells with easily usable energy. Proteins provide amino acids, the building blocks of body tissues and many active biochemicals. The fats provide lubrication and protection as well as fuel for the body. An excess or deficiency of any of the macronutrients can generate problems, so the art of nutrition is to create a diet with the right balance. The biggest concern, of course, is with the excessive amount of fats,

---

Primary Macronutrients of Common Foods

Proteins	FATS		CARBOHYDRATES		
	Saturated	**Unsaturated**	**Complex**	**Simple**	**Refined**
Eggs	Coconut	Vegetable oils	Grains	Fruit	Refined flour
Milk	Palm oil	Mayonnaise	Legumes	Honey	Bread
Cheese	Animal fat	Nuts	Hard squash	Maple syrup	Cookies
Nuts	Butter/lard	Seeds	Whole grains	Sweeteners	Doughnuts
Seeds	Mayonnaise		Breads/pasta		Candy
Legumes	Whole milk				Soft drinks
Fish	Cheese				Sugar
Poultry	Eggs				Pastry
Meats	Meats				
	Bacon				

particularly saturated fats, that are consumed by so many people. Second is the high amount of refined sugar eaten. Excessive protein intake may contribute to some congestive, degenerative problems as well. On the deficiency side, the most important is the low amount of complex carbohydrates and fiber commonly eaten in the United States diet. Deficient intake of usable protein, although less of a concern in our culture, is still a factor for many people. When we balance these key areas, we can greatly enhance nutrition and prevent future problems.

In 1999 and 2000, the average American diet contained 51% carbohydrates, 15% protein, and 34% fat, as shown in the table below, "Macronutrients in the Diet—Old Balance and New Goals." The table also suggests a healthier balance among these macronutrients, with 60% carbohydrate, 15% protein, and 25% fat. The staples of this type of diet are the vegetables and grains, with some fruits and protein and fat foods. The traditional diets of many cultures around the world may have contained approximately a 60:20:20 balance among carbohydrates, protein, and fat, with some meat, milk, nuts, and seeds consumed to provide a higher protein level. The naturally hunted range animals and fish eaten in these cultures had a much lower fat content than today's heavily fed, penned animals. Such oils and fatty processed foods as bacon and potato chips were not available either, so the protein level could be in-

creased without adding much fat. Today, that is more difficult to do.

Fat has more than twice the calories of protein and carbohydrates, so a little can greatly increase its percentage of the diet. In my analyses of people's diets, 40% to 50% dietary fat is not uncommon. **Decreasing fat consumption to between 25% and 30% fat may be among the hardest goals to attain for many people.** Yet, when we follow the guidelines outlined in this chapter, we can attain and maintain a healthy balance.

BALANCE—MICRONUTRIENTS

There are about 53 essential nutrients—those substances that the body needs to carry out its many functions but that it does not make, at least in sufficient amounts to provide for our needs. In other words, these are substances that we need to obtain from food or additional supplements. These include the vitamins and minerals as well as the essential amino acids from protein foods and the essential fatty acids from oils. Alongside of these 53 micronutrients are literally hundreds of critical phytonutrients also provided by the foods we eat. All of the substances that give plant foods their unique colors, flavors, and smells are substances that provide us with health benefits. When we are balancing the diet for micronutrients, we need to keep phytonutrients in mind as well.

Macronutrients in the Diet—Old Balance and New Goals

	AVERAGE AMERICAN DIET	NEW GOALS*
Carbohydrates	51%	60%
	27% complex	45% complex
	7% natural sugars	10% natural sugars
	17% refined sugars	5% refined sugars
Protein	15%	15%
Fat	34%	25%
	9% polyunsaturated	8% polyunsaturated
	13% monounsaturated	10% monounsaturated
	12% saturated	7% saturated

*This may range from 55% to 70% carbohydrates, 10% to 25% protein, and 20% to 35% fat.

Essential Nutrients

Amino Acids	—————— Minerals ——————		Vitamins
Isoleucine	Calcium	Nickel*	A—retinol and carotene
Leucine	Chloride	Phosphorus	B₁—thiamin
Lysine	Chromium	Potassium	B₂—riboflavin
Methionine	Cobalt	Rubidium*	B₃—niacin
Phenylalanine	Copper	Selenium	B₅—pantothenic acid
Threonine	Fluoride	Silicon	B₆—pyridoxine
Tryptophan	Iodine	Sodium	B₁₂—cobalamin
Valine	Iron	Strontium*	Biotin
Arginine**	Lithium*	Sulfur	C—ascorbic acid
Histidine**	Magnesium	Tin*	Choline
	Manganese	Vanadium	D—calciferol
Fatty Acids	Molybdenum	Zinc	E—tocopherol
Linoleic acid			Folic acid
Linolenic acid			Inositol**
			K—quinones
			P—bioflavonoids
			PABA—para-aminobenzoic acid**

*These may not be essential.

**These are "semiessential"—that is, they are needed in special times of growth and development, or at times may be synthesized by the body.

To obtain all of these nutrients from food, we need to eat a variety of natural, fresh, tasty, and nutritious foods. Still, it is not easy in this day and age, with the diminishing nutrients in the soil and the high amount of food processing, to obtain all of our nutrients from food. That is why I often suggest a general supplement for those who are not eating a completely balanced and wholesome diet or who have any signs or symptoms of a possible deficiency. Many people choose to take a general vitamin-mineral supplement and even additional amino acid formulas or essential fatty acids as insurance that they are obtaining all of these needed nutrients.

I would like to add a further thought about meeting our nutrient needs. Nearly all nutrients—whether included in my essential list or not—may require special attention depending on our health and lifestyle. For example, a nonessential amino acid, glycine, is considered by most authorities to be the simplest of all amino acids for the body to make and therefore the least likely to be needed in terms of diet. However, this simplest of amino acids may rise to the top as a nutrient of special need under certain circumstances. Glycine is needed, for example, to detoxify the food

additive sodium benzoate, as well as one of the three most commonly used over-the-counter pain relievers—namely, aspirin. So we need to stay aware of our own individual circumstances when we are working on our nutrient balance.

BALANCE—FOOD GROUPS

"Food groups" is a broad term that can mean many different things, such as the basic food groups discussed earlier in this chapter or specific classifications of foods, such as the cruciferous vegetables (broccoli, cauliflower, brussels sprouts, and cabbage) discussed in chapter 8, Foods. In this case, I use the term to refer to the larger categories of food, such as fruits, vegetables, grains, and legumes, also discussed in chapter 8. We need to obtain a proper balance among these foods to support the other components of this healthy diet. Our ideal food group balance will not be the same all year round; even the proportions of the different macronutrients will vary with the seasons. But the tables on this page provide good general guidelines, ranking the groups from those we should consume most to those we should eat least. Note:

This ranking does not necessarily indicate the relative importance of the food groups, because many foods that may not be eaten in great quantity are needed to make our bodies work or to provide vital nutrients.

BALANCE—FLAVORS AND COLORS

The concept of the five flavors of food representing a balanced diet comes from the laws of the five elements in traditional Oriental practice. According to this philosophy, each of the five flavors is associated with a different element and supports different organs and functions of the body. In the Chinese philosophy, eating a variety of foods that contains all of these different flavors is an important part of a balanced diet. An excess or deficiency of a certain flavor can cause an imbalance of energy in the body and thus lead to specific symptoms and diseases. Excesses of salt and of sweet are two common examples; low intakes of bitter or sour foods may lead to other difficulties.

All the flavors are not necessarily eaten in equal proportions. The flavor focus may vary from season to season, as the elemental dominance changes and according to our individual balance. Many naturally sweet foods are available, and these are consumed more plentifully than sour, salty, bitter, or spicy ones. Making a meal that contains all the five flavors is a challenge for any artful chef. The "Nutrition and the Elements" table on page 504 provides examples of foods associated with the different flavors. Another way of viewing this balance is in terms of the colors of the foods, with a different element associated with each color. These colors may act like the flavors in stimulating certain organs and functions. Thus the red foods (such as meats, cayenne, and tomatoes) may stimulate blood and circulation; green foods (such as many vegetables) may help purify us and support metabolism or strengthen the liver. This view actually seems to have a physiological basis in many instances, and in fact, the whole idea of color balancing is highly consistent with the explosion of information coming to us about food and its phytonutrient composition.

A more common approach to dietary color balance is the "rainbow diet" approach: eating foods from all colors of the rainbow—red, orange, yellow, green, blue, and violet. This makes for beautiful and colorful meals, and when we look at the various foods that

Food Group Priorities: Omnivorous

Vegetables	Eggs
Whole grains	Dairy products
Fruits	Fish, freshwater
Legumes	Poultry, nonorganic
Fish, saltwater	Shellfish
Poultry, organic	Meats
Seeds	Nuts

Food Group Priorities: Vegetarian*

Vegetables	Eggs
Whole grains	Dairy products
Legumes	Nuts
Fruits	Seeds

*With the exception of eggs and dairy products, this list also applies to vegans.

fit into this color spectrum, we can see that this can be a way of balancing nutrients in the diet. Gabriel Cousens, MD, has specifically addressed this diet in his book *Spiritual Nutrition and the Rainbow Diet.*

BALANCE—ACID-ALKALINE

This concept, discussed briefly in chapter 10, Nutritional Habits, and more thoroughly in my first book, *Staying Healthy with the Seasons,* fits in well with many of the other aspects of a healthy diet. To put it simply, foods are classified as basically acid or alkaline, not according to their taste but to the residue left after they have been metabolized in the body. If the human body is decomposed or burned, the final ashes are slightly alkaline—that is, they have a pH of above 7.0, the neutral pH of pure water. When foods are completely combusted, they are broken down into an alkaline or acid ash.

Human blood has a normal pH of 7.41, which is fairly stable. When this shifts, because of respiratory changes or metabolic changes via the kidneys, the body goes through further metabolic and respiratory

Nutrition and the Elements

	Wood	Fire	Earth	Metal	Water
ORGANS	Liver Gallbladder	Heart Small Intestine	Spleen Stomach	Lungs Large Intestine	Kidneys Bladder
COLOR	Green	Red	Yellow	White	Blue/black
FUNCTIONS	Purification Metabolism	Circulation Vitalization	Digestion Distribution	Elimination Mental	Storage Emotional Circulation
FLAVOR	Sour	Bitter	Sweet	Spicy/pungent	Salty
FOODS	Lemons Other citrus Sauerkraut Pickles Vinegars Buttermilk Yogurt Preserved foods	Lettuce Spinach Chard Other greens Celery Asparagus Eggplant Some nuts Herbs	Grains Potatoes Carrots Beets Squash Peas Corn Yams Sweet potatoes Most fruits Sugarcane Honey Maple syrup Milk	Onions Garlic Radish Mustard Cayenne Chile peppers Horseradish Chives	Seaweed Ocean fish Celery Olives Salted foods Miso Capers Soy sauce Brined foods

responses to try to recreate our acid-alkaline balance. **A diet that is too acidic affects blood and tissues, and the body will try to clear unwanted elements through enhanced elimination via the colon and kidneys and secondarily through the skin, sinuses, or other mucous membranes.** The congestion of mucus we experience in different body areas may often be caused in part by this acid-alkaline imbalance, usually because of too much acid food intake.

This is a difficult concept for many people to accept, because it is just that—a concept or theory. However, based on my experience and on good sense, I encourage people to eat more alkaline foods and reduce acid ones because, on many levels, this fits into a more balanced diet. It is also consistent with my basic belief that we need to consume more vegetables

and fruits (generally more alkaline foods), with some whole grains (more midrange foods) and smaller amounts of the meats and milks or refined sugar and flour products (the main acid foods). The list on the opposite page gives examples of alkaline, balanced, and acid foods.

Usually I suggest 70% to 80% alkaline and balanced foods in the spring and summer months. During later autumn and winter, at least 65% to 70% alkaline and balanced foods would be all right. In very cold climates, a higher percentage of richer-acid-forming foods may be tolerated, as these foods are higher in fats and burn hotter as body fuel. Also, fewer vegetables and far fewer fruits are available at these times. By and large, whenever possible, we need lots of vegetables and whole grains to keep the body balanced.

Acid-Alkaline Foods

Alkaline	Balanced	Acid
All vegetables	Brown rice	Wheat
Most fruits	Corn	Oats
Millet	Soybeans	White rice
Buckwheat	Lima beans	Pomegranates
Sprouted beans	Almonds	Strawberries
Sprouted seeds	Sunflower seeds	Cranberries
Olive oil	Brazil nuts	Breads
Water-soaked almonds	Honey	Refined flour
	Most dried beans and peas	Refined sugar
	Tofu	Cashews, pecans, and peanuts
	Nonfat milk	Butter*
	Vegetable oils	Milk*
		Cheeses*
		Eggs
		Meats
		Fish
		Poultry

* Some people place whole-milk products in the balanced area; I do not.

A REVIEW OF RECOMMENDED DIETARY CHANGES

It is likely that the poor farming people of developing nations have a better diet than North Americans do. The typical U.S. diet is far from the local seasonal vegetable and grain diet of many poorer cultures. Instead of the traditional fare, many of us dine regularly on prefabricated, processed, or treated foods with increased amounts of meat, fats, sugar, salt, and the many additives that help to flavor the refined foods.

With this all-too-popular American diet, there has been a huge decrease in the complex carbohydrate fiber foods and in the naturally high-vitamin and high-mineral whole foods, as well as deficiencies of the essential fatty acids while intake of many unnecessary and damaging fats has increased. The high amounts of refined oils and saturated fats can cause much disease. The decrease in the nutrition per calorie ratio with the increase in simple sugar and refined food intake has led to a strange combination of obesity and malnutrition. Many of the vital nutrients—such as vitamins A, C, and E, the B vitamins, calcium, mag-

nesium, chromium, and zinc—may be missing from the diet. This is of special concern in teenagers and the elderly, who tend to limit their diet more than other segments of the population.

A primary focus of this book is to help the reader shift his or her diet from the standard American diet to a healthier one. For this we first need to reject the processed foods, high-fat foods, lunch meats, and high-sugar foods that are so prevalent. Many Americans consume close to half of their dietary calories as fats, nearly twice the level that is healthy. Jane Brody, prolific author in the field of nutrition and widely-read health columnist, has pointed out in her *Nutrition Book* that additives are also a dominant part of our consumption. The average American in recent years annually consumed 128 pounds of sugar, 15 pounds of salt, 9 pounds of 33 common additives, and 1 pound of the other 2,600 food additives, for a total of 153 pounds—yes, the average human weight.

Changing the diet may be a difficult task. It takes guts and a lot of work. Our taste for fats, sweets, and processed foods is so ingrained. And our image is at stake. The meat and potatoes, beer and pretzel man could not possibly eat those sissy salads and wholesome natural foods such as rice and vegetables with beans or tofu. Some of us still think we need our hunk of animal protein, but evidence to the contrary is building. Many American now know that we have to get more basic and natural and less salty and sweet or fatty foods into our diet. We need to begin by selecting healthful foods, as Dr. Rudolph Ballentine has pointed out in *Diet and Nutrition*—when shopping, when cooking, and in restaurants. We should not shop when we are hungry. When we do shop, we could skip many of the aisles with those fancy, colorful boxes and cans. We want to choose foods as close to their natural state as possible.

Brody and many others have suggested that these changes may decrease the death rates from cardiovascular disease and diabetes by 25% to 30% and also reduce the cancer rate. A diet such as this will most assuredly affect both the vitality of newborn babies and our longevity. We are sure to feel better in our later years. The increase in chronic disease is primarily related to diet, and with more farsighted vision, we can be growing both older and healthier simultaneously.

Now, here are a couple of summary lists of how to make improvements in the general Western, industrialized diet. Make healthier choices and experience the positive results.

Suggested Dietary Changes

Decrease		Increase	
Calories	Refined sugar	Fresh vegetables	Complex carbohydrates
Fats	Refined flour	Fresh fruits	Fiber
Saturated fats	Salt	Sprouts	Whole grains
Cholesterol	Processed foods	Drinking water	Legumes
Red meats	Soda pop	Exercise	Vegetable oils
Dairy foods	Ice cream	Love	

Unhealthy	Healthier	Ideal
Sodas	Fruit juice	Water, mineral water
Refined sugar	Honey, raw sugar	Small amounts of honey, molasses, date sugar
Saturated fat	Unsaturated fat	Low-fat diet
Refined oils	Vegetable oils	Cold-pressed olive oil
Shortening and margarine	Butter or chemical-free margarine	Other cold-pressed vegetable oils, such as flaxseed, canola, or sunflower
Refined flour	Whole-grain flour	Home-ground flour
Refined grains	Whole grains	Organic whole grains
Processed foods	Naturally prepared foods	Whole foods
Additives and preservatives	Natural foods	Whole foods
Enriched or fortified products	Natural nutrients	Whole foods

Chapter 13

The Ideal Diet

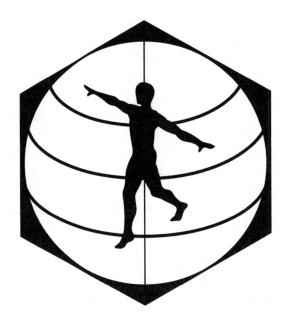

Dare I even attempt to discuss "the ideal diet"? To call any single diet "the diet" is to misunderstand the basic aspects of nutrition and to mislead ourselves that we can find a diet, stick with it forever, and not give it further thought. In this chapter, I first deal with principles and then lay out the basic foods that we can apply to these patterns. The ideal diet is the individual diet that adapts and fluctuates with our needs. It correlates with our activity level, our state of health, where we live, the time of the year, and even the daily weather. And even more important, it correlates with *how* we live.

All too often, we tend to put food into a tidy little category and assume it is somehow disconnected from the way we live our lives. But eating does not work that way. Eating is part of how we see ourselves, what we believe our life is all about. For example, later in this chapter, I provide a profile of my own ideal diet, exactly how I go about doing things during the course of my day. This diet is ideal for me, not only because it correlates with my activity level, state of health, and time of year, but also because it is in sync with the way I live. It is matched up with my life values and my sense of purpose. If I were to make other kinds of commit-ments, in either my professional or private life, my ideal eating might also change. It is easy for me to imagine a person who makes a commitment to construction and manual labor, living in a hot climate, eating in such a way as to detour around the midday heat. Or a person making a commitment to work a graveyard shift having to eat quite differently than what is ideal for me.

Let us assume that we are healthy and we expect this diet to maintain our good health. (Diet programs for illnesses and special needs are discussed in chapter 17, Medical Treatment Programs.) Learning to listen to our individual needs, or better stated, nurturing our basic ability to sense what the body needs through our inherent intuitive knowledge, is vital to both maintaining and adapting our own "correct" diet. The biggest problem in this, of course, is that our current lifestyle and busy environment take us out of this sensitive mode, and most of us get caught up in what the technological society has to offer instead of creating what we need to nourish ourselves and our families. The essential food is already available, but it takes time to gather (shop) and prepare it, and we may not wish or choose to take this time when we could be working or doing other things to support ourselves.

We must realize that to create our ideal diet, we need to make nourishing ourselves a high priority, because without that basic support (good nutrition) for health and vitality, the rest of our life has less meaning. If we can momentarily step back from our day-to-day existence and take an honest look at our lives, we will realize there is not a lot of joy in simply dragging ourselves around to a job and working by caffeine stimulation. Learning to nourish the body to give it the best possible chance for optimum energy makes sense from the standpoint of physical productivity, mental clarity, emotional contentment, and religious/spiritual well-being, as the body is a holy temple to house the spirit.

The best life diet, as Daniel Reuben, MD, has pointed out in his book *Everything You Always Wanted to Know About Nutrition,* begins with mother's milk. Because a mother is the sole source of nourishment to her baby, she has the responsibility to also take the best possible care of herself. I notice that many mothers make a real effort to cultivate better habits during pregnancy and lactation, often eating home-prepared nourishing foods more regularly and eliminating harmful habits, such as drinking alcohol or coffee and smoking cigarettes. We should all nourish ourselves as if our life, activity, and purpose here on Earth were important not only to our immediate friends and family but to the entire world. I believe we have that responsibility. When we move beyond our own individual scope and dilemmas to a more cosmic reality, we will realize that each of us is an important and necessary cog in the giant wheel that turns the universe—and we can choose not to break down, because it affects everyone else.

Listening to and supporting our individual needs in regard to nourishment takes an effort to keep this inherent ability alive, and some of us rediscipline ourselves to redevelop this quality, which is so easily lost in the technological age, and with poor examples from those who raise us and from the media that is so pervasive. A variety of individual processes that keep us more attuned to this natural process might include relaxation exercises, meditation, dream awareness, planting a garden, working the earth, and watching Nature's rhythm. Following these natural practices allows our true nature to resurface.

The beginning years of our nutrition significantly affect lifelong eating patterns and particular likes and dislikes for food. Early family relationships and parental examples may set us up for potential addictions to particular foods or flavors. These factors definitely influence us and often may interfere with healthier eating patterns or restrict us from developing better eating habits in later years. Most babies begin to eat some solid or pureed foods as early as 4 to 6 months. It is best, in my opinion, to feed them initially the fresh fruits (particularly noncitrus fruits, like pear and plum), vegetables (like squash and yam), and whole grains (especially rice, oatmeal, and millet)—all in the right form for an infant. This combination provides babies with both good nourishment and a basic sense of the natural and wonderful flavors of food. Avoiding cans, boxes, and jars of baby foods that may have additives or extra sweet or salty flavoring is essential so as to not desensitize their very alive taste buds to simple, less concentrated flavors.

Avoiding cow's milk and formulas, as Reuben suggests, is helpful in the first year to reduce the potential problems, such as allergy and digestive difficulties, that these more complex protein foods can generate. Other proteins, such as eggs and animal meats, might also be withheld for a few months to allow the baby's digestive tract to mature. Babies need simple foods first, and chemical-free foods at that. When these new protein foods are finally used, buy organic poultry, deep-sea fish, chemical-free eggs, and (if red meat is used) organic, range-fed beef. All of these can be prepared so that the baby can handle them. As much as possible, grow or purchase organic produce and wash it well to minimize pesticide exposure. It is likely that the cancer potential of chemicals is increased in infants, with their undeveloped immune systems, so we should be even more careful about chemicals in foods and environmental exposure than usual. **Be aware of the environmental and home chemicals that are so commonly used nowadays.** This is not meant to instill fear; the healthy baby or child is resilient and can handle most of what society has to offer, but it is best to reduce the exposure to potential toxins as much as possible.

As children grow, it is wise to continue to nourish them with wholesome foods and to not create patterns of using candy, cookies, and ice cream as rewards for "being good." This leads to a confused relationship to these foods. Remember, as-close-to-natural-as-possible is a priority in the ideal diet. Protecting our children from the processed and fast food industry pushed by street advertisements and television is next to impossible, but we must find this balance. Keep emphasizing the basic foods and the fact that these fruits, vegetables (the most difficult parental task), grains, legumes, and simple protein meals are essential. Occasionally the less wholesome foods may be consumed, but they should never become a regular part of the basic diet.

As children begin school, it is best, given the current state of nutrition in public schools, to create their menu as much as possible. Yet, some school districts across the country are making wonderfully welcome changes in this regard; the Seattle school district, for example, sets strict nutritional standards for all vending-machine products and actively promotes consumption of organic foods. Marketing campaigns on the part of manufacturers of soft drinks and other junk foods have brought required advertising of junk foods into some of the nation's school districts, through commercial-based programming in classrooms, like Channel One, and through other marketing campaigns, like Labels for Education. A special term called "pouring rights" has been developed to describe the soft drink company battles for representation in public schools. But some school districts are also voicing concern, and taking nutritional countermeasures. In Washington State, for example, the Department of Agriculture supports Farm to School programs in 2 school districts and 19 schools, and the number is growing. **Organic salad mixes, apples, pears, and other nutrient-dense, natural, whole foods are brought to school cafeterias through these programs. There is also a national Farm to School Program which can be reached through its website at www.farmtoschool.org.**

Packed lunches, if they are not swapped for less nutritious foods, can provide a varied diet and the continued support of parental nutritional guidance. Home cooking is an essential part of nutrition. Restaurant meals should be limited and considered as special dietary treats, although now there seem to be more restaurants offering natural and wholesome foods from which to choose.

In addition to this critical area of child rearing and school nourishment, there is another general area of our lives where food quality remains on particularly shaky grounds. That area also involves hospital food. If hospitalized, it is wise to avoid hospital meals, which offer commercialized poor nutrition in most cases. One of the basic conundrums in Western medicine is why hospitals feed people as if they want them to remain ill. I guess it makes economic sense, but it sure does not make health sense. If we need to spend time in a hospital, we would best make sure to have water and food (in harmony, of course, with the recommended diet) brought in unless we can get fresh and vital foods from the hospital, which fortunately is becoming more possible. We need the vitality of good nourishment to help heal the body. (In part 4, I look more at detoxification and the high-fruit-and-vegetable and juice cleansing diets that might be beneficial in treating a large number of illnesses.) When we are sick, even more than when we are healthy, we need to stop and listen to the body's needs for the best advice on how to move us along the path toward health.

BUILDING THE IDEAL DIET

So, of what might our ideal diet consist? When we talk about a diet or anything as "ideal," we seem to place it a little out of our reach, as if we were seeking to attain perfection. And even then, the ideal may be only a momentary experience. There is really no universal perfect or ideal diet, but individually, we can come as close as possible to an optimum diet by following some important guidelines. We must endeavor to obtain and consume (and even grow) the most wholesome, fresh, and organic (chemical-free and not genetically modified) foods. Meals should be simple in the number of foods, the amount consumed, and the way we combine them. The diet also needs to vary with activity level (usually in quantity and type of foods), local climate, time of year, and, of course, with the best foods available. Finding the best and freshest foods at local stores, in our garden, or at farmers' markets and creating meals around them is a much better plan than the opposite approach of planning a meal and then searching for the appropriate foods.

Preparing more natural foods and redeveloping a taste for the basic food flavors while avoiding the more processed foods and minimizing the amount of cans, boxes, and already prepared meals is a good beginning. Fresh-frozen foods, especially vegetables, are the most acceptable second choice over fresh ingredients. Rich meals with fatty foods or sauces can be reduced. Many other positive changes that can be made were discussed in the previous chapter.

As I have emphasized throughout this book, in the long run, a diet centered around whole grains and vegetables would best serve us individually as well as contribute to greater planetary harmony. The whole grain-legume mixture with abundant vegetables, both cooked and raw, is the main diet of the majority of Earth's people and, I think, the necessary beginning of our ideal diet. We must assume that following our instincts to nourish ourselves with what is available on our planet makes for the best diet. There is some order, I believe, to this universe, and we will have a lot less difficulty if we attune ourselves to that, as well as to our own individual participation in it.

The Ideal Diet will vary somewhat with the seasons, so that, for example, our fruit intake may rise in the summer, with lesser amounts of meats and possibly even fewer whole grains and beans. In winter, we need warmer foods, and there are not as many fresh vegetables available, although the hard, starchy squashes and the cold-weather cruciferous vegetables are good choices in this season. Fruit intake in winter is usually also at a minimum. Sprouted grains, seeds, and beans can bring a few more fresh and vital foods into the winter diet. I like the term "omnivarian" to describe this new diet, which is primarily vegetable based, in contrast to the more typical carnivorous/omnivorous diet.

I currently eat a limited omnivarian and "seasonal" diet, with more raw foods as fresh fruits and vegetables, nuts, and seeds as a basis during the warmer spring and summer months, along with some fish (salmon is my favorite). As the weather cools into the winter months, I might consume small amounts of dairy products, mainly as yogurt or butter, and more oils, with a bit of animal foods, solely as fresh fish and organic poultry, typically about 3 or 4 times per week. Overall, I focus more on a raw and vegan diet, especially when I wish to stay clean and light, and then as I said, adapt that when it is colder and my body needs a bit more concentrated fuel. (I also know I will be cleansing several times a year to help balance my tendency to easily gain weight.) We may feel comfortable to move anywhere along the spectrum from the omnivorous plan to the pure vegan diet, yet a diet of balanced and fresh food (higher vitality foods) will give us more vibrancy and energy. The ideal diet for the modified omnivore also has a new organization of food groups.

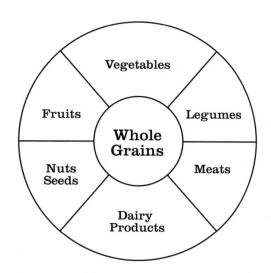

A General Guideline for the Percentage of Foods in Different Types of Diets

	Omnivore	Lacto-ovo Vegetarian	Vegan
Whole grains	25% to 30%	25% to 35%	30% to 40%
Vegetables	25% to 35%	25% to 35%	30% to 40%
Legumes	5% to 10%	10% to 15%	10% to 15%
Fruit	10% to 15%	10% to 15%	10% to 20%
Nuts and seeds	5% to 10%	5% to 10%	10% to 15%
Dairy products and eggs	5% to 10%	10% to 15%	
Meats, poultry and fish	10% to 15%		

New Dietary Guidelines

1. **Produce:** 5 or more servings per day of vegetables and fruits. Fresh is best.

2. **Starches:** 4 or more servings per day of whole grains and other starches, such carrots and beets, hard squashes, and some potato.

3. **Proteins:** 2 to 3 servings per day of sprouted legumes or seeds, cooked legumes, fish, eggs, seeds, nuts, poultry, lamb, beef, or pork—pretty much in that order of preference, in my opinion.

4. **Calcium foods:** 2 or more servings per day but no more than two of the dairy foods (if tolerated), and fewer is probably best. These calcium foods include nuts, seeds like sesame seeds, and green leafy vegetables for any diet; milk, cheese, and yogurt for lacto-ovo or omnivore diets.

5. **Oils:** 1 or 2 servings per day of vegetable oils. Olive, safflower, flaxseed, canola, and sunflower oils are the best choices. Nuts and seeds will also provide some vitamin E and the essential fatty acids.

Individual Needs

How can we decide what our individual dietary needs are? First and foremost, we can always attempt to listen to our body. If we have forgotten how to do this, we can relearn. We may need to avoid certain foods or food groups and eat differently to see if we feel better. We can then bring that food back to see if we notice any ill effects; this takes some planning and effort. But many people cannot or will not take the time or change their lives to reconnect with this instinctual process, so we need to have some basic knowledge. When we get the basic, simple concepts down, the fine-tuning of the diet then really becomes the art and adventure of our personal nutritional quest.

Besides listening to ourselves, it is well to listen to Nature, the great teacher. Nature provides us with the information and nourishment as we need it. Watching the seasons and the growing cycles of plants is obviously the beginning and the basis of creating the individual diet. Working in a garden or planting our own food with family or friends is the best way to stay connected to Earth and its secrets of health. When not eating from our garden, we should be aware of where and how these foods are produced, as well as how the body uses and recycles them (as digestion, assimilation, elimination). Another way to support our individual needs is to be aware of our own state of health. Part 4 of this book suggests specific programs for various problems and stages of life. These diets are usually a marked improvement over what most of us have been eating. This often makes a difference in our health and reduces the incidence of many degenerative disease processes.

Constitutional Typing

One aspect of our individual needs can be clarified by our constitutional type. Many people are not familiar with this idea, yet it is one of the oldest in all of health care. **The concept of constitutional typing goes back more than 5,000 years to the subcontinent of India, with the tradition of ayurveda.** *Ayurveda* is a Sanskrit word meaning "science of life." In ayurveda, the entire universe is described as evolving around the dynamic interplay of three forces or principles, and these same three principles also determine our individual constitution. The principles—called *vata, pitta,* and *kapha*—also bring with them consequences for eating. They affect our taste, digestion, and overall nutritional needs. To give you a better feel for this fascinating and popular approach to nourishment, next I provide a few examples of ayurveda in action.

Imagine that you have been experiencing impatience, irritability, hotheadedness, sharply increased thirst, heartburn, skin inflammation, and bad breath. From the perspective of ayurveda, you may be experiencing excess pitta—the *dosha* or constitution associated with fire, heat, anger, and excitement. Under these circumstances, you would want to avoid beef, pork, lamb, white sugar, raw onion, grapefruit, dry ginger, garlic, and cayenne in your diet, because these foods are said to increase pitta. Instead, you would want to focus on pitta-balancing foods, which are considered cooling, like celery, cilantro, cucumber, pears, plums, adzuki and mung beans, sunflower seeds, and if eating animal meats, chicken or turkey rather than beef. In general, you would also be emphasizing foods that taste sweet, bitter, or astringent, because these tastes would help decrease pitta. You would also be avoiding foods that tasted pungent, sour, or salty, because these foods tend to increase pitta. As you can see, the ayurvedic approach can be very sensory and can take us into a whole new realm of experience regarding food balancing and our everyday health.

One proponent of the ayurvedic approach who has gained a great deal of popularity in the United States is Deepak Chopra, a medical doctor, prolific author on ayurvedic medicine, and founder of the Chopra Center for Well Being in La Jolla, California, particularly through his book *Perfect Health*. Traditional Chinese medicine involves the theories of yin and yang as well as the five elements, and this provides guidance for eating based on our elemental balance or need to rebalance our fire, earth, metal (air), water, and wood. This system is explored a bit more below, as well as on page 503 in chapter 12, The Components of a Healthy Diet, and more thoroughly in my first book, *Staying Healthy with the Seasons*. Furthermore, there is a brief description of the ayurvedic diet and a few recipes in my *A Cookbook for All Seasons*.

The ayurvedic approach to constitutional typing is quite fascinating; however, it may be a bit more difficult to incorporate into the mainstream way of eating in the United States than the traditional Chinese medicine (TCM) approach. In that approach, itself more than 2,000 years old, there are really only two polar forces—yin and yang—and the interplay between these two forces gives rise to the single, unbroken wholeness of the universe. It also gives rise to our individual health and to our dietary needs. In TCM, unlike ayurveda, though, we do not always have a fixed constitution that consists of an absolutely predetermined amount of yin and yang. We may definitely tend to be more yin or more yang, but our yin-yang balance can also continuously shift, and our foods may need to shift accordingly. Let me give a quick food example.

In TCM, salt is highly yang—active, warm, and expansive. Sugar is the opposite—highly yin—inward, contracting, and cold. We may not directly experience these attributes of sugar and salt, but we know how they can roller-coaster us up and down: some salty chips, then a sip of sweet soda. Then back to the chips. Then back to the soda. A handful of pretzels, then a little chunk of chocolate. Then back to the pretzels.

Then back to the chocolate. From the TCM perspective, we are simply bouncing back and forth here between the extremes of yin and yang. And the remedy is always finding a less extreme balance—that is, foods that are not so lopsidedly sweet and salty. Sometimes the difference between yin and yang extremes can be subtle and unexpected. Short grain brown rice, for example, is cooling and yin from a TCM perspective, whereas long grain brown rice is more heating and yang. A person whose constitution was naturally on the hot side would thus do better with the short grain version.

The TCM approach to constitution is much more complicated than I have just described. It has been the subject of many books, some of which are even longer than this one. Given the scope of this book, I cannot cover the whole range of issues, but there is a final TCM topic I want to discuss: acid-base balancing, which is also important in Western and natural medicines. In Western science, there is a special scale for measuring the acidity of things. That's the pH scale (standing for "pressure of hydrogen"). The 0 end of the scale represents the most acidity possible; 14, the highest possible pH, represents the least acidic (or the most basic, or most alkaline) value. Everything has a pH. Lemons and limes, of course, are very acidic and score around 2. Pure water is right in the middle (neutral) and scores 7. Salt pushes more in the alkaline direction at 7.5. The fluids in our body also range widely from 1.5 in our stomach juice (from hydrochloric acid production) to 8.8 in our pancreatic fluid (with more alkaline enzymes).

Persons with a yin tendency generally need to eat foods that are yang acid or yang alkaline forming. Persons with a yang tendency generally need to focus on yin acid or yin alkaline-forming foods. I believe this kind of acid-base balancing belongs in the ideal diet and can greatly improve the body's response to stress as well as more specific kinds of problems, like mucus formation. The table "Yin-Yang and the Acid- and Alkaline-Forming Foods" on the opposite page gives a basic blueprint for the different types of acid- and alkaline-forming foods.

In addition to the age-old practices of ayurveda and TCM, a new way of thinking about constitutional typing has also gained popularity in the nutrition world. This approach, based on blood type, has been

---

Yin-Yang and the Acid- and Alkaline-Forming Foods

Yang Acid-Forming Foods
grains, all animal foods

Yin Acid-Forming Foods
candy, soft drinks,
beans, nuts, alcohol,
sugar

Yang Alkaline-Forming Foods
pickled foods, soy sauce,
miso, salt

Yin Alkaline-Forming Foods
fruits, vegetables, seeds,
honey, coffee

---

popularized by Peter D'Adamo, ND, in his book *Eat Right for Your Type*. Each of us has one of four basic blood types: O, A, B, or AB. Along with each type comes a recommended food list. Type O individuals are thought to need more meat and perhaps even more saturated fat and cholesterol than other blood types. The food recommendations for each blood type are based on an interpretation of human evolution. D'Adamo argues that the blood types evolved along with human evolution, so that type O, the earliest blood type, evolved when humans were primarily hunters and consumed larger amounts of meat.

From this blood-type perspective, we run into trouble when we eat foods not compatible with our blood type, because proteinlike molecules in food called *lectins* trigger inflammatory, allergy-like reactions that compromise our health. Because most foods contain lectins, it is possible to create fairly comprehensive lists of foods that are allowed and prohibited for each specific blood type. The health benefits of food avoidance, especially of the common reactive ones like wheat and cow's milk products, are what I believe to be the basis of some individual success. This process is described quite fully in my book *The False Fat Diet*.

Although I do not see any particular approach to constitution typing as being a mandatory part of an ideal diet, we might consider our constitution in some respect with our food choices to formulate an ideal plan. I personally tend more toward the acid-alkaline balancing approach and see it as playing an important role in my health. In other areas of this book, I discuss the importance of eating a more alkaline diet higher in fruits and vegetables and avoiding too much refined food and heavier meat and dairy foods, which create a more acid imbalance in the body. I believe that over time the latter style of eating leads to much of the chronic disease and aging of the body that many people living in industrialized societies experience.

CHANGING YOUR DIET

Eating seasonally provides us with foods from Nature when they are available, which provides us with the most nourishment and subsequent vitality from our foods. Ideally, the natural flavors of wholesome foods is what appeals to and satisfies the palate and the body. From day to day and season to season, this diet also provides a variety of foods and nutrients. It is important to point out that the variety in the diet is not being forced by anything complicated, like our combining a wide range of foods into a single meal. In this new diet, meals and snacks are simple. There is a balance throughout the day, rather than at each meal, as many people eat now. Not eating large amounts of fruit or the many sweet foods that are concentrated sources of simple sugars at the same time as more complex-to-digest foods, as well as

---

The Ideal Diet

Natural
Seasonal
Rotational
Balanced
Moderate
Well-combined

Sample Diet

TIME OF DAY	FOOD	EXAMPLES	PORTION	REASON
Morning 6:00–7:30 a.m.	Fruit	Orange or grapes	$1/2$–1 whole 10–20 grapes	A simple carbohydrate to break our fast and kick-start the engine (digestive tract).
Breakfast 7:00–8:30 a.m.	Starch	Whole-grain cereal or hard squash	unlimited 1–2 bowls $1/2$–1 whole	A complex carbohydrate breakfast is our time-release energy capsule.
Snack 10:00–11:00 a.m.	Nuts or seeds	Almonds or sunflower seeds	our own handful	This fat/oil primes the engine and stimulates HCl and pancreatic enzymes, such as lipase.
Lunch 11:30– 1:00 p.m.	Protein and green vegetable	Chicken with broccoli, or spinach salad with tomato and garbanzo sprouts	moderation to satisfaction	This combination offers more nutrient (fuel) intake and chlorophyll to further support digestion.
Snack 3:00– 4:00 p.m.	Fruit, vegetable, or starch	Apples, carrot sticks, or rice cakes	1 portion	A simple food to provide some energy lift for late afternoon.
Dinner 5:30– 7:30 p.m.	Starch and vegetable	Brown rice with mixed vegetables or pasta primavera	moderation to satisfaction	A basic complex carbohydrate meal to provide energy and nourishment, and light enough to allow proper digestion before bed.
Optional Snack 7:30– 9:00 p.m.	Fruit, vegetable, or starch	Apple and dates, celery, or popcorn	1 portion	A light snack if needed, depending on other foods consumed and individual metabolism.

minimizing overloads of either starch or protein, aids digestion and allows the best utilization of the nutrients coming from this wide variety of foods.

I suggest that we organize the daily diet according to the food groups that we consume at certain times, also taking into account the day's activities, including exercise, work, and relaxation. A sample day's plan is presented above. Those with special work or sleep schedules, or with varying types of productivity or cycles, should adapt this plan to meet their schedules.

Obviously, this diet varies with the seasons and climate as well as with one's activity level, individual needs, and metabolism. If we are trying to gain or lose weight, we should make modifications. If we are weight training, for example, and trying to increase bulk and muscle mass, we need bigger meals and more protein for dinner. If we want to drop some weight, however, eating a light dinner (ideally in the light of day, not too late) is probably the key (without later snacks), as well as eating moderately at all meals and increasing physical activity. It works if we actually do it.

Depending on our work schedules and specific metabolism, we may want to switch the lunch and dinner meals (see the "Seasonal Menu Plans," starting on page 539 in chapter 14, Seasonal Menu Plans and Recipes) and have the main meal at dinner instead of lunch. Overall, though, it is generally healthier to consume more food earlier in the day, when it can be digested and assimilated more completely, and to eat more lightly if at all after nightfall. In the next section, I go through a day's sample schedule for liquid and food intake, general activities, and other healthful tips.

IDEAL SCHEDULE

Morning

- Wake up with the sun. Go to sleep early enough to awaken without an alarm. Try to arise at least 1 hour before you must leave home.

- Sit quietly or lie propped up in bed and meditate and/or plan your day. Let any concerns or frustrations settle and visualize clearly how you would like to see your day.

- Drink 2 cups of purified or springwater. One may have a quarter or half of a fresh lemon squeezed into it to help with morning purification.

- Do some stretches and light exercise.

- Eat 1 or 2 pieces of fruit.

- A more vigorous exercise period may be included in this time period as well, either before or after fruit, depending on your needs.

- Shower or bathe and get ready for the day.

- A whole-grain or starch breakfast (single or double portion) can be consumed within 30 to 60 minutes after the fruit. Some tea can be taken at this time or even earlier with the fruit.

- If supplements are taken, this can be done now.

- In 1 to 2 hours (midmorning, or 10:00–11:00 a.m.), a handful of one type of nut or seed may be consumed.

- More water or tea can follow, up to about half an hour before lunch.

Morning note. You have started your body slowly and moved into a work pace. You have taken several cups of liquids (not caffeine), done some exercise, cleaned and nourished your body (first with simple fruits, then more complex carbohydrates), followed with some fat or oil-containing protein food. This allows early light eating and allows the digestive tract time to "break fast."

Afternoon

- The midday meal (on the early side, especially if you start your day early) can be substantial, to nourish you for the afternoon, and may consist of a protein food and vegetables, including at least 1 green vegetable.

- A brief period (15–20 minutes) of relaxation and recharging may follow lunch. A short walk outdoors would be helpful as well, to air out the brain, especially for indoor workers.

- Supplements can be taken at this time.

- A midafternoon snack may consist of a fruit, vegetable, or starch, or even a protein food, depending on your needs and food organization plan.

- Later afternoon might include another cup of tea or 1 or 2 glasses of water, in preparation for exercise.

- After work might include exercise or relaxation, also depending on individual needs and previous activities. Your main exercise may be at this time, as it is for many individuals.

Evening

- Dinner may consist of a starch and vegetables or a protein and vegetables.

- It is best to follow a good meal with a relaxation period.

- Supplements can also be taken at this time.

Daily Dietary Schedule

Diet Activity	Possible Time	Food Choice
Preparation	6:00–7:00 a.m.	Water
Breakfast	6:30–7:30 a.m.	Fruit
Breakfast	7:30–8:30 a.m.	Starch
Snack	10:00–11:00 a.m.	Nut or seed
Lunch	12:00–1:00 p.m.	Protein and/or vegetable
Snack	3:00–4:00 p.m.	Fruit, vegetable, or starch
Dinner	5:30–7:00 p.m.	Starch and vegetable or protein and vegetable
Snack	8:00–9:00 p.m.	Fruit, vegetable, or starch

In food groups, this is broken down into the following, depending, of course, on the size of portions consumed:

Meal	Food Choice and Quantity
Breakfast	1–2 fruits, 1–2 starches
Morning snack	1 nut or seed (1 protein, 1 calcium, and 1 oil food)
Lunch*	1–2 proteins, 2–3 vegetables
Afternoon snack	1–2 vegetables or 1 fruit
Dinner*	1–2 starches or 1–2 proteins, and 2–3 vegetables
Evening snack	1 fruit, 1 vegetable, or 1 starch

The breakdown of our "new" food groups gives us the following totals:

Food Group	Number of Servings
Produce	6–8 servings on the average
Starches	4–6 servings
Proteins	2–3 servings
Calcium foods	2–3 servings, including green vegetables, nuts or seeds, and some protein foods
Oil foods	1–2 servings of nuts or seeds or vegetable oils

* Fresh cold-pressed vegetable oil might also be consumed with lunch or dinner; in that case add 1 oil food.

- Then some type of mild activity may aid digestion and assimilation. A short walk with the kids, the dog, a friend, or alone is a good idea.

- The evening brings relaxation through reading, working, or romancing, depending on your wishes. The evening is a good time to nourish yourself in other ways besides eating food.

- A light evening snack of a fruit, vegetable, or starch may be consumed. This is optional. Fruit may be preferred, as it is sweet—a common flavor choice after dinner—and simple to digest.

- Some relaxing tea, warm lemon water, or a glass of plain water can be imbibed in the evening.

- Certain before-bed supplements, such as calcium and magnesium, can also be taken.

- A good night's sleep is now in order.

- Be aware of your dreams and open to remembering them in the morning to learn a little more about yourself.

SUPPLEMENTS TO THE DIET

Even when we eat an ideal diet for an extended period of time, it is hard to maintain an entire balance of nutrients from day to day, and our utilization of the nutrients from these wholesome foods is dependent on a generally healthy digestion and absorption and a minimum of stress or special, extra needs. When we are healthy, with strong, consistent energy, and we sleep well, live in an unpolluted natural environment, do not hustle and bustle about to work and play, eat a variety of wholesome foods from the Earth, and have good digestion and assimilation, we probably need little, if any, additional supplements. If anything, some extra minerals may be required, particularly those that might be deficient in the soils where we live. Yet, we do not often know what these actual or potential deficiencies are.

However, most of us living in the early twenty-first century do not live or eat in this ideal fashion. We may eat on the run, drive on freeways, breathe in polluted air, drink contaminated water, come in contact with various chemicals, and have a lot on our minds. In other words, we have a lot of stimuli, stress, and energy needs. Those of us who fit into this more realistic lifestyle category need a stabilizing, nourishing program of vitamins, minerals, and other supplements. Throughout this book, I have discussed most of the nutrients we could possibly take, why they are needed, by whom, in what special situation, and how to take them. In this section, I suggest an optimum supplement plan to accompany a basically healthy diet for the average adult male or female with a mild amount of activity and stress.

There are two amount columns in the table "General Adult Insurance Daily Supplement Program," on the following page: one column shows the suggested supportive intake level to supplement the basic diet, and the other offers a possible daily intake range to take into account the various supplement preparations and individual variances. In part 4, Nutritional Application: 32 Special Diets and Supplement Programs, there is a series of programs for increased stress situations, for different people and life stages, and for various medical conditions. Each of those programs includes specific supplement suggestions for that particular situation.

The table lists basic essential nutrients. There are, of course, many more vitamins, minerals, amino acids,

Nutrient	Unit of Measure	Daily Values
Protein	g	50
Total fat	g	65
Saturated fatty acids	g	20
Cholesterol	mg	300
Total carbohydrate	g	300
Fiber	g	25
Vitamin A	IU	5,000
Vitamin D	IU	400
Vitamin E	IU	30
Vitamin K	mcg	80
Thiamin (B1)	mg	1.5
Riboflavin (B2)	mg	1.7
Niacin (B3)	mg	20
Pantothenic acid (B5)	mg	10
Vitamin B6	mg	2
Vitamin B12	mcg	6
Folate	mcg	400
Biotin	mcg	300
Vitamin C	mg	60
Calcium	mg	1,000
Chloride	mg	3,400
Chromium	mcg	120
Copper	mg	2
Iodine	mcg	150
Iron	mg	18
Magnesium	mg	400
Manganese	mg	2
Molybdenum	mcg	75
Phosphorus	mg	1,000
Potassium	mg	3,500
Selenium	mcg	70
Sodium	mg	2,400
Zinc	mg	15

Chart of Government (FDA) Daily Values

fatty acids, herbs, and so on that could go into a general formula. For example, hydrochloric acid as betaine HCl is often added to help digestion and utilization of many of the minerals. Many formulas contain other products, such as acidophilus culture, amino acids like tyrosine or tryptophan, different glandulars, more

General Adult Insurance Daily Supplement Program

Vitamins	Form	Suggested Daily Amount	Possible Range
Vitamin A	palmitate	5,000 IU	3,000–10,000 IU
Beta-carotene or mixed carotenoids	vegetable	15,000 IU	10,000–25,000 IU
Vitamin D	D3—ergocalciferol	400 IU	200–600 IU
Vitamin E	d-alpha tocopherol with mixed tocopherols	400 IU	200–600 IU
Vitamin K	phylloquinone	100 mcg	50–200 mcg
Vitamin B1	thiamin HCl	10 mg	10–50 mg
Vitamin B2	riboflavin	10 mg	10–50 mg
Vitamin B3	niacin or niacinamide	20 mg 50 mg	20–100 mg 10–100 mg
Vitamin B5	calcium pantothenate	100 mg	50–100 mg
Vitamin B6	pyridoxine HCl or pyridoxal-5-phosphate	25 mg	10–100 mg
Vitamin B12	cyanocobalamin or cobalamin	100 mcg	50–500 mcg
Folic acid	folacin	400 mcg	400–1,000 mcg
Biotin	biotin	250 mcg	150–500 mcg
Choline	choline bitartrate	500 mg	100–1,000 mg
Vitamin C	ascorbic acid	1,000 mg	500–3,000 mg
Bioflavonoids	mixed complex	250 mg	100–500 mg

phosphorus, various bioflavonoids, inositol, glutamic acid, or herbs, like ginseng or ginkgo. Not all of these products have been clearly shown to do all they claim to do, which is the case even for some of those items listed in the table—although almost all are at least known to be essential to life. Some of the B vitamins are also usually manufactured in the healthy human colon.

The amounts suggested in the table are usually at or above the dietary reference intakes (DRIs) but not at the much higher levels that might be suggested by nutritional doctors for a more stressed or imbalanced, symptomatic individual, or that might be used in specific therapeutic situations. Remember, this insurance formula is for the basically healthy man or woman. There are some slight variations, such as for iron or zinc intake, between the needs for men and women;

these are discussed in chapter 15 (under "Adult Men" and "Adult Women"), along with recommendations for other life stages. Chapters 16 and 17 discuss special programs for the prevention and treatment of many medical conditions.

Herbals. Many multinutrient formulas will throw in a few herbs, such as ginseng, ginkgo, milk thistle, and others. Often this is to make the formula appear higher-quality, more cutting-edge, and more effective, yet typically the levels of herbs used are not enough to be in the naturally therapeutic range. This is often the case with joint supporters like glucosamine or chondroitin sulfates, and coenzyme Q10 as well. Note: Supplements should be hypoallergenic—not made from milk, yeast, wheat, corn, or soy—and contain no sugar, preservatives, or artificial colors.

General Adult Insurance Daily Supplement Program

Minerals	Form	Suggested Daily Amount	Possible Range
Calcium	dicalcium phosphate, calcium aspartate or citrate	700 mg	500–1,200 mg
Chromium	amino acid chelate or picolinate	200 mcg	50–500 mcg
Copper	sulfate or chelate, such as gluconate	2 mg	1–3 mg
Iodine	potassium iodide	150 mcg	50–200 mcg
Iron	citrate or chelate	15 mg	10–18 mg
Magnesium	citrate, gluconate, malate, or aspartate	350 mg	300–600 mg
Manganese	sulfate or chelate	10 mg	2–10 mg
Molybdenum	sodium molybdate or chelate	100 mcg	50–200 mcg
Potassium	chloride or chelate	400 mg	100–1,000 mg
Selenium	selenomethionine or sodium selenite	200 mcg	50–200 mcg
Silicon	equisetum/horsetail	20 mg	10–50 mg
Vanadium	pentoxide or chelate	100 mcg	50–200 mcg
Zinc	sulfate, gluconate, or picolinate	30 mg	15–45 mg

Other Possibilities

Flaxseed oil	balanced omega-3 and omega-6 combination	2 tsp or 4 caps	1–3 tsp 3–6 caps
Omega-3 fatty acids	EPA and DHA oil capsules	1,000 mg	500–1,500 mg
Coenzyme Q10	Coenzyme Q10	50 mg	25–150 mg
Lactobacillius and other probiotic cultures	powder or capsules	1 billion count	50 million to 10 billion organisms per dose

Chapter 14

Seasonal Menu Plans and Recipes

with Eleonora Manzolini

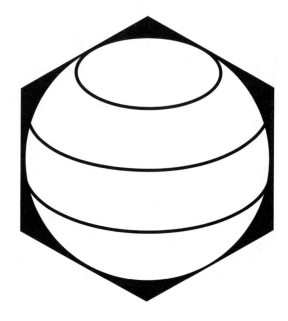

This is a nutrition book and therefore it would not be proper to provide dietary information without providing the basics of the kitchen, as well as instructions on how to prepare some key healthy foods and cuisine, how to keep a safe kitchen, and how to equip it. Be like the best Mediterranean chefs and find the freshest foods and then make the creations in your own cucina, with the spices and tastes you and your family will enjoy. Blessings from Nature are yours to experience as it provides the most vital and tastiest of foods. From my book *Staying Healthy with the Seasons,* Sunny Seasons, MD chef, has written: "The best Nutrition comes from staying close to the Garden of Life. Every step away from the orchard and garden bring a loss of vitality and food energy that is our potential Human Fuel."

The ideal diet menu plans in this chapter consist of 4-day rotation diets, one for each season. This diet/eating plan may require some new attentiveness and adaptation from our usual way of eating, yet, as with any new eating plan, it helps to learn what it takes, shop for what is needed, and have the foods that fit the plan available for our daily intake. For some people, following a natural and seasonally based diet may be a difficult shift, because it essentially includes little or no already prepared or prepackaged foods, such as pizza or the many boxes and cans that fill the typical grocery shelves. For others, including the food-combining principles might feel limiting because they are used to consuming more foods per meal, more variety, and especially the commonly consumed protein-starch meals (even a sandwich with the bread starch and any protein meats), which personally I find the most challenging change to make in my diet.

But this diet is also potentially highly therapeutic for a variety of food-generated health issues, such as digestive problems. It is also helpful in normalizing weight and beneficial for the average person with some food reactions or allergies. Those who have typically eaten a variety of fresh foods and who are healthy and have good digestive function probably do not need to follow strict food combining or a strict rotation diet. It is wise, though, to continue to eat simply of a great many foods and to avoid the daily eating of specific foods, especially such commonly allergenic ones as milk, eggs, wheat, corn, soy, peanuts, tomatoes, and oats.

It is helpful if you take the suggestions offered in this chapter and add your own tastes and creativity.

There are, of course, many other possibilities; feel free to adapt them to feed your heart, mind, soul, and, of course, your body. Creativity is an important part of nutrition. I have included some basic recipes that follow the menu plans as well as the common seasonal foods. Given the primary scope of this book, however, I suggest you take a look at my companion recipe book, *A Cookbook for All Seasons,* for more ideas. I offer the sample menu plans here primarily to educate and inspire readers to follow the principles of simple, regular, wholesome meals combined so as to best promote digestion and utilization. However, due to size constraints of this text, the recipes from the menu plans are found in my cookbook.

In reviewing the meal guidelines outlined in chapter 13, we see that breakfast is a meal composed of a simple carbohydrate (fruit) followed by a complex carbohydrate, such as whole grains. Some of the breakfast menus are even a little more involved, with some fruit, grain, and even nuts combined. Often we may give more than 1 breakfast suggestion, and those wanting to follow stricter guidelines and eat lighter can just consume fruit in the morning, which may be followed in 1 or 2 hours by some starchy food or some nuts or seeds. In the summer, this may be even more apropos. Even our complex breakfasts are still simpler than many people may currently eat, containing much less protein or fat, and this allows the body to prepare for those heavier foods later.

However, if our jobs require strenuous physical effort or we feel our bodies require more substantial foods earlier in the day (this may be true when we do not eat much food after dark), some proteins can be used for breakfast. Eggs (poached or soft-boiled are best; over easy with a small amount of butter or oil is okay) can be eaten with toast or tortillas and some vegetables. One of my favorite (and heavier) breakfasts is two eggs over easy served on tortillas with alfalfa sprouts, diced tomatoes, a slice of avocado, and some salsa. I definitely do not support the typical American breakfast of bacon or sausage (no cured or lunch meats ever) along with eggs, potatoes, toast, and juice; this is excessive in quantity of food, fats, and protein. Instead of that extra meat protein, vegetables are a better balance, as with a vegetable stir-fry with a couple of eggs added toward the end. Overall, the menu plans outlined in this chapter pro-

vide a modified, not strict, rotation diet. If a strict rotation diet is desired to help with food allergies, it will only take a little more discipline and adaptation from these plans. Clearly, though, no foods are suggested at all meals, or even daily.

With the common American 8:00 to 5:00 work lifestyle, it may be difficult to have the main meal at lunchtime. The typical business schedule does not allow a 1:00 to 4:00 p.m. break for lunch and siesta time as in many other countries. Because of this, some of the menu plans allow switches between the lunch and dinner meals, but they are still written as the main meal at midday because I believe this is best nutritionally. As an example, on day 3 of the spring menu plan, the fish lunch would need to be prepared the night before and taken to work. If this is not practical, the couscous dish can be eaten at lunch and the fish and vegetables prepared fresh for dinner.

Following each sample menu is a seasonal food list. The foods included are primarily from the vegetable kingdom. Most animal foods are available year-round, and in many parts of the world, with modern technology and improved storage systems, a lot of fruits and vegetables can be found outside their season. If we can consume about 50% to 75% of our foods as fresh and seasonal, that is a good beginning.

I am very supportive of vegetarianism, but I realize that most people in the U.S. culture and the world at large do not choose to eat this way. To be realistic and also supportive of the omnivorous diet, some of the meals in the menu plans contain fish and poultry; I have included no red meats, however. If we keep our priorities and food groups in the right perspective, an omnivorous diet can be equal to or healthier than a vegetarian one. An omnivorous diet is often easier to follow, primarily because it is easier to acquire all the essential nutrients. These menu plans are also low in milk products and eggs, foods that are best eaten only moderately by most adults. To help with creative cookery, I have cited some other popular recipe books throughout the chapter.

It is more common now for both vegetarians and omnivores to be finding a new balance that combines many of the wholesome foods of the strict vegetarian with the avoidance of land animals and their by-products, specifically milk and eggs. Instead, they consume the nourishing water animals, both freshwater and ocean fish. The quality of usable protein in fish is excellent, the nutrient content is high, and the digestibility is good for most people. I have termed this diet "pescaveganism"—fish and strict vegetarianism—and it is the main diet I have followed for many years. Because of recent concerns with ocean pollution and mercury toxicity of fish, I encourage people who eat fish to use a variety and not overdo any specific species, such as tuna or snapper. The smaller fish, like sardines, tend to have lower mercury levels.

Furthermore, I encourage people to maintain conscious and conscientious shopping and seasonal food awareness. Many foods—such as the grains, legumes, nuts, and seeds—store relatively well and are used commonly throughout the year by most people. Our selection of fruits and vegetables should bring out our seasonal awareness, and the eating plan should reflect that we are shopping for fresh, local produce as much as possible. I suggest people eat more fresh and uncooked fruits and vegetables, a more raw food diet that also includes seeds, nuts, and sprouts, during the warmer months of spring, summer, and autumn.

In my *Staying Healthy with the Seasons,* based on the Oriental five element theory, five seasons are discussed. Yet in this chapter I have outlined only four seasonal menu plans. The fifth season the Chinese call the *doyo,* meaning "transition." It relates both to late summer as well as to the 2 to 3 weeks of seasonal change around the solstices and equinoxes. These are the times that I take a closer look at my diet and ask myself whether it needs any changes to best support my energy and health and adaptation to the next season. Often I write down a plan encompassing what I am doing and outlining the changes I wish to make.

The equinoxes—moving into spring and autumn—appear to be the most significant shift periods of the year. At these times I usually do a cleansing diet to rest from food and lighten myself up so I can be more aware of shifts happening in my life. In spring, I do a 10-day Master Cleanser fast. The Master Cleanser is a spicy lemonade that is quite tasty and energizing, and it contains fresh lemon juice, pure maple syrup, cayenne pepper, and water. You can read more about this in "Fasting and Juice Cleansing" section on page 769 of chapter 18. In autumn, I usually take a few weeks of detoxification along with my nutrition work-

shop groups, utilizing programs found in my book *The New Detox Diet.* Participants focus on a cleaner diet and cleansing with fresh fruits and vegetables and their juices. Most people, unless they are too nutrient deficient, weak, or ill, can follow this type of program. The basic principles and guidelines for this process are outlined in chapter 18, Detoxification and Cleansing Programs, and more specifically in my book *The New Detox Diet.*

Before covering the menu plans and seasonal food lists, I provide some basics to help in creating a healthy diet. My colleague Eleonora Manzolini, a "cuisine artist" in her own right, helped me with this section. Simple utensil and shopping lists, basic cooking and storing ideas, as well as general tips and shortcuts are included here. The chapter ends with a glossary of new and unusual foods that may be found in some supermarkets and most health food stores. Natural food products have grown by leaps and bounds in recent years, and there are some good products available as well as some junk. I hope this information helps you on your path to a new way of eating, or allows you to fine-tune your already health-oriented diet. Enjoy!

INTRODUCTORY NOTE FROM ELEONORA MANZOLINI

In today's postindustrialized countries, people are eating more than ever before, yet most are receiving less nourishment. Real food, for the most part, is virtually unknown; yet fortunately, more and more people are becoming conscious that both shelved and perishable products in supermarkets contain a wide array of chemical additives and contaminants, and that their food choices have an impact not only on their health but on that of the entire planet.

Food is the earliest form of addiction; it may be more controversial than sex, politics, or religion. People in general have become out of touch with nature and possess little instinctual or rational basis for their diet, and as a result they can become emotional about it. Thus they may defend their diet and resist suggestions for change. Many people in the United States are not familiar with natural foods and do not know how to maintain good health; they eat mainly what is marketed by corporate America. Doctors in general may know a lot about disease yet little about health-promoting factors such as nutrition.

Today there are many philosophies around diet and many choices of foods and their preparation. I have examined diets from many perspectives and have come to the conclusion that since we are all different, genetically and otherwise, this predisposes the body to choose certain foods. In a natural setting, we would instinctually choose foods that provide just the right amount of energy and nutrients for our needs and for the level of consciousness and life adventure we would like to experience.

There are no "good" and "bad" foods per se, just as there are no correct and incorrect ways of preparing them (although definitely some foods and preparations may support health more than others). Rather, it is a matter of personal choice that has to do with our unique makeup. Moderation and balance are the keys. Our bodies are perfectly well equipped to handle everything in small amounts, and if we understand that we are part of the Earth just like the plants and animals, we will naturally have more respect for these other creatures and gravitate toward a more frugal and simple lifestyle. This will not only protect our health but also the entire ecosystem.

My advice, then, is, Do not fight your bad habits; be kind to yourself, nourish yourself well, and they will eventually fall away. Do not make food an end in itself, or an obsession. Construct a diet as healthy, that is, as wholesome and balanced, as your head can tolerate without losing the joy of living. And remember, everyone's needs are different and different stages of life require different nutrition (see chapter 15, Life Stage Programs). I feel in alignment with the philosophy of Dr. Elson Haas, and I like his direct and practical way of explaining things. In keeping with this simplicity, before the seasonal menu plans in this chapter, I provide a few time-saving tips for the busy person, as well as basic shopping and utensil lists.

The sample basic recipes in this chapter are all simple and quick to prepare. I believe it is important to eat well on a daily basis, and to be able to do this realistically in our busy lives, cooking cannot be too much of an ordeal. We have to learn to put together a healthy, well-balanced meal in a half hour with a few fresh ingredients and without having to give up taste or resort to lifeless, chemical, or processed foods. I hope my contribution to this book helps you accomplish this.

Basic Utensils

The size and number of pots and pans you need depend on how many people you are serving. The following basic collection should take care of up to 12 people. I prefer stainless steel materials, and also use cast-iron, glass, Corningware, and enamel.

Basic Utensil Collection

- one 1-quart saucepan
- one 2-quart saucepan
- two 3-quart saucepans
- one 9-inch skillet
- one soup pot
- one pressure cooker (could be the same as a soup pot)
- one 3- or 4-quart covered, ovenproof baking dish
- two shallow lasagna-style baking dishes
- two glass pie plates
- one cookie sheet
- six wooden stirring spoons of various sizes
- one set of measuring cups
- one set of measuring spoons
- two rubber spatulas
- one grater
- one hard brush for scrubbing vegetables
- one wire whisk
- two paring knives
- one good knife for chopping vegetables.
  Note: This is the most important purchase. Make sure that the weight is comfortably distributed and that the blade is thin so that it cuts easily. It may take several purchases to find "your" knife. My favorite is a Mac knife.

Shopping List for the Beginner

Choose organically grown products whenever possible. This list is organized by food category, in order of relative importance, with starches and grains at the beginning (even though we realize some people are currently choosing a low-grain and low-carbohydrate diet), followed by protein foods (vegetarian and non-vegetarian), vegetables, and fruits and other foods, such as oils and condiments, sweeteners, and snack foods, and, finally, substitutions for the most common allergens.

STARCHES

Grains. A few different varieties of rice, such as short grain brown rice, jasmine rice, basmati, and wild rice. Also included are millet, buckwheat, and quinoa.

Quick-cooking grains. Couscous, polenta, and rolled oats.

Noodles. Long and short noodles, such as spaghetti and penne; durum and whole wheat are best. Look for wheat-free alternatives, which include corn elbows, quinoa pasta, or soba (buckwheat) noodles.

Breads and flours. Sprouted whole-grain breads and tortillas, unyeasted breads, Wasa crackers, Essene or manna bread, and whole wheat pastry flour (keep in freezer).

PROTEIN FOODS (VEGETARIAN)

Beans. A variety of beans that may include pinto, adzuki, mung, garbanzo, and navy beans.

Quick cooking beans. Lentils, red lentils, and split peas.

Soybean products. Tofu (plain and marinated), tempeh (plain, marinated, and tempeh/grain mixtures), tofu and tempeh burgers.

Seitan. A wheat protein that is easy to use in grain and vegetable dishes, or in sandwiches.

PROTEIN FOODS (ANIMAL)

These are best purchased fresh and organically raised, but if necessary, can be bought frozen. Chose fish from cold, deep waters, and avoid farmed fish. Exceptions are sardines, anchovies, and anchovy paste; these are easy to keep on hand and can be added to many dishes. They are a great and tasty source of protein.

VEGETABLES

These are best purchased fresh and seasonal, as well as organically grown. If that is not possible, dehydrated and dried is better than canned, as is fresh frozen. Tomatoes and onions, as well as many herbs, are available dried. They can be soaked in water and used in stir-fries or added to sauces, soups, and casseroles.

Sea vegetables. Kombu, agar-agar, nori, arame, and hijiki. These are an acquired taste, but many have health-promoting qualities. They usually come in dehydrated form and keep indefinitely. The easiest ones to start out with are kombu (add a strip to soups, stews, and in cooking beans; remove before serving); dulse (mild tasting, can be shredded into any dish before serving; do not cook); and nori (used to make sushi rolls or crumbled into soups or over any dish).

FRUITS AND OTHER FOODS

Fruits. Again, these are best purchased fresh, organic, and seasonal. A selection of dried fruits might include unsulfured apples, apricots, prunes, and raisins. They make excellent snacks.

Oils. Extra-virgin olive oil, toasted sesame oil, safflower oil, corn oil, coconut oil, and red palm oil. Quality brands include Spectrum, Eden, and Sciabica's olive oil.

I am partial to olive oil, which is what I use for practically everything except frying. There are now so many varieties of good olive oil on the market that it is difficult to suggest any one in particular. Keep in mind that excellent olive oils are made in California. Toasted sesame oil is good to keep around for Oriental dishes. Fried foods are not the healthiest, but if you do fry, then use a light sunflower or rice bran oil.

Condiments. Good soy sauce or tamari, miso paste (used to make miso soup or in any soup or salad dressing), aged balsamic vinegar, apple cider or brown rice vinegars, Dijon mustard, soy-based mayonnaise, tahini (ground sesame seeds used in dips and sauces), and gomasio (a mixture of toasted sesame seeds and sea salt).

Herbs and spices. Dried thyme, marjoram, basil, oregano, and parsley. Garlic, ginger (fresh and powdered), onion, cayenne, and red chile flakes. Cumin powder, curry powder, cilantro (coriander), cinnamon sticks and powder, and cloves.

Sweeteners. Maple syrup, honey, rice syrup or agave (from cactus), and the herbal sweetener stevia (no calories).

Snack foods. Rice products such as mochi, rice cakes, and various rice crackers; fresh and dried fruit, like apples; vegetables such as carrots, celery, or radishes; grain-sweetened cookies; and raw nuts (especially almonds or walnuts).

SUBSTITUTIONS

For dairy. Soymilk, amazake (sweet rice drinks), nut milks, and nutritional yeast to sprinkle over foods instead of cheese.

For wheat. Rye flour breads and crackers, soy and rice noodles, quinoa pasta, buckwheat noodles (soba), and corn elbows (they fall apart easily, but are good in soups).

Kitchen Basics

Washing grains. I like the swirling method I learned from Annemarie Colbin, author of many popular natural cooking books. This is more effective than running water over the grains in a colander. Put the grains in a bowl and cover with twice the amount of water. Swirl thoroughly and pour off all the floating debris and stray grains. Catch the rest in a colander. If the water is very dirty, repeat the procedure. Quinoa, amaranth, and millet need to be washed more carefully, several times at least.

Cooking brown rice. Combine 1 cup rice to 2 cups cold water and a pinch of salt. The salt is important even if you are on a salt-free diet because it brings out the full flavor of the grain. Bring to a boil, adjust the flame to low, and cook the rice for 50 to 60 minutes (it may take less time, depending on the heat). If you are making rice with steamed vegetables, you can lay the cut-up vegetables on top of the rice during the last 10 minutes and they will cook with the steam from the rice. Rice connoisseurs suggest cooking the rice undisturbed for 1 hour over low heat. The pot must have a tight seal so the steam does not escape, and to tell it is done, listen to the pot. It will stop bubbling and you will hear a slight crackling or popping sound of rice toasting. Many rice lovers prepare the rice with more salt, about 1/4 to 1/2 teaspoon per cup of uncooked rice, and 1/2 to 1 tablespoon of oil or butter.

Cooking barley. Cook with the same amount of water as you would rice. I have found it takes slightly longer, 60 to 70 minutes.

Cooking quinoa. Use 1 cup of quinoa to 2 cups of water and a pinch of salt. Cover, bring to a boil, and simmer for 15 minutes.

Cooking millet. Another trick I learned from Annemarie Colbin is to dry roast this grain in a cast-iron or stainless steel skillet until a few grains begin to pop, about 5 to 10 minutes. Then add 2 cups of water for each cup of millet and the usual pinch of salt. Cover, bring to a boil, lower the heat, and simmer for about 30 to 40 minutes. Fluff with a fork before serving. If you are just cooking millet in water, rinse it well to remove any unseen dirt.

Cooking kasha. Bring 2 cups of water and a pinch of salt to a boil. Add 1 cup of kasha, lower the flame, and simmer for 15 to 20 minutes.

Proportions and Cooking Times for Various Grains		
Grain	**Ratio (grain to water)**	**Cooking Time**
Brown rice	1:2	50–60 minutes
Millet	1:2–2$\frac{1}{2}$	30–40 minutes
Oats	1:2	15–20 minutes
Kasha	1:2–2$\frac{1}{2}$	15–20 minutes
Barley	1:2$\frac{1}{2}$	60–70 minutes
Couscous	1:1$\frac{1}{2}$–2	10 minutes

You may wish to use a pressure cooker for some grains to shorten the cooking time. In that case, add less water, about 1½ cups of water to 1 cup of the grain. (Warning: Do not cook any cracked grain in a pressure cooker because it may clog up the escape valve and cause an explosion.) Pressure-cooked grains have a totally different texture and taste, especially rice, which tends to stick together. It is wonderful for making sushi but not appropriate for a rice salad or pilaf. If you make rice often, you may wish to buy an automatic rice cooker.

Washing and soaking beans. Beans that are bought in bulk need picking over because they often contain stones. This is common with lentils and garbanzo beans, so you might consider buying them packaged and already cleaned. The following beans do not need soaking: all kinds of lentils, split peas, and adzuki beans. All other beans are best soaked overnight in twice the amount of water. Throw away the soaking water. This will shorten the cooking time and also reduce the gas-producing effects. If you do not have time to soak the beans overnight, you can use a quick method. Boil them in twice the amount of water for 5 minutes, let them sit covered for 1 hour, and then change the water for further cooking.

Cooking beans. Black-eyed peas, lima beans, small white or navy beans, and adzuki beans can be cooked together with rice in the same pot because they have similar cooking times. Just add more water. Pressure-cooking reduces the time to about half those listed below, but be careful not to cook lentils and split peas in a pressure cooker because they may clog the escape valve and cause the pressure cooker to explode.

Always salt your beans at the end, about 10 minutes before they are done. This is important because adding salt at the beginning will cause the beans to remain tough. If you prefer not to use salt, remember that beans cooked with no salt at all tend to disintegrate. This may be okay for soups and stews but not if you are making a bean salad. Beans, like grains, can be cooked in an oven or slow cooker. Place the beans and water (add an additional cup of water per additional cup of beans) in an ovenproof bean pot or casserole dish. Put the covered dish in the oven and cook overnight or all day at a low setting, 200°F degrees to 220°F. The beans will be more tasty, tender, and thicker than if you use the quicker cooking method.

For more flavorful, spicy beans, cook with lightly sautéed onions and garlic. Dice a large onion and a few cloves of garlic and lightly sauté with 2 teaspoons of olive or other light oil in the pot. Add 2 cups of beans and about 6 cups of water, and simmer until the beans are tender. To avoid the oil, just add all the ingredients to the pot and cook.

To enhance and vary the flavor of the beans, a variety of herbs and spices can be added to the pot at the start or midway through. If beginning with 2 cups of beans, try one or more of the suggestions in the table on the opposite page, following your inspiration and taste.

Proportions and Cooking Times for Various Beans		
Bean	**Ratio (beans to water)**	**Cooking Time**
Red lentils	1:2	15–20 minutes
Lentils and split peas	1:2–2½	30 minutes
Black-eyed peas, lima beans, small white or navy beans, mung beans, and adzuki beans	1:3	60 minutes
Kidney beans, pinto beans, soybeans, and black beans	1:3½	90 minutes
Garbanzo beans	1:4	120 minutes

Possible Flavor Enhancers for Beans

Vegetables	Dried Herbs	Fresh Herbs
Garlic, 2–4 cloves, minced	Bay leaf, 1 or 2	Cilantro, 4–6 tsp
Onion, 1 medium or large, chopped	Oregano, 1/2 tsp	Parsley, 2–3 sprigs
Carrot, 1 or 2 chopped	Basil, 1/2–1 tsp	Sage, 2–3 leaves
Bell pepper, 1 chopped	Cumin, 1–2 tsp	Rosemary, 1 sprig
Jalapeño, 1 sliced, seeded	Cayenne, 1/4 tsp	Thyme, 2 sprigs
Tomatoes, 2 fresh, chopped	Chili powder, 1/2–1 tsp	
	Sage, pinch	
	Rosemary, 1/4 tsp	
	Thyme, 1/4–1/2 tsp	

Cleaning vegetables. If you buy organic root vegetables (carrots, radishes, turnips, and so on), there is no need to peel them; just scrub them with a stiff brush. Vegetables from commercial sources often have been treated with chemical pesticides and are waxed; therefore, peeling them first reduces the chemical exposure. To peel tomatoes, drop them in boiling water for 10 to 15 seconds. Allow them to cool and the skin comes off easily. To peel garlic, place your knife flat on the garlic clove and whack it with your other hand. The covering will burst open and the clove can be easily removed. For leafy greens, cut off the root end and plunge into a sink full of cold water. Swirl around a few times and let them sit for awhile. The sand, dirt, and other debris will settle to the bottom, and the leaves will float to the top and can be removed. Repeat the procedure if the greens (such as spinach) are very dirty.

Some tips about fish. When buying a whole fish, make sure it has firm flesh, red gills, and bright eyes. Steaks or fillets should be moist and not flaky. Also, it is a good idea to get your fish from a dependable source (like an organic grocer), not a supermarket, where it may be dipped in a solution of nitrites and nitrates to cover up any smell. Some stores use paper that is saturated with chemicals to lay the fish on to preserve the color. Before cooking, it is best to rinse the fish under cold running water. Do not use a wooden cutting board for chopping up fish or meat, because the wood absorbs the juices and becomes a breeding ground for bacteria.

Seasoning. By seasoning I am not referring to just salt, even if that is an important ingredient. I like to use true sea salt, which is free of additives, and use it only in cooking, not at the table. Earth mineral salts (from evaporated seawater) have more nutrients and are more healthful choices for human consumption than common table salt. Herbs and spices can lend a great deal of taste to even the simplest dish, but it is important to use just the right amount that will enhance and not overpower the flavor of the food. This is especially true for strong-tasting ones such as garlic, cayenne, sage, and tarragon. It is best to start with a little and then add more if necessary. For best results, fresh herbs should be added at the end of the cooking time, while dried ones should be added at the beginning. Cayenne and freshly ground black pepper can be added individually at the table, because not everybody likes a hot taste.

Suggestions for Flavor Repair

Too salty. Wash off the salt or add oil or butter. When cooking grains or pasta, if the water is too salty, add a whole potato.

Too sweet. Add salt or increase the liquid.

Too bitter. Avoid salt and add something sweet.

Too spicy. Add a whole potato or some grains, or something sweet.

Too sour. Add salt or liquid.

For giving such basic dishes as rice, vegetables, or chicken an international flavor, **a simple seasoning list might include the following:**

Italian. Basil, oregano, thyme, marjoram, garlic, and olive oil.

Chinese. Ginger, soy sauce, cayenne or chile oil, scallions, and toasted sesame oil.

Mexican. Cumin, cilantro, cayenne or chile pepper, garlic, and salsa.

Indian. Curry, coriander, cumin, saffron, cardamom, turmeric, and ghee (clarified butter).

French. Dill, tarragon, thyme, rosemary, mustard, butter, walnut oil, and wine.

East European. Paprika, poppy seed, caraway, dill, onion, and sour cream.

A Few Tips and Shortcuts

- Soak beans overnight to cut cooking time; throw away the soaking water.

- Soak nuts and seeds overnight and they will become easier to digest because the fats in them become more available as fatty acids. Soaked nuts and seeds also make wonderful additions to salads and can be stored in the refrigerator for a few days. Minimize your intake of roasted and salted nuts and seeds.

- Pressure-cooking beans and grains cuts the cooking time by approximately a third. I like to pressure-cook a big batch of beans at a time and then store them in the freezer in small containers, each about enough for 2 people. This way I can prepare a bean dish in no time at all, and besides, freezing helps get rid of the agents that cause flatulence in many people.

- Wash salad and other leafy greens when you buy them; let them dry and then keep them in plastic bags in the vegetable compartment of the refrigerator so you do not have to waste a lot of time when you want to use them. I also like to keep the basic vegetables—chopped onions, garlic, carrots, celery, and parsley—all

---

Seasoning Mix

A general seasoning mixture can be made from your own favorite choices or from the following recipe of dried ingredients:

1–2 tsp sea salt
2 tsp basil flakes
1–2 tsp onion powder
1 tsp parsley flakes
1/2 tsp garlic powder
1/2 tsp thyme
1/2–1 tsp mustard powder
1/2 tsp marjoram
1/4–1/2 tsp cayenne powder
1/2 tsp celery seeds
1 tsp paprika
1/2 tsp curry (optional)
1/2 tsp powdered kelp (optional)

---

ready to use. It's best to keep these in a plastic container with a lid.

- Keep a few basic sauces ready in the refrigerator, such as tomato sauce. Just simmer fresh or canned peeled tomatoes for about 20 minutes with a little salt. For a quick tomato sauce, you can then sauté onion, garlic, celery, carrot, and parsley and a little chile pepper in a small amount of olive oil and add it to the tomatoes. It takes about 5 minutes to put the whole thing together. Store in glass or stainless steel, not in aluminum or pottery ware.

- Miso-tahini is also a basic condiment that keeps well. Just blend miso and tahini with a little rice vinegar and water. You can add garlic, ginger, or mustard to it to make it different every time. Use it as a salad dressing by adding more water, or as a dip or creamy sauce over grains if you keep it thicker.

- Flavored oils add zest to any dish. I am partial to olive oil, but you can use any oil you like. Make small bottles and add a different herb to each— garlic, hot chile pepper, tarragon, sage, rosemary, thyme, and so on.

- If you do not have time to marinate things, here is a way to quick marinate. Bring your marinade to a boil and drop whatever you want to marinate into it for a few minutes.

- Instant pizza can be made by using tortillas or pita bread. Place them in the oven for a few minutes to crisp, spoon on some tomato sauce, your favorite toppings, and a little grated cheese, and put them into the oven again for a few minutes until the cheese melts.

- Quick-cooking grains are couscous, millet, quinoa, and polenta.

- Frozen grapes and cherries make wonderful alternatives to candy, or fun "ice cubes" for drinks.

- Almost any juices, fresh or bottled, can be placed in Popsicle containers and frozen to make warm-weather treats for children of all ages.

- For thickening sauces and gravies, there are many substitutes for wheat flour. Equivalents to 1 tablespoon of wheat flour include 1/2 tablespoon of arrowroot powder, rice or potato flour, or cornstarch.

- For those avoiding salt, lower-sodium substitutes include kelp, regular or low-sodium tamari, light miso, lemon juice, celery salt, various vegetable "salts," and the seasoning mix on the opposite page.

For Those Who Wish to Avoid Fats

- Substitute fish, chicken, or vegetable stock for half or all of the oil called for in a recipe.

- Water-sauté food instead of stir-frying it in oil. Put about 1/2 to 1 cup of water or stock into a wok or skillet and bring it to a rapid boil. Quickly add vegetables and keep stirring over a high flame until done. A small amount of oil can be added toward the end for flavor and fatty acid nutrition.

- Onions sautéed in their own juice and pureed with light miso make a wonderful onion butter that is great on toast or bread instead of using real butter. The same thing can be done with most vegetables.

- Apple butter is a great nonfat spread for those with a sweet tooth.

- Puree a loose oatmeal (about 1 cup of rolled oats to 4 cups of water). Use this instead of milk to make cream soups, gravies, and any dish that calls for milk.

- Tofu pureed with lemon juice makes a great mock sour cream.

Tips for Storing

- Cooked grains may be kept in a porcelain or wooden bowl in a cool place but out of the refrigerator. Covered with a napkin, they will keep for about 3 days. In the refrigerator they should be stored in airtight containers or they will absorb the flavors of other foods.

- Dried beans can be kept in jars on shelves or inside a cupboard. Cooked beans are best stored in the freezer in small containers.

- Mushrooms should be kept in a brown paper bag in the vegetable compartment of the refrigerator.

- Fresh herbs keep best in a glass of water in the refrigerator, like flowers.

- Once opened, oils should be refrigerated. The only exception is olive oil, which should be kept in a dark place, such as a cupboard.

- Nuts and seeds are best refrigerated or even frozen.

- Flour should be kept in the refrigerator or freezer.

- Fruits, potatoes, tomatoes, onions, and garlic are best not refrigerated but kept in a basket in a place in the shade or in a pantry.

SOME BASIC RECIPES

Here are a few simple recipes to follow the basic rice and beans discussion and the food preparation tips. With the help of all the diet and recipe books now on the market, once you learn to cook, you may use these basic ideas to create your own recipes in the kitchen. For many people, grains, beans, and vegetables—both raw and cooked—make up the major part of their diet; recipes are often used to learn new preparations or dishes for special occasions.

General Salad Ingredients

(LIMIT TO 4 TO 6 CHOICES)

mixed lettuce (red or green leaf, romaine, or butter head lettuce), shredded

spinach, broken

green or red bell pepper, diced

carrots, sliced or grated

cabbage (red or green), shredded

mushrooms, wiped and sliced

green onions, sliced

alfalfa sprouts

bean sprouts (mung, green peas, garbanzo, or adzuki)

sunflower or pumpkin seeds, raw and organic ideally

Any greens should be washed carefully and dried. Remove spinach stems. The sprouts, sunflower seeds, and mushrooms add some protein to the vegetable salad. Toss with a salad dressing of your choice.

Mixed Sprout Salad (SERVES 4-6)

Sprouts and fresh vegetables are some of our vital foods, active with enzymes, vitamins and minerals, and the important phytonutrients.

1 cup each fresh alfalfa, lentil, and mung bean sprouts

1/2 cup adzuki, green pea, or garbanzo sprouts, or a mixed-bean preparation

2 tbsp sunflower seeds

1/2 cup chopped green onions

1/2 cup diced green pepper or cucumber

1-2 tbsp chopped fresh herbs (optional), or 1 tbsp dried salad herbs

2 ripe tomatoes, or 12 cherry tomatoes

Toss everything but the tomatoes together and then decorate with tomatoes. Serve with a dressing of olive oil, lemon juice, and salad herbs, or a dressing of your choice. This high-protein, nutritious salad is filling.

Vegetable Broth/Soup (SERVES 6-8)

2 cups potatoes, cut in small chunks

1 large onion, sliced top to bottom

2 carrots, medium, sliced

1-2 stalks of celery

1 clove garlic, minced

4-6 shiitake mushroom stems (optional)

1-2 zucchinis, sliced

2 cups green cabbage, sliced (or other greens, such as spinach or kale)

1/2 tsp sea salt

cayenne or black pepper, pinch or to taste

6-8 cups purified water

1 cup yellow or green split peas (optional)

1 strip kombu

Place the first 10 ingredients into a pot with the water, cover, and bring to a boil. Lower the flame and simmer slowly for 1 to 2 hours, adding water if necessary. The shiitake mushrooms stems will give a richer broth flavor, yet should be removed when the broth is done.

For vegetable soup, cook the harder vegetables first, about 20 to 30 minutes depending on the size of the chunks, and then add zucchini, cabbage or greens, if used. For a thicker soup, add a cup of yellow or green split peas. Other herbs and spices can be used if desired. Blend part or all of cooled soup for a thicker broth or a rich soup. Serve with chopped green onion or cilantro, or eat the vegetables and save the broth for other recipes, such as for sauces or gravies.

You could keep the scraps from onions, carrots, celery, and other vegetables in a plastic bag in the freezer until you have enough to make a vegetable stock. Then simmer all of it with a strip of kombu and use this broth as a base for other soups or for cooking grains.

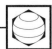

Thick (Spicy) Vegetable Soup
(MAKES 5–6 CUPS)

1 pound small or medium potatoes, or cauliflower pieces
4 cups water
$^1/_4$ tsp cayenne, or to taste (optional for spicy)
$^1/_2$ tsp dried basil
$^1/_2$ tsp cumin
3 tbsp sesame oil or corn oil (for a buttery flavor)
$^1/_2$–1 tsp sea salt
1 small onion, chopped
2 cloves garlic, chopped (optional)
$^1/_2$ cup tomato, diced
$^1/_2$ cup of several of the following vegetables: carrot,
*   celery, green pepper, zucchini, broccoli, cauliflower,*
*   beets (for pink soup)*
$^1/_2$ cup green onions, chopped

Scrub and wash potatoes or cauliflower and boil in the water in a medium-sized pot or saucepan for 15 to 20 minutes. Allow this to cool a bit and blend the vegetables with the water in which they were cooked, adding the seasonings, the oil, and the salt. Rinse the assorted vegetables and chop into bite-sized pieces. Place the blended mixture and chopped vegetables into the pot or saucepan, cover, and cook over a low heat for 10 to 15 minutes. Top with green onions and serve.

For a specific vegetable soup, such as potato or broccoli, use primarily that vegetable. For a cream soup, use milk (preferably low-fat), or for a milk-free cream soup, blend in an appropriate amount (1 cup in this recipe) of well-cooked, moist oatmeal.

Low-Fat, Low-Salt Vinaigrette
(MAKES ABOUT 1 CUP)

This variation of a recipe from Dean Ornish's *Stress, Diet, and Your Heart* is a healthy and tasty vinaigrette. There are even some decent oil-free dressings available in most stores.

2 tbsp safflower, sunflower, or olive oil
1–2 oz rice or apple cider vinegar, or $^1/_2$–1 lemon,
*   juiced*
1–2 cloves garlic, minced or pressed
$^1/_2$ tsp dried mustard
$^1/_4$ tsp dried tarragon, $^1/_2$ tsp salad herbs, or 1 tsp
*   chopped fresh herbs*
$^1/_4$ tsp dried basil or marjoram
$^1/_2$ cup nonfat yogurt, unsalted tomato juice, or water
pepper to taste

Mix the ingredients together well, or place in blender for a short blend (15 to 30 seconds) on low speed. Achieve desired thickness with water.

Joe Terry's Magic Miso Dressing
(MAKES ABOUT 2 CUPS)

3–4 cloves garlic
$^3/_4$ cup balsamic vinegar
$^1/_2$ cup water
6 oz unpasteurized white miso
1 tsp prepared mustard
2 tbsp olive oil

This is also a low-fat, cholesterol-free, yet spicy, flavorful dressing for salads or other dishes, such as grains or vegetables. It needs a long, slow blender ride to make it really creamy and mix all the flavors. Blend garlic cloves in vinegar and water. Slowly add miso, mustard, and olive oil.

Guacamole (SERVES 4)

3 medium avocados
1 small tomato, chopped and drained (optional)
2 green onions, chopped fine (optional)
$^1/_4$ cup of Spanish, Bermuda, or yellow onion, diced
*   (optional)*
2 cloves garlic, minced
$^1/_2$ lemon or 1 lime, juiced
$^1/_4$ tsp cayenne or chili powder, or to taste, or 1 small
*   jalapeño pepper, chopped finely, seeds removed*
$^1/_4$–$^1/_2$ tsp salt, or to taste

Mash avocados in a bowl and mix in other ingredients. Serve cold with chips and salsa or with vegetables. Add water and lemon to make avocado salad dressing in blender. Add miso paste to taste for miso-avocado dressing. Blend in a block of tofu (with more water) for avocado-tofu dip or dressing. A simple guacamole consists of only avocados, lemon, and salt. For a creamy version, add yogurt or sour cream.

Tostadas (Tortilla Meals)

tortillas, corn or wheat
grains (traditionally, this is rice, which works best,
    either brown, white, wild, or a mixture)
refried beans
cheese, grated (Jack, cheddar or soy)
chopped onion
sprouts or iceberg lettuce, shredded
avocado slices or guacamole
black olives
salsa
sour cream (optional)

Oil skillet and heat (on low) one side of tortilla. Turn and lay in grain or refried beans, sprinkle with cheese, and cover to melt. Serve with toppings. For a taco, fold in half and heat, flipping to other half if necessary. Remove and add vegetable ingredients of choice and seasonings.

Salsa (MAKES 3–4 CUPS)

3 cups chopped ripe tomatoes
1/2 small onion, chopped
1 small jalapeño or chile pepper, seeded and chopped
    (1/4 cup chopped bell pepper for milder salsa)
2 cloves garlic, minced
1/2 tsp chili powder, or 1/4–1/2 tsp cayenne
2 tsp fresh lemon or lime juice
2 tbsp chopped cilantro (optional)
1/4–1/2 tsp cumin (optional)
1/4 tsp salt (optional)

Mix everything together. Using a blender or a food processor will make creamier salsa.

Steamed Veggie Platter

Use several or all of the following vegetables:
    new potatoes, unpeeled
    carrots, half-length strips
    beets, quartered
    broccoli florets with a little stem
    cauliflower florets
    zucchini, steam whole, then slice lengthwise

For a dip, use guacamole, salsa, or hummus—all of which can be made or purchased from most stores.

Steam vegetables until only slightly soft, about 10 to 15 minutes (zucchini, 5 minutes). Arrange all on a platter and season with melted butter or olive oil, lemon juice, and salt or herb seasoning. Garnish with cherry tomatoes if available. May also serve around a bowl with an herbal butter or any dip of your choice. Raw celery sticks, carrot sticks, and tomatoes can be used as well. In summer, a lightly steamed vegetable platter really brings out the natural flavors.

Baked Veggie Platter

Fresh vegetables that are sliced and lightly oiled, and then baked in an oven at about 325°F to 350°F, bring out some unusually good flavors of this most important food category. As adapted from my book *The False Fat Diet*, the seasonal vegetable medleys listed below offer some tasty nutritional mixtures to go with any meal. Steaming and water sautéing are other healthful ways to prepare fresh vegetables. Good ones to include are zucchini, onions, carrots or yams, peppers, and potatoes. Making them warm and tender, rather than overcooking, keeps more of the nutritional energy alive. Of course, eating veggies raw, which takes more time and chewing power, releases the most nutrients, enzymes, and vitality, and eating veggies raw should be a good portion of your total vegetable intake. Buy them fresh and organic, ideally, whenever possible.

Preheat the oven to 350°F. Cut up vegetables into bite-sized pieces or strips and put them all in a large bowl. Massage lightly with olive oil and sprinkle with a little of your favorite seasoning salt and

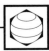

herbs. (You can also add the oil and seasonings after cooking.) Place the vegetables on a baking dish and then into your oven for 20 to 30 minutes, turning them about midway as they start to brown. You can turn the heat to broil for a few minutes to make them a bit crispier.

The vegetables in these medleys are listed seasonally. Some are more suited for baking or steaming. Pick your favorites. More seasonal foods are available in the "Seasonal Menu Plans" section on page 539.

Spring Medley. Asparagus, baby carrots, chard, spinach, spring garlic or green onions, leeks, beets, brussels sprouts, wild greens (mustard or sorrel), and artichokes.

Summer Medley. Green beans, zucchini, beets and beet greens, new potatoes, yellow and other soft squashes, peppers, eggplant, corn, and snow peas.

Autumn Medley. Hard squashes (acorn, butternut, and others), cauliflower, bell peppers, broccoli, carrots, celery, spinach, potatoes, okra, fresh corn, and Jerusalem artichokes.

Winter Medley. Onions, kale, cabbage, leeks, bok choy, Jerusalem artichokes, potatoes, chard, broccoli, cauliflower, and sweet potatoes.

Tomato Sauce (MAKES ABOUT 3 CUPS)

1/2 onion, chopped

1 clove garlic

2 tbsp olive oil

1 small carrot, grated

2 tbsp chopped green pepper

1 bay leaf

1/2 tsp oregano

1/2 tsp thyme

1 tsp basil

2 tbsp chopped fresh parsley

2 cups coarsely chopped tomatoes

1 6-oz can tomato paste

1/4 tsp honey

1 tsp salt

1/8 tsp pepper

This is a tasty tomato sauce. Use vegetable broth or water to thin it to the right consistency for spaghetti, or use it as is for dishes like pizza. Fresh tomatoes are wonderful, of course, but if they are not in season, use canned. (Be sure to check the label to avoid added salt and sugar.)

Sauté the onion and garlic clove in oil until the onion is soft. Crush the garlic with a fork. Add carrot, green pepper, and herbs. Stir well and then add the tomatoes, tomato paste, honey, salt, and pepper. Simmer 15 to 20 minutes. Remove the bay leaf.

Mexican variation. When the onion is nearly done, stir in 1 teaspoon cumin and 1 teaspoon chili powder, or to taste.

Italian variation. Add a pinch of fennel. Increase the oregano to 1 teaspoon.

Cold Rice Salad (SERVES 6)

6 cups cooked brown rice

1 cup chopped green or red pepper

4 green onions, chopped

4 radishes, sliced

1/2 cup fresh parsley chopped

1/2 cucumber, peeled and diced (optional)

1/2 cup roasted sunflower seeds

8–10 lettuce leaves

2 cups alfalfa sprouts

2 tomatoes, sliced

1 whole lemon, wedged

Mix rice with pepper, onions, radishes, parsley, cucumber, and sunflower seeds. Place rice mixture in the center of the lettuce leaves, surround with alfalfa sprouts, and top with sliced tomatoes. If desired, sprinkle with salad herbs. Serve with lemon wedges. An olive oil vinaigrette or a nonfat yogurt vinaigrette would be an ideal dressing.

Rainbow Rice (SERVES 6–8)

$^1/_2$ cup onion, chopped

$^1/_2$ cup red pepper, chopped

$^1/_2$ cup carrot, chopped

$^1/_2$ cup yellow squash, chopped

$^1/_2$ cup zucchini, chopped

$^1/_2$ cup purple (red) cabbage (or beet or eggplant), chopped

$^1/_2$ cup green onions, chopped

2 tbsp sunflower or sesame oil (or olive or canola)

2 tsp soy sauce or to taste

$^1/_2$ cup water

6 cups cooked rice

1 cup parsley (without stems), chopped

cayenne pepper to taste (optional)

Cut vegetables lengthwise and then dice. Sauté the vegetables in oil in this order: onion, pepper, carrot, squashes, cabbage (eggplant or beet), and green onions, adding water and soy sauce and stirring. Add cooked rice in clumps, stir into the vegetables, and heat gently for 5 minutes. Leave covered and serve warm. Before serving, add parsley (and cayenne if desired). Good with a tofu or miso-tahini dressing (see the recipe in *A Cookbook for All Seasons*). This is a good cold salad as well.

Chop Suey (SERVES 8–10)

$^1/_2$ cup oil (soy, canola, or sesame [toasted optional])

1 cup green pepper, diced (or celery, sliced)

1 cup onion, sliced in crescents

2 cups button mushrooms, sliced top to bottom

1 cup water chestnuts, sliced

2 cups green cabbage, shredded

1 cup Napa or Chinese cabbage, shredded

1 cup bok choy

2 cups mung bean sprouts

3 cups water

$^1/_2$ cup arrowroot powder

$^1/_2$ cup soy sauce

cayenne pepper or chile oil to taste (optional)

6–8 cups cooked rice

1 cup raw or toasted almonds, slivered or chopped (optional)

Use a heavy, large skillet or a wok for this chop suey dish. Heat the wok or the skillet first on medium heat. Add oil and then immediately add the vegetables, at 1- to 2-minute intervals, first adding the pepper and onions, then the mushrooms and water chestnuts, then the greens, and then bean sprouts, adding splashes of water up to 1 cup as needed. Have ready the arrowroot (a thickener), soy sauce, cayenne or chile oil if desired, and 1 to 2 cups cool water, whisked together until the powder is dissolved. Stir the liquid into vegetables, cover, and remove from heat. Serve over rice.

If toasted almonds are desired, bake in an oven on a cookie sheet for 15 to 20 minutes at 300°F or buy already-roasted almonds. For additional flavor, sprinkle some tamari soy sauce over the almonds before roasting.

Additional foods to add or substitute for this Chinese meal are tofu in cubes, bamboo shoots, snow peas, green beans, celery, green onions, sliced carrots, broccoli florets, cauliflower, zucchini, and minced garlic or ginger—or just any interesting veggies you might have on hand.

Also, a sukiyaki dish can be made in a pot using about half the portions of the listed ingredients and about a cup or more water, leaving out the almonds, substituting carrots for the green pepper, and adding some clear rice noodles and chunks of tofu. Simmer about 10 minutes and then add the greens, mung sprouts, and the arrowroot powder. For a richer flavor, sauté the hard vegetables lightly in oil before adding them to the pot.

Sesame Salt (Gomasio)

This is a tasty seasoning for soup, salads, or grain and vegetable dishes. Roast sesame seeds in a dry skillet, stirring continuously, until a few begin to pop. Blend with sea salt, 1 part salt to 8 to 10 parts sesame seeds. Place in a closed container and use as a table seasoning.

Wheat-Free Pie Crust (MAKES 1 PIE CRUST)

1 cup brown rice flour
1 cup oat flour
1/4 tsp sea salt
2 tbsp sesame oil
2/3–3/4 cup water

Lightly roast the flours in a skillet, stirring to toast but not brown. Combine all ingredients into a bowl and mix. Press the mixture into an oiled pie dish, spreading from center to edges to make a thin crust. Prebake for 10 to 15 minutes at 350°F, remove and cool before adding the pie filling. This recipe can also be used with whole wheat pastry flour and chopped walnuts.

Milk- and Egg-Free Sour Cream and Mayonnaise

The Tofu Sour Cream and Tofu Mayonnaises recipes from *The New Laurel's Kitchen* are milk- and egg-free recipes for those with allergies. They are also low in fat for individuals who like creamy sour cream or mayonnaise but are watching their waistlines or cholesterol levels.

Tofu Sour Cream (MAKES 1 1/2 CUPS)

1/4 cup lemon juice
2 tbsp oil
1 tbsp light miso
1/4 tsp mustard
2 tbsp water
1 tbsp shoyu (or other flavoring)
1/2 pound tofu

This makes a tasty substitute for plain sour cream. You will not need the water with soft tofu, but with firm tofu you probably will. When using a blender, place all the ingredients except tofu in the blender. Add the tofu bit by bit, blending smooth with each addition. If the mixture stops moving, turn off the blender and stir, then blend again. Add tofu and repeat until all is included. When using a food processor, put it all in and process until creamy smooth.

Tofu Mayonnaises

Follow the directions for Tofu Sour Cream, using the ingredients listed.

Russian

1 tbsp white miso
1 tbsp prepared mustard
2 tbsp oil
3 tbsp cider vinegar
pinch of black pepper
pinch of chili powder
1/2 tsp dill weed
1/8 tsp paprika
1/2 pound tofu

Oriental

1 tbsp shoyu or dark miso
3 tbsp rice vinegar
white part of 2 green onions, minced
2 tsp ginger, minced
2 tbsp oil
sliver of fresh garlic, minced
1/2 pound tofu

French Onion

2 tbsp oil sautéed with
1/2 small onion, minced
1 clove garlic
1/2 small carrot, grated
pinch of chili powder
1/8 tsp paprika
2 tbsp cider vinegar
1/8 tsp black pepper
1/2 pound tofu

Butter-Free Spreads

Here are two tasty, low-fat, butter-free, spreadable vegetable butters by Kristina Turner from her book *The Self-Healing Cookbook:* Sweet Carrot Butter and Sesame Squash Butter.

Sweet Carrot Butter (MAKES 1 SMALL BOWL)

4 cups carrots, sliced
$1/2$ cup water
pinch of sea salt
1 heaping tbsp kudzu, dissolved in 2 tbsp water
1–2 tbsp sesame tahini (optional)

Sweet, creamy, and super as a spread on whole wheat toast, rice cakes, or even waffles. Slice the carrots in 1-inch chunks and place them in a pressure cooker with water and salt. Bring to pressure, turn down, and simmer for 10 minutes. (If you do not have a pressure cooker, steam them for 20 minutes.) Puree the carrots in a blender with $1/2$ cup liquid from pressure-cooking or steaming. Dissolve kuzu in cool water, mix with carrot puree, and reheat. Stir until it bubbles (kuzu must be heated thoroughly to thicken). For a buttery flavor, stir in sesame tahini.

Sesame Squash Butter

(MAKES 1 SMALL BOWL)

1 cup mashed, cooked buttercup or butternut squash
3 tbsp sesame seeds*
1 tsp mellow white or chickpea miso
dash of cinnamon
water

Carrot butter was my number-one favorite until I invented this! Steam, bake, or pressure cook the squash, then mash. Roast the sesame seeds by stirring in a skillet over medium heat until they smell toasty and crumble easily between thumb and forefinger. Grind into a butter in a blender or food processor. Mix in the squash, miso, and cinnamon and add just enough water to make a creamy spread.

*Fresh roasted and ground sesame seeds add a special taste and aroma. In a rush? Substitute tahini.

Bean Spreads or Dips (MAKES 2 CUPS)

Basics

2 cups cooked beans, mashed
1 tbsp oil
1 small lemon, juiced
1 clove garlic, pressed
$1/2$ onion, chopped
cumin
salt

Herbs and Seasoning Choices

green pepper or chile pepper, chopped
parsley, chopped fine
green onions, chopped
$1/2$ –1 tsp chili powder
1 tsp basil
$1/2$ tsp oregano
$1/2$ tsp coriander
$1/4$ tsp thyme
1 tsp mustard
1–2 tbsp red wine vinegar
1–2 tbsp sesame tahini

You may use garbanzos, white beans, split peas, black-eyed peas, or pinto, kidney, or black beans. This recipe can be made into spreads with a variety of tastes, using many different ingredients. To make a dip, add a little more water, lemon juice, and oil.

Mash or blend the beans with oil, lemon, garlic and onion, then add cumin and salt to taste and 2 or 3 other herbs and seasonings. Add any other ingredients of choice. This can be used as a sandwich spread or served with crackers and vegetable sticks; celery and cucumber are good choices. As a sandwich with sliced tomato and sprouts or lettuce, it provides a nutritious meal.

Special Snacks for Kids (and Their Folks)

Because the best nutritional plan starts with childhood and this book addresses nutrition for all ages, here I include some more healthful recipes for kids. It is best to avoid or to use minimally as an occasional treat the junk food that is available literally all over the world. The concerns with so many of the poor-quality "foods" available for kids these days are the high amounts of sugar, refined flour, and preservatives, and the synthetic artificial colors. Try these more natural snacks and treats and see how they work at home or at school for the whole family. Other healthy snacks that most children appreciate are popcorn, granola, and dried fruits. Minimize use of dried fruits, however, as they can be constipating. Soaking dried fruits overnight allows them to be hydrated and often more tasty. Fresh fruits are, of course, a better choice.

Kids and most anyone will love "natural" french fries or baked fries. Cut potatoes into strips. Place on a pan and bake for 10 to 15 minutes at 350°F until golden brown (bake with a little olive oil and salt or garlic salt and cayenne for more spicy baked fries). Other vegetables, like carrots, zucchini, and even onions and garlic, can be baked in this way, and they are often tastier than other vegetable preparations (see Baked Veggie Platter on page 532). There are many fatty or sugary meals and snacks that can be made in healthier ways. Have fun in the kitchen and let your children play and create with you; you and your children will love it.

Frozen juice pops. Preferably, use bottled, non-sugared, naturally pressed juices. Choices of juices: orange, papaya, orange-papaya mix, tropical punch (a good one), apple, or apple mix (such as apple boysenberry, apple grape, and so on). Some juices, such as grape, will work better diluted with a little water; in general, for less sweet juice pops, add some water to the juice. Pour the juice into ice-cube containers, or any of the newer containers now available in various shapes, and freeze. A great summer treat!

Dr. Elson's Nice Cream. Frozen desserts made of fresh fruit can only be made in certain types of juicers or food processors. I used to make "nice cream" in a Champion brand juicer, which was also good for nut butters. Use the hookup that pushes out every-thing that goes in. Freeze peeled bananas, then push whole bananas through the juicer; they will come out as creamy banana "nice cream," a real taste treat. Carob powder, carob chips, coconut pieces, or walnuts can also be run through with the bananas for a "nice cream" variation. Fresh frozen peaches, strawberries (trimmed), or other berries can also be used straight or mixed with bananas. I have even thrown in some frozen kiwis, peeled first of course.

Yogurt freezes. There are also many choices for these frozen yogurt treats. Many fruits work well. Either mash the fruit and add the yogurt, or puree the fruit in the blender with a little honey or pure maple syrup, and add water or lemon juice for a tangy taste. Use plain regular, low-fat, or nonfat yogurt. Mix the yogurt in with the pureed fruit or blend it all together. If desired, add chopped walnuts or almonds, coconut flakes, carob powder, or natural flavorings for variations. Pour the mixture into freezable cups or scoop into ice-cube containers. Here are some sample yogurt freezes:

- **Banana yogurt freeze.** Mash 2 ripe bananas with 1/2 tsp of honey or maple syrup and 1/2 tsp lemon juice; mix in 1 cup of yogurt and freeze. For carob or cocoa banana, mix in 2 tbsp of carob powder or 1 tbsp pure cocoa.

- **Banana-papaya.** Mash 1 medium banana with 1/4–1/2 fresh papaya and 1/2 tsp lemon juice—or blend to puree. Mix in 1 cup yogurt.

- **Apple.** Puree 1 cup fresh apple without skin or use 1 cup applesauce, add 2 tsp honey, a pinch of cinnamon, and mix in 1 cup yogurt.

- **Strawberry.** Puree 1 1/2 cups strawberries with 1 tbsp honey and a splash of water. If using frozen, thawed berries, do not add water. Mix in 1 cup yogurt and freeze.

- **Other berries or fruits.** Peaches or nectarines can also be used. Take 1–2 cups fresh or fresh frozen fruits and blend with 1 tbsp honey and 1 cup of plain yogurt. Freeze in cups or ice-cube containers.

Nut Milks (MAKES 1–2 CUPS)

*¹/₄–¹/₂ cup nuts, preferably unsalted, raw whole nuts,
    or fresh coconut pieces (chopped or broken pieces of
    nuts or shredded coconut can also be used)*
1–1¹/₂ cup purified water
1–2 tsp pure maple syrup
1–2 pinches sea salt

Some milk-free, nutrient-rich beverage treats can be made in a blender with a variety of nuts, water, and a touch of maple syrup and sea salt. Almonds, Brazil nuts, cashews, or coconut can be used. Put the nuts in a blender or food processor, grind to a pulp, then cover with twice the level of water. Blend about 30 seconds, adding half of the maple syrup and salt. Pour nut milk through strainer into bowl and transfer to a storage jar. Place nuts back into blender and repeat blending with the remaining water, maple syrup, and salt. You may vary the proportions according to taste. Strain out the liquid "nut milk." Refrigerate and serve as a drink or on cereal. The mixture lasts several days, refrigerated (use pure coconut milk within 24 hours, however). The leftover nut pulp can be used in cooking, such as in grain or vegetable dishes, or in baking.

Halvah (MAKES 15–20 PIECES)

*1 cup ground sesame seeds or 1 cup raw tahini
    (sesame seed butter)*
3–4 tsp honey (hardened, crystalline works best)
¹/₄ cup raisins (optional)
2–3 tbsp shredded coconut (optional)

This is a rich, high-protein, high-oil, and high-nutrient treat. Mash the ingredients together in a small bowl and roll into balls or make into small bars. Roll on shredded coconut if desired. If desired, mix in 1–2 tsp of carob for carob halvah. Or mash in banana for a tahini-banana mix that is also tasty.

Tahini Candy (SERVES 4)

This recipe is from Annemarie Colbin's *The Book of Whole Meals.*

¹/₄ cup almonds
¹/₂ cup tahini
¹/₄ cup maple syrup
¹/₄ tsp almond extract
1 tbsp carob flour
¹/₄ cup grated coconut

Preheat the oven to 425°F. Spread the almonds on a baking sheet and roast in the oven for 5 minutes. In a small mixing bowl, blend the tahini, maple syrup, and almond extract, beating vigorously for 3 minutes until a stiff ball forms and the oil begins to separate; stir in the carob flour. As the mixture stiffens, press the dough against the sides of the bowl with a spoon to expel the oil, then pour it off. Allow the dough to sit for 1 to 2 minutes. Remove the almonds from the oven. Press and drain the dough again and place in a napkin or paper towel; squeeze to absorb the excess oil. Chop the almonds and add to the mixture. Place the mixture on a piece of wax paper (so it will not stick to the chopping board) and roll it into a cylinder shape. Slice the roll into bite-sized pieces and cover with grated coconut.

Fruit Bars (MAKES 10–12 BARS)

¹/₂ cup honey
1 cup rolled oats
¹/₂ cup raisins
¹/₂ cup sunflower seeds
¹/₄ cup chopped dates or dried apricots

Heat the honey in a saucepan and stir in the other ingredients. Press into a pan and let dry. Cut into bars and refrigerate or serve.

SEASONAL MENU PLANS

This section is divided into the four seasons and includes a specific 4-day menu plan for each. The recipes that are correlated with this book's nutritional philosophy are oriented to each particular season, and they are found in my complete recipe book, *A Cookbook for All Seasons.** The seasonal menu plans offer some variety and adaptability for the vegetarian and omnivore alike. A nutritional analysis of these four diets follows the winter recipes, on page 547. The italicized food selections in the menu plans offer a specific recipe after the 4-day menus. Enjoy!

SPRING MENU PLAN

Spring is the purification season, as we typically eat more fresh foods, especially greens, and take in more liquids. Start each day with some stretching exercises and 2 glasses of purified water, 1 with half a fresh lemon squeezed into it. This is a good time to lighten the diet and get things in proper perspective for the year; clean up all areas of your life and make new plans.

DAY 1

Fruit: 1 or 2 oranges
Breakfast: Cream of wheat or rye, plain or with some honey and oil or butter
Snack: One handful of soaked almonds
Lunch: *Pasta and Garbanzo Salad* or a salad of mixed lettuces and spring greens (cilantro, watercress, miner's lettuce, dandelion, sorrel), and a sliced red radish with *Avocado Dressing*
Snack: Glass of orange juice or whole wheat crackers
Dinner: *Pureed Carrot Soup* (with lemon, miso, and dill); steamed artichokes with *Tofunaise*
Snack: Herbal tea with honey

DAY 2

Fruit: Grapefruit
Breakfast: Cream of rice or puffed rice with yogurt or soy milk
Snack: Handful of raw or roasted pumpkin seeds
Lunch: Chicken breast with *Tomato-Caper Sauce* and a spinach salad with *Miso-Tahini Dressing*
Snack: Rice cakes
Dinner: *Vegetable Minestrone* (with rice) *Pesto Sauce*
Snack: Rice or soy ice cream (such as Rice Dream or Ice Bean)

DAY 3

Fruit: 1 or 2 apples
Breakfast: Oatmeal cooked with raisins
Snack: Handful of sunflower seeds
Lunch: Broiled fresh fish (halibut, sea bass, or salmon); oven-roasted potatoes with rosemary; a salad of mixed greens with vinaigrette of olive oil, balsamic vinegar, garlic, mustard, and sea salt
Snack: Carrot and celery sticks, or granola
Dinner: *Couscous Salad*
Snack: Baked apple with raisins

DAY 4

Fruit: Strawberries
Breakfast: Corn puffs or flakes with soy milk
Snack: Handful of soaked filberts (hazelnuts)
Lunch: *Polenta* with *Tomato-Lentil Sauce* and grated Parmesan cheese (optional); small green salad with vinaigrette
Snack: Raw carrot and celery sticks
Dinner: *Watercress Bisque* and *Sweet and Sour Tempeh or Tofu*
Snack: *Strawberry-Rhubarb Pudding*

---

* Please note that most of the recipe section published in the first edition of *Staying Healthy with Nutrition*, in 1992, has not been included in this second edition to make room for all of the new material in the book. I expanded and published that original recipe section in 1995 under the title *A Diet for All Seasons*. In 2000, I republished this as *A Cookbook for All Seasons*. Please use that cookbook as a companion to the recipes listed here, especially if you wish to follow these menu plans. I have included one or more recipes per season in this chapter as an example as well as the entire list of common seasonally available foods. The italicized recipes in the menu plans denote that the particular recipe is found in *A Cookbook for All Seasons*.

Watercress Salad with Pollution Solution Dressing (SERVES 4)

These two recipes are adapted from *The Airola Diet and Cookbook* by Paavo Airola.

1 bunch fresh watercress
1/4 pound fresh mushrooms, washed and sliced
1 cup mung bean sprouts
1/2–1 cup other sprouts, such as lentil and garbanzo (optional)
1 tbsp chopped fresh parsley
1 green onion, chopped
3 tbsp cold-pressed olive oil
1 tbsp red wine vinegar
1/8–1/4 tsp sea salt
pinch of cayenne pepper

Wash the watercress and tear into bite-sized pieces. Combine the watercress with the sliced mushrooms, sprouts, parsley, and green onion. Make a dressing with the olive oil, red wine vinegar, sea salt, and cayenne and pour it over the salad or use the Pollution Solution Dressing (see next recipe).

Pollution Solution Dressing
(MAKES ABOUT 2 CUPS)

1 cup mayonnaise or Tofu Mayonnaise (see recipe on page 535)
1 ripe tomato, chopped
1 small dill pickle, chopped
2 tbsp chopped onion
2 tbsp chopped green pepper
3 cloves garlic, minced
2 tsp honey
1 tbsp plain yogurt
1 tbsp lemon juice
1 tbsp algin powder (sodium alginate)
1 tbsp brewer's yeast flakes
2 tsp lecithin granules
1 tsp kelp
1/2 tsp sea salt
pinch of cayenne pepper

This salad dressing may help lower risks from environmental pollution. It contains nutrients that have been shown to be effective in protecting the body from the toxic effects of heavy metals and X-rays as well as other sources of harmful environmental radiation. Use it with any salad. Combine all the ingredients and mix well. Use a hand blender briefly, for a more creamy texture. Store in the refrigerator.

Spring Foods

Fruits	Vegetables			Sprouts	
				Grains	**Beans**
avocado	artichoke	comfrey	nettle	barley	adzuki
date	asparagus	dandelion greens	parsley	buckwheat	fava
grapefruit	beet	green garlic	radish	corn	garbanzo
jicama	beet greens	green onion	rhubarb	rice	lentil
lemon	bok choy	green peas	sorrel greens	rye	mung
lime	broccoli	kale	spinach	sprouted	sprouted
loquat	brussels sprout	leek	sprouts	wheat	
olive	cabbage	lettuces	sugar peas		
orange	carrot	butter	watercress		
plum	cauliflower	green leaf		**Seeds**	
strawberry	celery	iceberg		alfalfa	radish
tangelo	chard	red leaf		clover	sunflower
tangerine	chickweed	romaine			
	chicory	miner's lettuce			
	chives	mint			
	cilantro	mushroom			
	collard greens	mustard greens			

These foods are naturally available in springtime. This list may vary slightly between locales. Some are the winter crops, such as cabbage or cauliflower, and others are not available until later spring, after the early growing time. Of course, foods that can be dried after their harvest or that are naturally contained in a protective coating for storage are available throughout the year in most areas. These include the whole grains, beans, seaweeds, seeds, and nuts. Although they are often used, they would not be classified as "spring foods," however. For more information on the seasonal diets, see my *Seasonal Food Guide* poster, available from Celestial Arts, Berkeley, California.

SUMMER MENU PLAN

In summer, we typically consume more liquids as well as more raw, fresh fruits and vegetables and salads. We eat a lighter diet in general, and we are usually more active. It is wonderful to be outdoors exercising and getting that fresh air. This is a good season to experiment with special diets, such as fasting or a raw food diet. Fresh, vital eating is the way to go. The recipes for the italicized food selections in the menu plans below are included in my *Cookbook for All Seasons.*

DAY 1

Fruit: Fresh berries

Breakfast: *Breakfast Rice* or puffed rice or rye flakes with yogurt

Snack: Soaked almonds

Lunch: Salad of mixed greens, raw spinach, chives, grated carrots, tomatoes, and tuna fish (or a mixture of bean sprouts or tofu salad for the vegetarian) with vinaigrette of avocado or olive oil, lemon juice, Dijon mustard, herb salt, and cayenne pepper.

Snack: Peaches

Dinner: *Stuffed Bell Peppers* and steamed Swiss chard sprinkled with roasted pumpkin seeds, minced garlic, olive oil, and soy sauce or tamari

Snack: Rice cake with apple butter, or papaya

DAY 2

Fruit: Plums

Breakfast: Cream of wheat, *Crepes with Fruit,* or *Scrambled Tofu*

Snack: Wheat crackers or sprouted-wheat toast with tahini

Lunch: Cold pasta salad with fava beans, fresh basil, lightly steamed asparagus tips, baby (or sliced) carrots, and black olives with garlic oil, sea salt, and cayenne, served over a bed of lettuce

Snack: Cherries

Dinner: *Chicken en Chemise;* steamed artichoke with dilled tofu mayonnaise. watercress and baby lettuces with safflower oil, balsamic vinegar, and sea salt

Snack: *Fruit Sorbet*

Summer Foods

Fruits	Vegetables
apricot	artichoke
avocado	beet
berries	bell pepper
blackberry	cabbage
blueberry	celery
boysenberry	chile pepper
loganberry	chive
olallieberry	corn, fresh
raspberry	cucumber
strawberry	eggplant
fig	green beans
grapefruit	green peas
lemon	lettuce
lime	okra
melons	parsley
cantaloupe	radish
casaba	rhubarb
crenshaw	spinach
honeydew	squash (soft)
musk	crookneck
Persian	scallop
watermelon	zucchini
nectarine	sugar peas
orange	tomato
peach	watercress
pear	
plum	**Beans**
prickly pear	green beans
tangelo	sprouted beans
tangerine	
tropical fruits	**Nuts and Seeds**
banana	sprouted
cherimoya	
guava	**Grains**
mango	sprouted
papaya	
passionfruit	
pineapple	
sapote	

DAY 3

Fruit: Oranges
Breakfast: Granola with *Fruit Kanten*
Snack: Walnuts
Lunch: Broiled halibut basted with marinade of tamari, sesame oil, garlic, fresh thyme, and fresh marjoram; vegetable mélange of lightly steamed sweet peas and carrots served with fresh arugula and a vinaigrette of olive oil, lemon juice or balsamic vinegar, and a pinch of sea salt
Snack: Apricots
Dinner: *Moussaka,* salad greens with vinaigrette
Snack: Strawberries, blackberries, or fresh figs

DAY 4

Fruit: Grapefruit
Breakfast: Corn flakes with soymilk, or cornbread with *Peanut-Apple Butter*
Snack: Sunflower seeds
Lunch: Fresh corn on the cob with sweet, unpasteurized butter, and *Mexican Salad Bowl*
Snack: Banana
Dinner: *Baked Dill Wild Salmon,* green beans, and *Salad of Belgian Endives*
Snack: Fresh berries

Spicy Coleslaw (SERVES 4)

2 cups grated green cabbage
1 cup grated red cabbage
1 cup grated carrot
1/2 cup diced black olives
1/2 small onion, diced, and/or 2 cloves garlic, minced and pressed
1/2 cup almonds, slivered (optional for crunch)
2 tbsp mayonnaise or Tofu Mayonnaise (see recipe on page 535)
1 tbsp olive oil
1 tsp apple cider vinegar, or juice of 1 medium lemon
salt to taste
1/4 tsp black pepper
1/4 tsp red pepper flakes (more for very spicy)

Combine the cabbage and carrots in a bowl and mix in the olives, onion, garlic, and almonds, if desired. Mix together mayonnaise, oil, vinegar or lemon juice, and seasonings, and stir into the coleslaw. Refrigerate to cool before serving. I served this at my birthday party and it was a big hit!

Baked Dill Wild Salmon (SERVES 6)

This is a simple and nutritious recipe for the summer's wild salmon catch.

2 tbsp soy sauce
2 tbsp lemon juice
6 salmon fillets
6 lemon slices
6 tomato slices
6 sprigs fresh dill

Preheat oven to 375° F.

Mix together the soy sauce and lemon juice, and dip salmon fillets in mixture to coat both sides. Place the fillets in a large baking dish; place a lemon slice, a tomato slice, and a sprig of dill on top of each and then cover with a lid or foil. Bake about 20 minutes.

AUTUMN MENU PLAN

Autumn gives us richer and denser foods that require more heat to prepare; these include whole grains, dried legumes, and hard squashes. Thus there are more cooked foods, more calories, fats, and protein, fewer liquids, and often a few added pounds. Regular exercise, including stretching to maintain or improve flexibility, is important during this more contractive time. Recipes for the italicized food selections in the menu plans below are available in my *Cookbook for All Seasons.*

DAY 1

Fruit:	Apple
Breakfast:	Oatmeal with yogurt, raisins, and maple syrup
Lunch:	*Fillet of Sole Florentine,* baked or steamed carrot and beet mélange served over steamed beet tops with a splash of olive oil, lemon juice, and sea salt
Snack:	Granola
Dinner:	*Lasagna* and salad greens with vinaigrette
Snack:	Baked apple

Autumn Foods

Fruits	Vegetables		Grains (cooked)	Nuts
apple	bell pepper	potato	amaranth	almond
berries	broccoli	pumpkin	barley	Brazil
blackberry	burdock root	rutabaga	buckwheat	cashew
cranberry	cabbage	shallot	corn	filbert
date	red	spinach	millet	macadamia
fig	green	squash (hard)	oat	pecan
grape	Napa	acorn	quinoa	pine nut
mandarin orange	carrot	banana	rice	pistachio
melon	cauliflower	buttercup	rye	walnut
pear	chayote	butternut	wheat	
persimmon	corn, fresh	delicata		
plum	cucumber	Hubbard	**Beans**	**Seeds**
pomegranate	daikon radish	spaghetti	adzuki	flax
quince	eggplant	squash (soft)	black	pumpkin
rosehips	garlic (dried)	sweet potato	black-eyed pea	sesame
	ginger root	tomato	carob	sunflower
	horseradish	turnip	garbanzo	
	Jerusalem	yam	great northern	
	artichoke		kidney	
	jicama		lentil	
	leek		lima	
	lettuce		navy	
	okra		peanut	
	onion		pink	
	parsnip		red	
			soy	
			white	

DAY 2

Fruit: Grapes

Breakfast: Twice-cooked rice with *Prune and Apricot Compote*

Snack: Pumpkin seeds

Lunch: Baked potato with *Avo-Miso-Tofu Topping*; grated carrot and red and green cabbage salad with vinaigrette sprinkled with toasted sunflower seeds or sliced hard-boiled egg

Snack: Soaked prunes

Dinner: Brown rice with adzuki beans, and steamed broccoli and cauliflower with *Walnut-Miso Sauce*

Snack: *Carob-Tofu Mousse*

DAY 3

Fruit: Cantaloupe or other melon

Breakfast: Cornflakes, cooked millet, or *Millet Breakfast Cake with Orange Sauce*

Snack: Filberts or pecans

Lunch: *Turkey Breast* and *Wilted Spinach Salad*

Snack: Blackberries

Dinner: *Millet Croquettes, Brazilian Feijoada* (black beans), and salad greens

Snack: Popcorn

DAY 4

Fruit: Pear

Breakfast: Cream of Wheat or whole wheat toast with peanut-apple butter

Snack: Walnuts

Lunch: *Grilled Halibut with Pineapple Mustard* and *Warm Red Cabbage Salad*

Snack: Apple

Dinner: *Pasta alla Boscaiola* and salad greens with lemon and olive oil

Snack: *Pears in Black Cherry Juice*

Warm Red Cabbage Salad (SERVES 4–6)

1 head red cabbage

1 small onion, sliced

5 tbsp olive oil

1/2 cup sweet peas

3 tbsp rice vinegar

1 tbsp ume vinegar, or sea salt to taste

1/2 cup roasted walnuts (optional)

1/4–1/2 cup feta cheese, goat's or sheep's milk ideal (optional)

Cut cabbage lengthwise into 4 pieces, then slice into thin strips. Steam until soft, about 3 to 5 minutes. Sauté the onion in a bit of the oil until limp and transparent and add to the cabbage together with the peas. Combine the remaining olive oil, rice vinegar, and ume vinegar or sea salt and toss with the cabbage. Sprinkle roasted walnuts and crumbled feta cheese on top and serve warm.

Walnut-Miso Sauce (MAKES 2 CUPS)

We never have enough tasty and nourishing sauces to use on grains and veggies. Here's a good one.

1 cup roasted (or raw) walnuts pieces

1 tbsp light miso, or to taste

1 tbsp rice vinegar

1/2 tbsp stone-ground mustard

1/4 cup water

1/2 tsp maple syrup or honey

Blend all ingredients together until smooth.

WINTER MENU PLAN

The winter diet is often the richest, warmest, and heaviest of the seasonal diets. It includes more cooked, warming foods to support the body's need for heat and protection from the colder environment. And, of course, with this more calming and heavier diet, we may need more rest and dream time to tune us into the winter. Recipes for the italicized food selections in the menu plans below are available in my *Cookbook for All Seasons.*

DAY 1

Fruit: Pear
Breakfast: Sweet potatoes, cream of wheat, or *Cracked Wheat with Raisins and Walnuts*
Snack: Sunflower seeds
Lunch: *Cream of Broccoli Soup* (optional), *Roasted Turkey with Mushroom Sauce*, and steamed greens, such as kale or chard
Snack: Mandarin orange
Dinner: *Stir-Fried Vegetables with Tempeh or Tofu*, served over whole wheat pasta
Snack: *Oatmeal Spice Cookies*

Winter Foods

Fruits

apples	persimmon
Granny Smith	pomegranate
pippin	tangelo
Red Delicious	tangerine
cranberry	watermelon
date	
dried fruits	
apple	
apricot	
coconut	
mango	
papaya	
pear	
peach	
pineapple	
prune	
raisin	
grape	
kiwifruit	
kumquat	
mandarin orange	
navel orange	
pear	
Anjou	

Vegetables

bok choy	spinach (New Zealand)
broccoli	sprouts
brussels sprout	squash (hard)
burdock root	acorn
cabbage	butternut
carrot	delicata
cauliflower	Hubbard
chard	spaghetti
daikon radish	sugar pumpkin
garlic	sweet potato
ginger	turnip
Jerusalem artichoke	yam
jicama	
kale	
leek	**Nuts and Seeds**
onion	same as autumn
parsnip	
potato	
rutabaga	**Beans and Grains**
seaweeds	see autumn
agar-agar, kelp,	
arame, kombu,	
dulse, nori,	**Sprouts**
hijiki, wakame	seeds, grains, and beans

These foods are naturally available in many areas during the winter. For the colder and snowy climates, most winter foods must have been dried and stored to provide nourishment. My *Seasonal Food Guide* poster and booklet, published by Celestial Arts, provides further information on the seasonal diets.

DAY 2

Fruit: Orange

Breakfast: Oatmeal or 7-grain cereal with stewed fruit

Snack: Filberts or pistachios

Lunch: *Curried Chicken Breast* and coleslaw

Snack: Granola

Dinner: *Millet, Squash, and Adzuki Bean Stew,* steamed kale with olive oil, garlic, and soy sauce

Snack: *Apple-Raisin Compote*

DAY 3

Fruit: Apples

Breakfast: Baked acorn squash with sesame salt, or buckwheat cream (ground buckwheat, boiled) with raisins and sunflower seeds

Snack: Soaked almonds

Lunch: *Snapper Parmentière, Arame Carrots, Scallions, and Corn,* and steamed greens

Snack: Popcorn

Dinner: *Lentil Soup with Barley and Dulse* with salad greens and sprouts

Snack: *Pumpkin Pie*

DAY 4

Fruit: Kiwifruit

Breakfast: Cream of rice with yogurt and honey

Snack: Walnuts

Lunch: *Butternut Bisque* and poached fish with steamed broccoli and cauliflower, or *Norimaki Sushi* as a vegetable substitute

Snack: Dates or rice cakes with apple butter

Dinner: *Rice-Lentil Loaf with Green Sauce,* and steamed kale or chard with caraway seeds

Snack: Baked apple

Basmati Rice 'n' Eggs (SERVES 4–6)

Recipe contributed by Bethany Argisle.

3 cups basmati rice

5 cups water

6 eggs

6 green onions, chopped fine

1 small bunch cilantro, chopped fine

3 ripe tomatoes

1/4 cup olive oil

3 tbsp low-salt soy sauce

1/4 tsp cayenne pepper

2 tbsp toasted sesame oil

Basmati is known in the East as the "rice of kings." It is light with a flowery fragrance. Rinse the rice thoroughly until the water is clear. Add fresh water 2 finger breadths above the rice and boil rapidly over moderate heat. Do not burn. Soft boil the eggs 3 to 4 minutes; then run them under cold water and peel. Wash and chop separately the green onions, cilantro, and tomatoes; place them in individual bowls for personal serving garnish. Add the rice, eggs, oil, and all seasonings to a large bowl and mix lightly. Taste and balance the seasonings as desired. Add garnish according to individual taste.

Leftovers are a lot of fun and can be planned the day before by making more of this dish than needed. Get out your wok or skillet and heat it over a hot flame. Then add first 1/2 cup of purified water or 1/4 cup of olive oil or rice bran oil. Immediately add the rice and eggs with any lightly steamed vegetable (such as green or red bell or chile peppers), or you can pre-broil fresh, organic turkey sausage or soy sausage, chop, and add to the dish. Add some green onions a minute before the dish is done. Cilantro and tomatoes can be used for garnish.

Nutritional Analysis of the Seasonal Diets

Constituents	Recommendations	Spring	Summer	Autumn	Winter
Calories	1,300–2,000	1,500	1,500	1,650	1,880
Carbohydrates (g)	200	190	180	200	225
Cholesterol (mg)	under 300	100	160	105	130
Fats (g)	25–75	55	48	54	65
Protein (g)	56	60	65	70	76
Fiber (g)	NE(10)*	10	10	12	15
Water (liter)	2.5	2.6	2.9	2.7	2.8
Vitamins					
Vitamin A/beta-carotene (IU)	5,000	14,000	14,000	18,000	22,000
Vitamin E (IU)	15	14	10	12	15
Vitamin K (mcg)	300	340	240	500	320
Thiamin (B1) (mg)	1.4	1.5	1.3	1.4	1.7
Riboflavin (B2) (mg)	1.6	1.6	1.4	1.6	1.8
Niacin (B3) (mg)	18	20	19	18	24
Pantothenic acid (B5) (mg)	5	6	6	9	11
Pyrodoxine (B6) (mg)	2	3	3	2.6	3.4
Cobalamin (B12) (mcg)	3	0.6	1.0	0.6	1.3
Folic acid (mcg)	400	450	400	460	480
Vitamin C (mg)	45	175	200	180	240
Minerals					
Calcium (mg)	800	500	640	490	800
Copper (mg)	2.0	3.1	7	3.4	38
Iron (mg)	10–18	16	18	16	18
Magnesium (mg)	350	340	340	360	440
Potassium (g)	2.5	3.2	3.1	3.5	4.4
Phosphorus (mg)	800	1,150	1,200	1,100	1,400
Sodium (g)	2	1.4	1.5	1.4	2.4
Zinc (mg)	15	12	20	13	16

* NE — Not established.

Note: Values, of course, will vary with the quality and amount of food consumed. The seasonal diets, mostly vegetarian and low-fat, reveal slightly low values for certain nutrients in these analyses. Vitamins and minerals to watch include most of the B vitamins, especially B12, calcium, zinc, and iron for women. These diets are high in vitamin A and potassium levels and low in cholesterol and sodium. You can do an analysis of your diet using a book that includes food values or with a practitioner who uses a special nutritional service.

RECIPE GLOSSARY

Agar-agar. Flakes made from sea vegetables used to jelly desserts (aspics) and dressings. One tablespoon agar flakes will gel 1 cup of liquid.

Amazake. Creamy sweetener or beverage made from sweet brown rice; rich in flavor and easy to digest. Great over cereal instead of milk.

Arrowroot. Starch flour made from the root of the manioc plant. Used in sauces and desserts as a thickener.

Barley malt. Dark brown, complex carbohydrate sweetener made from sprouted barley. Similar to honey.

Bulgur. Whole wheat that has been cracked, partially boiled, and dried; used to make tabbouleh.

Carob. The pod of the tamarind tree, or St. John's bread; used as an alternative to chocolate.

Couscous. Cracked, partially cooked wheat. Different from bulgur in that it is cracked smaller and traditionally made from refined wheat. Whole wheat or even rice couscous is sometimes available.

Daikon. Long white radish with a sweet-pungent flavor. Cooked daikon helps dissolve fat and reduce mucus; fresh daikon helps in the digestion of oily foods.

Dulse. Mild-tasting purple sea vegetable, high in protein, natural iodine, iron, and other minerals. Must not be cooked as it becomes slimy and difficult to chew.

Fig pep. Water extract of dried figs, high in iron and minerals; used as a sweetener like molasses.

Gomasio. Dry-roasted sesame seeds and sea salt; used as a seasoning.

Kombu. Thick, wide, dark green sea vegetable used in making soup stock or cooked with beans to make them more digestible.

Kudzu. Rocklike starch made from the kudzu plant. Used as a thickener for sauces or gravies. Also called the "macrobiotic aspirin." A drink made from 1 cup of hot water, 1 tablespoon of kudzu (dissolved first in 2 tablespoons cold water), and 1 umeboshi plum will reduce flu or hangover symptoms.

Mirin. Sweet cooking wine made from whole sweet rice.

Miso. Protein-rich fermented bean and/or grain paste made from soybeans, brown rice, or barley. Miso is used in soups, main dishes, sauces, and dressings. It aids digestion and circulation. It is best bought unpasteurized and should not be boiled.

Mochi. Sweet brown rice pounded into a cake. It may be baked in the oven or layered with vegetables in a casserole. It can also be added to soups in small pieces.

Nori. Crispy thin sheets of pressed sea vegetable. Nori contains several minerals and B vitamins. It is mostly used in making sushi.

Polenta. Coarse ground whole corn used in many Mediterranean dishes.

Ponzu. Sweet and pungent condiment made from soy sauce, citrus juices, and mirin. Great over grains and vegetables or for marinating fish or tofu.

Quinoa. The mother grain of the Incas; a complete protein grain similar to millet. Cooks in 20 minutes.

Rice syrup. Sweet, thick syrup made from brown rice. A complex carbohydrate sweetener similar to honey in consistency and color, but a little less sweet.

Seitan. A hearty, high-protein food made from whole wheat gluten. It has a meatlike, chewy texture and is commonly used in many Asian dishes. It is made without salt, is low in fat, and has no cholesterol.

Shiitake. Flavorful mushroom used in traditional Japanese cuisine and folk medicine. Shiitake mushrooms are complete proteins and are a rich source of B vitamins.

Soymilk. Milklike liquid made from soybeans. Good for use on cereals, for cooking, or as a drink. Common packaged brands include Edensoy and Vitasoy. Fresh soymilk should not be used in cooking.

Stevia/sweetleaf. The best of all sweeteners, it is made from the stevia plant, is 10 times sweeter than sugar, and has no calories. Good for diabetics and hypoglycemics alike, as well as people with candida concerns.

Tahini. Smooth butter made from hulled and ground sesame seeds. Sold raw or roasted. Can be used as a snack on bread or crackers, or for dips and dressings.

Tamari. Rich natural soy sauce, a by-product of making miso. Used as a salty seasoning for foods.

Tempeh. A high-protein, whole-grain, cultured food made from soybeans and often brown rice or other grains. Easy to digest, low in fat, and cholesterol free. Apart from plain, there are now many marinated tempehs on the market, as well as tempeh burgers of various kinds.

Tofu. High-protein soybean curd, versatile and with no cholesterol.

Umeboshi plums. Zesty sour and salty pickled plums that stimulate digestion. They are used in some macrobiotic cooking. They are suggested to balance the blood and may help in motion sickness, too.

Unrefined oil. Vegetable oil that has been mechanically cold-pressed and has not been filtered. It retains its natural color, aroma, and nutrients. It has not been chemically bleached, deodorized, or deflavored and contains no preservatives, additives, antifoaming agents, or antioxidants. Some excellent brands include Spectrum and Eden.

Wasabi. Light green Japanese horseradish powder that is mixed with water and made into a paste. It is a pungent condiment traditionally eaten with sushi.

Part 4

Nutritional Application: 32 Special Diets and Supplement Programs

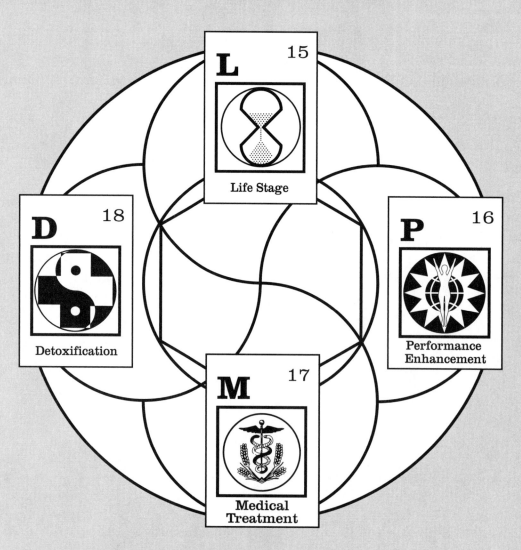

Introduction: Infancy to Immortality

This is an important section of the book for those interested in the life-supporting and therapeutic application of nutrition during the various states and stages of life, when we are afflicted with certain conditions or when we want to help change and enhance our health. In the following 32 programs (outlined in chapters 15 through 18), I offer some simple, basic guidelines regarding food and diet choices as well as special supplement suggestions to help heal a variety of problems and to support stressful periods in our individual evolution. With all of the basic information I have provided up to this point, part 4 of this book provides the nutritional application to take your health into your own hands.

The first goal of these programs is to avoid nutrient deficiencies. The second goal is to help provide all the nutrients in the right amounts to maintain healthy function. This may be more than the dietary reference intakes (DRIs) in many cases. The third goal, which is especially important to the nutritionally aware physician and individual, is to use nutrition in a way that supports optimum health. In this book I call this more orthomolecular approach a *performance enhancement program* (PEP). The idea

is to have sufficient levels of all of the necessary nutrients available in the blood and tissues so that these nutrient-rich fluids bathe the cells with all of the nutritional-biochemical metabolites required for an efficient and balanced metabolism. Also, higher amounts of some nutrients may provide some additional functions that lower levels do not; examples of this include the anti-inflammatory and antiviral effects of vitamin C or the cholesterol-lowering effect of niacin at levels of intake much higher than the DRI. Although researchers do not really know whether certain supplements are always necessary, many clinicians and scientists believe that such support adds an extra measure of safety to one's health program, particularly to avoid deficiencies.

My overall goal is to help you to be your own doctor as much as possible. Unfortunately, the Western medical system does not currently work this way. Rather, it is primarily oriented to the diagnosis and treatment of disease using drugs and surgery; it is not centered around evaluating people's lives in relation to their health and educating them in living healthfully. If this were done, medical practices and hospitals would focus more on preventive and nutritional medicine, lifestyle and stress management, and supportive encouragement to eat well, exercise, curb excesses and abuses, normalize weight, and stop smoking, as well as choosing other ways to live that generate optimum individual and planetary health. **Keeping people healthy offers the greatest economic advantage (savings) to our very stressed healthcare system.** The more we do to understand our needs, our growth, and the necessary changes to support our health and correct any minor or recurrent malfunctions of our magnificent bodies, the easier our lives will be. The key to preventive medicine is education. Nutritional application is a key component of self-care. Using vitamins, minerals, oils, and herbs, as well as special foods and diets (including fasting and milder forms of detoxification), can all help in the process of healing and wellness. Part 4 of this book can help you apply this nutritional know-how to your life and to share it with friends and family.

Preventive medicine and nutrition are now growing rapidly in popularity. They have moved, I believe, out of their infancy and toddler years into childhood and adolescence, when the acquisition of new knowledge is very exciting. This growth in knowledge and its practical application to health care and longevity is a result of the blending of science and Nature. Combining new research in clinical biochemistry and nutrition with the resurgence of pesticide-free natural foods grown in healthy soils and with more natural remedies available for healing, nutritionists and all health-care providers now have a chance to improve the field of nutritional medicine and overall health care. In this way, we can improve our health as individuals and as a population.

Unfortunately, however, I believe a large percentage of doctors are still limited by a lack of basic and clinical nutritional knowledge. The practice of nutrition in mainstream medicine is primarily carried out by registered dietitians (RDs), who consult with or for doctors or who work within the country's hospitals. There are about 70,000 RDs in the United States, and 34% of them work in hospital settings. Another third practice in clinics, extended-care facilities, and public health programs. Dietitians can treat disease only by referral from a primary care practitioner, and in many hospital and extended-care facilities, this often means helping the physician in charge achieve compliance with

a preestablished dietary protocol. This combination of circumstances seems to have worked against early adoption of new information and approaches to nutrition on the part of RDs. Because fewer than 4% of RDs work in private practice settings, room to initiate new protocols has been quite limited. (See my discussion of RDs and nutritionists on page 4 of this book's introduction.)

A 1994 study of RDs in Utah and Nevada indicated that 28% had not recommended a dietary supplement to any patient in the past 6 months. I am not surprised at this finding, even though I believe that many RDs have a strong interest in learning more about nutritional supplements and believe they can play a role in supporting health. (One reason I am convinced of this interest is because every survey taken of RDs since 1990 shows at least 50% to be taking supplements themselves on a regular basis.) It is difficult for most RDs to bring dietary supplements into their work settings, likely because they are typically not trained in the use of supplements and because there is often unfamiliarity and skepticism in the workplace about dietary supplementation. In addition, I do not think RDs should be expected to offer more supplement recommendations without having some solid evidence of effectiveness in their hands. This kind of evidence (and experience) takes some time and effort to obtain, and without some support on behalf of their hospitals and clinics, I can understand the stagnation in this area.

The American Dietetic Association (ADA) has most recently identified five key areas of interest in which it seeks to provide leadership:

1. Obesity and overweight

2. Aging

3. Complementary care and dietary supplements

4. A safe and nutritious food supply

5. The human genome and genetics

Unfortunately, I see the ADA's philosophy of health as getting in the way of its leadership capacity in all of these areas. More specifically, dietetics, the practice of diet therapy, has focused on five main disease areas: (1) weight loss and gain; (2) treatment of deficiencies, as with iodine for goiter and vitamin D for rickets; (3) support or rest for specific organs, such as a low-fat diet for gallbladder problems or avoiding spices for stomach ulcers; (4) special diets for metabolic problems, such as low sugar for diabetes or low salt for hypertension; and (5) elimination of harmful substances, such as caffeine and alcohol. Even though I believe that nutrition in practice has much greater value in preventing problems than in treating them, basic dietetics, like medicine, is mostly disease-oriented and often focuses on short-term therapeutic diets to be followed until the patient feels better, when he or she then returns to a "normal" diet and lifestyle.

This is a very limited approach, however. It overlooks the fact that some of the things we do or eat may play a part in creating our basic health problem in the first place. The concept that when we are sick, we need to totally reevaluate our life and create a new plan—which I believe is essential to good medicine and healing—has not been fully embraced by the general public, physicians, or insurance companies. More and more people are approaching their lifestyle and health in this way, however. With the new information becoming available through research and clinical experience, the future of nutritional medicine looks exciting. Nutrition professionals are realizing that there may be a big difference between treating and preventing deficiency, on one hand, and providing optimum levels of dietary macronutrients and micronutrients, on the other.

The standard American diet, as I have written in previous chapters, is not healthy. The concept of what *diet* is should be based on more wholesome, fresh foods, rather than meaning a special, temporary therapeutic plan that achieves some immediate nutritional goal through changes that cannot hold up over time. After many years of digestive abuse, these more natural foods may feel foreign and appear hard to digest and utilize. With a little time, however, this type of diet will feel much better to the body.

Current dietetic policies and applications are responsible for public school and hospital food, which are notoriously poor, even though they attempt to apply the established concepts of good nutrition and a balanced diet. These diets fall far short of supporting children's optimal learning abilities or the healing process of ill people. All of us need good, vital nutri-

tion to grow, to heal, and to thrive. The schools and hospitals are where we need the health-conscious master chefs. Surrounding these institutions should be beautiful gardens full of fresh foods to nourish the professional staff and workers, as well as the students and patients.

Some of the current choices in a standard hospital menu include: (1) a regular diet, which could run the spectrum from good to atrocious; (2) a soft diet of overcooked and pureed foods; (3) a liquid diet, which is low in fiber and includes strained gruel, broth, juices, coffee, tea, and gelatin; and (4) a clear diet, consisting of only broth (from bouillon cubes), canned juices, and coffee or tea. There also might be modifications of the regular diet, such as a calorie and carbohydrate restriction for diabetes, a low-salt diet for high blood pressure, or a low-fat or low-cholesterol diet for heart disease. These modifications are important, but they are really just a first step. If medicine is not aimed at helping people to change in order to treat or prevent future problems, it will only correct the immediate difficulty so that we can continue our health-threatening lifestyle with the least interruption necessary. This is both shortsighted and very costly.

This book, and especially part 4, is oriented toward changing old habits and advocates thinking and living in new ways, with the programs detailed herein geared toward healthful goals. These often include long-range lifestyle habits or foods and nutritional supplements required to attain and maintain these health goals. Many of the suggestions in this section are based on scientific research and population studies, while others are based on my own or other practitioners' experiences, or more on common sense, logic, or intuition. Some of these programs encompass my latest theories.

Overall, these programs should be safe for most anyone; however, if there are specific medical concerns, please consult your doctor or a practitioner who can be a judge of a nutritionally supportive program. Many of the diets and supplement plans are not oriented to the long term; I note that where appropriate. Most of the nutrient suggestions are estimates of the best levels, based on both research and experience, but definitely in safe ranges regarding potential nutrient toxicity. Most people handle these supplement levels well. Occasionally, however, some people (such as those with allergies, food intolerances, chemical sensitivities, or certain digestive disorders) experience such symptoms as headache, diarrhea, nausea, or flushing in response to particular nutrients. These people should adjust their program. Discontinuing the supplements for a few days and then restarting, adding a new one daily, can help isolate the supplement that elicits the negative response.

The programs here offer a basic plan. Ideally, work with a doctor or other experienced practitioner to have an evaluation and then to set up a carefully designed program to meet your individual needs. Often, specific tests (such as a biochemical profile, diet and digestive analyses, mineral or vitamin blood levels, an immune system analysis, or allergy tests) should be performed to help assess any of your special needs. **Also, remember that even with all the new and creative nutritional supplements available, nothing replaces a good diet.**

Not everyone has to take the supplements as suggested. With normal levels of nutrients in the body, a solid balanced diet of wholesome foods, low stress, and minimal pollution exposure, supplementation may not be necessary all the time. Maybe a few times a year, such as at seasonal transitions or with certain problems, a specific supplement program can be used for a month or so. With many health problems, additional nutrients at higher levels may be helpful; these can often be tried as a first level of treatment before prescription drugs. Following some of the other guidelines or trying some of the herbs mentioned in the programs may be helpful as well. Overall, though, because of the problem that many people have in finding wholesome foods, especially because of soil depletion of minerals and the loss of nutrients in the storage and cooking of foods, some basic level of supplementation is needed most of the time.

It is usually best to take vitamin and mineral supplements after meals, as they are naturally part of foods and are best tolerated and utilized in this way. Herbal remedies are often taken between meals to assist their medicinal activities; however, if they are not tolerated well, they can also be taken after meals. Vitamin C can be taken following meals if it is used only a couple of times a day, as it can help the absorption of many minerals, especially when taken as ascorbic acid. Usually some of the vitamin C we take should contain the bioflavonoids, which work together with vitamin C (synergistically) in its antioxidant role. If vitamin C is taken many times daily, it can easily be taken between meals or at bedtime as well. Buffered vitamin C powders or tablets with alkaline minerals such as calcium or magnesium are usually taken alone at bedtime, between meals, or 1 to 2 hours after meals so as not to weaken hydrochloric acid's digestive function. In general, I am more in favor of simple supplement tablets or powders than the big time-release tablets, which may not be digested well, especially in people with weak digestion. Also, I prefer that supplements be taken 2 or 3 times over the course of a day; this gives the body a better chance to assimilate the nutrients and improve utilization. After breakfast and dinner are good times to take general nutrients. For some people, however, lunch and evening are more convenient. Most of us can adapt these general guidelines to fit into our lifestyle.

If we wish to initiate any of these programs, we should first look at what we are currently doing and what may need to be adjusted. We can then implement more of the suggestions as we feel comfortable with them or as the situation warrants. The recommendations also take into consideration the fact that people are different. That is why ranges of intake levels are sometimes given, or amounts higher than the RDA or DRI are listed, so that they will cover those who are weaker or need increased nutrient levels.

With some of the more serious medical conditions for which we might be under a doctor's care, please consult with your doctor (ideally a knowledgeable, integrated physician) first and get his or her advice. We all seek open-minded physicians, but some may be unreceptive to anything that differs from their viewpoint or "current medical thinking." If we are open to exploring nutrition and supplements for our condition or lifestyle and our physician is not, we might consider finding someone who will work with us toward the goals we want to pursue. By doing this, we will positively influence the medical system by helping to inform physicians of new public interests and stimulate them to seek more knowledge of nutrition and natural medicine. That is how I initially became interested in this field—through patient requests and demands, and my own needs for better health.

Medicine has always been changing, and there has always been a strong force of tradition trying to hold it back. This is also the situation in each of us who tries to change. There is usually an evolutionary part of us that is trying to stimulate and guide us toward our new self, lifestyle, or work, while another part of us is used to the old habits and tries to hold us back with fears or reasons not to change. These fears, which may also come from a spouse, a parent, or a friend, can take over and stop the process of personal evolution, or at least slow it temporarily. Eventually, we will realize that the old self does not really die; it merely becomes incorporated into the new, healthier person that we become.

Any change in medicine, just like change in each of us, is difficult. The more support we have, the better. This book and others, my medical practice and others like it, are intended to offer support and guidance for change. The following 32 programs offer some specific ways for us to incorporate nutritional medicine into our lives and health care. These diets and supplements should fit into what we are already doing to improve our health. They are not meant to take the place of a doctor's advice or prescribed medications. But if, after a time, we feel better, we may then be able to let go of our medicines and then maybe even of our exterior doctor, over our inner healing guide. Going from a state of health where we need a doctor's care to one where we can use a doctor to help us evaluate and support our health is a big step. Cooperative health care involves an evolutionary step that empowers us to become an important part of the decision making regarding our health. Good luck!

Note: The suggestions in this part of *Staying Healthy with Nutrition* are not meant to replace your doctor (or your own intuitive guidance), and specifically, are not meant as medical treatment. Also, please realize that the same nutritional plan, much like the same medicine, does not work the same for every individual. You are a unique person, not a disease. Thus, medicine is always experimental (sounds optimistic?), or really experiential, meaning we do not know for sure how any specific remedy or program will work for any given individual. For example, many people with asthma, a disease that is often difficult to manage, will respond to my nutritional and supplemental program to different degrees, yet I am confident that most shall see significant benefit. Hopefully, you can use the guidance contained herein to inspire and support you along the important path of improving and optimizing your health, which I have done in my own life.

---

32 Nutritional Application Programs

1. Infants and Toddlers (Birth through 3 Years)
2. Childhood (4 through 12 Years)
3. Adolescence (13 through 18 Years)
4. Adult Men
5. Adult Women
6. Pregnancy
7. Lactation
8. Menopause and Bone Health
9. The Later Years (65 Years and Older)
10. Antiaging: The Longevity Program
11. Antistress
12. Skin Enhancement
13. Sexual Vitality
14. Athletes
15. Executives and Healthy Travel
16. Vegetarianism
17. Environmental Pollution and Radiation
18. Immune Enhancement
19. Cancer Prevention
20. Cardiovascular Disease Prevention
21. Fatigue
22. Viral Conditions
23. Weight Loss
24. Weight Gain
25. Yeast Syndrome
26. Allergies
27. Birth Control Pills
28. Premenstrual Syndrome
29. Pre- and Postsurgery (and Injuries)
30. Mental Health: Depression, Anxiety, and Attention-Deficit/Hyperactivity Disorder
31. General Detoxification and Cleansing
32. Fasting and Juice Cleansing

Chapter 15

Life Stage Programs

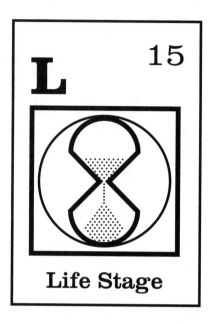

Life Stage

This initial set of programs applies to the different life stages, with special sections on the hormonal changes that most women experience. I offer simple discussions of the various age groups to help you understand the changing nutritional needs during growth and development. The emphasis is to support a positive and healthy lifestyle with some reference to potential poor habits that could lead to health difficulties.

Witin each program, I list the suggested amounts of essential nutrients. These are my personal recommendations for daily nutrient goals. In some cases they are double or triple the DRIs. Throughout the chapter, however, I have used the age and gender brackets common to the DRIs, which may be useful to anyone wishing to compare them. Many nutrients can be obtained from foods; often, however, additional supplementation may be desired to ensure that we acquire all the nutrients we need to support optimum health. Many common vitamin supplements contain at least the recommended dietary allowance (RDA) levels—which are now referred to more commonly at Dietary Reference Intakes (DRIs)—while other products contain higher levels than are commonly accepted as necessary (and possibly more adequate to an individual during increased stress or illness). With a healthy diet in a healthy individual, these supplement programs may not necessary all the time, but more during transition or with such symptoms as fatigue. As I have discussed in other areas of this book, it is wise for most of us to use some daily insurance supplementation, given the stresses under which most of us live and the potential deficiency of nutrients in even the natural, unrefined foods.

This section on life stage programs is really about diet and health for the family, so I have kept it fairly simple, suggesting what to avoid in your diet and emphasizing healthful plans. The programs for infancy through adolescence are relatively short discussions of basic needs and concerns for those years rather than detailed examinations of all the potential problems. The same is true for the adult programs, which are followed by discussions of special issues for women—pregnancy, lactation, and menopause. The chapter ends with a thorough discussion of nutrition regarding the aging process and the later years; however, the program on antiaging is in chapter 16.

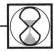

1. INFANTS AND TODDLERS (BIRTH THROUGH 3 YEARS)

I begin this chapter with the beginning of life. The time preceding birth, when the baby is still inside his or her mother, is an important period of growth and development. Prenatally as well as after birth, the baby's health is largely dependent on the mother's nourishment. Even the year or so *before* a woman becomes pregnant is important. *Preconceptional nutrition,* as it has come to be called, is a growing area of research. Studies have looked at the supplementation of folic acid, for example, in the year before the baby is conceived and have found this supplementation to be related to decreasing the risk of neural tube defects. (For more, see "Pregnancy" and "Lactation," on pages 569 and 575, respectively, later in this chapter.)

Nutrition is the key to growth and development. Ideally baby's first food is mother's milk, which is uniquely formulated to meet his or her growth needs, provided the mother eats an adequate diet. The colostrum the mother first produces has the fluid and nutrient levels, such as zinc, that correlate precisely with the baby's initial needs. As the first milk comes in, it is higher in fat and fatty acids, important to early developmental needs of the brain as well as the immune and nervous systems. Later, its fat content decreases and the protein and carbohydrate levels increase to meet the nutritional needs for general growth and development. With a good diet, mother's milk exclusively can support the baby for 6 months or more. Besides eating well, the mother should also avoid pharmaceutical drugs when possible as well as such chemicals as nicotine, alcohol, and caffeine. Occupational and even home chemical use should be avoided too. Pesticides, such as DDT and more recently used chemicals, may contaminate food and get into breast milk, so whenever possible, buy and eat organic or homegrown produce.

Breastfeeding is the best thing for both mother and baby. For the newly postpartum mother, breastfeeding stimulates uterine contractions, reducing bleeding and bringing the uterus back to its normal size. It provides intimate bonding for the mother and baby, so connected for the previous 9 months. It is convenient because the mother always has her baby's food with her; it is also less expensive. Also, the mother's output

of calories to baby helps bring her weight back toward its pre-pregnancy level. But above all, **breastfeeding is the healthiest choice for the child.** For the baby, breast milk provides the right nourishment ("as Nature intended"). It has more available iron, vitamins A and C, niacin, and potassium (and the right amino acids for growth) than any natural or formulated substitute. Breast milk not only has nutritional advantages but immunological ones as well, as the mother can pass her protective antibodies to her child. Recent studies show that breastfed babies are healthier than bottle-fed babies—they have fewer allergies, they are leaner, and they have lower cholesterol levels; this remains true in later years as well.

Many other aspects of breast milk and its health advantages for the baby are often overlooked. The sugar found in cow's milk (lactose) is also found in human milk, and nursing babies get this sugar just like babies being raised on cow's milk formulas. However, mothers send lactase, the enzyme for digesting lactose, along with the lactose in their milk content, so that the nursing baby gets both the milk sugar (lactose) and the enzyme needed to digest it (lactase). This breastfeeding combination is important, because the baby's liver cannot make lactase during the first months of life.

Most women are physically able to breastfeed if they wish. Breastfeeding support groups such as La Leche League are available in most cities for those who have trouble nursing; many hospitals also have lactation consultants on staff. Nursing mothers can also find help and reassurance from a midwife, a friend, or a neighbor who has breastfed a child. Relaxation and increased fluid intake facilitate breastfeeding. Luckily, the number of mothers who breastfeed has been increasing since the mid-1970s, even among women who work outside of the home, thanks to a desire on the part of many women to incorporate breastfeeding alongside of work, more willingness on the part of some employers to accommodate this desire, and availability of milk pumping and storage devices for women who would like to make use of them.

Unfortunately, there are really not many good substitutes for mother's milk. Although some research studies demonstrate the general safety of soy formula with respect to allergy, I am skeptical about these studies. I am concerned about soy formula for other reasons.

Without certified organic soymilk, I am worried about contaminants and genetically engineered soybeans. I also have some concern about the phytoestrogen content for a nursing infant. If you are planning to use any soy formula, I suggested holding off to at least 4 months or so to give the infant more time to develop more metabolic capacity with respect to soy. Several studies on colic show real benefits with 100% whey formulas. The benefits here make sense to me, and some of them apply to the use of whey-based supplements for adults as well. Goat's milk, slightly diluted, can also be used if the whey formula is not tolerated. Cow's milk is best avoided; it has a different amino acid balance than other substitutes, has more fats, and is more allergenic. Formulas may be used in an emergency, but I generally do not recommend them because of their unnatural and synthetic makeup.

A common problem during an infant's first 6 months is colic. It is more common in first children but may occur in children of any birth order. Some psychological stresses may influence colic, but it may also be affected by the nursing mother's diet. Cow's milk consumed by the mother may be a factor; excessive sugar or salt intake may also worsen colic. Often a decrease in the mother's milk product consumption reduces the colic symptoms. Some extra B vitamins, calcium, magnesium, and potassium taken by the mother may help reduce colic in the baby as well as reduce the mother's intestinal gas. Several fennel and chamomile oil products are available for herbal-based treatment of colic, and many mothers have reported success with these products. Also, mothers must constantly remember to eat well so that they do not become nutritionally depleted during nursing.

Babies need more calories and protein per pound than any other age group. Goat's milk, and even cow's milk, with their protein, fat, and calorie content, are potentially valuable foods in moderation (if tolerated well) for rapidly growing babies (after 8 to 10 months) and children. The "dairy" problem comes in when adults continue to use milk and its products as a regular part of their children's diet. Lifelong use of milk is among the biggest misconceptions and mistakes in nutrition. Consumption of dairy products should be greatly curtailed by the adult population, and by those children and teenagers sensitive to cow's milk. If infants and children develop any recurrent congestive problems, such as excessive nasal mucus or ear infections (often just fluid), I suggest they go off all cow's milk products for a time (several weeks) to see if their problems improve.

When and What to Feed Infants

This is a rather controversial issue. Some parents try to feed solid foods to their babies at 4 months or sooner—a big mistake. Infants will do fine on breast milk alone. The trend is returning to later rather than earlier feeding, fortunately. Premature feeding can lead to poor digestion, increased allergy, other immune problems, and obesity. There may appear to be increased growth, but it could be just increased fat. Skin-fold measurements are used now, along with growth and development charts, to show whether this is the case. Increased fat at this time can lead to increased numbers of fat cells, which may increase the likelihood of adult obesity. Premature feeding may also influence later eating habits. At about 5 to 6 months is the earliest time to begin feeding such little beings any solid foods. **Waiting until six months of age gives the baby time to develop his or her digestive tract and immunological system to reduce the likelihood of allergy and other reactions to food.**

First foods should be simple, natural, and pureed to assist digestion. The true flavors of food are best; avoid the use of sweetened or salted foods, especially refined-sugar and refined-flour foods. First foods may be pureed or cooked fruits (although not citrus; it is best to focus on pears, plums, and apples), cooked and pureed vegetables (yams and squashes work well), and cooked cereal grains (especially oatmeal or rice, formulated for babies). These foods along with mother's milk provide the proper nourishment for this time of rapid growth. Egg yolks can also be added to the diet, but avoid egg whites for now, as the albumin protein is more allergenic.

At 7 to 8 months, a few teeth may start to appear. Toast can be used for teething. Some meats, preferably organic, can be added now; these should be baked or broiled and then finely chopped or pureed. Potatoes (baked, boiled, and mashed), along with other vegetables, may also round out the menu. From 8 months to 1 year, babies may do some serious eating. They may be more independent, adventurous, and enthusiastic with food. They are likely to try more new foods, and the diet can become more well-rounded. Whole eggs may be used as a good source of protein now. Milk consumption may be reduced, but it is still a regular source of nourishment. Some infants may wean at this time, although many mother-baby teams continue nursing for another year or more, especially with the aid of a breast pump for working mothers. The average age of weaning, worldwide, is actually much, much later; some studies estimate that it occurs just after 4. I know of no scientific reason not to let a child nurse until he or she decides not to. Many other factors come into play, of course, and every mother and father have to weigh this balance for themselves. Foods and meals should be simple. Make as much of your own baby food as possible; prepackaged jars and cans of foods should not be used exclusively.

After 1 year, the baby's diet may shift. Food needs for growth are fewer now as the rate of growth slows down. Many parents become concerned because it appears that the child is not eating, but this is usually fine. Eating habits may change and food likes and dislikes develop. Try not to make eating a battle, and avoid

Daily Nutrient Program—Infants and Toddlers

Nutrient Amount	Age: Birth–6 Months	7 Months–1 Year	1–3 Years
Calories	108/kg	98/kg	102/kg (1,000–1,400)
Protein	2.2 g/kg	1.6 g/kg	1.2/kg
Vitamin A	2,000 IU	2,500 IU	2,000 IU
Vitamin D	400 IU	400 IU	400 IU
Vitamin E	5 IU	6 IU	8 IU
Vitamin K	4 mcg	5 mcg	30 mcg
Thiamin (B1)	0.4 mg	0.6 mg	0.8 mg
Riboflavin (B2)	0.5 mg	0.7 mg	0.9 mg
Niacin (B3)	6 mg	8 mg	10 mg
Pantothenic acid (B5)	3 mg	3 mg	4 mg
Pyridoxine (B6)	0.4 mg	0.6 mg	1.0 mg
Cobalamin (B12)	1.0 mcg	2.0 mcg	2.5 mcg
Folic acid	65 mcg	80 mcg	150 mcg
Biotin	10 mcg	12 mcg	16 mcg
Vitamin C	40 mg	60 mg	100 mg
Calcium	400 mg	600 mg	800 mg
Chloride	0.6 g	1.0 g	1.2 g
Chromium	50 mcg	60 mcg	80 mcg
Copper	0.4 mg	0.5 mg	0.6 mg
Fluoride	0.3 mg	0.6 mg	1.0 mg
Iodine	110 mcg	130 mcg	190 mcg
Iron	1 mg	11 mg	10 mg
Magnesium	70 mg	90 mg	150 mg
Manganese	0.7 mg	1.0 mg	1.5 mg
Molybdenum	5 mcg	10 mcg	40 mcg
Phosphorus	300 mg	500 mg	800 mg
Potassium	0.7 mg	1.0 mg	1.5 mg
Selenium	40 mcg	60 mcg	80 mcg
Sodium	0.3 g	0.6 g	0.9 g
Zinc	4 mg	6 mg	10 mg

games and rewards. Let the child eat; he or she will communicate his or her needs. Offer nourishing foods and avoid sweet treats. Balance the diet over days, not at each meal, so that meals can be simple. Most healthy children eat only what their bodies need.

Regarding supplements to the diet in the first 2 years, most parents are more comfortable with a moderate insurance formula that at least covers the child's recommended daily allowances (RDAs). (Note: When the RDAs were revised in 2000–2002, a broader phrase called dietary reference intakes (DRIs) was put into use to refer to the nutritional guidelines that contain the RDAs. I have used this new term throughout this chapter.) Some parents and pediatricians feel that for healthy babies on breast milk and infants eating a good diet, additional supplements are not really needed.

When a vitamin formula is used, however, it is often a liquid supplement in the first year, and after that a flavorful chewable. For toddlers, the multiple should contain all of the B vitamins as well as vitamins C, E, and A. Basic minerals such as calcium and iron as well as zinc, magnesium, manganese, and even a little chromium and selenium can also be included. I suggest more natural, chemical-free supplements, without sugar and artificial food colorings and flavors. The bigger companies with inexpensive vitamins may not believe that synthetic, treated chemical formulas are of concern, but many doctors and parents nowadays would certainly rather avoid those products.

The "Daily Nutrient Program—Infants and Toddlers" on page 559 shows the levels of vitamins and minerals suggested for this age group. Some values are higher than the DRIs to provide that extra margin of safety, particularly to cover those infants who may need more of some nutrients or for those who might be sick and need higher amounts of certain vitamins or minerals. Later sections in this chapter suggest what nutrients might be needed in higher amounts in specific health situations; do not, however, use the levels suggested for adults for your children. Talk to your doctor or refer to specific literature to find appropriate dosages for specific age groups. Unfortunately, some parents have misunderstood the suggested amounts and have given excessive and unhealthy amounts to their infants. Vitamin A toxicity is proba-

bly most common. Do not overuse vitamin A or D or cod liver oil, or the minerals calcium, phosphorus, or iron. Breastfed babies can get a bit deficient in vitamin D unless they get a little sunlight exposure. Babies need a balanced diet and lifestyle, too.

Breast milk is usually low in fluoride, and although fluoride use is still debatable, it appears relatively safe to supplement, and thus many parents and doctors use fluoridated vitamins to protect against tooth decay. However, if the nursing mother drinks fluoridated water, it is now recommended *not* to give fluoridated vitamins to breastfed babies because it comes through the milk. No fluoride supplements should be used at any age if the water is fluoridated.

2. CHILDHOOD (4 THROUGH 12 YEARS)

It is important for parents to instill good eating habits in their children and to avoid overindulgence in refined sugars and flours and high-fat, fried fast foods. Children need a lot of nourishing foods to provide them with all of the important nutrients for growth; although physical growth is a little slower during this period than it is in infancy or during the adolescent years, mental growth is relatively rapid. Creating healthy eating patterns begins with encouraging the consumption of good-quality, wholesome foods, which is a lot easier when parents themselves eat this type of diet. Setting a good example is my number-one tip for feeding kids healthfully. Children's tendencies are toward the sweets, treats, and salted snacks and away from vegetables, the important food group that in many cases offers the greatest nutritional challenge for parents. Try to be creative with veggies; most children prefer raw vegetables to cooked, so try more raw veggies. Offer whatever vegetables the child likes and maintain the fruits, grains, and protein foods. And with this, you'll be healthier, too, as you set a good nutritional example.

Many children like to help with and be part of their nutrition. Support this by reaching agreements and creatively inspiring their food choices. Teach them to prepare food and feed themselves at an early age. Avoid soft drinks and excessive poor-quality, "treat" foods, and offer more-nourishing snacks, such as fruits, cheese or yogurt, nuts, crackers, or popcorn. Avoid nutritional adversity—battles and hassles around mealtime and rewards of such sweets as ice cream, cake, or candy for eating their vegetables. **Bribery and rewards may emphasize the treats and lessen the value of the more healthful foods.** Again, getting children involved in meal planning and preparation as they get older is often helpful. Having them assist in preparing their school lunch will give them more pleasure in eating it. Good eating habits generate good nutrition.

For preschool kids, **ages 2 to 5,** this is often a time of slower growth, and sometimes these children decrease their food intake. Parents may be concerned, but usually these kids are fine. Offer them wholesome foods. Avoid bribing. Just keep offering them the foods they need, and be a good example yourself. Keep their diet low in refined foods, chemical foods, and sweet, salty, or fried foods. Children this age like to eat with their hands, especially finger snacks, so give them small pieces at meals when appropriate.

For schoolchildren, **ages 5 to 13,** it may get a little tougher. Often likes and dislikes limit their diets. Food games lose their charm, and rebellion may begin. However, many kids in this age group become more cooperative and want to be helpful and accepted, and thus they may really attempt to eat well. A good breakfast is essential for these children going off to school. Eating hot, whole-grain cereals provides a good source of morning energy (the sugary cereals may be more stimulating, but the boost is short-lived and may be followed by a depressed period); some protein, such as eggs, also provides sustaining energy. Adding some nuts or seeds to their grains offers better long-term energy and nutrients.

Given the current level of institutional (school) nutritional awareness, it is best to sack a good lunch for your child and encourage him or her to eat it at lunchtime. I am hopeful, however, that a bagged lunch might not always be necessary from a nutritional standpoint. There has been a concerted effort in several states to bring more-nourishing food into our schools, and even organically grown produce and dairy products. One source of information about this effort is the national Farm to School Program (www.farmtoschool.org).

There are always outside influences at this age, such as other children or television, that attempt to

> **General note to readers about age groupings and DRIs throughout the age groups:** The developmental stages described in this chapter do not exactly correspond to the DRI age groupings, which are 0–6 months, 7–12 months, 1–3, 4–8, 9–13, 14–18, 19–30, 31–50, 51–70, and >70. In addition, our lists are NOT DRI LISTS. We have some higher values on our lists suggested for support, even double and triple the DRIs. Yet, it makes sense for us to match our developmental language closer to the DRI age brackets. This step will enable readers to more directly compare our recommendations to the DRIs. In the case of childhood, we would have to define this term as 4–13 years to match the DRI brackets. Similarly, "adolescence" would have to be defined as 14–18 years. The overall ranges of nutrients involves more liberal thinking and experience in the support of more optimal levels of some vitamins, minerals, amino acids, and herbs to be utilized in more health-enhancing programs. And remember that the ages at the higher and lower parts of the ranges are merging into each other, so we need to adapt, just as we do throughout our life.

undermine the healthful eating habits you have worked to develop in your children. Again, setting a good example (to not only do as we say, but also as we do) is the best influence parents have on the overall nutritional patterns of their young ones.

Many parents overestimate their children's needs and the amount of food required (which we do for ourselves as well). It is best to create simple meals and serve smaller portions more frequently throughout the day. Needs for calories and many of the basic nutrients vary from ages 2 through 10. Obviously, with increased size and activity, the older children need more food, which they naturally eat when it's provided. The more we can support them in avoiding empty calories, the better chance they have of optimum growth and less obesity. During the middle years, the average youngster gains between 5 and 8 pounds and grows about ½ inch per year, provided they have the nutrients they need. Support a healthy amount of physical activity in place of laziness or too much TV, computer games, and phone use.

As insurance to prevent nutrient deficiencies, many parents want their children to take some supplements. Chewables are still a favorite, although as children become older, many can swallow tablets and capsules. Alternately, powdered formulas can be added to foods. The nutrient levels shown in the "Daily Nutrient Program—Childhood" table below reflect the DRIs plus a little insurance for the special needs of children between the ages of 4 and 13. In a few cases, I recommend amounts at 2 to 3 times the DRI level. Also, the 2002 edition of the DRIs arrived at different recommendations in some instances for boys and girls, and in the table I have included the values for both genders combined in the ranges.

3. ADOLESCENCE (13 THROUGH 18 YEARS)

The teenage years are trying times in a lot of ways, especially in terms of nutrition. Adolescence is a period of high nutritional risk, when the increased demands for nutrients are often met with poor choices of foods, unhealthy eating habits, and deficient intakes of calories and protein as well as many vitamins and minerals. Adolescence usually begins at age 10 to 12 in girls and 12 to 14 in boys. There are not only new demands but also many physiological changes because of the sexual hormones being released. Body composition also shifts, with girls increasing their percentage of fat and adding curves, while boys tend to increase protein and muscle development. During these years, young men may gain 15 to 20 pounds and 4 to 5 inches in height per year, while girls may add 13 to 18 pounds and grow 3 to 4 inches a year. The main years of growth are between ages 11 and 16 for girls and 13 and 18 for boys.

The nutritional problems of adolescence are probably related to the rebellious nature of these years. Teenagers eat what they want, when they want; they are hard to feed and harder to influence regarding dietary changes. Peer pressure is great. They often have limited food intake and poor nutrition, with a diet high in sweets and refined foods, fried foods, fast foods, and junk foods. The adolescent diet is often high on the glycemic index, meaning there are more rapidly absorbing sugars. A diet higher in the complex carbohydrates, such as whole grains and legumes, can help to balance this. Luckily, though, for many teenagers the great demands for nutrients to support growth increases their appetite for more concentrated protein foods and nutrient-rich foods. Some active adolescent males in particular may easily consume 4,000 calories daily.

Boys generally tend to eat enough food, but they may be deficient in nutrients because they often avoid vegetables, whole grains, and other whole foods. **Teenagers who eat more refined foods without taking supplements commonly develop deficien-**

Daily Nutrient Program—Childhood		
Nutrient	**Age: 4–8 Years Old Amount**	**9–12 or 13 Years Old Amount**
Calories	1,600–2,000	2,000–2,400
Protein	30–35 g	35–45 g
Vitamin A	3,000 IU	4,000 IU
Vitamin D	400 IU	400 IU
Vitamin E	20 IU	25 IU
Vitamin K	55 mcg	60 mcg
Thiamin (B1)	1.0 mg	1.5 mg
Riboflavin (B2)	1.2 mg	1.6 mg
Niacin (B3)	12 mg	17 mg
Pantothenic acid (B5)	4 mg	5 mg
Pyridoxine (B6)	1.5 mg	2.0 mg
Cobalamin (B12)	3 mcg	4 mcg
Folic acid	250 mcg	350 mcg
Biotin	25 mcg	50 mcg
Vitamin C	75 mg	135 mg
Calcium	800 mg	1,300 mg
Chloride	1.5 g	2.0 g
Chromium	45 mcg	75 mcg
Copper	0.8 mg	1.4 mg
Fluoride	2.0 mg	2.5 mg
Iodine	120 mcg	120 mcg
Iron	10 mg	8 mg
Magnesium	250 mg	300 mg
Manganese	2.5 mg	3.0 mg
Molybdenum	50 mcg	75 mcg
Phosphorus	800 mg	1,250 mg
Potassium	2.0 g	2.5 g
Selenium	90 mcg	120 mcg
Sodium	1.3 g	1.8 g
Zinc	10 mg	16 mg

cies. Teenage girls tend to eat less, as they are often concerned about their weight, and the changes in their fatty tissue increase this concern. Thus they also may consume a diet deficient in nutrients. With the beginning of the menstrual cycle, there are greater demands for iron and other nutrients. Problems of bulimia and anorexia nervosa are more common in teenage girls, which will be discussed further under "Weight Gain" on page 695 in chapter 17, Medical Treatment Programs. Teenage pregnancy can be a huge problem because of poor nutrition and deficiencies existing before pregnancy begins, let alone the challenge to a developing emotional system. Poor nutrition during pregnancy or prior to it greatly increases the risk of complications.

Obesity in adolescence usually results from poor food choices and laziness or lack of exercise, and is a major problem. Other habits can also lead to weight gain. For example, more average daily time spent watching TV is associated with higher weights, resulting from less activity and more snacks. With increased calorie intake during these growth years, there is an increase in the number and size of fat cells. This can lead to lifelong weight problems. Diet changes, sensible eating, and exercise are the best ways to counteract excessive weight gain, even in youngsters. Like eating habits, exercise habits are often created early in life and, once set, are harder to change. This is also true for attitudes toward health and life in general. These factors are all important in generating long-term health.

Teenagers need to realize the importance of good nutrition, which can help a great deal in promoting nice-looking skin and general good looks. Dental caries are more common in adolescence, probably because of hormonal changes, a poor diet high in refined sugars, and mineral deficiencies. A more wholesome diet along with regular brushing and flossing also promotes healthy teeth. Parents can help adolescent children best by being understanding and supportive. Our advice should be mild, with suggestions for avoiding certain foods and trying others. Parents can be good influences by being good examples themselves, eating well and not buying junk and refined snack foods for the home. Keep such nourishing snack foods as fruits, nuts, and yogurt on hand and prepare wholesome meals—these practices will help youngsters make the best food choices, at least at home.

Daily Nutrient Program—Adolescence (13–18 Years)

Nutrient	Amount	Nutrient	Amount
Calories	boys, 2,800–3,150	Vitamin C	300 mg
	girls, 2,000–2,400	Calcium	1,200 mg
Protein	boys, 56 g	Chloride	3 g
	girls, 46 g	Chromium	200 mcg
Vitamin A	5,400 IU	Copper	2–3 mg
Vitamin D	300 IU	Fluoride	2.5 mg
Vitamin E	30 IU	Iodine	150 mcg
Vitamin K	150 mcg	Iron	18 mg
Thiamin (B1)	1.5 mg	Magnesium	400 mg
Riboflavin (B2)	2 mg	Manganese	5 mg
Niacin (B3)	18 mg	Molybdenum	100 mcg
Pantothenic acid (B5)	10 mg	Phosphorus	1,200 mg
Pyridoxine (B6)	2.5 mg	Potassium	4 g
Cobalamin (B12)	5 mcg	Selenium	200 mcg
Folic acid	400 mcg	Sodium	3 g
Biotin	200 mcg	Zinc	15 mg

A big concern is the wide availability of fast foods. This problem has unfortunately spilled over even into some public school cafeterias, where some school districts have signed "pouring rights" with soft drink companies and other fast food providers. Fast foods contain high levels of salt, fat, and additives and low amounts of fiber and other vital nutrients. Protein is usually adequate, and sugar levels may be excessive. If fast foods are not eaten too frequently (more than once weekly), they are not a big cause for concern. Now some fast food restaurants are offering healthier salads and nonfried foods. A regular diet of soda pops, breads, cheese, sweets, and snack foods (which can be eaten at fast food places or at home and school) can be more of a problem, however. The protein content of such a diet may be low if too many heavily processed snacks take over for the meal-type staples, and the B vitamins and vitamins C, A, and E are often deficient. Minerals may be the biggest problem. Calcium and iron are needed in higher amounts in these growth years, and they are frequently not obtained in adequate amounts from diet alone. If soft drinks are substituted for milk, both calcium and vitamin D may be low. Zinc and manganese are also concerns, as are the trace minerals chromium and selenium. Those foods extra high in nutrients such as brewer's yeast, molasses, wheat germ, and nuts can be added to fruit smoothies to increase the dietary nutrients. Teenagers may accept these kinds of suggestions.

The recommended diet plan is a balanced one containing vegetables, including some greens, nuts, whole grains, fruit, and higher-protein foods (dairy and meats) to provide the needed B vitamins, C, calcium, zinc, and iron. Vegetarian teenagers need to be even more conscious nutritionally, making sure they obtain many high-nutrient and wholesome foods. (See "Vegetarianism" on page 624 in chapter 16, Performance Enhancement Programs.) To assure that growing teenagers obtain all the nutrients they need to support their heavy growth demands, a general multiple vitamin and mineral supplement is highly recommended. Girls especially need extra iron. Other needs may also be increased under certain circumstances, such as calcium, vitamin D, and other bone-support nutrients when bone growth is an issue of concern.

The "Daily Nutrient Program—Adolescence (13–18 Years)" on page 563 suggests the DRIs (or levels up to twice as high) for 13- to 18-year-olds. After that, the adult programs are used. There are, of course, nutritional supplements for young people that contain higher levels of vitamins and minerals that can also be used as additional support. Many teenagers do well on these products as they ensure good levels of most nutrients.

4. ADULT MEN

Adult males, like all other segments of the American populace, have their own special needs. Much of the information in this book relates to both men and women; in this section let's look at the differences between the genders regarding nutrition. In this program, I review the requirements for an adult male's optimum physical, mental, and sexual functions, as well as his specific nutritional needs.

Everyone wants a long, healthy, and happy life, but how do we create that? Heredity and nutrition are probably the most influential factors governing longevity. Other aspects of lifestyle—such as work, activity, exercise, environment, stress levels, and chemical exposure—are also important. More subtle aspects—such as purpose, creativity, attitude, and even spiritual awareness—may also be key factors for many men. I believe that the state of our nutrition, our general attitude toward life, and how we handle stress can influence our health and longevity more than anything else; these factors can maximize our potential or hasten our demise. In addition, many specific nutrients protect us and enhance our energy and physiological potential.

Men (and humans in general) in this modern age have departed from the basic aspects of supportive, natural living. Most of us have moved away from the land and manual labor to a frenetic lifestyle in cars and offices, eating on the run, and working more with our minds than with our bodies. These increased stresses require greater nourishment than we have needed under low-stress conditions. Unless we fill this vital nutrient gap, our energy, stamina, and productivity can be diminished. Obtaining quality foods and taking the relaxed, receptive time to eat them need to be more of a life priority. **Most active, productive men need a good supplement program to protect them from**

illness and deficiency symptoms and increase their longevity by reducing chronic degenerative disease patterns.

Many parts of this book deal with nutrition's effect on major diseases—cancer, cardiovascular disease, and diabetes. Even though the average life span in the United States has increased greatly (from 47 years for males born in 1900 to 77 years for those born in 2000), much of this is due to better prenatal and infant care, immunizations, and the use of antibiotics to treat acute infections. Now, many adult chronic, degenerative diseases result from regular overeating and from choosing the wrong foods (those high in fat and sugar) and too many refined or chemical-laden foods. At the same time, consumption of too few of the wholesome, nutritious foods may contribute to suppressed immunity, increased infection rates, and susceptibility to cancer.

It is important that men (and all people) find the right balance in diet and lifestyle. This includes all of the nutritional suggestions discussed throughout this book—eating more fresh fruits and vegetables, whole grains, legumes, nuts, seeds, fresh fish, and, if desired, occasional lean poultry or animal meats that are free of (at least low in) chemicals and antibiotics. Limiting the fatty, refined, and sugary foods—such as milk products, processed meats, fried foods, breads, candies, and pastries—while minimizing the use of caffeine, alcohol, and nicotine will help produce a healthier and longer life.

Most men with good energy levels can use regular detoxification periods (discussed in detail in chapter 18, Detoxification and Cleansing Programs). Regular fasting or cleansing—done yearly (in springtime), seasonally, monthly, or even 1 day weekly—is a great preventive medicine tool; it may also help to reenergize the will and the instincts. Difficulties may arise when we overwhelm our capacities to handle our foods, chemicals, emotions, thoughts, and so on. We may also begin to feel backed up when our abilities to digest, assimilate, and eliminate these many potential life stressors are reduced. Constipation, back pain, allergies, and sinus congestion, as well as certain cardiovascular diseases and gastrointestinal problems are the results of this type of lifestyle autointoxication. Many of these problems respond well to a cleansing program. See General Detoxification and Cleansing on page 741 in chapter 18.

These cleansing periods offer us a good chance to reevaluate our life and make a new plan for health, work, or whatever else we may need to renew ourselves. Most men do not usually consider this practice, but those who do, respond very well. In my experience, women are more likely to embrace these more evolutionary (or traditional) aspects of cultural medicine, hygienic practices, and healing; women are also usually more receptive to change and learning. Women require fasting programs less frequently, because their problems more commonly result from nutritional deficiencies. Men, of course, need these renewing processes as well. Ultimately, both men and women need to find a balance, ever-changing of course, that will keep them well and not require much detoxification.

Sexual energy and vitality are important male issues, especially when we are committed to getting along well with our mates, lovers, or friends. Safe sex is a big concern today, but if we do not have the energy for sex, we can forget these more adventurous subjects. Sexual function is supported by good diet and nutrient intake. The healthy diet should provide adequate protein and essential fatty acids as well as some cholesterol (eggs, dairy foods) or plant sterols, as are found in olive oil; these foods provide some of the precursors of certain sex hormones.

Several endocrine organs aid in normal sexual function. The thyroid gland, necessary for proper energy level and metabolism, is supported by iodine and B vitamins, particularly thiamin and pantothenic acid. Testicular function is vital to normal production of testosterone, the hormone most essential to male sex drive. Adrenal androgen hormones also support testicular activity and sexual development in men. Vitamin E and zinc may be the big two when it comes to sexual energy support. Vitamins A, C, and E as well as folic acid and the essential fatty acids are all important to sperm production. The minerals calcium, magnesium, zinc, and sulfur as well as vitamin B_{12}, inositol, and vitamin C are found in healthy sperm; they also may be necessary to fertility. Many nutrients support healthy adrenal function—vitamins A, C, and E, the B vitamins, especially pantothenic acid, and the essential fatty acids. Factors such as stress, worry, excess mental activity, and regular sugar and caffeine use may contribute to weaker adrenal function.

Adult Men's Nutrient Program (Minimum to Possible Optimum Safe Levels)

AGE: 19–70 YEARS OLD

Nutrient	Amount	Nutrient	Amount
Calories	2,100–3,500	Calcium*	1,000–1,200 mg
Fiber	40–70 g	Chloride*	2–5 g
Protein	50–75 g	Chromium	50–500 mcg
Fats	50–75 g	Copper	1–3 mg
Vitamin A	5,000–10,000 IU	Fluoride*	1.5–4.0 mg
Beta-carotene	5,000–20,000 IU	Iodine*	150–300 mcg
Vitamin D	400–600 IU	Iron*	8–15 mg
Vitamin E	30–800 IU	Magnesium	420–800 mg
Vitamin K*	150–600 mcg	Manganese	3–10 mg
Thiamin (B1)	1.4–50.0 mg	Molybdenum	50–500 mcg
Riboflavin (B2)	1.6–50.0 mg	Phosphorus*	800–1,200 mg
Niacin (B3)**	20–200 mg	Potassium*	2–6 g
Pantothenic acid (B5)	7–250 mg	Selenium	100–400 mcg
Pyridoxine (B6)	2.5–100.0 mg	Sodium*	1.0–3.5 g
Cobalamin (B12)	3–200 mcg	Zinc	15–60 mg
Folic acid	400–800 mcg		
Biotin	50–500 mcg		
Choline	550–750 mg		
Inositol	50–500 mg		
PABA	10–50 mg		
Vitamin C	90–2,000 mg		
Bioflavonoids	125–500 mg		

* These nutrients are noted because they are required for health; for men, however, they are usually adequate in the diet and do not require supplementation. Some calcium or iron may be taken occasionally in a multiple or if the man is a strict vegetarian.

** Mixed niacin and niacinamide; 50 mg or more of niacin may cause nausea, tingling, and flushing initially but could help to lower the cholesterol levels. (See Vitamin B3 on page 115 in chapter 5, Vitamins).

If a man has a decreased sex drive, some extra zinc, magnesium, and vitamin B6 may be helpful. (Stress, sleep, and a balanced diet are also crucial.) With impotence, vitamins C and E, B complex, and calcium, plus some counseling to explore the psychological factors, can provide support. Such herbs as ginseng root, which is a good tonic herb, can raise general and sexual energy levels. Also, reducing the use of sedative-type drugs, such as alcohol, and nicotine, which interferes with circulation, and generally reducing stress may all help. **Much sexual dysfunction has to do with mental stresses and fears of intimacy.** Massage and body therapy give an important balance to a busy lifestyle, as does regular exercise. All of these may be helpful in improving both energy levels and sexual vitality.

For men who experience premature ejaculation, there may be many factors involved. Among these are not enough practice or enough sex, poor circulation, and even allergies. Histamine, a chemical in our cells and blood, controls ejaculation. If this chemical is too high, as it often is with allergies, ejaculatory rate may be increased. Low histamine levels may slow this rate and in some men may even cause problems with ejaculating. Niacin and fatty acids tend to increase the release of stored histamine, while calcium and the amino acid methionine may lower it. Thus extra calcium and amino acids with higher methionine levels could help in certain cases of premature ejaculation. (For more on sex and nutrition, see "Sexual Vitality" on page 609 in chapter 16, Performance Enhancement Programs.)

Men, like women, have special nutrient needs to maintain their energy and sexuality. Men usually need at least the DRIs for all nutrients, with less iron and more magnesium and B vitamins than women. Otherwise, the requirements for a good nutritional foundation are really not very different. **Men should be particularly careful about iron. Anemia, a vegetarian diet, and problems with bleeding may make iron supplementation necessary. But researchers know that iron excess is much more common in men than iron deficiency.** Iron excess can lead to heart irregularity, joint pain, chronic fatigue, depression, and other chronic health problems. The risk here is particularly high for men routinely consuming beef alongside of supplements containing iron. A man's decision about iron may therefore require some lab work or other assessment by an informed health-care practitioner. (Transferrin saturation and serum ferritin are commonly used tests to determine the likelihood of iron overload.)

Men also obviously need more calories and protein to support their generally larger size and often higher activity levels. The number of calories they need varies with their desired weight and activity level. The male couch potato may need to reduce his caloric intake by eating fewer munchies, drinking less beer, and restricting his intake of foods high in fats and sugar.

The "Adult Men's Nutrient Program" on the opposite page offers guidelines for men "on the go" between the ages of 19 and 70. The values listed range from minimum requirements to more optimum levels. (The basic DRIs are listed on page 517 at the end of chapter 13, The Ideal Diet.) For certain nutrients (such as calories, fats, iron, and sodium), the lower numbers may be more appropriate. These values represent a combination of diet and additional supplements, and certain essential nutrients (such as sodium, chloride, fluoride, phosphorus, and vitamin K) are not usually taken above dietary levels, although vitamin K probably should be as it may help reduce cardiovascular risk. If such nutrients as iron, calcium, copper, iodine, and potassium are sufficient in the diet, these are not usually added unless there are specific problems with digestion and/or assimilation. Important extra support for men may come from B vitamins, vitamins C and E, beta-carotene, magnesium, manganese, selenium, and zinc.

5. ADULT WOMEN

Adult women also have special needs. On a basic level, they need to love and be loved, to create, and to express their feelings and their being. (Men, of course, share these basic needs.) Women also have special nutritional needs. During the menstruating years (generally between the ages of 13 and 50), their need for iron to replace lost red blood cells is high. They also need adequate amounts of other nutrients, such as the B vitamins, iodine, calcium, and magnesium—more, I think, than the DRIs suggest. One of the main concerns with women is that their food intake may not be adequate. Physical activity levels may be low, and often there is inadequate calorie intake related to dieting to stay thin. This may result in deficient nutrient intake to meet nutritional requirements. Very active women may also eat lightly to keep their weight down, and without adequate supplements, this can lead to deficiencies.

Some women put on weight very easily, however, and have a difficult time losing it. Even low-calorie diets may not do the trick. Changing food quality (to high vegetable, lean protein) may help more than calorie counting, as will significantly increased exercise. Verifying a good match between food intake and weight loss might also mean having a blood draw to check thyroid levels and measuring lean body mass. Also, a basic multivitamin plus additional supplements (particularly extra B vitamins, such as B6 and B12, plus potassium, calcium, and magnesium) will also be helpful. (For more on this, see "Weight Loss" on page 684 in chapter 17, Medical Treatment Programs.)

Sexual vitality is also important to women. A number of nutrients are important in supporting the sexual organs, sexual functions, and a normal menstrual cycle. Normal thyroid function is needed to provide sexual energy and motivation. Adrenal support and function are important for women as well as for men. The adrenal glands help us deal with stress and give us sexual energy. Stress, allergies, and high amounts of sugar intake can weaken these important glands, and this may be exacerbated by nutritional deficiency. The adrenals need adequate levels of vitamins A, C, and E, essential fatty acids, and B vitamins, particularly pantothenic acid. Chromium and adequate levels of amino acids will also help reduce sugar cravings and thus help support the adrenals.

Adult Women's Nutrient Program (Minimum to Possible Optimum Safe Levels)

AGE: 19–70 YEARS OLD

Nutrient	Amount	Nutrient	Amount
Calories	1,500–2,500	Bioflavonoids	125–500 mg
Fiber	20–40 g	Calcium	1,200–1,500 mg
Protein	45–65 g	Chloride**	2–4 g
Fats*	40–70 g	Chromium	40–400 mcg
Vitamin A	4,000–10,000 IU	Copper	1–3 mg
Beta-carotene	5,000–20,000 IU	Fluoride**	1.5–3.5 mg
Vitamin D	400–500 IU	Iodine**	150–300 mcg
Vitamin E	30–800 IU	Iron	18–30 mg
Vitamin K**	100–300 mcg	Magnesium	350–700 mg
Thiamin (B1)	1–30 mg	Manganese	2.5–10 mg
Riboflavin (B2)	1.2–30.0 mg	Molybdenum	40–500 mcg
Niacin or Niacinamide (B3)	15–100 mg	Phosphorus**	800–1,200 mg
Pantothenic acid (B5)	7–250 mg	Potassium**	2–5 g
Pyridoxine (B6)	2–50 mg	Selenium	100–300 mcg
Cobalamin (B12)	3–200 mcg	Sodium**	1.5–4.0 g
Folic acid	400–800 mcg	Zinc	15–30 mg
Biotin	50–500 mcg		
Choline	550–650 mg		
Inositol	50–500 mg		
PABA	5–50 mg		
Vitamin C	75–1,000 mg		

* Total fats include olive oil and fish/salmon oil with eicosapentaenoic acid (EPA) and docosahexaenoic acid (DHA) but a low amount of saturated fats.

** These nutrients are listed because they are required in the diet (they have RDAs), although they are not usually added to formulas or taken as extra supplements.

The female ovaries secrete estrogen and progesterone, which control the menstrual cycle. These hormones are influenced by the pituitary gland in the brain; the pituitary is influenced by higher brain centers, which are in turn affected by emotions, moon cycles, weather, and the seasons. This female hormonal balance is therefore delicate and needs a lot of support. It requires sufficient levels of B vitamins, especially folic acid and niacin, plus zinc and vitamin E. Certain fats and cholesterol are important precursors of female hormones, mediated through the liver's biochemical processes. Drug and alcohol use (and most chemicals), which can stress the liver, may weaken this sensitive hormonal function. Some women's cholesterol levels are too low, especially those who are strict vegetarians, and this may be related to low hormonal levels and early menopause.

During the actual menstrual cycle, women tend to lose iron in the red blood cells; there are also tendencies to lose calcium and zinc. Copper levels usually increase, as they do with the use of birth control pills, which contain estrogen. During and after menstruation, women can take a little extra iron, magnesium, calcium (vitamins D and C help absorption), zinc, and vitamin B6. Copper should be avoided above dietary levels or above the usual 1 to 2 mg in a general supplement. A good protein diet with extra B complex and vitamin C is also recommended. Additional calcium and magnesium, ideally in the citrate or aspartate forms, may be helpful for menstrual cramps. Niacin (50–100 mg) might also be beneficial. Although it may not be easy, women should try to avoid too many sweets during the pre- and postmenstruation times.

When women become pregnant or breastfeed, they have greatly increased requirements for calories, protein, and many vitamins and minerals, especially calcium, magnesium, and iron. If birth control pills are taken (not recommended), many nutrients are needed in greater amounts. (See a more detailed discussion in "Birth Control Pills" on page 717 in chapter 17.) More zinc and less copper and iron, more vitamin B6, a basic B vitamin formula, and vitamins E and C should be taken.

Menopause can be a stressful time, filled with hormonal effects and changes, stresses, and various symptoms—fatigue, irritability, hot flashes, headaches, cramps, and depression are a few. Continuing to take estrogen hormones helps reduce these symptoms, but there are also many possible aids to be found through diet, lifestyle, nutritional supplements, and herbs. Vitamins E and A as well as the minerals calcium, magnesium, and zinc, plus the B vitamins may help. So-called female herbs such as black cohosh, red clover flower, and dong quai (angelica root) have been shown to reduce symptoms too.

After menopause, calcium needs and bone health are the greatest concern unless extra hormones are taken. (See "Pregnancy" on this page, "Lactation" on page 575, and "Menopause and Bone Health" on page 577 in this chapter for further discussions of these subjects.) **Natural, bioidentical hormones derived from plant sources are now available; these may be tolerated better and carry fewer risks.** Talk to your health-care practitioner about this as well as the latest saliva testing, which may more accurately assess hormone status. (See Appendix A, "Laboratories and Clinical Nutrition Tests.")

In my experience, most women do best on a low- to moderate-calorie diet that includes a good amount of protein and vegetables, some whole grains as well as nuts and seeds for good oils, and fairly few fruits and sweet foods. Milk products are tolerated by some people, but they can be weight-increasing foods, especially cheese. Some low- or nonfat milk and plain yogurt (goat's or cow's milk) seem to be the best utilized. Women also need to exercise and stay fit, especially if they are thinking about having babies or working at a high-stress job. A good exercise program maintains energy, vitality, and your figure better than TV and munchies.

Women need fewer calories than men, but only slightly less protein and the same amount or more of many of the essential nutrients. They need a more compact (a good nutrient-to-calorie ratio), nourishing diet of high-quality foods. **The requirements for most minerals are the same, but women need more iron, almost double men's level, until the menopause years, when the need drops back down to men's level.** Vegetarian women must focus more intently than others to get adequate iron in their diet, because the foods containing the most available iron are meats and liver. But iron can be obtained from many other foods and supplements, or by cooking in cast-iron cookware.

In general, women need a little less magnesium than men, but I find that many women actually require even more calcium and magnesium, especially when they exercise. The "Adult Women's Nutrient Program" on the opposite page lists the nutrients needed by the average active, healthy woman as insurance to maintain her health. The amounts shown range from the DRIs to optimum levels and include a combination of dietary intake and additional supplements. Such nutrients as protein, fats, vitamin K, chloride, fluoride, phosphorus, potassium, and sodium are not usually taken above dietary levels. Most others will be part of basic supplements. In the fats category, women should be particularly careful to get at least 3 grams of omega-3 fatty acids each day.

6. PREGNANCY

Nutrition during pregnancy is probably the most important aspect of this magical creation of life. Good nutrition before and during pregnancy can make the difference between health and sickness and support the general constitution of the child for life. The key word for pregnancy is *eat*—and that means to eat well, to eat highly nourishing foods, not to overeat or eat junky, high-calorie, empty-nutrient, or high-fat or salty foods. **The pregnant woman's body needs more of everything—calories, protein, calcium, iron, zinc, B vitamins, and most other vitamins and minerals, as well as rest and activity.**

The woman's pre-pregnancy condition is an important factor in a healthy pregnancy. The risk of nutrient depletions is greatly enhanced during pregnancy and nursing. To enter this demanding period with illness, bad habits, or any nutritional deficiency, such as anemia, may mean a troublesome pregnancy and years of recovery. So if you are thinking about having children, even vaguely considering the possibility, begin early to care for yourself. This applies to men as well. Nutritionally healthy men provide healthier, more functional sperm and probably healthier children. My advice to people planning a pregnancy is to prepare themselves by having a complete evaluation—physical, general biochemistry, diet and nutrient analyses—and then get on a good diet and supplement program. Getting off health-damaging habits (such as smoking, regular alcohol or caffeine use, and other drug use) is definitely a wise move.

In *Nutrition in Health and Disease*, Myron Winick, MD, calculates that it takes an estimated 75,000 calories to make a baby, or about 350 to 450 extra calories a day. The average woman needs 2,400 to 2,800 calories a day during pregnancy, and even more in the last trimester. This means about 20% to 25% more calories than usual. An extra few hundred calories can be consumed pretty easily, but if they come from sweets or other empty-calorie foods, they will not provide the extra nourishment needed. Wholesome foods are a necessity, and concentrated or nutrient-dense foods are crucial if a mother-to-be wants to get much of her requirements from food. Women need a higher nutrient-to-calorie ratio during pregnancy. The following topics are especially important regarding nutrient deficiency and a healthy pregnancy.

Protein. Besides more food and more calories, pregnant women need about 50% more protein than the 45 grams usually required; 70 to 85 (and sometimes even up to 100) grams of protein are needed daily during pregnancy. Some preliminary research, however, points out that too much protein intake during pregnancy can lead to some problems, such as larger babies and thus more difficult births and postmature babies. This area needs further study. During pregnancy, women need adequate good-quality protein within a balanced diet. This protein supports the tissue growth of both the fetus and the new tissues made by the mother. Common protein foods are meat, fish and poultry, eggs, and dairy foods. Nuts, seeds, grains, and legumes are also important.

The lacto-ovo vegetarian needs sufficient grains, legumes, seeds, nuts, eggs, and dairy foods. I do not suggest strict veganism during pregnancy. Although it can be done, it does not have the same degree of safety as eating a wider range of protein foods, let alone the

added calcium and iron needed. Even though vitamin B_{12} may be absorbed better by vegetarians than by meat-eaters because of their needs, it is not found in many vegetable foods. Traces may be found in such foods as kelp and other seaweeds as well as in some soybean products, particularly tempeh, miso, and soy sauce. However, the presence of B_{12} in these products depends entirely on the way they were produced, because vitamin B_{12} can only be made by microorganisms like bacteria and fungi; unless these microorganisms have been used in the fermentation or culturing process, B_{12} is not present in the food. This vitamin has disappeared from products all too often as companies have switched over from traditional practices to mass production, or have responded to governmental regulations requiring high-heat food "sanitation." In comparison with the above foods, however, seafood has much higher levels of vitamin B_{12}.

Calcium. I am concerned that the importance of calcium in a pregnant woman's diet may be overlooked in the future, because in 2000–2002, when the new DRIs were created for calcium and other minerals, the calcium requirement was revised and set at the same amount as during nonpregnancy. (For women age 18 and under, the requirement remained 1,300 mg per day, and for women 19 and older, 1,000 mg per day.) However, the fact that total calcium requirements may not be increased during pregnancy does not mean that the importance of sufficient calcium does not increase. If the mother is not obtaining sufficient calcium, her body will pull it from her bones to nourish the growing fetus. (In fact, for women with lifelong exposure to environmental toxins like lead, pulling too much calcium out of bone may also result in too many toxins being pulled out of bone and passed on to the fetus.) So it is important to get the 1,000 to 1,300 mg needed daily, and this amount may be difficult to obtain from the diet alone unless more dairy products and fish are eaten. Calcium helps form the baby's bones and teeth and aids muscle and heart function, blood clotting, and nerve transmission. Besides fish and milk products, calcium foods include nuts and seeds, leafy greens, sea vegetables, whole grains, and many vegetables. Meats contain some calcium, but their high phosphorus levels may interfere with calcium utilization.

Iron. This crucial nutrient is needed to help build blood cells in the mother and the fetus. A mother's blood volume has to increase by about 50% during her pregnancy. Iron also aids in disease resistance and elimination. For pregnant teenagers, the iron requirement practically doubles from 15 to 27 mg per day. For women 19 years and older, who already have a recommendation of 18 mg, the pregnancy requirement goes up by 50%, to 27 mg. It is not easy to get that much iron. Three cups of steamed chard, 1.5 ounces of pumpkin seeds, 3 cups of whole wheat pasta noodles, and 1.5 tablespoons of blackstrap molasses would do it, but these are some pretty carefully selected foods that may or may not fit with a mother's desires or appetite. Thirty ounces of steak would also do the trick, but this would be 1,750 to 3,000 calories and 50 to 100 grams of fat.

If the mother-to-be does not obtain enough iron from her diet, she will deplete her iron stores. With these reduced, her demands to make more blood cells will not be met, and anemia will occur, usually accompanied by fatigue and poor endurance. Thus almost all pregnant women take an iron supplement with their vitamin program. Using 2 or 3 iron tablets to spread out delivery of this nutrient over the course of the day can be helpful (and better tolerated) in comparison to a single large dose. Some women have trouble handling iron supplements; certain formulas may be handled more easily than others (see "Iron" on page 188 in chapter 6, Minerals). Good animal sources of iron include beef liver, red meats (beef, lamb, and pork), eggs, chicken, and salmon. Vegetable sources are seaweed, brewer's yeast, molasses, millet, prunes, raisins, mushrooms, chard, and spinach, as well as most nuts, seeds, and legumes.

Zinc. Women can be deficient in this important mineral during pregnancy. It is needed to aid normal development of the immune system in the fetus. Zinc is found in the same foods in which iron is found, with additional amounts in shellfish, especially oysters.

Folic acid. A crucial nutrient during pregnancy, folic acid is needed to help form red blood cells, to aid the growth and reproduction of other cells, and to support the development of the nervous system in the fetus. Folic acid also helps stimulate the mother's appetite. Deficiency of folic acid has led to congenital neurological defects in babies. **Needs are increased by 50% during pregnancy, to 600 mcg daily, and taking 800 to 1,000 mcg daily is wise because**

there is virtually no toxicity of folic acid. This vitamin is found in leafy green vegetables, whole grains, yeast, fish, dairy foods, and organ meats.

Other nutrients. Other nutrients are also needed at increased levels. The needs for vitamins A, C, E, and B6 all go up. **I do not suggest megadoses of vitamin C during pregnancy,** however, because the effects of this have not been clearly determined. In fact, a current controversy and debate is going on concerning vitamin C over a potential problem called *rebound scurvy,* which may occur with regular high usage of vitamin C. What happens in this situation, questioned by some clinicians as being a real phenomenon, is pretty simple. During pregnancy, the baby gets used to unnaturally high levels of vitamin C in his or her bloodstream, because this vitamin C is passed on from the mother. When the baby is born, the vitamin C level drops too far down unless the mother continues to take the same megadoses while breastfeeding her baby. By comparison with its life in the womb, the newborn baby feels deficient in vitamin C and develops some of the symptoms of scurvy, the vitamin C deficiency disease. Of course, this problem is easily remedied by having the mother breastfeed and gradually taper down her level of vitamin C supplementation. Not everyone agrees that this problem actually occurs, but it is a good reminder that pregnant women should not just megadose willy-nilly during this important time. That being said, however, I believe that regular intake of 50 to 100 mg of vitamin C several times daily will help utilize iron, calcium, magnesium, folic acid, zinc, and vitamin A.

Other minerals, such as iodine, magnesium, and sodium, are also needed in increased amounts. For years, obstetricians advised pregnant women to avoid sodium, but now they are suggesting that they use it as usual. For most women, some added salt is fine, and they can eat foods that naturally contain sodium, such as celery, beets, red meats, cheese, eggs, seaweeds, and seafood. The craving that some women have for pickles, olives, or sauerkraut may be related to a need for sodium. While more salt is needed to build the blood volume, there are limits, and very salty foods, such as potato chips and pretzels, should be avoided. **Excessive salt intake can lead to problems of water retention, elevated blood pressure, and further risks to the mother and baby.**

Another change that has been suggested in the field of obstetrics involves the healthy level of weight gain during pregnancy. As recently as the mid-1980s, doctors suggested that women limit their weight gain to 20 pounds, and even a limit of 10 to 15 pounds was sometimes suggested. Now the goal is more like 20 to 25 pounds, or about 20% of the mother's ideal weight. It has recently been shown that women who gain even 30 to 40 pounds, especially from good food, deliver larger and very healthy babies. The average weight gain is around 25 pounds, but 25 to 35 is fine. Most of the weight (13–20 pounds) is gained in the last trimester, about 8 to 12 pounds during the middle trimester, and only 3 to 4 pounds during the first 3 months.

As emphasized, the mother needs more of everything during pregnancy because she has to make a new being. And Mother Nature has provided the fetus with the mechanisms to get what it needs from the mother whether she has extra supplies or not. The baby can pull minerals, vitamins, and protein from the mother's bones, organs, tissues, and other storage areas. This can leave the mother depleted, however, a condition that can take a long time, even years, to correct. Besides making a new baby, these nutrients are needed to form the placenta, to increase the size of the uterus and breast tissue, and to create amniotic fluid. Mothers' blood volume increases by 25% to 50%, and more fluids, iron, B12, folic acid, zinc, copper, calcium, magnesium, and proteins are needed to support this new blood. Storage levels of most nutrients must be obtained from the diet as well.

So what is the best diet for a pregnant woman? First, she should eat a well-balanced diet containing all the food nutrients, with an increased amount of calories, usually about 350 to 450 more per day than usual. Weight-reduction programs during pregnancy are definitely taboo except for obesity concerns and should be done only with medical supervision. (The weight-loss support group Weight Watchers actually has a program for pregnant and nursing women.) There is much less worry about weight gain and sodium use now than there was years ago, as both factors may contribute to a healthy pregnancy and child when present in the right proportion. It is really the quality of the weight gain that is important—that is, the building of the necessary tissues rather than just adding fat, which can arise mostly from no-nutrient calories.

A wholesome diet is crucial to avoid wasted calories from junk foods and sugary snacks and to provide plenty of nutrient-rich foods to satisfy the increased needs for most of the vitamins, minerals, and protein. More dairy products, animal meats, whole grains, and vegetables are key. Nutrient-rich foods for pregnancy that also help guard against dietary deficiencies include eggs, fish, poultry, organ meats, milk products, red meats, whole grains, wheat germ, nuts and seeds, yeast, molasses, seaweeds, and leafy green vegetables. Some of these should be eaten daily. For a more specific food plan during pregnancy, see page 576.

A high-fiber diet with whole grains, fruits, and vegetables is important for good bowel function to avoid constipation, a common problem during pregnancy. At least 6 to 8 glasses of good drinking water should be consumed daily besides some milk and herbal teas. The top herbal choice is raspberry leaf tea, which is thought to tone up the uterus. **Herbal folklore claims that a cup of raspberry leaf tea drunk daily during pregnancy will assure a strong uterus and healthy labor.**

Exercise is important during pregnancy, as during all life stages. Keeping the body limber, loose, and toned is necessary to a healthy pregnancy. Do exercise; do not get lazy. It is important for good circulation and can help prevent constipation, varicose veins, and a flabby tummy. Regular stretching, movement classes, and even aerobic-type activities, such as indoor

---

Nutrient-Rich Foods That Will Help Guard against Dietary Deficiencies during Pregnancy

Eggs	Poultry
Fish	Red meats
Leafy green vegetables	Sea vegetables
Milk products	Wheat germ
Molasses	Whole grains
Nuts and seeds	Yeast
Organ meats*	

* Please only use organ meats from organically raised animals; these foods are really more like medicines and have higher concentrations of hormones and nutrients.

and outdoor bicycling, swimming, and hiking, will help maintain vitality. If you have not been exercising much before becoming pregnant, however, begin slowly with stretching and light activities. Avoid impact aerobics, jumping rope, and horseback riding, but keep moving. Regular, quiet internal "exercises," such as meditation and visualizations, are also important to prepare for all the bodily changes, emotional shifts, and a smooth labor and healthy baby. Breathing practice, walking, and warm baths are all a good foundation.

It is particularly important during pregnancy to avoid drugs of all kinds. Caffeine and alcohol should be minimized to occasional use only and are better avoided completely. Nicotine use is best eliminated, as it is associated with many problems in pregnancy, birth, and the health of the infant as well as the mother. It is also wise to avoid chemicals of all kinds—in foods, at work, and in the home. Many chemicals pass through the placenta to the baby. Although the placenta protects the baby from many harmful substances, there are very few that it blocks completely. Pesticides or metals can become concentrated in the fetus. Sugar substitutes such as aspartame and saccharin as well as artificial flavors, food dyes, and nitrites should all be eliminated from the diet. Nitrosamines formed from nitrates and nitrites (found in hot dogs, bacon, and lunch meats) have been shown in animal studies to produce cancer in the offspring. Good levels of vitamin C in the body can help prevent nitrosamine formation.

Any pharmaceutical drug use should be carefully monitored by the doctor or midwife. All drugs would be best avoided if possible. Many drugs may interact with body nutrients and increase the risk of deficiency. Pregnant women need to be careful to avoid drug and chemical exposure, because it is more difficult with all the body demands to keep up with healthy detoxification during pregnancy. The body is in a building-up, gathering state and will utilize most everything that comes into it or store it away for later use.

Nutritional changes and support may help remedy some of the common problems of pregnancy. Morning sickness with nausea and vomiting is especially common during the first few months. This problem is likely a result of biliary or liver activity. During

---

The Pregnancy Shake

Blend together
- $1/2$–1 cup apple juice
- 1–2 tsp blackstrap molasses
- 1 banana
- 1–2 tsp nutritional yeast
- $1/2$–1 cup yogurt
- 1 tbsp wheat germ or fresh-ground flaxseeds
- 1–2 tbsp honey or pure maple syrup
- $1/2$–1 cup low-fat milk
- $1/3$ tsp powdered kelp

This shake can be adapted to the pregnant woman's special desires and the flavors she can tolerate. If something in the drink does not appeal, avoid it and try something else. Other fruits or juices can be used, or no juice and just milk (cow's, goat's, almond, or rice milk), a banana, or another fruit as a base. Adding water will dilute the shake, which some women tolerate better. Such flavorings as vanilla or almond or a handful of raw almonds, coconut, or sunflower seeds can be added and blended. There are also some organic brown rice and soy protein powders now on the market that work nicely in the blender and can provide an incomplete but substantial protein boost to blenderized morning shakes. Regarding food combining, when different foods are blended together as a drink, they often seem to be better tolerated. However, if the pregnant woman does not handle this mixture well, simplify the drink and just use a banana, yogurt, and milk or water, along with some yeast or wheat germ or flaxseed and a little sweetener. Overall, the Pregnancy Shake can be very tasty and nourishing.

---

the night, the liver works to eliminate toxins, which are thus in the system on awakening. **A good diet and avoidance of fatty foods, alcohol, and other liver-irritating drugs before pregnancy is helpful in minimizing morning sickness.** Vitamin B6 aids liver metabolism. The active metabolic form is the pyridoxine precursor, pyridoxal-5-phosphate (P5P), because it enters directly into the functioning metabolic cycle. Usually, supplementing 25 to 50 mg of B6 3 times daily

Nutrient Program during Pregnancy (Minimum to Possible Optimum Safe Levels)

AGE: ALL PREGNANT WOMEN

Nutrient	Amount	Nutrient	Amount
Calories*	2,500–3,200	Chromium	50–400 mcg
Fiber	25–45 g	Copper	2–3 mg
Protein*	75–90 g	Fluoride+	1.5–3.5 mg
Vitamin A*	6,000–10,000 IU	Iodine*+	290–350 mcg
Beta-carotene	10,000–15,000 IU	Iron*#	30–50 mg
Vitamin D	400–600 IU	Magnesium*	450–1,000 mg
Vitamin E*	50–400 IU	Manganese	2.5–15.0 mg
Vitamin K	100–400 mcg	Molybdenum	150–250 mcg
Thiamin (B1)	1.5–50.0 mg	Phosphorus*+	1,200–1,600 mg
Riboflavin (B2)	1.5–30.0 mg	Potassium+	2–5 g
Niacin (B3)	16–100 mg	Selenium	150–300 mcg
Pantothenic acid (B5)	7–250 mg	Sodium*+	2.5–4.0 g
Pyridoxine (B6)	2.6–100.0 mg	Zinc*	20–40 mg
Cobalamin (B12)	4–200 mcg	Essential fatty acids**	2–3 tsp
Folic acid*	800–1,200 mcg		
Biotin	200–500 mcg		
Choline	450–500 mg		
Inositol	50–250 mg		
PABA	10–50 mg		
Vitamin C*++	80–1,000 mg		
Bioflavonoids	100–250 mg		
Calcium*	1,200–1,600 mg		
Chloride+	2–4 g		

* Requirements for these nutrients are increased during pregnancy.

+These nutrients are required for health but are not usually taken as additional supplements.

\# Iron intakes include diet plus additional supplementation of 30 mg to 50 mg daily.

++ More vitamin C can be used for short periods for colds, flu, and so on.

** Fatty acids come from olive oil, flaxseed oil, or other nutritious cold-pressed vegetable oils.

will help reduce the symptoms of morning sickness. Occasionally, higher amounts are needed. If these higher levels are used, it is wise to continue smaller amounts for a while to prevent pyridoxine withdrawal in the mother or the baby; higher dosages, however, are usually not required all the way up to delivery time, because intestinal symptoms decrease after the first few months. Other supplements helpful in alleviating morning sickness include vitamins B12, C, and E as well as extra magnesium and potassium. On occasion, I have seen vitamin injections provide much-needed relief for problems associated with morning sickness. Herbs are often helpful as well. Raspberry leaf, peppermint, or ginger root teas have been effective for some women.

Dietary changes are usually the best way to handle morning sickness, however. A reduction of fatty food intake and an increase in carbohydrates may be helpful. A higher fiber intake keeps the intestines moving, which helps elimination and detoxification. Acidic foods, such as citrus fruits or juice, and iron supplements or milk may increase nausea and vomiting. Small, frequent meals and snacks of carbohydrate or protein can be best tolerated. Munching on a few soda crackers or dry toast upon awakening may help alleviate early morning nausea. Some women feel it makes a difference when these crackers are eaten before even sitting up in the bed. Don't worry, this too shall pass. Breathing and relaxing can help.

Pregnant women and their husbands and families need to be understanding and adaptable during this period, especially regarding diet. Food cravings can be wild, food consumption goes up, and sometimes a woman's whole life becomes centered around food.

These can be obstacles. The digestive tract is more sensitive, and as the pregnancy progresses, the size of the stomach shrinks because of the growing womb. Often food intolerances or many new likes and dislikes develop. To adapt, the diet may shift to frequent small and simple but nourishing meals. Nutritious liquid meals are a good choice. From protein powders to fruit or vegetable smoothies, these drinks can be packed with nutrients. One possibility for building and nourishing mother and baby is the Pregnancy Shake on page 573, an adaptation of the "Pregnancy Cocktail" described by Fred Rohè in *The Complete Book of Natural Foods.*

Later in pregnancy, when labor is just beginning, take some extra calcium and magnesium to help reduce the pain of contractions and muscle aches and spasms. About 1,500 to 2,000 mg of each has been helpful to some women. This can be repeated later if labor is extended. If a caesarean section is going to be done, it is wise to take extra tissue-healing nutrients (vitamins A and C as well as the mineral zinc) before and after the procedure, for several days to several weeks if possible. (See "Pre- and Post-Surgery" on page 724 in chapter 17, Medical Treatment Programs.) As for regular supplements during pregnancy, usually a high-potency multiple or special prenatal formula with plenty of iron should be taken. If nausea occurs with the supplement, try to take it later in the day and with meals. The "Nutrient Program during Pregnancy" on the opposite page gives the ranges for nutrient intakes that I consider to be minimal to optimal during pregnancy.

For special problems, such as anemia, more iron may be needed. Consult your doctor or midwife. Of course, not all of these nutrients will be used as supplements. Many of them, such as sodium, chloride, fluoride, and potassium, are obtained from the diet. However, depending on the dietary intake of various nutrients, such as calcium, zinc, or B vitamins, or individual blood measurements, any specific nutrient can be further increased by supplement use to give the necessary intake. (Note: more specifics of the pregnancy diet are discussed in the next section, "Lactation.")

7. LACTATION

Breastfeeding is an important follow-through to the pregnancy and birth process and the best way to nourish the new infant. It is also helpful for the mother to balance her pregnancy. Nursing not only is a calorie and fluid outlet, helping the mother to reattain her pre-pregnancy weight, it is often vital to her emotional and psychological well-being and to the bonding with the new baby. In addition, the hormone released during breastfeeding, oxytocin, helps contract the uterus back to normal size and health.

Nutritional requirements are much the same as during pregnancy, with even higher requirements for many nutrients and reduced needs for a few. After all, the mother is feeding a growing baby. An infant requires about 2 to 3 ounces of milk per pound of weight, so a newborn of 7 pounds needs about 18 ounces of milk daily; as he or she grows, more milk is required. Each ounce of milk has about 20 calories, so the mother is giving out 300 to 400 calories a day initially, more as the baby grows. The extra calories needed for pregnancy do not drop off during lactation. Some mothers consume fewer calories after birth in order to lose weight, but this is not wise. **Too great a reduction in calories can diminish milk production, as can resuming cigarette smoking or not drinking enough fluids.** The nursing mother should naturally lose weight during breastfeeding, and as she reduces her level of nursing, she may also lessen her calorie intake.

Water is the main ingredient of mother's milk, so adequate fluid intake is essential. At least 3 quarts of liquid are recommended daily, including water, juices, and milk. The nursing mother's diet should be high in nutrients, mainly from eating good, wholesome foods. High protein levels are still required, although a little less is needed than during pregnancy; calcium, magnesium, and iron requirements are also similar. Vitamins C and A, zinc, and iodine are needed in higher (but not megadose) levels. Folic acid requirements decrease by 25% as the mother's blood volume decreases. Extra B vitamins may be helpful (for stress and fatigue related to sleep deprivation), as breast milk is fairly low in them, but high-dosage B vitamin pills are best avoided during lactation. Specifically, high amounts of vitamin B6 can reduce milk production.

General Pregnancy Nutritional Plan

(SERVINGS PER DAY)

	Nonpregnant	Pregnant	Nursing
Milk foods—low-fat milk (avoid skim), cheese, yogurt, butter (1 serving = 1 cup milk or yogurt, or 3–4 oz. cheese)	2	3–4	5–6
Cereal grains (1 serving = about 1 cup grain or 1 slice of bread)	3	4–5	5
Vegetables—raw yellow or dark green (1 serving = 1 cup)	1	2	2
Other vegetables (1 cup)	1	2	2
Vitamin C foods—citrus, berries, peppers, tomato (1 serving = 1 cup)	1	2	2
Eggs (1 serving = 1 egg)	1	1–2	1–2
Meats—fish, poultry, or lean red (1 serving = 3–4 oz.)	1	1–2	2–3
Legumes (1 serving = 6 oz.)	1	1–2	1–2

Nutrient Program for Nursing Mothers (Minimum to Possible Optimum Safe Levels)

AGE: ALL LACTATING WOMEN

Nutrient	Amount	Nutrient	Amount
Calories*	2,500–3,200	Bioflavonoids	125–250 mg
Fiber	25–45 g	Calcium*	1,200–1,600 mg
Protein*	65–90 g	Chloride+	2–4 g
Vitamin A*	7,000–10,000 IU	Chromium	50–400 mcg
Beta-carotene	5,000–15,000 IU	Copper	2–3 mg
Vitamin D	400–600 IU	Fluoride+	1.5–3.5 mg
Vitamin E*	60–400 IU	Iodine*	290–400 mcg
Vitamin K	100–400 mcg	Iron*	30–50 mg
Thiamin (B1)	1.6–25.0 mg	Magnesium*	450–1,000 mg
Riboflavin (B2)	1.7–25.0 mg	Manganese	2.5–15 mg
Niacin (B3)	18–100 mg	Molybdenum	150–250 mcg
Pantothenic acid (B5)	7–250 mg	Phosphorus*+	1,200–1,600 mg
Pyridoxine (B6)	2.5–100 mg	Potassium+	2–5 g
Cobalamin (B12)	4–200 mcg	Selenium	150–300 mcg
Folic acid*	600–1,000 mcg	Sodium+	2.5–4.0 g
Biotin	200–500 mcg	Zinc*	25–40 mg
Choline	100–250 mg		
Inositol	100–250 mg		
PABA	25–100 mg		
Vitamin C*	120–2,000 mg		

*These nutrients are needed in higher than usual amounts during lactation.

+These nutrients are required in the diet, although they are not usually supplemented.

Good nourishment is essential to prevent depletion in the mother and to provide the right nutrients for the baby. Remember, the food that the nursing mother eats provides the nutrients in her milk and thus the infant's nutrition. Many of the nutrient-rich foods suggested for pregnancy should be consumed—dairy products, eggs, fish, other animal foods, whole grains, vegetables (especially leafy greens), and vitamin C fruits. Standard food-group orientation suggests more portions of most everything. The summary of food group needs for nonpregnant, pregnant, and nursing women in the "General Pregnancy Nutritional Plan" on the opposite page is adapted from *Mowry's Basic Nutrition and Diet Therapy,* by Sue Rodwell Williams.

For vegetarian women, it is wise to eat the recommended amount of the dairy products and eggs to meet protein and calcium needs, as well as to eat more whole grains and legumes. If milk consumption is minimized, more tofu, legumes, nuts and seeds, and leafy greens and a calcium supplement are recommended. More care in balancing the diet is usually necessary whenever the diet limits specific food groups. Additional protein powder or supplemental amino acids (free form), as powder or capsules (750–1,500 mg daily) may be useful if the protein intake is not sufficient.

For healthy breastfeeding, mother's comfort is important. To maintain good milk production, use both breasts regularly and relax before and after nursing. Remember, good fluid and nutrient intake is essential for successful nursing and thus for the growth and development of the baby. Many women tell me that using olive or coconut oil on their nipples keeps their skin healthier and aids nursing. (See "Infants and Toddlers" on page 557 of this chapter for further discussion on nursing.)

The "Nutrient Program for Nursing Mothers" on the opposite page gives values for what I consider to be the minimal-to-optimal requirements for nursing mothers. Refer to the table on page 574 under "Pregnancy" for comparison with the nutrient needs listed here. The program for nursing mothers refers to the combined intake of diet and nutritional supplements. Chloride, fluoride, phosphorus, potassium, and sodium are not usually supplemented unless shown by testing to be needed.

8. MENOPAUSE AND BONE HEALTH

Menopause represents a major transition in the lives of most women, thus it is often called the "change of life." Women experience a decreased production of sex hormones by the ovaries, and many times there are symptoms representative of estrogen deficiency and withdrawal. Men may also experience some "change of life," consisting of physiological and hormonal as well as social changes, but usually this is fairly mild compared with what women experience.

Most women enter menopause between the ages of 45 and 50, but it may occur anywhere between 40 and 55. (There may in fact be a trend for women to begin experiencing these events even earlier, in some cases as early as 35 to 40 years old, and the term *premature ovarian syndrome* is now being used to describe some aspects of this situation.) Those whose ovaries are surgically removed before they have entered menopause will almost immediately experience menopausal symptoms and often are placed on estrogen alone or hormone replacement therapy (HRT), using estrogen and progesterone, to simulate their natural cycle.

Although estrogen therapy or HRT is helpful to most women, there are potential risks and side effects, so many women eventually go off synthetic hormones and shift to a more natural program (or switch to bioidentical hormone therapy). **Natural, bioidentical hormones that are exactly the same as what the body has always produced are now available and are typically used by health practitioners who wish for safer, yet effective programs.** These hormones can be tried to see their effectiveness with less risk of side effects and cancer. This approach usually uses low levels of a variety of hormones, such as estriol and estradiol, progesterone, and testosterone (yes, women need testosterone, too), and also evaluates and balances thyroid and adrenal functions using DHEA (dehydroepiandrosterone) and natural hydrocortisone for the latter. If you are interested in this approach, you will need to see a physician who is knowledgeable in testing and using appropriate bioidentical hormone therapy. In this program, I will focus on what you can do yourself. This discussion is therefore oriented toward a natural program of diet, nutritional supplements, and herbs to minimize menopausal symptoms and enhance vitality.

The symptoms of menopause include a change in the frequency or volume of blood flow of the periods (or actual cessation of menstrual periods), irritability, hot flashes and night sweats, emotional swings, headaches, depression, insomnia, loss of sex drive, and weight changes. Vaginal dryness and a weakening of the vaginal area tissues may also occur. More-internal metabolic shifts, such as bone loss, may also occur. There are many factors that influence the intensity of symptoms and probably even the time they appear. A poor diet, emotional stress, and lack of exercise may lead to an increase in symptoms, particularly when these lifestyle habits have been going on for years. Women who become aware of these relationships before menopause and change their habits to help build themselves up with diet and supplements and deal with their stressful issues most assuredly have an easier time. Not all women have a difficult menopause; some may not even experience symptoms at all, just a loss of their periods.

A good diet along with supportive nutritional supplements and stress management may help to delay the onset of menopause and reduce symptoms when they do occur. Of other positive lifestyle habits, regular exercise is the most important. It strengthens the bones and improves calcium metabolism. It may also help mobilize some stored estrogen from the fatty tissues, which may make for an easier transition. Outdoor exercise, such as walking, bicycling, swimming, golf, or tennis, adds sunlight and thus aids the body's vitamin D production, which improves calcium utilization.

During menopause, it is also wise for women to get adequate sleep and even take naps if they feel tired. Menopause can often be a time of lowered energy. Stress reduction and dealing with the concerns and worries about aging are important. Embracing maturity and wisdom adds a positive attitude and supports this process. Drinking plenty of water helps keep the body vital and young, with the internal processes functioning best, as does the intake of essential fatty acids while avoiding excess saturated and hydrogenated fats and chemical toxins.

A diet that contains vital and wholesome foods supports a stronger life force and the ability to better handle changes. As I have emphasized throughout this book, the optimal diet includes fresh fruits and vegetables, whole grains, nuts, seeds, and legumes; with fish, poultry, eggs, milk products, and cold-pressed oils used in moderation and sugar, refined-flour products, other refined and processed foods, cured meats, fried foods, and chemicals avoided whenever possible.

A diet with good quantity and quality of protein and one high in B complex foods may help delay the onset of menopause by supporting the pituitary gland, which regulates the ovaries and the female cycle. (It appears that vegan women and those with low cholesterol levels have an earlier menopause than more omnivorous women; further research in this area may help us to understand more about diet, cholesterol, and menopause.) Some of the protein foods suggested are fish, such milk products as yogurt and cottage cheese, eggs, whole grains and legumes, nuts, and seeds (ideally raw, organic nuts and seeds). Foods high in B vitamins are green vegetables, whole grains, wheat germ, and yeast. Good levels of pantothenic acid, choline, and inositol also aid the adrenal and pituitary functions. Special foods that offer high amounts of vitamins, minerals, and energy include brewer's yeast, molasses, lecithin, and kelp or other seaweeds, which are a rich source of minerals, especially calcium. These can be used with milk or juice to make a high-nutrient drink.

Osteoporosis is a loss of bone minerals, density, and bone strength, particularly of the spine and long bones of the arms and legs; it is a common problem of menopausal women and difficult to diagnose. Regular X-rays are not that sensitive, and they reveal bone loss only after it is fairly significant. The newer techniques available to measure bone density, such as dual photon absorptiometry, are more sensitive at assessing early osteoporosis. These are most valuable as a reference to see whether bones are losing minerals (matrix) over the years. Serial measurements are most helpful. There are no easy ways to observe early warning signs; therefore it is important through life, even starting as children, to prevent the risk of osteoporosis with a good diet and exercise. Some scientists believe that osteoporosis is a "pediatric disease," as we first build our bone strength as children. Women should also be aware of observable warning signs, such as periodontal disease, loss of height, or changes in the curvature of the spinal column, such as a so-called dowager's hump. The most important factor is preventing the loss of bone matrix; this is much easier than correcting bone loss after it occurs. A good diet and regular exercise, including muscle building with weights, is most helpful.

There are other components to maintaining healthy bones, including adequate intake of the minerals magnesium, manganese, phosphorus, strontium, and silicon. Also, vitamin D levels are more deficient around the time of menopause than previously thought, and researchers know that vitamin D helps the absorption and utilization of calcium. Getting adequate sun exposure, at least 15 to 20 minutes daily (without sunscreen) is important for adequate production of vitamin D. Furthermore, two other nutrients help in bone health. These are vitamin K and boron, which aid the incorporation of calcium into bones. Ipriflavone, a bioflavonoid that is being studied as well as utilized as a supplement, may help in bone building. The hormone testosterone may also support bone health, and testosterone deficiency in women may contribute to osteopenia (an earlier stage of bone loss) and osteoporosis. Speak with your health-care practitioner about these areas for appropriate testing and treatment.

To prevent osteoporosis, it is wise to eat a good diet and maintain an adequate calcium intake through foods and supplements in the years before menopause. Many people eat a diet that is much higher in phosphorus than in calcium. This can lead to improper bone metabolism and loss of bone calcium. Meats, nuts, seeds, poultry, boneless seafood, and even whole grains have a higher phosphorus than calcium content. Soda pops have added phosphates, increasing their phosphorus level. One advantage of using milk products is that they have a good calcium-to-phosphorus ratio, with actually slightly more calcium. Eggs and many vegetables, especially the green leafy veggies, also have lower phosphorus content. **It helps to squeeze a little lemon or vinegar, like apple cider or balsamic, over the greens because calcium is best absorbed in an acid medium.**

Premenopausal women should regularly consume at least 1,200 to 1,500 mg of calcium a day from food and supplements. Supplementing some calcium without phosphorus usually balances out these nutrients. Adding about 250 to 500 IU of extra vitamin D (in supplement form) and about 300 to 450 mg of supplemental magnesium a day helps the calcium be best utilized and protects against osteoporosis. Adequate boron, a

trace mineral, may also be deficient in the diet, and supplementing at the 2 to 3 mg level may help with calcium utilization. A diet containing good amounts of fish, leafy greens, whole grains, and dairy foods supports healthy bones. Phosphorus, zinc, copper, and manganese are also important to building strong bones. **If osteoporosis is present, research suggests that estrogen therapy may help slow its progress and even improve the bone health, although it also poses risks.** (See the discussion above on bioidentical hormones.) Fluoride, 2 to 4 mg per day in foods or even taken as a supplement, has been shown to strengthen bones, but it may present other concerns, including attention-deficit disorder in children, and in adults, fertility problems and potentially increased risk of cancer. While there is no definitive research in this area, there are definitely unanswered questions that give rise to concern. **In general, I do not recommend fluoride supplementation for anyone regularly consuming fluoridated tap water (which I also do not recommend), especially in adults.** See chapter 6, Minerals, page 218 for a detailed discussion of fluoride. Also see page 264 in chapter 7, Special Supplements, for a discussion of ipriflavone, a bioflavonoid that supports bone metabolism and strength.

When estrogen is used during or after menopause, it is wise to follow a program similar to that suggested for users of birth control pills. If the woman still has a uterus, a progesterone agent should also be used to simulate the natural cycle and to protect the uterus from increased cancer risk. Extra vitamins C, E, and B_6, extra zinc, and minimum copper intake are the main suggestions. **It is clear that appropriate estrogen or HRT does prevent osteoporosis, possibly better than any other program, especially with a good diet, adequate calcium intake, and plenty of exercise.** Again, speak with your practitioner to see about natural, bioidentical hormone support. Regular exercise has clearly been shown to minimize bone loss, especially postmenopausally. Weight-bearing exercises, such as walking, tennis, or golf, help to strengthen the bones, probably more than swimming. When taking estrogen, usually less calcium is needed than when no hormones are used. Still, a natural program will help prevent osteoporosis and ease the symptoms and transition of menopause. (For more on osteoporosis, see "Calcium" on page 154 in chapter 6, Minerals.)

Younger women can also develop osteoporosis, usually because of a poor diet, low calcium intake, and excessive vigorous exercise. Dancers, gymnasts, and long-distance runners have this problem most commonly, and it is exaggerated with anorexia and weight loss. These young women often have associated low body fat, low estrogen levels, and irregular or non-existent menstrual periods. A more nourishing diet, reduced activity, and calcium-vitamin-mineral supplements can help to correct this problem and prevent future ones.

For menopausal hot flashes, irritability, and night sweats, supplemental calcium and vitamins D and E often help. Certain herbs that work are the cohosh herbs, unicorn root, and licorice root. The popular black cohosh product Remifemin has given relief to many women in menopause. Red clover flowers are made into an extract (one such product is Promensil)

that can be helpful with menopausal symptoms. Motherwort is another helpful herb for hot flashes. The female formulas described in "Premenstrual Syndrome" on page 719 of chapter 17, Medical Treatment Programs, may also be helpful in menopause, as they seem to support estrogen production by stimulating the female organs.

Dong quai has also benefited many women with those symptoms. Research suggests dong quai may work best in combination formulas. Two capsules taken 2 or 3 times daily is the standard usage in this regard. Ginseng has also been helpful, especially when there is associated fatigue. Sarsaparilla root has been used as a so-called female herb, and valerian root can be used for insomnia and irritability. The amino acid L-tryptophan can be useful for aiding sleep and lessening depression and food cravings, as well as providing some relief for hot flashes. Calcium and magnesium

Menopause Nutrient Program

AGE: MENOPAUSE

Nutrient	Amount	Nutrient	Amount
Protein	45–80 g	Iodine*	150–300 mcg
Vitamin A	3,000–5,000–IU	Iron	10–18 mg
Beta-carotene	15,000–20,000 IU	Magnesium+	600–1,000 mg
Vitamin D	400–1,000 IU	Manganese	2.5–15,0 mg
Vitamin E	800–1,000 IU	Molybdenum	150–500 mcg
Vitamin K*	150–400 mcg	Phosphorus*	800–1,000 mg
Thiamin (B1)	50–100 mg	Potassium	3–5 g
Riboflavin (B2)	25–50 mg	Selenium	100–300 mcg
Niacinamide (B3)	50–100 mg	Zinc	15–30 mg
Pantothenic acid (B5)	100–750 mg		
Pyridoxine (B6)	50–100 mg	**Optional**	
Cobalamin (B12)	30–100 mcg	Lecithin	500–1,000 mg
Folic acid	400–800 mcg	Primrose oil	1,000–2,000 mg
Biotin	50–500 mcg	or other GLA-	1,000–2,000 mg or
Choline	500–1,000 mg	containing oil	4–6 capsules
Inositol	500–1,000 mg	Hydrochloric acid	1 or 2 tablets
PABA	200–400 mg	(with meals)	
Vitamin C	1–3 g	Digestive enzymes	1 or 2 tablets
Bioflavonoids	250–500 mg	(after meals)	
Boron	2–3 mg		
Calcium+	1,000–1,500 mg		
Chromium	150–400 mcg	*These are not usually be supplemented in the diet.	
Copper	1–2 mg	+The dietary levels of calcium and magnesium should also be considered in these totals.	

are helpful for muscle and back pains or cramps. Kelp tablets have been used to support thyroid function, which helps women through the changes of menopause. Iron is still needed in premenopausal amounts until there is no more bleeding; then the iron requirements decrease from 18 to 8 mg per day.

The "Menopause Nutrient Program" on the opposite page includes dietary plus supplemental needs. Such nutrients as chloride, phosphorus, fluoride, sodium, and potassium are usually not supplemented but obtained from diet. The ranges allow for individual comfort in using the higher amounts, which may be best for this program. (See "The Later Years," below for further information. The "Antiaging" and "Antistress" programs detailed on pages 588 and 597, respectively, in chapter 16, Performance Enhancement Programs, may also provide assistance to the menopausal woman.)

9. THE LATER YEARS (65, 70, AND OLDER)

This program is designed primarily for people over 65, an age group that continues to increase in numbers in U.S. society. In 1990, there were 31 million people over 65; in 2000, there were 35 million—a 12% increase in just 10 years. In fact, it is estimated that by the year 2010, another 10 million adults will jump into this age group, so that 15.8% of the total U.S. population will be 65 years or older. We need to care for ourselves in our younger years so that we can stay healthy in our older ones. Also, our society needs to learn to better care for our elders and to incorporate them into a meaningful life to keep them feeling useful and youthful.

Being old or aging is as much a state of mind involving how we live and our attitude toward life as it is a physical condition. Of course, genetics are also important. Some people become old in their 50s and 60s, while others only really start to age (or degenerate) 1 or 2 years before they die in their 80s or 90s. Even some young people are old psychologically. They are limited and resist change and lose the positive energy and love of life. Youth, like age, is really a state of mind.

With regard to nutritional status, elderly people are sometimes even more difficult to nourish than teen-agers. Many are resentful or rebellious and eat an unbalanced diet consisting of a limited number of foods. Malnutrition is fairly common in the elderly, with low calorie and protein intakes, as well as many deficiencies of important vitamins and minerals. Many elders eat less because of such reasons as apathy, diminished sense of taste and smell, poor teeth, low income, or inability to obtain or prepare foods. They typically have reduced digestion and absorption, which makes their intake needs even higher than usual. The government DRIs become relatively meaningless for the elderly—they simply need more nutrients!

Many old-age problems—such as insomnia, anorexia, fatigue, depression, diminishing eyesight and hearing, fragile bones, and fractures—are a result of poor diet and nutritional deficiencies. This can also lead to a weakened immune system and more infections. The thymus gland, which produces the important T lymphocytes that mediate the cellular immune system and help to regulate antibody formation, tends to diminish in activity with aging—especially in those who have a low-vitality diet, who are living under stress, and who are suffering possible emotional factors, such as loss of friends and relatives, anxieties of aging and loneliness, and depression. All of this can lead to problems of weakened resistance, infections, and sometimes cancer. Tissue weakness because of the lack of cellular support can lead to decreased skin protection and increased aging of the skin. Free-radical formation and a reduction of neurotransmitter chemicals, such as acetylcholine, gamma-aminobutyric acid (GABA), glycine, L-glutamine, norepinephrine, and serotonin (caused by deficiencies of amino acids and the B vitamins, including inositol and choline) all may contribute to aging, internally and externally, mentally and physically. (This is discussed further in "Antiaging" on page 588, in chapter 16, Performance Enhancement Programs.)

Most elderly people have reduced production of gastric hydrochloric acid, which minimizes the breakdown of complex carbohydrates, fats, and proteins. The general function of the other digestive organs, such as the pancreas, which produces digestive enzymes, is also reduced. Often the digestive lining does not function as it once did, and the absorption of nutrients, particularly minerals, decreases.

Many elderly people simply do not obtain enough calories. Calorie count can be easily increased with more food, but it is important that it be more nutrient-rich food, so that the important vitamins and minerals are also provided. Less protein may be needed for tissue production, but because of poorer assimilation, as much protein as usual is needed. Amino acid intake is necessary to build cells, for energy, and for tissue repair.

Fiber, in foods and as a supplement, is important to colon health and function, and thus reduces the common problem of diverticulosis, little outpockets from pressure and weakness in the colon wall. It also reduces the incidence of colon cancer and possibly other types of cancer, as well as pulling some chemical toxins from the body. Eating more natural fiber foods, such as vegetables and whole grains, offers many other benefits as well. Extra bran (insoluble fiber) or psyllium (soluble fiber) will help bowel function when natural fiber foods are not eaten in sufficient quantities. Constipation, a common problem in the elderly, can be reduced and eliminated with adequate fiber and water. Fluid intake by older people may be low. **Drinking enough clean water is crucial to good internal organ function for clearing impurities and for waste elimination.** It also keeps the skin healthier and prevents dehydration, which may lead to all kinds of problems.

A number of common vitamin and mineral deficiencies occur in the elderly, mainly from not consuming enough fresh, nutrient-rich foods. Vitamin A is commonly low, and this can lead to poor vision, dry skin, and weakened immunity. Thiamin (B1) and riboflavin (B2) may not be adequate in the diet because of low intake of whole grains, and this may affect the skin and energy level. Pyridoxine (B6) is often low, especially with avoidance of whole foods and with eating refined-flour products. Folic acid may be deficient because of avoidance of leafy greens, and vitamin B12 may be inadequate because of both low intake and poor absorption (mainly from low stomach acid). Folic acid and vitamin B12 are important for building blood cells and for energy. Supplemental B12, even through injections, is often helpful for enhancing energy levels in the elderly. Research has shown that the need for additional B vitamins is often overlooked in seniors. Those who care for the elderly should consider supplementing them, perhaps as a routine practice. Vitamin C intake may also be inadequate because of avoidance of citrus fruits and fresh, raw vegetables; this deficiency may lead to poor tissue health, healing abilities, and disease resistance.

Deficiencies of minerals and hydrochloric acid (HCl)—needed for adequate absorption of most minerals, such as iron, calcium, and zinc—are very common among the elderly. This inadequacy of digestion by limited production of HCl (and digestive enzymes) may in fact be among the most common health factors affecting the elderly, although it may be less obvious than some more-externalized problems. Vitamin B12 absorption may be low because of weak intrinsic factor, which is produced by the stomach in the same parietal cells that produce HCl.

Calcium intake is one of the biggest concerns. Calcium deficiency is more common in women than in men. Low-calcium foods, lack of exercise, low hydrochloric acid, and poor digestion lessen calcium availability. Antacids, especially those containing aluminum, are best avoided because of their interference with calcium absorption and the possibility of aluminum toxicity, which has been implicated in Alzheimer's disease and other types of senility. Avoiding both aluminum cookware and the storage or heating of foods in aluminum foil are also good ideas. Imbalances among calcium, phosphorus, and magnesium and possibly low levels of vitamin D also affect calcium bone metabolism.

Magnesium, present in whole grains, nuts, and seeds, may be low in the typical diet of the elderly. Phosphorus intake is often normal or elevated, and excess phosphorus may allow even more bone loss

Common Deficiencies in the Elderly

Calcium	Potassium	Water
Calories	Protein	Chewing
Chromium	Vitamin A	Enzymes
Copper	Vitamin B1	Hydrochloric
Fiber	Vitamin B2	acid
Fluids	Vitamin B6	Touch
Folic acid	Vitamin B12	Love
Iron	Vitamin C	Massage
Magnesium	Zinc	

when calcium is deficient. Occasionally, older people with arthritis avoid calcium with the support of their doctors. There is no reason for that, however. With arthritis, calcium is being lost from the bones and may precipitate in the joints, but this is a result of the mineral imbalance. Calcium is needed in balance with phosphorus, magnesium, boron, and vitamin D. (See more about bone health in the previous section, "Menopause and Bone Health," on page 577.)

Decreased absorption and limitations in the diet may affect the levels of most of the minerals as well. Iron may be low, but fortunately there is less need for it in the elderly. If anemia is present, check for iron levels as well as B12, folic acid, copper, and protein. Such iron-rich foods as red meats, even liver, may be used occasionally for their good protein and other nutrient contents. Copper, important to many energy and enzyme systems, can be obtained from whole grains, nuts, seeds, and many vegetables, and is found in high levels in oysters. Zinc, which is necessary for immune function, acid-base balance, tissue healing, and the prevention of premature aging, is also often inadequate in the diet. Low immune function because of zinc deficiency is frequently a factor in infections, cancer, and cardiovascular problems. Zinc is present in many of the same foods as copper, including oysters and most nuts.

One of the most commonly deficient minerals is chromium, which can be sparse in the soil and foods, and is often poorly absorbed. Chromium is important to the proper use of blood sugar, working along with glucose tolerance factor (GTF) to support the function of insulin. Supplemental chromium is often helpful, and brewer's yeast, if tolerated, is among the better foods for supplying this mineral. Potassium may also be deficient because of low intake of vegetables and higher intake of salt. Sodium, chloride, and potassium are the body electrolytes that help balance acid-base chemistry and fluid movement. With weakened kidney function, which is not uncommon in the elderly, electrolyte imbalances occur. Adding potassium in food and supplements and diminishing salt intake can help restore the balance.

Many medicines may interfere with mineral absorption and function. Antacids may bind calcium, as mentioned earlier, as well as other minerals, such as zinc or magnesium. Many diuretic drugs stimulate the kidneys to clear more potassium, lessening body stores. When these drugs are prescribed by a physician, this is often carefully watched, and potassium may then be supplemented. But the diuretics, which are commonly used by the elderly, also increase clearance of zinc, magnesium, and other minerals, and these are not always replaced, so that deficiencies of these minerals can result. Antibiotics can reduce colon flora, a source for the production of B vitamins and vitamin K. This can limit many intestinal functions in any age group. Laxatives can also cause loss of nutrients, and mineral oil, used more frequently years ago, can bind the fat-soluble vitamins A, D, E, and K.

Dietary factors that should be monitored include excessive consumption of simple sugars and total fats. Intake of sugar, refined foods, and other nonnutrient calories should be minimized. High intakes of sugar increase blood fats, which speed up aging and atherosclerosis. Dietary fat is also best kept at a minimum. Lower levels of stomach acid and reduced production of digestive enzymes make fat harder to process. There are more-nutritious foods than the fatty foods, although some dairy products, if tolerated, may be helpful. Low-fat or nonfat milk is probably better than whole, unless we are trying to gain weight. Other milks, such as goat's, almond, soy, oat, and rice can also be used. However, the essential fats found in raw nuts and seeds or good quality oils, such as olive or flaxseed, should be included in the diet. If chewing nuts and seeds is a problem, nut or seed butters can be used on crackers or good breads.

The prevention of aging is important. There are many aspects to this, although the psychological ones are the most significant. The time to prevent growing old is between 40 and 60, when a good, well-balanced diet high in vitamins, minerals, and other basic nutrients and low in fats and refined foods is crucial. Of course, this type of supportive nutrition does not become less important in the senior years (nor is it less important between birth and 40). How we lived yesterday affects us today, and what we do today influences our tomorrow. I am talking about our whole attitude toward life and how we live our days. The way we feed ourselves is an outcome of our self-image, knowledge, conditioning, education, self-love, and desire to live and be healthy.

The diet of the elderly should contain a variety of foods. This is often a challenge because of past experience, eccentric likes and dislikes, economics, and the state of the teeth and the oral cavity. Good teeth or dentures are important to a healthy diet. Sometimes whole food groups have been omitted because of an inability to chew certain foods. If chewing is a problem, more fresh vegetable juices should be drunk; pureed foods, particularly vegetables, and cooled whole-grain cereals add a lot of nutrition. Even balanced protein-nutrient drinks may be better than not eating those foods. All of these juices and drinks add water content to the diet as well.

Sufficient fluids and fiber are crucial to any elder's diet. Fluids are important to prevent constipation and dry skin. Keeping everything moving in the tissues, circulatory system, and intestinal tract is a vital part of feeling good. Stagnation due to poor flow and dehydration can shut us down physiologically and psychologically. Good flow on all levels is essential to regaining health and staying well. Fluid intake should be enough to produce 3 to 4 pints of urine a day. More water, herbal teas, juices, and soups, as well as fresh fruits and vegetables (all high-water-content foods), help in this regard. Prune juice, psyllium fiber, and bran are common laxative foods to help keep the elimination regular and avoid the problem of constipation. A morning or evening drink made with 4 to 6 ounces of prune juice, 2 to 4 ounces of water, a quarter or half lemon, and 2 tablespoons of wheat or oat bran should do the trick.

An older body usually uses fewer calories, while the percentage of body fat may rise. Problems of being both underweight and overweight may commonly occur in the elderly and are often harder to correct at this time of life. At this age, a little excess weight (5–10 pounds) is probably healthier than being underweight. Being too heavy, though, is hard on the bones; in addition, obesity increases the risk of cardiovascular disease and cancer. Blood pressure, cholesterol levels, and weight are the 3 health monitors that should not rise too much as we age. To maintain weight, it is wise to eat a diet containing the calories required for our ideal weight at 25 to 30. A nutritionist, dietitian, or doctor should be able to help with the calculation of these caloric needs.

Remember, though, those calories must contain plenty of nutrients. Some meats and dairy products may be used to obtain appropriate amounts of protein and vitamin B12. Supplemental amino acids with good levels of methionine and lysine are helpful for protein building when protein food intake or energy is low,

because they may be more easily utilized as they do not need to go through digestion. It is important to include plenty of fresh fruits and vegetables (raw and steamed, and even vegetable juices and soups), as well as the whole-grain cereals and legumes. These high-nutrient foods contain some calcium and other nutrients that are helpful to bone health.

Older people who are not currently on a wholesome diet can make a slow transition over 1 or 2 months to more natural foods. This means replacing refined foods, canned and packaged foods, and devitalized foods with new choices. It may be helpful to make these changes gradually, to allay the threat of upheaval. Although it is more difficult to change our ways as we age, these positive changes are still possible and helpful. Remember, if we eat vital foods, we will *be* vital!

Avoiding overeating and underactivity is important, because this nondynamic duo can be disastrous. Likewise, a poor appetite can result from a lack of exercise with poor utilization and circulation of previously obtained nutrients. Exercise is necessary at all stages of life, and it is no different for the elderly. Not only will it improve the appetite and the desire for better foods, it may significantly improve our attitude toward life. Exercise is a key to bone health, helping prevent osteoporosis. It will also improve other functions—digestion, assimilation, and circulation, as well as muscle tone. Walking, swimming, and dancing are probably the best all-around exercises for older folks, although any exercise may be suitable depending on past history and present condition. If you are not exercising regularly, it is wise to build up endurance slowly to a good active program. It will help in all walks of life.

Sometimes there may not be as much enthusiasm for good nutrition, exercise, and life in general in the elderly. When the body is not working as well, it is not as much fun to take it out for a spin. That is why it is so important to care for ourselves well in earlier years so that we can maintain our vitality and spirit as we age. Creating more support programs for the elderly, plus training programs for those who care for elders, will help our society and each of us individually in our later years. Loneliness and isolation from family and other loved ones are common for the elderly. Death of a spouse may leave the remaining partner without the enthusiasm or capability to care for him- or herself. Encouraging and supporting these folks to attend

> Think of a few people in their 60s, 70s, or 80s. What has led to their degeneration or to their health and vitality? What are you planning for *your* antiaging program? Have you already begun? Begin now!

group or community meals and find new friends can make a big difference.

Sharing meals and visiting with relatives may have a special meaning and be a primary encouragement to living. Extended family and local community meetings and meals, especially if they have good food, can be supportive to many elderly people. Engaging one another in exercise activities, such as walking, hikes, or classes, will help in socializing with peers and boosting morale. Interactive, nurturing therapies, such as counseling or massage, can also be helpful at reducing resistances and enhancing physical energy and flexibility. Society also needs to learn how to better incorporate this growing age group into the functioning community. Connecting the elderly with the support or care of young children, for example, is an ideal approach. Young children and elderly people often seem to have special magic together.

For single people who cook mainly for themselves, I offer some suggestions to economize, be practical, and eat well. Sharing cooking and meals with friends allows easier preparation, easier shopping, and reduced costs, especially if the friends take turns shopping and cooking. The more people that food is prepared for, the lower the cost per person. If you are cooking just for yourself, buy smaller quantities of food and prepare simpler meals. With many foods, it is wiser to make extra portions, enough for a few days. Soups, grains, and casseroles refrigerate well and can be used over 2 or 3 days. Meat dishes and other foods can be packaged in individual meal sizes and frozen for later use. If the appetite is not too good, it is still wise to eat regularly, with smaller, nutritious meals. Many quick-fix foods—such as eggs, yogurt, and instant whole-grain cereals—should be on hand. Nutritional yeast and molasses can be used in blender fruit drinks, with or without milk and 1 or 2 pieces of fruit, such as banana or pear (if this is supported by the digestion; it is not perfect food combining). Organic brown rice or soy protein powders, as well as the green

powders with algae and herbs, can also boost the nourishment in these drinks.

Overall, good nutrition is a vital part of any senior's health plan—one of the best buys in the health insurance market. Maintaining regular activity and exercise is equally important. Drinking plenty of pure water, avoiding processed and chemical foods, and eating lots of fiber foods, such as the fruits, vegetables, and whole grains, are basic nutritional guidelines for staying healthy. Avoiding or minimizing the use of unnecessary pharmaceutical medications and other drugs, such as nicotine, caffeine, and alcohol, is also important. Following these suggestions will help to prevent or slow the aging process. Additional antioxidant nutrients are a good idea. Many of these free-radical scavengers are included in this program (they are further discussed in "Antiaging" on page 588 in chapter 16, Performance Enhancement Programs). **In general, it's easier for seniors to stay healthy when they incorporate regular meals in a low-fat, high-fiber diet along with regular exercise and the wise use of nutritional supplements.**

There are many **herbs** that may be helpful to aging people, including ginseng root (as panax or Siberian ginsengs), ginkgo biloba, and gotu kola leaf. Ginseng has long been used in the Orient to relieve fatigue and strengthen people. Known as the "longevity herb," it is used regularly by elderly Chinese men and women to slow the aging process. Ginseng tea bags, powder, or concentrate can be used in hot water to make tea (2 cups daily is ideal). Taking 1 or 2 capsules of powdered ginseng root twice daily can give a feeling of greater strength. Raw pieces of the hard root can be sucked or chewed, but this is not as potent as the tea. Be aware that excessive use of ginseng root can elevate the blood pressure (as can licorice root) and possibly irritate the gastrointestinal mucosa. Siberian ginseng is good for balancing stress and giving energy that can be helpful without being overstimulating. Tinctures or capsules can be used. The trace mineral germanium has been found to be in high concentration in ginsengs. Ginkgo biloba, another popular Asian (and international) herb from the leaves of an ancient tree, has been more recently used in this country to help with circulatory problems, senility, and hearing disorders. (See chapter 7, Special Supplements, for further discussion of these herbs.)

Gotu kola herb is more popular in India, where it also has an ancient tradition. It acts as a brain stimulant, strengthening the memory and other mental powers. Gotu kola can be taken as a tea or in capsules, by itself or with other herbs. In Western medicine, a drug that has been fairly popular among the elderly population (as well as with young men who want to appear alert and quick-witted) is Hydergine. It is a cerebral stimulant that improves memory and mental clarity, with very few side effects. It is now commonly used in people with senility and poor memory. There are also new drugs that help reduce symptoms of senility. The nutrient acetyl-L-carnitine may help support brain function and is being looked at as a possible prevention of Alzheimer's disease. Antioxidant support, including lipoic acid, may also be useful, along with the more typical antioxidants vitamins C and E, selenium, and zinc.

As men age, prostate enlargement affecting urine flow and possibly leading to prostate surgery (especially if untreated) is surprisingly common. *Benign prostatic hypertrophy* (BPH) is conventionally used to describe this condition. For men in their 30s, the likelihood of BPH is 1 in 10. But for men in their 80s, the likelihood is an astounding 9 in 10. A swelling of the fibromuscular prostate gland can be related to a variety of dietary and lifestyle factors, such as a high-fat, excess-animal-protein diet and lack of physical activity, along with too much sitting. Thus regular exercise and stretching, especially yoga-type inverted positions, and maintaining some sexual activity also offer preventive benefits. Such nutrients as vitamins A, C, and E and other antioxidants, especially zinc, may be helpful in reducing or preventing prostate problems. Such herbs as saw palmetto berries, corn silk tea, parsley, ginger root, marshmallow root, juniper berries, and uva ursi have also been helpful to many men with prostate problems. Palmetto prostate formula with *Pygeum africanum* can also be helpful for prostate protection and prostate problems. Usually 1 or 2 capsules taken twice daily is the appropriate amount. There are also herbal teas that can be drunk 2 or 3 times daily. Refer to an herbal text or a practitioner for further information on these and other herbs related to the prostate or the aging process.

Most people in their later years would be helped by an easy-to-digest, well-balanced vitamin and mineral formula for nutritional insurance. There are few people over 60 who do not have some symptoms of early chronic illness—the body degenerates slowly, blood vessels get clogged, senses may diminish, and digestion and assimilation may weaken. So it is wise to use a nutritional supplement to ensure the best chance for the body to get plenty of what it needs for proper functioning. Many of the nutrients offer some protection against inflammation, regulate blood clotting, improve immune function, and improve fat metabolism by helping the body to handle cholesterol and triglycerides. Several high-quality powdered and encapsulated general formulas, which are easier to digest and assimilate, are available from such companies as Nutricology, Karuna Corporation, and Twinlab. For more listings, see Appendix B, "Nutritional Supplement Companies."

As with the other programs, the nutrient ranges in the "Dietary Nutrient Program for the Later Years" on the opposite page are from minimum needs, which may be obtained through diet or a basic daily supplement, to optimum insurance levels, which may require higher-dose formulas or even vitamin injections. For the elderly, because of poor digestive function, a powdered general formula taken a few times daily improves the chances of absorbing sufficient amounts of many important though hard-to-assimilate nutrients. Many seniors are also helped by digestive aids such as extra hydrochloric acid before or with meals and pancreatic enzymes right after meals to improve the breakdown of food.

When high amounts of supplemental fiber, such as psyllium seed husks or wheat or oat bran, are used (I recommend eating more high-fiber foods), more vitamins and particularly more minerals may be needed to make up for those pulled out through the colon by the fiber. Extra B vitamins are often needed to support function. Usually, double levels of most of the B vitamins are suggested. I think doubling the intake of most of the hard-to-absorb minerals, such as chromium and zinc, can help as well.

THE FUTURE OF ELDERS

Some of the areas concerning seniors must of course address healthy aging. When people live longer and stay healthier, it's going to save huge amounts in our disease-focused health-care system. Let's learn more about healthy aging in regard to healthy lifestyles, and this includes dietary patterns over the decades, exercise approaches and activities, chemical issues and vitalizing detoxification practices, and natural hormone support. Many antiaging doctors believe that one of the best ways to stay healthy and slow down aging is to maintain or create earlier hormonal states with plant-based "natural" and bioidentical hormones (just like the ones our body makes and not synthetic hormones), and this is helpful for men and women. Look for new and exciting studies on healthy aging.

On a more social note, isolation and loneliness in seniors is one of the great travesties in our modern Western cultures. In many Asian countries, the elders remain part of the families, which is much easier when people don't move and change locations so frequently as we do in the West. What we can do is to involve elders more in child care. The young and old are such a good fit and the joy involved is so visible; the elders have the patience to be and to play, and the youngsters really appreciate attention and focus upon them. Feeling useful and worthwhile is important for our health at all ages.

Dietary Nutrient Program for the Later Years* (Minimal to Optimum)

AGE: 65 AND OLDER

Nutrient	Amount	Nutrient	Amount
Calories		Copper	2–3 mg
Men	1,900–2,600	Fluoride*	1.5–4.0 mg
Women	1,600–2,200	Iodine*	150–300 mcg
Protein	60–80 g	Iron	10–20 mg
Vitamin A	5,000–10,000 IU	Magnesium	400–800 mg
Beta-carotene	10,000–20,000 IU	Manganese	3–15 mg
Vitamin D+	200–600 IU	Molybdenum	150–500 mcg
Vitamin E**	60–1,000 IU	Phosphorus*	800–1,200 mg
Vitamin K	100–300 mcg	Potassium*	2–5 g
Thiamin (B1)	1.5–50.0 mg	Selenium	150–300 mcg
Riboflavin (B2)	1.5–50.0 mg	Silicon	50–100 mg
Niacin (B3)	16–100 mg	Sodium*	1.5–3.0 g
Niacinamide (B3)	50–100 mg	Zinc	15–60 mg
Pantothenic Acid (B5)	7–500 mg	Hydrochloric acid	5–10 g
Pyridoxine (B6)	2.5–50.0 mg	(as betaine or glutamic acid,	1–2 capsules
Pyridoxal-5-phosphate	20–50 mg	before or with meals)	
Cobalamin (B12)***	10–500 mcg	Digestive enzymes	1–2 tablets
Folic acid	400–800 mcg	(pancreatic enzymes,	or capsules
Biotin	150–400 mcg	after meals)	
Choline	250–1,000 mg	Flaxseed or cod liver oil	1 tbsp
Inositol	250–1,000 mg		
PABA	25–100 mg		
Vitamin C	60–3,000 mg		
Bioflavonoids	125–500 mg		
Boron	1–2 mg		
Calcium	800–1,500 mg		
Chloride*	2–4 g		
Chromium	200–500 mcg		

* As with other life-stage support programs, nutrients easily available—such as sodium, chloride, phosphorus, sulfur, and potassium—are not usually supplemented unless there is a deficiency. Of these, potassium may be more commonly supplemented because of poor nutrition or medication.

** Can go up to 1,600–2,400 IU for insufficient circulation.

*** Vitamin B12 is commonly used as an injection in the elderly, at least several times a year, to help build up tissue stores.

+ Many elders appear to need more vitamin D, at least 1,000–2,000 IU.

Chapter 16

Performance Enhancement Programs

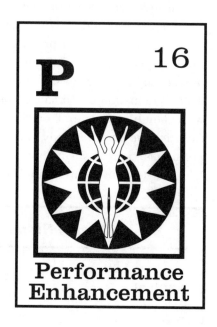

Performance Enhancement

Yep, this is the chapter for PEP! These special performance enhancement programs (PEPs) focus on optimizing the immune function or such body areas as our skin; preventing problems in special situations, such as when traveling, doing extensive exercise, or eating a vegetarian diet; protecting us from such chronic conditions as the negative effects of pollution or from developing cancer or cardiovascular disease; and supporting such life processes as our sexuality, minimizing the aging process, or reducing stress. **So much of our health is up to us. The more energy, work, and commitment we put into our health and well-being on all levels, the better body and function (that is, performance) we will manifest.**

These PEPs are designed to give you the information and know-how to take the best care of yourself, to have your body perform optimally, and to help you be your own best diagnostician should certain problems occur. Chapter 17, Medical Treatment Programs, is more geared to fixing health problems; for those programs, you will need to learn more medicine to understand better how your beautiful body-machine works so you know what is going on when it is or is

not running right. Some of medicine is mechanical, but much is not. An intuitive art can never be replaced by technology. Your own self-awareness regarding your spectrum of health is part of the goal. Learning to listen to what is out of sync and to adapt your lifestyle—by changing your diet, taking certain supplements, reducing or increasing your activity level, or changing your life's direction in some way—are your basic tools for healing. Believe me, they can aid your body to repair many existing and potential problems. Just being able to listen to your inner self and make the necessary shifts based on motivational messages you receive is the beginning and the foundation of true healing—and being your own doctor.

10. ANTIAGING: THE LONGEVITY PROGRAM

This section explores the basic process of physical and mental aging as it relates to many of the chronic degenerative, and sometimes fatal, diseases. This program can be used in conjunction with others detailed throughout this chapter (see "Antistress" on page 597,

"Skin Enhancement" on page 604, "Sexual Vitality" on page 609, "Immune Enhancement" on page 633, "Cancer Prevention" on page 640, and "Cardiovascular Disease Prevention" on page 651). For example, because this antiaging plan may help to prevent cellular and DNA changes, to reduce the level of mutagenic cells, and to decrease the impact of environmental chemicals, it may also help us prevent the twenty-first-century plague: cancer.

This program can also take us beyond just learning to be healthy; it can lead to an enhancement of vitality in our elderly years so that we can experience the fruits of our years of labor and further embrace the wisdom and joys of life. Aging is not inevitable. To live to be older than 100 in a healthy state is not out of the question if we just take care of ourselves regarding diet, exercise, and the many other factors discussed in this book. Although building a healthy foundation may be challenging in our younger years, we will look back and know the worth of our efforts as we enjoy feeling good and staying youthful. The goals of this program are twofold: first, to increase longevity by preventing and decreasing the potential for and the progression of degenerative disease and, second, to improve the vitality and tissue health of the body through proper nutrient support.

There is, of course, wide individual variation in the aging process. Genetics and constitutional factors make some people more predisposed to problems in such areas as the cardiovascular system and circulation, skin, or memory. But with better care and by following some of these guidelines, those less fortunately genetically endowed can increase their potential health and longevity. The aging process does not have to reach a level that interferes with function. In fact, the Baltimore Longitudinal Study of Aging, initiated in the 1950s, has shown that many healthy older people can have cardiovascular systems and memories as functional as those of much younger people. To keep the body fit, we need to exercise it, and to keep the mind sharp, we must also give it a regular workout. Unless there are specific health problems, particularly with the circulation, the memory should not really diminish until a late stage of life. Similarly, sexual hormones, particularly in men but also in women, are present and active in the later years, most assuredly in those who have been sexually active and

who have maintained their activity into their 60s, 70s, and 80s. In fact, maintaining hormone levels similar to levels found in our 20s and 30s using bioidentical plant-based products may offer the "best anti-aging medicine" as stated by Thierry Hartough, MD, fourth-generation endocrinologist from Belgium.

This antiaging program can be employed by anyone older than 40, especially those who wish to begin the protective, antiaging process early, although it is clearly still applicable in later years. The program can also be useful to those under stress or with demanding jobs, as well as people who push themselves in work or have trouble dealing with day-to-day demands. People who live in cities and those whose work or life exposes them to chemicals may benefit from many of these suggestions. Those on diets of processed foods, red meats and cured meats, and other chemical foods would do well to change these habits and follow the antiaging plan for at least 6 months to experience the benefits. Smokers, alcohol drinkers, and those who have used other drugs that contribute to body breakdown are also candidates for this program, which can reverse some of the damaging effects. Specific programs for most of these groups are detailed in chapter 18, Detoxification and Cleansing Programs and in my book *The New Detox Diet*.

Problems of the Aging Process

The most common problems of aging affect the cardiovascular and nervous systems, manifesting themselves in atherosclerosis and senility. Other problems include arthritis and chronic pain due to injuries, cancer, diabetes, certain immunological diseases, gastrointestinal problems (such as diverticulosis), and skin diseases. Here I explore some of the common physiological effects of aging that generate many of these diseases. Most of these lifestyle-related diseases, of course, come about when we do not take the best care of ourselves. **Many subtle and gross changes in the cardiovascular and respiratory systems lead to poor delivery of oxygen and nutrients to the tissues. In conjunction with an insufficiency of the necessary nutrients coming into the body, this is the most important underlying factor in most problems of aging.**

Many other changes occur in the heart and circulation before the diminished nutrient supply. A reduction in heart pumping action with decreased lung capacity reduces oxygen delivery and increases carbon dioxide buildup. An increase in blood vessel stiffness and blood pressure with age also diminishes circulation. Smoking, a high-fat diet, and lack of exercise severely affect these changes. Other diseases, such as diabetes and hypertension, contribute to the additional problems of atherosclerosis, abnormal heart function, and reduced circulation.

The nervous system can also be affected, with a slowing of nerve conduction, a loss of brain weight, reduced reflexes, and a decrease in memory and learning capacity. Dementia or senility may result from the diminishing nervous system function along with the cardiovascular effects of reduced circulation. Brain neurotransmitters are vital to nerve conductivity and brain function. Acetylcholine, norepinephrine, and serotonin, the three main neurotransmitters, are all produced and affected by such dietary nutrients as choline, pantothenic acid, and the amino acids tyrosine, phenylalanine, and tryptophan. Acetylcholine supports brain function, memory, and sexual activity; norepinephrine also affects sexual and general energy levels, memory, and learning; and serotonin aids relaxation and sleep.

Alzheimer's disease, a common form of senile dementia, has received a lot of attention since the mid-1980s. It often begins earlier (in the 50s) than other types of senility. Some recent theories about the cause of Alzheimer's have focused on the breakdown of the myelin sheath that serves as the outer wrapping around the nerves. Many different factors may directly or indirectly contribute to the breakdown of this nerve wrapping, including high cholesterol levels, accumulation of certain proteins (amyloid proteins), excess

formation of free radicals, head trauma, and perhaps aluminum exposure. Cigarette smoking also clearly increases the risk of Alzheimer's. Microscopic brain cell and brain tissue changes described as *neurofibrillary tangles* are classic in Alzheimer's disease; the diagnosis is most often accomplished by excluding other possibilities. The main effect seems to be on the cholinergic system, which is governed by the neurotransmitter acetylcholine, but other neurotransmitters are probably affected as well. Many treatments have been tried without much success, however. Clearing excess aluminum and reducing aluminum intake may be helpful. Lecithin or choline supplements have been helpful in some people for strengthening cell membrane function and communication between cells.

Other body systems affected by aging include the musculoskeletal system and the gastrointestinal, genitourinary, and endocrine organs. There is often a loss of muscular strength and coordination with aging. There may be some thinning of spinal disks and bones in general, degeneration of cartilage and ligaments, and loss of tissue elasticity and flexibility. With aging there is a loss of height and an increase in bone fractures. Arthritis becomes more common and leads to greater joint wear and tear. The hips are a typical site for both joint pains and arthritis in the elderly.

Good digestive function is important to proper assimilation of nutrients. This begins with good teeth. Teeth are made up of minerals, nutrients that are not well absorbed when there is low stomach acid and pancreatic digestive enzyme function. Good colon function and elimination are also important to prevent constipation and diverticular disease. Kidney function may also diminish with aging, inhibiting clearance of excess nutrients, chemicals, and toxins. The prostate and sexual organs also need good blood and energy supply to keep them functioning properly.

Many hormonal changes also occur with aging. The basal metabolic rate and thyroid hormone function may diminish, thus decreasing the energy level. Weakened glucose tolerance can lead to more problems with diabetes. Body fat percentages usually increase with age, even with the same dietary intake. Immune functions may also be reduced with the "scavenger" white blood cells becoming less effective, allowing an increase in infections. Cell repair and elimination of

Aging Theories	
Stagnation and toxicity	Errors in DNA replication
Aging clock and hormones	
Telomerase inactivity	Changes in brain function
Cross-linking of proteins	
Free radicals	Autoimmunity
	Stress

defective cells may lessen, leading to an increased incidence of cancer. Autoimmune problems from a misguided immune system may also occur.

And of course, the male and female hormones all go down and this quickens the aging process. Men and women both have all the hormones: testosterone and estrogen, progesterone and pregnenolone, cortisol and DHEA. These important substances have so many functions. They can be measured and supported with plant-based bioidentical hormones, and monitored over time to see health improvement as it relates to changing hormone levels. There are many more physicians who are incorporating this important anti-aging field of medicine, as my colleague Philip Lee Miller, MD, is his 2005 book, *The Life Extension Revolution: The New Science of Growing Older without Aging.*

Many habits and activities affect these common changes of aging. Factors that increase aging and degeneration include smoking, excess alcohol, fats and chemicals in food, poor or deficient diet, overeating, stress, pollution, and inactivity. Psychological factors influencing aging include extreme emotions, negativity, resisting positive suggestions and support, getting trapped in ruts, and hanging onto depression, loneliness, anger, and grief. A positive attitude and psychological health greatly increase longevity and delay "getting old."

> Loneliness is a symptom; aloneness is an achievement. —Bethany Argisle

Theories of Aging

My own combined theory of aging is that stagnation is the key—stagnation of bioenergy circulation and stagnation of the digestive tract and bowels. Good colon function to prevent toxin buildup, regular exercise to stimulate energy production and circulation of the blood and lymph, dealing properly with extreme emotions and stresses, and maintaining a positive attitude all help to support vitality and circulation. Chemical irritants and nutritional deficiencies accelerate the aging process. We need to maintain proper food acquisition, digestion, assimilation, and elimination to have good health long-term and to minimize the aging

process. We also need to have all the nutrient building blocks available to the cells and tissues when they need them. This requires eating wholesome, nutritious food, as well as maintaining proper digestion, assimilation, and elimination.

The **aging clock theory** refers to the aging process as programmed by an inherent, preset number of possible cellular divisions. Our individual set of cell divisions and the time between them determines our life span. Different cells have different division rates. Such lifestyle factors as stress and nutrition, degenerative changes, and immunological and hormonal health can affect our inherent cell division potential or the length of time between cell divisions. Our genes are most closely influenced by nucleic acids, RNA and DNA. When RNA is affected, it may influence cell activity, protein building, and tissue repair and healing. Basic wear and tear and random insults to our genes can speed up our individual aging process. Chemicals, microorganisms, random toxins, and nutritional or functional deficiencies (such as reduced digestive enzyme production) all affect this important cellular process.

One closely related and fascinating theory of aging in this DNA/RNA genetic area is the **telomerase inactivity theory.** Telomeres are the repetitive stretches of DNA found at the ends of chromosomes, like the little plastic caps on the ends of a shoelace that keep them from fraying. But telomeres shorten every time a cell divides. After about 50 times, the cell runs out of steam and stops dividing, possibly because the telomeres become too short and allow the DNA to "fray." An enzyme called *telomerase* can sometimes remold the ends of the chromosomes and give the cell new life. Researchers have yet to understand the dietary and lifestyle factors that influence telomerase activity, but expect to hear more about this in aging research in the years to come.

As far as scientists know, currently there is no hormone or code that causes death or self-destruction. But there are many subconscious, self-destructive tendencies, such as not taking care of ourselves in the best ways possible. As we age, we must attend to minimizing internal aging to maintain vitality and tissue health. This is accomplished in part by eating light and staying light but also by eating well. The synergy of nutrient inadequacy and emotional deficits and depletions contributes to both aging and the subsequent dying process.

The **cross-linking theory** suggests that molecular changes occur in the protein molecules of body tissues, causing microfibers to be laid down against the normal direction of other tissue fibers. This creates aging through loss of elasticity, stiffness, and degeneration. This may always be going on as the underlying mechanism for tissue change, inflammation, and degeneration, but it is more likely a result of the biochemical process of free-radical formation.

The **free-radical theory,** currently among the most accepted aging hypotheses, offers an explanation of the basis of degenerative disease. It suggests that free radicals—unstable, reactive molecules with a free electron—seek to latch onto whatever they can find. When they are not countered by antioxidant nutrients, they may interact with cell membranes, fat molecules, or tissue linings. Free radicals are generated by the metabolism of oxygen and other chemicals. They are a normal part of body function, and in and of themselves, are not bad. But too many of them can result in damage throughout the body. Singlet oxygens, hydroxyl ions, peroxides, and superoxide molecules are some of the products of oxidation. Environmental pollutants can increase our exposure to these reactive molecules, as can smoking cigarettes. Contaminants in food and water can also add to the oxidative load (called *oxidative stress*).

In food and in our bodies, unsaturated fat is most likely to undergo unwanted oxidation. Unsaturated food fat largely means nuts, seeds, and vegetable oils; in our bodies it means parts of fat that make up our cell membranes. The nuts and seeds have their own natural antioxidant protection, so they can do fine as long as we keep them refrigerated and tightly sealed. The oils need the same treatment to be safe, plus some protection from light in the form of a dark-tinted glass bottle. **Our cell membranes can be protected only through a diet that is rich in antioxidant nutrients.** The antioxidants, also termed "free-radical scavengers," protect us by binding the free radicals.

When we get sufficient levels of these antioxidants, such as vitamins E and C, selenium, and beta-carotene (a vitamin A precursor) in the diet or as supplements, we can neutralize the free radicals and prevent cellular and tissue damage. The body produces superoxide dismutase (SOD) and glutathione peroxidase, enzymes that also help counteract free radicals. These enzymes, however, are themselves unstable and are not specifically helpful as supplements because they are metabolized rapidly and are not readily absorbed. An exception to the enzyme rule would be use of supplements for the digestive tract. Supplemental enzymes have been shown to be active in the digestive tract and can be helpful in improving digestion and lowering digestive tract inflammation for that reason. By keeping the liver and its cells functioning well, we can support the production and function of these important antioxidant enzymes.

Other aging theories include **errors in DNA** (which could be generated by free radicals), chemical exposure, general toxicity, and basic genetics. **Changes in brain function** and the regulation of balance in the hormonal and nervous systems may also be at the core of the aging process. **Autoimmunity** and a general breakdown of immune function is another theory of degeneration; **stress,** which likely increases free-radical formation, may itself be at the heart of the aging process, as well as other diminishing vital physiological processes. The general process of aging probably involves combinations of all of these theories working together in varying ways within each individual.

Diet and Supplements

The diet and supplement plan that best provides us with the basic and special nourishment we need **to maintain health and prevent aging includes the following guidelines:**

- **Regularly undereat.** Avoid obesity; eat more low-calorie foods, such as vegetables, especially colorful ones high in carotenoids and flavonoids. By *undereat,* what I am really recommending is something like eating the most nutrients for the least calories. Most of us overeat and choose foods that have too many calories and not enough nutrition. When I lead detox groups, the participants consistently tell me that they realize how little they need to eat to feel their best, and they often alter their eating choices long-term as a result. There is a fascinating phenomenon in research on longevity called "undernutrition without malnutrition." Basically, there is a relationship between diet and life span in which the longest-lived animals are those that get the most nutrients in their diet while taking in the fewest amount of calories. This phenomenon makes perfect sense, because a situation is created in which the body gets optimal support while paying the minimal price in terms of metabolic load and demand.

- **Minimize fat intake.** The diet should be low in saturated and animal fats and hydrogenated oils, with only moderate intake of vegetable-oil foods and cold-pressed vegetable oils and low intake of fried fats or oils. Overall, not more than 25% of the calories in the diet should come from fat.

- **Focus the diet on foods containing complex carbohydrates** to acquire more fiber and sustained energy without overconsumption and congestion. Complex carbohydrates such as whole grains (specifically, brown rice, millet, oats, quinoa, barley, buckwheat, and whole wheat), legumes, root vegetables, and squashes can be major contributors to longevity.

- **Protein intake should be moderate**—no more than 50 to 70 grams daily—with an increase in such vegetable proteins as nuts, seeds, and whole grain and legume combinations to about 75% of the dietary protein intake. The popular high-protein diets may help initially with weight loss, but they are not good for long-term health and longevity other than the benefits from weighing less. (See "Weight Loss" on page 684 in chapter 17, Medical Treatment Programs, for healthy plans.)

- **Eat a chemical-free diet as much as possible.** Most chemicals have some toxic properties, and many generate free-radical production. Some, such as certain pesticides and the nitrates and nitrites in cured meats, can even be carcinogenic in the body. Choosing organically produced foods is one of the best ways of accomplishing a chemical-free meal plan.

- **Moderate salt, sugar, alcohol, nicotine, and caffeine.** Each of these has specific irritating properties; however, regular nicotine use is the worst in regard to aging.

- **Drink plenty of good drinking water** (see chapter 1, Water for further discussion), free of toxic pesticides and other chemicals. Proper hydration is important to skin health, digestive function, proper elimination, and all bodily functions.

- **Follow the antiaging program for micronutrients and antioxidants** presented in the "Antiaging Nutrient Program" on page 596.

- **Use periods of detoxification, or cleansing,** to balance and rest the body's systems. Fasting or cleansing is the missing link in Western nutrition. It is important to regenerate optimum function and to enhance elimination. It helps improve many body functions, including the important digestion-assimilation-elimination cycle (see "General Detoxification and Cleansing" and "Fasting and Juice Cleansing" in chapter 18, Detoxification and Cleansing Programs, on pages 741 and 769, respectively, for more information).

Supplements are important to the antiaging program. I recommend a general and complete multivitamin and mineral formula. There are now more high-quality multivitamins that contain additional antioxidants; these extra nutrients counteract many disease processes as well as stress, likely the underlying cause of many problems. In addition to a general formula, the following nutrients are specific to the antiaging program (the first 8 are antioxidants):

Vitamin C. This crucial antioxidant and anticancer nutrient has been shown to reduce cervical dysplasia, an early stage of cancer, and to prevent the conversion of nitrites to the carcinogenic nitrosamines. Ascorbic acid specifically protects cell membranes from viruses and may prevent chemical irritations. It also helps to lower blood fats, thus decreasing cardiovascular disease risk, and reduces irritation from cigarette smoke and air pollution.

Vitamin E. This important antioxidant nutrient, when taken in amounts well above the RDA (usually at least 400–1,000 IU daily), protects cell membranes and in particular prevents lipid irritation and breakdown. It also counteracts some of the negative effects of air pollution chemicals and metals. Mixed tocopherols and tocotrienols combined are the most comprehensive delivery form for vitamin E.

Selenium. This antioxidant mineral works synergistically with vitamin E; together they have a better effect than when each is used separately. The selenium-containing enzyme glutathione peroxidase protects cellular membranes and reduces irritation from metals. Selenium deficiency is associated with an increased risk of cancer, and adequate selenium intake is correlated with a reduced incidence of malignancy, particularly of the breasts, colon, and lungs—common sites of cancer.

Beta-carotene. Another antiaging and cancer-preventing antioxidant nutrient, this form of vitamin A is better than retinol (from animal sources). Beta-carotene is a dual vitamin A molecule that can be split easily in the small intestine or liver. **Vitamin A deficiencies are associated with an increased risk of cancer, particularly cervical and lung cancer.** Although the cancer-preventive effects of beta-carotene have come into question from studies like that on male Finnish smokers, in which researchers found increased risk of cancer in some smoking subjects who supplemented with beta-carotene, I believe that a close look at the details of this study and others actually vindicates beta-carotene while raising other questions about the relationship between cancer and diet.

Bioflavonoids. Found in many vitamin C foods, these also have antioxidant properties. Adequate amounts of bioflavonoids in the diet can help strengthen and protect blood vessels, improve enzyme activity, and may even help reduce the incidence of cataracts. Vitamin C supplements should contain some bioflavonoids.

L-cysteine. This sulfur-containing amino acid acts as a free-radical scavenger, binding and neutralizing those irritating molecules. It aids detoxification, in part by supporting the liver in producing and storing glutathione, a tripeptide (protein) that is part of an important antioxidant enzyme system. L-cysteine gives us cellular and tissue protection from chemicals as well. This amino acid is usually taken with vitamin C to protect the kidneys from forming stones made of cystine (a by-product of cysteine metabolism). The recommended dose is 250 mg of L-cysteine with 1 gram of vitamin C twice daily. If this amino acid is taken regularly, it is wise to also take a general formula containing the other required amino acids.

Zinc. This also has important antioxidant effects through its function in the enzyme superoxide dismutase, a free-radical scavenger. Zinc also contributes to immune support. A daily dose of 30 to 60 mg, including diet, is part of the antiaging plan.

Manganese and copper. These also act as antioxidants, mainly as support, along with zinc, of the superoxide dismutase (SOD) enzymes, which metabolize the superoxide free radicals.

Fiber. Necessary as part of the diet (and may be taken as a supplement), fiber helps colon elimination and may reduce the likelihood of cancer, especially in the breast and colon. Low-fiber, high-fat diets have been associated with an increased incidence of colon cancer. So, reach for some broccoli, apples, an artichoke, or other fruits, vegetables, and whole grains.

Water. A vital part of the "fountain of youth" program, it helps all the body functions, nourishes the skin, and is necessary for good elimination. See chapter 1, Water.

Calcium. This protects against carcinogenic changes of the cells in the colon lining. It is also important to energy (ATP) production, heart and nerve function, good teeth, and bone health, protecting against osteoporosis.

Magnesium. This protects the cardiovascular system by supporting heart function and preventing vascular spasms. It also aids in relaxation by reducing nervous tensions, an important part of staying healthy. Magnesium is also necessary for amino acid metabolism and energy (ATP) production.

Chromium. This supports glucose tolerance, often reducing sugar cravings and possibly the incidence of diabetes. It also may help to lower blood cholesterol, thereby helping to prevent the main degenerative disease, atherosclerosis.

Molybdenum. This trace mineral may play a role in inhibiting cancer. Researchers now know that this mineral is required for proper function of the enzymes xanthine oxidase, aldehyde oxidase, and sulfite oxidase—all of which may participate in deactivation of toxic substances, some of them potentially carcinogenic.

Niacin. The active circulatory stimulant form of vitamin B_3, this nutrient helps improve circulation and also lowers cholesterol, both factors that reduce the risk of cardiovascular disease.

Vitamin B12. This helps keep energy up and protects nerve coverings. B12 is needed in the production of red blood cells and in the synthesis of DNA and RNA, important rebuilding processes in the body.

Folic acid. This also helps in RNA and DNA (and red blood cell) production, but only in dosages higher than the 400 mcg RDA. A dose of 1 to 2 mg twice daily is commonly prescribed in Canada for this supportive function. Even higher amounts of folic acid, like 5 to 10 mg twice daily, are quite safe.

RNA. As found in such foods as the blue-green algae chlorella, spirulina, and wheat grass—all high in chlorophyll as well—RNA may help slow the aging process. RNA supplements have not been shown, however, to be effective in actually increasing RNA in the tissues.

Choline. Found in lecithin, choline supports production of cell membranes and the important neurotransmitter acetylcholine.

Omega-3 fatty acids. Fatty acids such as EPA and DHA, help reduce cholesterol and cardiovascular disease risk. Flaxseed oil contains both these omega-3 essential fatty acids as well as omega-6s, yet fish oils are still the best source of omega-3s as long as the products are free of the chemicals that are now often found in ocean fish.

L-carnitine. This nonessential amino acid helps to balance fat metabolism (utilization) and support energy production within the cell and in the muscles. L-carnitine may also reduce body fat and weight, which is important to longevity.

Coenzyme Q10. Also called *ubiquinone*, this improves the function of the cardiac muscle, the body's most important pump for longevity. It also may enhance specific immune functions and is critical for energy production by the all-star energy producers—the mitochondria in our cells.

***Lactobacillus acidophilus* and other intestinal bacteria.** These are also important to support the normal colon ecology and for the breakdown of food and the production of vitamins in the colon. Reimplanting healthy bacteria may also help reduce other organisms, yeasts, or parasites.

Organo-germanium (trace mineral complex, germanium sesquioxide). This oxygenating nutrient has been show to have detoxifying ability (in relation to heavy metals), free-radical-scavenging effects, and a potentially enhancing impact on the immune system.

Mucopolysaccharides. Also called *glycosaminoglycans* (GAGs), these are important components of connective tissue. Maintaining integrity and flexibility in this type of tissue is critical for healthy aging, because it is part of the lining inside the joints. Glucosamine sulfate and chondroitin sulfate are the two best-studied of the GAGs, and they have been shown to be effective as supplements for restoring joint tissue integrity, in speeding up postinjury healing, preventing injury in the first place, and potentially decreasing risk of chronic joint-related problems like osteoarthritis. Foods containing GAGs include mussels and oysters.

Hydrochloric acid. Such digestive enzyme support may be helpful, particularly if this substance is deficient in our bodies. Proper breakdown and use of food nutrients are essential to staying healthy. Poor digestion can lead to many problems, including increased incidence of allergy. Furthermore, improper assimilation of undigested foods can ultimately lead to increased nutrient deficiencies as well as free-radical formation from food reactions.

Herbs

Herbs have long been known for their benefits in cleansing the body and blood, protecting us from irritants and cancer cells, and supporting longevity. I think the best for these purposes are garlic, ginseng root, capsicum (also known as cayenne pepper), and gotu kola.

Garlic. This has some antiviral, antifungal, and antibacterial properties. It also has some anticancer functions. Garlic helps to stimulate liver and colon detoxification and aids in reducing both blood pressure and cholesterol levels, which reduces the risk of cardiovascular disease.

Ginseng root. Known as the "longevity herb," ginseng has been used for centuries throughout Asia to improve energy, especially in the elderly. It seems to support the adrenal glands and the immune function, although further tests are needed to confirm this. There are many kinds of ginseng; the red may lead to a mild increase in blood pressure, while the white varieties may help reduce it. Siberian ginseng has an energetic quality as well as a stress-reducing component (an *adaptogen* in herbology terms). Ginseng should not be used regularly in an antiaging program unless there is fatigue. It may be used 3 or 4 times a year, with a few capsules taken daily for 1 or 2 weeks or as a tea prepared from the root, drunk over several days.

Capsicum. This is an interesting herb. A spicy bush berry, cayenne helps to stimulate both circulation and elimination. It also acts as a mild diuretic, increasing kidney cleansing. Cayenne is a natural energy stimulant that, unlike coffee, helps to reduce the blood pressure as well as the cholesterol level.

And it is one of the ingredients—along with lemon, maple syrup, and water—of my favorite cleansing drink, the Master Cleanser (see "Fasting and Juice Cleansing" on page 768 in chapter 18, Detoxification and Cleansing Programs.)

Gotu kola. This has long been used by Indians for a variety of conditions. It is used in an antiaging program as a memory and brain stimulant and has been known as a longevity herb, likely for its effect on mental and physical vitality. Gotu kola has a diuretic effect and has been used as a glandular tonic in both men and women.

Antiaging Nutrient Program

Nutrient	Amount	Nutrient	Amount
Calories	1,600–3,000	Iron	
Protein	50–75 g	men and postmenopausal women	8–15 mg
Fats	40–70 g	(depends on blood count and	
Carbohydrate	250–400 g	iron stores)	
Fiber	10–20 g	menstruating women	18–30 mg
Water	1.5–3.0 qt	Magnesium	600–800 mg
Vitamin A	10,000 IU	Manganese	5–15 mg
Beta-carotene	25,000–50,000 IU	Molybdenum	100–500 mcg
Vitamin D	400 IU	Selenium, preferably as	
Vitamin E	400–800 IU	selenomethionine	200–300 mcg
Vitamin K	300 mcg	Silicon	100–200 mg
Thiamin (B1)	10–50 mg	Zinc	
Riboflavin (B2)	10–50 mg	men	30–60 mg
Niacin (B3)	50–100 mg	women	25–50 mg
Niacinamide (B3)	50–100 mg	L-amino acids complex	1,000 mg
Pantothenic acid (B5)	250–500 mg	L-cysteine	500 mg
Pyridoxine (B6)	25–200 mg	L-carnitine	250–500 mg
Pyridoxal-5-phosphate	25–50 mg	Coenzyme Q10	30–60 mg
Cobalamin (B12)	50–250 mcg	Flaxseed oil	1–2 tsp
Folic acid	1,000–2,000 mcg	Organo-germanium	75–300 mg
Biotin	500 mcg		
Choline	250–1,000 mg	**Others**	
Inositol	500–1,000 mg	Hydrochloric acid	5–10 grains
Vitamin C	2–6 g	(with protein meals)	(1–2 tablets)
Bioflavonoids	250–500 mg	Digestive enzymes	2–3 tablets
Calcium	800–1,200 mg	(including bromelain,	
Chromium	200–500 mcg	after meals)	
Copper	2–3 mg	Wheat germ oil	4 capsules
Iodine	150–200 mcg	Mucopolysaccharides	100–500 mg

In the future, more and more specific nutrients and herbs will be used to slow down the aging process and enhance health, mainly by reducing stress and supporting immune function. Immune enhancement and a greater understanding of the relationship between immunology and health will probably be a cornerstone of our future medicine. (See "Immune Enhancement," on page 633 in this chapter for more.)

Unless there is more research involving the cloning of cells and tissues or in *cryobiology* (the freezing of cells, tissues, and whole bodies to prolong or regenerate life), it is going to be up to each of us to live according to the health-sustaining laws of Nature and the universe. A total revamping of the diet, with nutrient-rich, wholesome foods and a focus on regular undereating, will support us best. Reducing chemical exposure by cleaning up the environment is necessary for greatest longevity. Learning to reduce and manage stress in our daily lives and generate an attitude of enthusiasm and love for life is crucial to our future health and happiness.

The specific nutrient program I recommend for antiaging is shown in the table on the opposite page. The values given are averages for men and women of different sizes and shapes. Ranges are shown for most values to allow for some flexibility in individual application. Unless otherwise noted, these amounts are to be taken daily, usually divided into 2 or 3 portions over the course of the day. Amounts consumed in the diet can be taken into consideration for such nutrients as folic acid, calcium, or iron; excess iron should not be taken unless you are being treated for iron deficiency or are monitored by a nutritional specialist. This supplementation program may be used for 1 month several times yearly for healthy people in their 40s and 50s and then more regularly in the later years or with particular aging concerns. For specific medical conditions, using more specific programs discussed in chapter 17, Medical Treatment Programs, may be more relevant.

11. ANTISTRESS

In the future, stress may come to be seen as the primary contributing cause of most disease. Research continues to link stress to more and more symptoms and diseases, both acute and chronic. Stress is inevitable in today's world and, of course, we need a certain amount to func-

tion. The key is to be able to manage our level of stress. Stress is our reaction to our external environment as well as our inner thoughts and feelings. Stress in essence is the body's natural response to dangers, the fight-or-flight mechanisms—the body's preparedness to do battle or flee from danger. This response involves a complex biochemical-hormonal process (discussed shortly).

Stress in today's world is mainly a result of continuous high demands that are imposed on us by work, family, and lifestyle, or that we impose on ourselves because of our desire to accomplish. Mild stress acts as a useful motivation for activity and productivity. But when the stresses in our life are too extreme or too many, this may result in all kinds of problems. Some people consistently overreact to their day-to-day life. However, most of us might be overwhelmed only when we have an increased intensity or number of stresses, such as excessive demands all at once leading to a continuous feeling of not having enough time or energy to do what we feel we must do. Others respond stressfully to intense emotional experiences, personal changes, extreme weather, or overexposure to electronic stimuli, all of which can weaken us. Stress can generate many symptoms and diseases, mediated by changes in immune function, hormonal response, and biochemical reactions, which then influence body functions in the digestive tract and the cardiovascular, neurological, or musculoskeletal systems. A wide variety of problems—such as headache, backache, infection, and even heart disease or cancer in the long term—may result.

The brain and pituitary gland respond to stress by releasing adrenocorticotropic hormone (ACTH). This stimulates the adrenals to increase production of the hormones epinephrine, norepinephrine, and cortisol. Other hormones that affect metabolism and water balance may also be released. Epinephrine and norepinephrine, known as the adrenalines or catecholamines, are the main stimuli to the stress response. They stimulate the heart, increase blood pressure and heart rate, and constrict certain blood vessels to increase blood flow to the muscles and brain and to decrease blood flow to the digestive tract and internal organs, preparing us for the "battle" with the "danger," wherever it is. Adrenaline also raises blood sugar, as it stimulates the liver to produce and release more glucose (and cholesterol) into the blood so our cells will have the energy we need. All of this results in an increased rate of metabolism. **Stress experienced around the time of eating thus diverts the energy needed for efficient digestion.**

During times of increased stress and greater demand, the body's nutrients are used more rapidly to meet the increased biochemical needs of metabolism, so we require increased amounts of many of these nutrients. The diet and nutrient plan presented in this program is specifically designed to reduce the negative biochemical effects of stress. There are also many other important aspects of handling this modern-day problem, primarily psychological and lifestyle approaches to stress management. A whole field of medicine, called *psychoneuroimmunology*, has looked in depth at stress-induced diseases. In fact, most specialties now have some set of symptoms or a diagnosis in their field of expertise related to these psycho-emotional/stress-induced diseases. But most doctors are not trained to do more than diagnose them, and often these diagnoses—such as "irritable bowel syndrome" (sometimes called "spastic colon"), tension headaches, or neurogenic bladder disease—are made primarily by excluding the "real diseases." Often only tranquilizers, psychotherapy, or

biofeedback are available in most circles of medicine, and these approaches may be limited. There is a lot more that each of us can do to better manage our stress, such as learning relaxation and meditation practices.

Who will benefit from this antistress program? It is mainly for those who are routinely subjected to high demands, particularly mental demands, and who suffer from intellectual performance anxiety. People in this group are mostly executives or office workers, people who must sit and be productive for eight to ten hours a day with little physical outlet. Others who might benefit from this plan include salespeople, flight attendants, mechanics, nurses, and journalists. The antistress program is also suitable for people undergoing short-term periods of increased stress because of personal changes or other events that increase energy demands, such as divorce or a new marriage, the death of a loved one, a relocation, a job change, or travel.

Many of the conditions discussed in this chapter are related in some way to stress—for example, athletes experience extra physical stress and executives experience more mental stress; stress is also a factor in the aging process. Stress can occur at all levels of our being. There are physical, emotional, mental, and spiritual stress factors involved in almost all diseases. Particular medical conditions that have a high stress component include asthma and allergies, cardiovascular and gastrointestinal diseases, arthritis, and cancer. Surgery, viral conditions, and environmental chemical exposure may be short-term problems with high-stress components. Thus aspects of this anti-stress program may apply to many of the other programs.

Please realize, though, that stress is not the situations or incidents themselves; rather, real stress comes from the way we react to these events or experiences. (We all need to learn to respond rather than react. *Response* means to take in any issues, process them, and then come up with appropriate interactions.) For stress to arise and negatively influence our health, we must experience something as a danger. When we do, anxiety is generated, which we often experience as fear or a feeling of threat to our survival. If we view stress positively, we see it as simply a survival response. But if we cannot handle the stress, we may experience the symptoms and diseases of stress. Learning to adapt our attitude and find suitable outlets for our stress is an important long-range plan.

As stated earlier, the normal biochemical response to a sense of danger is the stimulation of the adrenal glands to release increased levels of hormones, particularly the catecholamines—epinephrine (adrenaline) and norepinephrine (noradrenaline). The catecholamines are cardiovascular stimulants that increase heart rate, constrict blood vessels, stimulate the brain, and affect every other body system to prepare it for fight or flight. The problem comes when there is really no physical danger but our body reacts as if there were. In that case, if greater physical demands and activity do not provide an outlet for the increased adrenal activity, it may be turned inward and play havoc with our physiology and organs, as well as with our emotions and our mind, and also our relationships with family and friends.

All parts of the body are affected by stress, but certain areas seem to be more sensitive than others. In my estimation, the digestive tract is the most easily influenced, followed by the neurological and circulatory systems and the muscles that accumulate some of the tensions and toxins from metabolism. An individual's psychological outlook and welfare are strongly affected by acute and chronic stress. How the damage comes about involves the mechanisms of constant adrenal stimulation along with free-radical production (see "Antiaging" on page 588 for a full discussion) and immune suppression. Stress produces irritating molecules that generate immunological changes, damage cells, and inflame organ and blood vessel linings. Stress responses also eat up more important nutrients, which can lead to deficiencies

and allow the other stress-response changes to damage the tissues even more. **Stress has been shown to decrease protective antibodies and reduce the important T lymphocytes that function in the cellular immune system. Chronic stress is clearly**

Common Stress Factors

Attitude toward self

Demands at the office

Emotional challenges—personal relationships, fear, anger, loneliness

Family changes—marriage, divorce, separation, a new baby

Health challenges—illness, injury, surgery, chemical exposures

Job and career challenges

Life changes—adolescence, aging, pregnancy, menopause

Meeting someone new

Moving

Personal financial state

Physical challenges—weather changes, extreme climates, athletic events

Promotion, job loss

Public speaking

Raising children

Tests in school

Traffic tickets

War and the fear of war

Stress-Related Symptoms and Diseases

Allergies	Eczema	Muscle tension
Anorexia nervosa	Fatigue	Neck and back pains
Arthritis	Headaches	Nutritional deficiencies
Asthma	High blood pressure	Peptic ulcer
Atherosclerosis	Indigestion	Premenstrual symptoms
Cancer	Infections	Psoriasis
Constipation	Insomnia	Psychological problems
Depression	Irritability	Sexual problems
Diabetes	Irritable bowel	Weight changes
Diarrhea	Loss of appetite	

a culprit in the generation of aging and degenerative diseases.

In addition to the increased demands on the adrenal cortex, certain mechanisms affect the stomach and pancreas and thus digestion. Stress initially increases stomach hydrochloric acid production, leading to indigestion, heartburn, gastritis, and ulcer problems. With increased acid levels, however, the pancreas is stimulated to release alkaline enzymes to help balance the acidity. With chronic stress, this can lead to hypochlorhydria (low stomach acid) and reduced function of the pancreas. This may result in poor digestion and assimilation of nutrients and thus vitamin and mineral deficiencies—as well as the development of food reactions because of the improper breakdown of the bulk foodstuffs and the subsequent absorption of larger molecules, which may be immunogenic.

There is also a weakening of the adrenal response with chronic stress, whether the stress is from regular sugar intake (adrenaline helps rebalance blood sugar) or from other physical or emotional demands. When the adrenals do not respond, the body has a more difficult time coping with the stress, and when this inability to cope sets in deeply, the body may feel like giving up. We might experience depression, hopelessness, or even death, which can result from the serious diseases that arise with a severely weakened immune system. That is why it is so important to avoid the vicious cycle of trying to meet high demands by pushing ourselves with poor nourishment, poor sleep, and lack of fun. Psychoneuroimmunology deals with the relationship between stress, immunity, brain functions, and disease, examining such problems as AIDS, cancer, and chronic viral conditions. Although scientists have learned a lot about stress and its influence on disease in recent years, there is still a great deal more to learn regarding the physical mechanisms involved in immune interaction. This is going to be a dominant medical field of the future.

For people with elevated stress levels, I suggest a variety of stress-reducing activities to minimize the dangers of this underlying cause of disease:

- **Have more fun.** Do things that you enjoy and that help you to relax.

- **Express your feelings.** Emotions need regular venting; unexpressed emotions are the building blocks of stress, pain, and illness.

- **Get good sleep.** Poor sleep or sleep habits do not let your body really rest, discharge tensions, and recharge.

- **Learn relaxation exercises.** These can help a great deal in reducing stress through letting go of mental stresses and experiencing moments of inner peace. This quiet, "nothing happening" space is where, I believe, the healing process begins.

- **Exercise.** Regular physical exercise is one of the best ways to clear your tensions and feel good, with more energy and a better attitude toward life.

- **Develop good relationships.** It is important to have friends in whom you can confide and find support. Those who love and accept you and will advise but not judge you are your true friends. It is also very meaningful to be a true friend to another.

- **Experience love and satisfying sex.** A primary relationship that is loving, sensual, and sexual can also be a major stress reducer. Having an understanding, accepting, and warm being to receive your hardworking body and mind can be the best therapy available. However, if you do not have this in your life, there are many other therapies that are helpful. These would include all bodywork involving massage, as well as movement and dance therapy. Also, having a loving pet offers comfort and stress reduction. Often, an intense relationship can also be a stressor. It is important to find a balance in all you do, in each endeavor and in your life as a whole.

- **Change perceptions and attitudes.** When ideas or views are not serving you, it is wise to examine and adapt them. It is important to learn to respond to life's situations and not react. This is a true "response-ability" (the ability to respond and not react)! Hanging onto frustrations, holding grudges, and accepting the victim-blame game are not in your best health interests. It serves you to look at the big picture and step out of the little struggles. Ask why you might need to experience these challenges and try to view them as opportunities for growth and learning. Applying more spiritual principles to life is useful and often helps solve many of the conflicts involved in finding greater peace of mind and heart. Find and experience self-love, self-respect, and self-worth. Remember to take your daily dose of vitamin L (the love nutrient); see chapter 5, page 146, for a full discussion.

Diet and Stress

There are many positive things to do with regard to diet and nutrition, as well as many things to avoid. This program is designed to counteract and reduce the negative biochemical and physiological effects of stress and to minimize the specific stressing agents, such as the wide variety of drugs, both over-the-counter and prescription. Caffeine, nicotine, and alcohol are all irritating drugs. Many over-the-counter and prescription drugs may also cause physiological problems and irritate us physically or mentally.

A diet of high-nutrient foods is essential for people under stress, because stress increases cellular activity, which leads to increased nutrient usage. The resulting depletions may aggravate the damaging effects of stress. Also, less food may be consumed during times of stress, as the digestive tract may be a little upset; and the higher-nutrient foods make up for lower consumption. Some people who are stressed tend to push themselves and not take good care of themselves, avoiding meals, especially wholesome ones, and snacking on quick-energy or fast foods. They may be martyrs who feel that they must serve the cause and that there is no time for such things as eating properly, or they may just be too busy and forget to eat. These people are usually not overweight; on the contrary, they need to be reminded to eat. This unrelenting push without feeding the stomach (and every cell) can lead to acid irritation of the digestive organs and ulcers. Then the cycle of antacids starts and further poor digestion and assimilation is the final outcome. There are many more-natural therapies to use, such as chamomile tea, peppermint tea, licorice, and others discussed shortly.

Probably the best type of diet for the fast-track people with intellectual performance anxiety is 3 to 5 small but wholesome meals a day, like the Warrior's Diet discussed on page 366 in chapter 9, Diets. Lots of water is important to keep us well hydrated and to help counteract stress by circulating nutrients. Avoiding stress around meals is also important. Try to rest and relax before and after eating, even if just for a few minutes placing your body in a receptive state for the nourishment coming in—rather like clearing the computer of its active program so that it can receive new information. If there is time, take 10 to 15 minutes before and after meals, especially after large meals. Listening to relaxing music also helps.

A detoxification-type diet may be useful at times of intense stress, and it is often a natural response to these increased demands. Drinking lots of liquids, such as water and juices, and reducing heavier meals that may not be handled well can help us lighten up when life gets too heavy. A response of overeating and food abuse can only make matters worse. Juices, soups, and salads, for example, can nourish us well without creating great demands on the body and digestion, which may not be working well at the time. Our energy level and productivity may rise with lighter eating and simpler meals. A lighter, cleansing diet may help us through times of short-term stress. Some food intake may enable the body to assimilate the supplements that can also be of value. A good supplement plan is imperative to an antistress program. Stress depletes so many of the body's nutrients that it is difficult to obtain the levels we need from food alone unless we spend 8 hours a day shopping, preparing food, and feeding ourselves—and that is not too realistic.

Nutrients and Stress

Nutrients that are commonly depleted by stress include the antioxidant vitamins A, E, and C, the B vitamins, and the minerals zinc, selenium, calcium, magnesium, iron, potassium, sulfur, and molybdenum. Because of increased metabolism and use of energy, the stressed body uses more carbohydrates, proteins, and fats, especially the fatty acids. Unrelenting stress, however, is not the basis for a healthy weight-loss program.

The B vitamins and vitamin C are the main constituents of many antistress formulas. They are all significantly depleted by stress, and the stress-related problems may be compounded by deficiencies resulting from poor nutrition before the time of increased stress. All of the B vitamins are important here. Pantothenic acid, or vitamin B5, may well be the most important antistress nutrient of the B complex. Along with folic acid and vitamin C, it is necessary for proper functioning of the adrenal glands. Niacin, enough to generate the so-called niacin flush, may be useful in counteracting some of the biochemical effects of stress. "Niacin flush" is a shorthand phrase for describing the impact of this vitamin on our nervous and cardiovascular system. Working through the nervous system, high amounts of niacin cause our small blood vessels to open wider, bringing more blood to the skin surface and causing it to redden and tingle. Vitamins B1, B2, B6, biotin, and PABA are also helpful. I recommend taking higher than the dietary reference intake (DRI) of all of the B vitamins, spread out in 2 or 3 portions, all taken before dark, because they can be stimulating; it is wise to let the mind and body relax toward bedtime. I suggest more minerals in the evening, as they tend to help in relaxation. However, if evening work is important or there are evening meetings, a good B complex supplement can be taken after dinner.

The B vitamins may even have a relaxing effect on some people, and they could be used in the evenings to calm the nerves. A regular B vitamin, with 25 to 50 mg each of most of the Bs, for example, will be used and eliminated by the body within a few hours. Such tablets or capsules can be taken several times daily. Time-release B vitamins, which do not have to be taken so often, are also commonly used. Many people do better with hypoallergenic or yeast-free and wheat-free B vitamins. Although the body will use some of the B vitamins taken at any time, most vitamin and mineral supplements are best assimilated after a meal.

Vitamin C supplementation is also important during times of stress. **Vitamin C, or ascorbic acid, may indeed be the single most essential antistress nutrient.** It offers cellular protection, immune support, and adrenal support to produce more cortisone and epinephrine. Vitamin C is also an important antioxidant that helps protect against fat peroxidation,

including restoring vitamin E after it is oxidized. Vitamin C is rapidly utilized and minimally stored in the body. Therefore, regular usage, even 4 to 6 times daily, is ideal. A dosage of 1 to 2 grams a day is recommended, although as much as 8 to 10 grams may be used for severe problems related to stress. One or two of the vitamin C dosages taken each day should contain the bioflavonoid C complex, including rutin and hesperidin. In addition to extra B vitamins and C, I suggest an antioxidant program such as described on page 596 for the antiaging program. Vitamin A and beta-carotene, vitamin E and selenium, and the amino acid L-cysteine are all part of this. As with vitamin C, these antioxidants sacrifice themselves (through oxidation) to balance out the free radicals.

Minerals are also important, with potassium, calcium, and magnesium leading the antistress list. Potassium is essential for most crucial physiologic activities. Calcium is vital to nerve transmission as well as regular heartbeat and immune function. It aids both relaxation and muscle tone. Magnesium is a tranquilizing mineral that helps balance the nervous system and support heart function. Adding 1 cup of Epsom salts (magnesium sulfate), to a bath can be very relaxing. In general, a dosage of 600 to 1,000 mg of calcium and 400 to 800 mg of magnesium daily, in addition to that eaten in the diet, is recommended, with most of it being taken in the evening before bed. Calcium and magnesium can also be used to balance the stomach acid. For acute or early stress with hyperacidity, these alkaline minerals taken before meals can be a helpful antacid. With chronic stress, when stomach acid is more often low, taking them before bed is better. Pancreatic function is often low as well with chronic stress, and additional pancreatic enzymes after meals may be helpful.

Minerals that are helpful for their immune and enzyme support, such as superoxide dismutase, include zinc, copper, manganese, and selenium. Chromium may be useful in allaying sugar cravings, while potassium is important to prevent heart irregularities and muscle cramps and to balance the hypertensive effects of sodium when salt is used in excess. Like vitamin C and the Bs, minerals are best taken in several portions for optimum absorption and utilization. Taking the important ones (calcium, magnesium, iron, or zinc) by themselves reduces competitive absorption between them and produces higher levels of each in the blood.

Supplemental amino acids may allow better protein utilization and energy balance, especially when digestion is poor. The powdered, L- form amino acids are easily utilized by the body, much more easily than steak, although the meat has other nutrition (and possibly other toxins). The antioxidant amino acid L-cysteine promotes liver function and detoxification. L-glutamine is helpful for proper brain function, especially with stress, and may reduce sugar cravings, which many stressed people have. Methionine may also be protective against stress through its support of fatty acid metabolism and other functions. L-tyrosine and L-phenylalanine may help reduce stress-induced high blood pressure, while L-tryptophan can be used for relaxation and sleep (see the "Sleep-Aid Nutrient Cocktail" recipe, below). Tryptophan is available again through compounding pharmacists and doctors. More readily available in natural food stores and pharmacies is 5-hydroxytryptophan (5-HTP).

Herbs may be useful in the antistress program as well. Licorice root and its active extract deglycyrrhizinated licorice (DGL) have a soothing and anti-inflammatory effect and may be useful for stress. Valerian root, by itself or in combination with other herbs, has a tranquilizing effect and can be used before sleep or as a muscle relaxant, either as a tea or in a capsule. Catnip leaf can tame that wild or ferocious feeling and is a safe herb to improve the recharging quality of our catnaps. Ginseng root, as a tea or in capsules, is often thought of as a stimulant but is commonly used as an antistress herb, especially as Siberian ginseng. It strengthens deeper energies and the ability to handle life, and it is definitely better in the long run than coffee. White ginsengs, such as northern or white Siberian, tend to be safer for the blood pressure (too much red ginseng can elevate it). Gotu kola leaf is a good herb for mental stress. Like ginseng, it is popular in the Eastern cultures. Two formulas that I have used for patients are made by Professional Botanicals: RLX ("relax"), which contains skullcap, passion flower, celery seed, musk root, lupulin, and hops, and RST ("rest") or Sleepeaze, which contains passion flower, valerian root, black cohosh root, German chamomile flowers, lupulin, and lemon balm. There are other similar formulas available at pharmacies and natural food stores.

Some practitioners use adrenal glandular tablets to support the extra adrenal demands during stress. Many people respond well to this treatment if they feel comfortable taking beef adrenals. I personally do not. Adrenal cortical extract (ACE) had once been a popular injection for a number of years among alternative doctors for stimulating energy and treating a variety of problems, such as allergies, hypoglycemia, and fatigue. This appears to be less commonly used and harder to obtain, likely because of medical politics. It was not particularly unsafe; its effectiveness and safety were not well enough established to satisfy the FDA.

Some of the freeze-dried blue-green algae products have also been useful because of their mild detoxifying and energizing effects. They also seem to reduce some mental stress. I personally like how I feel when I take chlorella or spirulina. They provide protein and all the essential amino acids as well as many vitamins and minerals.

The "Antistress Nutrient Program" on page 604 shows the total day's intake of the recommended nutrients (in addition to the diet), which I suggest be split into three portions. Where ranges are shown, these are to accommodate individual needs and ability to handle higher amounts of these nutrients.

Sleep-Aid Nutrient Cocktail

Nutrient	Amount
Vitamin C*	500–1,000 mg (helps mineral absorption)
Calcium	500–750 mg
Magnesium	350–500 mg
Potassium	300–500 mg
L-tryptophan	500–2,000 mg (if available) or
5-HTP (5-hydroxy-tryptophan)	50–200 mg

*A mineralized ascorbic acid powder with calcium, magnesium, and potassium can be used in a drink.

Relaxing herbs, such as valerian, chamomile, vervain, catnip, hops, or linden flowers may also be added. Begin with just the C, calcium, and magnesium. If that does not work, add 500 mg of L-tryptophan (or 5-HTP), increasing the dosage if necessary by 500 mg every 3 days, up to 2,000 mg. If you still have no relief, try an herbal sleep-inducing formula, beginning with 1 or 2 capsules and building up if needed. Celestial Seasonings Sleepytime tea has helped many people. Drinking a warm cup of it or another nighttime relaxant tea is a helpful addition to a calming-down routine. Some people also enjoy a warm cup of whole milk before bed for its tranquilizing effect, if the digestion will handle it.

Antistress Nutrient Program	
Nutrient	**Amount**
Water	2–3 qt
Vitamin A	7,500–15,000 IU
Beta-carotene	10,000–25,000 IU
Vitamin D	400 IU
Vitamin E	400–1,000 IU
Vitamin K	200–400 mcg
Thiamin (B1)	75–150 mg
Riboflavin (B2)	50–100 mg
Niacin (B3)	50–150 mg
Niacinamide (B3)	25–100 mg
Pantothenic acid (B5)	500–1,000 mg
Pyridoxine (B6)	50–100 mg
Pyridoxal-5-phosphate	25–75 mg
Cobalamin (B12)	50–250 mcg
Folic acid	500–1,000 mcg
Biotin	150–500 mcg
Choline	500–1,000 mg
Inositol	500–1,000 mg
PABA	50–100 mg
Vitamin C	4–8 g
Bioflavonoids	250–500 mg
Calcium	600–1,000 mg
Chromium	200–400 mcg
Copper	2–3 mg
Iodine	150–200 mcg
Iron	10–20 mg
Magnesium	350–600 mg
Manganese	5–10 mg
Molybdenum	300–800 mg
Potassium	300–500 mg
Selenium	200–400 mcg
Zinc	30–60 mg
L-amino acids	1,000–1,500 mg
L-cysteine with vitamin C	250–500 mg

Optional

Hydrochloric acid with meals for chronic stress	5–10 grains
Pancreatic enzyme tablets	1–2 (after meals)
Adrenal glandular	50–100 mg
Chlorella	1–2 packets or 6–12 tablets daily
Licorice root	2–4 capsules

12. SKIN ENHANCEMENT

In this section let's discuss what it takes to keep the skin looking young and healthy—what we can do for it, what to avoid, and some dietary guidelines and supplement suggestions. Many aspects of lifestyle, including stress, cigarette smoking, and sunbathing or ultraviolet (UV) tanning may lead to premature aging of the skin. I also review some of the many acute and chronic skin disorders that occur at various ages or throughout life. Fortunately, most of these problems eventually heal on their own. I examine these briefly with a focus on nutritional influences and treatment, trying to be a bit more helpful than the lighthearted maxim of the dermatologist: "If it's dry, wet it; if it's wet, dry it out. If that doesn't work, use cortisone."

The skin is the largest organ. It functions as a protective covering, a key sensing organ, an oil producer, and an important organ of elimination. Through regular evaporation and perspiration, the skin can clear all kinds of toxins to help maintain internal balance. The skin must be well nourished to stay healthy. It needs good circulation through its millions of tiny capillaries, good nerve function, and a ready supply of nutrients to aid its rapid growth. The skin's surface is the intermediary between the external and internal environments and reflects the health of the underlying organs and the internal body function. By looking at the skin, tongue surface, eye tissue, and hair quality, I can get a good idea of an individual's general health, vitality, and internal balance. In Chinese medicine, the skin coloration or hue around and under the eyes reflects the subtle balance among the Chinese five elements. For example, a greenish hue may suggest a liver/gallbladder imbalance. In this system, the colors are related to different organs as shown in the following table.

The Chinese Five Elements		
Color	**Organ**	**Element**
Green	Liver, gallbladder	Wood
Red	Heart, small intestine	Fire
Yellow	Spleen, stomach	Earth
White	Lungs, large intestine	Metal (air)
Blue	Kidneys, bladder	Water

The condition of the skin and tissue around the eyes can suggest certain other problems. Signs of fatigue and increased aging lines or dark circles under the eyes may indicate stress; the Chinese would diagnose weak adrenal-kidney energy. Water or kidney imbalance may show up as puffiness, while colon congestion or imbalance might be represented by wrinkled bags under the eyes or a white coloration. Allergies may be revealed by slightly puffy or pitted dark circles, even looking like black and blue "shiners" under the eyes when severe. As the skin is an eliminating organ, the general skin health may tie into functions of the lungs, colon, kidneys, and liver. In Chinese medicine, many skin problems are treated by strengthening the function of these organs.

To keep our skin healthy, it is most important to take good overall care of ourselves, as the skin's well-being is dependent on the health of the rest of the body. Drinking adequate amounts of water may be the single most important factor in healthy skin and good eliminative functions. Two quarts of quality drinking water per day is the suggested average, but this may vary for different individuals, according to a number of factors. More water is needed with a rich, fatty diet than with a diet high in fruits and vegetables; more with a greater activity level than with a sedentary lifestyle; more with hot, dry weather than with cold and damp more in summer than in winter; and more with constipation than with normal bowel function. We must each find our own balance of fluid intake. It is wise to drink regularly upon awakening, between meals up to about a half hour before eating (it keeps the appetite down, too), and whenever thirsty. **Water is the best liquid for us, followed by herb teas, fruit juices (ideally diluted some), and mineral waters; avoid caffeinated beverages, sugary drinks, and soda pops.**

NO SMOKING! for healthy skin. The smoke and chemical irritation, besides causing a variety of serious medical conditions, causes rapid aging of the skin, especially around the mouth and eyes. Smokers notoriously have many more age lines around those areas than nonsmokers of the same age. The effect of tobacco smoke on the aging process is due mainly to an increase in free radicals, which are damaging to the skin cells in the dermis as well as to the cells in the inner organs and tissue linings. Smoking has a drying effect

Increased Water Needs	Decreased Water Needs
Rich, fatty diet	Diet high in fruits and vegetables
Activity and exercise	Sedentary
Hot, dry climate	Cold, damp climate
Summer	Winter
Constipation	Normal or loose bowels

and also exposes smokers and others to many toxic chemicals (such as carbon monoxide) and metals (such as cadmium), which may cause more chronic irritation internally. For similar reasons, avoiding or protecting ourselves from other chemicals—at home, at work, and especially in foods and pharmaceuticals—is also important to healthy skin.

Ultraviolet light, including sunlight, is known to be damaging to the skin and results in more rapid aging and dryness of the skin, as can be seen in many a farmer, construction worker, or sun worshiper. The ever-growing changes in the ozone layer over the past 50 to 60 years make sun exposure more dangerous than ever. Care must be taken with sunbathing or using sun lamps, because excessive ultraviolet light exposure can eventually reduce skin elasticity and tone. Along with dehydration or nutrient deficiencies, this may lead to rapid skin aging.

Skin care with moisturizing and beauty products requires a fine balance between nurturance and chemical exposure. I recommend natural products whenever possible. A number of companies now produce natural skin care products that can help rehydrate dried skin, relubricate skin with oils, and protect the skin from heat, cold, chemicals, and the sun. Sunscreens are popular now, but I have a concern about the damaging and carcinogenic effects of excessive use of chemically based sunscreens. Here again, the natural and skin-nurturing products may be better overall. Beauty creams with aloe vera, clay packs, herbal wraps, honey or egg white facials, and dry-brush massaging are some ways to clean, detoxify, and nurture the epidermis. Saunas and sweats are also helpful in clearing impurities through the skin. Herbal facials and steams are great for opening and cleansing facial pores.

Diet and Supplements

The diet that supports healthy skin includes high-nutrient, high-water-content foods such as fresh fruits and vegetables. These important foods should be consumed daily, as fresh fruits eaten alone in the morning and vegetable salads at lunch or dinner. Cooked vegetables with proteins or starches are also recommended. The essential fatty acids found in the vegetable oils, seeds, and nuts are also necessary to nourish the skin and keep the texture and vitality strong. Cold-pressed olive oil and flaxseed oil are some of the best sources of essential fats. Olive oil is stable to moderate heat; however, flaxseed should only be used uncooked. Some of the cold-pressed polyunsaturated oils, such as safflower, soy, and sunflower, can also be used in moderation (and should be used fresh; oils go bad with age) but should not be used for frying or cooking; sesame oil can be used in cooking, sparingly. (Some manufacturers make refined and/or conditioned, organic versions of these oils, and their use in frying and high-heat cooking may not be as problematic.) Some cholesterol-containing foods, such as eggs, poultry, and occasionally even meat, may be used. Fresh fish is one of the better, slightly lower-fat (on average) animal foods, and also contains healthful oils.

Water is important to help carry nutrients throughout the body and to flush out toxins. Adequate protein intake, along with good protein digestion and assimilation, is essential to make available the amino acids vital to tissue building and rapid cellular turnover in skin. Two amino acids, L-cysteine and L-proline, are especially important here. A high-fiber diet consisting of whole grains, legumes, and vegetables is helpful to detoxify the colon regularly and prevent accumulation of toxins going through the body causing tissue toxicity, which can lead to problems in the skin. Vitamin A and beta-carotene foods are helpful to skin health, as are zinc- and silica-rich foods. (See chapters 5 and 6.)

Supplements for healthy skin include a multivitamin and mineral, antioxidant nutrients to counteract free-radical damage, and the essential fatty acids. Fiber, such as bran or psyllium seed husks, helps prevent colon stagnation and general body toxicity, which easily affect the skin. Vitamin A and beta-carotene are

Skin-Supporting Nutrients	
All amino acids	L-proline
B vitamins	Olive oil
Beta-carotene	Omega-3 fatty acids
Biotin	(including EPA)
Calcium	Selenium
Cod liver oil	Silica
Essential fatty acids	Vitamin A
Fiber	Vitamin B6
Flaxseed oil	Vitamin C
Gamma-linolenic acid	Vitamin E
(GLA)	Water
L-cysteine	Zinc

important to in preventing acne, blemishes, and dry skin and may help to prevent skin cancer. Vitamin A deficiency can lead to all kinds of skin problems. The antioxidant function of beta-carotene is useful as well. Ascorbic acid (vitamin C) provides more antioxidant free-radical protection in the blood and body fluids and helps to reduce some of the aging effects of smoke or chemicals. Vitamin E and selenium also perform this function, especially with regard to fats. Selenium may also reduce the risks of skin and other cancers. Zinc is needed in cell repair, for DNA, RNA, and enzyme production, and to keep the immune function strong. Silica is thought to strengthen the skin, hair, and nails; after all, it is highly concentrated in the coverings (skins) of most fruits, vegetables, and grains.

The B vitamins are also essential to healthy skin. Niacin, pyridoxine, riboflavin, and thiamin deficiencies are all associated with skin disorders. Biotin supports skin health, as it helps the body synthesize fats and proteins and utilize carbohydrates. Vitamin B6, or pyridoxine, is needed for cell division and protein synthesis, both important skin functions. Essential fatty acids are vital to skin tissue health; these are found in many oils, such as olive and flaxseed oils. Cod liver oil is high in vitamins A and D and other nutrients, but it also may concentrate impurities. Eicosapentaenoic acid (EPA), the main omega-3 fish oil, also has some nourishing qualities for the skin, besides protecting against cardiovascular disease. Gamma-linolenic acid (GLA), as found in evening primrose and borage seed oils, does the same and has been used successfully for some cases of eczema and as a mild anti-inflammatory. **The amino acids are essential to protein building, cell division, and tissue health and repair and are certainly important to well-functioning skin.** The sulfur-containing amino acids, such as L-cysteine and methionine, are especially important skin amino acids. Tyrosine and copper help in skin and hair pigmentation.

Common Skin Conditions

Skin problems include dry skin, dandruff, acne, poison oak or ivy and other types of contact dermatitis, and psoriasis. There are, of course, a variety of bug bites or infections that generate self-limited skin eruptions. Some, like staphylococcus infections, which commonly cause painful boils, may require the use of antibiotics or a more long-range detoxification/blood-purifying program in addition to topical care of the problem. See *The New Detox Diet* book for specific guidance in this area.

Dry skin. This fairly common problem can give rise to painful cracks and fissures, or at least a look of low vitality. Dry skin may result from poor nourishment, dehydration, or soap and chemical exposure. Certain hormonal problems, such as low thyroid function, could also lead to xeroderma (dry skin). With dry skin, more water is usually indicated, as are the essential fatty acids. Supplemental olive or flaxseed oil internally and externally is usually helpful. A supplement formula with vitamin A and beta-carotene, the B vitamins, and zinc is also useful.

Dandruff. This is a form of dry skin of the scalp. It often results from an improper diet high in certain fats, such as hydrogenated fats and fried fats, and deficient in important essential fatty acids, which are found in the vegetable oils and fresh nuts and seeds. Poor water intake and lack of proper oils usually underlie a dandruff condition, which is also more common in people who overuse their minds with a focus of energy in the head (from a Chinese medicine perspective, this makes the head too hot and dry). Food allergies/reactions or deficiencies of the B vitamins, beta-carotene, and such minerals as zinc are also possible causes. Seborrheic dermatitis is a specific oil-based irregularity of the skin and scalp. Selenium sulfide shampoos (such as the

brand Selsun Blue) are often helpful in the treatment of dandruff. An overnight olive oil wrap may remoisturize the skin and clear the snowstorm. To apply such a wrap, shampoo and let hair almost dry, or just dampen it slightly. Apply cold-pressed olive oil and massage it into the scalp. Wrap with a towel and sleep, then shampoo in the morning. Additional amounts of such nutrients as vitamins A, B6, C, E, zinc, selenium, and essential fatty acids may help correct the dandruff problem from the inside out.

Acne. This common problem in teenagers results from a combination of hormone stimulation, production of irritating fatty acids by certain bacteria, stress, and poor diet. Acne vulgaris (the medical name) is tied to an overproduction of the oil in the sebaceous glands of the skin. More water intake, eliminating fried foods and hydrogenated fats from the diet, and taking extra vitamin A and zinc will often reduce acne outbreaks. Food allergies and intestinal yeast overgrowth also seem to increase acne problems (possibly from the biotoxins produced in the gut and absorbed into the body). Extra essential fatty acids, such as 1 or 2 tablespoons of cold-pressed flaxseed oil daily, plus the B vitamins, extra pantothenic acid, calcium, and sulfur, may help. Aloe vera gel applied to the skin, and goldenseal powder and comfrey compresses may protect and help heal the acne sores. Such oral antibiotics as tetracycline (the most commonly used), a topical erythromycin gel, or a dangerous pharmaceutical, Accutane, can be effective in more serious, nonresponsive cases of acne. The latter is a last resort, since it has more health risks with its use.

Insect bites or contact (allergic) dermatitis. From plants, chemicals, or metals, contact dermatitis may respond to local application of various poultices, such as baking soda or clay or goldenseal root powder, applied to the skin and covered with a bandage. This is often beneficial for poison oak sores, for example. Increased levels of vitamin C, often with additional A and zinc, may be helpful for insect bites. Higher levels of thiamin, or vitamin B1, such as 50 to 100 mg 2 or 3 times daily, may repel insects such as mosquitoes or fleas as they dislike the thiamin odor that is eliminated through the skin. The other B vitamins should be taken along with B1 to prevent imbalances.

Psoriasis. This more complex problem, associated with well-demarcated raised red patches on the skin with a silvery scale, most commonly occurs around the elbows and knees—that is, at the hard or stressed surfaces. It may also appear around the scalp and, in fact, can occur anywhere. Its exact etiology is not known, although psoriatic skin does show rapid cell division—it is skin that is growing too fast. Whether this is an immunological, genetic, or stress problem (or a combination) is not known for certain, although stress definitely seems to aggravate psoriasis. A recommended treatment plan for this condition includes relatively a low-fat and low-protein diet; more high-water-content, high-nutrient foods; extra vitamin A and/or beta-carotene, zinc, vitamin C, bioflavonoids, good quality fish oils for EPA and DHA, and liquid lecithin; in addition, use a sulfur-based ointment reg-

ularly on the lesions with alternate applications of aloe vera gel. Light therapies may be a helpful treatment as well. Following some of the guidelines in the antistress program may also be helpful.

Herbs

Herbs useful in maintaining healthy skin or treating some conditions include comfrey leaf and root (not readily available nowadays), topical aloe vera gel, yellow dock, horsetail (in springtime), licorice root, parsley, cayenne pepper, and garlic. Comfrey's healing properties help strengthen tissues of the skin, tendons, ligaments, and bone. This herb can be used both internally and externally. Yellow dock and cayenne

---

Skin Enhancement Program

Nutrient	Amount	Nutrient	Amount
Water	2–3 qt	Copper	2 mg
Protein*	50–75 g	Iodine	150 mcg
Fats*	40–65 g	Iron	10–18 mg
Fiber	10–15 g	Magnesium	300–500 mg
Vitamin A	5,000–10,000 IU	Manganese	10 mg
Beta-carotene	15,000–25,000 IU	Molybdenum	500 mcg
Vitamin D	400 IU	Selenium,	200–300 mcg
Vitamin E	400–600 IU	as selenomethionine	
Vitamin K	150–300 mcg	Silicon	200 mg
Thiamin (B1)	25–50 mg	Sulfur	400–800 mg
Riboflavin (B2)	25 mg	Vanadium	200 mcg
Niacin (B3)	50 mg	Zinc	45 mg
Niacinamide (B3)	100 mg	L-amino acids	1000 mg
Pantothenic acid (B5)	250 mg	Essential fatty acids	1–2 tbsp
Pyridoxine (B6)	50 mg	from olive oil and on	
Pyridoxal-5-phosphate	50 mg	food through the day	
Cobalamin (B12)	100 mcg	Flaxseed oil, or evening	2 tsp as supplement
Folic acid	800 mcg	primrose oil	4–6 caps
Biotin	500 mcg	EPA/DHA omega-3s	2–3 caps twice daily
Choline	500 mg	from fish oil	
Inositol	500 mg	*Lactobacillus*	1 billion or more
PABA	100 mg	*acidophilus*	organisms per
Vitamin C	2–4 g		dosage
Bioflavonoids	250 mg		
Calcium	600–800 mg		
Chromium	200 mcg		

* With increased caloric needs, and for bigger and more active people, these numbers may be higher to maintain 30% fat (9 calories per gram) and 12–15% protein (4 calories per gram).

work mainly to help detoxify the liver and blood. Parsley acts as a diuretic and may help clear toxins as well. Licorice aids the digestive and adrenal functions. The cortisone-like activity from the adrenal glands helps the skin tissue maintain its tone and elasticity. However, excess cortisone, usually from medicines, may cause very bad stretch marks (striae) and many other side effects. Garlic is also a purifier, and it is known to reduce skin cancer potential.

In his fascinating book *The Scientific Validation of Herbal Medicine,* Daniel B. Mowrey recommends an herbal skin formula for general cleansing or itching and dry skin of many disorders, such as acne, eczema, and psoriasis. It includes chaparral to cleanse and decrease mutagenic cells; dandelion root for liver and blood detoxification; burdock root and yellow dock root for blood purification (these are often helpful for eczema); echinacea for immunological support (it also reduces boils and skin ulcers, helps cleanse lymph, and stimulates white blood cell production); licorice root; kelp; and cayenne. This is a powdered formula taken in capsules, from several a day for maintenance or purification up to 10 to 12 a day to treat particular skin conditions. A steam facial using flowers such as rose petals is cleansing and relaxing. Boil a pot of water, drop some rose, calendula, or marigold flowers in it, and sit over the steam with a towel over your head for 10 to 15 minutes. Follow with a little lotion or your preference of skin care products.

The general program for skin enhancement shown in the table on the opposite page is intended for people with dull or lackluster skin, dry skin, or a chronic skin condition. Aspects of other programs, such as the antistress program (see page 597), the antiaging program (see page 588), or the detoxification programs outlined in chapter 18, may be combined with this program. Smokers should follow the very specific nicotine detoxification program that is provided in my book *The New Detox Diet.* Remember, too, that worry and extreme emotions tend to increase the aging process and wrinkle the skin. To take good care of our skin, we should take care of the whole body. Focus on this program for a few months. Evaluate your skin and general health before and after, and work to incorporate healthy habits, such as drinking adequate amounts of good-quality water, exercising, and eating well.

13. SEXUAL VITALITY

Although most species use the sexual act for procreation, humans may be the only one for which sex is a pleasure, a sport, and, for some, an obsession. Along with money, hunger, and desire for power, sex is a primary motivating force. It is a basic instinctual urge that all humans experience at some time, and the sexual/sensual component of a relationship is often necessary to keep it strong and healthy. Many changes have occurred in the sexual focus since the late twentieth century. It is no longer oriented just to erections, marathon sex, and multiple partners, although those aspects might be the interest for some. We now have more responsibilities for our own and each other's health. Safe sex—not transmitting diseases or creating unprepared-for pregnancies—is definitely both sensible and in vogue. Condoms are back, birth control is important, and knowing your partner is crucial to health. There have always been some built-in dangers with sexual activity, from syphilis to gonorrhea to herpes and AIDS. As the dangers grow, often so do the mystique and adventure of sexuality.

People are more monogamous today, attempting to focus on loving and supporting one another, looking more for growth and learning and less for control and dependency. Sexual vitality is important and often secondary to relationship vitality; love that bonds us must reach many levels, emotional and spiritual as well as physical. Few relationships last over the long term that are based on good sex alone, just as few endure without a decent sexual relationship. Ultimately, love is the overriding principle, and with love, physical sharing and enjoyment are humanifest.

Stress and nutrition are important factors in sexual vitality. Stress, particularly mental stress in the form of worry, overwork, and financial concerns, can interfere with sexual energy and expression. Sexual problems themselves can be a source of anxiety and unhappiness. Resolving relationship problems and getting over relationship changes or loss of a loved one often requires some psychological assistance to come out of isolation into the comfort of intimacy. Guilt can also be a big psychological block to adequate sexual energy. In many situations, there has not been a clear emotional separation from a parent or a previous loved one, and subconscious feelings of incest or adultery may be undermining the experience. Fears of certain fantasies becoming reality may also create anxiety interference. There are all kinds of potential sexual problems. In this section, however, I concentrate more on supporting a healthy sexual function rather than the wide range of sexual dysfunctions and infertility.

The so-called sexual potency drugs—including Viagra, Levitra, and Cialis—have gotten quite popular with some men. These add, for the user anyway, a decreased anxiety over erection failure and a strengthened comfort with sustainability in the pleasure of lovemaking. Well, maybe here it is not fully about love but about performance. Of course, love has a lot more to do with chemistry, caring, and sharing; many people in loving relationships go on to bear offspring, further solidifying and creating a life of partnership. With this comes more issues and challenges along with more joys and successes and the mutual responsibility of caring for the children in a positive, loving way and as good examples of healthy living, physically and emotionally.

These erection-enhancing drugs that affect blood flow to the genitals and penis clearly work, and the use of these drugs has certainly altered men's sexual interactions with women and/or other men. As with other drugs, they can sometimes bypass the real correction of the cause that generates the problem in the first place. For example, a drug like Viagra (sildenafil) works by allowing nitric oxide to continue acting on the blood vessels to the penis, keeping them dilated and maintaining the increased blood flow that is necessary for erection. But this blood flow and the activity of nitric oxide are also influenced by stress, and by diet, and by long-term lifestyle practices that may need to be addressed. I am concerned that science is failing to address some of these root-level issues when people can gravitate so quickly to a drug to "solve" a problem. There can also be side effects with the use of drugs, including heart stimulation, headaches, and gastrointestinal upset. Some men report that their wives and partners are not as excited as they are about their better and longer-lasting erections. Many of these women wish for a more balanced lovemaking, with more heart and hands, lips and love. Used in their lower dosage levels, however, these drugs are bringing more fun in the bedroom to pleasure-seeking

humans. My motto is always "Use the minimum meds to get the desired effects."

For normal sexual function, we need healthy organs and a balanced, working endocrine system that produces the necessary hormones. Low pituitary function may lead to decreased development of the sexual organs, early menopause in women, and impotence in men. Weak adrenals may reduce the desire and strength for sex and increase sensitivity to stress. Low thyroid may cause a lack of desire or capacity for sex. In men, low testicular function decreases sex drive and sperm production. In women, low estrogen slows sexual maturity, decreases breast size, and retards egg maturation. Estrogen-progesterone imbalance can create many menstrual cycle variations and symptoms.

For a fulfilling sexual relationship, women particularly need to feel love and to have energy without fatigue, a hormonal balance that allows peaceful emotions, and some level of relaxation with a good sex drive. Men need good circulation to create a penile erection, physical vitality, and good hormone function. Lust often encourages more passionate sex. This is most common early in a relationship, when fantasy and sensuality arouse the sexual desires of both partners. But for a longer run and repeat performances, some other qualities must be present in the relationship. A big obstacle to a sexual relationship that is satisfying long-term is boredom or complacency. Becoming used to each other, along with the little day-to-day irritations or conflicts, can easily interfere with the sexual energy of either or both partners, and soon, sex may be a rare occurrence, decreasing in frequency from daily or weekly to monthly, or even less often. Bringing a feeling of freshness, fantasy, romance, and new energy into the relationship and bedroom can often revive the sex life. Creativity in a relationship is important.

There is no reason why sexual activity has to decrease as we age, although for most people, it usually does become less frequent. The changes that come with age still allow sexual function; realistically, however, it is not the same as it is in a young person. Women have lower hormone levels later in life, unless they go on hormone replacement therapy, but they can still maintain sexual vitality and drive, with or without hormones. Men usually have less decrease or a less distinct cutoff in hormone levels, which are

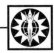

more necessary for their sexual function. As long as there is good circulation and cardiovascular health, both sexes can maintain a good sex life. Obesity, poor diet, mental and emotional stress, and cardiovascular disease are some common conditions that can interfere with sexual vitality.

The Chinese have a concept about the frequency of ejaculation and orgasm for men and women, which is described in the fascinating book *The Tao of Love and Sex,* by Jolan Chang. According to this theory, men are meant to have frequent erections, lots of sex, and only rare orgasms. Regular ejaculations drain the kidney/adrenal chi (energy) and possibly lead to fatigue, decreased vitality, or lower and mid-back tightness and weakness in men. When the adrenals are weakened, there is also lower ability to handle stress. Men can learn to have more complete orgasms without ejaculation with special techniques described in the book. Women are meant to have as many orgasms as they wish, which are energizing to them. And if the man is not releasing all the time, he will have more sexual vitality to satisfy his partner. Sound or feel intriguing?

Many other factors seem to affect sexual desire and performance. Alcohol, nicotine, coffee, marijuana, and sugar are some of the so-called pleasure drugs that may reduce sexual vitality, as can many pharmaceuticals, such as tranquilizers, antihypertensives (particularly beta-blockers), and birth control pills or hormones. Genetics, childhood upbringing, personal attitudes, and basic hormone levels may also influence sexuality, as can stress and an overfocus on TV. Men with higher testosterone levels and better adrenal function usually have more sex drive. For men and women, there are newer and apparently better testing methods to assess current hormone function; these involve using saliva measurements to look at tissue levels of progesterone, testosterone, cortisol, dehydroepiandrosterone (DHEA), and the estrogens: estradiol, estriol, and estrone. Ask your natural health practitioner about this testing as well as treatment with bioidentical hormones.

Stress levels also can interfere directly with sexual function and drive. Often, underlying worries about money, job, and so on, take our minds off sex. One study revealed that men who received raises or promotions at work increased their sexual frequency; the reverse happened to those who were demoted or whose pay was decreased. (For a deeper understanding of these stress aspects, see "Antistress" on page 597, earlier in this chapter. Further discussion of sexuality is found in the programs "Adult Men" (page 564), "Adult Women" (page 567), and "The Later Years" (page 581) in chapter 15, Life Stage Programs.)

Diet and Supplements

Nutrition also has a lot to do with sexual vitality, which clearly decreases with malnourishment. The focus of the diet for sexual vitality is on antiaging and a healthy cardiovascular system. A wholesome diet low in fat and high in fiber and complex carbohydrates is a good place to begin. Any diet (and lifestyle) that maintains good circulation and normal weight and contains high-vitality fresh foods will lead to better sexual function. A good protein intake is important, but excessive protein may interfere with sexuality. Likewise, adequate dietary fats and fatty acids are required for normal hormonal function. Cholesterol is a precursor of several sexual hormones, and if it is too low, this may lead to impaired sexual function and vitality. Regular exercise is also important to reduce stress and anxiety and support a healthy heart. Beware, however, that excessive exercise, especially in women, can reduce fertility, hormone levels, menstrual periods, and sex drive. Balance is important here as well.

Many of the foods traditionally believed to improve sexual function are from the ocean. Fish are thought to be good for brain and sexual function, especially shellfish, such as oysters and clams. This may be because of their high levels of zinc. High-zinc foods have been thought to support male prostate function; pumpkin seeds, an old prostate helper, are high in zinc. Also from the ocean come the very high-mineral seaweeds, which seem to support sexual function. Celery, especially celery root, is thought to be a mild aphrodisiac. Alternatively, such milk products as cheeses and ice cream may have a sedative effect on sexual energy. And many people, especially women, crave chocolate as their most sexually satisfying food, maybe more in the emotional sense rather than the physical.

There are many specific supplements that influence sexual vitality, particularly vitamin E and the just-mentioned zinc. Vitamin C, niacin, and the amino acid arginine also seem to support sexual function. Many glandular formulas are available, and some men and women may experience improvement with them. The idea that if we eat the organs or organ extracts from other animals to offer some essential help to our own corresponding organs is not a new concept and does make some sense, but there is no good research to substantiate the effectiveness of doing this. Animal organs eaten in this way would include brains, heart, stomach, and liver. In the natural products industry, glandular extracts—primarily from cows—include adrenal gland, thymus gland, and pancreatic gland products.

As for many other programs related to age and stress, a general multivitamin and antioxidant formula is a good idea. Extra vitamin E may be helpful for sexual vitality and fertility, but this has not yet been proven in humans. The essential fatty acids are important to tissue strength and membrane integrity and fluidity. Niacin, one of the active forms of vitamin B3, acts as a vasodilator, increasing blood flow to the skin and many other parts of the body. Some people also experience sexual stimulation from this niacin flush. Zinc seems to be especially related to male fertility and sex drive. Low zinc levels may lead to impotence, a low sperm count, and a loss of sexual interest. Taking more than 100 mg daily, however, is not recommended as this can reduce immune function and absorption of other minerals, such as copper and manganese. Prostate health and testosterone hormone production may also be influenced by zinc.

Vitamin C is associated with sperm motility, and male infertility has been related in part to vitamin C deficiency. Besides vitamin C, the bioflavonoids, along with vitamins A and E and the mineral zinc are important to healthy mucous membrane tissue and function. There is some good evidence that arginine, an amino acid, can be helpful with male infertility, because it acts to protect the sperm from oxidative damage and it simultaneously revs up some of the energy production processes in the sperm, making it more mobile. Like most amino acids, arginine needs to be supplemented in gram doses (2–4 grams a day) to achieve these kinds of therapeutic effects. Selenium may mildly stimulate sexual energy; manganese may also be related to sex drive; and molybdenum may have an as yet undetermined influence on sexual function. Pantothenic acid provides pituitary and adrenal support and thus indirectly improves testosterone production in men. Folic acid is a B vitamin helpful for both ovarian function and sperm production, and it, along with beta-carotene, vitamin E, and selenium, may reduce the production of abnormal cells. Iodine supports the thyroid gland function, which improves both the desire and the capacity for sexual activity.

A number of herbs seem to influence sexual function and enhance sexual vitality, in addition to the many botanicals that have been used for treating various sexual maladies. **Ginseng root is the classic example of a sexual strengthening herb.** It is used more for men than for women, although when the lack of sexual energy is a result of fatigue, ginseng may help

---

Nutrients for Specific Sexual Organs

Brain	Pituitary	Adrenal	Thyroid	Testes and Sperm*	Ovaries
B vitamins	B vitamins	Vitamin A	Iodine	Vitamin E	B vitamins
Choline	Pantothenic acid	B vitamins	B vitamins	Zinc	Niacin
Calcium	Niacin	Pantothenic acid	Thiamin	Vitamin A	Folic acid
Magnesium	Vitamin E	Niacin	Vitamin E	Vitamin C	Vitamin E
Potassium	Zinc	Thiamin	Tyrosine	Folic acid	Zinc
L-amino acids	Vitamin C				
Tryptophan	Vitamin E				
	Essential fatty acids				

* Sperm contains calcium, magnesium, zinc, sulfur, vitamin B12, vitamin C, and inositol, so these are likely important also. ATP (energy) is an absolute requirement for sperm motility, so nucleic acids, especially inosine, are important for fertility.

Sexual Vitality Nutrient Program	
Nutrient	**Amount**
Water	2 qt
Protein	50–70 g
Fats	50–75 g
Fiber	15–20 g
Vitamin A	5,000–8,000 IU
Beta-carotene	20,000 IU
Vitamin D	400 IU
Vitamin E	800 IU
Vitamin K	300 mcg
Thiamin (B1)	50 mg
Riboflavin (B2)	50 mg
Niacin (B3)	50 mg
Niacinamide (B3)	50 mg
Pantothenic acid (B5)	500 mg
Pyridoxine (B6)	50 mg
Pyridoxal-5-phosphate	50 mg
Cobalamin (B12)	100 mcg
Folic acid	800 mcg
Biotin	500 mcg
Inositol	500 mg
Choline	500 mg
Vitamin C	2–3 g
Bioflavonoids	250 mg
Calcium	650 mg
Chromium	200 mcg
Copper	women—2 mg
	men—3 mg
Iodine	225 mcg
Iron	women—18 mg
	men—10 mg
Magnesium	350 mg
Manganese	10 mg
Molybdenum	500 mcg
Selenium	200 mcg
Silicon	100 mg
Zinc	women—30 mg
	men—60 mg
Flaxseed oil	1–2 tsp
L-amino acids	1,000 mg
Inosine	150–300 mg

in both sexes. The aphrodisiac and sexual power capacities of ginseng, however, are only anecdotal and not supported by research; its main benefit may be its effects in supporting general vitality. Dong quai (*Angelica sinensis*) and fo-ti tieng (*Polygonium multiflora*) are two other herbal roots used in traditional Chinese medicine. Dong quai is a female herb that acts a blood purifier, an antispasmodic for cramps, and as a hormonal tonic. Fo-ti tieng is used more in males as a kidney tonic and diuretic and to enhance fertility. It is also used for blood sugar programs. Both herbs can be taken in capsules or boiled to make tea. Damiana leaf has a historical reputation as an aphrodisiac and a stimulant of sexual activity. Good-quality (fresh, dried) damiana has helped many people stimulate their sexual appetites. Saw palmetto herb is best known for its treatment of male prostate problems. It and damiana have been used together to enhance sexual health. Both are also employed for respiratory difficulties. Licorice root seems to possess some estrogenic properties and has been used in many female tonifying formulas. It may be useful for reproductive health and for treating infertility. Sarsaparilla root contains "building block" chemicals that stimulate the synthesis of steroid sex hormones. Maca, a South American herb, has some supportive qualities for improved sexual energy.

The "Sexual Vitality Nutrient Program" on this page lists the supplement suggestions for maintaining or strengthening sexual energy. Following this, along with a good diet, a low anxiety level, a little romance, and a springtime picnic with the one you love, will keep all your body parts alive from the top down and from your toes up. Keep loving yourself and others to feel young and lively.

14. ATHLETES

I am really excited about this program, partly because I like to think that I am an athlete. This program can really make a significant difference in the fine-tuning and longevity of the competitive athlete. The nutritional misconceptions among sports people are great, and the diets, protein concoctions, and vitamins they are taking might even be dangerous. Although there may be some differences between the bodybuilder and the marathon runner, they are both required to push their bodies to the limit. Increased activity levels, sweating, and tissue wear and tear require special support. Any intelligent athlete also should know how important it is to balance workouts with proper stretching exercises to maintain flexibility, and with toning exercises as well as some aerobic activity for cardiovascular health. Aerobic exercise—continuous, repetitive movement of large muscle groups (legs or the whole body) for more than 10 to 15 minutes—uses oxygen more efficiently, plus it burns fat. **Our maximum aerobic exercise heart rate (calculated simply) is 220 minus our age. Depending on our physical state, we will usually exercise at a range from 70% to 85% of our maximum.**

A concern I see in my practice is the ex-athlete, the retired sports professional or the college jock who was in training for years on a special high-protein, high-fat diet. Such people usually handle this type of diet well enough in their early years because of the high amount of exercise they did. When they enter the work world instead of professional sports and change their lifestyle but not their diet, however, they gain weight and clog their arteries. Changes in activity levels require changes in diet, both in total calories and in the types of food eaten. Ex-athletes need to keep exercising as well as change their diets to reduce the chances of early death from cardiovascular disease. No one should ever really become an ex-athlete anyway—exercise is for life, as it represents a commitment to health and longevity.

One of the big problems with athletes is that regular training and vigorous workouts allow them to get along with the worst kind of diet. The body uses up everything and needs more. Exercise is as important as (or more important than) a good diet, but implementing both together is the optimum; this duo is the best plan for weight reduction and maintenance. **Regular exercise improves metabolism and calorie/nutrient use and reduces risks of cardiovascular disease, osteoporosis, and diabetes, while it improves oxygenation and psychological attitude.** Competitive or professional athletes also require a balanced exercise program supported by proper nutrition.

Athletics is affected by a lot of nutritional controversies, and it may be hard for athletes to know what is good for them. High-protein diets, lots of meat, protein powders, salt tablets, special vitamin pills, and carboloading to prepare for endurance and competitive efforts—these are just a few of the topics. I do not support high-protein diets or protein powders, although in some cases these may be helpful. People in active training do have some increased protein needs, but too much animal protein and protein powders can stress the kidneys and contribute to toxic metabolic products in the colon and body. Salt tablets are almost always unnecessary—water and high-nutrient foods and occasional salted snacks will replace what is needed. Potassium and magnesium are required as much as (or more than) sodium chloride. High-fat diets are also contraindicated. Muscles need glycogen (a carbohydrate) for their fuel, and carbohydrates give us the sustained energy we need for athletic activity. Thus a basic complex carbohydrate diet is the healthiest focus, with some added special dimensions for training.

Regular vigorous exercise obviously increases the body's demands for most everything, particularly calories and nutrients. Exercise improves elimination and metabolism, which means the body needs to nourish itself regularly. Physical exercise is also a stressor that may increase free-radical formation, so that additional antioxidant nutrients may be required. The physical stresses of vigorous exercise may also cause tissue irritation and breakdown, which can be counteracted with natural anti-inflammatories, such as vitamins E and C and the enzyme bromelain, and with amino acids to build up the tissues again as well as with glucosamine products, which support joint tissue health. Regular sweating also causes the loss of many nutrients, particularly water, vitamin B_1, and some minerals—sodium, potassium, chloride, and magnesium are probably the most significant.

If all of these processes and nutrients are not balanced, nutritional deficiencies may result. Then injuries can occur more easily (and heal more slowly), and bone or muscle loss or breakdown may result—all of which interfere with athletic performance. We prevent injuries with proper care in nutrition, adequate stretching and warm-ups, proper cooldowns, and sufficient liquid intake. In the competitive world, the slightest changes may make a great difference—sometimes the difference between losing and winning. For professional athletes, of course, this could affect their livelihood.

A good diet for the athlete in training and for performance is centered on the complex carbohydrates—whole grains and their products (such as pasta), legumes, potatoes, and other starchy vegetables—along with some good-quality vegetable and/or animal protein, fruits, and a low-to-moderate fat intake. Nuts and seeds, ideally organic and raw (so the oils will not be damaged) are useful in the diet for the necessary and essential fatty acids; these can be eaten as snacks for sustained energy or with meals, such as sprinkled on a salad or stirred into oatmeal. Athletes, like everyone else, need a well-balanced diet with a high nutrient intake. The increased activity generates the need for a higher amount of calories, protein, and other nutrients than the less active person requires. For weight control or maintenance, the athlete needs to vary his or her calorie intake with the specific activity level. When the season is over or the athlete takes time off or just stops exercising for whatever reason, he or she needs to change the diet, consuming fewer calories, fats, and proteins.

A high-fat diet is definitely out for athletes. It slows them down and can increase the body fat percentage, something taboo for the active athlete. For many of us, the fatty flavor of foods is the more addictive aspect of the diet, and with any lessening of physical activity, the higher-fat foods will begin to clog the blood vessels and increase cholesterol and heart disease risk. **Athletes should definitely avoid fried foods, high-fat meals, lunch meats, bacon, ham, and any foods cooked in animal fats.** The higher-protein, lower-fat foods like fish and poultry are better than the red meats. Some nuts and seeds, high in essential fatty acids, nutrients, and protein, can be used as well.

Protein is important for athletes, but the subject of how much and which proteins are best needs clarification. Protein intake in general should be less of a focus in the diet. Excess protein intake can produce minor problems, including clogging of the colon and stress on the kidneys. More protein than is needed for tissue building and its other functions merely gets used for energy or must be eliminated. The complex carbohydrates, though, are used much more efficiently for energy needs or for storage for later use. So, for best efficiency and performance, I believe that a diet based on complex carbohydrates with adequate but not excess protein is ideal.

Athletes (and regular exercisers), however, need some extra protein with increased activity, but it should be increased in proportion to calories. People who are trying to gain weight, those wanting to build muscle, or those in heavy training need additional protein, sometimes up to 150 to 200 grams daily, to stay in positive protein balance, especially when the calorie intake goes up near 3,000 a day. Some protein powders and amino acid formulas can be used to augment the protein balance. Aerobic-type exercises may slightly increase protein needs but not as much as bodybuilding activities. Some extra protein intake, still along with a higher-complex-carbohydrate, low-fat diet, supports muscle bulk while maintaining body fat levels. Young athletes need even more good protein foods than adults but should still focus on the complex carbohydrates for proper development. Again, avoid high-protein diets that exclude other important foods, particularly the complex carbohydrates, fruits, and vegetables. For building muscle, it may be better in many cases (especially when extra calories are not needed) to use good-quality supplemental amino acids or protein hydrolysates containing peptides to provide the cells and tissues with what they need to build and repair, rather than eating an excess of heavier flesh-food proteins. Protein powder drinks and smoothies can also be nutritious.

Complex carbohydrates provide the sustaining long-term energy, proteins the tissue building, and fats (as the essential fatty acids) the lubrication and tissue support. This type of diet is also high in fiber, which allows good elimination. It is wise for serious athletes and health-conscious people to avoid excessive use of alcohol, regular cigarette smoking, and such stimulants as caffeine in coffee, tea, and cola beverages. Some iron-rich foods are especially important for female athletes or active runners, as their red blood cells may be broken down more rapidly. High-iron foods include red meats and liver (organic only), such shellfish as oysters, leafy greens, prunes, and mushrooms. With anemia, higher doses of supplemental iron are usually needed.

Carbo-loading is not a new concept in the athletic world, but many people still do not understand exactly how this process works. It is based on the fact that complex carbohydrates (such as grains, pastas, pancakes, and whole-grain breads) increase available energy, improving the stamina and ability to work. For example, 4 or 5 days before an endurance-type event, we increase our exercise and reduce our complex carbohydrate intake to about 40% to 50% of the diet and eat more protein, fats (such as dairy products and eggs), and fruit. This depletes the glycogen in the muscles and liver. Then, 2 or 3 days before the event, we increase complex carbohydrates to 70% to 75% of the diet, eating at least three big meals of carbohydrates plus some proteins and fats. This increases the stored glycogen in the liver and muscles. Glycogen, the storage form of glucose, is easily converted to the simple sugar that is used by all cells and tissues for energy. Glycogen is then burned first for energy; if more energy is needed, fat will be utilized, and that works well too. If there is very low body fat, proteins in tissues may also be converted to energy. All of these macronutrients will need to be replaced. Some athletes report that carbohydrate loading increases sexual energy too. For any athletes with fatigue, carbohydrates will often help. Adding more grains, pasta, cereals, breads, vegetables, and fruits may also add strength and endurance.

One of the biggest nutritional and health concerns in athletes is water depletion. With heavy training, be it strenuous or extensive activity, large water losses can occur, and drinking water is the only way to remedy this. Long endurance events also increase the need for fluids. Any activity where sweating occurs sets up an even higher requirement for water than the usual 1½ or 2 quarts per day. Water, which should be our main liquid, has many essential

functions. It supports the whole process of sweating and elimination of toxins, it nourishes the skin and other tissues, and it is the medium in which the blood cells circulate and everything in the body lives. Dehydration from low fluid intake leads to weakened tissue perfusion (circulation of blood with oxygen and nutrients), fatigue, and poor performance.

In addition to water, extra minerals must be replaced, especially the sodium, potassium, and magnesium that are lost in sweat. These can be added to the water or replaced with food consumed after exercise. Prepared fluid-replacement drinks are good in theory, but many contain chemicals and are overly sweet. For fluid replacement, it is best to avoid sugary drinks with artificial colors or even lots of fruit juices. Diluted fruit juices with minerals would be helpful. I use a vitamin C powder with calcium, magnesium, and potassium designed by Allergy Research Company/Nutricology and Emergen-C by Alacer (see Appendix B, "Nutritional Supplement Companies"), sometimes adding some powdered amino acids.

For long events, a little sweet liquid, such as fruit juice, can be added to water to provide some calories and energy. Some exercisers handle foods well and perform better during marathons and other activities, while others may not perform as well or may experience indigestion. Water should be drunk in the couple of hours before an event to hydrate the tissues and then, if there is extended competition or workout, sipped throughout the activity. **No colas, caffeine, or alcohol should be consumed before or during a race or any exercise. Salt tablets are also best avoided.** Nutritional supplements are often helpful in improving athletic performance. A good-quality, high multivitamin/mineral dosage is crucial, one whose total daily dosage is contained in 3 to 6 capsules or tablets, which are best taken several times daily to ensure regular availability. Many B vitamins, such as thiamin, riboflavin, niacin, and pantothenic acid, are lost more rapidly with exercise and need more frequent replacement.

Minerals are of major importance, as many are eliminated and need replacement to prevent muscle cramping, reduced cellular support, and other weakened physiological functions. Potassium chloride is lost through sweat during exercise. It is an important electrolyte for nerve conduction and muscle and heart function and is often useful in preventing

---

General Balanced Diet for Athletes

Carbohydrates—50% to 60% of total calories.
   10% to 20% simple—fruits, most vegetables,
      and any special "treats"
   40% to 50% complex—whole grains, legumes,
      and starchy vegetables
Proteins—15% to 20% (maximum 25%) of total calories.
   Animal—fish, poultry, meats, eggs, and dairy
   Vegetable—nuts, seeds, and legumes
Fats—25% to 30% of total calories.
   Saturated—meats, eggs, and dairy products
   Unsaturated (more than 50% of total fats)—
      nuts, seeds, vegetable oils, and avocado

---

spasms. Extra potassium, about 100 to 200 mg, is helpful after periods of exercise, along with potassium-rich foods eaten throughout the day. Calcium and magnesium are also important, a bit more so for women than for men. The calcium-magnesium cellular exchange supports muscle contraction and relaxation, nerve conductivity, cellular and bone strength, and delivery of oxygen to the muscles. From 600 to 1,000 mg of calcium and 400 to 600 mg of magnesium daily (above the diet) in two portions is suggested. Taking these supplements after exercise and before bed is the minimum. Iron is especially needed by women to maintain the red blood cells' hemoglobin to carry oxygen; iron is also part of the muscle protein myoglobin. Without enough iron, energy and endurance are usually poor. Chromium is also lost in higher amounts during exercise; at least

Nutrients and Exercise

- **Water.** Essential to cell respiration and circulation.
- **Antioxidants (vitamins A, C, and E; selenium, L-cysteine).** Protect against tissue, joint, and cell irritation by reducing free radicals and oxidation of fats.
- **Bioflavonoids.** Improve vitamin C effectiveness; serve as anti-inflammatory agents.

B VITAMINS

- **B1.** Generates energy.
- **B2.** Improves cell oxidation.
- **B3.** Energy metabolism.
- **B5.** Adrenal support; boosts energy.
- **B6.** Enhances performance by metabolism of amino acids and proteins.
- **Folic acid and B12.** Red blood cell formation; adequate oxygen delivery.
- **Biotin.** Carbohydrate metabolism; generates energy.
- **Choline.** Supports brain and nervous system.

MINERALS

- **Calcium.** Bone metabolism; muscle and nerve function.
- **Iodine.** Thyroid support.
- **Iron.** Blood cells and oxygen.
- **Magnesium.** Muscle and nerve function; with potassium, improves endurance.
- **Manganese.** Tissue strength and cellular function.
- **Potassium.** Muscle and nerve function; improves endurance.
- **Zinc.** Improves performance; growth and tissue repair.

AMINO ACIDS (ALL L- FORMS)

- **Leucine, isoleucine, valine.** Muscle energy.
- **Carnitine.** Fat utilization; energy generating.
- **Arginine.** Growth hormone; muscle building.
- **Lysine, ornithine.** Work with arginine.
- **Tyrosine.** Thyroid hormone and neuro-transmitter.
- **Tryptophan.** Good sleep.
- **Phenylalanine.** Improves mental performance; may reduce pain of exercise.
- **Aspartic acid.** Brain support.
- **Proline.** Tissue support.

OTHERS

- **Enzymes (trypsin, bromelin, papain, pancreas, superoxide dismutase).** Reduce inflammation.
- **Coenzyme Q10.** Supports heart function, aerobic energy production.
- **Octacosanol.** Increases stamina by sparing muscle glycogen and increasing the oxidative capacity of the muscle tissue long-term.
- **Liver.** Boosts energy.
- **Adrenal, heart, thyroid extract.** Individual organ support.
- **Dimethylglycine.** Improves oxygen utilization.
- **Gamma-linolenic acid.** Anti-inflammatory.
- **Inosine.** Energizing through ATP formation.
- **Organo-germanium.** Energizing through facilitating electron transport.

200 mcg is needed daily to help prevent or reduce any risk of sugar metabolism problems.

The antioxidant nutrients are important to reduce tissue irritations, inflammations, and loss of energy caused by free radicals. Vitamin A and beta-carotene, vitamin E, selenium, and vitamin C are all part of the athlete's performance enhancement plan. Loss of vitamin C, essential to connective tissue strength, is also increased with exercise. Joggers need extra C to prevent bone and ligament injuries, and ascorbic acid may be helpful in reducing all kinds of musculoskeletal irritation and injury. The vitamin C–mineral formula mentioned previously is not only useful for assimilating the vitamin C, it is also an easily absorbable formula that replaces several important minerals. A complete mineral tablet can also be taken with it. Silicon or silica, usually derived from the horsetail herb *(Equisetum arvense)*, is important for maintaining elasticity and flexibility in the tissues.

For adequate amino acids, a general formula of the L- forms (not D- or DL-) is best. Usually, 2 or 3 portions are taken daily, after exercise or after meals. An L-amino formula higher in L-tyrosine and L-phenylalanine may be more stimulating and physically energizing. L-proline supports the syntheses of collagen for membranes, ligaments, and tendons. Some extra magnesium and pyridoxal-5-phosphate (P5P), the active form of vitamin B6, may improve the metabolism of the amino acids in the liver and could be used as well after a workout. Other amino acids useful for athletes could be used only in addition to the general formula. L-carnitine is an important one. It is peculiar in that it is not used in the formation of body tissues and can be made in the liver and kidneys from other amino acids, methionine and lysine, along with niacin, vitamins B6 and C, and iron. It is found in few foods other than animal meats. Carnitine is thought to be helpful in preventing cardiovascular disease, aiding weight loss, and improving athletic performance. It aids in fat metabolism and energy production in the cells' mitochondria by improving utilization of fats. It is a good amino acid supplement for people who exercise.

The combination of L-arginine and L-lysine has also been shown to improve exercise endurance and strength, according to Rita Aero and Stephanie Rick in their book *Vitamin Power.* Taken together, 2 to 3 grams of arginine and 1 gram of lysine stimulate growth hormone and protein building. Other authors, such as Dirk Pearson and Sandy Shaw in their book *Life Extension,* have suggested an arginine-ornithine combination. These combinations help put the body into a positive nitrogen balance, meaning that more protein is being made in the tissues than is being broken down and eliminated. These can be taken together in an amount of about 1,000 mg each at night after days of heavy workouts, up to 4 or 5 times a week, when the other amino acids are taken as well during the day.

The branched-chain amino acids (BCAAs) are leucine, isoleucine, and valine—all of which are essential. In our bodies, these comprise about one-third of our muscle tissue. For people working on muscle building, supplementing the BCAAs can be helpful to this process. Having enough of these amino acids can prevent tissue wasting (protein loss) with exercise. Taking 1 to 3 grams of each of these amino acids has an anabolic (building) effect on muscle tissue similar to that experienced with steroid treatment, but without the risks and side effects (although they are also not as potent anabolically). When the BCAAs are used, it is necessary to take them together, about half an hour to an hour before a workout. Taking 50 mg of vitamin B6 or pyridoxal-5-phosphate, its active metabolite, aids the utilization of the BCAAs. It is also wise to take additional amino acids, including extra L-tryptophan and L-tyrosine, because the BCAAs are so rapidly used that they can interfere with the absorption of these other amino acids. A number of other supplements have been associated with increased athletic strength and endurance. None has been clearly shown to be effective by the little research done, but many an athlete has described feeling better when using these products. I leave it up to you to try these "bioenergetic boosters" and see what they do for you.

Octacosanol increases endurance by bolstering the oxidative capacity of the muscles and by helping us hang on to our glycogen stores as long as possible. It is obtained mainly from wheat germ oil, where it is found in high concentration. Bee pollen and other bee products, such as royal jelly, definitely provide some simple carbohydrate energy, and many people feel uplifted and supercharged when using them. They also provide various minerals plus possibly some yet-to-be-discovered power agents. Pangamic acid (see

"Vitamin B15" on page 136 of chapter 5, Vitamins) is no longer available in the United States, but it is highly touted in Russia for its healing powers and endurance enhancement. Dimethylglycine (DMG) is the form that people take now to get some of the pangamic acid precursors. Although it is not really clear how this product works, many people describe benefits from its use. Another precursor nutrient that I really like is inosine; used at a dosage of 300 to 500 mg daily, inosine helps to release oxygen from hemoglobin. It is the precursor of adenosine, which is the building block for production of ATP, the energy molecule for cellular metabolism.

I use OxyNutrients by Nutricology (also known as Allergy Research Group), based in San Leandro, California; see Appendix B, "Nutritional Supplement Companies" regularly and before exercise. It contains 150 mg of inosine per capsule, plus tridimethylglycine, L-carnitine, organo-germanium, coenzyme Q10, and more nutritional energizers. One capsule taken 2 or

Athlete's Nutrient Program

Nutrient	Amount	Nutrient	Amount
Calories*	2,000–3,500	Molybdenum	500 mcg
Water*	2–3$\frac{1}{2}$ qt	Potassium	2–3 g
Protein*	75–150 g	Selenium	250–400 mcg
Fats*	60–100 g	Silicon	100–200 mg
Vitamin A	5,000–10,000 IU	Zinc	women—15–30 mg
Beta-carotene	15,000–25,000 IU		men—30–60 mg
Vitamin D	400 IU		
Vitamin E	400–1,000 IU	**Optional**	
Vitamin K	300 mcg	L-amino acids	1,500 mg
Thiamin (B1)	75 mg	L-carnitine	500–1,000 mg
Riboflavin (B2)	25–75 mg	L-arginine	1,000–1,500 mg
Niacin (B3)	50 mg	L-lysine	1,000–1,500 mg
Niacinamide (B3)	100 mg	L-proline	500 mg
Pantothenic acid (B5)	1,000 mg	Branched-chain amino	1,000 mg each (before
Pyridoxine (B6)	50 mg	acids (leucine, isoleucine,	workouts with
Pyridoxal-5-phosphate	100 mg	valine)	50 mg vitamin B6)
Cobalamin (B12)	100 mcg	Bromelain	100–200 mg
Folic acid	800 mcg	Pancreatic enzymes	200–400 mg
Biotin	500 mcg	(after meals)	(1–2) tablets
Choline	500 mg	Lactobacillus	1–2 billion organisms
Inositol	500 mg	Dimethylglycine	25–50 mg
Vitamin C	2–5 g	(before exercise)	
Bioflavonoids	250–500 mg	Coenzyme Q10	30–60 mg
Calcium	600–1,000 mg	Flaxseed oil	2–3 tsp
Chromium	250–400 mcg	Gamma-linolenic acid	160–400 mg
Copper	2–3 mg	(GLA)	
Iodine	150–250 mcg		
Iron	women—20–25 mg	Octacosanol	2–4 capsules
	men—10–15 mg		(250–500 mg)
Magnesium	400–650 mg		
Manganese	5–15 mg	*Varies from women to men and with the extent of exercise.	

3 times daily or 2 to 3 capsules taken 30 minutes before exercise really makes a difference. I also use it in patients with fatigue or viral problems and typically receive positive reports.

Of course, inosine, CoQ10, carnitine, and other nutrients can support energy use in cells, which helps during all athletic performance. See "Energy Boosters and Stress Reducers" and "Metabolic and Cellular Aids" in chapter 7.

Various body therapies—such as massage, acupressure, and chiropractic skeletal alignment—have helped many athletes perform better. Sexual activity also may add that extra charge for better performance, but this is controversial. Many athletes avoid sexual relations before competition. It is, however, a very relaxing and energizing practice for some people.

Herbs have been used in many ways for the various problems encountered by athletes as well as for increasing performance. Ginseng root has been known to increase stamina. It is a general tonic and also has some antistress properties. Cayenne pepper is a natural stimulant that may raise the metabolism and increase energy levels. Comfrey is a common herb for musculoskeletal injuries. Used topically, it has some mild anti-inflammatory effects, and I have seen comfrey leaf work "magically" for healing sprains. To use it for this purpose, wrap lightly steamed leaves (or chew them and make a poultice) over the wound and then cover with a cloth. Leave on, if possible, for a few hours. Also, drinking an herbal tea containing comfrey leaf and the silica-containing spring horsetail can support the healing process. White willow bark contains natural salicylates and thus possesses anti-inflammatory properties. It is available in tablets or capsules and can be used like aspirin for sore joints or muscle aches. The enzyme bromelain, from pineapple, is available as a supplement; it too has mild anti-inflammatory effects and aids digestion of vegetable protein in the gastrointestinal tract.

Vigorous workouts cause muscle and tissue irritation and inflammation, which can lead to soreness after exercise. This is commonly due to lactic acid buildup and free-radical formation. Antioxidant nutrients, more water, and some anti-inflammatory nutrients and herbs may help reduce some of that soreness when it is bothersome. Also, warm baths, massage, and a long, slow walk can help restore the feeling of being loose and ready for more vigorous exercise. The research on the use of glucosamine sulfate (and glucosamine chloride) shows it helps in joint pain and stiffness, as it appears to be used by the body to support and build normal cartilage. It is taken at 500 mg 3 times daily and can be used at once, or in two portions as well. I have seen higher amounts, up to 2 or 3 grams daily help reduce other peri-joint inflammations like tendinitis and bursitis; chondroitin sulfate is also used often in formulas combined with glucosamine. Although some users find improvement, the research on chondroitin is less convincing as it does not appear to be very highly absorbed from the gut.

The "Athlete's Nutrient Program" on page 619 is designed for the serious athlete, as well as anyone who is regularly working out, to achieve top physical condition by improving strength, flexibility, and endurance. When we work out this way, it affects every other aspect of our life. The amounts listed for each nutrient are the day's total suggested intake, usually taken in several portions throughout the day. Good luck and keep exercising—it is worth it!

15. EXECUTIVES AND HEALTHY TRAVEL

This program is specifically for businesspeople with persistently high-stress lifestyles. I call it a program for "executives" because most of us associate executives with a busy life with lots of responsibilities and tight travel schedules, but any of us may fit into this category—we are all the executives of our own lives. While similar to the antistress program on page 597, this one focuses on a particular kind of stress—the high mental and physical demands placed on the "work athlete." These demands often include regular or varied chemical exposures, like inhaling carbon monoxide and other chemicals when driving on freeways; working in smoke-filled (not so common anymore) environments or offices with exposure to chemicals and poor ventilation; or flying in airplanes sprayed with chemicals. Such a lifestyle also may mean frequent eating out, creating a need for special nutrient protection (and enhancement), and regular travel by car or airplanes, especially across time zones, where jet lag may be a problem. **This program is for anyone whose**

demanding lifestyle means having peak energy and a clear head for longer hours than 9 to 5.

Many of the habitual stimulants add to already existing stresses. Coffee and doughnuts, let alone cigarettes, play havoc with all the body's systems and deplete its energies. Driving in traffic, exposure to smog or chemicals at work, quick snacks on the run, fast foods, sugary treats, big meals at meetings, a little extra alcohol—all are added stressors. With a poor diet, being too busy to exercise regularly or being out of touch with our own rhythms and needs, and the many stresses of work, we may soon be lying in bed trying to recover our energy and see where we fell off of our healthy life path. We all need to be aware of how the many factors of our lifestyles affect us, and then recover our balance through change. Anyone who smokes or drinks too much coffee or alcohol can refer to information about those particular problems in chapter 18, Detoxification and Cleansing Programs, and create a plan to stop, or at least reduce, the excessive use. This program will also help counteract some of the deleterious effects of those drugs and habits. **As a practicing physician, I often see that my first important role is getting overly stressed workers or martyred mothers to make their own personal health a higher priority, because they cannot do their best jobs working and parenting if their health is not strong.**

Most of us find ways to handle our lifestyle stresses from day to day or week to week. We may take little vacations every month or so. If we are strong and healthy to start with and take decent care of ourselves, we should be able to sustain a hardworking schedule almost indefinitely; from a spiritual perspective, though, we all need that special time, even a few weeks, every so often to reevaluate and reprogram our lives. For most of us, this occurs only every few years; for some it takes place yearly; others may always be in this process. Part of staying healthy is learning to listen to our inner voice and timing and to keep nourishing our essential being so that we do not need to break down or get sick to reattune.

The general executive nutritional plan includes food low in fat and high in nutrients and water content, with substantial amounts of fresh fruits and vegetables, whole grains, some animal or vegetable proteins, and adequate good-quality drinking water. It is wise to maintain the real energy

sources instead of relying on fake caffeine or nicotine stimulation, excess alcohol, and such sugary treats and sweets as candy or doughnuts. Occasional use is okay, but when any of these become a regular habit or a crutch, there is potential for trouble. It is also smart to avoid high-fat and fried foods, such as burgers, hot dogs, and other cured meats, as well as non-nutrient, chemical foods, such as soft drinks and refined baked goods. Basically, we need something more like the ideal diet discussed in chapter 13—a balanced diet of wholesome meals, with plenty of the fresh foods, especially in the spring, summer, and early autumn.

Eating out at restaurants, where lots of hidden chemicals or potentially dangerous substances, such as excess fats, salt, germs, or additives, may be in the food can be a real challenge. When traveling, I usually carry some of my regular foods with me on the plane and use them for snacks and nourishment over the first 1 or 2 days away, which is my danger zone for getting off my basic diet plan. I also carry water with me, as I do not drink airline or tap water, and drink lots of it. This helps prevent me from getting out of tune in bowel function and sleep patterns. If I will be eating in restaurants, I limit myself to one main meal daily and eat light snacks at other times. I also ask for sauces on the side and order some extra lemon wedges and olive oil. See more about safe and healthy travel in my book *The Staying Healthy Shopper's Guide.* It is also wise for the busy executive to take a moment to relax before and after meals, to let go of tensions or worries that may affect digestion. Gastrointestinal problems are not at all uncommon with the busy executive types. Because you may not have much time to go to the doctor, are you not better off taking care of yourself?

Regular exercise is, of course, essential for any hardworking executive. It reduces stress, helps clear toxins through sweating, and keeps us fit to continue our endeavors. And we would best adapt our attitude to view exercise as fun, convenient, and lifelong, rather than as a chore or hassle. There are a multitude of excuses that can interfere with the lifesaving and life-generating benefits of regular exercise. Qualities that we develop internally through exercise may also help us in our external life. For example, flexibility developed through stretching and yoga is essential to handling life's stresses. Strength gained from weight lifting, Nautilus machines, or calisthenics and endurance from

Healthier Choices for Dining Out

Meal	Avoid	Choose
Breakfast	Fried and scrambled eggs Omelets Bacon Sausage Baked goods Sugar products	Fresh fruit juice Fruit and yogurt Oatmeal Other whole grains Granola Soft-boiled eggs
Lunch	Hamburgers Hot dogs Fried foods Lunch meat sandwiches Alcohol	Fish Pasta Salad Fruit Cottage cheese
Dinner	Steak Ham and pork chops Heavy sauces Alcohol Rich desserts	Big salads Whole grains Pasta Vegetables Fish or poultry
Snacks	Soft drinks Candy bars Coffee Salted, roasted nuts	Mineral water Fresh fruit Vegetable sticks Raw, organic almonds

such aerobic activities as dancing, running, bicycling, or swimming will help get us through some of those tougher days. Swimming is especially nice because the water also has a tranquilizing effect.

All executives need a relaxation plan. Wisdom suggests an occasional weekend or at least a day away from it all to recharge, play, let go, and get our minds off business. Whatever helps us relax is worthwhile, whether it be reading, a walk in the woods, healthy exercise, going to museums, or hot baths. Plan ahead for this time, and keep the schedule! Good sleep is essential to staying on top of a demanding lifestyle. If sleep is a problem, check the antistress program on page 597 for advice. With extensive travel, a bath or hot shower, a steam, or occasional massage can be useful for staying fit. Massage can clear tensions and bring relaxation; I think it is an absolute necessity for a busy lifestyle.

When we feel stuck and want to change any area of our life—be it job, relationship, or location—counseling often facilitates the process of looking inward. It helps us get a clearer picture of our needs and desires and set up a new plan; therapists also may assist us to learn relaxation and stress-management skills. It may be that we need an update in our attitude so that we do not feel so trapped, or we may really need to change our life externally to create improved health and happiness.

The stress of a busy lifestyle increases the demands for many nutrients, so I recommend a multivitamin supplement. Extra B vitamins are essential for anyone under stress. Whereas the exercising athlete needs more minerals and amino acids, the "work athlete" needs more B vitamins to meet the different kind of mental stress and demands. The Bs are best taken 2 or 3 times daily, mainly after breakfast and lunch.

Vitamin C is also important, as stress eats up C as well as the Bs. Ascorbic acid, or buffered vitamin C if there are acid stomach symptoms, is best taken regularly 3, 4, or more times daily, 1 gram after each meal and before bed, along with extra calcium and magnesium at bedtime to help relax the nerves and calm the sleep. Calcium and magnesium are alkaline minerals, and they can buffer the mildly acidic ascorbic acid. There is also increased need for pantothenic acid as well as vitamin C to support the adrenal glands. Digestive enzymes may be helpful to aid digestion and the assimilation of nutrients. With long-term stress, adrenal glandulars may help support the counterstress functions. With exposure to chemicals and the general stress-induced, free-radical toxin production, the antioxidant nutrients are also needed daily. Vitamin A, beta-carotene, vitamin E, selenium, and zinc are all helpful for their protective functions. Amino acids may be helpful for busy executives on the go. A formula with a higher amount of tryptophan and less tyrosine and phenylalanine will be more relaxing, which may be particularly helpful when there is a lot of air travel. L-cysteine aids the body's detoxification processes and can be added as needed with travel.

A nutrient (supplement) program is important for busy people who fly regularly, including airline pilots and flight attendants. We must counteract the effects of many potential hazards, such as ozone and radiation exposure at high altitudes, cigarette smoke (less so now), lower oxygen levels, air pollution, alcohol, food chemicals, pesticide sprays, airport stress, and time-zone changes. Water intake to avoid dehydration is most important. The air inside a plane is dry and dehydrates us rapidly. Alcohol consumption adds to the problem, and coffee and nicotine are mild dehydrating agents as well. Thus constipation, headaches, and fatigue can result from the dehydration as well as from the stress effects of flying. Increasing fluids and vitamin C before, during, and after plane flights will definitely help. I usually take an herbal laxative (such as aloe vera capsules, a laxative tea, or a mixture of laxative herbs) when I fly. My whole life seems to back up when my bowels slow down. I often get a colonic irrigation (colon hydrotherapy treatment from an experienced practitioner using modern and sterilized equipment) before I leave for long trips. That usually makes the trip smoother, plus

I feel lighter and more positive. I also take extra B vitamins for travel stresses and additional antioxidants to balance out chemical and radiation exposures.

Flying across time zones, particularly from west to east against the sun, affects the body's natural biorhythms, nature's time clock. It changes the usual light cycle and thus affects the pineal and pituitary glands, which influence most of the hormonal and energy systems. Extra L-amino acids along with B vitamins and vitamin C help counter jet lag. A meal high in complex carbohydrates and additional tryptophan or 5-HTP along with extra water intake provides relaxation and good sleep. It is best to reattune our bodies to the new time zone, including eating, sleeping, and activity cycles, rather than to live in the old time. An L-amino acid formula with a high proportion of tryptophan is more relaxing, especially to the brain, than a formula with more tyrosine and phenylalanine, which compete with tryptophan in the brain and are more likely to be stimulating. But many people find that the tyrosine-phenylalanine combination, 1,000 mg of each, works better for them for jet lag. In *The Immune Power Diet,* Stuart Berger, MD, has noted that this amino acid combination, along with 1,000 mg vitamin C and 100 mg vitamin B6, taken before sleep, is what works best for him, especially after flying from west to east.

Extra L-tryptophan (500–1,000 mg) taken at night (or 5-HTP, 100–200 mg) along with vitamin C, calcium, and magnesium will help us to relax and get a good night's sleep. Melatonin is even more popular for handling jet lag and rebalancing with new time zones and proper sleep. Carrying a tape or CD player with some relaxing music can be useful during the flight and for sleep. Also, doing some exercise and stretching after landing, followed by a warm bath or sauna, a massage, and a light meal, is a great way to recharge in a new city and does wonders for jet lag. These approaches are integral parts of a jet-set lifestyle. Give them a try!

Some herbs may also help provide a calming effect during travel and with a highly stressed, busy lifestyle in general. There are two phases to this program—energizing and relaxing. To strengthen the active part of this cycle, such herbs as ginseng, a general tonic, or gotu kola leaf, a mental energizer, can be used. I might also suggest various coffee- or caffeine-substitutes rather than using and abusing coffee. Yerba mate is a mildly caffeinated herb that may be part of some

Executive's and Traveler's Nutrient Program

Nutrient	Amount
Water	2–3 qt
Fats	under 70 g
Vitamin A	5,000–10,000 IU
Beta-carotene	15,000–30,000 IU
Vitamin D	400 IU
Vitamin E	400–800 IU
Vitamin K	300 mcg
Thiamin (B1)	75–150 mg
Riboflavin (B2)	25–75 mg
Niacin (B3)	50–100 mg
Niacinamide (B3)	50–100 mg
Pantothenic acid (B5)	500–1,000 mg
Pyridoxine (B6)	100 mg
Pyridoxal-5-phosphate	50 mg
Cobalamin (B12)	100–200 mcg
Folic acid	800 mcg
Biotin	300 mcg
Inositol	500 mg
Vitamin C	4–6 g
Bioflavonoids	250–500 mg
Calcium	600–800 mg
Chromium	200 mcg
Copper	2 mg
Iodine	150 mcg
Iron	10–18 mg
Magnesium	350–500 mg
Manganese	10 mg
Molybdenum	500 mcg
Selenium	200 mcg
Zinc	30 mg
L-amino acids	1,500 mg
L-tryptophan (before bed)	500–1,500 mg
or 5-HTP	100-200 mg at bed
or Melatonin	1–3 mg

Optional

Adrenal glandular	100–200 mg
or ginseng root powder	250–500 mg AM
or Siberian ginseng	250–500 mg AM
Herbal relaxing formula	2 capsules or as directed

herbal stimulating formulas, such as Celestial Seasonings' Morning Thunder blend. Various mixtures of roasted roots, such as barley or chicory, are mildly stimulating but have no caffeine; Cafix and Pero are flavorful examples. The more calming herbs that may be helpful for the busy executive include valerian root and chamomile. These can be made into a tea or taken in capsules.

There are many possible nighttime relaxing teas or encapsulated formulas available. These are often a lot more helpful and healthful than using alcohol or sleeping pills, and they produce no hangover! A cup of warm chamomile tea or a mixture such as Celestial Seasonings' Sleepytime (even 2 bags per cup) drunk before bed often makes for a pleasant sleep. Catnip leaf tea is sometimes tranquilizing, as are linden flowers and hops. A homeopathic remedy called Calms Forte (available at most health food stores) also works well for aiding sleep; use as directed on the bottle. The "Executive's and Traveler's Nutrient Program" on this page can be used either on a regular basis or during periods of high stress. The total amounts can be spread throughout the day in 2 or 3 portions.

16. VEGETARIANISM

Some aspects of vegetarianism have been discussed in chapter 3, Proteins, and this type of diet was more fully described in chapter 9, Diets. In this section I explore the particular nutrient needs of those following a vegetarian diet. I also review briefly the many advantages and a few disadvantages of this most humane diet. Vegetarianism has a long history, and a primarily vegetarian diet is still the most common type on the planet. Even in the United States, most people's diets were mainly vegetarian until the turn of the twentieth century, when beef consumption began to increase; it has continued to increase steadily until only recently.

A change to a vegetarian diet automatically reduces intake of both protein and saturated fats unless there is a marked increase in the consumption of dairy foods and eggs. **One of the biggest problems with the contemporary American diet is the focus on (or obsession with) protein as the staple of the diet.** Although a protein-focused diet may help in the short term for weight reduction (mainly by filling up on meats and limiting higher-calorie carbs), this is probably responsible for the increase in cardiovascular diseases and cancer because it also naturally increases the intake of saturated fats. We can decide to return to a focus on whole grains, legumes, and vegetables to give us the high-complex-carbohydrate, high-fiber, high-nutrient, and low-fat diet that is so essential to good health and longevity.

Vegetarianism is indeed becoming more popular again. It has support from the American Heart Association and the American Cancer Society, who in their own subtle ways are finally acknowledging that diet is an important component of health and disease. Many more diet books and cookbooks now focus on the vegetarian diet, and more athletes, businesspeople, and others are adopting this diet and life-style plan. Vegetarianism makes a statement about both health and planetary consciousness. In his groundbreaking book *Diet for a New America,* EarthSave International founder John Robbins discusses the inhumane treatment of animals and the waste of resources (water and land) by the cattle and poultry industries. Our diet says a lot more about us than just our personal tastes, as Robbins pointed out in the book's subtitle, "How Your Food Choices Affect Your Health, Happiness, and the Future of Life on Earth." We could all stand to be a little more vegetarian even if we are not exclusively vegetarian. Supporting the current carnivorous planetary program creates pollution, economic imbalance, and relative starvation. I believe we must change this for the health and peace of future generations.

In my experience, vegetarians often adopt many other positive health habits in addition to eating more naturally. Those who are vegetarians more for health than for religious reasons tend to eat wholesome foods, avoiding the refined flour and sugar foods and other empty-calorie treats that are also vegetarian "foods." Even the Seventh-day Adventists, the most celebrated group of vegetarians, at least in the medical literature, could have a much healthier diet and better statistics if they would adopt these principles. Still, as a group, they have lower triglyceride and cholesterol levels and a lower incidence of cancer, heart disease, and obesity than the meat-eating population. A decrease in chronic diseases and an increase in longevity go hand in hand with vegetarianism.

Among the potential disadvantages of vegetarianism is that a diet without flesh foods often makes it more difficult to balance the intake of all the necessary nutrients, particularly protein, vitamin B12, iron, and zinc. Calcium deficiency, in general a big concern, seems not to be as common in vegetarians as had once been thought. Adequate protein can easily be obtained, as discussed later in this section. Vitamin B12, or cobalamin, is consistently a problem for vegetarians, especially for the pure vegetarian, or vegan, who eats no animal foods at all. Vitamin B12 is most plentiful in red meats, and some is found in other animal foods, but most plant proteins are fairly low in this "red vitamin." Brewer's yeast, tempeh (fermented soybeans), and some sprouts have small amounts of B12. Vitamin B12 deficiency leads to poor metabolism of protein, fats, and carbohydrate; problems in building the coverings of nerves; and a low red blood cell count, called *pernicious anemia.* Fortunately, though, B12 is stored in the tissues at levels high enough to last for several years of low intake. A vegetarian's body, or the body of anyone who has a particularly low intake of a nutrient, will naturally develop better absorption of that nutrient. Few long-term vegetarians whom I have evaluated have had low blood levels of vitamin B12. Extra B12 as a supplement (the sublingual tablets or liquid are currently the best source of oral B12) usually prevents any deficiency unless there are problems with the stomach making the substance known as *intrinsic factor* or with the liver's ability to store this vitamin (see the discussion of vitamin B12 on page 125 in chapter 5, Vitamins).

A vegetarian diet can also be an important part of a good therapeutic plan for many problems. It is more cleansing or detoxifying than the usual higher-fat and higher-protein diets, because it usually contains a greater percentage of dietary fiber and the watery fruits and vegetables. In terms of the body's nutritional cycles of cleansing, building, and balancing, the vegetarian regime is effective in cleansing, beneficial in balancing if it is well-planned and implemented, and generally less effective in its building powers. For that reason, **I do not recommend a vegan diet for children or teenagers or during pregnancy or lactation,** periods during which I feel more building and strengthening are needed. The lacto-ovo type of vegetarianism, though, should work fine. It might be wise for all of us to eat a vegetarian diet every so often, such as 1 or 2 days a week, 1 week a month, or even more often during spring and summer. Variations of the vegetarian diet can be used for detoxification as discussed in chapter 18, Detoxification and Cleansing Programs. A fast or cleansing diet may be a useful remedy for many types of congestive problems. With sickness, though, I usually suggest more complex carbohydrates in the diet, with higher intake of water and water-containing foods; this helps avoid dehydration and usually improves vitality.

Some people choose vegetarianism for spiritual reasons, however, feeling that it elevates them to their higher vibrational levels, more finely attuned to the universe and its energy, and enhances sensitivity. These folks belief that eating meats and animal foods pulls them down into the earthly realms of sexual instincts, aggression, and desire for power. Often, someone eating a completely vegetarian diet may choose to move away from the busy, active life of the city, where the hustle and bustle requires a more aggressive energy. When I lived for years in the country as a vegetarian, the locals used to describe going into San Francisco on business as a "meat loaf" day.

The vegetarian diet composed of organically grown foods comes the closest to following the general nutritional guidelines recommended throughout this book. **A high-fiber, high-complex-carbohydrate, nutrient-rich diet composed mainly of whole grains, legumes, vegetables, fruits, nuts, and seeds provides all the nutrients we need.** Whether vegetarian or not, this should be the basic foundation of all health-oriented diets. It is also more alkaline and higher in most vitamins and minerals than any other type of diet. Only small amounts of milk products, eggs, or various animal fleshes might be added to the vegetarian diet to make it easier to obtain the necessary calcium, iron, zinc, and B12.

Protein is always the big topic of discussion when it comes to vegetarianism. Eating complementary proteins, such as grains or seeds with legumes, or eggs or dairy foods with any of the vegetable proteins, is the usual suggestion for obtaining adequate protein. Each specific vegetable protein is low in 1 or 2 of the essential amino acids, and when eaten alone it does not provide equivalent levels of all the essential amino acids required to build tissue proteins. When we eat some legumes (which are high in lysine and isoleucine and low in tryptophan and methionine) with grains (which

have the opposite strengths and weaknesses), we obtain all of the essential amino acids in more equal levels. If the digestion of proteins and the assimilation of amino acids and peptides are normal, then a minimum daily requirement of protein should be in the range of 40 to 50 grams (about 32 ounces of a bean like navy bean, or 6–7 ounces of a fish like halibut).

Several noted authors have suggested that we do not need to be as concerned about complementary proteins as was previously thought. Frances Moore Lappé, who proposed the idea of complementing proteins in her 1971 *Diet for a Small Planet*, now suggests that the body can find the needed amino acids when any plant protein food has been eaten over the course of the day. Although I have felt that this might be true, I have not seen any conclusive research, which might be hard to conduct, about this issue. But it would seem that when there is any malnutrition and subsequent deficiency or low body stores of certain nutrients, in this case amino acids, it would be more difficult to manufacture necessary body proteins from consistent meals containing incomplete proteins eaten over several days. In that situation, or when food intake analyses or blood tests suggest inadequate protein intake or assimilation, we then must focus more on protein consumption and possibly digestion. Otherwise, a balanced vegetarian diet should pose no concerns about the adequacy of protein intake.

Given the current knowledge and an attitude of better safe than sorry, I still suggest combining vegetable proteins at meals or at least in the same day to create a complete profile of essential amino acids. Protein deficiency, although much rarer than most people fear, can cause some problems. With a more stressful lifestyle or a high level of athletic activity, protein needs may be increased, and thus more high-protein foods are required. **Fatigue is a common problem in vegetarians with low-protein diets.** Weight loss and low body weights are also more likely with this type of diet. Another concern I have is that amino acids and proteins are important to the immune system. I commonly see lower white (and red) blood cell counts in vegetarians, likely because they do not have all the cell-building nutrients, particularly protein. If the immune system is weakened by a low nutrient availability, especially in combination with high stresses, infectious disease is much more likely.

In the digestive analyses of my patients, I also see a higher amount of parasites and intestinal yeast overgrowth present in the vegetarians. This may be because of the lower-protein and higher-sweet diet that appears more common with inadequate protein intake—more vegetable-based foods are higher in carbohydrates and sweet flavors, plus many vegetarians crave sweet foods. It may also result from a more alkaline system, which supports growth of parasites and yeasts, or low immunity. In most of these cases, I recommend a higher-protein, wholesome-food diet. I may even suggest the additional L-amino acids to ensure that all are present for immune functions, although most amino acid formulas are not "vegetarian derived." There are also many good-quality protein powders from milk or whey, soy, or rice (even hemp protein from the seeds) that can be used in smoothies to enhance the nutritional intake.

There is also some concern that a high-fiber vegetarian diet does not provide enough of such important minerals as zinc, manganese, copper, iron, and calcium, or that the phytic acid in grains combines with these minerals in the intestinal tract and reduces their absorption. Several studies have confirmed the fact that our bodies adapt when we shift over to high-fiber vegetarian diets, however, and our absorption of minerals like zinc, iron, calcium, and copper can increase as the body adjusts. Nevertheless, I recommend a good mineral supplement program to ensure that the vegetarian ingests enough of these nutrients. The mineral intake should be in balance, because a high amount of one mineral may interfere with the absorption of the others; this is especially true for zinc and copper or calcium and magnesium.

As part of the supplement program, I suggest a general multiple-nutrient formula, from vegetarian sources, of course. I suggest additional calcium and magnesium if there is low intake of dairy products. Extra vitamin D will enhance calcium absorption, and this is particularly important during the less sunny months and for those who avoid the sunshine. I encourage taking extra zinc (and copper and manganese to balance with zinc) because it is so important and dietary deficiencies are common, even in vegetarians. I often suggest additional iron, especially if the red blood cell count is low; menstruating women frequently need higher amounts of iron. It is wise for vegetarians to have

Vegetarianism Nutrient Program

Nutrient	Amount
Calories	1,800–3,000*
Protein	50–70 g
Vitamin A	5,000–8,000 IU
Beta-carotene	10,000 IU
Vitamin D	400 IU
Vitamin E	400 IU
Vitamin K	150–300 mcg
Thiamin (B1)	25 mg
Riboflavin (B2)	25 mg
Niacin (B3) or	50 mg
Niacinamide (B3)	50 mg
Pantothenic acid (B5)	100 mg
Pyridoxine (B6) or	50 mg
Pyridoxal-5-phosphate	50 mg
Cobalamin (B12)	100–250 mcg
Folic acid	400 mcg
Biotin	500 mcg
Choline	250–500 mg
Inositol	250–500 mg
Vitamin C	2 g
Bioflavonoids	250 mg
Calcium	500–800 mg
Chromium	200 mcg
Copper	2 mg
Iodine	150 mcg
Iron	men—15 mg
	women—25 mg
Magnesium	350–500 mg
Manganese	5–10 mg
Molybdenum	300 mcg
Selenium	200 mcg
Silicon	100 mg
Zinc	30 mg
Lactobacillus	2 billion organisms

Optional

L-amino acids	1,500–3,000 mg

* Depends on the size, age, and activity level of the individual.

blood counts done occasionally (every 1 or 2 years) to make sure that anemia is not developing.

Regarding supplemental vitamin B12, I suggest it for all strict vegetarians. It is contained in almost all multiple formulas, although even higher amounts are often wise, at least several times yearly for a month or so. Vitamin B12 may often help with problems of fatigue. If there is any problem with absorption (this can be checked by monitoring blood levels), vitamin B12 injections would be indicated—or at least the sublingual variety, which has better absorption through the oral mucosa. An amino acid formula or protein powder may also be useful if there is any fatigue, excessive weight loss, or concern about inadequate protein ingestion, digestion, or assimilation.

The "Vegetarianism Nutrient Program" on page 627 offers a basic supplement plan as insurance for those on a vegetarian diet. Some naturalists do not like to take vitamins, as they are not whole foods (they are extracts of foods or synthetic preparations), but in many instances I feel they are indicated. Vitamins are suggested here as a means for prevention of depletions and deficiency diseases. If we eat very well, balance our foods, maintain low stress levels, stay attuned to the body's functions, and occasionally test body nutrient states and biochemical functions, then we might be able to avoid supplementation. However, I recommend at least short-term periods, several times yearly, of more intense nutrient intake to ensure proper availability of all the micronutrients.

17. ENVIRONMENTAL POLLUTION AND RADIATION

There are many reasons for concerns about environmental pollution and radiation exposure in this day and age. This is more true around big cities, but even in the rural sections of the United States, air and water contamination is spreading, and pesticides are a danger everywhere. Unless we want to live in the wilderness, we need to be aware of many environmental toxins and learn how to protect ourselves from them; unfortunately, even the wilderness is likely to be contaminated these days. The air and waterways transport industrial and agricultural pollutants, and radioactive fallout may affect living things anywhere.

Environmental pollution has become a major political and health issue. There is a focus on short-term profits versus the health of the planet and its people. Many of the specific issues and individual environmental toxins, as well as the politics involved, are discussed in detail in chapter 11, Food and the Earth. Here I examine some of the specific toxins, but primarily I offer a general program on how to minimize, handle, and protect ourselves from the many environmental pollutants and their effects. Exposure to environmental pollution is inevitable. A healthy human can adapt to mild and periodic exposure to pollutants in the air, water, and food. Some chemicals are easier to avoid (or process) than others. We have more control over what we take into the body than what goes into the air and water. Making healthy food choices, such as organic produce and purified water, and avoiding food additives, cigarettes, and home chemicals can certainly diminish the risks.

Our immune defenses, gastrointestinal and liver functions, and other systems of elimination all play an important role in handling and clearing body toxins. With increased or prolonged exposure or with a diminished ability to handle chemical contamination for a variety of reasons, such as a weakened immune system or a liver overworked with excessive demands from processing certain drugs or consuming too much fat in the diet, our interaction with these toxins can have many damaging effects. The damage may range from mild tissue irritation or immune suppression to an increase in the formation of carcinogenic cells. If these processes continue unchecked, cancer could develop. (See chapter 11, Food and the Earth, for a discussion of chemical carcinogenesis and "Cancer Prevention" on page 640 in this chapter.)

Understanding the hazards and where and how we are exposed to these environmental dangers is an important beginning. Our greatest insurance is maintaining a healthy, functioning body and immune system through positive lifestyle habits, such as eating a wholesome diet, exercising regularly, minimizing stress, having good and refreshing sleep, and maintaining positive attitudes. Many nutrients in the diet as well as extra nutritional supplements can support needed functions and protect against possible dangers. This program is designed for people subject to regular (daily) environmental exposure, such as those living in a smoggy industrial city, as well as for people who are chronically or acutely exposed to particular chemical agents. These include artists, chemical workers, metal workers, electronics workers, people who use pesticides, printers, those exposed to X-rays (either as technicians or as patients), those who work around or at nuclear or other power plants, and those who work in department stores amid the perfumes, colognes, and cleaning chemicals.

The basic guidelines for staying healthy in an increasingly polluted environment involve avoiding certain subtle dangers, protecting ourselves against others, and taking positive personal and political actions. It is wise to live, if possible, where the air is relatively clean, or if we cannot do that, to invest in a home air purifier and to take protective supplements. Stopping smoking and avoiding others' cigarette smoke are also important steps. Making sure our water is clean wherever we live means testing it and possibly investing in a good-quality, solid carbon block filter or reverse osmosis water purifier to ensure that water, the most important nutrient, does not add to our contamination (see chapter 1, Water, for more information).

Buying and eating certified organic foods as much as possible will also help to minimize further exposure to pesticides and other chemicals used to treat food. Growing our own garden is an even better idea and will orient us toward eating more fresh, wholesome, and seasonal food. Avoiding overuse of chemicals at home is also a good idea, as is reducing exposure at work whenever possible. Commonly used steroid drugs can suppress the immune function and reduce the body's natural defenses in protecting us from toxins and microorganisms, leading to slower healing as well. These steroid drugs with their complex and suppressive effects should be avoided, and if possible, natural healing should be supported and encouraged.

Avoiding excessive sun exposure, especially of the face and particularly in fair-skinned individuals, is important. There has been a marked increase in skin cancer in recent decades, thought to be a result of the thinning of the ozone layer caused by air pollution with chlorofluorocarbons. This means that the sun's ultraviolet rays are less filtered and more dangerous now than they were in 1980. I suggest sunscreen (at least 30 SPF) whenever sun exposure will

last longer than an hour. Many natural sunscreens contain PABA, a B vitamin. (For more ideas on healthy survival, see the "88 Survival Suggestions" on page 785 in the Futureword.)

Our nutritional plan to counteract exposure to environmental pollutants and radiation begins with a diet that will keep us healthy and not compromise our immune functions with irritating or allergenic foods. That means a diet that provides adequate, balanced protein, is high in complex carbohydrates and low in fat and sugar, and includes plenty of fresh fruits and vegetables. A minimum of 4 to 6 glasses of purified water, as well, helps keep everything moving and favors elimination of toxins. Remember, dilution is the solution to pollution.

Taking "medicinal" baths can also be used for detoxification of certain pollutants and radiation exposure. Try a **salt-soda bath** following airline flights or long hours at a computer. Add 1 pound each of sea salt and baking soda to a hot bath; soak until the bath is cool. For an **energizing detoxification bath,** add 2 cups of apple cider vinegar to a hot bath; soak 15 to 30 minutes. This can be used for radiation exposure in place of salt-soda. **Bath therapy salts** are available in stores to add to bath water for relaxation and relief of muscle aches.

Because chemical bombardment can lead to a weakened immune system, an increase in allergies, and more symptoms and disease, avoiding foods high in chemicals is definitely part of the plan. Some people become hypersensitive to the chemicals in the environment as a result of chemical exposures, and foods can be a major factor. The most important food additives to avoid are the food colors found in so many artificial foods and the nitrates and nitrites used in cured meats, such as bacon, ham, bologna, and salami. Artificial flavors and other food additives, such as sulfites and MSG, should also be avoided.

Chlorophyll-containing foods, such as the greens—lettuces, spinach, chard, and kale—are good choices, as are the cruciferous vegetables, such as cabbage, cauliflower, broccoli, and brussels sprouts, which are thought to be anticancer foods (these should all be organically grown, however, as these skinless vegetables may concentrate chemicals). All of these foods, as well as most sprouts, are good sources of vitamin K. Foods rich in beta-carotene, like the cruciferous vegetables as well as carrots and sweet potatoes, will add more of this antioxidant nutrient. Some freshly made vegetable juice mixtures daily can be a vitalizing and purifying drink. Miso, a fermented soybean paste used for soup broth, is known to protect against pollution and radiation. Seaweeds, high in natural metal-chelating algins, are likewise useful antipollution foods. They are also high in minerals. Some authorities believe that yogurt and other fermented milk products help protect against pollution. Extra kelp (seaweed powder), brewer's yeast, or liquid lecithin may also give additional support.

Many vitamins, minerals, and other nutrients (in the form of a good-quality multiple) can counteract some of the actions of environmental toxins. The antioxidant nutrients decrease the potential of free-radical toxicity. Vitamin A provides immune support and tissue protection. Beta-carotene specifically reduces the carcinogenicity of many chemicals, especially airborne ones and the chemicals in cigarette smoke; it

---

Antiradiation Soup (Serves 2)

Created by Bethany Argisle

4 oz tofu, cut in small squares

1 oz kombu or nori, cut in strips

3 cups purified water

1 tbsp miso paste (or to taste)

1 lemon

1 tbsp toasted sesame oil (optional)

green onions, chopped (optional)

cilantro, chopped (optional)

1 1/2 cups cooked brown rice

Add the tofu and seaweed (kombu or nori) to boiling water and simmer for a few minutes. Stir in some miso paste for flavor (do not boil the miso), add lemon juice and the optional ingredients if desired, cover, and let sit for 15 to 20 minutes. Remove kombu; serve with brown rice—eaten separately or stirred into the soup. This macrobiotic dish was shown to reduce radiation sickness after the Hiroshima bombing and will probably protect us from some of the hazardous effects of X-rays and metal exposures.

---

also helps decrease the negative effects of ionizing radiation. Vitamin C protects the cells and tissues against the effects of water-soluble chemicals such as carbon monoxide, metals such as cadmium, and metabolic by-products such as carcinogenic nitrosamines made from nitrites. At least several grams of ascorbic acid daily are needed for this protection. Vitamin E (400–800 IU) and selenium (200–300 mcg) work together to protect the cells from pollutants including ozone, nitrogen dioxide, nitrites, and metals, such as lead, mercury, silver, and cadmium. For environmental protection, the sodium selenite form of selenium may not be as effective as the more direct-acting selenomethionine (selenium chelated with an amino acid), especially regarding its detoxifying function.

Many minerals are useful in this program. Zinc is probably most important as an immune strengthener and tissue healer necessary for the functioning of many detoxifying enzymes, thus helping to protect the cells from pollutant toxins. Zinc, as well as copper and manganese, function in the superoxide dismutase system to detoxify oxygen free radicals that might be generated from ozone and photochemical smog. Calcium and magnesium help to neutralize some colon toxins and decrease heavy metal absorption from the gastrointestinal tract.

The B vitamins are also important. A B complex formula with sufficient thiamin, pantothenic acid, and niacinamide is usually helpful. Niacin, the B_3 "flushing" form, has an interesting role in the purification process, especially with many chemicals and pesticides. A combination of taking high amounts of niacin and other vitamins and minerals, taking long saunas, drinking fluids, and engaging in a healthy amount of exercise offers a very purifying process. There have even been claims of improvement of symptoms from Agent Orange (a combination of 2,4-D and 2,4,5-T—a common herbicide and war agent used to defoliate jungles) toxicity with the use of this kind of detoxification program, which is usually carried out over periods of about 2 or 3 weeks. It can even be done on occasion after recent exposure or excessive drug intake (see "General Detoxification and Cleansing" on page 741, in chapter 18, Detoxification and Cleansing Programs).

Lipoic acid, a cofactor in the metabolism of pyruvate and an important antioxidant nutrient in its own right, is another interesting relative of the B vitamins.

It is not essential in humans, but it does have some medicinal effects and is safe. It helps protect the liver and aids in detoxification, particularly for the effects of radiation. On the antioxidant front, lipoic acid is tied in with the recycling of glutathione—a critical component in both detoxification and prevention of oxidative stress. This vitamin can be taken at levels of about 100 mg daily for these effects.

The sulfur-containing amino acids have a protective and detoxifying effect as well. L-cysteine, the primary one, may help neutralize many heavy metal toxins and toxic by-products (aldehydes) of smoking, smog, alcohol, and fats through its precursor role in the formation of glutathione, a tripeptide essential to the action of several important enzymes, particularly glutathione peroxidase. Because glutathione itself is not very stable or thought to be well utilized as an oral supplement, L-cysteine appears best utilized for this protective purpose. The NAC (N-acetyl-cysteine) version of cysteine is also an excellent choice here; 500 mg 3 times daily may support and protect the lung membranes. Methionine, another sulfur-containing amino acid, also has critical detoxification and protective functions. This role for methionine is based on its ability to act as a methyl donor—to provide a small organic compound, called a *methyl group,* which can be linked onto certain toxins and neutralize their impact in the body.

Fiber, both the insoluble type (such as wheat bran) and the more soluble (like psyllium husks) encourage natural detoxification in the colon, binding toxins and reducing absorption of metals. Another chelating fiber is the algin molecule sodium alginate, which comes from seaweeds. It can be utilized as a supplement to decrease absorption of minerals, especially the heavy metals and radioactive metals used in nuclear power plants and medical testing. The chlorophyll-containing algae, such as chlorella and spirulina, also provide this chelating effect, although more mildly than the alginate extracts. Several studies have shown a decreased absorption of radioactive strontium (Sr 90) as well as barium, silver, mercury, cadmium, zinc, and manganese with the use of oral alginates. Two other nutrients that are popular in antioxidant and antistress energizing formulas are the enzyme superoxide dismutase (SOD) and dimethylglycine (DMG). Although there has been little supporting research on the oral use of these nutrients (a bit more with DMG), many people who take them describe improved energy and mental clarity.

Regarding radiation exposure, the first suggestion is to avoid it whenever possible. Minimize irradiating medical tests. Particularly avoid medical body scans, which may require injection of radioactive metals such as cobalt 60, iodine 131, or technetium 90. With X-rays, shield the genitals and the thymus gland, an important immunological organ in the upper chest. When dental X-rays are taken, ask the dental technician for a thyroid (neck) screen. The dentist should have a lead "thyroid collar" available. Do not live near a nuclear power plant or an industry that employs radioactive wastes or toxic chemicals. Also do not eat fish caught from waters containing effluents from these factories. Frequent high-altitude airline flights increase radiation exposure. Avoiding irradiated food is also worthwhile, if for no other reason that to discourage ongoing use of radioactive materials like cesium 137 or cobalt 60 in our everyday lives. We don't yet know the lifelong effects of consuming irradiated food, but there are at least potential risks here that need more research follow-up. (See "Food Irradiation" on page 478 in chapter 11, Food and the Earth; see also my "88 Survival Suggestions" on page 785 in the Futureword.)

With any radioactive iodine tests or exposure to iodine fallout, take kelp or iodine for several weeks before and after the test to occupy the iodine-binding sites (unless, of course, this interferes with the test) so that the least amount of the radioactive element will stay in the body. Strontium 90 competes with calcium and also lowers vitamin D. Taking extra vitamin D, calcium, and magnesium plus kelp and algin, pectin and lecithin, and L-cysteine may reduce absorption and speed elimination to prevent strontium 90 from getting stored in the bones. Radiation causes many undesirable internal reactions, especially in the most prolific tissues, such as the gastrointestinal tract and skin. Radiation therapy may affect the appetite, tastes, and the ability to eat. Radiation is cumulative, and many things may add to it, from color TV and microwaves to X-rays and fallout exposure. We need a good protective program! When living in areas with high background radiation, it is wise to take higher amounts of antioxidants regularly.

Several writers have offered guidelines for protection against the effects of radiation. In *How to Get Well,* the pioneering natural-health author Paavo Airola in suggests a plan of high amounts of vitamin C with rutin (a bioflavonoid), extra pantothenic acid, brewer's yeast, yogurt, vitamin F or essential fatty acids, inositol and lecithin, and lemon juice or lemon peel. Another popular author, now deceased, Stuart Berger, MD, presents guidelines in *The Immune Power Diet* that include extra potassium, 1,200 mg of calcium, and 800 mg of magnesium in addition to his usual environmental protection plan of 4 to 6 grams of vitamin C, 600 IU of vitamin E, 100 mg of zinc, and 20,000 IU of beta-carotene. In *The Complete Guide to Anti-aging Nutrients,* Sheldon Hendler, MD, medical-school faculty member at the University of California San Diego, recommends vitamins C and E, niacin, and copper to protect against the effects of X-rays and environmental toxins. There is also some interesting research on potassium iodate (KI), a form of potassium that can prevent the thyroid gland from uptaking various forms of radiation. In 2002, for example, the county government in Westchester County, New York, handed out free KI supplements to anyone living within a 10-mile radius of the Indian Point nuclear power plant in that county.

In addition to mitigating damage from radiation, this program also helps against environmental pollutants, including a number of toxic chemicals, such as carbon monoxide, ozone, sulfur dioxide, and nitrogen dioxide from the air; various pesticides and volatile hydrocarbons; food additives such as nitrites and sulfites; and toxic heavy metals such as lead, cadmium, and mercury. Cigarette smoke is a big problem, mainly for those who choose to smoke or cannot quit, but also for the air supply and the production of these chemical-laden "cancer sticks." (See "Nicotine" on page 756 in chapter 18, Detoxification and Cleansing Programs.)

A number of herbs and food extracts can be used to help detoxification and decrease the risks from environmental pollution. The algins, mentioned earlier, help clear metal and radiation toxins. Fibers such as wheat (or oat) bran and psyllium seed husks help to increase toxin elimination. Alfalfa, rich in chlorophylls and vitamin K, may help reduce tissue damage with radiation exposure. Apple pectin also helps bind and clear intestinal metal and chemical toxins. In *The*

Environmental Pollution and Radiation Program

Nutrient	Amount
Water	2–3 qt
Fiber*	12–18 g
Vitamin A	5,000–10,000 IU
Beta-carotene	15,000–30,000 IU
Vitamin D	400 IU
Vitamin E	800–1,000 IU
Vitamin K	500 mcg
Thiamin (B1)	25–75 mg
Riboflavin (B2)	25–75 mg
Niacin (B3)	150 mg
Pantothenic acid (B5)	1000 mg
Pyridoxine (B6)	50–100 mg
Pyridoxal-5-phosphate	25–50 mg
Cobalamin (B12)	100–200 mcg
Folic acid	800 mcg
Biotin	500 mcg
Choline	1,000 mg
Inositol	1,000 mg
PABA	100 mg
Vitamin C	6,000 mg
Bioflavonoids	500 mg
Calcium	600–1,000 mg
Chromium	400 mcg
Copper	3 mg
Iodine	150–300 mcg
Iron	15–20 mg
Magnesium	350–650 mg
Manganese	15 mg
Molybdenum	600 mcg
Selenium, as selenomethionine	300 mcg
Silicon	100 mg
Zinc	60 mg
L-amino acids	500 mg
L-cysteine+	500 mg
L-methionine+	250 mg
Lipoic acid	100 mg
Chlorophyll	6 tablets or 2 tsp
Sodium alginate	300–600 mg

* A high-fiber diet and/or 6 g each of oat bran and psyllium husks.

+ Take with 3 times the amount of vitamin C.

Scientific Validation of Herbal Medicine, Daniel Mowrey, a PhD-level researcher with training in psychopharmacology, recommends a formula for environmental pollution including alfalfa, algin (from seaweed or algae), wheat bran, apple pectin, and kelp. These help to decrease the toxicity of chemical and metal pollutants; in addition, this high-fiber formula helps to reduce cholesterol levels and is often useful in treating colds and flus, where bowel elimination is so important. Extra vitamin E and fish oils containing DHA and EPA, as well as an antioxidant formula with additional vitamin C, may make this formula work even better. Of course, we as a culture must pay heed. Even our potential healing sources (water, food, oils, and so on) can become toxic when we do not care for Earth's environment.

The "Environmental Pollution and Radiation Program" on the opposite page concentrates on the nutrients that protect against damage by toxins and free radicals. These nutrients offer protection by providing immune support, antioxidant and anticancer effects, and detoxification. The amounts listed in the table are daily totals, usually taken in several portions over the course of the day.

18. IMMUNE ENHANCEMENT

The immune system is the most dynamic body component in determining our state of health or disease. It will be the basis, I believe, of future breakthroughs in medicine. There is a great deal of evidence from research demonstrating life's effects on human immune function and the immune system's influences on health. These investigations provide a continuous flood of knowledge about the sensitive balance and many levels involved in wellness. Psychoneuroimmunology, which provides a bridge between psychology and the nervous and immune systems, plays an essential role in medicine.

Our immune system constantly interacts with our internal environment, protects us from our external environment, and provides the inherent knowledge to sense the difference between friend and foe. For many reasons, including genetics and individuality, some of us may be overactive or not active enough in our defenses, which can create a variety of

health problems, such as allergies, infections, and cancer. There are many components to the immune system—organs, bone marrow, cells, antibodies, chemicals, and the nutrients that help nourish and generate them. The immune system protects us from viruses, bacteria, yeasts and fungi, foreign proteins, and cancer cells. It provides two kinds of protection: **innate (inborn) nonspecific immunity** and **specific learned or acquired immunity.** Specific immunity depends on humoral (antibodies and chemicals carried in the blood) and cellular (white blood cells) responses, which can be immediate or delayed.

The thymus-derived lymphocytes (T lymphocytes or, simply, T cells) run the cellular defense and the delayed immune reactions. T cells, specifically T-helper lymphocytes, guide the B cells to produce antibodies (each cell produces only 1 specific antibody), a process that takes a 3- to 5-day induction period, often the time of infection by new viruses. Reexposure to the same virus creates a more rapid antibody response. This is our important immune memory, and so-called memory B cells circulate in the blood to respond to subsequent infections. The T-helper cells stimulate immune activity, especially B cell activity, whereas the T-suppressor cells slow down certain functions such as antibody formation, usually after a problem has been handled.

Another important cell, which is neither a T or a B cell, nor a phagocyte, is the NK (natural killer) cell. The T lymphocytes also send messages to (and receive messages from) the macrophages and other phagocytes to attack virus-infected cells and foreign organisms, by either engulfing or marking them. Other T cells can also be cytotoxic (cell killing) to virus-infected cells. **All of these important T lymphocytes originate in the bone marrow and mature in the thymus gland, the "king" of the immune system.** B lymphocytes also originate in the bone marrow and may mature there, and in the spleen, lymph nodes, and elsewhere; they are programmed to become the antibody factories or the plasma cells, which are formed from B cells and also produce the specific antibodies.

Explaining the entire immune anatomy and interrelationships goes beyond the scope of this book, but a few relevant and explanatory notes are important here. The skin and mucous membranes, including the

633

Immune Anatomy and Functioning Components

Organ Tissues	Nonspecific* Defenses	Antigen-Specific** Defenses
Skin	Skin	Macrophages
Thymus gland	Mucous membranes	T cells
Bone marrow	Mucus secretions	T-helper cells
Spleen	Cilia	T-suppressor cells
Lymph nodes	Neutrophils	Natural killer cells
Tonsils	Lysosomes	B cells
Adenoids	Iron-binding proteins	Plasma cells
Peyer's patches	Other chemical mediators,	Antibodies—IgA, IgE, IgG, IgM, IgD
(small intestine)	stomach acid	Complement system
Appendix	Lysozymes in tears, saliva	Interferon
Liver		

* Not mediated by antigenic stimuli. ** Mediated through antigenic stimuli.

cilia (tiny hairs) lining these membranes and the mucus itself, are all first lines of nonspecific, physical defense by providing a physical barrier against invasion. The lymphatic system is the secondary circulatory system that removes foreign cells and proteins, eventually dumping them into the blood to be broken down and eliminated. **The lymphatic system itself has no pump and thus relies on muscle activity and exercise for the lymph to circulate.** That is a key reason why I believe that physical stagnation increases the chance of infections and, conversely, that exercise improves resistance.

Lymph nodes are storage sites for cells along the lymphatic system. There are hundreds of these nodes throughout the body. When infection is present, these nodes can commonly be felt in the area closest to the infection. Predominant lymph nodes are in the neck, groin, or axillary regions. The tonsils, adenoids, appendix, and Peyer's patches along the small intestine are other important lymphoid tissues. The lymphoid tissue in the digestive tract is known as GALT (gut-associated lymphatic tissue). The thymus, bone marrow, and spleen are all sites for immune cell maturation. The liver is also important to immune function, because it helps to detoxify many substances in the body that could be taxing to the immune system.

The phagocytic white blood cells are important in immune surveillance first as the frontline of defense patrolling the body. They engulf foreign substances and microorganisms and then can kill or dissolve them by their chemicals. The neutrophils and macrophages work through oxidative destruction. The NK cells kill by secreting a phospholipase enzyme, which dissolves the lipid protection of cells containing viruses or other germs. The NK cells may also release a series of chemicals called *interleukins,* such as interleukin 2 (IL-2), which act as mediators in T lymphocyte functions and proliferation as well as other possible functions. Neutrophils can use their niacin-related NADP oxidase enzymes to produce superoxide radicals and damage the bacteria to disable them. (This process is called *phagocytic burst.*) They can also use their myeloperoxidase enzymes to make equally lethal hypochlorite ions.

Zinc may help in the production and function of NK cells as well as T and B cells. Methods for measuring immune function continue to evolve. Traditionally, cell ratios have been used to measure function. (The ratio of T-helper cells to T-suppressor cells would be a good example here.) More recently, specialized tests like the measurement of IL-2 receptor–positive cells, have also become available. Leukotrienes and prostaglandins (E_2 series) are other chemicals implicated in inflammatory and allergic reactions. More of these are produced when the diet is high in arachidonic acid, found mainly in saturated animal fats. The complement system releases chemicals in the serum that can lyse, or break apart, antibody-coated cells and microorganisms. Lysozymes and enzymes in tears and saliva can also lyse certain microorganisms. Interferon is an antiviral substance produced by T lymphocytes and macrophages. Iron-binding protein in phagocytic cells also plays a role in protecting against certain infections.

As with other body systems, **immune balance is the key.** A number of important factors in life influence immune health; unfortunately, there are many more factors that suppress it than enhance it. The basic aging process usually reduces immune competence. Allergies and infections may do this also, although initially these may stimulate immune activity. Surgery, radiation, and chemotherapy, all standard Western cancer treatments, as well as some antibiotic therapy, can weaken immune function, which is not ideal for healing or future prevention of cancer. Stress responses, such as that caused by business activity or travel, can lower immunity, as can all varieties of intense emotional and psychological experience. Low self-esteem, emotional extremes, or loss of a loved one may reduce lymphocyte and NK cell numbers and function. Many drugs and chemicals can be immune suppressors—from steroids (and possibly steroid-like agents, such as excess vitamin D or progesterone) and other anti-inflammatory agents to sugar, alcohol, and marijuana. The external environment can also be detrimental to the normal functioning of the immune system. Photochemical smog, industrial chemicals, pesticides, and certain antibiotic residues in meats as well as a high-fat diet may tax the immune system further. Even excess intake of the polyunsaturated fatty acids (PUFAs) from vegetable oils may increase free-radical formation and affect immunity. Nutritionally, low protein intake and vitamin A and zinc deficiencies are most relevant to immune suppression; a deficiency of essential fatty acids and other essential nutrients (such as pyridoxine, pantothenic acid, selenium, and copper) may also contribute.

A major concern is that immune suppression or weakness can predispose us to infections as well as cancer; these diseases may generally deplete our energy level and vitality. Overwork, multiple stresses, and lack of rest, exercise, and sleep tend to deplete our energies, our strength, and our ability to defend ourselves, which leaves us more vulnerable to outside influences. I believe that these imbalances of lifestyle, along with emotional and other psychological factors, are the basis of immune weakness. Besides immune compromise, problems of hyperimmunity seem also to be more common nowadays. Allergies are the main example of immune overactivity; however, the autoimmune diseases appear more prevalent as well. In these diseases, such as thyroiditis (Hashimoto's), rheumatoid arthritis, and lupus erythematosus, the immune system aberrantly makes antibodies to the body's own tissues, which then leads to inflammation, pain, or malfunction of those organs or tissues, as the case may be. Researchers have a great deal more to learn about these autoimmune diseases (and allergies, for that matter) in the coming years.

A balanced and optimistic attitude, healthy lifestyle habits regarding diet, and basic care of the human body support the optimal function of not only the immune system but the entire body as well. There are not many specific agents that are clearly shown to increase immunity. Immune function is optimal when we supply the body with the necessary nutrients, take time to relax and recreate, and do not block and weaken our natural vital energy circulation with immune suppressors. Adopt more of these lifestyle-related immune supporters!

For whom is this immune enhancement program best suited? It can be employed by people with chronic fatigue, particularly secondary to viral infections, or by anyone with repeated illnesses or infections who needs a stronger immune defense system. People under stress, both physical and psychological, need to strengthen their immune systems. Anyone subject to several immune suppressors might benefit from this immune enhancement program, which is not really dissimilar from the programs for antiaging and cancer prevention. People who have cancer or have had cancer should include many of the recommendations in this program as well.

Our immune functions can be evaluated in a variety of ways. If we are healthy and full of energy and do not get many infectious diseases, it is not likely that we need any blood tests for our immune system; it is probably normal. But if we are easily fatigued or get recurrent colds, flus, or other infections by viruses, bacteria, yeast, or parasites, the immune system may be out of balance or deficient in one or more functions. The most common blood test that indicates immunological activity is a simple, inexpensive complete blood count (CBC). Particularly important is the white blood cell count (WBC). The differential count provides the percentages of the basic WBCs—polymorphonucleocytes (PMN-phagocytes), bands (PMN-precursors), lymphocytes (the immune directors, including T and B lymphocytes, although they are not specifically noted), and the other less common monocytes (scavengers), eosinophils (allergy cells), and basophils.

The specialized T and B cell study provides a sensitive index of the immune system. A complete test provides absolute levels and relative percentages of T cells and B cells, T-helper (TH) cells, T-suppressor (TS) cells, natural killer (NK) cells, and the helper-to-suppressor (TH-to-TS) ratio. This TH-to-TS ratio is currently the most generally used monitor of immune function. It may be elevated in problems such as infections or allergies, or decreased in other infections or in acquired immune deficiency syndrome (AIDS), where the T-helper cell counts are most crucial. The TH-to-TS ratio can be monitored over the course of certain illnesses to determine the effectiveness of treatment.

In healthy people, it is also thought to be among the better objective monitors of more subtle immune status. More specialized tests for evaluating immune status include cytotoxic tests measuring the cytotoxic activity of NK cells; memory lymphocyte immunosorbent assays in which lymphocytes can be tested to determine whether antibodies are produced in response to toxic agents, including heavy metals and other chemicals; and T cell response tests in which the stimulatory effects of toxins or drugs are examined. Other tests that may also be relevant in an immunological evaluation include antibody (immunoglobulin) levels, complement, interferon, routine blood and liver function tests, and allergy tests for both environmental and food allergens.

Reducing any active allergic response through avoidance, desensitization, and detoxification may help to reduce the immunosuppressant effects of existing allergies. More generally, avoiding chemicals and other immune suppressors may also minimize any immune function weaknesses. Further measures for immune support include the ideas presented under "Antistress" (page 597) and "Executives and Healthy Travel" (page

620). Intense as well as chronic, unrelenting stress and emotions are real concerns in weakening immunity. Preventive care in lifestyle, diet, and supplements is ultimately most important. The immune-supporting diet plan includes the commonsense suggestions discussed in chapter 13, The Ideal Diet, as well as suggestions from "Allergies" (page 704) in chapter 17, Medical Treatment Programs, as well as in "Antistress" (page 597) and "Cancer Prevention" (page 640) in this chapter. **A low-chemical, low-sugar, and low-fat diet is mandatory!** Regarding fats, avoid the saturated and hydrogenated oils and eat mainly the essential fatty acid foods, such as raw nuts and seeds. A rotating diet, without regular use of milk or its products, eggs, wheat, corn, sugar, and yeast or other specific foods to which one may be reactive/allergic is suggested.

Wholesome foods free of chemicals and pesticides are the best. Care must be taken to prevent food expo-

---

Immune System Suppressors

Aging

Airplane travel

Allergies (pollens, dust, food)

Chemicals in the diet and environment (phenol, formaldehyde, hydrocarbons, air/water pollution)

Chemotherapy

Drugs, recreational (alcohol, amphetamines, cocaine, marijuana, nicotine)

Drugs, therapeutic (cortisone and other steroids, anti-inflammatories, adrenaline, insulin)

Emotional extremes (depression, loneliness)

Excess iron

Food (overeating, high-fat diet including excess PUFAs, sugar)

Infections (viruses, bacteria, yeasts and fungi, parasites)

Lack of sleep

Malnutrition (especially in infants and the elderly) nutrient deficiencies (vitamins A, C, and E; B vitamins, especially B_5, folic acid, B_6, and B_{12}; zinc and selenium; essential fatty acids; protein)

Radiation

Stress (social, work, financial)

Surgery

sure to microorganisms, including parasites, as they may have a deleterious influence on immune health. Low chemical intake is important. This means avoiding both chemicals in foods and chemical consumptive habits, such as alcohol, caffeine, cocaine, marijuana, and nicotine—as is always the case for optimal health. A water purification system that removes chemicals is also a good investment for health (see chapter 1, Water).

Care must be taken to obtain sufficient dietary proteins and L-amino acids, which help form the immune tissues and antibodies. For proper protein production, adequate amounts of pyridoxine, pantothenic acid, folic acid, magnesium, and zinc are important. The essential fatty acids are also required for cell and tissue health. Excess protein and saturated fats, however, are clogging to the vascular and lymphatic systems and may suppress immunity. **Fasting and detoxification diets can strengthen immune functions and reduce immune overload and reactions, as can be seen in allergies and infections or autoimmune problems such as rheumatoid arthritis.** The reduced intake of allergenic substances and the cleansing of potentially allergenic materials from the body can reduce many symptoms and allow the T lymphocytes to restore balance and reduce their hyperreactivity.

Nutrients and Immunity

Regarding specific supplements, it is most important to prevent deficiencies of many vital nutrients, such as vitamins A and C and zinc, by following the previous suggestions and eating foods high in these nutrients. Additional supplements, if not excessive, are insurance, possibly in the face of poor digestion and assimilation, to provide adequate nutrients to the cells and tissues. Useful supplements for immune enhancement begin with a basic multiple that includes the essential vitamins and minerals plus the important antioxidant nutrients. If the multiple does not provide adequate amounts of the antioxidants (such as vitamin C, vitamin E, beta-carotene, zinc, and selenium), then an antioxidant formula or additional specific nutrients are needed to reach the optimum levels. Of course, this program is designed for those with some immune suppression or those who want to

---

Immune System Supporters

Adequate digestive function and digestive
    enzymes (bromelain, papain, trypsin)

Allergies, infections, and fever*

Amino acids (arginine, carnitine, ornithine, cysteine
    and glutathione, possibly lysine and taurine)

Breathing for best oxygenation and relaxation

Chemical-free diet

Chemical-free home and work

Dimethylglycine

Exercise, yoga

Fasting

Filtered, purified water

Herbs (garlic, licorice, echinacea, goldenseal,
    ginseng)

Immune-boosting vitamins, minerals, and other
    nutrients: vitamins A, B12, C, and E; copper,
    iron,** selenium, zinc, beta-carotene, bio-
    flavonoids, coenzyme Q10, dietary protein,
    essential fatty acids, folic acid, pantothenic
    acid, and organo-germanium)

Interpersonal love

Laughter

Low-fat, low-sugar diet

Meditation

Positive affirmations ("My body is healthy
    and vibrant")

Positive attitudes

Pyridoxine

Relaxing

Rotating diet

Self-love

Thymus glandular***

Wholesome foods

---

* May initially stimulate immune activity and then be suppressive.

** Excess iron can increase oxidation and weaken immunity.

*** Possibly also spleen, thyroid, and adrenal glandulars as long as these are free of pesticides and viruses that could cause disease.

---

enhance a sluggish immune system. **Vitamin C is probably the most important of the antioxidant nutrients.** A higher level of intake than usual, about

---

Immune Problems Related to Nutrient Deficiency

Nutrient *	Immunologic Problems Related to Deficiency
Vitamin A	Reduced cellular immunity, slow tissue healing, increased infection rate, lowered IgA levels (which affect defense at the mucous membranes).
Vitamin C	Decreased phagocyte function, reduced cellular protection, and slow wound healing.
Vitamin E	Decreased antibody production and response; with selenium deficiency, lowered cell membrane integrity.
Vitamin B5	Lowered humoral immunity, increased irritation of stress.
Vitamin B6	Lessened cellular immunity, slow energy metabolism.
Vitamin B12	Decreased lymphocyte proliferation and PMN bacteriocidal activity.
Folic acid	Reduced blood cell production, perhaps increased cervical cancer.
Zinc	Decreased T and B cell function and thymic hormones, increased infection rates, and slow healing.
Iron	Decreased cellular immunity and neutrophil activity. (Excess iron can also impair bacteriocidal activity.)
Selenium	With vitamin E deficiency, antibody response is lowered; increased cellular carcinogenosis.
Copper	Lowered resistance to infection.

* Adequate levels of these nutrients will support or enhance these immunological functions.

---

4 to 10 grams if tolerated, can help in antibody response and in some white blood cell functions. Vitamin C has been shown to increase production of interferon, a substance with antiviral and possibly anticancer effects. Vitamin C levels have been found to be commonly decreased in the presence of such situations as surgery, stress, and progressive disease, as well as colds and other infections, especially those of viral origin. In these situations, C is needed in increased amounts. The vitamin C complex nutrients, such as rutin and other bioflavonoids, may also have mild antioxidant, synergistic effects. Bioflavonoids appear to act with C to potentiate its anti-inflammatory properties and to improve cellular defense against various microbes. Quercetin, a type of bioflavonoid, has also recently been found to function as an immune supporter and antihistamine.

Two nutrient pairs—vitamin A and zinc, and vitamin E and selenium—are also essential. Selenium (as sodium selenite or selenomethionine) and vitamin E (as natural mixed tocopherols) stimulate antibody production and strengthen cellular immunity. Zinc and vitamin A are also needed for cellular immunity, increasing T cell activity and the function

of the phagocytic white blood cells. Both are important to tissue healing. Beta-carotene is useful as a vitamin A precursor, also aiding in wound healing and protecting against carcinogenesis.

Some B vitamins are particularly helpful. Vitamin B6 aids immunity and antibody formation and is probably the most important of the B vitamins. Vitamin B12 may help stimulate immune function, more readily when injected, as oral absorption is slow. Pantothenic acid is helpful in combating stress, and B1, B2, and B3 may give subtle immune help by providing a balanced complement of the B vitamins. This helps the overall antibody production. Folic acid is also needed for normal cellular function.

In addition to zinc and selenium, the most important minerals are iodine, iron, copper, and magnesium, although basic levels of manganese, molybdenum, and chromium are also important. Iodine is required in the neutrophil killing of microbial invaders. Iron improves resistance against infection by increasing cellular metabolic efficiency and immune activity; it supports the lymphocytes and neutrophils (phagocytes) and can improve bacterial killing. **Excessive iron intake, however, can also be immunosuppressive (it**

Immune Enhancement Nutrient Program

Nutrient	Amount	Nutrient	Amount
Water	2 1/2–3 qt	Iodine	150 mcg
Calories	1,500–2,500	Iron	10–20 mg
Protein	60–80 g	Magnesium	300–600 mg
Fats	50–75 g (20% to 30% of caloric intake)	Manganese	5–10 mg
		Molybdenum	300 mcg
Fiber	10–20 g	Selenium, as selenomethionine	300–400 mcg
Vitamin A	5,000–10,000 IU	Zinc	45–60 mg
Beta-carotene	15,000–30,000 IU	L-amino acids	1,000 mg
Vitamin D	400 IU	L-cysteine	250 mg
Vitamin E	600–800 IU	L-arginine	500 mg
Vitamin K	150–300 mcg	L-carnitine	500 mg
Thiamin (B1)	50 mg	Thymus gland	100 mg
Riboflavin (B2)	25–50 mg	Essential fatty acids or flaxseed oil*	3–6 capsules
Riboflavin-5-phosphate	25–50 mg		
Niacinamide (B3)	50 mg	GLA (using evening primrose or borage seed oil)**	3–6 capsules or 200–400 mg
Niacin (B3)	50 mg		
Pantothenic acid (B5)	500 mg	EPA (using fish oil)***	2–4 capsules or 200–400 mg
Pyridoxine (B6)	50 mg		
Pyridoxal-5-phosphate	50 mg	Organo-germanium	100–250 mg
Cobalamin (B12)	200 mcg	Dimethylglycine	50–100 mg
Folic acid	800 mcg	Coenzyme Q10	30–60 mg
Biotin	500 mcg		
Vitamin C	4–10 g		
Bioflavonoids	250–500 mg		
Calcium	600–1,000 mg	* Not necessary if 2 or more teaspoons of fresh (uncooked) cold-pressed vegetable oils are consumed daily.	
Chromium	200 mcg	** Use with allergies or inflammatory problems.	
Copper	3 mg	*** Use if blood fats are relatively high.	

increases oxidation), enhance microbial growth, and reduce phagocytic cellular activity. Copper also improves resistance to infection and should be increased to balance out zinc intake. Like iron, too much copper can have deleterious effects, so careful monitoring is important.

Water, fiber, adequate protein, and essential fatty acids (EFAs) are all crucial to a healthy body and immune system. Water helps to flush out impurities and, with fiber, helps to clear colon toxins. EFAs found in nuts, seeds, and vegetable oils, as well as gamma-linolenic acid (GLA), help increase the anti-inflammatory prostaglandin E1 (PGE1). EPA (eicosapentaenoic acid) can decrease the level of PGE2 prostaglandins, which can be inflammatory and irritating and may produce a false or unnecessary immune response that is part of many illnesses. A mixed-oil formula with a high proportion of EPA and GLA is probably best used here.

The antioxidants and other nutrients help counteract the free-radical irritants. These unstable, free-radical molecules include superoxides, peroxides, hydroxyls, singlet oxygens, and hypochlorites. Vitamins C and E are helpful modulators of free radicals in general; along with zinc, copper, and manganese, they help reduce superoxides through superoxide dismutase enzymes. Selenium supports the production of the enzyme glutathione peroxidase, which counteracts peroxides, stimulates immune response, and protects against many toxins. Riboflavin subtly assists at maintaining electron balance.

The sulfur-containing amino acids L-cysteine and L-methionine also trap free-radicals and part of a general antioxidant program. Other amino acids that are useful for immune enhancement include L-arginine and L-carnitine. L-arginine stimulates thymus activity and the number and activity of the T lymphocytes. L-carnitine, which can be synthesized from lysine with the help of vitamin C, also helps enhance immunity, possibly by stimulating the utilization of fats, thus increasing energy (ATP) production while preventing oxidation and free-radical formation.

For either immune suppression or protection from colds and flus, vitamins A and C and zinc are recommended. Together these nutrients activate the thymus gland and increase production of thymosin, one of the thymus hormones, which in turn improves T cell and natural killer lymphocyte numbers and activity. Thymosin injections can also be used to stimulate the cellular immune response. If stress is the key element that weakens immunity, then additional adrenal or thyroid glandular support may help. Other possible immune supporters we may wish to use include organo-germanium (Ge-132), tridimethylglycine (DMG), and coenzyme Q_{10}. OxyNutrients, formulated by Dr. Stephen Levine of the Nutriology Company (see "Appendix B, "Nutritional Supplement Companies"), includes all these plus other energy-enhancing nutrients.

When we are sick with an infection or we feel like we are getting sick, I suggest increasing the supplemented levels of vitamin A to 25,000 to 50,000 IU (just for a few days), vitamin C to 4 to 8 grams, and zinc to 50 to 100 mg. I would also add garlic, which is a natural antibiotic, and goldenseal, which is thought to improve immunity, to help clear wastes through liver tonification, and to have antimicrobial properties. When we are feeling better and ready for recovery, we can add ginseng root to help rebuild our energies. Licorice root is another herb that can be used for stress-related immune problems. It seems to support energy and adrenal balance and has been shown to improve interferon production.

It is a good idea not to reduce fevers unless they are high (over 103 degrees Fahrenheit). Fevers have a purpose, in both children and adults. They help in detoxi-fication, immune stimulation, and increasing metabolism and, in some cases, killing the microorganism. Intake of fluids and minerals needs to be increased with fevers to counteract the body losses. Exercise is also important to immune function. Regular activity increases the circulation of nutrients and the cellular immune components. And remember, muscle activity is necessary to circulate the lymph fluid. Circulation of blood, lymph, energy, thoughts, and feelings is important to the vitality and health of the body, mind, heart, and spirit, as well as to the immune system.

The "Immune Enhancement Nutrient Program" on page 639 provides you with a range of the many nutrients that support your health.

19. CANCER PREVENTION

Because cancer has become the plague (and big business) and among the greatest fears of the modern technological, chemical age, and because cancer treatment in general, other than for certain malignancies, has not to date been very successful, **prevention of cancer is the only sensible approach.** The relationship of diet to cancer came of age in the 1980s. With this new knowledge, we can clearly now do something about the threats of cancer for our future. Caring for ourselves and others as if we really love life and have a desire to live must be a centerpiece of our approach to preventing cancer! This involves avoiding toxins and making wise choices in our eating and other habits.

Chapter 11, Food and the Earth, contains a fairly detailed discussion of cancer—its genesis, potential offending agents, dietary concepts, prevention ideas, and so on. Here I focus more on general nutrition and supplements and their importance in preventing cancer. In the mid-1970s, it was difficult to find any major institutions, doctors, or groups like the medical associations or the American Cancer Society who would admit that there were any ties between cancer and nutrition. Today, the nutritional and environmental influences on the genesis of cancer, the second-biggest killer of the American adult population, have been fairly well accepted as key components in this disease.

The breakthrough came with the 1977 *Senate Select Committee's Dietary Goals for the United States,* which listed cancer as among the major degenerative diseases linked to improper diet (cardiovascular disease and diabetes are others). The committee's suggestions of lower fat, higher fiber, and more natural foods are definitely a part of the cancer-prevention diet today. An important report called *Diet, Nutrition, and Cancer,* compiled by the National Academy of Sciences and released in 1982, gave further credence to the relationship between diet and cancer and offered more specific dietary suggestions. And in 1988, the U.S. Department of Health and Human Services published a major manuscript by C. Everett Koop, MD, entitled *The Surgeon General's Report on Nutrition and Health.* It discussed the relationships between nutrition and our common degenerative diseases, including cancer. In 2003, the National Academy of Sciences, through its Institute of Medicine (IOM), related in their lengthy report *Fulfilling the Potential of Cancer Prevention and Early Detection* many nutrition-related factors as possibly associated with cancer and requiring our foremost attention. These factors included inadequate intake of fruits and vegetables, excessive intake of red meat and possibly dairy foods, too little fiber, too much trans and saturated fat, and a long list of nutrient deficiencies (of vitamins A, D, and E, beta-carotene, folate, selenium, and calcium). Soil depletion from agricultural practices leads to mineral depletions in food. But cancer is a multifactorial, multidimensional disease. Although nutritional and environmental influences are definite components, physiological, social, emotional, psychological, and spiritual factors are also important. Therefore, the prevention and treatment of cancer must deal with all of these aspects of life.

The aging process itself increases cancer risk, particularly if we have not taken good care of ourselves. Poor nutrition can lead to many functional problems, such as lowered immunity and slower cell repair. The increased exposure to carcinogens is no help either. (See more on this under "Antiaging" on page 588). To most of the medical profession, cancer prevention means primarily early detection—more exams, X-rays, mammograms, and biopsies—so that the necessary surgery, drugs, and radiation can be applied sooner to prevent an untimely death. Prevention of cancer is much more than early detection, however. It means not creating the disease in the first place. A good diet and stress management are important cancer preventives. A strong, healthy immune (defense) system

is also an essential part of this plan (see the previous section, "Immune Enhancement," on page 633). With a strong immune system, even the few cancer cells that might be regularly generated would be easily removed from the body. Put simply (according to current thinking), it takes both the disease of the cells and the failure of the immune system together to create cancer—in other words, the effect of potential carcinogens on an already unstable body.

Michio Kushi, author of the in-depth book *The Cancer Prevention Diet,* believes that cancer is caused not so much by carcinogens per se as by the imbalance in the body caused by improprieties of diet that allows the agents to create problems. He advocates the "unified theory of disease," which sees the internal imbalance between yin and yang as the primary cause of cancer and most diseases. It is this "duality" or seeing of body parts or diseases as separate from our entire being, that allows us to treat even the mildest of symptoms as an enemy and not as an ally trying to guide us in a new direction. As we continue to approach our health in this way, says Kushi, we create further diversions from unity and manifest more-difficult-to-treat acute and chronic problems. Cancer itself, as is true of most disease, can be seen as a lack of harmony with our environment and a diversion from our inner truth.

This cancer prevention program is suitable for most everyone, especially those in a high-cancer-risk group. That includes men and women older than 40 or 50 years old and people with a family history of cancer, especially women with a family history of breast cancer. Smokers, people with a dietary history that includes cancer risks, and those who have been exposed to known carcinogens will also benefit.

What really causes cancer? Is it a virus or genetic code, the effect of chemical carcinogens on cellular growth, or a weakened immune system? Is it a poor, cancer-promoting diet? Or does it have to do with the psychological factors influenced by stress, poor attitude, or low self-esteem? Scientists do not really know; cancer seems to be linked to all of these factors. Family history is definitely a factor, and if someone in our family has had cancer, that should increase our watchfulness for this disease and encourage us to use early detection procedures.

Discussion of cancer risks and promoting factors could easily fill a book. Here I keep it simple. The

"11 Key Cancer Risk Factors" table below lists the 11 main cancer risks. Next is a more extensive discussion of various factors that may add to our chances of developing cancer sometime in our lives. One of the difficult tasks in researching many cancer risks is that cancer can often take 30 to 40 years from the time of exposure to a carcinogen for it to manifest as a physical tumor. But the table clearly shows that the promotion of cancer involves almost exclusively diet, environment, and lifestyle. Problems that result from pharmaceutical medicines or viral conditions that weaken immunity and allow cancer to develop more easily are probably rarer. Usually we have some control over the factors that predispose us to these conditions. I was walking through an airport recently and the TV channel blurted out, "If you died from cancer, it was 70% likely that it was your fault." This stopped me in my tracks, so I listened as the report pointed out that most of the factors linked to cancer were ones we have control over—mainly diet and cigarette smoking.

---

11 Key Cancer Risk Factors

1. **Smoking.**
2. **Dietary excesses.** Fats (mainly saturated oils, fried polyunsaturated oils, and cholesterol); protein; and obesity (calories).
3. **Undernutrition.** Deficient fiber and nutrients such as vitamins C and E, beta-carotene, and selenium.
4. **Occupational chemicals.** In such high-risk fields as farm work, work in plastic manufacturing plants, and so on.
5. **Food chemicals.** Pesticides, additives, and hormones.
6. **Air and water pollution.**
7. **Excess sunlight and radiation.**
8. **Certain pharmaceutical drugs.** Estrogen, metronidazole (Flagyl), lindane (Kwell), or griseofulvin.
9. **Alcohol.**
10. **Viruses.**
11. **Psychological influences.** Such as personal changes, loss of loved one, grief, and divorce.

Smoking. Smoking, mainly of cigarettes, is a primary cancer risk and is correlated with nearly all lung cancer. It is also a factor in cancers of the mouth, throat, and larynx and possibly others. Pipe and cigar smoking produce higher incidences of mouth cancer but less of lung. Cigarette smoke acts synergistically with alcohol, asbestos, and other carcinogens in air, water, and food to further increase cancer risk and rates. It is likely that naturally grown tobacco rolled in untreated paper poses less cancer risk; the chemical production and treatment processes involved in manufacturing a pack of cigarettes are definitely an added cause for concern. Regular marijuana smoking may also be a factor in cancer, although more research on this is needed. **Cigarette smoking is clearly the largest and most preventable cancer risk.**

Dietary excesses. Excess fats in the diet definitely increase the incidence of breast, colon, and prostate cancer and possibly others, such as uterine or ovarian cancer. The fats of most concern include saturated animal fats, as found in meats and dairy products; fried or rancid oils; hydrogenated and refined oils, and cooked polyunsaturated fatty acids (PUFAs). Rancid oils and foods cooked in oils cause more free-radical irritation (as do high amounts of PUFAs), mainly from lipid peroxides, and these act as mutagens and carcinogens. Excess protein in some studies correlates with cancer rates, but most of the higher-protein foods also contribute to higher fat levels, and this type of diet often leads to more general body congestive and degenerative processes. **Obesity** is definitely correlated with higher cancer rates. Colon, rectum, and prostate cancer rates are higher in obese men, while obese women have increased risks of cancer of the breast, cervix, uterus, ovary, and gallbladder. It is not totally clear whether the risk is posed by the obesity itself, higher caloric intake, or by the many associated factors, both nutritional and psychological (overweight people tend to hold things in).

Undernutrition. Deficiencies of many nutrients are implicated in some cancers. Low fiber in the diet is probably the biggest culprit, mainly in the increasing problem of colon cancer. Slow transit time through the intestinal tract, allowing more contact with carcinogens, may be the main factor here. Many specific nutrient deficiencies have been correlated with various cancers. Vitamin A and beta-carotene deficits increase the incidence of lung and mouth cancer, especially among cigarette smokers, and are also implicated in cancers of the skin, throat, prostate, bladder, cervix, colon, esophagus, and stomach. Also of concern is selenium deficiency, which researchers now know may increase the risk of many cancers, mainly of the breast, lungs, colon, rectum, and prostate, as well as skin, pancreas, and intestinal cancer and leukemia. Vitamin C may reduce the carcinogenicity of nitrosamines and other chemicals; vitamin C deficits may increase cervical, bladder, stomach, and esophageal cancers, as well as the general carcinogenic process. Vitamin E deficiency definitely weakens the body's ability to balance rancid oils and free radicals, and this increases cancer risk. Other mineral deficiencies implicated in cancer include molybdenum deficiency in esophageal and stomach cancer; zinc deficiency in cancer of the prostate, colon, esophagus, and bronchi, as well as general immune system weakening; and possibly iodine and iron deficiencies.

Occupational chemicals. These are a topic of great concern. Many workers at home or in the workplace are exposed to a wide range of chemicals with varying carcinogenicity. Possible agents include nuclear radiation and fallout, chemicals used in dry cleaning and other cleaning supplies, benzene, coal tar and its derivatives, asbestos, arsenic, PVC, gasoline and petroleum products and other hydrocarbons, pesticides, cosmetic chemicals, and many others. A more detailed discussion is included in chapter 11, Food and the Earth. Cigarette smoking also increases the risks from these occupational hazards.

Food chemicals. These are another big topic. There are many possible carcinogens, most of minimum risk but often cumulative, and researchers still have much to learn about possible interactions of multiple carcinogens. Chemicals may be added to food during growth, manufacture, or preparation, and some are even made by the foods themselves or in combination with other microorganisms.

Air and water pollution. This may involve a great many chemicals; metals, pesticides, PCBs, vinyl chloride, carbon tetrachloride, and gasoline are a few examples. Contamination of underground water tables may spread rapidly. Air pollution may also contain many carcinogenic substances from the nitrous and sulfur gases to hydrocarbons, carbon monoxide, and so on.

Possible Food Carcinogens

Additives. Food colors, flavors, nitrates, and nitrites.

Saccharin. Implicated (still unclearly) in bladder cancer.

Hormones. In animal meats, particularly beef, although the use of hormones is decreasing. Possibly even DES (diethylstilbestrol), which was banned for use in food production and animal raising in 1979. However, other estrogens and growth-enhancing hormones are still in use, and their effects on humans are still of concern.

Pesticides. Sprayed on foods before and after harvesting.

Aflatoxin. Produced by molds on peanuts, other legumes, and possibly other foods; may cause liver cancer.

Coffee. Questionably implicated in bladder cancer. Decaffeinated coffee may be treated with such carcinogens as trichloroethylene or methyl chloride.

Sugar. May weaken immunity and increase cancer risk.

Nitrates and nitrites. Common in preserved and smoked meats, such as ham, bologna, salami, corned beef, hot dogs, and bacon; may convert to carcinogenic nitrosamines.

Pickled or salt-cured foods. May influence stomach and digestive lining.

Barbecuing. Creates protein changes and production of benzopyrene, a mild carcinogen. Charbroiled meats and burnt toast may also be concerns.

Mushrooms. May contain toxic hydrazines.

Potatoes. When bruised or green, because of increased toxins.

Other foods. Cottonseed oil, cocoa, mustard, black pepper, horseradish, fava beans, parsley, celery, alfalfa sprouts, parsnips, and figs all may naturally contain mild carcinogenic substances. (Some of the agents produced by these plants may act as natural pesticides.)

Excess sunlight and radiation. Excessive sunlight is implicated in skin cancer and excess radiation for cancer in general. Light-colored skin, cosmetic chemicals, and nutrient deficiencies, as well as the changes in Earth's ozone layer because of pollution, may also be factors in skin cancer. In some cases, medical X-rays can increase the risks of leukemia and other cancers, and this risk may be worsened by other precipitating factors, such as exposure to other carcinogens and/or low levels of necessary antioxidant nutrients. Mammograms, used to detect early breast cancer, have also been implicated as a factor in generating breast cancer with the radiation exposure directly to the breast tissue.

Certain pharmaceutical drugs. Some have a cancer-producing potential that has been well studied, at least in animals. Taking estrogen hormones, for postmenopausal use or as birth control pills, is a factor of concern in women, although the latest research suggests less correlation with both breast and uterine cancers than was previously thought. Researchers now believe that the more natural and bioidentical hormones have lower risk. When a combination of estrogens are used with less estradiol (the most carcinogenic of the three) and more estriol and estrone, there appears to be a lower cancer risk. Adding natural progesterone may be helpful as well in protecting the female tissues. Metronidazole (Flagyl), a commonly used antibiotic for bacteria and parasites, poses cancer risks, as does lindane, a pesticide used on the skin for mites and lice and found in such medicines as Kwell, Gamene, and others. Griseofulvin, an antifungal agent, also poses mild cancer risks. In my opinion, steroid drugs, commonly used for suppressing all kinds of natural and unnatural body responses, have definite potential through immune suppression for increasing cancer risk. I believe there should be more research done regarding the implication of steroid use in the incidence of postinfections and cancer.

Alcohol. This has also been implicated in some cancers, such as cancers of the mouth, larynx, esophagus, and pancreas. These risks are increased when alcohol use is combined with cigarette smoking. Alcohol abuse is also often associated with poor diet and many nutritional deficiencies.

Viruses. Viral diseases have been implicated in a variety of cancers. For years, genital herpes infections were thought to increase cervical cancer rates. It is now shown that the human papilloma virus responsible for common venereal warts is more closely tied to cervical cancer than are herpes viruses. Vitamin A, folic acid, and selenium deficiencies may also be involved in cervical cancer. Cytomegalic and Epstein-Barr viruses have been considered as factors in cancer, possibly through mutagenic cellular effects, and may contribute to certain lymphomas or leukemias.

Psychological influences. Psychological factors and the role they play in cancer is a fascinating topic; an increasing amount of research is being done in this area. Some studies have shown that a significant loss or perception of loss of a loved one occurred between 1 and 2 years before the diagnosis of cancer. This gives us another insight into the idea that it may take years, even 30 to 40, for a cancer to develop; cancer can also be a rapidly occurring and progressive disease.

There may indeed even be a cancer-type personality. The cancer disease process may be more prevalent in individuals who do not easily form close bonds or love relationships and do not easily express their feelings (such as anger or frustration) or who internalize most of their feelings, not necessarily aware that they even have any. These people might also show passive, compliant, or overly nice behavior and have low self-esteem. When such people experience unresolved loss of a loved one through death or divorce, a sense of helplessness or hopelessness may set in and weaken the immune system. Research seems to indicate that the feisty, tough scrappers who do not easily accept others' opinions or condemnation of themselves and can readily express their own feelings do much better with cancer, recovering more rapidly and more commonly than the more passive, accepting types.

Bernie S. Siegel, MD, discusses this area of personality and cancer extensively in his wonderful book *Love, Medicine, and Miracles*. He reported that children who developed cancer also had shown some of the aforementioned traits, with a definite correlation with loss or perceived loss of a loved one—usually a parent but possibly a sibling or even a pet—in their early years. Excessive stress and psychological traumas influence immunity and increase cancer risk. It is possible that the relationship between cancer and psychology can be summarized by the statement that cancer or any stress-related illness can result from a deep or chronic challenge or threat to personal identity, roles, or relationships.

It is clear that cancer is not a simple disease to understand, diagnose, or treat. There are many types of cancer, each with its own set of predisposing factors, growth rates, treatment options, and so on. What is common to all, though, is the uncontrolled growth of aberrant cells that endangers healthy tissues, function, and life. Still, each person with cancer is an individual, and in most situations, many factors are involved in the genesis of the cancer. My focus here, however, is to minimize the risks and prevent cancer, which now afflicts more than 1 in every 4 people at some time in their life and eventually touches nearly every family in the Western world.

It is obvious that avoiding smoking and second-hand smoke, minimizing the use of carcinogenic chemicals at home and work, and doing our best to breathe clean air and drink good water may help to prevent some cancers. We should also minimize exposure to radiation. Reducing time in front of the television and computer screens will lower our exposure. Not living near nuclear power plants is important; limiting airline flights may help. Exposure to medical, dental, and chiropractic X-rays can be decreased. Many practitioners in each of these professions overuse regular radiation to follow patients. Routine chest X-rays for hospital admissions, for detecting tuberculosis or other lung or heart disease, or for employment are often unnecessary. Routine dental X-rays can be taken every 5 years instead of at the usual 2-year intervals. Chiropractors often X-ray the entire spine; this can be helpful, but it should not be done more than once or twice in a decade. Care can be taken to use the best equipment with the least radiation exposure and leakage. Whenever possible, X-ray films should be shared among practitioners, rather than each one taking new films. In recent years, many more women and practitioners are supporting thermography as a means of cancer detection in the breast. It appears to have some advantages in addition to lower radiation exposure.

Positive Action

In addition to all of these things to avoid, there are also many positive things to emphasize to reduce cancer risks. Diet (low fat, high fiber) and nutrients (extra vitamins A, C, and E, and selenium) can be very helpful. Although healing from cancer may be difficult, it is clear that the earlier it is found, the better the chances for survival (although this viewpoint is not universal). The current consensus is still that regular breast self-exam, Pap smears, prostate exam and PSA tests (prostate blood tests for cancer detection), sigmoidoscopy, colonoscopy, and possibly routine mammography may be to our advantage in early detection. Of course, these tests are advantageous only to those who have cancer; the high percentage of people with normal results have gone through the expense of time and money, radiation exposure in some, and often some pain.

It is important to keep ourselves physically and psychologically fit through exercise and working on maintaining a positive attitude. Regular exercise definitely improves attitude and energy for life and supports a good immune system. When we are distressed or confronting important issues, dilemmas, or crises, it is wise to seek appropriate support to process our feelings if we are not able to handle them fully ourselves. A good friend and confidant can help, or a trained therapist may be beneficial. We all need to break the association of seeing a psychologist or therapist with being "crazy" and instead look at therapy (or at least emotional counseling and support) as an important part of preventive medicine. Being able to deal with life's stresses as a challenge (and adventure) rather than with despair, helplessness, hopelessness, or other internalized feelings that make us feel that there is no escape is essential, not only in preventing cancer but for general health as well. Most of us still play out childhood patterns, and our individualized attitudes of trust and self-image affect our adult relationships and everyday life. This does not serve our best or most-evolved interests. Astute, interactive therapy and/or hypnotherapy can help point out these old patterns and replace them with new, more helpful ones to improve our potential for experiencing love, health, and success in most areas of our lives.

Stress management techniques, relaxation and visualization exercises, and meditation are all useful self-help processes that may be learned. Developing a spiritual or universal perspective about the world and our involvement with life is also important for interpreting and coping with challenging experiences such as cancer. Founder of the Kushi Institute in Becket, Massachussetts, and macrobiotic pioneer Michio Kushi has suggested that a complaining, arrogant, rigid, and competitive character makes one more susceptible to degenerative disease, while a healthier approach to life might include being more peaceful, grateful, flexible, and cooperative.

The Cancer Prevention Diet

This usually involves a moderate to major change in the average person's dietary habits. Even the most traditional nutrition books now suggest the following as the main components of the cancer-prevention diet:

- Lower fat intake to about 20% of total calories (25% to 30% is more realistic; the average has been more than 40%). A maximum of 65 grams of fat per day is suggested; 50 grams is better. That represents 450 calories of fat daily, or 20% of a 2,250-calorie diet. More of the fats should be the mono- and polyunsaturated types, with a reduction of saturated fat intake, and little or no consumption of refined and heated oils.

- Increase dietary fiber to improve colon function mainly by increasing complex carbohydrates in the form of whole grains and lots of vegetables, along with some fruits, all of which contain high amounts of many of the important nutrients.

- Increase fresh fruits, vegetables, and whole grains.

- Maintain ideal weight and avoid obesity.

- Avoid smoking.

- Avoid smoked, salted, pickled, and barbecued foods.

The 7 dietary suggestions of the American Cancer Society are similar:

1. Avoid obesity.

2. Cut down on total fat intake.

3. Eat more high-fiber foods, including whole grains, fruits, and vegetables.

4. Include cruciferous vegetables, such as cauliflower, broccoli, and cabbage.

5. Include foods rich in vitamins A and C.

6. Lower alcohol consumption.

7. Lower intake of salt-cured, smoked, or nitrite-containing foods.

Let us begin with a high-nutrient, low-fat, high-fiber diet. More specifically, protein intake should be about 15% of the diet—from 12% to 18%, and not more than 20%, or 100 grams (400 calories) per day of a typical 2,000 calorie diet. Complex carbohydrates could make up about 60% of the diet, which would greatly increase the fiber intake. Up to 40 grams daily of fiber is not unrealistic. Foods high in fiber and water content to promote good bowel function and a diet and lifestyle supportive of healthy adrenal glands (minimize stress and sugar), liver (minimize chemicals and alcohol), thyroid (less stress and radiation exposure), and thymus/immune system (see "Immune Enhancement" on page 633) to review immune suppressors and supporters) are all important in keeping cancer risks low. In addition to vitamins A and C, increase dietary intake of the B vitamins, especially folic acid, vitamin E, selenium, beta-carotene, and zinc. The diet should be low in alcohol, salt, coffee, and, obviously, chemicals and preservatives in foods.

The low-fat, cancer-prevention diet focuses on starches, such as whole grains, legumes, potatoes, pastas, and squashes, along with fruits and vegetables and some other protein foods, such as small amounts of meats, preferably fish and poultry, nuts and seeds, and occasional eggs or milk products if tolerated. The overall best foods for cancer prevention include organic white meats of poultry and fish, whole grains, vegetables, especially organically grown cruciferous ones, and fruits, such as citrus fruits.

Cancer Prevention: Dietary Suggestions

Emphasize* | **Avoid**

Emphasize*
Cruciferous vegetables
Other vegetables, and especially green vegetables
Whole grains
Fruits
Poultry
Fish (untreated)
Legumes
Some nuts and seeds
Seaweeds/sea vegetables

* Buy organic when possible.

Avoid
High-fat foods
Hydrogenated fats
Synthetic or high-chemical foods
Smoked foods
Pickled foods
Barbecued foods
Excess polyunsaturated oils
Alcohol
High-calorie diet
High-cholesterol diet
Low-fiber diet
Environmental chemicals
Excessive proteins

Phytonutrients and Cancer Prevention

Mechanism of Prevention/Phytonutrient	Food Sources
STIMULATE DETOXIFYING ENZYMES	
Isothiocyanates	Cruciferous vegetables, onion, garlic
Sulforaphane	Cruciferous vegetables, onion, garlic
Limonene	Lime, lemon, guava, mango, root vegetables, oats, grapefruit
Terpenoids	Teas, many vegetables
Curcumin	Turmeric
N-acetyl-cysteine (NAC)	Cruciferous vegetables, onion, garlic
INHIBIT ENZYMES THAT CREATE CARCINOGENS	
Isothiocyanates	Cruciferous vegetables, onion, garlic
Diallyl sulfide	Cruciferous vegetables, onion, garlic
Ellagic acid	Berries, guava, walnuts, chestnuts
Ferulic acid	Cantaloupe, honeydew, pineapple, cabbage, spinach
INHIBIT FORMATION OF CARCINOGENS	
Caffeic acid	Cassava, strawberry, avocado
Ferulic acid	Cantaloupe, honeydew, pineapple, cabbage, spinach, olives, many other vegetables

A primarily or exclusively vegetarian diet is generally helpful in preventing cancer. All studies of people on vegetarian diets showed reduced incidences of a variety of cancers, including the common ones of the colon, breast, and prostate. The macrobiotic diet (primarily cooked grains and vegetables) and vegan diet (avoiding eggs and milk) probably pose even a lower risk than the classically researched Seventh-day Adventist diet; although both these diets contain wholesome foods, they must be watched for deficiency problems. A macrobiotic diet has become popular among people who are suffering from cancer or concerned about preventing it. Such a diet focuses on whole grains (50% to 60%); vegetables (25% to 30%), mainly cooked; soups (5% to 10%); and beans and sea vegetables (5% to 10%). Michio Kushi discusses the macrobiotic diet and its application to cancer in great detail in his book *The Cancer Prevention Diet*. Also refer to chapter 9, Diets, in this book.

No area of nutrition has become a greater hotbed of research than the area relating phytonutrients to cancer. A tidal wave of interest continues to be awakened in relationship to foods, their unique phytonutrient composition, and cancer prevention. Particularly important in this regard are the sulfur-containing cruciferous vegetables like broccoli, brussels sprouts, and kale. Also getting attention are the chlorophyllic greens and sulfur-containing onions and garlic. I have highlighted some of this new information about phytonutrients and cancer prevention in the "Phytonutrients and Cancer Prevention" table on page 647. Please refer back to chapter 8, Foods, for additional details on foods containing these particular phytonutrients.

Detoxification and Diet

I consider the genesis of cancer to be largely a result of autointoxication, chemical exposure, stagnation, and congestion (physical, mental, and emotional), thus I believe that periodic detoxification diets and fasting are appropriate for most people as a preventive to degenerative disease and to generally improve clarity and vitality. Juice fasting or a fruit and vegetable detoxification diet also helps us reflect on and reevaluate our diets, attitudes, life priorities, and personal path. This enhances our evolutionary process, which is essential to staying healthy. For more information

on fasting and detoxification, see chapter 18, Detoxification and Cleansing Programs.

The ideal diet, as discussed in chapter 13, is basically a good anticancer diet. It is a moderately low-fat, low-calorie, high-fiber diet that includes many of the nutrient-rich foods, such as fruits, vegetables, whole grains, legumes, seeds, nuts, and the low-fat animal proteins if desired. It is adapted to the seasons, which allows better availability of organically grown local produce, extremely important in minimizing intake of potentially dangerous chemical carcinogens. I am impressed with the American Institute for Cancer Research's 4-volume series *An Ounce of Prevention*. There is a volume for each season, presenting a low-fat, high-fiber, chemically light, appealing diet with a focus on practical recipes that contain naturally grown foods. For more than 25 years, I have been an advocate of this seasonal back-to-nature diet, a commonsense approach that clearly supports our greater nutritional health and vitality.

Anticancer Nutrients

Let us now explore some of the anticancer nutrients. There are three main avenues for defense against cancer, and each has specific nutrients that support a particular function:

1. **Strengthening the immune system.** Vitamins C and E, vitamin A and beta-carotene, zinc and copper, and the B vitamins folic acid, riboflavin, pyridoxine, and pantothenic acid.

2. **Avoiding or neutralizing carcinogens.** Vitamins C and A, selenomethionine, and the amino acid L-cysteine.

3. **Preventing DNA and cellular damage.** Vitamin A, vitamins C and E, beta-carotene, and the minerals selenium, zinc, and manganese.

The diet suggested here will provide adequate levels of most of these nutrients if the foods are digested and assimilated. High amounts of fruits and vegetables will provide lots of vitamins C and A (as beta-carotene), and some of the B vitamins. Whole grains will give us more B vitamins, some vitamin E, and many minerals. Good-quality proteins will provide amino acids and cysteine. With a more vegetarian and low-fat diet, there can be slight deficiencies, such as vitamin E. Zinc and selenium depend more on the soil content, and both of these minerals may require supplementation.

Vitamin A and beta-carotene also support normal cellular differentiation of the tissues and internal linings. Vitamin A may prevent cancer cell formation by inhibiting the binding of carcinogens to the cell wall; similarly, beta-carotene may protect the DNA in the nucleus of the cell by decreasing the bonding of chemicals to the membrane around the nucleus, which contains the DNA, our basic life material. Both of these nutrients are antioxidants that scavenge free radicals, particularly singlet oxygen molecules. Decreased levels of vitamin A are associated with increased rates of cancer of the lungs especially, and also of the mouth, esophagus, bladder, cervix, and stomach.

Beta-carotene has been shown to be deficient in a large proportion of smokers who develop lung cancer, as it seems to specifically protect cells of the mucous membranes. It has also been shown to be low in people who develop cancers of the throat, skin, prostate, and colon and is probably protective against those cancers as well. Because of its stronger antioxidant functions, beta-carotene is likely the better anticancer nutrient than the retinol form of vitamin A. Zinc, which is needed to form the retinol-binding protein (for vitamin A), may also be low in people who develop cancer. Vitamin A and especially beta-carotene are found mainly in fruits and vegetables, such as carrots, sweet potatoes, squashes, greens like spinach and broccoli, seaweed and blue-green algae, bell peppers, apricots, and cantaloupe. Vitamin A in the retinol, or animal, form is found in fish, eggs, and liver.

Vitamin C is involved in all three of the cancer defense functions and is obviously an important nutrient. It is among the main antioxidant nutrients, protecting cell and mucous membranes and vascular linings from free radicals generated by carcinogens and other molecules. Even though the use of ascorbic acid in cancer treatment is controversial, it is important to use for cancer prevention. This vitamin is abundant in such foods as citrus fruits, cruciferous vegetables, and peppers. With the current stresses and chemical exposures in our society, and the inability to acquire high levels of vitamin C from our diet, I usually suggest some regular supplementation, at least

> ### 6 Anticancer Aspects of Vitamin C
>
> 1. Is an antioxidant.
> 2. It stimulates T lymphocytes to produce interferon, which decreases virus reproduction.
> 3. It supports thymus function, specifically in strengthening the cytotoxic and killer T lymphocytes, and it supports antibody responsiveness.
> 4. It reduces the production of nitrosamines (a strong carcinogen) from dietary nitrates and nitrites from the soil and those added to smoked or processed meats, as well as those we produce through our own digestion and metabolism.
> 5. It reduces stomach, esophageal, and bladder cancers by means of its multiple protective effects on mucous membranes (this needs more research).
> 6. It has been shown, along with folic acid and vitamin A, to minimize cervical dysplasia and cancer, where these nutrients have been measured at reduced levels.

2 to 3 grams daily, although even 500 to 1,000 mg is probably sufficient for most of its protective functions. Rutin, a nutrient in the vitamin C complex, or bioflavonoids, found in various foods and herbs, may also have some anticancer properties.

Vitamin E functions best with adequate levels of selenium as selenomethionine, and vice versa, as antioxidants and cell membrane protectors. Vitamin E is found naturally in vegetable oils and nuts and seeds, with a little in the germ of such whole grains as wheat and rice. It reduces carcinogen production and strengthens immune cells and cell membranes against the penetration of viruses and toxic chemicals. Selenium helps regulate glutathione peroxidase, a strong antioxidant enzyme. Low selenium levels in the soil and in the body are clearly associated with increased rates of leukemia and cancers of the breast, lungs, colon, rectum, prostate, ovary, skin, and pancreas. If soils are low in this mineral, the foods grown in them will not contain much selenium. It is wise to increase selenium-rich foods, such as the whole grains and legumes or brewer's yeast, if tolerated, as well as to take a supplemental 100 to 200 mcg per day to be safe. High copper levels can reduce selenium absorption and utilization as well.

Zinc is another important mineral. It is an immune supporter and is important to the formation and function of many enzymes that work on detoxifying chemicals. Low levels of zinc in the body have been associated with higher rates of prostate, bronchial, esophageal, and colon cancers. Low levels of molybdenum in the soil have also been shown to be associated with increased levels of esophageal cancer. Calcium protects against colon cancer by protecting and correcting irregular cells in the colon. Other minerals that may have anticancer qualities include iron and iodine.

Fiber is another important anticancer substance and is a part of many foods and can also be taken as a supplement, such as psyllium seed husks or the bran of wheat or oats. Adequate dietary fiber improves intestinal transit time and binds carcinogens, thus reducing exposure to them. **A high-fiber diet clearly reduces the incidence of colon cancer and diverticular disease (and may lower blood cholesterol), whereas a high-fat, low-fiber diet increases the risk of colon, breast, and other cancers.**

Lactobacillus acidophilus is, I believe, a useful anticancer agent, mainly to prevent colon cancer. Lactobacilli cultures in the colon decrease other bacteria that can change bile salts into irritating carcinogens, as well as reduce yeast overgrowth and inflammation that result from these organisms, which also contribute to allergies and immune suppression. A few other immune-supporting nutrients include gamma-linolenic acid (GLA), extracted from evening primrose oil or other sources; GLA helps increase certain prostaglandins that support lymphocyte immune

Cancer Prevention Nutrient Program

Nutrient	Amount	Nutrient	Amount
Water	2 qt	Calcium	850–1,200 mg
Calories	1,500–2,500	Chromium	200–400 mcg
Protein	50–75 g	Copper	2–3 mg
Fats	40–65 g	Iodine	150–200 mcg
Fiber	15–30 g	Iron	10–20 mg
Vitamin A	5,000–10,000 IU	Magnesium	300–600 mg
Beta-carotene	15,000–30,000 IU	Manganese	5–10 mg
Vitamin D	400 IU	Molybdenum	250–500 mcg
Vitamin E	400–800 IU	Potassium	300–600 mg
Vitamin K	150–300 mcg	Selenium, preferably	200–300 mcg
Thiamin (B1)	50–100 mg	as selenomethionine	
Riboflavin (B2)	25–75 mg	Silicon	100–200 mg
Riboflavin-5-phosphate	25–50 mg	Vanadium	150–300 mcg
Niacin (B3)	50 mg	Zinc	30–60 mg
Niacinamide (B3)	50–100 mg	Lactobacillus	1–2 billion organisms
Pantothenic acid (B5)	250–500 mg	Garlic oil or powder	2–3 capsules
Pyridoxine (B6)	50–100 mg	Essential fatty acids,	2–4 capsules
Pyridoxal-5-phosphate	25–50 mg	or flaxseed oil	1–2 teaspoons
Cobalamin (B12)	100 mcg	Gamma-linolenic acid	4 capsules
Folic acid	800 mcg		or 200–300 mg
Biotin	500 mcg	L-amino acids	1,000 mg
Vitamin C	3–6 g	L-cysteine	250 mg
Bioflavonoids	250–500 mg	L-carnitine	500 mg

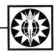

activity, and there is some indication that it has an anticancer effect. More research is also needed on the anticancer or procancer effects of L-arginine, a semi-essential amino acid. L-carnitine may also be helpful for improving fat utilization, as poor fat metabolism and free-radical fat molecules can cause cellular and tissue irritation. Organo-germanium may also be effective in cancer prevention, although it is more clearly useful in cancer treatment. BHA and BHT are antioxidant food chemicals (preservatives) that some researchers feel have potential to lower chemically induced cancers; other authorities believe these chemicals are too toxic to use as supplements. I prefer the natural antioxidant nutrients that are commonly found in foods.

Garlic and echinacea are thought to help support immune function and thus may play a role in preventing cancer. Aside from garlic, no herbs have been studied well enough to determine their possible cancer-preventive effects. There may be other herbs, both Western and Eastern, that have anticancer effects. Among those that may have properties effective in preventing cancer development are intestinal detoxicants, such as the algins and kelps; herbal blood cleansers (alteratives) such as chaparral, cayenne and chile peppers, burdock and yellow dock roots, and blue flag root; colon cleansers such as rhubarb root and black walnut; diuretics and kidney cleansers such as cleavers, uva ursi, and dandelion; lymph cleansers such as echinacea; and nutritives, such as alfalfa.

The "Cancer Prevention Nutrient Program" on the opposite page is particularly geared to protect those with added cancer risks, although it may also be used periodically, for 1 or 2 months several times yearly, for the average individual. With aging, or during times of stress or emotional traumas, this program may also be helpful. The values in the table can include nutrients in the diet and/or additional supplements.

20. CARDIOVASCULAR DISEASE PREVENTION

This is the biggie! With a little effort on each of our parts and a willingness to change, we can make a big difference in the incidence of this nation's number-one killer, cardiovascular disease (CVD). Heart and blood vessel diseases are not inevitable; in fact, they are preventable in most cases. It is clear from every major study since the mid-1990s that diets high in saturated fats and cholesterol, which would consist of regular intake of red meats, dairy foods, and eggs, are directly correlated to the incidence of CVD and its complications, whereas a low-saturated-fat, low-cholesterol diet greatly lowers the risk of these diseases.

The main disease process at the base of the cardiovascular diseases is atherosclerosis, or hardening and clogging of the arteries. (*Arteriosclerosis* is the generic term referring to hardening of the arteries. *Atherosclerosis* refers to the disease process of artery plaquing and is the term used in this section.) The main underlying factor in atherosclerosis is inflammation, which comes from bad foods as with chemicals and junky fats, as well as stress and other factors. Atherosclerosis involves the thickening and narrowing of the blood vessels, which occurs somewhat in most people, but with certain risk factors it can progress rapidly and lead to early demise, in some cases as early as the 40s or 50s. Atherosclerosis commonly affects the coronary arteries, which deliver blood to the heart muscle itself. This biggest cardiovascular concern causes a great deal of limitation and chest pain, or angina pectoris. When advanced, this coronary artery disease can result in a myocardial infarction (MI), otherwise known as a heart attack or a "coronary." Heart attacks are clearly the most common cause of death in the United States and the Western world. Other areas of the body may also be affected with atherosclerosis. Disease of the carotid arteries of the neck affects our mental faculties; atherosclerosis of the leg arteries decreases the ability to walk without pain; and clogging of the pelvic arteries affects sexual performance.

The inflammatory process, so common in today's society, is the result of a toxic lifestyle. The best approach to prevention may be in minimizing blood vessel inflammation, which may begin the disease process. There are many factors of concern. The first prevention approach is to follow a primarily alkaline diet higher in fresh fruits and vegetables, with their many nutrients and phytonutrients. **The acid chemistry in the body causes much inflammation and illness, and this comes from the food toxins and chemicals and the choices of acid-forming foods,**

Common Cardiovascular Diseases and Their Results

Cardiovascular Diseases	Results
Atherosclerosis	Angina pectoris (chest pain)
Hypertension	Limitation of movement
	Intermittent claudication (pain in legs with activity)
Coronary artery disease	Memory loss
	Decreased sexual function
Carotid artery disease	Cerebrovascular accident (stroke)
Peripheral artery disease	Cardiac arrhythmias
Heart disease	Myocardial infarction (heart attack)
	Congestive heart failure
	Valvular heart disease*

* Especially mitral and aortic disease from high blood pressure.

such as breads and baked goods, sugar and refined-flour products, animal proteins, and dairy products. **This balance may be the key to preventing or delaying disease.**

Avoiding cigarette smoke and other chemical fumes is crucial, because nicotine is a blood vessel inflammatory agent. Avoiding inhaled chemicals used so commonly in homes, gardens, and the workplace is also useful. Learning to relax and release stress, getting regular exercise for better peace and energy in the body, and taking a protective supplement program offers a good start to cardiovascular protection. Hypertension, or high blood pressure, is often a hidden multifactorial problem and the most common CVD; a key pathologic process involved in hypertension is atherosclerosis. The narrowing and hardening of the arteries increase their resistance and pressure and makes the heart work harder, which can then wear down this vital muscle. Untreated hypertension may lead to further heart disease, including heart attacks and congestive heart failure, as well as to cerebrovascular accidents (strokes).

The primary component of cardiovascular disease (heart and coronary artery disease) remains the number-one cause of death in the United States, and the second principle component (stroke) is the third leading cause. At the turn of the nineteenth century, it was not even in the top ten. In underdeveloped countries, where people live on a more natural or "native" diet,

there is a low incidence of CVD. In the United States, however, the many CVDs now account for more than 50% of all deaths. Of course, people live longer now, which allows for the development of more degenerative disease, but there is also more middle-age weight gain in a more sedentary population that eats more fats and refined foods than in the past. These factors are fairly easy to change (if change is ever easy) and form the basis of preventing these now-common diseases.

Hypertension and heart disease are not inevitable results of aging. In countries where populations eat a diet low in fats, cholesterol, and salt, there is little or no hypertension in comparison to countries whose people eat those richer foods. The 90-year-olds in Hunza society in the Himalayan mountains of northern Pakistan, for example, appear to be free of CVD and have normal blood pressure, although legitimate scientific studies do not exist to document this observation. **To keep the blood pressure low with age and to minimize the atherosclerotic process, we need to do the following:**

- Eat a diet low in saturated and hydrogenated fats, cholesterol, salt, and processed, refined foods (both fats and sugars).

- Eat high-fiber foods.

- Eat plenty of whole grains, fruits, and vegetables.

- Exercise or have a regular, active lifestyle, especially including walking.

- Keep body fat low.

There has already been some progress. The previous rapidly rising death rate from CVDs began leveling off and decreasing in the mid-1980s, likely due to better coronary care, CPR education, public education, and drug control of high blood pressure. Since 1968 and the beginnings of the natural medicine revival, there has also been greater dietary awareness, a growing interest in regular exercise, and an effort to diminish cigarette smoking. It is clear that a good (lower-fat, more-vegetarian) diet, regular exercise, weight reduction, and stress modification can reduce the symptoms of atherosclerosis, hypertension, and angina pectoris as well as decrease the risk and incidence of CVD in general.

So why is CVD still so prevalent? Often, people must be hit over the head before they will acknowledge new information and change long-term patterns. On both an economic and educational level, the big industries fight changes that might affect their status and income. The meat, dairy, and egg megabusinesses still try to deny the relationship between their foods and high cholesterol levels and cardiovascular disease—advertising their products as being good for everybody and providing literature to young children to encourage the regular use of their foods. Now other businesses, such as fast food chains, have gotten heavily into the educational act, claiming that a hamburger, fries, and a milkshake comprise a balanced meal. Kids are already influenced enough by advertising for sugary and refined-food products.

Despite some improvement, however, there are still more than 500,000 deaths per year from heart attacks and strokes (down from the previous 1 million annually). About a third of the 1.5 million people who have coronaries each year die from those attacks. Nearly 61 million Americans have some CVD, mostly high blood pressure (more than 50 million) and coronary artery disease (CAD, about 11 million), with many more people who are undiagnosed. Our cholesterol profile, a key contributing factor in CVDs, can only be determined with a blood chemistry analysis, while hypertension often does not reveal itself before being found during a physical exam. When either ele-

vated cholesterol profiles (lipids—triglycerides, cholesterol, and LDL and HDL cholesterol fractions) or high blood pressure are found, cardiovascular damage may already have begun. Because it is difficult for people to know if they have high blood pressure, it has been labeled the silent killer. In this section, let's first look at the many risk factors for CVD, and then examine the underlying disease process—atherosclerosis.

The cardiovascular risk factors are commonly classified into the primary factors, of which there are three (cigarette smoking, high cholesterol values, and high blood pressure) and the secondary concerns, of which there are many. Some of these significant factors in the genesis of CVD include obesity and being overweight, genetics, stress, a sedentary lifestyle, diabetes, and alcohol abuse. Many authorities feel that even more than the moderate or high fat and cholesterol intake, it is the many nutritional deficiencies that arise from our present-day nutrition and that affect the cholesterol metabolism that lead to increased atherosclerosis. Deficiencies of vitamins C, E, and B6 as well as selenium are the main concerns. Other relevant nutrients are magnesium, chromium, niacin, the essential fatty acids, and fiber.

The types of fats consumed in the diet and the deficiency of the essential fatty acids, linoleic and linolenic, are felt by some authorities to be the source of the CVD problem. Udo Erasmus, well-known popular press author in the area of dietary fat quality and related dietary supplements, has described this in his book *Fats and Oils,* in which he has also suggested that the heated and hydrogenated modern oils (like margarine) used for cooking and frying are a big concern. The increased consumption of homogenized milk fat in the standard milk appears to be linked with cardiovascular problems. And it has become clear since the mid-1990s that elevated cholesterol, as such, is not responsible for our heart-related problems. Rather, heart health is undermined due to an overall diet (and lifestyle) that fails to keep the blood vessels in good health, the fat transport mechanisms protected, and the immune system on even keel.

Regarding minerals, the calcium-magnesium interchange and the sodium-potassium relationship affect hardening of the arteries and blood pressure. Even copper and zinc deficiencies and imbalance may

---

Cardiovascular Disease Risks

Primary	Secondary	Others
High cholesterol*	Family history of hyperlipidemia	Caffeine
Hypertension	Male gender	Soft water
Smoking	Obesity	Hypothyroidism
	Stress (type A)	Cadmium toxicity
	Lack of activity (heart exercise)	Aging (with other risks)
	Diabetes	Nutritional deficiencies:
	Nutritional deficiencies:	vitamin B6
	folate (folic acid)	vitamin B12
	vitamin E	vitamin C
	selenium	niacin (B3)
	chromium	fiber
	fatty acids	zinc
	magnesium	copper
	potassium	

Another way of categorizing these risk factors is:

Personal Factors	Disease Relationships	Behavior Patterns
Family history	Diabetes	Smoking (nicotine)
Gender	High blood pressure	Diet (high- or low-fat)
Age	Hyperlipidemia	Overweight
Stress level	(types II and IV)	Stress, overwork
Personality (type A)	High cholesterol	Exercise (low to high)
Overwork, time	Elevated lipoproteins	Nutrient deficiencies
pressure, etc.	(high LDL to HDL ratio)	Water choices
Overweight	High triglycerides	Substance abuse (sugar, alcohol,
	Hypothyroidism	caffeine, and other drugs)
		Regular use of homogenized milk,
		margarines, and hydrogenated fats

* Due to heredity and/or a diet high in fats and cholesterol.

---

be related. It is clear, however, that the saturated fats and cholesterol in the diet are linked to CVD in all animals studied, including humans. Carnivorous animals, such as dogs and cats, seem relatively immune to high-fat diets. Possibly understanding their protection will give us further insight into CVD prevention.

It used to be that cholesterol took center stage in the cardiovascular disease arena. Thanks to the Framingham, Massachusetts, studies, begun in 1948, researchers have had a closer look at cholesterol levels and their relationship with heart disease. This area continues to be controversial. Initially, we believed that high amounts of total cholesterol—whatever the form in the body—could be problematic. The large Framingham study showed that people with a blood cholesterol level of 260 mg had three times the incidence of myocardial infarctions than those with levels of 195. Lowering cholesterol levels by whatever means—diet, weight loss, exercise, and even drugs—decreased the risk of heart attacks. However, fairly quickly, this viewpoint shifted as researchers took a more careful look at the different forms of cholesterol. The LDL form (a low-density lipoprotein molecule that contains cholesterol) was quickly determined to be more problematic when elevated, in contrast to the HDL (high-density lipoprotein) form, which was found to actually be *beneficial* when increased. Now, the ratios of total cholesterol to HDL as well as LDL to HDL are considered important parameters in evaluating cardiovascular risk.

LDL became the "bad" cholesterol and HDL the "good," because the latter was viewed as picking up used cholesterol and carrying it back to the liver for eventual processing and elimination from the body. Many researchers still feel that increasing the HDL cholesterol as much as possible (a process that occurs primarily through increased exercise and increased intake of dietary fiber) and decreasing LDL cholesterol as much as possible (by reducing saturated animal fat intake, as well as the trans fat intake) are still some of the best ways of lowering heart disease risk.

Current thinking about cholesterol and heart disease has progressed far beyond the HDL/LDL level, however. There is now a fairly conclusive body of evidence to suggest that it is not the total amount of cholesterol—or any particular type of cholesterol—that in and of itself triggers heart disease. Rather, it is the degree to which the cholesterol is protected from damage, particularly by oxygen. Once the cholesterol has become oxidized, the immune system kicks in, spotting a potential danger in the bloodstream. The immune system sends out its macrophage cells to scavenge and clean up the oxidized cholesterol "debris"—but too much of it can overwhelm the macrophage cells and the result is a gummed-up mess that leads to the formation of foam cells that start to adhere to the blood vessel walls and disrupt blood vessel function. Preventing cholesterol oxidation through optimal intake of antioxidant nutrients—including the traditional vitamins like E and C, the traditional minerals like zinc, selenium, manganese, and copper, but also the wide range of phytonutrients found in fresh fruits and vegetables—has therefore become a new focus in dealing with cholesterol problems. **In general, we want to keep down free radicals and inflammation.**

Even with the increasingly sophisticated understanding of cholesterol, however, this area of research no longer takes center stage in the heart disease arena.

That role has quickly shifted over to homocysteine. Since 1969, Kilmer McCully, a cum laude Harvard-trained MD, has been working and publishing from his posts at Harvard (where he was eventually dismissed because of the radical nature of his ideas about homocysteine) and Brown Universities to understand more about the relationship between cholesterol and heart disease. All along, McCully has viewed cholesterol problems as a symptom of heart disease rather than its cause. Through a series of case reviews, he landed on the problem of high homocysteine as the cause he was looking for.

Homocysteine is an amino acid that is naturally produced in most of the body's cells. When homocysteine is produced, it usually gets converted into other molecules, including the amino acid methionine. Three vitamins are especially important for the conversions of homocysteine to take place—B_6, B_{12}, and folate (folic acid). Without adequate amounts of these vitamins, homocysteine can rise to problematic levels in the bloodstream and increase the risk of heart disease. (High homocysteine has also been linked to increased risk of diabetes, Alzheimer's disease, and rheumatoid arthritis.)

There is every reason to pay attention on both sides of the equation. On one hand, **preventing cholesterol oxidation is critical. We can do that by:**

- Not overdosing on high-cholesterol foods in the diet

- Restricting saturated fat intake, trans fat intake, and hydrogenated oil intake

- Keeping up our antioxidant protection, primarily through ample intake of fresh organic fruits and vegetables

We can also pay close attention to our B_6, B_{12}, and folate intake by making sure to include plenty of green leafy vegetables, whole grains, and other foods rich in B complex vitamins (like nutritional yeast) in the diet as well as making sure that these important B vitamins are in our supplement regimen.

I personally believe it still makes sense to monitor total cholesterol-to-HDL cholesterol levels, and LDL-to-HDL cholesterol ratios, along with routine checks on homocysteine levels, particularly for men

Dietary Fats and Oils

Cholesterol-Rich Foods	Saturated and Trans Fats	Monounsaturated Fats	Polyunsaturated Fats
Egg yolks	Butter	Olive oil	Vegetable oils:
Liver	Cheese	Olives	sesame
Other organ meats	Milk	Almonds	safflower
Pâtés	Red meats	Pecans	sunflower
Milk fat	Poultry	Peanuts	corn
Fatty meats	Coconut oil	Cashews	soybean
	Palm oil	Avocados	walnut
		Margarine	Fish

Other fats contained in foods that have beneficial effects on cholesterol are the omega-3 fatty acids EPA and DHA, found in such coldwater fish as salmon, mackerel, and sardines. This fairly important discovery, as well as other essential nutrients, especially magnesium and pyridoxine, is discussed in more detail in the text.

and women over 50. While total cholesterol intake needs to be watched, this task is not usually as difficult as people make it out to be. By limiting dairy fats from cheeses and other dairy products, eating only 4 to 6 eggs per week, and limiting fat-containing meats (especially lunchmeats), we can keep our cholesterol levels in check.

Smoking, being sedentary, and consuming saturated fats in the diet lower protective HDLs. Exercise, a high-fiber diet, and alcohol increase HDL, although alcohol also produces irritating effects on the liver and the vascular system and may increase total cholesterol. Increased LDL levels can be caused by increased consumption of saturated fats and sugar, deficient levels of vitamin C or chromium, and high copper or iron levels. The various fats have different effects on cholesterol. Saturated fats lead to more LDL and VLDL. (VLDL stands for very low-density lipoprotein, another form in which cholesterol and triglyceride fats get circulated around the bloodstream.) The monounsaturated fats tend to have a neutral influence on cholesterol levels, while the polyunsaturated fats tend to lower total cholesterol but may also likewise lower the good HDLs.

Smoking is another crucial factor and an instigator of not only our number-one killer, cardiovascular disease, but also our number-two life destroyer, cancer. Day-to-day smoking sensitizes the vascular system and heart to irritation and inflammation. Nicotine damages the vascular lining, increases heart rate, and decreases oxygen delivery, with further carbon monoxide intoxication. Smoking also increases LDL cholesterol levels and possibly poses an additional risk of increased levels of beta-VLDL (currently under research). Cadmium, which is a blood pressure elevator, and other toxic minerals are also found in cigarette smoke. Nicotine also increases arterial constriction, which further limits oxygen and nutrient delivery to the cells and tissues. Chronic cigarette smoking clearly increases the chances of having atherosclerosis and hypertension with all of their complications. **Thus cigarette smoking by itself includes all three primary risk factors for CVD.**

Hypertension is not only another major risk factor, but it also occurs as a result of atherosclerosis itself. High blood pressure is defined as being over 140/90 mm Hg (millimeters of mercury, a pressure reading). Normal blood pressure (BP) should range from 100/70 to 120/80. The higher number represents the systolic BP, the BP while the heart pumps; while the lower number represents the diastolic BP during the rest between beats. The blood pressure itself is basically the pressure that the blood exerts on the arterial walls. An elevated diastolic pressure has a worse effect on the genesis of atherosclerosis than does a high systolic pressure. Even a diastolic pressure between 80 and 90 is associated with an increased risk. More commonly, elderly people have primarily high systolic pressure, and this is also a concern, yet sometimes harder to manage with blood pressure medicines. Overall, high blood pressure puts strain on the blood vessels, the heart, and the kidneys (especially important in controlling the BP).

Many doctors consider a BP in the range of 140/90 to 160/95 to be only mildly elevated, although it definitely increases risk. We can do most about this area of borderline hypertension. Hypertension, like CVD in general, is affected by a number of risk factors. Weight, diet, family history, gender, race, stress, smoking, and lack of exercise are some of the main ones; there are many more, such as excessive sodium dietary intake over potassium. Suffice it to say that hypertension is a major disease, limiting and shortening the lives of nearly 50 million people in the United States and many more times that in the entire world. It is a disease we can do something to prevent. The CVD prevention program applies to high blood pressure as well, and lowering elevated blood pressure by whatever means possible (even drugs) reduces the risk of heart disease, heart attacks, and strokes.

Sodium and potassium intake play out a little differently in the case of hypertension than researchers previously thought. Even though a processed-food diet is high in sodium, this excess only appears to affect about 12% of the population in terms of directly increasing the risk of high blood pressure. The majority of us are not directly salt-sensitive in this way. However, the ratio of sodium to other minerals, including potassium, seems important. So we need to keep a balance here, with approximately equal amounts of both, instead of a lopsided combination that favors sodium over potassium.

One final point I would like to make about hypertension is the close involvement with three macrominerals and one important vitamin: calcium, magnesium, phosphorus, and vitamin D. The highly processed diet has a poor balance in the mineral area. There is vitamin D coming from required fortification of cow's milk, calcium is voluntarily added to a wide variety of products ranging from orange juice to breakfast cereal, and phosphorus crops up in soft drinks in the form of phosphoric acid. But there is not any equivalent manufacturing process that adds magnesium, which has been shown to be a key regulator of blood pressure. Increased calcium and magnesium have both been shown to decrease blood pressure more consistently than reduction of sodium, and I would like to see us clean up our processed food supply to bring these nutrients into better balance. Also, there are important roles for coenzyme Q and EPA in helping to get our hypertension problems under control.

Obesity is another major risk factor in CVD, contributing to both atherosclerosis and hypertension. Being overweight raises blood pressure, increases blood fats, reduces HDL, usually minimizes exercise, and adds to the incidence of diabetes. This all speeds up the atherosclerotic process and increases the occurrence of coronary artery disease. By decreasing obesity, we can decrease many of the CVD risk factors all at once. Stress factors also contribute to CVD. The type A personality has an increased risk, more indirectly, through poor diet, caffeine use, and increased adrenaline output—all of which raise blood pressure. The hard-driven, ambitious type A person is constantly creating his or her life under the pressure of time, with the attitude that there is never enough time to do it all, or that it should be done faster. Some authorities further attribute to this personality a low awareness of spiritual or philosophical values, with a perspective basically geared toward work and running around. These type A people could benefit from stress reduction to help them relax, and from exercise, especially with a sense of fun, to aid in letting go of the ever-riding tensions. Yet ultimately it is up to each of us to order our values and priorities in life. My goal is for everyone to put health into their top two or three priorities. What are yours?

Lack of exercise is also a problem. The heart and circulation need regular, even vigorous exercise, to keep them strong. Remember, the heart is a muscle that needs to work out. We will look more at exercise as a positive practice for preventing cardiovascular disease later in this section. Drinking soft water is another risk. It replaces the minerals calcium and magnesium in normally CVD-protective water with sodium mainly, which has a tendency to increase blood pressure and worsen atherosclerosis. Areas where people drink soft water have higher incidences of CVD and heart attacks. It is best to drink spring or well water for its beneficial minerals as well as to prevent chemical exposure. Water is definitely better for us than caffeine and alcohol. Caffeine increases heart rate and blood pressure and adds the risk of cardiac arrhythmias. Alcohol is a suppressant but also an irritant and is a minor risk factor itself in CVD.

Family history is not something we can do much about, but our knowledge of it can motivate us to take extra special care of ourselves and more diligently apply this CVD prevention program. Certain genetic traits may influence cholesterol metabolism and levels of production of cholesterol and other fats. It appears that some people actually make more cholesterol (or perhaps clear less or use less) than others. This increases their risk of vascular problems. Specific genetic (familial) problems of fat levels are described in medicine. These are termed *hyperlipidemias* (meaning elevated fat levels), the lipid disorders, and include five types. Types II and IV cause high cholesterol and high triglyceride levels, respectively. Type IV is the most common and is thought to result more from familial eating patterns than from genetics. It also can proceed to problems in sugar metabolism. These disorders can be revealed by a blood test, specifically a lipoprotein electrophoresis.

A history of hyperlipidemia disorder or a family history of coronary heart disease, high blood pressure, diabetes, or obesity puts us at increased risk for developing some type of CVD. This means we need to enhance our prevention efforts, which may require many changes, depending on our current lifestyle. Cardiovascular disease really needs to be prevented in childhood. Atherosclerosis often starts in children, as can hypertension. Avoiding the typical high-fat, high-sugar, and high-salt foods and snacks and fried oils can make a big difference. Keeping the weight normal and getting plenty of exercise is the way to go. In some manner, television is a cardiovascular disease risk as it encourages a sedentary life and poor food choices, which are highly advertised. Dietary suggestions for children with CVD risk and obesity are discussed later in this section. It is important to remember that the effects from risk factors are cumulative. Just being overweight is not a big problem if cholesterol and diet are okay or if we do not smoke. If we are an overweight, sedentary smoker with high blood pressure and a poor diet, however, we will not be living on that path very long.

Next I discuss the process of atherosclerosis, the hardening of the inner arterial walls with lipids (mainly cholesterol), smooth muscle cells from the blood vessel walls themselves, fibrin, and calcium. This process, which is stimulated and added to by platelets and white blood cells, forms the plaque, or atheromas. Atherosclerosis can begin early with these fatty streaks in the blood vessel walls. Many teenagers with high-fat diets have plaque in their arteries. The fries, shakes, burgers, and hot dogs that are so prevalent in our culture's diet, along with the deficiencies that arise from the high intake of sugar and refined foods (there often is not much room left for many nutrient-rich foods), predispose our youth to this early hardening of the arteries.

The basic process of atherosclerosis is thought to begin with minor microinjuries to the vascular linings. These tiny wounds stimulate the overgrowth of muscle cells and attract and attach the fat/cholesterol and platelet aggregation along with calcium precipitation to eventually form a small fibrous scar that begins to narrow the opening of the artery. (Cholesterol is a waxy fat/sterol that is attempting to heal the irritated or injured tissues—it is really trying to help!) This arterial plaque reduces the blood flow and also decreases the strength and elasticity of the vessel wall. This can predispose us to increased blood pressure and aneurysm (ballooning of the artery), which can then lead to bleeding, strokes, or other, milder consequences. These tiny injuries to the blood vessels involve many contributors, but the mechanism by which they occur is via free-radical pathology, not dissimilar to most inflammatory and cellular changes.

Atherosclerosis can be a slow process. The disease may not cause problems for many years, and then the symptoms can begin and progress rapidly, as a blood vessel usually must be more than half (more like 70% to 80%) closed before it creates difficulty. A full clot—that is, a thrombosis—will lead to blocked circulation and often death of the tissues to which the blood vessel leads unless collateral circulation already exists to that area. This is how a heart attack develops, with atherosclerosis in the significant coronary arteries. In coronary artery disease, 70% to 80% closure will more likely lead to chest pain, the symptom of angina pectoris. If an atheroma or clot breaks off from its blood vessel attachment, it will move through the blood until it reaches a vessel that it is too large to pass through and then clog up that vessel, which can be disastrous.

Clots in the blood vessels also can stimulate arterial spasm, which often worsens symptoms.

Atherosclerosis affects the vascular, mainly the arterial, system and commonly leads to problems in the heart, kidneys, brain, ears, and sexual organs. The heart, or coronary, blood vessels are the biggest area of concern. The effect on the kidney (renal) circulation can lead to hypertension. Carotid artery disease directly influences brain circulation, which can lead to memory problems, hearing loss, perhaps dizziness or vertigo, senility, and strokes. Transient ischemic attacks (TIAs) affect the state of consciousness with intermittent loss of blood flow. **Poor circulation is the biggest cause of decreased sexual function and impotence in middle-aged or older men.**

The best way to evaluate the presence or state of CVD is by a thorough workup. A medical history will describe any possible symptoms tied to circulatory compromise or blockage, the result of atherosclerosis. A physical exam will not usually tell much unless there is some heart abnormality, poor circulation, or elevated blood pressure. The blood pressure should ideally be under 120/80 in adults and about 110/70 in children. Any elevation puts a patient at higher risk and calls for closer follow-up. The blood pressure can go up just from the nervousness of being in a doctor's office, so it needs to be checked under more normal circumstances if it is abnormal. If it goes up under the stress of visiting a doctor, however, it likely goes up with other stress also.

An electrocardiogram (EKG) is a measurement of the heart rhythm and electrical activity. This is positive only after problems already exist. Neither an EKG nor a chest X-ray is preventive; they simply show the presence of disease after it occurs and offer few clues that would point out potential future problems, as can the blood pressure or blood levels of cholesterol, HDL, and LDL. Increased blood levels of triglycerides, sugar, and uric acid are also of concern. Many doctors are encouraging patients to treat cholesterol levels over 200 mg/dl with diet, exercise, and even drug therapy. This has become even more popular with the studies that show reduced heart attacks in people with CVD who take the statin drugs, especially the brand name Lipitor. Keeping check on levels of homocysteine in the blood is also high up on the list of many practitioners. Another test that is being used commonly now measures an inflammatory marker and is called a cardio CRP (C-reactive protein). The main problem with this test, however, is that any inflammatory condition can cause the result to be elevated.

A more extensive test for the heart is an echocardiogram using ultrasound, which can pick up more subtle changes in the heart muscle and its internal valves. And a stress echo includes exercise (treadmill) intended to challenge the heart and look at it when it is beating fast from the demands of exercise. Angiography, the injection of dye into the blood to study the circulation through the heart or any area of the body, is done more commonly these days to measure the circulatory status. It is performed before cardiac bypass surgery and is itself very risky (deaths do occur during this procedure), expensive, and sometimes painful.

The best approach to cardiovascular disease is, of course, prevention. To prevent CVD, the overall plan includes not smoking; preventing and/or controlling obesity, high blood pressure, and diabetes; exercising and staying fit; eating a low-fat, more vegetarian diet; and monitoring cholesterol levels and keeping them low, both in our diet and in our blood. For high-risk people, the program needs to be more vigorous. They need clear dietary guidelines and good follow-up care if they are to have a good chance of reducing development of CVD potential and its associated morbidity and mortality in later years. Not smoking; more aggressive control of obesity, hypertension, or diabetes; and a more strict low-fat diet are really mandatory.

Goals for Decreasing CVD Risks

- Quit or minimize smoking.
- Lower and control blood pressure.
- Lower total cholesterol.
- Lower high homocysteine.
- Lower LDL cholesterol.
- Increase HDL cholesterol.
- Lower weight if overweight.
- Increase aerobic exercise.

Improving Cholesterol Balance

To Lower Cholesterol and LDL

Decrease total fats in diet.

Decrease saturated fats in diet.

Decrease cholesterol in diet.

Increase essential fatty acid foods
(polyunsaturates) in diet.

Use more monounsaturated oils, such as olive or canola.

Increase fiber with more fruits, vegetables,
and whole-grain foods.

Use psyllium husks.

Add oat bran.

Increase complex carbohydrates.

Decrease caffeine and nicotine.

Supplement nutrients: Vitamins B_6, B_{12}, B_3, and C, folate,
chromium, EPA, garlic.

To Increase HDL Cholesterol

Get regular aerobic exercise.

Do not smoke.

Decrease weight.

Supplement nutrients: essential fatty acids,
niacin, EPA, fiber, garlic, L-carnitine.

Atherosclerosis is clearly reversible. Science owes a debt of thanks to Dean Ornish, MD, who has published rigorously in this area since the mid-1990s. Ornish has shown that a combination of diet, exercise, and lifestyle changes can predictably help unclog clogged arteries. His book *Dr. Dean Ornish's Program for Reversing Heart Disease: The Only System Scientifically Proven to Reverse Heart Disease without Drugs or Surgery* describes his intervention program in detail. I fully recommend it.

Many of the significant risk factors contributing to CVD can be lessened through dietary influences. These risks include high blood pressure, high cholesterol (especially high LDL levels), high triglyceride levels, and obesity, as well as many early cases of diabetes. High fat consumption, low fiber intake, and excess salt and sodium intake are influential nutritional risks. **Proper diet alone can decrease cholesterol levels by 30% or more, although this usually requires some radical dietary shifts.** (For some people, genetics are stronger and they may still have high cholesterol even with an excellent, low-fat diet.) Smoking and lack of exercise, the main nondietary cardiovascular risk factors involved, often require similar changes of willpower as does diet; and furthermore, we need a feeling of positive self-worth to even gather the force to make these successful changes.

The primary dietary focus of the cardiovascular disease prevention diet is fat intake. The diet should be low in fat in general and particularly low in saturated fats (animal fats plus palm oil) and the hydrogenated fats (all margarines) and oils such as those used for frying foods. These are mainly poor-quality vegetable oils used so commonly in commercial food preparation and restaurant cooking. I highly recommend avoiding these oils. It is clear that a diet high in saturated fats and cholesterol leads to increased blood cholesterol levels and increased atherosclerosis. In my clinical experience, homogenized, pasteurized milk and dairy fats seem to drive cholesterol to high levels. A quart or more of whole milk daily or regular intake of ice cream can lead to cholesterol levels over 300 mg/dl; thus, going off these foods can dramatically lower the cholesterol.

To prevent atherosclerosis, a low-fat, low-cholesterol, and high-fiber diet is recommended. Fiber reduces CVD risk in many ways. It binds cholesterol and fats and lessens their absorption. It subsequently decreases blood cholesterol and LDL and increases protective HDL cholesterol. Increased fiber levels—at least 20 to 30 grams daily, which often requires supplemented fiber—will also help reduce blood pressure levels in those with elevations. Fat intake should be reduced from the average 40% to 45%

to a maximum of 25% to 30% of total calories; even lower levels, 15% to 20%, are suggested. With supplemental fatty acids or the use of good-quality cold-pressed vegetable oils to obtain the necessary linolenic acid, even lower fat intake can be consumed safely. This, however, is difficult unless we eliminate a wide variety of common foods, including all fried foods, meats, milk products, butter, cheese, eggs, nuts, and seeds, which also clearly reduces protein intake.

Currently, the average American fat intake ranges from about 100 to 150 grams per day. Of course, men usually consume more than women, and many people with some food awareness consume less. In diet analyses, however, I commonly see this range, even up to and over 200 grams daily. At 9 calories per gram, 125 grams means 1,125 calories a day of fat. If that represents the average of about 40% of total calories, it would mean a diet of about 2,800 calories a day, which would add weight to most folks other than athletic men. If we eat 100 grams (900 calories) of fat daily, and that is one-third of our total calories, that means a total of 2,700 calories a day. If fats are a more healthful 25% of the diet, that means a total of 3,600 calories, more than most people consume. Realistically, fat intake levels must be no higher than 50 to 75 grams a day to create a calorie range of 1,800 to 2,700, with a diet containing 25% fat.

The types of fat consumed are also important. More unsaturated (poly- and monounsaturated) than saturated fats are suggested; that means a higher intake of vegetable oils and foods containing polyunsaturated fats. Beef, for example, has a ratio of saturated to polyunsaturated fat (S:P) of around 15:1, whereas the ratios in poultry and fish are closer to even. Vegetable fats found in nuts or seeds have an even lower S:P ratio. The polyunsaturates tend to be more beneficial to our levels of fat and cholesterol than the saturated fats found in milk, eggs, and meat. However, the polyunsaturated fats are unstable and not only lower total cholesterol but may also reduce the important HDL; the monounsaturated fats are probably better. Be careful of the hydrogenated polyunsaturates (many margarines and cooking oils)—they have increased saturated fats and unusable, trans-fatty acids (mirror image molecules of the natural cis-fatty acids). Cis-fatty acids are the most common form found in foods and have a unique chemistry in which hydrogen

atoms line up in a special way; trans-fatty acids are even less desirable than the fats from butter, milk, or meat. Excess polyunsaturates also have added cancer and heart disease risks, possibly because of oxidation and the potential formation of free radicals. **Overall, a minimum of fats is suggested, with avoidance of many of the less healthful unsaturated fats, such as refined cooking oils, margarines, mayonnaise, and artificial dressings and creamers, which also contain questionable chemicals.** Many chips, crackers, and cookies contain higher amounts of hydrogenated and polyunsaturated oils. It is fairly clear that the total fat intake has an important influence on blood cholesterol, as does the proportion of saturated fats or cholesterol-containing foods, so this needs to be an important area of focus.

Particularly helpful oils are contained in such cold-water fish such as salmon, mackerel, sardines, and herring. These contain EPA (eicosapentaenoic acid)

Dietary Suggestions to Reduce CVD Risk

- Eat more fruits and vegetables.
- Eat more whole grains.
- Use low-fat snacks.
- Reduce fat intake to 25% to 30% of the diet.
- Reduce cholesterol intake to fewer than 300 mg per day.
- Reduce consumption of egg yolks to 3 to 5 per week.
- Minimize use of whole milk and its products; use low-fat or nonfat milk products.
- Avoid red meats; eliminate all cured meats and lunch meats.
- Limit the use of nuts and seeds to not more than 1 or 2 handfuls daily. These are generally healthy foods.
- Avoid excess intake of avocados, olives, crab, and shrimp.
- Eat more coldwater fish, such as sardines and salmon.
- Use fresh, monounsaturated, mechanically pressed oils, such as olive or flaxseed oils, to provide the essential fatty acids.

and DHA (docosahexaenoic acid), which have a positive effect on lowering cholesterol and triglycerides. These are considered CVD-prevention nutrients and consuming these oil-containing fish 2 or 3 times a week is beneficial to our cardiovascular health. EPA can also be used as a supplement to the diet.

A low-salt and low-sugar diet is also suggested. Avoiding salted and pickled or cured foods, especially meats, is suggested for health. Excess sugar, because it increases calories, weight, and blood fats, is an indirect risk factor in CVD; it is not healthy for many other reasons. More complex carbohydrates, including mostly whole-grain and vegetable foods, are definitely in our favor for CVD prevention. The starch-centered diet, along with exercise, is the basis of the well-known Pritikin program to reduce and prevent CVD. Nathan Pritikin was one of the more vigorous proponents of this excessively low-fat diet.

Children and Cardiovascular Disease

CVD prevention may need to start in young people, even preteens and adolescents, particularly if there is early obesity or a family history of heart disease. Weight, blood pressure, and cholesterol levels can be followed in these higher risk children. Diet modifications may be begun early with a lower-fat diet, primarily by reducing the animal fat and fried food consumption; this is accomplished by minimizing the intake of such foods as burgers, hot dogs, french fries, chips, and excessive cheese, ice cream, and even milk products overall. Low-fat or nonfat dairy products can be used with these young people while still providing a diet that contains adequate levels of protein, essential fatty acids, calcium, and even eggs, although these should not be consumed excessively. Encouraging more fruits, vegetables, whole grains, nuts and seeds, and some low-fat dairy foods will provide an adequate-fiber, lower-fat diet with adequate calcium and calories. Some fish and poultry and occasional meat will support the protein needs well, yet there are now many more vegetarian-oriented teenagers and young adults in our society who do fine.

With children who eat a lot of fast foods, ice cream, pizza, cookies, chips, sodas, and other exciting modern-day treats, the challenge is to get them to eat more wholesomely. Parents should provide these "treat"

foods to their children only after they eat their more nutritious foods, and then only occasionally. Wholesome suggestions include replacing some soda and cookie snacks with low-fat milk, yogurt, and crackers; adding oat bran to cereals, meat loaf, or casseroles; using whole-grain cereals in place of sugary ones as well as using cooked whole grains at meals; substituting Popsicles and fruit juice bars for fattier ice cream; using some low-fat cheeses such as cottage cheese or mozzarella (pizza with cheese and vegetables, not with fatty meats, is acceptable, even once or twice weekly); encouraging vegetables and fruits (with skins), even green salads when possible; and buying cookies and treats with low saturated fats and low sugar, such as fig bars, animal or graham crackers, ginger snaps, or fruit juice–sweetened cookies. We as parents also need to set a good example ourselves with healthy food choices, having these good foods at home, and by not overeating. Also, not snacking while watching television is suggested.

There is some controversy among authorities regarding the diet for the young in regard to CVD risk. Some believe that all children should be on a low-fat diet, at least lower than the current 40% national average. Most definitely, many of the poor-quality, refined foods should be avoided. Clearly, children who are obese or who have cholesterol levels over 200 mg/dl should work to correct these states, and those who have families with CVD should be watched more closely. But overall, the higher-protein, higher-fat diet so consistent throughout the Western world does lead to increased growth and size of children and adults. Many cholesterol-rich foods, such as milk, cheese, meats, and eggs support the growth spurts. Yet consumption of these foods is also associated with reduced longevity secondary to degenerative disease. One possible approach is to feed children this richer diet with more protein and fat foods, although it would still need to be a wholesome one, avoiding the junk, sweets, and fried oils. Then, as they move into their later teens and early adulthood, prepare them to shift their diet focus to a more natural, lower-fat, more vegetarian plan, with regular exercise supported along the way.

Herbs and Supplements for Cardiovascular Health

In addition to the oily coldwater fish, specific foods can help prevent CVD, including garlic, which can lower cholesterol and blood pressure, and onions and cayenne pepper, which have milder effects. These three foods are also herbs that are used in blood cleansing and thinning; garlic specifically lowers blood clotting potential. Soybeans and soy products such as tofu and tempeh may have a positive effect on cholesterol and atherosclerosis; besides, all are low in fat and higher in protein. Natural-health advocate and popular author, the late Paavo Airola suggests other good foods for reducing CVD risk, including the grains millet and buckwheat, sunflower seeds, okra, potatoes, asparagus, apples, and bananas, as well as yeast, lecithin, and Flaxseed oil. Flaxseed oil has a high amount of the omega-3 fatty acids, such as EPA and DHA, and is a less expensive supplement to help reduce cholesterol levels. Flaxseed oil also contains the essential fatty acids (EFAs) linoleic and linolenic acid, which may help reduce blood fat levels and fatty deposits. Cold-pressed flaxseed oil is also readily used by our bodies in the important EFA functions, but it is a fragile oil and must be fresh and then protected from light, heat, and oxidation.

Most of the common vegetable oils are high in the omega-6 fatty acids, as are borage seed and evening primrose oil, although they contain mainly gamma-linoleic acid (GLA). Soybean oil and walnut oil are higher in the omega-3s, and flaxseed oil is highest. All

Fatty Acid Percentages in Commonly Used Plant Oils		
Oils	**Omega-3 (%)**	**Omega-6 (%)**
Flaxseed	50–60	15–20
Walnut	5–10	20–30
Soy	5–10	40
Safflower	0.5	70
Sunflower	0.5	65
Corn	0.5	60
Cottonseed	0.5	50
Olive	0.5	10

of the EFAs, both omega-3 and omega-6, help in cell membrane support and prostaglandin synthesis. They also help in the transfer of oxygen in the lungs and are essential to growth in the young.

I also recommend fruits, as they have some nutrients and are high-water-content cleansing foods that make the diet more alkaline. A diet of only fruit and vegetables for 1 or 2 weeks is a good way to realkalinize the body and blood, which aids detoxification and lowers blood fats. A more acidic, richer diet creates more mucus as well as thicker, more viscous blood and lymphatic congestion. I think of atherosclerosis as being much like the crud that builds up in water pipes because of various chemical or mineral imbalances that allow particle precipitation. I then think of fasting on juice or water as a means of cleaning that sludge from the blood vessels and organs. Fasting definitely reduces blood

The Effects of Diet and Lifestyle on Cholesterol and LDL-to-HDL Ratios		
Agent	**Cholesterol Effect**	**Effect on LDL-to-HDL Ratio***
Saturated fat	↑	↑(↑ LDL)
Monounsaturated fat	↓ or =	= HDL
Polyunsaturated fat	↓	= or ↑(↓ HDL)
EPA	↓	↓(↓ LDL)
Lecithin	↓ (possibly)	=
Smoking	↑	↑(↓ HDL)
Exercise	↓	↓

* Lower ratios have a lower risk of CVD.

Cholesterol-Lowering Nutrients

Chromium	Niacin
EPA	Policosanol
Fiber	Red yeast rice
Garlic	Vitamin B6
L-carnitine	Vitamin C

Other Nutrients That Reduce CVD Risk and Complications

Beta-carotene	Magnesium
Calcium	Potassium
Choline	Selenium
Coenzyme Q10	Vitamin B2, B6, B12, and folate
GLA	Vitamin E
Inositol	Zinc

---

fats and blood viscosity so that blood flows better. It also reduces weight and blood pressure, and I believe fasting is useful in the prevention and treatment of CVDs. Of course, fasting is not a diet but a supervised therapy. See "Fasting and Juice Cleansing" on page 769 in chapter 18, Detoxification and Cleansing Programs.

There are a number of important nutrients, both in the diet and as supplements, that help prevent cardiovascular disease. Three of these important aids to reducing cholesterol and CVD risk are fiber, garlic, and the fish oils EPA and DHA. Fiber has been shown to have several positive effects. It reduces blood pressure, cholesterol, and LDL and raises HDL. Apple pectin, oat fiber, psyllium husks, and locust bean gum have all been shown to reduce cholesterol and LDL. By reducing LDL while maintaining or raising the HDL cholesterol, this reduces the LDL-to-HDL ratio and therefore lowers the CVD risk. Alfalfa seed meal is high in saponin, an agent that is thought to be lipotropic—that is, it improves the utilization of fats.

Garlic, as a supplemental powder or oil, or used freely in the diet, has a positive effect on reducing triglycerides, cholesterol, and LDL while raising HDL. Studies have shown that higher amounts of garlic, such as 10 to 15 grams daily, produce these effects without tox-

icity and that garlic reduces platelet stickiness and clotting. The sulfur-containing amino acids and other sulfur components of garlic may be what helps to reduce these fats by their effect on cholesterol synthesis.

Omega-3 fatty acids—marine lipids, fish oils, EPA and DHA, or whatever other names they are known by, and alpha-linolenic acid (found in some vegetable oils)—have a number of positive effects for both CVD prevention and treatment. EPA helps reduce lipid blood levels and plaque formation, thereby lessening atherosclerosis. It thins the blood and reduces platelet aggregation, a process that is relevant in atheroma progression and thrombosis. Fish oils reduce cholesterol but not the important HDL, whereas most vegetable oils lower both. EPA probably works by reducing platelet thromboxane secretion and increasing the prostaglandin E3 series, which are anti-inflammatory agents. It also has been shown to have an effect on decreasing the activity of monocytes, which are phagocytic white blood cells involved in atheromas through adherence to the blood vessel wall. Aspirin, commonly used in medicine in low dosages to reduce clotting risks, decreases platelet stickiness and stimulates prostaglandin synthesis, but it also reduces platelet function and can have various side effects.

Animal fats, in contrast to fish oils, increase platelet stickiness, which tends to clog the blood, reducing circulation and oxygenation. In addition to a low-fat diet and exercise, EPA helps reduce cardiovascular risk through its just-described effects. Its ability to lower cholesterol and LDL is not dramatic, although in some people it may be the best agent. The higher amounts of EPA oil needed to lower lipid levels can be caloric, cause intestinal upset, and may adversely affect carbohydrate metabolism. Clearly, a low-fat diet can offer the most dramatic effect on cholesterol levels initially.

Two relatively new products are red yeast rice and policosanol. Both have been shown in research to make positive alterations in all the lipid levels, raising HDL while lowering total cholesterol, LDL, and triglycerides. Red yeast rice was discovered in China many years ago and the active substance grown on the rice is similar biochemically to the drug Mevacor, a statin used to lower cholesterol. The company that makes Mevacor has sought repeatedly to ban the substance from market as a patent infringement on their drug;

they lost initially through the courts but have recently had some success. The product is still available over the counter, and the needed amount is 1 to 2 600 mg capsules taken twice daily, at breakfast and dinner. **Red yeast rice alters (slows) cholesterol production and thus lowers blood levels. Policosanol is another interesting waxy oil that comes from sugarcane and beeswax.** It alters cholesterol metabolism and production. The amount needed for lipid-lowering effects is 5 to 10 mg twice daily.

A number of other nutrients help reduce cholesterol. Chromium supplementation has been shown to lower LDL and raise HDL, reducing CVD risk. Pyridoxine (B6) deficiency may increase plaque formation, as may vitamin C deficiency. Vitamin C treatment improves cholesterol metabolism and can also reduce total cholesterol and LDL levels, as well as the incidence of postsurgical clots. Niacin in dosages higher than 100 mg clearly has a cholesterol-lowering effect and has also been shown to reduce risk of recurrence of heart attacks and to improve the circulation in general. Supplementing niacin (vitamin B3) has become a popular therapy for reducing cholesterol. Increasing amounts up to 2 to 3 grams daily definitely helps to lower blood fats; however, many people do not tolerate well the niacin flush and other symptoms often associated with niacin supplementation. Also, certain niacins may irritate the liver. A commonly used "no-flush" niacin is the hexanicotinate form that binds the B vitamin inositol to vitamin B3 molecules. It does have some cholesterol-lowering effects, although the circulatory flush has some benefits in my opinion, so if that is tolerated, use some of the straight niacin. (See "Vitamin B3," on page 115 in chapter 5, Vitamins.)

L-carnitine helps in fatty acid metabolism. One study suggests that it increases prostacyclin, a prostaglandin that dilates coronary arteries, possibly as a result of decreased platelet thromboxane levels. A dosage of 250 to 500 mg of L-carnitine twice daily is suggested as a CVD preventive. Coenzyme Q10 is another favorable nutrient for cardiac and lipid function. This can be taken in dosages of 30 to 100 mg twice daily.

Antioxidant nutrients are also important to protect tissue and vascular linings from free-radical irritants. Vitamin E is a strong antioxidant, especially for preventing the oxidation of fats. Low vitamin E levels have been associated with increased platelet stickiness. Studies to determine its cholesterol-lowering and cardiovascular-protection effects have been inconclusive, but I feel that it should definitely be a part of a CVD prevention program for its protection against free radicals. A daily amount of 800 to 1,000 IU can be taken in 1 or 2 doses. Selenium, vitamin E's functional partner, helps protect the cells and tissue linings, as well as decreasing cadmium's blood-pressure-raising effect. Low selenium levels have been associated with an increased incidence of heart disease, strokes, and cancer. About 100 mcg of selenium can be taken with each dose of vitamin E, up to 250 to 300 mcg daily. Beta-carotene is also protective of tissue linings and may improve oxygen utilization and reduce platelet clumping, thus decreasing clotting potential. Zinc may also be protective against CVD, as it aids tissue healing and immune function, but high amounts (more than 100 mg per day) may raise cholesterol levels.

Other nutrients that may play a role in CVD prevention are vitamins B6, B12, B5, B2, folic acid, and several minerals. Pantothenic acid (B5) and riboflavin (B2) help in lipid metabolism. B6, B12, and folate help to metabolize and reduce homocysteine, thus reducing CVD risk. Calcium is needed for normal heart function and nerve transmission. Low calcium, especially in combination with increased sodium, as is found in soft water, increases blood pressure. For this reason, excess sodium in the diet should be avoided. Like calcium and magnesium, potassium is an important nutrient for normal heart function; it helps to balance out some of the detrimental effects of elevated sodium. (See more about this on page 169 in chapter 6, Minerals.)

Depletion of copper may also increase the risk of CVD, so it is needed in sufficient, although not excessive, amounts. Inositol and choline may help reduce blood pressure and atherosclerosis. There has also been some suggestion that gamma-linolenic acid (GLA) from evening primrose oil or other sources helps reduce blood clotting potential. Lecithin is another nutrient often recommended for CVD prevention. High amounts of it have been shown to decrease cholesterol levels, but in these amounts, this oil is highly caloric and contains high levels of phosphorus, which can affect calcium metabolism. Lecithin can be obtained naturally from whole grains, soy products, nuts, seeds, and vegetable oils.

Magnesium may be the single most important nutrient in CVD protection, especially when it is deficient. Magnesium, which is found readily in the whole grains, nuts, seeds, and many vegetables, is important to heart function and tissue health. It can actually dilate coronary arteries (and thus reduce angina) and increase the collateral circulation. Low heart tissue levels of magnesium have been found in heart attack victims and may contribute to coronary artery spasm, which reduces or closes off blood flow. Magnesium also helps normalize the heartbeat (a deficiency increases sensitivity to arrhythmias), the blood pressure, and the heart's sensitivity to toxins and to the effect of norepinephrine. I am certain that sustained, adequate magnesium levels reduces the incidence of fatal heart attacks. Another important function of magnesium is that it helps keep calcium in circulation so that it does not precipitate in tissues, a big factor in atherosclerosis, as well as in kidney stone formation and other problems of abnormal calcification. Along with calcium, magnesium helps maintain the electrical stability of cells, especially in the heart muscle. **Alcohol causes a loss of magnesium through the kidneys, as do diuretic drugs.** Magnesium in foods and as supplements is a good tranquilizer and also aids in blood pressure control.

Some herbs, including the aforementioned garlic and cayenne pepper, can be helpful in cardiovascular disease prevention. Ginger root helps with circulation, while hawthorn berries are the safest effective heart tonic. Many herbs can be used in CVD as heart tonics, as diuretics in hypertension, and for improving general circulation, including ginkgo (for general circulation), garlic and gugulipid (for the prevention of heart disease), and Asian ginseng (for blood pressure).

Lifestyle factors helpful in reducing CVD, besides reducing smoking and avoiding excessive caffeine and alcohol, are exercise and stress management. Before the technological age, exercise was part of everyday life; now it must be a special activity. The reality is that to be healthy, we must trade all the time we save in faster travel, mechanical devices, and easier cooking and cleaning and put that time into exercise.

In a healthy person, the resting heart rate may range from 50 to 65 beats per minute (bpm) for men and 55 to 70 for women. An unfit person may have a rate in the 80s or 90s. A good exercise program strength-

---

Exercise Benefits in Cardiovascular Disease Prevention

- Strengthens heart muscle.
- Improves oxygen delivery.
- Lowers pulse rate.
- Lowers blood pressure.
- Lowers blood fats, cholesterol, and triglycerides.
- Raises protective HDL cholesterol.
- Reduces stress.
- Enhances healthy sexuality.
- Improves attitude toward life.

---

ens the heart muscle, helps to reduce the resting heart rate, lowers blood pressure and blood fats, and raises the "good" HDL cholesterol, thus lessening atherosclerosis risk. Regular aerobic exercise is crucial to maintenance of a healthy circulatory system with a strong heart, which can then deliver more blood and more oxygen to the tissues.

When starting an exercise program, walk more and monitor the pulse and blood pressure. It is important to find an exercise program that is enjoyable, as stress reduction is another advantage of exercise. It is a good idea to vary the activity and do proper warm-ups and cooldowns. Avoid big meals before exercising and stop if any pain develops during the activity and attempt to assess any problem. If the pain persists, check it out with a doctor. If it has been months or years since you've exercised, if you are overweight or out of shape, or if you have any health problems, please have a thorough checkup before beginning any serious exercise program. An exercise-treadmill test will indicate whether the heart and blood pressure respond normally to vigorous activity. (If interested, see a cardiologist.)

Managing stress is an important key to cardiovascular health. We all experience stress, and it has its uses; however, we must counteract its negative effects—increased blood pressure and heart rate and free-radical generation. We may also benefit from developing or maintaining a generally positive attitude toward life, whether that takes counseling, taking more vacations, learning relaxation techniques, or seeking a more fulfilling religious/spiritual life. Spend-

Cardiovascular Disease Prevention Nutrient Program

Nutrient	Amount	Nutrient	Amount
Calories	1,500–2,500*	Chromium	300–500 mcg
Fats	40–70 g	Copper	2–3 mg
Fiber	15–25 g	Iodine	150–225 mcg
Vitamin A	5,000–10,000 IU	Iron	10–20 mg
Beta-carotene	15,000–25,000 IU	Magnesium	400–750 mg
Vitamin D	200 IU	Manganese	5–10 mg
Vitamin E	600–800 IU	Molybdenum	300–500 mcg
Vitamin K	150–300 mcg	Potassium	300–500 mg
Thiamin (B1)	50–75 mg	Selenium	200–300 mcg
Riboflavin (B2)	25–75 mg	Silicon	100 mg
Niacin (B3)	50–1,000 mg**	Vanadium	200 mcg
Niacinamide (B3)	100 mg	Zinc	30–60 mg
Pantothenic acid (B5)	250–500 mg	Flaxseed oil	1–2 tsp or 2–4 capsules
Pyridoxine (B6)	50 mg	EPA/DHA (fish oil)	2–4 capsules (200–600 mg**)
Cobalamin (B12)	100 mcg	Coenzyme Q10	50–200 mg
Folic acid	600 mcg	L-carnitine	500–1,000 mg
Biotin	300 mcg	Garlic	4 capsules
Choline	500 mg		
Inositol	500 mg		
Vitamin C	3–6 g		
Bioflavonoids	250–500 mg		
Calcium	650–1,000 mg		

* Depends on size and activity level.

**The dosage can be increased slowly, and it depends on cholesterol level, taking more niacin or EPA for higher levels.

ing time with family and ourselves is usually relaxing. For many people, exercise is an important aid to stress reduction. When we are stressed, we often tend to eat a poorer diet with less-nutritious food choices. We speed through meals and may consume more caffeine to get going and more alcohol to slow down at the end of the day. These habits need to be changed. See "Antistress" on page 597 earlier in this chapter.

If all of these suggestions do not help reduce risk factors and cholesterol, there are some pharmaceutical drugs that may be used to at least reduce cholesterol. These are suitable mainly for people with high blood fat levels or those who will not change their diet. The cardiovascular drug cholestyramine (Questran) blocks cholesterol absorption. It is effective but does have side effects, such as indigestion, bloating, and constipation. The newer statin drugs—most prominently lovastatin (Mevacor) and Lipitor—have been widely used for cholesterol reduction. These drugs can be fairly effective, but their use should always be accompanied by supplemental doses of coenzyme Q10 (50–200 mg per day) because the drug blocks formation of this critical nutrient. There are also many drugs to control hypertension. If lifestyle changes cannot reduce blood pressure, these may be needed.

Some doctors offer chelation therapy treatments, which is controversial, to reduce atherosclerosis. This is a series of moderately expensive intravenous infusions of EDTA, a mineral-chelating molecule that binds calcium from the blood and possibly from arterial plaque and removes it through the kidneys. Some patients experience dramatic benefits, but research to date has not been promising. I personally would definitely try it before "the knife" if I were experiencing cardiovascular disease symptoms, but I am not enthusiastic enough about it to use it in my practice. We must work diligently in our earlier years to do all we can to reduce CVD risk. Although not everyone can prevent atherosclerosis and degenerative cardiovascular disease, many can. It is worth a try.

Chapter 17

Medical Treatment Programs

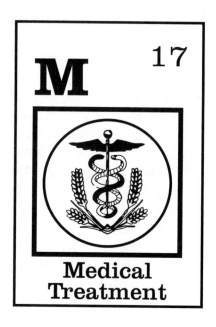

M 17

Medical
Treatment

Medical doctors are primarily trained in the diagnosis and treatment of disease. There is so much to learn about this highly technical science that it takes many years to learn to practice well. It may take even more years of experience (and personal growth), seeing what does and does not work, to progress into *the art of medicine*. Only recently has medical education (still limited in medical schools) returned to its roots and begun to show interest in nutrition, environmental medicine, natural remedies (such as herbs), healing arts, basic communication skills, and interest in how people's lives and attitudes both cause and influence their diseases and healing.

Much of this interest comes from public demand for more *health* care over disease care. As this occurs, it requires more personal experience and growth during medical training and practice to help develop the true art of healing. It is my belief that doctors who acquire interest and insight in these areas of training have more to offer their patients. Yet even with an increasing number of doctors interested in more humanitarian and natural medicine, it is still difficult to find practitioners who are willing to go beyond

symptom/disease treatment into correcting the causes of problems and healing lifestyles and lives.

Another crucial dimension of medical practice is giving patients more responsibility and involving, and even encouraging, them in self-healing care. Doctors who only diagnose and treat with drugs and surgery are ignoring an entire field of preventive medicine and patient education. In the same way, medical reactionaries to Western practices who refuse to accept the potential benefits and proven necessity, especially in acute cases, are also ignoring an entire field of value, such as crisis care, one of the greatest attributes of Western medicine. As more doctors (and individuals) experience the effects that dietary changes, natural therapies, herbal and nutritional supplements, and inner techniques have in stimulating healing (and improving overall health), it can only help health-care delivery and markedly reduce the costs involved.

There are many philosophies and dietary approaches, and much of this nutritional practice is outside the current standard (conventional) medical field. I am working to bring nutritional and medical practice together through more scientific assessment and individual treatment programs. This may require an in-depth evaluation of one's diet and nutritional status, specifically for vitamin and mineral levels, any food allergies (reactions of various kinds), and immune function. (See Appendix A, "Laboratories and Clinical Nutrition Tests" for specific tests.) With this information and the understanding, guidance, and support needed to carry it through, doctors can design a most effective and appropriate program for a given unique individual. Clearly, one's lifestyle (and environment and exposures to chemicals) affects personal health; nutrition is important, as are one's attitude and behavior, as well as proper sleep and rest, exercise, and stress levels. By addressing these areas, physicians could more easily prevent many problems. **It is easier to prevent disease than to heal the body after disease occurs, when much more energy, time, and money are needed to return to health.**

I often tell patients that what they experience as symptoms and disease are not the real problems; rather, they are a result of their lives—what they eat, do, and feel, and their deeper issues, attitudes, beliefs, and emotions. I believe that doctors and all healers who work with people as well as their lives—not just their diseases—are better health guides. As Bernie Siegel, MD, has pointed out in his book *Peace, Love, and Healing,* doctors need to learn how to treat people's whole lives; when we do that, their diseases heal more easily. I have long considered myself a philosopher-physician in the school of the ancient Chinese practice, guiding people in how to live in harmony with their environment, seasons, emotions, and lives. This becomes a more rewarding job when our J-O-B is also a J-O-Y.

This chapter brings together specific discussions of various medical concerns and the factors that contribute to these problems along with some philosophy in regard to the health conditions. I also offer a complete nutritional approach—using diet and natural remedies, nutritional supplements, and herbs—to work on the biochemical healing processes for these conditions.

In this chapter, I discuss only a few common nutritional medicine concerns, although there are many other potential medical problems that exist. This book focuses on disease prevention and stresses healthy nutrition and a symbiotic personal-planetary

lifestyle. I am currently conducting more extensive research and writing on such medical nutrition areas (some discussed here and in others of my books) as arthritis, asthma, gastrointestinal problems (including parasites), diabetes and hypoglycemia, cardiovascular disease, cancer treatments, and the nutritional factors of mental health. Some of this research is included in the book I am currently working on, *NOW Medicine,* which also includes paradigms of future health-care delivery systems. I have added several new and important programs to this chapter that were not included in the previous edition of *Staying Healthy with Nutrition:* "Fatigue" (including chronic fatigue syndrome), "Viral Conditions" (so common these days), and "Mental Health: Depression, Anxiety, and Attention-Deficit/Hyperactivity Disorder (ADHD)." Use this chapter's information to support your standard medical care or as your main therapeutic regimen, as the case may be.

21. FATIGUE

Fatigue, meaning tiredness or the feeling of having not enough energy, is a symptom that may result from a great variety of causes, and it is probably among the most common symptoms described to physicians and other practitioners. It may range from a mild loss of usual energy, to greater weariness at certain times of the day, to complete exhaustion and a near inability to move.

Chronic fatigue syndrome (CFS), or chronic fatigue immune dysfunction syndrome (CFIDS), is much less common and a more concerning and harder-to-correct problem. Practitioners and scientists are still working to figure out the cause. Even though my focus in this section is on fatigue in general, I begin by telling you a little more about CFS. Nearly any of the components in CFS, such as viruses, allergy, or nutritional deficiency, can contribute to general, everyday fatigue. Although I use the acronym CFS to refer to this specific type of fatigue diagnosis, please think of CFS and CFIDS as interchangeable. During initial investigations in the early 1980s, CFS was thought to be caused by a virus, specifically Epstein-Barr virus (EBV), a common virus that causes mononucleosis and other viral-type illnesses. Most people have been exposed to EBV and show positive antibodies to it, but not many people show it with chronic activity. Anyway, EBV was considered not a clear determinate of CFS and was disregarded as the cause. Then some doctors purported the yeast *Candida albicans* and the immune-allergic reactions that it causes in the body, as well as the disruption of proper digestion and assimilation, to be the cause in many of their patients. Although "candida," as we commonly refer to this concern, can be a problem (many doctors still do not think so, but I clearly do), it also is not "the" cause.

After more years of searching, researchers saw that many people have subtle problems in their immune cells and activities, and their resistance to disease (along with their sensitivity to foods and chemicals) and this caused yet another shift in the name, to chronic fatigue immune dysfunction syndrome. I believe that the cause of CFS and CFIDS is multifactorial, and thus I concur with the philosophies from the following books: *From Fatigued to Fantastic: A Proven Program to Regain Vibrant Health, Based on a New Scientific Study Showing Effective Treatment for Chronic Fatigue and Fibromyalgia*, by Jacob Teitelbaum, and *Living Well with Chronic Fatigue Syndrome and Fibromyalgia: What Your Doctor Doesn't Tell You . . . That You Need to Know*, by Mary Shomon.

Many factors contribute to chronic fatigue, including viral and yeast infections, some chronic; allergies and immune reactions to foods and environmental factors; nutrient deficiencies; chemical and metal toxicities; and stress and other life-issue conflicts. I believe that CFS represents a life challenge to clarify one's identity to oneself and to the world. When people with CFS address these many factors and improve their lifestyle, they often feel better, if not completely clear of this syndrome.

In evaluating general fatigue of a few weeks to months, a thorough medical evaluation may turn up 1 or more of the many possible underlying causes of fatigue. A good history, a physical exam, and a complete biochemical profile may reveal such concerns as anemia, a low-grade infection, or low thyroid function. (See the book *Thyroid Power*, by Drs. Richard and Karilee Shames.) Also, how well does the person sleep or how much stress is he or she under? These factors can be overlooked easily by looking for more exotic causes. Proper sleep is very important in restoring our batteries every night to recharge us for the next

day's activities. A diet evaluation in conjunction with an analysis of blood vitamins and minerals or a test for food allergies (reactions) may reveal additional findings that may be associated with fatigue. Other lifestyle habits like stress or overwork, or abuse of such substances as coffee, sugar, alcohol, or other drugs, may also lead to a loss or a lack of energy.

Changing our habits to find a better balance between work, play, and rest as well as creating a better diet, with supplementation of some additional nutrients and medicinal herbs, will often improve the energy level greatly. Frequently, a simple lifestyle and laboratory analysis followed by a nutritional and lifestyle program will be effective. However, there may be more complex issues at play, such as psychological or emotional conflicts or a difficult job or relationship or environmental impact; these issues require more understanding, time, and effort to sort out and to change.

Common underlying problems that I have found to be correlated with fatigue include low thyroid (hypothyroidism) and adrenal gland function, nutrient deficiencies (particularly of such minerals as magnesium, potassium, and iron); stress and overwork;

Factors Contributing to Fatigue

Allergies

Anemia

Cancer

Chronic diarrhea and nutrient loss

Chronic pain

Constipation

Depression (and persistent anxiety)

Environmental toxicity

Hypoglycemia

Immune suppression

Lack of sleep (or poor sleep and sleep apnea)

Low hydrochloric acid

Obesity

Poor digestion

Progressive disease

Sluggish liver

Stress and overwork

Structural misalignment

Toxicity from the colon

viral infections (which may also come from immune weakness, which may come from nutritional deficiency, stress, poor sleep, and poor dietary habits), yeast *(Candida albicans)* overgrowth, mold sensitivities, and a wide variety of intestinal parasites; other factors include food and environmental allergies and essential life-issue conflicts in the patient. There are often other symptoms that go along with fatigue that may help us better assess the underlying causes, whether physical, mental, or emotional (it is usually a combination). Whether the fatigue is acute or chronic will also point toward specific conditions.

The basic guidelines for anyone experiencing fatigue begin with getting more rest and better sleep and adding more positive lifestyle habits. Avoid any abusive drugs or foods, eat well, work less, and try to reduce stress in all areas of your life. Turning to stimulants, such as caffeine in coffee or sodas, is not the answer. Eating a well-balanced diet without overeating and getting adequate rest, even taking a few naps, can help rebuild energy reserves. Exercise is often helpful unless the fatigue is too severe. Up to a certain point, exercise can resolve fatigue by improving circulation and respiration (oxygenation), leading to both energization and relaxation; however, if the energy level is too low, increased activity aggravates the fatigue. One of the diagnostic features of CFS is postexertional fatigue. Most people feel better and build energy from regular exercise, whereas people with CFS feel worse, exhausted, and unable to function for a period after exercise. Analyzing our life—looking at why we do not have the energy to do what we want to do (or what we think or feel we want to do)—and resolving internal frustrations or developing a more creative work style or attitude can make a great difference.

Before we engage in this more subtle level of exploration, however, we should have a complete medical examination. Often a medical evaluation, at least the routine type of exam and the usual blood tests, will not really turn up many answers unless there is anemia, liver disease, an infection, or hypothyroidism. Nutritional evaluations may give more insight but also may not resolve everything. **Then we are left with these more subtle issues of energy balance (for which acupuncture or meditation, as examples, may be helpful), psychological states, other lifestyle habits, and some spiritual questions:**

- Am I really doing what I am meant to be doing?
- Do I have joy in my life?
- What is my inner truth?
- Am I living even close to my inner truth?
- If not, how do I begin to realign?

Some people who do not have as much energy as they wish try to correct the problem by fasting and juice cleansing. I do not recommend this because many people with fatigue are more nutrient-deficient

---

More Specific Causes of Fatigue and Chronic Fatigue

Yeast and mold infections and allergies. *Candida albicans.*

Viral infections (acute). Colds, flus, hepatitis, and mononucleosis.

Viral infections (chronic). HIV, Epstein-Barr, cytomegalovirus, and herpes. (See next program, on page 675.)

Parasite infections. Many possible, such as amoebas or worms.

Bacterial infections. Staphylococcus or streptococcus.

Hormonal deficiencies. Hypothyroidism, low adrenal function (often due to chronic stress and sugar abuse), and pituitary dysfunction, as well as menopause.

Nutritional deficiencies. Magnesium, potassium, iodine, iron, copper, calcium, vitamin B12, folic acid, other B vitamins, vitamins C and E.

Toxic mineral excesses. Lead, aluminum, mercury, nickel, and cadmium.

Metabolic disease. Such as of the heart, liver, or kidneys.

Substance abuse. Coffee, alcohol, sugar, food reactions, rancid oils, marijuana, and other drugs.

Environmental contamination. Fluorescent lights, chemical sensitivity.

Psychological problems. Boredom and depression, and overall unhappiness about life situations and progress.

than they are toxic or congested, and fasting can lead to further depletions. The only type of people with mild to moderate lack of energy (never with severe fatigue) to whom I would suggest fasting are those usually active people with other associated symptoms of congestion, such as sinus problems, constipation, or backaches. An evaluation of such people would show a tight body musculature with lots of sore muscles or tender acupuncture points, which indicates that there is more potential energy, which is trapped in the body channels and not circulating. Often, a detoxifying diet and herbal supplements or a juice fast with colon cleansing, acupuncture, and body therapy will stimulate that stored potential vitality to circulate freely. If other problems of toxicity are also present, I suggest following the general detoxification and cleansing program (see page 741, in chapter 18, Detoxification and Cleansing Programs) rather than this one, or trying the ideas in my book *The New Detox Diet*.

Diet and Supplements for Fatigue

The most appropriate diet for people with fatigue is high in easily digested complex carbohydrates and adequate amounts of protein foods along with at least 2 quarts of filtered, good-quality water daily. The whole-grain products and starchy vegetables are the foods that are utilized in the energy-producing cycle of glycolysis (using sugar for energy) and provide a more sustaining source of energy (ATP) for the body. (Many people with CFS have problems with energy production in the cell mitochondria, and they may not tolerate much carbohydrate in the diet.) This diet contains other vegetables for their nutrients and fiber content and good-quality proteins, but it should be moderately low in fats unless the person is underweight or lives in a cold climate. In that case, more vegetable oils could be consumed, but fried foods and hydrogenated fats should be avoided.

Some people with fatigue are too sensitive to sugars and starches to raise their energy on this diet; rather, they need to focus more on protein intake with lots of fresh vegetables, both steamed and as salad greens, with some nuts and seeds, sprouted beans (better in protein with less starch), and only some grains, starchy vegetables, and fruits. Starchy foods can be helpful in the initial healing of chronic fatigue. Indi-

viduals with chronic fatigue often have compromised energy production when it comes to breaking down fat and converting it into usable energy. This process, called *beta-oxidation,* happens in the mitochondria. Carbohydrate-based energy production that does not require mitochondrial activity may be important until these other fat-related processes can heal. I also recommend avoiding industrial and agricultural chemicals as well as most food additives, as they may place more stress on the probably weak or overworked liver. Staying away from sugar and refined foods is also wise.

There are also a large number of nutrients and supplements that are used to improve energy levels. Of course, what works depends on the cause of the fatigue. If it is due to low levels of certain nutrients, then, obviously, taking additional amounts of those particular nutrients can be helpful, provided there is adequate digestion and assimilation. In addition to specific nutritional deficiencies—such as iron, vitamin B12, folic acid, iodine, potassium, or magnesium—that can lead to fatigue, there can also be a milder form of deficiency, which I call nutritional "depletion disorders." This means that there may not be an adequate supply of nutrients regularly available to the cells and tissues for all the biochemical functions. This leads to a lower energy efficiency and vitality than potentially available with adequate diet, digestive function, and appropriate supplementation.

The nutrients suggested in this program will generally improve energy levels and energy use to provide enhanced vitality necessary to recharge and overcome fatigue. For example, extra vitamin B2 (riboflavin) has been shown to increase resistance to fatigue, particularly with exercise. Taking vitamin B2, even as little as 10 mg, before exercise can help to increase performance and endurance. Vitamin B12, the "red" or "energy" B vitamin, is the most commonly injected vitamin in medicine. Often, injections of hydroxycobalamin or cyanocobalamin in high amounts (500–1,000 mcg) twice a week can help relieve some physical fatigue, even when there is no measured deficiency of this vitamin. This may reflect an effect of vitamin B12 on nerve functions that has not yet been characterized.

I would also like to mention the Krebs cycle nutrients, including malic acid, succinic acid, fumaric acid, and others. Because this group of nutrients is essential when our bodies want to produce energy from fat, our energy supplies can become deficient when these nutrients are not around. Although supplements are available containing these nutrients themselves, some practitioners also like to use these Krebs cycle organic acids in their mineral chelates. For example, even though magnesium (a mineral that is frequently deficient in those with chronic fatigue) is available in many well-absorbed forms like magnesium gluconate, in the case of fatigue, it may be helpful to insist on magnesium malate or magnesium succinate as a way of getting in these Krebs cycle nutrients. I have seen magnesium malate products be quite helpful in many people with CFS and fibromyalgia.

A general multivitamin is usually recommended, as well as increased amounts of all the B vitamins, particularly B_2, B_{12}, and extra B_5 for stress. Also, because deficiencies of folic acid and B_6 have been correlated with specific instances of fatigue, they should be taken as well. Vitamins C and E add protection against further irritations.

Minerals are as important, and in certain people, they are perhaps even more important than the B vitamins. **Magnesium** and **potassium** deficiency is a common cause of low energy, as they support proper cell respiration and energy production. In whole blood analysis, these two minerals are commonly found deficient in my patients with fatigue. Blood test (serum) measurements of these two important minerals are often normal, because the test is only measuring small amounts of the body's stores since potassium and magnesium are mostly inside cells (intracellular minerals, whereas sodium and calcium are more extracellular, or outside cells, and more easily assessed in the serum). Magnesium deficiency is quite common; if you suspect it, ask your doctor to measure a red blood cell (RBC) magnesium level. Supporting the body with 150 to 300 mg of magnesium and 100 to 200 mg of potassium several times daily may help to correct the deficiencies and restore better energy levels.

Iron is essential to build red blood cells to carry oxygen and for ATP production, and increasing intake of this will correct iron-deficiency anemia. **Iodine** is needed for normal thyroid function, which supports proper metabolism and energy production. **Copper** is also necessary for blood building and for energy-producing enzymes, such as superoxide dismutase (SOD). **Zinc** and **manganese** are also essential components of many enzymes, as is magnesium, which is also involved in protein synthesis and ATP transfer—both important in muscle function and nerve conduction. In the case of fatigue, manganese may be especially important, because the manganese form of SOD is the only form that works inside the mitochondria, and the mitochondria are the place where all of our oxygen-based energy production takes place. **Chromium** may help in some cases of fatigue related to blood sugar abnormalities. Really, all of the macrominerals and trace minerals are needed in amounts greater than the RDA, especially if the digestion is slow or deficient and assimilation poor.

Speaking of digestion, it is sometimes helpful for people with fatigue to take additional hydrochloric acid temporarily with meals and supplemental digestive enzymes after eating or between meals. Better digestion and assimilation of nutrients often lead to improved energy levels and less sluggishness from poorly digested food sitting in the bowels. **Better digestion also decreases the potential for food reactions that can be caused by absorption of larger, undigested food molecules.**

Both the **essential fatty acids** and the **L-amino acids** can also be helpful to people with fatigue. The fatty acids are important to energy (ATP) production in the mitochondria of the cells. The amino acid L-carnitine is important to fatty acid metabolism and the efficient use of the fats in the cells. Many people experience improved energy and endurance with L-carnitine supplementation, 500 to 750 mg twice daily, usually taken between or before meals. A couple other nutrients, relatively new in the nutritional field, may also be helpful to many people with fatigue. **Coenzyme Q10,** or ubiquinone, is necessary for energy production and heart function as well as more subtle body activities. **Dimethylglycine** (DMG) also seems to be helpful for some people suffering from fatigue (see more about DMG on page 285 in chapter 7, Special Supplements). Trimethylglycine (TMG) is also available and has a similar effect.

A number of herbs can also be used to alleviate fatigue. Ginseng root and gotu kola have both been known in their respective cultures as antifatigue herbs. **Ginseng** is most helpful in relieving physical fatigue and is the most commonly used tonifying herb in the world. Its antifatigue and antistress effects seem to have been well verified by research. Either Siberian ginseng

(*Eleutherococcus senticosis*) or Chinese red ginseng (*Panax ginseng*) can be used; the red varieties are more likely to increase blood pressure, which may be helpful for weaker people who get cold easily and have lower blood pressure. I particularly like the Siberian ginseng extract in a tincture or glycerin (nonalcohol) extract, as this herb is energizing without being overstimulating and has a stress-reducing factor. It is often called an *adaptogen,* meaning it helps protect the body from adverse and stress effects. Drinking ginseng tea or taking 1 or 2 capsules twice daily, in the morning and at noon, is a way to raise energy with this herb. It usually takes a couple of weeks to produce a noticeable effect. **Most tonifying herbs are taken in low to moderate doses over extended periods of time, even for several months, to achieve best results.**

Gotu kola seems to provide more of a mental stimulation than the physical effect of the ginsengs, yet it too can reduce fatigue. Although it is not a caffeine-type stimulation, it seems to improve mental clarity and memory. **Cayenne pepper** is one of the true natural stimulants, and it works quickly. Using more cayenne in the diet or taking supplemental capsules can provide additional warmth, a mild diuretic effect, and an increase in energy. **Peppermint leaf** tea also seems to provide quick energy and is helpful to the digestion. **Ginger root** stimulates digestion and circulation, is a warming herb, and may help with headaches, nausea, or low energy. **Licorice root** is a balancer and has been used in many formulas for improving energy levels through enhanced body function.

Antifatigue Nutrient Program

Nutrient	Amount	Nutrient	Amount
Water	1 1/2–2 1/2 qt	Iodine	150–225 mcg
Protein	50–100 g	Iron	10–20 mg*
Vitamin A	5,000–10,000 IU	Magnesium	500–800 mg
Beta-carotene	15,000–30,000 IU	Manganese	10–15 mg
Vitamin D	400 IU	Molybdenum	300–500 mcg
Vitamin E	800 IU	Potassium	2–3 g
Vitamin K	300 mcg	Selenium	200 mcg
Thiamin (B1)	50 mg	Silicon	100 mg
Riboflavin (B2)	50–100 mg	Vanadium	200 mcg
Niacin (B3)	50 mg	Zinc	45 mg
Niacinamide (B3)	25–50 mg	Hydrochloric acid	10 grains or 1–2 tablets with meals
Pantothenic acid (B5)	1,000 mg		
Pyridoxine (B6)	50–100 mg, or	Digestive enzymes	2 tablets after meals
Pyridoxal-5-phosphate	50–100 mg	Omega-3 fatty acids	2–4 g
Cobalamin (B12)	250–500 mcg	L-amino acids	1,000 mg
Folic acid	1,000 mcg	L-carnitine	500–1,500 mg
Biotin	500 mcg	Coenzyme Q10	50–200 mg
Choline	1,000 mg	Dimethylglycine	50–100 mg
Inositol	1,000 mg	Ginseng root	2–4 capsules
PABA	100 mg	Licorice root	2–4 capsules
Vitamin C	2 g	Adrenal, glandular	50–100 mg
Bioflavonoids	250 mg		
Calcium	800–1,200 mg		
Chromium	200 mcg		
Copper	2 mg		

* Of course, with iron-deficiency anemia, more iron will be needed.

A combination of these various herbs can be used as powders in teas or in an encapsulated formula to support the treatment of fatigue. They can also help those with increased stress, decreased circulation, hypoglycemia, and weak adrenal function. Even for the emotional and mental "blahs," these herbs can offer a pick-me-up. Remember, with any problem of serious or chronic fatigue, an evaluation to discover the cause is essential! Your natural-health-care provider can get more results with less effort when he or she knows more about the cause(s) of your fatigue; the more the doctor knows, the better he or she can recommend the appropriate nutrients, rest, and therapies.

Many naturally oriented doctors and other practitioners take a multidisciplinary approach to treating problems like fatigue in general, CFS, and fibromyalgia. We look at understanding what is out of balance and supporting the body's health while also treating infections, reducing allergies, and balancing hormones. In his popular book *From Fatigued to Fantastic,* Jacob Teitelbaum, a medical doctor and director of the Annapolis Center for Effective CFS/Fibromyalgia Therapies, talks about the importance of sleep in healing fibromyalgia and CFS. He addresses additional issues in healing from these troublesome conditions (troublesome for both patients and practitioners alike). **A multifaceted approach to treating chronic fatigue and fibromyalgia could include:**

- Natural hormone support, including thyroid, adrenal, and sex hormones.

- Nutritional therapies with magnesium especially, B_{12}, other B vitamins, and amino acids.

- Herbal treatment with ginseng, ginger, turmeric, ginkgo, and so on.

- Avoidance of sugar, refined flour, caffeine, and alcohol.

- Avoiding allergenic foods and reactions to dairy, wheat, soy, and so on.

- Treating chronic infections of the bladder, vagina, prostate, and sinuses.

- Resolving intestinal dysbiosis (imbalanced microbes) and treating abnormal bacteria, yeasts, and parasites.

The "Antifatigue Nutrient Program" on the opposite page lists the daily levels of nutrients that can be used by people with fatigue. Spread the total amounts out throughout the day. If possible, try to take more B vitamins and the herbs earlier in the day, and more of the minerals, especially calcium and magnesium, later and into the evening. The effects of these nutrients can be different from person to person (some people get relaxed rather than stimulated from B vitamins). It is possible you may need to put several formulas together to acquire these levels.

22. VIRAL CONDITIONS

This is such an important area of modern health care because so many people are plagued by various viral conditions—acutely, repeatedly, and chronically. Young and old suffer from the hundreds, likely even thousands, of these microorganisms. The state of our immune system and overall health is quite important to preventing viral infections, and this ties into nutritional toxicity and deficiency, food and environmental allergies, stress and emotions, as well as many other factors. (See the "Conditions That May Reduce Immunity" table on page 678 in this program, as well as the section "Immune Enhancement" on page 633 in chapter 16, Performance Enhancement Programs.)

There are many specific viral conditions caused by these ubiquitous, obligate parasites (meaning they need our cells to reproduce). The viruses affecting human health range from new influenza viruses to common childhood and young adult viral diseases, such as chickenpox, measles, mumps, and mononucleosis. More chronic conditions include herpes viruses, affecting the mouth and lips or the genital area. Viral hepatitis infects millions of people worldwide and kills many thousands a year. And, of course, the HIV microbe alters many people's lives. We must understand these mysterious and powerful microbes that can interfere with our cellular and metabolic functions.

It seems that a virus is always going around. Some viruses cause vague and varying symptoms, while others, including many of the common childhood diseases, lead to similar symptoms from person to person. Viral conditions can be acute and short-lived, such as colds and most influenzas, or may lead to longer illnesses and chronic difficulties, such as *Herpes simplex* infections, hepatitis types B and C, Epstein-Barr syndrome, cytomegaloviral (CMV) disease, and AIDS, caused by the human immunodeficiency virus (HIV). Some of these viruses are difficult to heal and clear from our tissues and cells, and if they get the best of our body, they can even be fatal.

Viral infections seem to be part of the environment's natural "survival of the fittest" selection process. Both epidemic flus or colds and more severe, chronic viruses can be aggressive problems in those who are already sick, the elderly, those weakened by other stresses or illnesses, and those who may already have immune suppression. Some especially virulent viruses may also attack people who outwardly seem to be healthy.

The key area of the body in protection and healing from viral conditions is the immune system. Often a reduced immune defense system allows viruses to attack, to grow, and to spread without being checked by the phagocytes and T lymphocytes. Viruses usually spread in the body by first getting inside the cells, where they can use cellular mechanisms to grow and multiply and then they explode the cell, releasing thousands of viruses into the blood or tissues. **Cell membrane integrity is therefore essential in preventing the beginnings of a viral infection.** Until the viruses get into the cells for protection, they can be coded for antibody formation, which helps provide defense against the virus later on; also, the virus-infected cells can be eaten by the frontline phagocytic immune cells. **Cell integrity is supported mainly by vitamins C and E, plus vitamin A, selenium, and the essential fatty acids.**

The primary way we heal from viruses is through the immune response—by means of lymphocyte (natural killer cell) attack functions and through the formation of specific antiviral antibodies. The antibody response, however, may take from 3 to 14 days to reach adequate levels to counter the millions of viral organisms; often the virus has wreaked havoc during that time. Luckily for us, we usually do not come down with the same viral illness twice, because the antibody memory and rapid response will handle any reinfection with the same virus. But this response is specific to each virus on the never-ending list of viruses—new ones are being discovered all the time—and thus ongoing protection requires a healthy, functioning immune

Various Common Viral Conditions	
Acute Viral Conditions	**Chronic Viral Conditions**
Colds	Herpes
Flus	Viral hepatitis
Bronchitis	Epstein-Barr syndrome
Gastroenteritis	Cytomegalovirus
Herpes—genital and cold sores	Mononucleosis
HIV exposure	AIDS
Infectious mononucleosis	
Acute viral hepatitis	

system and strong, intact cellular membranes. For an antiviral program to be effective, it must support several areas of function simultaneously. **This program incorporates ways to reduce the number of viruses through detoxification and immune support, ways to enhance immune function overall, and ways to improve cell wall integrity and general health.**

Colds and flus are the most common viral problems, affecting nearly everyone at some time. Many are spread through the air by sneezes, by hand-to-mouth contact, or by kissing others. Their frequency may range from 1 or 2 infections every 5 years to repeated infections 5 or 6 times yearly, and symptoms may range from mild fatigue or sinus congestion to total debilitation requiring bed rest for many days. Colds, or upper respiratory infections (URIs), are caused by specific viruses and tend to be localized. Colds may be accompanied by sore throat, cough, weakness, sneezing, nasal congestion, and a mild fever and headache. Fortunately, they are rarely serious and pass within a week or so.

The flu, caused by a variety of changing influenza viruses, is a more acute, rapidly progressing, and systemic condition. It is more likely to be epidemic and can be more dangerous, especially in the weak, sick, or elderly. The flu viruses multiply rapidly, mutate frequently, and spread through the blood, causing higher fevers, generalized aches and pains, headaches, and sore eyes. Usually, we need to go to bed for 1 or 2 days with the flu. (One reason we may have gotten sick, or at least a contributor, is not enough rest and time for destressing.) It is often short-lived; however, it may also settle into the throat and bronchial tubes or the intestines and hang around, being a nuisance for weeks at a time without us really getting the amount of rest and nurturance that we need to heal. A viral bronchitis can lead to a mild mucus-producing or dry cough; gastroenteritis can cause mild to severe digestive upset and diarrhea. All of these flu illnesses are usually associated with some fatigue.

Acute (initial viral infections) **herpes, hepatitis, and infectious mononucleosis** all have their own sets of symptoms and often can be much worse than any long-term version of these problems. Herpes can lead to cold sores or fever blisters around the mouth or occasionally to a painful infection inside the mouth. Luckily, this version does not usually recur. Another acute form of herpes also caused by the *Herpes simplex* virus is transmitted through sexual contact with someone carrying the virus. It causes a sensitivity of the skin and a cluster of blisters on or around the genitals, often taking 1 or 2 weeks to heal, and it can be fairly uncomfortable and contagious. This herpes infection more easily becomes a chronic condition than infectious hepatitis (type A) or mononucleosis, both of which can be more severe in the initial phase.

Hepatitis is a viral infection of the liver that can be contracted through blood contact via intravenous drug injections or blood transfusions (hepatitis types B and C) or through body fluid/fecal contact (infectious hepatitis, type A). Acute infectious hepatitis A is associated with fatigue and a yellowing of the skin and eyes (jaundice) and possibly an initial period of dark urine and white- or gray-colored stools. Infectious mononucleosis, the "kissing disease," is spread through intimate contact. It typically causes significant fatigue/exhaustion, often a fever and a sore throat, and may also lead to a mild hepatitis and enlargement of the spleen. Both hepatitis and mononucleosis usually require extensive care, rest, plenty of drinking water and herbal teas, a good diet, and avoidance of such liver-irritating substances as alcohol and fats; full recovery may take 1 to several months.

Chronic viral conditions are specific types of infections where the virus remains alive and active in the body, often in quiescent states, possibly with occasional recurrences of the acute condition. **Such lifestyle factors as stress and diet, which affect acid-alkaline balance and seem to influence recurrences more than anything else, are the primary focus of this discussion.** With this approach, it appears that there are things we can do to reduce these more common and more serious chronic viral conditions.

Chronic genital herpes (and fever blisters or cold sores) is definitely a result of increased stresses and other hidden factors. Luckily, it is not usually as intense as the initial outbreak, but it definitely interferes with an intimate relationship; conversely, relationship issues and/or sexual stress often are psychological factors in persistent herpes. A number of nutrients can be helpful in reducing recurrences; decreasing stress is also important. There are several new medicines realted to acyclovir, or Zovirax (the original antiherpes drug) that are helpful in treating and preventing recurrent herpes infections, and they are usually well tolerated with few side effects. These newer drugs include Valtrex (valacyclovir) and Famvir (famcyclovir). Herpes is still not curable, at this point, although there can be long-term remissions. Oral lysine, 500 to 1,000 mg daily, commonly will prevent cold sore outbreaks; however, this amino acid appears to offer little help for people with genital herpes. Eating too many nuts and seeds, higher in the amino acid arginine, may precipitate recurrences of herpes infections. It is thought that the herpes virus stays in the nerves or nerve roots and when activated creates a mild neuritis and skin outbreak at the site of the infected nerves. A treatment I use for patients includes higher levels of vitamin C, 3 to 4 grams a day, and monolaurin containing Lauricidin, an extract of coconut oil, which may reduce the replication of the herpes virus.

Chronic hepatitis (B and C, and possibly other viruses) has become more common in U.S. culture and can be a significant health problem. It results from an acute infectious hepatitis type A, which apparently does not become chronic. Types B and C come from blood contact, although there may be some possible exposure with sexual activity (incidence of this is rare if at all). When there are torn tissues during sex and possible blood contact, this may be a contributing factor. There also may be various strains of these two chronic hepatitis viruses, some more virulent than others. I have many patients who experience long-term good health even though they have these viruses, and I have found that a healthy lifestyle of good diet, regular exercise, good sleep, stress management, and a positive attitude toward life all contribute to better outcomes in many conditions—especially viral problems like chronic hepatitis and HIV infections. The consistent supplementation with nutrients and herbs is quite important. I am not impressed with the medical treatment for chronic hepatitis, as the drugs cause many side effects and are typically not curative.

Epstein-Barr virus (EBV), HHV-6 (human herpes virus type 6), and cytomegalovirus (CMV) are several organisms that have been associated with chronic fatigue syndrome. However, even though a symptom of these viruses may be fatigue, they do not clearly appear to be the *cause* of chronic fatigue. The chronic form of EBV (a viral infection contained in the B cell lymphocytes, differing from herpes types 1 and 2, which hide out in the nerve roots) more commonly than CMV leads to fatigue, and HHV-6 is often associated with EBV. All of these viruses stress immune function and vary in their activity; this may account for wide swings in energy, including periods of extreme fatigue, experienced by people with these viruses, which may also affect antibody response to other agents. They often show signs of CFS and have to take time off from work to reevaluate their lives, as it can take months or even years to recover. They can be diagnosed and their progress followed through the use of blood tests of antibody titers, which measure levels of antibodies specific to each virus. Nutritional and stress management therapies are often helpful, in my experience, at speeding recovery time. Improving immune function, particularly of T lymphocytes, may help to remedy these problems. (See "Immune Enhancement" on page 633 in chapter 16, Performance Enhancement Programs.)

Acquired Immune Deficiency Syndrome (AIDS) is believed to be a viral infection of the T-helper cells (there are other theories as well), which both modulate and stimulate the human immune response. Initially a sexually transmitted disease primarily affecting gay men, it has crossed the boundaries of the homosexual population to heterosexuals, IV drug users, and people with hemophilia or others who require blood transfusions. It is possible that, as with other viruses, people who have had an initial contact may have mild symptoms or none at all initially—the immune system makes antibodies, and that is it, no further problem. But the once called HTLV-III (human T-lymphotropic virus)—now termed HIV (human immunodeficiency virus)—may exist in quiescent stages and create a problem later. Further research may show it to be a steadily growing virus that will eventually cause problems in most carriers. The development of new drugs has changed the course for many with AIDS, and more drugs are being researched; there may be more answers around the corner. (The discussion and use of the latest drugs prescribed for HIV can be done with your treating doctor.) People no longer need to accept a death sentence when diagnosed with HIV infection. As with other chronic viral issues, a healthy lifestyle often creates better outcomes. This should be evaluated more fully with research to motivate people with viruses like HIV, hepatitis B and C, and other chronic viral infections to focus on good self-care to protect their long-term health.

Conditions That May Reduce Immunity

Air pollution
Alcohol
Bacterial infections
Cigarette smoke
Environmental chemicals
Excess activity
Extreme emotions
Extreme weather
Lack of exercise
Negative attitudes
Nutrient deficiencies: fatty acid deficiency
    (weakens cell membranes, which allows viruses
    to get in); selenium; vitamins A and C
Overwork
Parasitic infections
Poor diet (a low-protein diet or a congestive "high-
    acid" diet)
Poor sleep
Steroid drugs
Stimulant drugs such as cocaine and amphetamines
Stress
Sugar overuse
Toxic heavy metals
Viral infections
Yeast infections

Some keys of nutritional therapy may help to prevent viral illnesses or at least slow their progress, and research to date has shown some benefits from high nutrient intake, particularly of vitamin C. Many knowledgeable authorities suggest additional supplements of other vitamins and minerals, particularly vitamins C, E, B5, B6, B12, and folic acid, as well as the minerals zinc, copper, manganese, and magnesium. More research is needed regarding nutritional support for people with AIDS and other life-altering viral infections. In dealing with viral conditions of all kinds, researchers are looking at another important chapter in immunology. A healthy immune system is essential to prevent viral problems. A decrease in immune protection can allow various viruses to get into the body and take hold, and most viruses are not easy to clear. Many changes in body environment allow easier "catching" of these ubiquitous germs. Many conditions, even other viral problems, lead to further decreases in resistance and immune function.

The key with viruses is prevention. We need to live healthfully, following the guidance in this book and others. Keeping the immune system strong by managing stress and eating well, making sure we obtain the immune-supporting and antioxidant nutrients—vitamins C, A (both preformed and as beta-carotene), and E, selenium, and zinc, as well as the amino acid L-cysteine. Avoid any regular intake of sugar, saturated and processed fats, refined foods, and allergenic foods that irritate the immune system. Regular exercise offers energy and relaxation and aids detoxification. Proper sleep is essential to high vitality and productivity. Regular elimination and good colon function are also necessary to prevent the stagnation that breeds disease. Congesting diets (higher in proteins, fats, sugars, and refined foods) and excessive stress create a more acidic body chemistry, which allows viruses to take hold and progress in the body.

To protect us from upper respiratory infections, the health of the mucous membranes, mucus production, and salivary antibodies (such as secretory IgA) are all important; these factors are similar in the protection against viral entry via the gastrointestinal route, with the secretory IgA from the cells an important defense. A balanced diet supports a balanced body chemistry; with congestion and a more acid chemistry, a diet higher in chlorophyll foods, water, good

oils (essential fatty acids), and high-fiber foods will help in maintaining adequate detoxification. Expressing feelings and handling intense emotional experiences, through taking time off and/or with counseling, are essential to prevent the immune suppression that can result from major stresses, changes, and challenges. And, of course, it is necessary to keep a positive attitude toward life—to ride the wave rather than get caught up in the flood, where little germs can invade us more easily. There are many individual keys to staying strong and healthy. The health quest is to know ourselves well enough to create the right path for us as individuals, and to keep on that path when we find it.

Diet and Supplements for Viral Conditions

The general dietary suggestions for times when we have viral infections vary somewhat depending on whether the infection is acute or chronic. For acute colds and flus, I usually suggest fluids and light eating, or even a fast or detoxification diet. A juice cleanse may be helpful but is not always indicated, particularly if there is much fatigue—in which case more nutrients are needed. **Almost always, a mild detoxification can be done by just decreasing consumption of congesting foods, such as meats, milk products, breads and sweet treats, while increasing liquids and the nutrient-rich water foods, the fruits and vegetables.** Soups are ideal for these conditions, with some salads or cooked vegetables. Water should be the main fluid, but herbal teas, fruit juices (such as citrus, apple, or cranberry), and some vegetable juices (such as carrot, celery, spinach or kale, and beet) are also nourishing and purifying. Some extra protein is needed, but not much over the minimum needs. Excess fats and oils should be avoided. High-chlorophyll green vegetables are a plus, and the whole grains or some whole-grain toast will provide more fiber. Especially when there is constipation or bowel sluggishness, emphasize the fluids, fruits, vegetables, and grains.

An enema or colonic irrigation may be helpful in these instances of acute congestion or chronic constipation. (See chapter 18, Detoxification and Cleansing Programs, for more advice in this area. A cleansed and healthy body does not get sick easily and is less prone to viral invasion.) Reducing stress, totally letting go if possible, taking time off from work or other responsibilities, and getting lots of rest and sleep will support the healing process. Having a cold, flu, or other acute viral problem is sometimes the only thing that will induce many people to take time off, to be quiet, and to rest. The keys for treating acute viral conditions are rest, fluids, and extra vitamin A and beta-carotene, vitamin C, and zinc.

For chronic viral problems, a more balanced diet is indicated. There is usually fatigue and some depletion in these situations, so detoxification is not often a primary approach; however, it could be appropriate for some people. If someone is already underweight or deficient in nutrients, a fast may make matters worse. A more nutrient-rich detoxifying diet may be helpful. To be safe, I do not recommend juice fasting with chronic viruses. Increasing higher-nutrient fresh vegetable juices is often helpful, but this should be in conjunction with a diet higher in good-quality protein than that used for acute viral conditions. Nourishing foods are always indicated in these cases, with an avoidance of refined foods, junk foods, and fast foods. Soups, whole grains, legumes, salads, and some fruits are great. For proteins, I suggest eating some fresh fish and poultry, legumes, sprouted seeds, and only a few nuts, eggs, or dairy foods, as they are the higher-fat proteins.

Reducing fried foods, saturated fats and oily foods as well as alcohol and stimulants is wise to keep the liver working to ensure slow detoxification and regeneration. Adding cold-pressed vegetable oils and flaxseed oil helps support the needed fatty acids. Both garlic and lemon water in the diet are helpful supporters of the liver. Avoid chemicals from food and the environment with any chronic disease, especially with viruses. **With chronic viral problems, the key is high-quality nourishment, individualized supplementation programs, and rest.**

A great many **supplements** have been used to treat viral infections, including vitamins, minerals, enzymes, amino acids, and many herbs. Herbs are the major medicinal components of nutritional or natural therapies. The treatment of viral infections is among the more appropriate uses of nutritional supplements in higher, orthomolecular, doses. In my opinion, they offer some benefits where Western pharmaceutical medicine has little to offer without cre-

ating further immune imbalance. For acute infections with viruses, primarily colds and flus, I often recommend a multiple vitamin/mineral and higher levels of **vitamin A and vitamin C.** Mixed carotenoids and beta-carotene, the vitamin A precursor, can be used, but the retinol form of vitamin A has the immune and anti-infection effect. I suggest 50,000 to 100,000 IU daily for a few days up to a week, and then about 25,000 to 50,000 IU for a few more days, tapering off over the week. The toxic side effects that could result from regular use of these dosages of vitamin A are uncommon when they are taken for short periods of time, and the body seems to handle much higher amounts when it is sick.

That is also true of vitamin C, perhaps the key nutrient in treating viral conditions. Ascorbic acid offers cellular protection by stabilizing cell membranes. In larger doses, it also has an antihistamine effect, and it stimulates bowel activity, which is often helpful for acute congestion by supporting better elimination. The bowel tolerance level of vitamin C is determined by finding out how much can be taken without causing diarrhea—that is, by taking vitamin C every 1 or 2 hours until the bowels are loose and then cutting back. Usually, pure ascorbic acid powder is best used for this purpose; however, it does contribute to an acid shift in body chemistry and can be irritating to the gastrointestinal mucosa at these levels. With this process, amounts of 30 to 40 grams or more per day might be used, which is what some doctors recommend, but I suggest up to 1 to 2 grams every couple of hours during the day, as the vitamin C is used so rapidly by a sick and healing body that it is needed almost every hour. I have used intravenous vitamin C drips, with 10 to 20 grams of vitamin C slowly infused over an hour, along with other vitamins and minerals, for treatment of acute and chronic viral infections. It is usually well tolerated and often quite effective. Sometimes the results are as dramatic as those from an IV dose of antibiotics to treat a sensitive bacterial infection. Orally, even a few grams daily can make a difference in symptoms and healing, as vitamin C offers extra antioxidant and cell membrane protection as well has some direct antiviral effect.

Zinc is useful in acute viral infections, especially with vitamin A, as the two enhance each other's effects in providing immune support. Amounts of zinc up to 50 to 100 mg daily are usually well tolerated when split into several doses and not taken for extended periods, although many people take these high amounts regularly with no complications (an upset stomach is the most common problem with zinc). **Be sure to take extra copper and manganese and possibly iron for several weeks after taking higher amounts of zinc.** Zinc gluconate or other chelated zinc, such as picolinate, are good orally, and special zinc throat lozenges have produced some remarkable results with acute viral sore throats and beginning colds. Sucking on zinc lozenges is also a good way to get extra zinc into the body.

Magnesium is usually depleted in acute infections, so more should be taken during these illnesses. Other minerals and vitamins can be taken as a general multivitamin. Extra B vitamins, especially B5 and B6, are helpful to some people. Additional L-amino acids in combination with a high-complex-carbohydrate, modified vegetarian diet is closer to the ideal plan than consuming lots of the heavier animal proteins and fats. **The L-amino acids can bypass the pancreas and digestive process and are easily used by the liver and body to perform the building functions needed.** Fresh vegetable oils (cold-pressed) and some raw seeds and sprouted seeds are the best of the fat-containing foods. Also, do not forget to continue drinking more good-quality water or herbal teas and fruit or vegetable juices.

A supplement program for chronic viral conditions should include a hypoallergenic multiple **vitamin-mineral supplement** without preservatives and artificial colors. Antioxidant nutrients have a higher priority in chronic viral syndromes; therefore, more carotenes, vitamin E, selenium, and L-cysteine are used in addition to the elevated levels of vitamins A, C, and zinc. Regular usage of vitamin C may range from 3 to 4 grams up to 20 grams a day or more. The amount of zinc can range from 50 to 75 mg; about 30,000 to 40,000 IU of vitamin A can be taken for short periods of time, such as 1 or 2 weeks and only if liver function is adequate. These are all smaller amounts than are used with acute infections but still greater than the normal amounts of these three important nutrients. Magnesium is also especially needed.

Some other interesting nutrients for viral problems are **organo-germanium and monolaurin,** a compound derived from lauric acid. Organo-germanium

has been shown to have antiviral properties. Early research shows that it both stimulates T lymphocyte production and increases levels of interferon, a protein molecule thought to help in the treatment and healing of viral diseases and cancer. The pure powder from Japan (or the tablets or capsules made from that) is still available. It can be taken in several doses of 50 to 150 mg. It is nontoxic and can be mixed easily into water and drunk. Therapeutic levels of organo-germanium may reach as high as many grams per day, and it is still being looked at regarding cancer therapy.

Monolaurin, a product supplied by Ecological Formulas (see Appendix B, "Nutritional Supplement Companies"), is more interesting and likely more effective, but further research is needed on it as well. It contains Lauricidin, which is an ester of lauric acid, a fatty acid found in coconut and canola oils. The Lauricidin compound has stronger antiviral properties than lauric acid by itself. Certain of the chronic viruses—EBV, CMV, herpes, and some influenza organisms—are termed "envelope" viruses, which means that the virus is protected inside a lipid-membrane coating. Monolaurin can disturb the lipid in the virus's protective membrane coating and thus prevent the virus from attaching to the host cells; thus, it cannot replicate. This product works best when taken on an empty stomach or following a low-fat meal. I recommend 3 to 4 capsules in the morning and later in the day for acute viral problems and usually 3 to 6 capsules once in the morning for chronic viral concerns.

Ecological Formulas also sells another lauric acid product called Viricidin. Each capsule contains 90 mg of Lauricidin and smaller amounts of BHT (butylated hydroxytoluene) and zinc for additional antioxidant and immune support. This formula is designed for people with herpes viral infections and Epstein-Barr virus, although the monolaurin formula has more Lauricidin (300 mg per capsule) and is better for problems of EBV. Viricidin can also be used by taking 3 capsules initially in the morning and then an additional 1 or 2 capsules several times over the day.

An innovative therapy used by some contemporary health-care practitioners for chronic viral problems is injections of adenosine monophosphate (AMP). It feeds directly into nucleic acid synthesis

Viral Conditions and Key Nutrients

Problem	Nutrients
Colds and flus	Fluids—water, herb teas, juice, soup
Bronchitis	Vitamins C and A, zinc, n-acetyl-cysteine (an antioxidant that protects respiratory membranes)
Gastroenteritis	Acidophilus and other probiotics, echinacea, garlic, goldenseal, grapefruit seed extract
Herpes simplex I (oral lesions)	L-lysine, acidophilus
Herpes simplex II (genital problems)	Lauric acid
Epstein-Barr, CMV, and mononucleosis	
acute	Vitamin C, zinc, lauric acid, L-lysine, organo-germanium
chronic	Antioxidants—vitamins C, A, and E, selenium, zinc, L-cysteine; lauric acid, organo-germanium
Hepatitis	
acute, active	Fluids, rest, low-protein, low-fat diet
acute, resolution	Balanced diet, vitamin C, antioxidant nutrients
chronic	Antioxidants, vitamin C, silymarin (milk thistle)

Acute Viral Nutrient Program

Nutrient	Amount	Nutrient	Amount
Water	3–4 qt	Calcium	600–1,000 mg
Protein	50 g	Chromium	200 mcg
Fats	30–50 g	Copper	4–6 mg
Vitamin A palmitate*	25,000–50,000 IU	Iodine	150–200 mcg
Beta-carotene and/or		Iron	10–18 mg
mixed carotenoids	25,000–50,000 IU	Magnesium	400–750 mg
Vitamin D	400–1,000 IU	Manganese	10–15 mg
Vitamin E	400 IU	Molybdenum	500 mg
Vitamin K	300 mcg	Selenium as selenomethionine	200–400 mcg
Thiamin (B1)	50 mg	or sodium selenite	150–250 mcg
Riboflavin (B2)	50 mg	Zinc	50–150 mg
or riboflavin-5-phosphate	50 mg		
Niacin (B3)	50 mg	**Optional**	
Niacinamide (B3)	100 mg	Garlic oil	4–6 capsules
Pantothenic acid (B5)	500 mg	Echinacea (freeze-dried or	2–4 capsules or
Pyridoxine (B6)	50 mg	extract) as directed on bottle	1–2 dropperfuls
or pyridoxal-5-phosphate	50 mg	Goldenseal (1–2 weeks at most)	6 capsules
Cobalamin (B12)	100–200 mcg	Monolaurin	6 capsules
Folic acid	800 mcg	Lactobacillus and bifidobacteria	1 billion–
Biotin	500 mcg		10 billion count
Vitamin C	8–20 g		
Bioflavonoids	500 mg	* limited to 1–2 weeks, then reduce	

pathways and improves energy levels; it may interfere in some way with the growing cycle of some viruses, such as Epstein-Barr or *Herpes simplex.* Injections 2 or 3 times weekly along with vitamin B12 have shown some helpful results for many patients; there are no adverse side effects known at the present time.

A number of **herbs** have therapeutic effects in the treatment of acute and chronic viral infections. **Garlic, echinacea, goldenseal, propolis, and myrrh** all offer some benefits for acute infections. Echinacea–vitamin C tablets and echinacea tinctures are popular, probably because they work well in alleviating some of the symptoms of colds and flus. Echinacea is an effective blood purifier, helping the body to eliminate toxins. More research is needed to see how this historically used herb works, but preliminary studies suggest that it improves white blood cell

function in destroying microorganisms and is a lymphatic cleanser. Use of garlic oil capsules or crushed garlic soaked in olive oil and increasing fresh garlic intake are also popular herbal treatments for acute and some chronic viral problems. Capsules of powdered goldenseal root can be used at the beginning of an illness, 1 or 2 capsules several times daily, to help strengthen the body's defenses, or during the recovery time for 1 or 2 weeks to help support liver detoxification and tissue building. Similarly, goldenseal extract in alcohol can be used as 1/2 to 1 dropperful several times daily.

Propolis and myrrh are often used during the initial phases of infections as mild "antibiotics" (although more often for bacterial infections) in lieu of using pharmaceutical antibiotics. Myrrh is more of a blood purifier, while propolis may have some antimicrobial

Chronic Viral Nutrient Program

Nutrient	Amount	Nutrient	Amount
Water	2–3 qt	Calcium	650–1,000 mg
Protein	75–100 g	Chromium	200 mcg
Fats	40–65 g	Copper	2–3 mg
Vitamin A (1–2 weeks on,		Iodine	150–225 mcg
1 week off)	10,000–20,000 IU	Iron	10–18 mg
Beta-carotene or mixed		Magnesium	450–700 mg
carotenoids	15,000–30,000 IU	Manganese	10 mg
Vitamin D	400 IU	Molybdenum	500 mcg
Vitamin E	800–1,000 IU	Selenium as selenomethionine	200–400 mcg
Vitamin K	300 mcg	or sodium selenite	150–300 mcg
Thiamin (B1)	50–100 mg	Silicon	50–100 mg
Riboflavin (B2)	50–100 mg	Zinc	45–60 mg
or riboflavin-5-phosphate	25–50 mg	L-amino acids	750–1,500 mg
Niacin (B3)	50–200 mg	L-cysteine	500 mg
Niacinamide (B3)	50–100 mg	L-carnitine	500 mg
Pantothenic acid (B5)	500–1,000 mg	Organo-germanium	150–500 mg
Pyridoxine (B6)	50–100 mg		
and/or pyridoxal-5-phosphate	25–50 mg	**Optional**	
Cobalamin (B12)	250–500 mcg	Monolaurin	600–1,800 mg
Folic acid	800–1,200 mcg	Pau d'arco	6 capsules or
Biotin	500 mcg		3 cups
Choline	500–1,000 mg	Dimethylglycine or	
Inositol	500–1,000 mg	trimethylglycine	50–100 mg
Vitamin C	4–8 g	Digestive enzymes	2–3 tablets
Bioflavonoids	250–500 mg		after meals

effects. A formula I have used for several years with positive results is ANI, made by Professional Botanicals in Utah (see Appendix B, "Nutritional Supplement Companies"). ANI includes propolis, myrrh, echinacea root, garlic, and goldenseal root. Another herb formula that can be used in both acute and chronic infections is a tea made from sage, garlic, and ginger root. **Ginger** is good for warming a chilled body, and **sage** is a blood purifier. Some lemon juice is also added to this tea, and a taste of honey if needed.

Other herbs that can be employed for various viral conditions include white willow bark—an anti-inflammatory herb for fevers, aches, and pain; peppermint leaf—soothing for fevers and upset stomachs; catnip leaf—calming to the nerves and gastrointestinal tract and helpful in bronchitis; mullein leaf—useful for respiratory problems; licorice root—for cough from bronchitis or intestinal upset; pau d'arco (taheebo)—a tonic herb that may be mildly antimicrobial and has been demonstrated to have antiviral properties. Oregano oil and grapefruit seed extract also have antimicrobial effects.

The two tables on pages 682 and 683 present programs for acute and chronic viral conditions. Each shows the basic components, with suggestions for optional treatments. There are many remedies and health-restoring programs available for treating viral infections in the realms of naturopathic and homeopathic medicine that also seem to be helpful. Many of the remedies, such as atomidine, echinacea extracts, and oscillococcinum or other specific homeopathics, can be purchased at most natural foods stores.

23. WEIGHT LOSS

This is a common and complex health topic, with staggering numbers of obese and overweight people in the United States and the Western world. Most Americans are heavier than their optimum weight, but they may not be obese—yet. The terms *obesity* and *overweight* can be defined in terms of percentage body fat, body mass index (BMI), as well as weight in pounds. The "Weight Problems and Body Mass Index" table below shows how overweight and obesity are currently defined by the U.S. Department of Health and Human Services.

Being overweight could also be defined in terms of what we think and feel about ourselves, as the psychological attitude toward our weight is so important. Some people, mostly young women, may think that they are overweight and eat sparingly, when they are actually malnourished and underweight. Most "overweight" people are fickle about their weight-control regimens. They will try any and many programs, mostly short-term crash diets that focus on calorie restriction or a single food group, such as a high-protein diet. The up-and-down weight syndrome may lead us to the path of lifelong obesity.

Quick weight loss is not the aim of the program discussed here. That is relatively easy to do time and again (yet less easy the more we do it). The only healthy and effective long-range weight-reduction plan is to have a balanced and healthy lifestyle and to find the diet and eating habits that allow us to reach and maintain the weight that is right for each of us. With moderate to active regular exercise, we can all be close to our optimum weight. This optimum weight may not be quite as low as that of the body we idolize or

Weight Problems and Body Mass Index (BMI)			
	Weight (lbs)	**% Body Fat**	**Body Mass Index (BMI)**
Overweight	164–195 (men)	—	25.0–29.9
	145–174 (women)	—	
Obesity	>195 (men)	>25% (men)	30 and above
	>174 (women)	>32% (women)	

Source: "National Health and Nutrition Examination Survey Data Briefs," July 2003, U.S. Department of Health and Human Services, Centers for Disease Control and Prevention, National Center for Health Statistics.

even as low as that listed in the ideal weight charts. Heredity, conditioning, and metabolism, as well as percentage of body fat, all influence what is ideal, or healthy, for each of us.

Significant excess weight—more than 30 pounds—and more extreme obesity are some of the bigger health concerns of the Western world. Both the overintake and the underutilization of food as well as the storage of excess fuel in the body as fat and waste create a serious nutritional disease. This problem contributes to many more serious diseases, such as cardiovascular disease, cancer, and diabetes—the three most life-threatening, chronic degenerative conditions in U.S. society. Obesity is an important risk factor in all of these conditions; in addition, it causes a general decrease in longevity.

The "3M" Keys to Weight Loss: Mother, Motivation, and Metabolism

Mother. Weight problems begin early; the majority of overweight adults had some problem with their weight as children or adolescents. Genetics clearly plays a part, but distinguishing its effects from those of conditioning and environmental stimuli is quite difficult. Children of overweight parents have a greater tendency to be overweight. Our mother is usually the first one to feed us, and early on we develop patterns of eating and relating that often influence us for life. For many, this pattern with our mother continues, with moms trying to nourish us on many levels throughout life. The sugary treats come with behavior interactions, with grandparents as well if they are involved, and this sweetness, in Chinese medicine, often relates to the relationship with the mother. Counseling concerning this relationship helps many overweight people clarify the issues and desires related to food and may allow new motivations to come forth.

Motivation. Most overweight people know that experiencing ups and downs in one's weight does not work as a weight-control method. Fad diets may be fun, but they are usually frivolous: 80% to 90% of people who lose weight on these diets regain their lost weight, sometimes even more; this is less healthy than just staying the weight we are. We need a lifetime plan, and this is where motivation comes in. Gathering our deeper strength by focusing on the long-range

Medical and Health Problems Related to Obesity	
Arthritis	Infertility
Atherosclerosis	Job stress
Cancer	Kidney disease
Diabetes	Liver disease
Gallbladder disease	Menstrual problems
Gout	Relationship problems
Heart disease	Strokes
High cholesterol levels	Varicose veins
Hypertension	

vision as well as the quick benefits, and continually telling ourselves that we can do it, will help to overcome our weight problem. Most people think more about the immediate benefits of the slimmer body or a better appearance than the lifelong health risks of being overweight. Emphasizing both may help improve motivation.

Overeating and poor habits are hard to change but easy to develop. I know from experience. It takes little to simply say change the diet, but without the motivation and the ability to break through our psychological barriers, it is difficult to make major changes. It is helpful to first change the types of foods one eats to a more natural-food diet. Sugars, fats, and refined foods can easily be replaced with more wholesome choices. Refined and rich foods may increase hunger as well as add low-nutrient calories. (Complex carbohydrates fill us with fewer calories and reduce the appetite.) Thus reducing their intake usually makes a difference in calorie and nutrient intake, and often in our metabolism and general health, which influences our weight. Then we can move on to deal with the more difficult habits. Isolating and eliminating allergenic/addictive foods is difficult only for a few days. Then eating a variety of foods will minimize other possible allergens in the diet. Our healthful aim is to create a new, stable lifestyle approach to give us the right body weight and energy as well as the effective level of metabolism to maintain them.

Metabolism. There are several theories regarding the effects of our metabolism on our weight, and I am convinced that they each describe important factors. The basal metabolic rate (BMR) is the rate at which the body burns calories to maintain its functions at rest. It is affected by gender, age, diet, activity level, thyroid function, amount of sleep, amount of body fat, body temperature, weight, and likely by genetics. We need a certain number of calories to maintain our weight with a regular exercise level. We can calculate our acceptable calorie intake by figuring the number of calories required to meet our basic needs and adding to it the extra calories used in exercise and mental activity. Formulas for doing this are provided in many nutrition books, but here is a simple way you can do it on your own:

First, take your weight in pounds and add a 0 on the end. For example, if you weight 140 pounds, add a zero on the end to get 1,400 calories. Second, take your right hand (if you are right-handed) or your left hand (if you are left-handed) and wrap your thumb and middle finger around your other wrist. Are your two fingers close to touching? If they overlap, you are most likely small framed (in terms of bone size); if they just barely touch, you are most likely medium framed; and if they do not come anywhere close to touching, you are most likely large framed. Large-framed persons should add another 10% to their calorie total. In my example, a large-framed person would add 140 calories to 1,400 calories to get 1,540 calories. A small-framed person would subtract 140 calories to get 1,260 calories. These amounts are definitely rough estimates, and do not include deliberate daily exercise. If you want to factor in exercise level, add another 5 to 10 calories per minute of exercise, moving toward 10 calories only if the exercise is intense and strenuous. For example, a person doing 30 minutes of walking might add another 150 calories to their daily total. Once again, these results are only ballpark estimates, but they should get you started in the right direction.

Set-point theory. One way of describing a complex metabolic process, this theory applies to what the body "thinks" is normal. The set point is actually the amount of body fat the body tries to maintain. Obese people have a higher set point than trimmer people. This may be related to the number of fat cells, which may in turn be tied to genetics and early eating patterns. The set-point theory suggests that the body works like a thermostat. When we diet and con-

---

Theories and Causes of Being Overweight

General	Specific
Metabolic rate	Excess calories
Set point	and/or fats
Fat cell type and number	Excess sugar and
	refined foods
Family Influences	Overeating
Heredity	Slow liver metabolism
Eating patterns	Nutrient deficiencies
Food choices	Low thyroid function
Family relationships	Lack of exercise
Food as a security	Food allergies/reactions
substitute	Yeast infections
Psychological attitudes	Parasites
Self-image within family	Insulin insensitivity
How we deal with stress	Emotional factors,
	such as depression
	Fat body self-image

---

sume fewer calories, the body reacts as if a starvation crisis is upon us, with compensatory responses, such as lowering the BMR, the rate at which we burn calories, in an attempt to conserve calories and weight. The end result is that we can maintain the same weight on fewer calories. This theory makes sense, considering our long-term experiences with weight reduction. However, it is unlikely that any of us actually has a set *point*. Rather, we are much more likely to have a set *range* in which we remain healthiest.

Regular dieting, especially the low-calorie starvation diet, is met with ever greater difficulty in maintaining weight loss and often results in faster rebounds. As our weight goes up and down, our metabolism seems to slow, as it does with age, and it becomes harder and harder to lose weight. Once established, our personal set point and level of body fat are not easily influenced. Our set point, and thus our weight, might even go up. The body really needs regular exercise and a long-term, steady, lower-calorie diet plan to adapt to a lower weight and better energy efficiency—in short, turning down our thermostat.

The fat-cell theory. This theory seems to correlate with the set-point philosophy. Research has shown that we each develop a specific number of fat cells in the body. This mainly occurs before birth, during infancy, and during the adolescent growth phase. This may be genetically determined, but it also appears that if we are overfed or overeat during these times, we may create more fat cells. At other times, as in our adult life, we increase only the size of our fat cells. When we take in more calories than we use, our fat cells and fat stores get bigger. So a trim person may have a lower number of fat cells than, or the same number of smaller fat cells as, a heavier person, but when we lose weight and become thinner, the fat cells become smaller.

This process involves primarily "white" fat found mainly in the fat cells that lie under the skin. This is our energy, or calorie-storage fat. The "brown" fat, or the "good" fat, actually burns calories for body heat. This fat is deeper and surrounds and protects our organs. Normal fatty acid metabolism supports and nourishes the brown fat. The storage, or white, fat is where the body puts the extra calories from dietary sources that we do not use. When we diet regularly or when our weight goes up and down, the internal weight control system fears starvation and will store more fat as energy for the future. With repeated weight loss and weight gain, the same number of calories in the diet may keep us at a higher weight because we have a higher set point.

When we have developed more fat cells during our growth periods (infancy and adolescence), we tend to have more fat, a slower metabolism, and a higher set point, and we are more likely to have a higher weight. Once this pattern develops, by being overweight early in life, for example, it is hard to change. It takes work and a new self-image! Regular exercise and increasing exercise capacity are the main physical ways to improve the set point and lose weight and then to be able to maintain our weight with a reasonable number of calories. This is a far healthier approach than taking diet pills or any of the many possible diet stimulants. Although there is research evidence about the attainment of a certain number of fat cells, and a set range in which our metabolism operates, none of this means that we are destined to be overweight, or that we are stuck with too many fat cells all screaming, "Feed me, feed me!" All of us can reach and maintain our ideal weight range regardless of our fat cell number and thermostat.

Other ideas about individual weight suggest two opposing views. One school says that people are thin because they do not overeat as much as fat people, because they are guided more by internal signals of hunger and the types of food that their bodies want. Overweight people, however, respond more to external signals, such as the presence of food or other people and social situations, or they may react more emotionally to the normal internal messages. Others believe that obese people do not really eat a great deal more than thin people; they just have a different set point and a slower metabolic rate. Heredity and early conditioning play a major role here. The food choices of some heavier people may not be as wholesome as those of thin people, with higher-fat and higher-calorie foods predominating. Malnutrition from nutrient deficiencies and food allergies can also be influential. Obesity is really a combination of these many factors, I believe. Of course, most of us know overweight people who eat a lot of food. Then again, we may know overweight people who eat lightly, as well as trim people who can really put it away. Most overweight people have overeaten at some point to develop their capacity for obesity, I believe, unless there is some hormonal imbalance, which is actually not very common.

We need to start as early as possible to achieve dietary control. Children need wholesome, nutritious foods as well as loving guidance. Only about 10% of elementary schoolchildren are overweight, yet between 20% and 30% of high schoolers are at least moderately obese, based on body mass index measurements. To lose weight and maintain it, behavior must change. Behavior modification can be practiced by us or with the help of a close friend, spouse, or diet buddy, with the assistance of a behavioral or other counselor.

An important beginning to this process is to try to get in touch with one's level of hunger. Many overweight people do not eat out of hunger; in fact, many of us rarely experience this natural guide to eating. Using a food diary to evaluate what, when, and where we eat, how much, the level of hunger experienced, and what else we are doing at the time can be very revealing. Keeping such a diary for several weeks can help us to see more clearly our relationship to eating. We can then make a plan incorporating new, positive habits and use new rules to change our behavior in weak areas. For example, if we snack while we make dinner or pick at the leftovers in the kitchen, we can make a commitment to eat food only at the dining room table and allow no eating in the kitchen or when standing.

It may be difficult at first; constant awareness is needed. Behaviorists claim that it takes 3 weeks to change a habit and create a new one, so keep at it. Part of our eating behavior is affected by psychological aspects, such as our self-image, relationships to our family or partner, sexuality, and general stress. Often, counseling is important to help change behavior to meet our dietary challenge. One book that is useful for addressing psycho-emotional eating habits is celebrity psychologist Dr. Phil McGraw's *The Ultimate Weight Solution: The 7 Keys to Weight Loss Freedom.* Successfully achieving a new weight means changing the diet, not "going on a diet." When we return to our old, "normal" diet, we will create the same body we had before—and likely add a few more pounds. First we change the diet by substituting wholesome foods for the more high-calorie and chemical foods in the diet. Next, we work to create good habits. Below I offer some suggestions for behavior patterns, food choices, and activities to help reach and maintain an optimum weight.

Before beginning a new diet plan, a health evaluation may be important, especially for those with recent weight gain or symptoms of medical problems. Before embarking on any low-calorie diet, please have a complete exam, a general biochemistry panel, and, if older than 45, an electrocardiogram. A complete thyroid hormone panel is often useful to rule out low thyroid function, which could be a cause of weight gain or difficulty in losing weight. Blood fats, protein, potassium, and calcium levels are also important monitors in the process of weight loss. A positive side effect of diet change and weight loss is reduction of blood cholesterol and triglycerides and high blood pressure; watching for mineral depletions, particularly of potassium, is a good idea.

An evaluation for food allergies (immune reactions to foods) may be a valuable step on the path to a trim and healthier body. For more details and programs about food reactions, see my book *The False Fat Diet.* Many people have internal reactions to foods, with increased immune response, cellular irritation, and many possible symptoms. These can cause inflam-

matory activity and water retention, as well as poor utilization of other foods. Currently, the best way to isolate problem foods is a blood test that measures levels of IgG antibodies to specific food antigens (the protein stimuli of the food). This reveals delayed or "hidden" food allergy or hypersensitivity. Measuring IgE levels can determine foods causing more immediate reactions, such as hives, asthma, or eczema, although these reactions are relatively uncommon, which is why skin tests (which measure the IgE reactions) are not very helpful.

Cytotoxic testing, looking at cellular reactions, is no longer used because interpretations of its results were too subjective. A more objective test called the ALCAT (the antigen leukocyte cellular antibody test) uses this same technology to measure our own cells' damage when exposed to foods. Immune antibody reactions and cell reactions are two common ways that we react to foods. Although this test remains unproven from a research perspective, it appears to be an improvement from earlier cytotoxicity approaches Although the IgG antibody testing is the most popular way to measure more subtle food reactions (separate from skin testing, which measures true allergy, an IgE response), antibody testing may show as much as a 25% false-positive rate (by some studies), meaning that it rates us as having a food reaction when we really don't about 25% of the time. It also may miss reactions when we might experience symptoms after certain foods. **Personal experience is still the most comprehensive way to evaluate this area of health.** (For labs that test for food reactions, see Appendix A.)

Testing food reactions ourselves by trying different foods in the diet and observing how we feel can be useful for the astute person, but the reactions may involve other variables besides the foods. Some practitioners feel that the ultimate method is double-blind testing—giving patients encapsulated dried foods as well as placebos, without the patient or tester knowing which is which, or even what food is being tested. This is a good method, but it is time-consuming and assumes that food reactions occur so dramatically and immediately that people can be aware of them. Some reactions do happen at once, but many are more subtle and occur 12 to 24 hours later. Avoiding the causes of these quieter internal reactions contributes to the body's fine-tuning and makes weight loss easier. Food allergy testing followed by a rotation diet avoiding the reactive foods plays an essential part in reaching and maintaining optimum weight and health (see more under "Allergies" on page 704 of this chapter).

Another method I recommend is elimination-challenge. In this approach, we go on a "hypoallergenic" diet in which the most commonly allergenic foods are totally eliminated for at least 2 weeks. Then begins a challenge phase in which the potentially suspect foods are reintroduced one by one, with two washout days in between, to see if any reaction occurs. If a reaction does occur, that food can be regarded as one to reduce, rotate, or perhaps eliminate from the diet altogether.

Behavior Patterns for Optimum Weight

It may be helpful to highlight or write out the important issues for you and work on 1 to 2 per week. Motivation is the key. Journal your journey.

- Focus on decreasing caloric intake and increasing calories out (exercise).
- Eat most foods early in the day for best use of calories.
- Drink 8 to 10 glasses of water daily, but not with meals.
- Drink 2 glasses of water 30 minutes before meals to reduce appetite.
- Eat slowly and chew food well.
- Limit treats and refined foods; avoid sodas and chemical foods.
- Eat lots of fruits and vegetables—as snacks, too.
- Walk a lot and exercise regularly.
- Avoid fats in the diet—they are more caloric.
- Use only low-fat or nonfat milk products.
- Minimize salad dressings, cream soups, and meats.
- Lessen or avoid alcohol and caffeine; minimize salt intake.
- Rotate foods—eat a variety; isolate allergenic foods and avoid them.
- Practice food combining.
- See a nutritionist to help with the eating plan or for food-habit counseling.
- Use smaller plates and portions.
- Fill up first on lower-calorie foods, such as soups or vegetable salads.
- Avoid high-calorie snacks and desserts.
- Wait 10 to 15 minutes before taking seconds—your hunger will decrease.
- At restaurants, avoid overeating and take any extra food home.

- Take at least 20 to 30 minutes to eat a meal, even snacks.
- Eat at only 1 or 2 places in the home.
- Sit and relax before eating.
- Avoid eating while watching TV, driving, or doing other things.
- Shop for food only after eating, not when hungry.
- Focus on eating only when hungry.
- Create a schedule for eating.
- Plan meals and food choices ahead, snacks included.
- Focus on what you are eating and not what you are avoiding.
- Make a list of your "good" (that is, healthy) foods, shop for them, and then carry them with you to work or when going out so that you have the right choices.
- Put snacks and sweet foods away at home.
- Stay out of the kitchen, cupboards, and refrigerator unless preparing food.
- Plan activities to occupy your free time when you might snack.
- Tell family and friends to support you and not push food.
- If you blow it, go right back to your plan, and do not make it an excuse to indulge.
- Weigh yourself only once every 1 or 2 weeks.
- Learn about food, fats, calories, and so on, so you know what you are doing.
- Keep a good self-image and positive attitude toward life.
- Allow yourself to indulge (within reason) once weekly without guilt or self-judgment.
- Realize that it is ultimately up to you.

This topic of food reactions and elimination diets is discussed in *The False Fat Diet.*

Several possible diets can be used as long-term plans for people who have problems maintaining their optimum weight. These are all generally healthier diets than those of the general population. There are literally thousands of quick-weight-loss, low-calorie, nutrient-deficient diets available to consumers, which are not recommended for achieving our goals. I do not usually recommend fasting for weight loss, but if someone wants to lose a quick 5 to 10 pounds in a short period of time, I will work with them, after an evaluation, with the overall intention of using that period to create a new eating plan to be used when the fast is over. Fasting is valuable at increasing food awareness and sensitivity to both bad and good foods and eliminating addictive food and eating patterns, so that people can come back to eating with new enthusiasm and attention. Fasting 1 day a week on water or juices can be a valuable tool for many people who want to lose or maintain weight. It reemphasizes the importance of food choices and food awareness.

The essential aspects of a healthy weight-loss diet are lean protein (for example, fish and poultry), low fat, and lots of vegetables. High-fiber foods, with some complex carbohydrates, are also helpful, especially with an orientation to vegetables and vegetable-protein combinations such as grains and legumes. Eating a variety of foods and rotating those foods every few days is important. Some raw and organic nuts and seeds provide the essential fats for maintaining health, but avoid eating too many as they are caloric. Including some important fish oils from salmon, mackerel, or sardines is also wise as these have been shown to be great health foods. Cold-pressed vegetable oils can be the main fats, with some low-fat dairy products if tolerated. Saturated and hydrogenated fats are minimized. Refined-sugar and refined-flour foods, including baked goods, candy, sodas, and other sweets, are avoided. Alcohol is out, and caffeine is minimized. Drink lots of water instead to support normal weight and healthy skin and internal functions.

Meals are restructured to include a moderate breakfast, a large lunch, and a light dinner. Snacks are low-calorie foods, such as fruits, vegetables, popcorn, or crackers. Overeating is prohibited. Take breaks during big meals to let the body balance and let you know whether it needs more food. It usually does not; we require a lot less food than our overweight mind tells us. Our satiation meter needs to be turned down, and that will take a golden key, which is not always easy to find. Patience (and slower eating and chewing) is required to maintain harmony between our taste buds, our brain (desires), and our stomach and digestive tract. It may require going through our past, and our emotional and psychological barriers, to find our creative spark and drive to be our best self and not let food interfere with this path of power. It takes responsibility and a commitment to our new body-to-be as well as a knowledge and belief that we can do it. We need to think/feel/know more about eating to survive and feeding our body with the best possible fuel. Taking the time to eat, chewing each bite thoroughly, is essential to short-term digestion and absorption and the long-term health of the whole digestive tract. Being aware of the process of eating and of what food is eaten is a must.

Eating Plans for Weight Balance

In this section I focus on four specific diets for weight loss and/or weight maintenance: the Fish, Fowl, and Green Vegetable diet, the High-fiber Starch diet, the Allergy-rotation diet, and the Haas plan—the Ideal Diet.

The Fish, Fowl, and Green Vegetable diet. This is a fairly healthy weight-loss diet that should be used for 1 or 2 months at the most. This is an example of a low-carbohydrate diet because it avoids grains and baked goods, sugars, and refined foods. Several pounds a week can be lost fairly easily with this diet, even with only moderate activity. It includes fresh ocean fish, tuna, shrimp, and trout, organic poultry, and green vegetables, both raw and cooked—all to be eaten in the quantity desired (within reason, of course). One piece of fresh fruit and 1 cooked egg daily are also suggested. This provides good balance, although the diet is fairly low in fiber. Some bran or psyllium can be used to support bowel function. Salad dressing should be limited to 1 or 2 tablespoons daily of quality vegetable oils, such as olive, with some fresh lemon juice or vinegar, particularly balsamic or apple cider vinegar. If no oils are used, an essential fatty acid supplement should be added. Herbal teas and springwater or filtered water are the main fluids. Some clear soup broths are acceptable. Daily fluid intake should be 8 to 10 glasses (8 ounces each), with 2 to 3 glasses being drunk first thing in the morning and 30 to 60 minutes before each meal. A general multivitamin or the "Weight-Loss Nutrient Program" on page 695 should also be used daily to ensure good health.

The High-Fiber Starch diet. Another weight loss/maintenance alternative, this diet is not exclusively starches. It includes some fruit, green vegetables, and protein foods, but the main foods are the whole grains, legumes, pasta, potatoes, and starchy vegetables, such as carrots and squashes. This diet can be a good weight-loss plan for overweight vegetarians, especially if they avoid excessive grains and sweets, or for meat and potato lovers as a switch to a more vegetarian or plant-based diet. These high-fiber complex carbohydrates when eaten at the beginning of a meal provide bulk and thus decrease the appetite and give a feeling of fullness. They are also relatively low-calorie foods because they are low in fat, but only if they do not have sauces, gravies, butter, or oil added to them. The complex carbohydrates also provide a consistent energy production and can stabilize the energy imbalance that some people experience.

Vegetables can be consumed as desired, at least several cups daily. They are also low in calories. A couple of pieces of fruit daily are suggested. Dairy foods, red meats, and any fried, fatty, or refined foods are avoided, as are sweets. One meal, early in the day, can include a concentrated protein, such as fish, poultry, eggs, or, for strict vegetarians, some tofu, nuts, seeds, or beans. Soups and salads are helpful. Water intake is 8 to 10 glasses daily for this diet also. A multivitamin product can be used, along with some extra B12. Care should be taken that iron and calcium intake are adequate; these and other minerals, like zinc, might be supplemented, although most should be found in sufficient amounts in this diet.

The Allergy-Rotation diet. This is becoming more popular for weight loss as well as for general health, especially when there are food allergies present. The ideal diet described in chapter 13 is a modified rotation diet; also see "Allergies" on page 704. My book *The False Fat Diet* focuses on this topic as well. When food allergies (or *food reactions* as a more general term because medical allergists refer to allergy as only 1 specific process rather than the many ways we

can react to foods) are suspected, we should be tested or guided by a doctor or nutritionist. Any foods shown to be a possible problem should come out of the diet for 1 to 2 months, depending on the degree of sensitivity. After that time, individual foods can be tested again (this is called a "challenge"), but only one per day. If we seem to be addicted to any foods—that is, we crave them and eat them every day, sometimes even at every meal—those foods should be completely removed from the diet for at least several weeks before testing them, although avoiding them even for only four days will allow the body to be more sensitive to their true effects.

If we can be aware enough of our diet to know which foods are doing what, then we can know which foods to eliminate. This rotation diet can be well-balanced because it includes a wide variety of foods. To desensitize to other possible food reactions, a rotating diet means setting up a 4-day rotation plan—any food eaten on one day must be excluded from the diet for the next three days. For example, if apples, corn, or peas are eaten on Monday, we would not eat them again until Friday. This diet is not easy to initiate, but once started is not too difficult to maintain. It does, however, require preparing most of our own foods and thus limiting restaurant eating. Just planning foods and meals and preparing food ahead of time creates better eating habits. Eliminating allergenic foods also reduces water retention through reduced immune reactions and secondary inflammation and may allow us to feel much better while we lower body fat.

The Ideal Diet. Discussed at length in chapters 12 through 14 of this book, this diet is good for weight reduction and maintenance for most people, provided we limit the quantities of food consumed. It is a well-balanced diet that incorporates aspects of all the previous diets. It is a rotation diet, good for food reactions; it has a high fiber content from the whole grains and vegetables; it is low in fat; and it contains good-quality protein. To reduce calories further, the morning nut snack can be replaced with another fruit.

In this diet, water should be consumed as usual—8 to 10 glasses per day, mainly about an hour before meals—and a basic multivitamin/mineral supplement could be used, including essential fatty acids or some fresh vegetable oil, 1 or 2 teaspoons daily. (Refer to "Seasonal Menu Plans" beginning on page 539 in

---

Basics of the Ideal Diet

Meal	Foods
Early morning	1 or 2 pieces of fruit
Breakfast	Starch, such as a cereal grain or hard squash
Midmorning snack	Fruit or a handful of nuts or seeds
Lunch	Protein and green and other vegetables
Midafternoon snack	Vegetable or fruit
Dinner	Starch or protein with vegetables
Evening snack	Vegetable or fruit, if needed

---

chapter 14, Seasonal Menu Plans and Recipes, for more ideas.) More water and fiber and more filling low-calorie foods can help in decreasing the appetite. Water and fiber are the two most useful and inexpensive nutrients for weight reduction and maintenance. They also support good colon function, which is helpful to detoxification and reducing food cravings. Lowering fat intake and absorption (fiber also does that) and increasing foods high in vitamins and minerals as well as supplemental nutrients will also support optimum metabolism and aid in weight loss.

Exercise is crucial. Few weight-loss programs are effective without increasing physical activity. To lose weight or mass, reduce intake and increase output. Reducing fat stores and adding muscle improves energy utilization by using more calories for active metabolic tissues. Exercise also improves general metabolism and vitality and lowers that important "set point," allowing us to maintain lower weight and body fat with the same food intake. At a good level of exercise, the body will burn more calories than usual, even 12 hours after exercising. **Regular, daily exercise is clearly needed to keep fat off.** When we are just starting out, we should first begin slowly and build to a regular daily program. When we make it a habit, we will really see the benefit. Then, at most we might skip it for 1 day a week, but only if we must, and then we should stretch and walk anyway. Some aerobic activity is ideal, even 20 to 30 minutes a day, 5 or 6 days a week.

Our body stores energy, not as calories, but mainly as fat. Aerobic-type exercise will burn and reduce fat stores without reducing muscle tissue (weight-loss programs without exercise can cause muscle loss). One to

2 hours daily of activity is fine; we must make the time to do it. We can add brisk walks to the more strenuous activity as we get into shape. A 30-minute walk about a half hour after lighter meals is just the thing to further help digestion and assimilation. With more exercise, our vitality, endurance, and ability to handle stress and life all improve. Try it!

Let me say a bit more about water and fiber. A 2003 study showed that the direct effect of water drinking on metabolic rate—6 to 7 eight-ounce glasses a day—is extremely small. In terms of its direct effect, water drinking only increases total calorie burn by a few calories a day. However, water is extremely important during weight loss for other reasons. One involves our sense of fullness—water definitely helps with this satiety factor. Keeping our appetite in check is definitely a plus when it comes to weight loss. Another benefit is water's ability to help us eliminate waste and toxins. During periods of weight loss, the body will be breaking down more tissue that needs recycling or elimination from the body. Toxins that have been stored in fat tissue can also be released in greater amounts during this time. Water helps us keep these toxins and breakdown products flowing out of us.

Finally, water is especially important for people who follow low-carb, high-protein diets that push their metabolism toward ketosis. In ketosis, when we are looking more to our fat stores for energy, we also tend to break down more of the body's protein. This breakdown of protein leaves us with more nitrogen to get out of our system. We depend on our kidneys to accomplish this elimination of excess nitrogen, but it takes a good bit more water for our kidneys to process this extra nitrogen. (By the way, the water loss that usually occurs during this process is often mistaken for real and dramatic weight loss, when in fact, this weight loss is only temporary and will end when the ketosis ends and the body water levels are no longer taxed by the need for extra nitrogen elimination.)

Sufficient fiber in the diet supports good colon function and, like water, can help to eliminate wastes that are released during weight loss. Especially if the diet is low in fiber foods, we may add supplemental fiber as psyllium seed husks and bran. Psyllium is a soluble fiber that increases bulk and can help reduce the appetite. Insoluble wheat or oat bran fiber can also help in detoxification as well as in stimulating the colon function. Although there is no direct impact of fiber on fat elimination from the body, increased fiber helps us keep our blood sugar well regulated, and our fat metabolism may also benefit from this carb-related improvement in our blood sugar regulation.

Other digestive supports include liquid chlorophyll. A teaspoon or so added to water twice daily can help nourish the intestinal lining and improve digestion. With better assimilation, the tissues and cells are more nourished and there may be fewer cravings and less desire for food. Ginger-lemon water can help with circulation and diuresis, as well as support liver and gallbladder function. Even just lemon water—half a small lemon squeezed into water—drunk 15 to 30 minutes before meals can help digestion and utilization of fats. The flavored mineral waters (no calories) can be used as a beverage, up to 2 or 3 cups daily. These drinks, because of the carbonation, are somewhat filling. Common flavors include lemon, lime, orange, and cherry.

Supplements and Weight Loss

Many other supplements can be helpful during and after weight loss. A general multivitamin/mineral supplement is important, especially when we are on special diets that may not be perfectly balanced (few are) or if we take in fewer than 1,500 calories daily. Extra minerals are essential to prevent deficiency, especially with high fiber intake, which may reduce mineral absorption. Amounts over the Dietary Reference Intakes (DRIs) are needed for iron, zinc, copper, manganese, and molybdenum. Calcium is especially important to prevent bone loss, as less calcium is also absorbed with the fiber. Magnesium is cleared in the gut as well as through the kidneys, so a good intake is vital. Vitamin B6 can help provide a diuretic effect during weight release.

Because weight loss involves a mild process of detoxification, with the body burning fat and other tissues (without proper exercise, the body loses muscle as well), some antioxidant nutrients are suggested to handle the extra toxin load. Vitamin C, 1 to 3 grams daily in 2 or 3 portions, and vitamin E and selenium, usually taken together in the morning, are suggested. L-cysteine can also be used; this amino acid helps liver and intestinal detoxification processes. Other amino acids have been recommended by some authorities. A general L-amino acid formula can be used; Dr. Stuart Berger, in *The Immune Power Diet*, suggests taking it about 30 to 60 minutes before meals, as certain amino acids, such as phenylalanine, may help reduce the appetite. In *Vitamin Power*, authors Stephanie Rick and Rita Aero cite research that suggests that a combination of arginine and lysine, 1,500 mg each, taken before bed can help weight loss by increasing growth hormone production and improving fatty acid metabolism and general energy. I am slightly more impressed with L-carnitine's help in weight loss, as it supports the efficient use of fats in the body. The usual plan is 500 mg taken twice daily, with the morning and evening meals.

Various fatty acids may also be taken to stimulate weight loss by improving fatty acid metabolism. An essential fatty acid formula can be used. Most obese people need more good polyunsaturated fats to balance their lipid metabolism. Gamma-linolenic acid (GLA) from evening primrose or borage seed oils and eicosapentaenoic acid (EPA) from fish oil are both precursors to different prostaglandins and may also be helpful. Some chronically obese people will respond to supplementation with essential fatty acids and evening primrose oil. Cold-pressed flaxseed oil is high in both omega-3 (alpha-linolenic) and omega-6 (linoleic and others) fatty acids and is a less expensive way to obtain these oils. Usually, 3 or 4 teaspoons a day are sufficient if fats are avoided in the diet. There is recent interest in conjugated linoleic acid (CLA) and its effects on weight reduction. Although the research is not there yet, some people experience benefit. In one preliminary study, the benefits of CLA appeared related to reduced appetite levels. When taking additional fatty acids, it is wise to supplement the many cofactors that help in fatty acid metabolism. These are zinc, magnesium, beta-carotene, and vitamins A, C, niacin, pyridoxine, and biotin. Vitamin E also aids metabolism as well as prevents oxidation of the other oils.

Two other nutrients have captured their share of the weight-loss spotlight: chromium and hydroxycitric acid (HCA). Chromium has some legitimate research supporting its weight-loss benefits. In some studies at the University of Texas Health Center, 200 to 400 mcg of daily chromium (in the form of chromium picolinate) helped beginning weight-training students in the study decrease their percentage of body fat. Interestingly, however, the same effect was not found in already

trained athletes who had little body fat to begin with and were already in good shape in terms of their physical conditioning. Researchers do not know exactly how chromium helped, but it is likely that its effect on fat was related to its impact on carbohydrate metabolism, especially the effectiveness of insulin in moving sugar out of the blood stream and into the cells. (See "Chromium" on page 177 in chapter 6, Minerals, for more information.)

The second nutrient is HCA, which is extracted from the Malabar tamarind plant *(Garcinia cambogia)*, native to Southeast Asia. HCA blocks the activity of the enzyme ATP citrate lyase, and for this reason can slow down the production of fatty acids and reduce fat accumulation. HCA may also work as an appetite suppressant. Although supplementing with these nutrients may help in some weight-loss plans, I would caution against treating them as substitutes for the much more important steps I have described regarding food, lifestyle, and attitude.

There are many herbs that can also be helpful during weight loss. Juniper berry is a good diuretic herb and helps in detoxification. Parsley leaf is also a diuretic, and peppermint leaf tea helps reduce the appetite for many people, as it is said to relax the stomach nerves. Chickweed herb, a spring green, has historically been known for reducing appetite and helping in weight loss. Bladderwrack is a type of sea vegetable; when taken with kelp, it will support thyroid function, and the high mineral levels of this herb aid general energy utilization. Garlic has also been used in weight-loss programs to help lower blood lipids and for detoxification.

In *The Scientific Validation of Herbal Medicine,* Dr. Daniel Mowrey has noted that he never suggests chickweed because of the lack of backup research on it. Plantain *(Plantago major* and *Plantago lanceolata)* is a green with much more scientific support. The plantain fiber aids in weight loss by reducing cholesterol and triglyceride levels, by lessening fat absorption, and by its appetite-satiating effect. Mowrey's herbal formula for weight loss includes plantain, fennel seed, burdock root, hawthorn berry (to support heart function), kelp, and bladderwrack.

Losing weight effectively and healthfully and maintaining a proper weight is a complex and multifaceted process. Finding a diet that works for the

---

Weight-Loss Support Plan*

- **Improving digestive effectiveness.** Poor breakdown of foods allows poor cell nutrition, which can lead to cravings and overeating. Adequate production (or replacement) of hydrochloric acid and digestive enzymes from the pancreas may help.

- **Improving metabolism** (utilization efficiency) of carbohydrates, fats, and proteins, particularly the burning of fats for fuel. Their suggested supplements include L-carnitine, vitamin B12, vitamin B6, folic acid, choline, inositol, methionine, taurine, liver and thyroid glandulars, vitamin A, dimethylglycine (DMG), and gamma-linolenic acid (GLA).

- **Stimulating energy levels** with vitamin C, pantothenic acid, adrenal glandular, potassium, magnesium, manganese, chromium, octocosanol, and the branched-chain amino acids—leucine, isoleucine, and valine.

- **Reducing cravings,** especially for sweets, by using the amino acid glutamine and chromium, and by avoiding allergenic foods.

- **Suppressing the appetite** with the amino acids phenylalanine and tryptophan.

---

* Adapted from Super Fitness Beyond Vitamins, *by Michael Rosenbaum, MD, and Dominick Bosco.*

Weight-Loss Nutrient Program

Nutrient	Amount	Nutrient	Amount
Water	3 qt	Iodine	150–225 mcg
Calories	1,000–1,800	Iron	10–20 mg
Fiber (includes diet plus bran		Magnesium	500–800 mg
and psyllium supplements)	20–40 g	Manganese	10 mg
Vitamin A	3,000–6,000 IU	Molybdenum	500 mcg
Beta-carotene	10,000–30,000 IU	Potassium	1–2 g
Vitamin D	400 IU	Selenium	200 mcg
Vitamin E	400–800 IU	Silicon	100 mg
Vitamin K	300 mcg	Zinc	30–60 mg
Thiamin (B1)	50–100 mg		
Riboflavin (B2)	50–100 mg	**Others**	
Niacinamide (B3)	50–150 mg	Digestive enzymes (after meals)	2–3 tablets
Pantothenic acid (B5)	250–500 mg	Adrenal glandular	50–100 mg
Pyridoxine (B6)	50–100 mg	L-amino acids	1,500 mg
Pyridoxal-5-phosphate	50–100 mg	L-carnitine	1,000 mg
Cobalamin (B12)	100–200 mcg	Phenylalanine (before meals)	500 mg
Folic acid	600–800 mcg	Flaxseed oil	1 tbsp
Biotin	500 mcg	Olive oil	2–3 tsp
Choline	500–1,000 mg	Psyllium (before meals)	1–2 tsp
Inositol	500 mg	Bran (after meals and	
Vitamin C	3 g	at bedtime)	8–10 g daily
Bioflavonoids	250–500 mg	Evening primrose oil	4–6 capsules
Calcium	800–1,200 mg	Coenzyme Q10	20–30 mg
Chromium	400 mcg	Dimethylglycine	50–100 mg
Copper	2–3 mg	Organo-germanium	100–200 mg

individual is important, and creating a good exercise program is essential for long-term weight control. Implementing a healthy diet almost always requires changes in various habits and relationships that affected our weight previously. Behavior patterns need to be altered in order to achieve a new relationship to food. Both behavior and motivation can be learned, but it takes work—repeated and sustained effort. Beginning to believe in ourselves and our success is a catalyst as well as a source of support in becoming who we want to be, with the body and energy we desire. We have to know we can do it, believe it, see it in our mind's eye, and feel it in our hearts—and then do the work it takes to maintain it. The "Weight-Loss Nutrient Program" plan above can be used during a weight-reduction plan when daily calorie intake is limited. The amounts for each nutrient are a daily total, which can be divided into three portions.

24. WEIGHT GAIN

This program is basically the opposite of the weight-loss program, but with similar emphasis on avoiding junk foods, excessive fats, and other poor nutritional choices. People who want to gain weight need to eat more calories and more food, yet they also need more nourishment. To most of the overweight population, this would be a dream come true, but for underweight people who have trouble gaining weight, it can be a real problem. Like obesity, being underweight involves many factors. Undernourishment during infancy and adolescence or nutrient deficiencies of the mother during pregnancy can lead to a lower number of fat cells and thus the potential for lower amounts of fatty tissue. Genetics and conditioning are also factors. Thinness, of course, runs in families, as does obesity. Poor eating habits and low food intake are other causes of underweight. Illness can cause weight loss. Flus or debilitating diseases such as cancer can lead to loss of weight, which can be hard to regain.

Stress and anxiety are often found with low body weight. High-strung people and worriers can have trouble putting on weight. During times of extreme emotional upset, it may be difficult to eat. People who use stimulants such as caffeine and cigarettes are more commonly underweight than those who do not abuse these stimulants. The caffeine-cigarette combination generates a lot of nervous energy and frenetic mental activity. It may be productive for office work but not for health.

Several medical problems can be associated with weight loss or the inability to gain weight. Thyroid problems, mainly hyperthyroidism, are the most common of these and are associated with many other symptoms, such as a rapid heart rate, sweaty palms, and insomnia. Some psychologically related medical problems are also associated with underweight. Bulimia and anorexia nervosa are two serious food-oriented maladies; they are, in fact, often symptoms of much deeper emotional, attitudinal problems. Treatment of bulimia—where binge eating is followed by some inappropriate method of compensating (for example, vomiting or excessively exercising)—may require a combination of medical and psychological care. This cycle is hard on the body, and when vomiting is the path taken, it can irritate the upper gastrointestinal tract with hydrochloric acid and cause a loss of potassium and other nutrients.

Anorexia nervosa—involving the refusal to maintain a minimally normal body weight and an intense fear of gaining weight—mainly afflicts young women ages 13 to 25. Women of other ages, however, as well as men, sometimes experience this kind of problem. Anorexics are often malnourished, deficient in both calories and nutrients. They may be involved in regular vigorous exercise, such as aerobics or ballet, and may use laxatives, both of which may lead to further

loss of body nutrients. They may become socially separated because of a fear of group pressure toward eating. People with this syndrome should receive immediate treatment with education, emotional support, understanding, and food. This problem is more common in the teen years, which is even more a concern because nutrient needs are very high and poor nutrition is more common in this age group. Fortunately, though, this eating avoidance (not really loss of appetite) usually passes with treatment. There should also be care not to overdiagnose or overtreat young people who may watch their weight and eat sparingly. Encourage eating of good-quality, lower-calorie foods and suggest a supplement program such as the "Weight-Gain Nutrient Program" on page 698 at the end of this section.

For underweight people, a medical evaluation is usually needed, especially if the problem is recent. A general physical exam and blood chemistry test may rule out medical problems such as anemia, abnormal thyroid function, or even cancer. Mineral tests and a diet profile may assist in isolating nutritional deficiencies. Usually, though, if both parents were trim and the individual has been thin most of his or her life, no medical problems will be revealed. A faster metabolism and lower potential for fat storage are usually the explanation.

People with low weight who have difficulty gaining weight often need a combined program. Working with a psychologist, stress counselor, or hypnotherapist to deal with some of the psychological, attitudinal, and emotional factors may be helpful. Stress reduction (such as through relaxation exercises, music, or meditation) can be important, especially for nervous or high-strung individuals. Learning to slow down internally and externally can improve metabolism and the assimilation of nutrients. Stopping smoking or the overuse of caffeine is helpful at adding a few pounds, as it will often slow the metabolism, at least initially.

The other primary focus for gaining weight is good nutrition—diet and supplements. In this area, the suggestions are the opposite of those for weight loss. Bigger portions, many meals along with extra snacks, and more healthy, easily digested, high-calorie foods are the plan's foundation. Increasing calories is the key; an extra 500 calories a day over and above body requirements can lead to 1 pound a week of weight gain. More yogurt and cheeses, nuts and seeds, avocados, rice, potatoes, and bread with some butter may be helpful and healthful for getting extra calories. This will also increase dietary fats somewhat; fats are more caloric than the complex carbohydrates or sweeter foods.

If there is a low cardiovascular risk, with a moderate cholesterol level (160–195) and good blood pressure, even more fats, especially monounsaturated fats such as olive oil, can be consumed. Smokers are at a slightly greater risk of developing cardiovascular diseases with this higher-fat diet, although additional oils, seeds, butter and other milk products, and even meats, if those are tolerated, may be used to add weight. It is still wise to avoid fried foods and hydrogenated oils; an increase in vegetable fats, especially cold-pressed oils, is wiser than adding more animal fats. It is also sometimes wise to avoid foods that are highly diluted in terms of calories, like brothy soups, because they tend to make us full more quickly than they provide us with calories.

Underweight people often experience symptoms of fatigue and coldness in the body. Fat helps to keep us warm, and low body fat with poor circulation will reduce vitality and warmth. Fatigue may also be related to nutritional deficiencies secondary to limited-calorie diets and low intake. Vegetarians and people who eat macrobiotic diets tend to have lower weights, but these may be healthier weights if these people consume reasonable amounts of calories, protein, and vegetable oils—and mostly nutrient-rich foods. Still, these diets can more easily lead to deficient calorie intake, because they are lower in fats, and most of the foods consumed are low-calorie foods (better for weight loss). In these cases, more animal proteins can be therapeutic. Deepwater fish and organic poultry are best; but even organic red meat and liver may be helpful for deficient and tired people.

Low thyroid function and anemia can produce fatigue and coldness; however, hypothyroidism usually causes some weight gain also. Most often, low weight with fatigue results from inadequate nutrition. In the Chinese energy system, the imbalance that is associated with "weak fire element" may lead to fatigue, low endurance, and coldness, although this symptom complex may be associated with either low or increased weight. These symptoms may also accompany anemia, a part of "weak fire" or weak blood, and

in this case more iron, as is found in the animal meats, poultry, and fish, or as supplements, is the appropriate medicine. Folic acid, vitamin B12, copper, and adequate protein intake, as well as regular exercise, also help to build up the blood and improve the energy, endurance, and weight.

Another dietary suggestion for weight gain is to increase the size and number of meals. Three main meals and three or four snacks will help keep calorie intake up. A decrease in the bulky low-calorie foods and a focus on the higher-calorie ones will also help. It is good to eat the main course first (the opposite of the weight-loss plan). Follow the richer foods with vegetables and salads, with lots of good dressing if there is room. Of the vegetables, eat mainly starchier ones, such as potatoes, carrots, beets, and squashes. Also, eat the starchy grains, such as rice, oats, and pastas. Sweets and desserts are really not very helpful; they tend to fill people with short-term energy without nutritional value and may actually lead to increased energy expenditure; yet they are more caloric. Fluid intake just before or during meals is not recommended, as it reduces the appetite, and you will want to eat more to gain weight. Some alcohol, maybe a glass of a good wine, before a meal occasionally is helpful as it promotes relaxation and improves the appetite. Even bedtime snacks are appropriate when it comes to gaining weight, as long as they do not interfere with sleep.

Adequate rest and deep sleep are important to help the body slow down and relax the nervous tension that can eat up calories. Warm milk before bed with a little treat such as toast or a cookie can be useful to improve sleep and add calories. Avoiding stimulants that increase nervous energy, especially in the evening, is a good idea. And again, stopping smoking is important to this program and life itself. A regular exercise program should be followed, but it should be oriented more to toning and conditioning exercise, such as working with weights, to build up the body muscle and tissue density, and thus increase weight. Vigorous aerobic activity, however, burns off more calories and may keep weight down (although some is useful to maintain endurance). Walks in the fresh air and Nature may help us to stay fit and relaxed enough to be more receptive to food.

Weight-Gain Nutrient Program	
Nutrient	**Amount**
Calories	2,500–3,500
Protein	65–125 g
Fat	60–110 g
Vitamin A	5,000–10,000 IU
Beta-carotene	20,000 IU
Vitamin D	400 IU
Vitamin E	400 IU
Vitamin K	300 mcg
Thiamin (B1)	50–75 mg
Riboflavin (B2)	25–75 mg
Niacinamide (B3)	100 mg
Pantothenic acid (B5)	100 mg
Pyridoxine (B6)	50 mg
Pyridoxal-5-phosphate	25–50 mg
Cobalamin (B12)	50 mcg
Folic acid	600 mcg
Biotin	250 mcg
Vitamin C	1,500 mg
Bioflavonoids	250 mg
Calcium	600–850 mg
Chromium	200 mcg
Copper	2 mg
Iodine	150 mcg
Iron	10–18 mg
Magnesium	300–500 mg
Manganese	5–10 mg
Molybdenum	200 mcg
Selenium	200 mcg
Silicon	50 mg
Zinc	30 mg
L-amino acids	
(500 mg before each meal)	1,500 mg
Essential fatty acids	6 capsules
or flaxseed oil	2 tbsp

Optional (if needed for better digestion)

Hydrochloric acid	5–10 grains
(with protein meals)	
Digestive enzymes	1–2 tablets
(after meals)	

Some supplements are helpful in improving the potential for weight increase. A general multivitamin is suggested to provide all of the essential nutrients. Additional B vitamins taken several times daily may also help; most of the B vitamins aid the metabolism and assimilation of food and proper generation of energy (ATP). Essential fatty acids, as a supplement or as additional vegetable oil in the diet, are helpful from both a caloric perspective and a metabolic one. Amino acids are also effective when taken before meals. They stimulate the appetite and provide good protein synthesis capacity, thus helping to build the body. Overall, a moderate supplement program (not high amounts) is indicated, just to cover the basic needs for nutrients; we are not trying to increase the metabolism in general. People with significant weight loss or people who generally have low weight, say 10% to 15% below their ideal, need to focus more on "living to eat" rather than their usual "eating to live" plan, at least for a while, to bring up their weight.

25. YEAST SYNDROME

The yeast condition from the organism *Candida albicans* (and other yeasts) is a medical concern that emerged during the 1980s and continues today. The problem was originally described by two prominent physicians—C. Orian Truss in *The Missing Diagnosis* and William Crook* in *The Yeast Connection*—and then more recently by Jeanne Marie Martin and Zoltan Rona in *Complete Candida Yeast Guidebook* and other books. I believe and see that this concept about yeast, commonly called "candida" problems, is a medical breakthough that is still awaiting its validation from the mainstream medical and scientific communities. What I have observed now for more than 20 years is that often the therapy for yeast, or candidiasis as it is commonly known, will positively and dramatically change lives. This somewhat complex, multilevel treatment program has been effective in a high percentage of the people I have treated, and I have worked with thousands with this problem since the mid-1980s.

The yeast syndrome is still a controversial topic. Most conventional doctors do not want to hear about

---

* Dr. Billy Crook, my friend and a wonderfully sweet man (and respected pediatric allergist) who really brought the Candida syndrome to the medical and health world passed on in 2002. His daughter, Elizabeth Crook, is carrying on his work and has completed the newest version of *The Yeast Connection and Women's Health* (Women's Health Connection, 2003), coauthored by Hyla Cass, MD, and a later version with Carolyn Dean, MD.

this condition and call it a fad disease, but those who will explore the possibility and look for it in their patients are hard-pressed not to accept this problem as real. **One of the reasons, in my estimation, for mainstream medicine not really accepting the yeast syndrome is because the problem arises predominantly as a side effect from the use of commonly prescribed drugs—antibiotics, birth control pills, and corticosteroids.** The problem originates when a common yeast, *Candida albicans,* begins to overgrow in the intestinal or genitourinary tract. It may be contracted initially through sexual contact. When other normal body microflora are killed off by antibiotics, the yeasts may then proliferate and coexist with the useful germs. Mild mucocutaneous infections (of the skin, vagina, throat, or bladder, for example) may develop in the yeast phase of this dimorphic (two structures) organism.

This common yeast is usually noninvasive (that is, it remains localized) except in the severely debilitated patient. However, with long-term infestation or with the weakened immune state that can result from a reduction of normal colon bacteria, the yeast can shift into its fungal form, wherein it develops rhizoids, or roots, that can be implanted in the intestinal wall or other mucosal linings. This allows absorption into the body of by-products (toxins) of fermentation and other antigenic material generated by the fungus. The body then makes antibodies to the *Candida albicans* organisms. This can lead to an immunological or hypersensitivity reaction that is manifested as the polysystemic disease for which this syndrome is now known.

The yeast problem thus occurs at two levels—the localized infections, of which skin rashes and vaginitis are the most common (intestinal overgrowth is also common), and the secondary and more serious systemic reactions. This problem can then produce such symptoms and conditions as recurrent skin fungus infections or nail problems; headaches; fatigue; cystitis or prostatitis; mental symptoms such as mood swings, poor memory or concentration, depression, or confusion; premenstrual symptoms; recurrent herpes infection; joint pains; cravings for sweets, bread, or alcohol; indigestion or food reactions; and sensitivity to molds, dampness, environmental pollution, cigarettes, and various smells. This yeast syndrome is much more common in women than in men and

---

Factors Common to Patients with Yeast Syndrome

- Frequent or long-term use of antibiotics, such as tetracycline for acne.
- Frequent use of broad-spectrum antibiotics for recurrent infections, such as in the ears, sinuses, bladder, vagina, or throat.
- Birth control pill use in women.
- Premenstrual symptoms.
- Recurrent vaginal yeast infections in women or prostate problems in men.
- Regular use of cortisone-type drugs.
- Cravings for (and overeating of) sweets, breads, or alcohol.
- Sensitivity (and exposures) to molds, dampness, and certain smells.
- Mental symptoms, such as depression, mood swings, or confusion.
- Chronic fatigue, indigestion, or food reactions.
- Recurrent skin fungus infections, such as ringworm, athlete's foot, jock itch, or nail problems.

---

seems to affect the hormonal balance, initially causing mild premenstrual symptoms of irritability, depression, fatigue, and swelling, and leading to actually abnormal and/or painful menstrual periods. I estimate that a significant number of women with PMS have a problem with *Candida albicans,* and probably more than half the women with candidiasis have some uncomfortable premenstrual symptoms.

Diagnosing polysystemic candidiasis may involve several tests. Most doctors who work with this problem use a questionnaire such as the one Crook provides in *The Yeast Connection.* The scores indicate the likelihood of a yeast problem, and while not exact, this is a fairly accurate tool. Many doctors suggest a trial treatment program merely on the basis of an interview, exam, and questionnaire score, as the response to therapy is often a good indication of the presence of the problem. I like to have more objective monitors, however, so I perform two main tests, both reasonably inexpensive. One is a culture of a stool specimen to both identify and quantify the amount of *Candida albicans* (or other yeast) organisms present. This can then be repeated to measure the effectiveness of the program. Also, a sensitivity test that finds what substances will actually kill (or inhibit) the yeast (in the lab, at least) can be done after the organism is isolated. The other test, which measures the blood levels of three antibodies (IgA, IgM, and IgG) to the *Candida albcans* organism, was developed by Ed Winger, MD, and is performed by LabCorp in California. (Note: People may have other yeast overgrowth and sensitivities that may not reveal elevated antibodies since they have different organisms, such as other *Candida* species, or various species of *Geotrichum* or *Rhodotorula*.) If these antibodies are elevated, this suggests that some systemic (immune and inflammatory) reaction is occurring in the body (the stool reveals only an intestinal overgrowth), which may be correlated with more widespread symptoms. This test also gives us the opportunity to monitor the body's status over time to measure treatment response. Reducing yeast organisms in the body and replacing friendly bacteria will usually reduce elevated antibody levels, but typically only after a couple years.

Other tests may be helpful in determining coexisting medical problems. A study of the stool for ova and parasites may show these to be more commonly present in yeast carriers than in the average population, as often the same predisposing factors, poor digestion and low stomach acid, are present. Treatment may also be needed to eliminate these parasites. Creating proper colon ecology is a crucial factor in health, disease resistance, and many important body functions. When normal colon bacteria are present in sufficient quantities (which they may not be when other invaders are taking their place), they will actually produce many vitamins using the nutrient fuel provided them. Vitamin K and most of the B complex vitamins—niacin, B12, pantothenic acid, B6, biotin, and folic acid—are among these. Intestinal bacteria also aid final digestion of food, such as proteins and milk. With low colon bacteria counts, poor digestion, and an unhealthy intestinal lining, more food allergies may develop. A blood test measuring specific antibodies to many commonly reactive foods may be indicated in some people with candidiasis, especially when there is a real problem with food intolerance. Frequently found reactions, indicated by greatly elevated IgG antibody levels, include reactions to both baker's and brewer's yeasts, wheat,

---

3-Faceted Approach to Treatment of the Yeast Syndrome

1. Do not feed the yeasts foods upon which they thrive.
2. Reduce yeast growth through natural and pharmaceutical agents.
3. Reestablish normal intestinal ecology.

---

milk, cheeses, mushrooms, and eggs. Many others are possible, yet these are the ones I have found to be most common and strongest.

The overall approach to treating the yeast problem is threefold. **The first facet is to refrain from feeding those "yeasty beasties" what they like to eat so they cannot thrive and divide.** They live on mostly simple sugars, yeast, and fermented foods, including fruits, fruit juices, dried fruits, sugary foods, refined-flour products, alcoholic beverages, cheese, vinegar, breads, and other yeasted or fermented food products, such as soy sauce.

What to eat? There are many recommended foods—fish, poultry, meat, lots of vegetables, some whole grains, nuts, seeds, and occasional eggs. (The antiyeast diet is more difficult for vegetarians but definitely possible with legumes, nuts, and seeds as the main proteins.) Some yogurt, especially with healthy bacterial cultures, is all right if milk is tolerated. (There are now goat's milk and soy yogurts available.) Oils are obtained from some butter and more cold-pressed vegetable oils, such as olive, flaxseed, sesame, and sunflower. Legumes are often limited because they add to intestinal gas. There are many versions of the antiyeast diet, depending on whose version you read. Some are stricter than others, but the basic ideas are the same. I have found over the years that what people tolerate is an individual experience and do not ask my patients to be overly severe if it does not make a difference in how they feel. Often, yeast elimination and probiotics help to resolve the issues with a basic diet that excludes sugars and refined flour, baked goods, alcohol, and vinegars. Because I believe fruit is a vital and healthy food, I encourage people to include a couple pieces daily if certain fruits appear to be tolerated. My overall diet approach follows.

Basic meals include proteins and vegetables or, occasionally, starch and vegetables. For the first few weeks, the carbohydrates, including pastas and especially breads, are limited, with only some whole-grain cereals being used. Brown rice, millet, buckwheat, and quinoa are some better tolerated whole grains. Avoiding all grains lowers fiber intake, but usually other aspects of the treatment help colon function. The Ideal Diet discussed in chapters 13 and 14, with certain modifications, makes a good anti-candida, diet. The rotation is a good way to reduce food reactions. Initially, the diet includes no fruit, or only 1 or 2 pieces a day, and fewer sweeter fruits, such as grapes, bananas, and melons. Apples and pears can be tried. The starches are limited to one portion a day, and the meals are oriented toward proteins and vegetables.

This is a special therapeutic diet, not necessarily a lifelong one, although many people like the way they feel on it. Intestinal symptoms decrease, energy improves, and itchy or irritated skin may start to heal with a decrease in sugar and yeasted foods. Also, some weight can be shed easily on this diet. This may be a problem for the already trim person, and lighter people need to emphasize regular eating to prevent weight loss and include more nuts and seeds in the diet to enhance the caloric intake. After a few weeks of avoiding some foods, we can test ourselves with fruit, bread, other grain products, or cheese—of course, one food at a time and only one daily—to see how we handle them. If they seem to cause no problems, we can then bring these foods into our diet on a rotating basis. Eventually, adding more whole grains and fiber provides a healthier diet. Different degrees of strictness with the diet may be necessary, depending on the severity of the problem. A more stringent diet might exclude all fruits; whole grains, particularly the glutinous ones—wheat, rye, barley, and oats; herbal teas and spices, which may contain molds; and many nuts, which can also carry molds.

The second facet of the treatment is to diminish the amount of yeast present. This is what Western medicine is so good at accomplishing. Nystatin powder is the most commonly used pharmaceutical for initial treatment of intestinal yeast (and the basis of many medications for the common vaginal yeast infections). Nystatin itself is made from a culture of

Anti-Yeast Diet Plan

Emphasize	Avoid
Vegetables—all	Sugar—all forms
Beans	Baked goods
Nuts and Seeds	Alcoholic beverages
Meats*	Vinegars
Butter	Fruit juices
Poultry*	Pickled vegetables
Eggs	Dried fruits
Cold-pressed oils	Cheese
Fish*	Refined flours
Lemon	Mushrooms
Whole grains	Breads
Fruit, fresh**	

* Vegetarians will need to use more whole grains, beans, and nuts and seeds, but this higher carbohydrate diet does not really curb yeast as well as a higher-protein and vegetable plan. Furthermore, vegetarians seem to be more prone to yeast overgrowth because their diet is more alkaline and sweet, which supports the yeast.

** Limited to 2 pieces daily.

certain bacteria and it will actually kill yeast. It is not readily absorbed through the intestinal mucosa, so basically it just handles the gastrointestinal yeast. Because it is most often given as pure powder dissolved in water, it will also kill some of the yeast in the oral cavity and upper gastrointestinal tract when it is gargled and swallowed. A solution can be used to wash the sinuses as well, by dissolving nystatin in saline solution and using a dropper or inhaling the solution.

I may prescribe a stronger antifungal agent, ketoconazole (Nizoral), for men with candidiasis and recurrent prostatitis or genital or skin symptoms of yeast, or for women with recurrent cystitis or other systemic symptoms, or for anyone with chronic yeast issues or elevated immune antibodies (showing allergy or hypersensitivity). This is effective for most yeast problems, but it can be irritating to the liver, so its use must be watched closely. For people who do not respond well to nystatin or other natural remedies, Nizoral may be indicated. I use Nizoral more commonly because it appears to be more of a broad-spectrum antifungal than the newer drugs. The usual dosage is one 200 mg tablet daily for 3 to 6 weeks if it is well tolerated. I usually start with 7 to 10 days and have patients take a break to assess the effects. A newer azole drug—fluconazole (Diflucan)—is more expensive yet has lesser potential toxicity than Nizoral. Other azole drugs are available from many European countries and Canada, many of which are now available through compounding pharmacies in the United States. These include clotrimazole, miconazole, tinidazole, and econazole. Tinidazole is now available in the U.S. in any pharmacy. They have similar systemic antifungal action (most are also mild amoebicides), are less expensive, and are also less toxic on the liver.

During yeast treatment, symptoms may arise secondary to killing the yeast. This occurs most with nystatin, at times with the natural therapies, and only occasionally with the systemic medicines. The symptoms might include headache, fatigue, a mild flulike syndrome, or an exacerbation of already existing symptoms. It may be helpful during die-off periods to clear the colon every 2 or 3 days with a water enema or have a colonic irrigation every 1 or 2 weeks for several treatments. Adding some nystatin to the water to introduce it directly into the colon may help clear some additional yeast.

Natural remedies that help to reduce yeast by killing it or by interfering with its growth include caprylic acid, fresh garlic and garlic extract, oregano oil, herbal products from the tannin-containing herb pau d'arco or taheebo, and the product Tanalbit. Caprylic acid is a natural fatty acid extracted from coconut oil. It interferes with the growing and duplicating process of *Candida albicans*. Caprylic acid does not actually kill yeast, but it may be effective in reducing intestinal yeast levels. It appears less effective since the mid-1990s, however; perhaps more yeasts are adapting, as microbes do. It must also be used for a fairly long period. I often prescribe the caprylates to follow a 2- to 3-month course of nystatin and use a caprylic acid product (there are many available) for a few months also. The length of treatment for yeast depends on the degree of the problem, the response to the treatment, and the results of tests.

Garlic has been shown to kill some yeast in sensitivity tests in the lab. It can be added to the treatment regimen and often helps. Two capsules several times daily is the usual dosage, although good garlic may

have a blood-pressure-lowering effect at that amount, which may detrimentally affect some people. Goldenseal root, and specifically its extract berberine, also has some antifungal properties. Pau d'arco, a Brazilian tree bark, has become a popular herb in the treatment of yeast, allergies, and other immune problems. It can be taken in capsules, or tea made from the bark can be drunk several times daily. It seems to tonify or strengthen the gastrointestinal tract and may help reduce yeast. Other possible natural yeast inhibitors include grapefruit seed extract, oregano oil, and undecylenic acid, made from castor bean oil.

The third facet of the yeast treatment involves restoring the colon to its natural state, mainly by reimplanting *Lactobacillus* species and other bacteria. Acidophilus-containing products are the primary ones used for this restoration. A couple of other bacteria are also helpful in the gut and used in some formulas. *Lactobacillus bifidus,* now referred to as bifidobacteria, adds a helpful function by replacing the once-present yeast typically found in youngsters. There are many formulas that contain these bacteria and are available in most natural food stores. I use a high-quality, milk-free product called Vital-Plex, which is produced and marketed by the nutritional supplement company ProThera, in Reno, Nevada. It can be taken as a supplement during the yeast treatment.

Another well-researched product is DDS-1, produced by UAS Laboratories. It is available in powder, capsules, and tablets. Although unpublished, studies at the University of Nebraska and Michigan State University have shown acidophilus DDS-1 to have many positive effects. This acidophilus in the colon can produce acidophilin, which has an antibiotic effect on a number of potentially pathogenic colon bacteria. It also has been shown to inhibit growth of *Candida albicans.* This product, as do most effective acidophilus cultures, helps restore bacteria that produce many B vitamins, including B_2, B_3, B_6, B_{12}, folic acid, biotin, and pantothenic acid. DDS-1 has also been shown to produce enzymes that help in digestion of proteins and milk sugar (lactose), and through its effect on fat metabolism, it has a mild cholesterol-lowering potential. Other research has revealed that DDS-1 and other lactobacilli may have antiviral effects with some viruses (herpes is one example) and anticancer effects, especially in the colon. I have seen lactobacillus treatment reduce the severity and recurrence of cold sores, genital herpes outbreaks, and canker sores, which may be a result of its correcting chemical or acid-base imbalance. By replacing putrefying bacteria in the mouth, throat, and upper intestinal tract, it has been seen to resolve bad breath as well as many symptoms of gastrointestinal upset, helping people's guts feel more settled.

DDS-1 *Lactobacillus acidophilus* has been studied more extensively than others. Other lactobacillus products likely have similar effects, however, and these are being researched as well. Potency of the product is probably important. Many cultures now contain billions of live bacteria per dosage, rather than the few million that were once common. This should make them more effective, because the higher counts will allow a greater number of bacteria to actually reach the colon. Replacing the diminishing yeast with these physiologically active bacteria will help restore the colon's normal functions. **Yeast organisms in the colon use up nutrients, rather than making additional ones, and they ferment foods, often leading to gas, bloating, abdominal discomfort, and flatulence. Reimplanting the colon with friendly bacteria helps to reduce many of the intestinal and digestive symptoms of candidiasis.**

There are a number of other supplements that can help in treating the yeast syndrome. Supplemental hydrochloric acid with meals (especially protein-containing meals) followed by digestive enzymes after eating can often help us to better break down and utilize our protein, fats, and food in general to make available the amino acids, essential fatty acids, and mineral micronutrients we need for healing. And they help to relieve digestive symptoms and make it easier for us to obtain the energy from the food. Healing the intestinal wall is an important part of clearing the candidiasis symptoms and reducing food reactions. Flaxseed or evening primrose oil and certain herbs can help with this.

For nutrient supplementation, a general multiple is used as a base, with some additional antioxidants to help handle certain toxic by-products, avoid immune suppression, and improve immune function. Organo-germanium may be used to aid in this immune support and to improve the gut mucosa. Although yet to be proven in research studies, vitamin A, beta-carotene, and vitamin C are useful in the regulation of the yeast and support of the immune function (as my clinical experience has convinced me). Extra magnesium is also a part of the program. Less zinc is suggested than in other programs, at least initially, as it possibly stimulates the candida growth. Extra B vitamins, including biotin, provide support by replacing some of those lost because of the diminished colon bacteria that produce them. Coenzyme Q10 has been shown to have positive effects in yeast treatment as well.

Some of the nutrient oils may be used in the treatment of the yeast problem. In addition to garlic oil and the caprylic acid formulas, essential fatty acids, fish oil (EPA/DHA), and evening primrose oil may be helpful, along with vitamin E. A product I have used that incorporates all of these oils is Samolinic, made and distributed by the Key Company in St. Louis, Missouri. I might suggest a product such as this or separate portions of some of these oils if there seem to be many inflammatory or allergic symptoms.

The type of herbal treatment suggested for the yeast condition depends mostly on the other coexisting problems. If there are premenstrual symptoms, diuretic herbs or female tonifying herbs may help (see "Premenstrual Syndrome" on page 719 later in this chapter). With intestinal symptoms or upset, soothing digestive herbs may be helpful. Peppermint or chamomile teas are beneficial; capsules containing slippery elm bark and licorice root powder can help heal the intestinal lining. Goldenseal root powder in short courses (1 or 2 weeks) strengthens the mucous membranes, but it also stimulates liver detoxification, which can cause an increase in symptoms. The tonic herb pau d'arco is often used in yeast treatment. Oregano oil offers some help at reducing yeast growth, and some patients claim benefits from that.

Evaluating and treating the yeast syndrome is a challenge for both doctors and patients. It takes patience and often requires a long therapy as the body uses its sensitive biofeedback process to let us know what is working. Often nystatin or other antifungal products must be taken for years but usually will produce, within a few months, a marked change in the symptoms and a reduction in colon yeast colonization and eventually reduced blood antibodies to the yeast.

Yeast Syndrome Nutrient Program			
Nutrient	**Amount**	**Nutrient**	**Amount**
Yeast-free diet	See page 701	Selenium	300 mcg
Vitamin A	3,000–7,500 IU	Zinc	15 mg
Beta-carotene	15,000 IU	Lactobacillus and other	
Vitamin D	400 IU	helpful microorganisms	4–10 billion
Vitamin E	800 IU		organisms
Vitamin K	300 mcg	Caprylic acid	300–600 mg
Thiamin (B1)	50 mg	Coenzyme Q10	20–40 mg
Riboflavin (B2)	25–50 mg	Essential fatty acids*	4 capsules
Niacinamide (B3)	100 mg	Gamma-linolenic acid, such	
Pantothenic acid (B5)	500 mg	as evening primrose oil	4 capsules
Pyridoxine (B6)	50 mg	Hydrochloric acid (with meals)	1–2 tablets
Pyridoxal-5-phosphate	50 mg		
Cobalamin (B12)	50 mcg	Digestive enzymes	2–3 tablets
Folic acid	800 mcg	(after meals)	
Biotin	1,000 mcg		
Vitamin C	3,000 mg	**Optional**	
Bioflavonoids	250 mg	Goldenseal root powder	2–3 capsules
Calcium	600–1,000 mg		(2–3 weeks)
Chromium	500 mcg	Pau d'arco	2–4 capsules or
Copper	2 mg		2 cups tea
Iodine	150–225 mcg	Garlic oil or garlic extract	4–6 capsules
Iron	10–18 mg	or oregano oil	2–4 capsules
Magnesium	400–800 mg	Echinacea	2–4 capsules
Manganese	5–10 mg		
Molybdenum	500 mcg		

* Flaxseed oil, 2–4 teaspoons daily, can replace these 2 products.

Many people experience a profound and positive change in their health with proper diagnosis and treatment of this condition. However, we must also be careful not to overtreat and turn this medical concern into nothing more than the latest designer disease, as the mainstream medical profession might like. I believe that yeast awareness is here to stay, and doctors and patients must be even more careful in their use of antibiotics, birth control pills, and the immune-suppressive corticosteroids. For more on the yeast syndrome, see my other books *The False Fat Diet* and *The New Detox Diet*.

26. ALLERGIES

The theories, problems, and treatments of allergies and hypersensitivities represent an enormous topic that could easily fill an entire book—in fact, many such books have been written by noted medical authors. My book *The False Fat Diet* deals with this very topic, focusing on clearing food and environmental allergies/reactions via elimination diets, nutritional supplements, and healing the gastrointestinal tract. This section discusses some of the basic concepts in the field of allergy, with an emphasis on new work related to this growing twentieth- and now twenty-first-century dilemma. It is not getting better either, with more people suffering from allergies and asthma because of the decades of pollution in our food, air, and water. I also explore the use of diet and supplements in treating allergies and reactions of all kinds.

Allergies are a result of our physiological and biochemical interaction with the world around us and within us—with the foods, chemicals, and natural substances in our immediate environment that we ingest, inhale, or physically contact, and with various internal microbes and body tissues. The body's immune system is designed to correctly identify and differentiate between self and nonself—that is, between what the body needs and what is foreign to it—and when it encounters foreign substances, it reacts by making antibodies or releasing certain chemicals, such as histamines. Of course, it is appropriate for us to make protective antibodies against infectious organisms, chemicals, and other foreign substances; pollens, molds, animal hairs, dust, and foods all contain protein antigens that stimulate some antibody response. The problem arises when we have an inappropriate response, or a hyperresponse. Then the antibodies attach to the antigens, causing a variety of internal reactions. Histamine and other chemicals are released into the system, causing an inflammatory reaction. These antigen-antibody (Ag-Ab) reactions affect the tissues and organs, mainly the skin, mucous membranes, lungs, and gastrointestinal tract. Symptoms commonly produced include itchy and watery eyes, runny and congested nose and sinuses, skin reactions, and rapid heart rate. Less obvious but still common allergic symptoms include fatigue, headache, intestinal gas or pain, abdominal bloating, and mood changes.

These allergic manifestations often are the result of multiple stressors and biochemical reactions. I often describe this to patients as the "cup runneth over" theory. Certain people may be reactive to specific environmental and food products, as I myself am. However, when the diet is relatively clean, the stress level is low, and the eliminative functions are working well, we will exhibit minimal, if any, symptoms. But if we have too many stressors going into our cup—a high-demand schedule; a few dinners out with more bread, cheese, and wine; a few extra worries; less exercise; and a little constipation—our cup may runneth over, and we may experience sinus or upper respiratory symptoms, a skin rash, or other "allergic" problems. From a naturopathic viewpoint, allergic symptoms represent detoxification of any overly congested body; the traditional Chinese viewpoint suggests an imbalance of energies and organs. Western medicine has its own theories, which I also discuss in this section.

Related to allergies are hypersensitivities, allergy-like reactions that result from the repeated sensitizing of the body by certain substances, usually a protein antigen of foods or specific chemicals. Hypersensitivities are distinguished from immediate allergies by the fact that hypersensitivity reactions are usually delayed, with symptoms appearing several hours or longer after exposure, even up to several days later. They are mediated through T lymphocytes of the cellular immune system and delayed-type IgG antibodies rather than the IgE/mast cell/histamine system of rapid allergic responses. Regarding other allergic-type reactions, the term *hypersusceptibility* describes the rapid symptoms associated with environmental illness or exposure to environmental chemicals. This is likely a neuro-endocrine interaction rather than a true allergy.

Primary External Factors Causing Allergies and Hypersensitivity Reactions

Natural environmental substances. Mold spores, pollens from trees and grasses, dust (actually dust mites), animal hairs, and insects. These commonly produce upper respiratory symptoms in sensitive individuals. Itching, redness, and fluid (water and mucus) may affect the eyes, nose, sinuses, throat, bronchial tubes, and lungs.

Foods. Any food may be allergenic or cause reactions. Common ones include wheat, milk, eggs, corn, yeast, coffee, and chocolate. Many people are sensitive to sugars and refined foods or chemicals, but these are less allergic reactions and more intolerances. Even herbs and teas may lead to allergic symptoms. Food allergies and reactions may affect most body systems, with the gastrointestinal, nervous, respiratory, and skin areas affected the most. I am also concerned about the allergy problems that we may be inviting through our increasing dependence on genetically modified foods.

Chemicals. Both environmental chemicals and food additives may create sensitivities. There are literally thousands of possibilities, including sprays, resins, hydrocarbons, pesticides, and so on. Some may weaken our immunity and allow further allergies to develop. Tobacco is a common allergen, containing substances to which many people are both addicted and allergic, a common duo according to the current understanding of allergies.

Pathways of Allergens into the Body

Depending on a variety of factors, some individuals are more sensitive to allergens that enter through a particular area. These are the most common pathways:

Nose and respiratory tract. Inhalation of environmental allergens.

Mouth and gastrointestinal tract. Ingestion of food and chemicals found in foods, water, and medicines. The GI tract has the highest level of immune activity of the body, thus food reactions are quite common, especially with the diet and stresses that many people experience.

Skin. Although this is not really an entry point, our skin is a site for allergic reactions that can definitely affect the body and health.

We may also have internal "allergies," where the immune system reacts to the body's tissues as protein antigens and actually forms specific antibodies to them. These antibodies then latch onto the antigen-coded organ tissues, where they may interfere with proper function and produce a wide variety of inflammatory symptoms and diseases. More common areas affected include the thyroid gland, blood vessels, and joints, causing problems such as Hashimoto's (autoimmune) thyroiditis, polyarteritis nodosa (inflamed arteries), and rheumatoid arthritis. These abnormal responses to normal tissues are termed *autoimmune diseases*. They are increasing in frequency and still represent a great mystery of modern medicine. They may also be connected to viral diseases (that the immune system tries to attack and conquer), toxicity issues and immunizations, genetic factors, and psycho-emotional-spiritual issues.

Common Allergy Problems

Common allergic problems include hay fever, hives, eczema, contact dermatitis (like poison oak), and bronchial asthma. **Hay fever,** or allergic rhinitis, is characterized by sneezing, runny nose, itchy eyes, and postnasal drip. It is caused by reactions to pollens such as ragweed, trees, dust, grasses, molds, animals, and foods. It can be diagnosed by skin testing or blood antibody levels. Treatment may include avoidance of, or desensitization to, the allergens, or drugs such as antihistamines, decongestants, cortisone sprays or tablets, and cromolyn sodium nasal spray. Hay fever tends to run in families and is usually seasonal. In sensitive people, there are also skin and respiratory reactions to external chemicals and irritants, such as washing and cleaning supplies, chlorine in pools and water, and hair and makeup products.

Hives, or urticaria, is characterized by red, itchy, and possibly painful wheals (bumps) on the skin. This condition may be caused by reactions to insect bites, chemicals (such as sulfites or food colors), drugs (such as aspirin or penicillin), or foods. Common foods causing hives are shellfish, nuts, citrus fruits, tomatoes, strawberries, chocolate, beef, pork, and mangoes. Avoidance is the key to treatment; antihistamines may relieve symptoms. When reactions are caused by drugs, more acute treatment may be needed. Genetics may play a role in this type of allergy, and prior sensitization to the specific agent is necessary for the reaction, as for most allergies.

Eczema (dermatitis) is characterized by dry, itchy skin, especially on the arms and legs. It is often hereditary, and it may be worsened by stress, sweating, or food allergies. Treatment involves lowering stress, avoiding strong soaps and detergents, use of cortisone creams and drugs, and an elimination diet with avoidance of allergenic foods. Desensitization is usually not very helpful for this problem. I have found that diet and supplements can improve the condition quite well.

Contact dermatitis is characterized by an itchy, red, raised rash that may blister. It can occur anywhere on the body where contact to the allergen has been made. Common allergenic agents are poison oak or ivy, such chemicals as nail polish or soaps, plastics, metals (nickel is common), and fabrics. Medical treatment involves avoidance of known allergens and the use of antihistamine and cortisone drugs to reduce symptoms.

Asthma is characterized by difficulty in breathing, wheezing, coughing, and production of bronchial mucus. It is caused by a combination of genetic, allergic, and stress factors. It is commonly treated with drugs, avoidance and desensitization, and stress management. Diet and supplements can offer some help, but often time helps the clearing for many asthma sufferers.

Headaches, alcoholism, and cigarette smoking may also involve allergy factors. Pain in the head, neck aches, and painful sensitivity to light, while they may be a result of stress or muscle tension, may also be caused by reactions to chemicals and foods.

In such cases, the treatment would include rest, relaxation, pain relievers, and the clearing of allergenic agents. Alcoholism often involves an allergic component with an addiction to grains and/or yeast. (Intestinal or vaginal yeast, skin fungus, or internal parasites or worms may also act as allergens as well as tissue irritants; see "Yeast Syndrome" on page 698.) Alcoholism may also be a psychological disease with possible genetic predisposition and may be related to a deficiency of the trace mineral chromium (see discussion of this mineral on page 177 in chapter 6, Minerals), which is a key component of glucose tolerance factor. Treatment involves avoidance and therapy, possibly with the use of drugs or counseling. Cigarette smoking often involves an allergic addiction to either tobacco or the chemicals added to cigarettes. Treatment of nicotine addiction incorporates the elimination of the addiction, which may require counseling, willpower, detoxification, and a change of lifestyle. See my book *The New Detox Diet* for a more thorough discussions of these common substance abuse problems.

Although there are a great many types of allergic reactions, almost all result from elevated levels of two different antibodies—immunoglobulin E (IgE) and immunoglobulin G (IgG), which occurs more often with foods. IgE stimulates the release of histamine, causing immediate physiological activities. The common histamine response includes swelling, redness, itching, and possibly pain. The IgG antibody causes more delayed and long-term reactions. Some of the problems caused by the IgE reaction are hay fever or pollen reactions, insect sting reactions, urticaria (hives) from ingested substances (such as foods or drugs), and atopic (hereditary allergy—mediated IgE) dermatitis or eczema. Many of these are fairly easy to observe and diagnose; however, reactions such as a change in energy level, decreased mental clarity, or digestive symptoms may be more difficult to acknowledge and to understand as allergic responses. IgG-mediated delayed types of reactions include many drug side effects, problems from exposure to chemicals (including tobacco), and most food reactions (that is why skin testing is not very useful for such allergies—it measures only IgE responses). Most allergy problems are a mixture of these different immunoglobulin-mediated reactions.

The main focus of traditional allergy practice is the diseases involving the IgE-histamine response—hay fever, eczema, and asthma. These are termed *atopies* (hereditary allergies); sensitive individuals have a genetic or at least familial propensity for experiencing these diseases sometime in their lives. These problems are more common in children and tend to regress with age. When such problems start later in life, they may be less genetically dominated and more related to other factors. Each of these conditions involves increased sensitivity to certain allergens. For example, an asthmatic or eczema sufferer may be allergic to eggs, wheat, or milk; hay fever sufferers are usually sensitive to pollen and environmental agents. Isolating the specific reactions and avoiding the agents that cause them, and/or using injection desensitization, may relieve the symptomatology. However, in all these cases, even with an elimination of symptoms, there is still the potential for the problem because of genetic or familial predisposition. Schools of natural healing or Chinese medicine may view these allergy problems in terms of body biochemical or energy imbalances and attempt to offer relief by correcting these difficulties. Nutritional medicine may have a lot to offer the allergic person by providing the optimum tissue and cellular nutrient levels that allow improved function and reduced allergic symptoms.

A deeper realm of allergy and immunology, now incorporated into the field of clinical ecology, has fascinated many physicians for years. It involves our interaction with the environment and its effect on human health and disease. Clinical ecologists are physicians who evaluate and treat chronic illness on the basis of allergy, immune response (and immune weakness), and nutrition. Therapy may involve isolation from allergens, dietary changes, and an orthomolecular approach to nutritional supplements—that is, using higher amounts of various nutrients to support the body's functions and to alter abnormal physiology and correct functional or metabolic nutritional imbalances. Such problems as chronic fatigue, rapid aging, recurrent infections, arthritis, headaches, asthma, and mental illness have been treated successfully with this approach. The theories of "cerebral allergy" and "allergy-addiction" have been set forth by these pioneering physicians.

Herbert Rinkel, MD, was probably the first to notice the problem of cumulative allergic reactions, which led to his initial work on the "rotary-diversified" diet. This diet, and variations of it, have been used since the mid-1950s, and each year more physicians employ the diet in their practices. The basic theory is that inappropriate immune responses produce antibodies to basically harmless and even usable macromolecules; these reactions may affect the normal body functions. Many of these reactions may be "hidden" or masked in the process of "allergy-addiction." In this case, foods may be acting on the body much like such agents as coffee, alcohol beverages, or tobacco—which are also common allergens. To avoid the withdrawal symptoms, we must regularly take in the specific substance. This type of reaction most commonly causes what are now called "cerebral allergies"—altered neurotransmitter reactions that affect the energy, emotions, and psyche.

The theory is that certain allergenic antigens or antigen-antibody complexes cross the blood-brain barrier and cause these unusual reactions. Common cerebral symptoms include headache, dullness, lightheadedness, dizziness, anxiety, irritability, confusion, incoordination, and depression. Lethargy, aggression, crying spells, insomnia, and even psychotic symptoms may also be experienced. The research of Herbert Rinkel, originator of laboratory methods in the 1940s still used in the field of immunotherapy, along with that of William Philpott, psychiatrist and founding member of the Academy of Orthomolecular Psychiatry, and Marshall Mandell, MD, a practicing allergist in Norwalk, Connecticut, has shown a fairly high percentage of food allergies in schizophrenic patients and those with other psychological disorders. Wheat, milk, and tobacco were most commonly found to be involved; these so-called cerebral allergies can be most significant with the cereal grains. Food allergies may occur as a fixed reaction (stable over time) or cumulative (increasing with repeated use and lessening with avoidance).

> ### Foods Commonly Associated with Specific Allergies
>
> - **Asthma:** wheat, eggs
> - **Cerebral symptoms:** corn, wheat, milk, soybeans
> - **Childhood allergies:** milk, wheat, eggs, artificial colors/flavors, salicylates, peanuts (less common: rye, beef, fish)
> - **Eczema:** eggs, citrus fruits, tomatoes
> - **Hay fever:** milk, wheat, nuts, chocolate, colas, and sulfites
> - **Headaches:** wheat, chocolate
> - **Hives:** strawberries, tomatoes, chocolate, eggs, shellfish, mangoes, pork, nuts
> - **Migraine headaches:** alcoholic beverages, cheese, chocolate, nuts, wheat, citrus fruits, tomatoes, MSG, nitrates, eggs, and milk

The allergy-addiction syndrome related to foods is common. These easily become "hidden" allergies, which may be involved in food cravings, binge eating, overeating, weight gain, and general ups and downs that come from eating food. Food cravings, even very subtle ones, often are part of this syndrome, but people who experience this might think that they just like a particular food and so eat it regularly. When they eat it, they may feel a lift. This is thought to be a result of stimulation of beta-endorphins in the brain, which give us an "up" or euphoric feeling, as occurs with prolonged exercise.

Most addictions, especially to foods (and some street drugs), involve some allergy, but the allergic reactions may be masked, with repeated exposures producing no symptoms. A positive identification of the allergenic food cannot be made until it has been eliminated for 4 or more days; although at times, avoidance for 24 hours might be enough to reveal the allergy reaction. After a few days, trying the food by itself may produce a marked, abnormal response, and then we can see more clearly what has been happening. Much like an alcoholic with allergies to yeast and grains, people with such food addictions may tend to binge on the allergenic foods, especially when they are under psychological stress.

A wide variety of symptoms are possible with food allergy-addictions. Theron Randolph and Ralph Moss's

An Alternative Approach to Allergies offers an advanced and somewhat complex analysis of the many theories and symptoms of food allergies, noting that the addiction occurs in two phases, stimulatory and withdrawal. During the stimulatory cycle, when we eat the food, we experience a decrease in symptoms; when we avoid it, we experience a "hangover" and an increase in symptoms. In the withdrawal phase, we experience initially a worsening of symptoms and then improvement. When we reexpose ourselves to the food, we often get a marked increase in symptoms and a clearer picture of the problem.

Children experience food reactions quite commonly. Cerebral symptoms may occur, leading to hyperactivity, poor attention, and difficulty in learning, as well as many other physical symptoms. Often, isolating the allergens, which may be foods and/or chemicals in foods, and eliminating them from the diet can make a huge difference in the life of the affected child and consequently in the lives of his or her parents and siblings. What foods are most commonly connected to these allergies? Dr. Rinkel's research led him to conclude that "the constant, monotonous intake of any food promotes the development of a food allergy (reaction) in a susceptible person." **The foods he found most frequently to cause reactions were wheat, eggs, milk, coffee, corn, yeast, beef, and pork.**

Although different practitioners report different lists of foods that they find to be commonly allergenic— for example, some include corn, soy products, cane sugar, or nuts, while others do not—all agree that wheat, milk, and eggs are the top three; yeast is another common allergen. All of these foods not only are consumed daily by most people but also are found as components of many other foods, giving us repeated exposures daily. In general, infrequently eaten foods are less likely to lead to allergies.

Causes of Allergies

The causes of allergies are, I believe, multiple. There is, of course, the genetic predisposition, which is clearly established in the atopic diseases of hay fever, asthma, and eczema but may also predispose us to many others. Eating habits during the first year of life may influence our potential for allergy more than anything else, even heredity. Feeding babies solid foods too early and not breastfeeding them is a primary way to cause allergies and thus produce many problems in infants. Cow's milk and baby formulas provide large molecules that are difficult for the infant's immature gastrointestinal tract and immune system to handle. Gluten allergy from early feeding of wheat is also common. The best way to prevent allergies, particularly childhood ones, is to breastfeed a child exclusively for 6 months before introducing solid foods. (See "Infants and Toddlers" on page 557 in chapter 15, Life Stage Programs.) Even in adults, poor digestion, with low levels of hydrochloric acid or pancreatic enzymes, is an underlying cause of many food reactions, as are the presence of abnormal or immune-stimulating microorganisms.

The digestive process is tied to allergies, particularly to foods. The problem starts with incomplete digestion that results from improper chewing (and choosing) of food and poor action of hydrochloric acid, pancreatic enzymes, and bile. These are influenced by stress and by excessive fluid intake around meals. The incomplete digestion along with the "leaky gut" that comes from inflammation in the gastrointestinal mucosa—resulting from stress, the intake of fried and fatty foods, as well as chemicals, and the presence of parasites or *Candida albicans*—allow absorption of larger molecules that then generate an immune reaction. Low-level infectious microorganisms may also create allergic (and immunologic) propensity; I believe this is common with worms, other parasites, yeasts, and certain bacteria. Chronic stress affects pancreatic and adrenal function, which are tied to digestion, energy level, and food cravings.

The key here is to minimize food allergies by enhancing digestion—chewing well, eating good foods, lowering stress, and supporting digestive juices. Decreasing inflammation and healing the gut, treating any abnormally present microorganisms, supporting immune and glandular functions, and stimulating proper detoxification will all help minimize food reactions and true allergies as well. Many nutrients, discussed beginning on page 715, can further support all of these functions.

Toxicity in the environment is another probable cause for the increasing numbers of allergic people. Exposure to many more irritating and allergenic substances also may adversely affect immune function. Today, many people are reacting to new synthetic products and pollutants in the air. Formaldehyde, hydrocarbons, and carbon monoxide in the air as well as many industrial or food chemicals found in food—such as antibiotics, certain food colors, sulfites, MSG, and sodium benzoate—may all stimulate allergic responses as well as lower our immunity. There are many other chemicals that are not easy to discover or avoid. Living as natural a life as possible, avoiding polluted areas and chemicals, is the best we can do.

Stress also plays a major role in allergies by disregulating immune functions and by weakening adrenal response. Stress can also directly influence our digestive function, which can be a core factor in allergies. Chronic stress may lead to a reduction of hydrochloric acid (HCl) output (initially it may raise HCl secretions) and digestive enzyme function, so that we do not break down our food properly. As stated earlier, absorption of larger food molecules into the blood may lead to increased antibody responses and subsequent allergies. Furthermore, the effects of stress on the immune system can lead to an increase in infections, which contribute to both environmental and food allergies. For example, parasitic intestinal infections may act as direct allergens and also increase other allergic responses. In addition, other aspects of stress, including emotional and mental stress, anxiety, and fatigue, all increase susceptibility to allergies. Menstrual stress (hormonal changes) also seems to increase allergic reactions.

Overexposure to chemicals and overintake of refined foods are other factors that can cause or exacerbate allergies. They can also enhance stress levels and weaken immunity and may lead to nutritional deficiencies—another problem that increases allergic sensitivity. Low nutrient levels of vitamin C, most B vitamins, vitamin A, and many minerals influence body function sufficiently to weaken allergic resistance.

Excess or repeated contact with particular foods and substances in the environment (like pets and some people) causes allergies. It usually takes a few days for the immune system, mainly our T lymphocytes, to be sensitized to an antigen and guide the formation of antibodies by B lymphocytes. After that, reactions to exposures are immediate and usually produce mild immune-inflammatory responses. Initially, histamine released by other cells causes some redness, swelling, and fluid release and also stimulates the T cell antibody activity. Also, repeated exposures create delayed antigen-antibody responses, which can have a variety of effects on the tissues and bodily functions.

Temperature extremes also influence many people's allergic problems and generally increase susceptibility to allergies. Quick changes of temperature, particularly going from heat to air conditioning, may themselves produce symptoms such as sinus congestion, skin rash, hives, or even asthmatic attacks. Hot and dry weather, or winds particularly, may make some people more allergic.

The causes of allergies are indeed a complex issue. Everything from our genes to our spiritual awareness is a factor, with diet and stress levels being especially important. The traditional Chinese medical viewpoint suggests that allergies reflect internal balance or imbalance, mainly of the wood (liver) and metal (lungs and colon) elements, as well as being a result of general energy congestion. If that is the case, then rebalancing these organs within the entire energy system will help improve allergic symptoms. I have seen improvement with acupuncture treatments along with some liver and colon detoxification through diet and herbs.

Genetically modified foods may also be an increasing cause of concern with respect to food allergy. Researchers do not yet know exactly what kinds of new proteins are being introduced into the food supply, or how the digestive tracts will respond. At the very least, this country needs some good labeling laws to enable us to identify foods that contain genetically engineered components, so that we can better understand how this unprecedented change in the food supply is affecting us.

Just as there are many causes, there are also many symptoms related to allergies, both gross and subtle, visible and invisible. Often such acute symptoms as fatigue, itching, or a runny nose can progress to a chronic problem with repeated exposure, especially to food allergens; such difficulties as headache, depression, or arthritis may follow. Really, any of the inflammatory "-itis" diseases—colitis, arthritis, dermatitis, bronchitis, for example—can come from allergies.

Allergy Evaluation

Evaluating allergies is another complex and controversial issue. There are a number of tests available to evaluate environmental and food allergies. Skin testing is probably the best way to isolate specific environmental allergens, because these are harder to detect ourselves, especially for substances such as pollens. Molds may be a bit easier to isolate, as by noticing our reactions upon going into a damp house or any moldy environment. Allergies to animals are often fairly simple to identify, though many of us deny our chronic reaction to a beloved cat or dog. There are many techniques for skin testing. I prefer the Rinkel method because it individualizes the analysis and treatment plan. Some doctors use group antigen testing, mixing a variety of pollens or animal danders together. This is simpler and usually less costly and time-consuming, although not always as effective, especially in patients with more complex problems.

When it comes to foods, the source of most allergies (sensitivities), skin testing is not as useful. Only a small percentage of reactions may be found through this method. That is why conventional allergists believe that all the brouhaha over food allergies is unwarranted. They have defined allergy as IgE immediate reactions, or those that respond to skin (scratch) testing. But many allergy-oriented family doctors know that food reactions are indeed important, and the basis of many problems. One of these is Dr. Theron Randolph, who set up an inpatient clinical ecology unit at a Chicago hospital, where he isolated people from most allergens and then tested them with one allergen at a time. He and his patients were able to see and experience more directly that many symptoms improved with food eliminations and were reactivated by exposure to specific food triggers. Many practitioners over these past decades, including myself, are able to corroborate these findings.

Some tests are fairly good for measuring food antibody reactions; techniques have improved since the

---

Possible Allergy Symptoms and Problems

Alcoholism	Eczema	Obesity
Anxiety	Edema	Overeating
Arthritis, juvenile	Emotional outbursts	Palpitations
Arthritis, rheumatoid	Fatigue	Poor thinking
Asthma	Frequent hunger	Postnasal drip
Binge eating	Hay fever	Recurrent ear infections
Bloating	Headaches	Recurrent vaginitis
Brain fog (fatigue and lack of clarity)	Heartburn	Regional ileitis
	Hives	Runny nose
Canker sores	Hoarseness	Seizures
Chest congestion	Hyperactivity	Sinus congestion
Cigarette smoking	Irritability	Sore throat
Constipation	Itching	Stomachache
Cough	Joint pain	Swelling of hands or feet
Dark circles under eyes	Learning disabilities	Tachycardia
Depression	Loss of sex drive	Tinnitus
Diarrhea	Mood swings	Ulcerative colitis
Disorientation	Muscle aches	Vaginal itching
Drug addiction	Muscle weakness	Vomiting
Ear congestion	Nausea	Weight gain
Earaches	Nonspecific rash	Weight swings

mid-1990s. **The radioallergosorbent test (RAST),** which measures IgG or IgE antibodies to specific food antigens, is probably the best. It is costly and not fool-proof by any means (people can react to foods in a variety of ways, as discussed in my book *The False Fat Diet*), but it can give us the most accurate results for a large number of foods all at once. Cytotoxic testing, which measures the cellular response (mainly of white blood cells) to food antigens, has fallen into disuse because of lack of accuracy of many labs due to the subjective nature of the test. A newer, computerized technique known as **ALCAT** measures white blood cell reactions to food antigens and may be a more useful test, as it picks up another way that people can react. For some of my patients who wish to invest in these studies, doing both an antibody test and the ALCAT offers the most information. The costs for this testing run from $400 to $1,000, depending on the extensiveness of each test.

Some practitioners are using more subtle and bioenergetic ways to evaluate and treat food reactions. These are the **NAET (Nambudripad's allergy elimination technique)** method using applied kinesiology (muscle testing) and an electromagnetic assessment by Dr. Ellen Cutler called the BioSET method. My overall sense is that the results depend much on the quality and energy of the practitioner. This process can be time-consuming with multiple visits, and thus costly, but it does propose to "clear" the reactive foods and allow people to still consume them. My patients who have done these treatments have reported very mixed results, from failure to great success.

There are other ways (maybe the best ways) to test in order to evaluate and correlate allergic reactions to food through actual patient experiences. **Self-testing (through avoidance and challenge, noting any reactions)** or a clinical form of self-testing is really the best method. These include a variety of techniques using a general method called **provocative testing,** where the patient receives sublingual drops of foods, ingests capsules containing powdered foods, or eats whole foods. Ideally, the patient does not know what food is being tested and has not eaten it for several days, for then reactions will be most clear. In a clinical setting, however, a patient may know what food is being tested, may have eaten it within the past 12 to 24 hours, and may have only 30 minutes to observe a

reaction. All these factors make this type of test less accurate. It may take longer than the time allotted to react to a food, and our psyche often influences our reactions when we know what food is being tested. In addition, when several foods are tested on the same day, overlapping reactions may occur.

The best practical testing involves following an elimination diet and then consuming various suspect foods and watching for reactions over 24 hours. This means that only one food a day can be tested if the results are to be accurate. **The absolute best test, of course, is a double-blind test,** where neither the patient nor the clinician knows what food extract is in those funny little capsules and the specific reactions are quantified over a period of at least 3 or 4 hours, and even up to 1 or 2 days. This, however, is not very practical. Food elimination testing is not easy, because it requires self-discipline, but it is fairly simple in technique. As mentioned earlier, many food allergies (as well as "intolerances" and "sensitivities") and symptoms are masked by addictive behavior, so a food elimination plan is needed to uncover them.

The advantage of food elimination or avoidance and retesting is that it helps the body release these addictions, so that retesting the food will reveal the actual allergy. It is also inexpensive and offers us a valuable direct experience of our food reactions. Its disadvantages are that it is time-consuming and sometimes difficult to fit into everyday life and that the results are based on our subjective experience, so that accuracy is dependent on a significant short-term reaction (many food reactions are not immediate) and high awareness of the body's functioning. Yet, overall, food elimination testing can be valuable. If it does not reveal clear findings and we still suspect food allergies, a blood antibody test can be done.

Another testing method involves doing a short fast on water or juices, which will clear addictive foods and resensitize the body. In my first book, *Staying Healthy with the Seasons,* a lengthy food elimination program is delineated whereby individual food groups are eliminated one by one until we get down to a few days of only juice and water before individual foods are tested. A simpler technique would be to eat a diet that contains only foods that are unlikely to be allergenic. These include all fruits except citrus; all

---

What to Eat for an Allergy Elimination Diet

- All fruits, except citrus
- All vegetables, except corn and tomatoes
- Brown or white rice
- Turkey
- Whitefish—halibut, sole, and swordfish
- Hazelnuts, walnuts, and sunflower seeds
- Water and herbal teas

---

vegetables except corn and tomatoes; brown or white rice (but no other grains; other starches could include hard squashes and sweet potatoes); turkey (and chicken if it is not regularly consumed); deep-sea whitefish, such as halibut, swordfish, or sole (no shellfish or salmon); as well as walnuts, hazelnuts (filberts), and sunflower seeds (in moderation). If any of these foods have been eaten regularly or craved, they should be avoided. If symptoms develop during the avoidance (or testing) period, 1 to 2 grams of vitamin C should be taken every couple of hours. The buffered ascorbates with minerals (such as calcium, magnesium, and potassium) or bicarbonate are usually helpful. Withdrawal symptoms are not at all common during the avoidance phase, but they may occur.

The best thing about food elimination is that it is usually an important part of the treatment as well as of the evaluation. After testing, the new diet becomes our individualized therapeutic diet. To test foods, though, only one food should be consumed at a time. This is termed a "challenge." Testing foods singly is the only way to really follow what the reaction, if any, will be. **Because it is possible to react to chemicals, preservatives, and pesticides on foods, it is wise to use whole organic foods whenever possible.**

There are two approaches to this testing method. The first is to eat "mono meals," consisting of a moderate to large portion of an individual food and then to monitor any reactions to that food over the next 3 or 4 hours. In this way, several foods can be tested in a day. I generally suggest this method following a short fast because the body is in a cleaner state and able to respond more clearly to food challenges. For basic food testing, it may be more appropriate and

simpler just to create a diet of foods found to be safe through the elimination phase and then build on that, trying new ones. Again, **only one new food should be added at a time;** adding only one per day is ideal rather than three or four, which could confuse the body's responses. Use the less potentially allergenic foods first, before attempting a wheat, egg, or milk challenge. Some people will want to try their most suspected foods first, and this can be all right, although it may interfere with further testing if there is a positive reaction.

If we do react positively to a food, we eliminate it again for 3 to 6 weeks before retesting. This will help to reduce the allergy and reduce antibody levels, so that we may not react as much or even at all. Certain food reactions are fairly fixed, and we may need to completely avoid the foods that cause them, some possibly even forever. However, we will be able to tolerate most foods if we eat them infrequently or work them into a new "rotary-diversified" diet, where most foods are rotated on a 4-day basis—part of the suggested food allergy diet therapy.

It is important to keep a journal during food testing and record any reactions—how we feel before, immediately after, and in the several hours (even up to 12–24) after consuming a food. And if possible, how we feel when we wake up the next morning because some of these delayed reactions take a day to cause some symptoms, such as congestion, foggy-headedness, or fatigue (or any energy and mood alterations). If we leave it all to memory, we may miss subtle reactions or forget what happened. This also increases our food awareness. Most of us have not been trained to observe how we feel after we eat a meal.

Monitoring our pulse rate is another aid to evaluating food reactions. If we take our pulse often enough to know the basic resting pulse and become efficient in the technique, we can record the pulse before and after consuming a food or meal. If it increases by more than 12 to 14 beats per minute after eating, one of the foods may be an allergen. We should check our pulse about five minutes after eating and at 15-minute intervals for the next hour. This so-called pulse test, devised by Arthur Coca, MD, can be used as a more subtle physiological evaluation as well as a way to monitor the pulse alongside actual symptoms.

Allergy Treatment

Treatment of allergies is also rather diversified and somewhat complex. The standard medical approach is to use antihistamine or immunosuppressive steroid drugs to reduce symptoms; a more corrective approach involves the isolation of specific allergens through skin testing and then doing desensitization through shots, as well as avoiding allergen exposure where possible. This is the usual procedure for environmental allergies and common problems (such as hay fever and asthma); however, as previously mentioned, this process is not useful for discovering or treating most food reactions. For hay fever or asthma, cromolyn sodium works well but must be taken regularly for several weeks to be effective. There are obviously hundreds of drugs available for allergic conditions, but my focus in this book is to try to be drug free. With drug or food reactions, the approach is usually avoidance of the allergenic agents, if they can be determined.

Most medical treatment for allergies is not curative but is aimed at reducing symptoms. Ideally, we want to correct and heal the body so that we become less congested and less allergic. Before even thinking about medical investigation and treatment, it is wise to do what we can ourselves first. Reducing stress, eating a good diet, and taking nutritional supplements will often work rapidly to reduce allergic symptoms. The elimination diet or even a short fast can help us identify and handle food allergies. Personally, I would begin with a detoxification program, use herbs and supplements, and have acupuncture treatments; I believe that this would give me the best chance for rapid recovery. For example, I cleared my allergies of many years during my first juice cleanse. If necessary, I will suggest skin testing and desensitization to my patients, and this is also helpful; it is just more time-consuming and expensive. To help in allergy treatment, it is also important to pay attention to the gastrointestinal tract. If yeast infections or parasites are present, treating for these problems is often helpful. Many allergic people have weak digestion and are low in hydrochloric acid and digestive enzyme production, and supplementing these is often beneficial.

I believe that changing the diet itself can aid in preventing and treating all kinds of allergies, espe-

> **Allergy Diet**
>
> - Eat whole, unadulterated foods.
> - Diversify the diet.
> - Rotate foods.
> - Rotate food families.
> - Eat only nonallergenic foods at first.
> - Of course, drink good-quality water regularly.

cially those to foods. Often, just eliminating "reactive" foods from the diet can reduce symptoms of other allergies, especially hay fever–type reactions. The most common diet for allergies is the standard 4-day rotation plan (one of the basics of the ideal diet discussed in chapter 13), emphasizing fresh, wholesome, unprocessed foods. For the sensitive person, or for those with difficult digestion, prepare foods in easily digestible forms, such as soups or fresh juices. It takes 4 days for the body to clear the food we have eaten. By rotating this way, we prevent the chronic buildup of antibodies and reduce possible allergic reactions. After antibody levels decrease and these "reactive" foods again become tolerated, they should not be consumed regularly because they may generate reactions as before. Other foods should also be rotated to prevent becoming sensitive to them as well.

The high-water-content nutritious foods in the Ideal Diet (see chapter 13) will support the body's detoxification and healing processes. Eliminating reactive foods reduces cravings and allows satiety to be reached sooner; smaller amounts of better-quality foods are usually easier to digest. This diet usually produces steady weight loss in people who are overweight; normal-weight or underweight people will usually have less or no weight loss on the ideal diet, but they may need to increase food intake for maintenance.

Fasting and detoxification programs are often beneficial for allergic conditions. A body that is less congested is less allergic. In working with hundreds of allergic patients throughout the years, I have found short fasts to be helpful for a vast majority of people. With allergies, the focus of the cleansing fast is the liver and the colon. Lemon water or the lemonade fast (see "Fasting and Juice Cleansing" on page 769 in chapter 18, Detoxification and Cleansing Programs) helps the liver, while general juice fasting with a cleansing of the colon through enemas or colonic irrigations can make an incredible difference.

For seasonal allergies that are fairly predictable, it is often helpful to do a fast 1 or 2 weeks before the usual onset of symptoms. This is most commonly in the spring, which is naturally the season for cleansing. The beginning of the spring is the best time to clear out bad habits and past addictions and to create a new diet and lifestyle plan. Of course, after the fast, it is important to introduce foods slowly and to be aware of any reactions.

Supplements for Allergies

There are many nutrients and supplements that may be helpful in reducing allergic symptoms. I have often seen improvement with a simple program of a multiple vitamin-mineral supplement with an extra 3 to 4 grams of vitamin C (in higher amounts, C appears to have some antihistamine effects), quercetin, and 500 mg of pantothenic acid (B5). The vitamins C and B5 help to ameliorate the impacts of stress by supporting the weakened adrenals; the adrenal corticosteroids released can then minimize the allergic-inflammatory response. Vitamin C can also be used for any withdrawal symptoms or for reactions secondary to food intake, and higher levels have an antihistaminic effect. The quercetin reduces histamine allergy reactions. Along with vitamin C, its supportive bioflavonoids could be added. Many have anti-inflammatory and antiallergy effects. Quercetin has been shown in research to reduce histamine levels and allergy symptoms. My personal experience and that of my patients is favorable. An amount of 250 to 300 mg several times daily is needed for the effect. There are many quercetin products available.

Other B vitamins are also helpful. Folic acid, B6, and B12 all support antibody formation. The pyridoxal-5-phosphate form of vitamin B6 may be particularly helpful in the allergic patient. It has an apparent anti-inflammatory effect, and as the active metabolite of pyridoxine, it works more directly. It is possible that allergy patients do not phosphorylate pyridoxine very easily (in other words, their metabolism has difficulty adding phosphorus to vitamin B6 so that it can function more actively). Repeated small doses of niacin

(10–50 mg) will cause release of histamine and may contribute to increased allergy symptoms initially. Regular niacin flushes, however, will within days reduce stores of histamine, which may then help lessen allergic symptoms; then continued niacin use will maintain those lower levels of histamine and allergy symptoms.

Vitamin A, about 20,000 IU a day (for 1 to 2 weeks only because this level of vitamin A can have some toxicity over time), and zinc, 50 to 100 mg, are both helpful in alleviating allergy symptoms and in preventing infections. They also help to heal the gastrointestinal mucosa, along with vitamin C, and they improve or normalize the antibody response to antigens, which is often "out of whack" in people with allergies. Other minerals besides zinc, particularly manganese, may also be useful. Magnesium, selenium, and chromium are also frequently beneficial.

The fat-soluble nutrients are also needed. Vitamin E, about 800 IU a day, is a helpful protectant of membranes. Gamma-linolenic acid (GLA) from evening primrose oil, borage, or black currant seeds is found to be an effective nutrient in the reduction of allergic symptoms. This is probably due to the anti-inflammatory effects of the series 1 and 3 prostaglandins that are formed from GLA. Taking 6 to 8 capsules daily (200–400 mg total GLA), divided into several portions, is usually effective. Other anti-inflammatory nutrients include the omega-3 oils EPA and DHA, vitamins A, B5, B6, and C, bioflavonoids, zinc, and the enzyme bromelain. The antioxidants—including beta-carotene, vitamin E, selenium, zinc, vitamin C, and dimethylglycine—may also help with inflammation and immune support.

L-amino acids can also be helpful by stabilizing energy levels and supporting immune components and functions. As mentioned earlier, people with allergies often have poor digestion, particularly of proteins; L-amino acids are a simple, quick way to obtain these building blocks. Digestive support is also useful in allergic patients. Better breakdown, assimilation, and metabolism of foods reduce allergic components and irritations in the gastrointestinal tract and have often been seen to reduce symptoms as well. Taking hydrochloric acid tablets with meals, followed by digestive enzymes after eating, is a good beginning plan; of course, for anyone with hyperacidity, ulcer symptoms, or other abdominal pains, this is not recommended. Many formulas are now available that combine both digestive enzymes and hydrochloric acid in 1 tablet. When such formulas are used, usually 2 or 3 tablets (depending on meal size) can be taken with or just after meals (especially after meals that contain high amounts of proteins and fats).

Additional fiber can provide mild colon detoxification. Supplemental psyllium and bran can be added to a good high-fiber diet. Garlic in the diet can also help with detoxification, as can the supplement sodium alginate, which lessens possible heavy metal toxicity. Betonite clay (montmorillonite) is a strong absorbent that binds chemicals, metals, and other impurities in the gut. It also, as do most of the fiber molecules, has the potential to bind such minerals as calcium and zinc. Because fiber and clay can be bulking and binding, and thus constipating in some people, it may be helpful to use a laxative herbal formula along with these colon-cleansing fibers.

A relatively recent formulated physiological sulfur, methylsulfonylmethane (MSM), has been shown to have anti-inflammatory effects on the mucous membranes. Thus it may be helpful for both food allergies (by helping to heal the gut) and for inhalant allergies. It also may be a useful nutrient for those with arthritis. MSM is a naturally occurring sulfur metabolite in human tissues and is present in high amounts in breast milk. A beginning amount is one 500 to 1,000 mg capsule daily, going up to 3 or 4 capsules daily.

Many people also try a glandular supplement approach in treating allergies. Adrenal is often the first choice to support the body's ability to handle stress and allergies. Thymus gland tablets may help strengthen cell-mediated immunity, although this is not well proven. Liver extracts are also used sometimes. Another approach is to conduct a general evaluation of organ strengths and weaknesses and then to use particular glandulars to create the proper balance. If glands or extracts of glands are chosen, they should be free of pesticides, herbicides, and other agricultural chemicals as well as free of viruses (in other words, through a reputable company that is using tested products).

Many herbs are commonly used and can be quite helpful in the treatment of allergies—to strengthen the immune system and lungs, to promote detoxification,

and to reduce inflammation and histamine-mediated allergy symptoms. A good herbal allergy formula consists of nettle leaf, echinacea, wild cherry bark, white willow bark, mullein leaves, cayenne pepper, and garlic. Nettle is a good tonic spring herb and has been shown to relieve congestion and reduce inflammation. Echinacea improves the white blood cell response and has been shown to lower IgE levels. Wild cherry bark has traditionally been used in formulas for the upper respiratory tract to calm irritated tissues. Coltsfoot leaf is also soothing to dry and irritated membranes, while mullein leaf is used for lung strengthening and to reduce inflammation. White willow bark is an anti-inflammatory and pain reliever; cayenne supports circulation and can help clear the lungs; and garlic reduces mucus in the lungs and bronchi and further assists in detoxification.

Some other lung-strengthening herbs include pleurisy root, horehound, and licorice root. Licorice supports the adrenals and soothes the digestive tract. Other soothing herbs include slippery elm bark and marshmallow root. Comfrey root, which contains the tissue-supporting nutrient allantoin, is useful for helping to heal the intestinal lining; this herb is no longer readily available because of some toxicity concerns, however.

Some people have reported experiencing a reduction of local hay fever and pollen-allergy symptoms by the use of small amounts of bee pollen. Eating 1 to 3 grains at first and increasing the number of grains slowly over a period of a few weeks seems to have benefited some pollen allergy sufferers. I do not recommend this, however, because the types of pollens present may vary, and some may cause a temporary worsening of symptoms. Other brave souls desensitize themselves (reduce their reactivity) to poison oak or

---

Herbal Allergy Formula

Nettle leaf	Mullein leaves
Echinacea	Cayenne pepper
Wild cherry bark	Garlic
White willow bark	

Mix equal amounts into "00" size-capsules or a tea. Take 2 capsules 3 times daily.

poison ivy by eating young spring leaves in small amounts, building up to larger amounts over a few weeks. This is not a supported medical treatment and should only be done with care and/or guidance from someone experienced.

The following "Allergy Nutrient Program" presents suggested daily amounts, taken in several portions daily, of the essential nutrients and other supplements for reducing allergic potential and minimizing allergy symptoms.

27. BIRTH CONTROL PILLS

Birth control pills (BCPs, also called OCs, for oral contraceptives) are both the most effective and the most hazardous form of contraception. Preventing pregnancy in this way is most commonly done by taking an oral dose of a combination of the hormones estrogen and progestin (synthetic progesterone) in amounts higher than the body's natural levels. This prevents the pituitary hormones that stimulate ovulation and fertilization of the egg from being released

Allergy Nutrient Program

Nutrient	Amount	Nutrient	Amount
Water	2–3 qt	Sulfur, as methyl-	
Fiber	10–15 g	sulfonylmethane	1,000–3,000 mg
Vitamin A	5,000–20,000 IU*	Silicon	100 mg
Beta-carotene	20,000 IU	Zinc	60 mg
Vitamin D	400 IU	L-amino acids	1,500 mg
Vitamin E	800 IU	L-cysteine	250–500 mg
Vitamin K	300 mcg	Gamma-linolenic acid	6 capsules or 240–480 mg
Thiamin (B1)	50 mg	Lactobacillus	1–2 billion organisms
Riboflavin (B2)	50 mg	Coenzyme Q10	50–150 mg
Niacin (B3)	100 mg	Dimethylglycine	50–100 mg
Niacinamide (B3)	50–100 mg	Hydrochloric acid	10–15 g
Pantothenic acid (B5)	1,500 mg	(betaine, with	
Pyridoxine (B6)	50–100 mg	protein meals)	
Pyridoxal-5-phosphate	50–100 mg	Digestive enzymes	2–3 tablets
Cobalamin (B12)	100 mcg	(after meals)	
Folic acid	800 mcg		
Biotin	1,000 mcg	**Optional**	
PABA	150 mg	Bromelain	100 mg
Vitamin C	4–8 g	(between meals)	
Bioflavonoids	250–750 mg	Adrenal glandular	100 mg
Quercetin	300–1,000 mg	Thymus glandular	100 mg
Calcium	600–1,000 mg	Liver glandular	100 mg
Chromium	200 mcg	Sodium alginate	300–450 mg
Copper	2–3 mg	Herbal formula with	
Iodine	150 mcg	nettle and others	
Iron	18 mg		
Magnesium	300–600 mg		
Manganese	10 mg		
Molybdenum	500 mcg	* Limit vitamin A to 6 weeks, then cut back to 5,000–10,000 IU daily.	
Selenium	200 mcg		

and thus prevents pregnancy. This goal can also be accomplished by using the "mini-pill," a progesterone-only product.

Although taking oral contraceptives regularly is 99% effective in birth control, there are many possible side effects. (Note: Being on birth control pills does not protect against STDs.) Weight gain, emotional swings, circulatory and vascular symptoms, and gastrointestinal upset are not uncommon. Blood clots, liver problems, and cancer (still controversial, this is not fully proven) are also possible, although relatively rare; these side effects were more common in the 1960s with the higher-dose pills. Many women have difficulty with oral contraceptives, but many others seem to tolerate them well. The use of birth control pills is more common in young women and teenagers, which adds another dimension of uncertainty regarding the nutritional effects of these drugs. Oral contraceptives may create certain nutrient deficiencies and excesses as well as increase the user's nutritional needs. Most of the B vitamins, particularly pyridoxine (B6) and folic acid, are needed in higher amounts when birth control pills are taken. The copper level usually rises, and zinc levels often fall. Thus more zinc is needed as well. An increased need for vitamins C, E, and K may also result from the use of birth control pills.

In *Nutrition and Vitamin Therapy*, Michael Lesser, MD, has pointed out that birth control pills cause an alkaline imbalance in the vagina that may lead to increased susceptibility to infection. Extra ascorbic acid, 1 to 2 grams per day, may help balance the pH and prevent this problem. He and other authors suggest that the increased blood levels of copper generated by oral contraceptive use may contribute to depression and emotional symptoms; additional manganese and zinc may reverse these symptoms. Others believe that the depression from BCPs is also a neurochemical reaction to artificial steroids (female hormones) and from a lack of a women's own superior hormones—estradiol and natural progesterone secreted with ovulation. Most of the unpleasant emotional side effects from OCs come from the synthetic progestin. Many of the women who experience these are able to tolerate the natural or bioidentical progesterone quite well. Iron levels may also rise, and less iron may be required because the pills often reduce the amount of menstrual blood loss as well.

Because BCPs are metabolized by the liver before being eliminated, a diet low in other liver irritants is suggested. Alcohol, cocaine, other drugs, pesticides, and preservative chemicals in food, as well as fried foods should be avoided. Cutting down on refined foods and sugary treats is also suggested; these foods are empty calories and may cause further nutrient depletion. Avoiding nicotine and fried foods is also a good idea to prevent further vascular irritation. Teenage girls on the Pill must also be particularly careful to avoid nutritional deficiencies, and all would be well advised to take a supportive nutritional supplement. Adequate intake of the antioxidant nutrients—such as vitamins C and E, selenium, and beta-carotene—can help reduce the potential toxicity of oral contraceptives. The herb milk thistle contains silymarin and may be especially helpful.

A high-nutrient diet is the best prevention for problems. Low-fat proteins and other nutritious foods (such as whole grains, vegetables, nuts, and seeds) are also important. Eating lots of vegetables is the best way to prevent many mineral deficits and also to maintain weight. Several teaspoons of cold-pressed vegetable oil, particularly olive oil, should be used daily to ensure the intake of the essential fatty acids. Eating all of these foods, along with protein intake from such foods as eggs, fish (especially oily fish like salmon and sardines with omega-3 oils), poultry, dairy foods, and legumes, is a sensible approach. In addition to the usual female adult or teenage levels, if taking oral contraceptives, it is recommended that intake of specific nutrients be increased.

Other B vitamins can also be increased to higher levels, such as an additional 25 mg of each, to balance out the B complex. More antioxidants can also help

Nutrient	Daily Amounts (in 1 or 2 doses)
Nutrients Needing Increased Intake with Oral Contraceptive Use	
Vitamin B6	50–100 mg
Vitamin B12	50–200 mcg
Folic acid	600–800 mcg
Vitamin E	400–600 IU
Vitamin C	1–3 g
Zinc	20–40 mg

Nutrient Program for Oral Contraceptives	
Nutrient	**Amount**
Water	1¹/₂–2 qt
Vitamin A	5,000–10,000 IU
Carotenes	10,000–20,000 IU
Vitamin D	200–400 IU
Vitamin E	400–600 IU
Thiamin (B₁)	25–50 mg
Riboflavin (B₂)	25–50 mg
Niacin or	
niacinamide (B₃)	25–50 mg
Pantothenic acid (B₅)	50–250 mg
Pyridoxine (B₆)	25–50 mg
Cobalamin (B₁₂)	50–200 mcg
Folic acid	600–800 mcg
Biotin	200–400 mcg
PABA	5–50 mg
Vitamin C	1–3 g
Bioflavonoids	250–500 mg
Calcium*	600–1,000 mg
Chromium	200–400 mcg
Copper	1–2 mg
Iron	15–20 mg
Magnesium*	400–600 mg
Manganese	5–10 mg
Molybdenum	150–300 mcg
Phosphorus	600–800 mg
Potassium	1–2 g
Selenium	150–300 mcg
Zinc	30–60 mg
Fatty acids, olive	
or flaxseed oils	1–2 tsp

* Calcium and magnesium are best supplemented as citrates or aspartates, amino acid chelates.

reduce the deleterious effects of the drugs. These include beta-carotene and mixed carotenoids, selenium, and possibly the amino acid L-cysteine to complement the additional vitamins C and E.

Copper intake in supplements should be limited to 1 mg, although the increased zinc intake will help lower copper levels. Whole grains, nuts, seeds, and vegetables will ensure that copper requirements are met. Iron supplements may be decreased somewhat with use of birth control pills unless the menstrual periods are heavy or there is anemia. Iron needs are probably reduced from the usual 18 mg to around 12 to 15 mg per day. All of these values can be checked occasionally by blood biochemistry profiles or evaluation of mineral levels to ensure proper individualized care.

28. PREMENSTRUAL SYNDROME

Premenstrual syndrome (PMS) is a recently described problem, since the 1980s. Although the history of symptoms that occur around the menstrual cycle is ancient, it is likely that modern-day women—with increased demands and stresses, changes in nutrition, and careers that take them away from their natural cycle and their connection to home, garden, and Nature—are particularly susceptible to such symptoms. Women might think about these symptoms as a "call of the womb and the moon" to be more attuned to their female cycle. It may not be easy, but it is possible for women to stay connected to their female cycles and still be active and productive in the outer world. This may require more care regarding nutrition and a supplement program that counteracts stress while supporting the female organs and hormone functions. Stress (and being out of touch with one's emotions or not following one's true emotions) is definitely a big factor in women's premenstrual symptoms.

The current medical theories about PMS, or as it is sometimes termed, *premenstrual tension (PMT)*, relate it to an estrogen-progesterone imbalance, particularly reactions to the increased estradiol levels. During the second half of the cycle, after ovulation, progesterone levels normally rise, while estrogen levels also rise slightly. These changes can influence water retention, causing some fullness of the uterus and other body tissues; this seems to be exaggerated premenstrually with the relatively deficient level of progesterone. Many of the symptoms—such as bloating, breast swelling and tenderness, fatigue, headaches, emotional irritability, depression, back pain, and pelvic pain—are probably a result of the water retention and subsequent emotional tension.

Other hormonal and physiological factors, or effects on the immune system, may contribute to the problem as well. Less common symptoms include dizziness, fainting, cystitis, hives, acne, sore throat, joint pains and swelling, and constipation.

Low progesterone levels seem to be the main factor in PMS symptoms. Why progesterone levels may be low has not yet been determined, but many women seem to respond to treatment with progesterone in the second half of their cycle, from just after ovulation to the usual time of menstruation. A common treatment is to use vaginal or rectal suppositories containing natural progesterone (or even topical progesterone) once or twice daily. The newer treatment is oral, micronized progesterone that is not destroyed by the gastrointestinal tract (because of the small particle size). It is still metabolized by the liver. Usually, however, progesterone therapy is not needed, because most women will respond to a nutritional and herbal approach to treating PMS. Many nutrients are needed, but probably the two most important ones are vitamin B6 (pyridoxine) and magnesium. B6 helps to clear water through a diuretic effect on the kidneys. Usually 50 to 100 mg once or twice daily will be effective. A complete B vitamin supplement is also necessary to prevent these higher amounts of B6 from causing imbalances of other B vitamins. It has been theorized and shown in some studies that magnesium deficiency within the cells is also correlated with some of the PMS symptoms. Supplementing magnesium at amounts equal to up to 1.5 times the calcium level (that is, about 800–1,200 mg) is helpful in reducing some PMS symptoms. Zinc is also an important mineral here. Some studies have shown a benefit (by decreasing symptoms) from raising serotonin levels, while others have looked at the improvement from higher calcium and magnesium intake.

Other possible menstrual irregularities have symptoms that may be related to low estrogen levels. Women with this problem often experience more of their symptoms after their period than before it. This low-estrogen state is far less common than the progesterone deficiency. Tests to measure hormonal levels can be done at specific times of the month. These are expensive, however, and not always easy to interpret (the range of normal is wide) unless done repeatedly. **Newer salivary hormone testing may be more representative of tissue hormone activity.** These can be ordered from your health practitioner. Generally, though, as long as there are relatively regular menstrual periods, these ovarian and pituitary blood hormone levels will typically be within normal values. Other blood tests that may be abnormal include thyroid hormone levels, thyroid antibodies, or antiovarian antibodies, which may represent some autoimmune problems.

Another common symptom, not only of PMS but of most women's premenstrual time, is a craving for sweets. This desire is often enhanced in those with PMS, which brings up another important point. Women with PMS often have other correlating conditions that may contribute to symptoms. These include hypoglycemia (low blood sugar), candidiasis (an overgrowth of and hypersensitivity to the common yeast *Candida albicans*), food and/or environmental allergies, moderate to severe stress, and vitamin and mineral deficiencies. Whether these problems contribute to or are a result of the premenstrual and hormonal problems is not clear, but it is important to evaluate women for these conditions when they either have significant PMS symptoms or do not respond well to treatment. PMS is definitely aggravated by low blood sugar generated by stress and an intake of refined-flour and sugar products.

From a dietary point of view, it is important to avoid the food stressors, irritants, and stimulants that, if they do not contribute to the PMS problem in the first place, definitely make it worse. These include sugars and refined foods, caffeine, alcohol, and chemicals. A diet that helps in reducing symptoms is balanced, wholesome, and high in nutrients, with lots of whole grains, leafy greens and other vegetables, good protein foods, and some fruits, but a minimum of fruit juice. A hypoglycemic diet of regular meals and protein-oriented snacks is often helpful. If there are yeast or allergy problems, a diet to help with those conditions (see "Yeast Syndrome" and "Allergies" on pages 698 and 704, respectively) would be beneficial. If these problems are not present, extra brewer's yeast, with its high levels of B vitamins and minerals, can be a supportive food. Eating a variety of foods and a modified rotation diet are also helpful in getting the wide range of important nutrients and maximizing food sensitivities. Some women also experience a reduction of symptoms through colon detoxification and a cleansing-type diet high in juices, soups, and salads. Intake of fiber as psyllium or bran started a week before symptoms usually begin will improve colon elimination, and an enema or colonic irrigation at the time symptoms begin might be helpful.

PMS is more common in women in their 30s and 40s than in those in their 20s and younger. Former faculty member at Stanford University Medical School and author Susan Lark, MD, has pointed out in her *PMS Self Help Book* a number of other factors associated with an increased likelihood of PMS problems; these include women who are or have been married, do not exercise, have had children, experience side effects from birth control pills, have had a pregnancy complicated by toxemia, experience repeated medical problems requiring antibiotic and other drug therapies, have a significant amount of emotional stress in their lives, or those whose nutritional habits lead to certain deficiencies or excesses. Dietary factors that worsen PMS include foods high in refined sugars and fats, processed or chemical foods, caffeine drinks (coffee, tea, colas), alcohol (especially wine and beer with their higher carbohydrate levels), chocolate products, eggs, cheese, red meats, and high-salt foods. In Chinese medicine assessment, eating a high amount of sugar in the diet is associated with more menstrual irregularities and PMS symptoms.

British physician Katherine Dalton, MD, was among the first to describe PMS in the early 1980s and offer some therapeutic help. Guy Abraham, an obstetrician-gynecologist, has further classified PMS problems, a system that Lark also discusses in her book.

Lark's *The PMS Self Help Book* provides specific treatment plans for the different types of symptoms. The recommendations for the different types, including diet and suggestions, are all similar. In Lark's programs, all include some form of stress reduction, exercise, supplementation, herbal therapy, acupressure massage, and yoga postures. For acne problems with PMS, extra vitamin A (20,000–40,000 IU, mainly as beta-carotene) and zinc (20–40 mg) are usually helpful. Choline and inositol, nutrients found in lecithin, may help nourish the skin; 500 mg of each daily are recommended.

Dysmenorrhea and other pain problems respond well to higher amounts of magnesium, about 500 mg more than calcium, as this has a nerve-tranquilizing

---

Five Types of Premenstral Syndrome

1. **Type A (anxiety).** A mixture of emotional symptoms: anxiety, irritability, and mood swings.
2. **Type C (carbohydrates and cravings).** Sugar cravings (chocolate), fatigue, and headaches.
3. **Type H (hyperhydration), also known as Type W (water retention).** Bloating, weight gain, and breast swelling and tenderness.
4. **Type D (depression).** Depression, confusion, and memory loss.
5. **Other groups of symptoms.** These include acne as well as oily skin and hair, and dysmenorrhea (painful periods), which can include cramps, low back pain, nausea, and vomiting. This was recently classified as **Type P**, for pain.

---

and muscle-relaxing effect. Vitamin E (400–800 IU) and vitamin B6 (100–300 mg daily) may also be helpful in reducing pain and reducing fluid retention. Extra B vitamins and a general vitamin and mineral program are usually also necessary.

Anxiety symptoms, such as mood swings and irritability, often respond to extra B vitamins, particularly thiamin (B1), 150 to 250 mg per day, and pyridoxine (B6), 200 to 300 mg per day, with about 50 mg each of the rest of the B vitamins. Using inositol and extra magnesium, such as magnesium glycinate (which causes fewer bowel symptoms, especially diarrhea, than other magnesium salts), about 400 to 600 mg daily, will help. Progesterone therapy may be most helpful for type A (anxiety) problems. A doctor could be consulted for this therapy, although these natural progesterone creams are now readily available over the counter. The late John Lee, MD, brought to light the need for women to increase progesterone levels for PMS and perimenopause in his book *What Your Doctor May Not Tell You about Menopause*. In this regard, he did a great service for women's health care. Also, phenylethanolamine (PEA), a substance found in certain foods (such as bananas, chocolate, and hard cheeses) may increase symptoms of anxiety. These foods should be avoided in this type of PMS.

For depression, added tryptophan (500–1,000 mg) before bed may be helpful. Use 5-HTP, 50 to 150 mg at bed and 50 to 100 in the day, as it may also work to lessen depression. Zinc, vitamin B6, and calcium/magnesium may be beneficial in reducing premenstrual depression. L-tyrosine, an energizing amino acid, may help restore a better mood with a dosage of 500 to 1,000 mg twice daily in the morning and early afternoon. For women with the type C (sugar cravings) pattern—often associated with stress, fatigue, headaches, confusion, or dizziness—a program that should help reduce these symptoms supplements the basic vitamin and mineral plan with additional B vitamins, particularly B6 (100–200 mg per day) and B1 (100–200 mg per day); chromium (200–400 mcg); vitamin E (800 IU); and vitamin C (around 6–8 grams per day). Eating frequent, small meals and avoiding sugar will also be helpful in reducing cravings.

For type H with water or bloating problems, which can be the most troublesome, causing weight gain, breast tenderness, and general emotional upset, the basic B vitamins (including high amounts of B6 and supplemental B1), magnesium, potassium, vitamin E, and evening primrose oil (with GLA as the active ingredient), 1 to 2 capsules taken 3 times daily, may be helpful. Also, with water retention problems, food allergy (particularly to wheat) may be a contributing factor. A trial of a month or so of avoiding wheat products can aid in providing relief of symptoms. Sometimes the response can be dramatic. Regular exercise is also important in reducing this type of PMS.

Many herbs are helpful in treating PMS. Angelica, or dong quai, is a commonly used herb that acts as an energizer and female tonic when it is taken regularly as capsules (2 capsules twice a day) or as a tea. Ginger root acts as a circulation aid and mild stimulant and is helpful in getting some of that retained water moving. Other diuretic herbs include parsley and juniper berry. Licorice root is a good balancer and seems to provide an "up" feeling when drunk with some ginger as a tea. Their flavors tend to combine well. Valerian root or catnip tea will provide some relaxation when there is general anxiety or irritability. Sarsaparilla is a tonifying (strengthening) herb that supports the hormonal functions and may actually contain some hormones itself. There are also many herbal formulas for treating PMS and for strengthening the female functions. One that I have found helpful to my patients contains black haw, licorice, false unicorn root (an estrogen-containing plant), ginseng root, ginger, and life root. I recommend 2 capsules 2 or 3 times daily, usually for 3 to 6 months if it appears helpful.

Perhaps the most helpful herb is vitex, which seems to support progesterone effects without raising hormone levels. It may also have the benefit of decreasing prolactin levels, which helps to lessen breast swelling and tenderness for some women. In the first 1 or 2 months, herbs tend to work more slowly and must be taken over a longer period of time than

Premenstrual Tension (PMT)		
TYPE	MAIN SYMPTOMS	KEY TREATMENT PLANS
Type-A	Anxiety	Magnesium 400–600 mg per day. Progesterone therapy. Low PEA (phenylethanolamine) diet—avoid chocolate, bananas, and hard cheeses.
Type-D	Depression	Zinc 30–60 mg per day. Vitamin B6 100–300 mg per day. Magnesium 400–600 mg per day. Tryptophan 1,000–1,500 mg before bed or 500 mg 2 or 3 times daily.
Type-H or W	Water retention	Avoid food allergens, particularly wheat. Potassium 1–2 grams per day, plus potassium foods. B complex vitamins with extra B6, 50–200 mg per day. Regular exercise.
Type-P	Pain	Vitamin E 400–800 IU per day. Magnesium 400–600 mg per day. Vitamin B6 100–300 mg per day.
Type-C	Cravings	Low-sugar diet. Frequent small meals. Chromium 200–400 mcg per day.

stronger pharmaceuticals. There are many similar formulas available now for PMS and other female problems. Some doctors also use glandular supplements in treating PMS. In *Super Fitness Beyond Vitamins,* Michael Rosenbaum, MD, has described his success with the use of pituitary, particularly anterior pituitary, extract in treating stubborn PMS symptoms. Brain and pancreas glandular supplements may also be helpful, Rosenbaum points out. Simplex-F by Standard Process (see Appendix B, "Nutritional Supplement Companies") is a good combination formula.

There are also many nutritional supplement formulas available for PMS. The "Premenstrual Syndrome Nutrient Program" below presents an all-encompassing nutrient program; most of these nutrients are best taken in 2 or 3 portions over the course of the day. This may be tailored for specific symptoms by application of the suggestions given earlier in this sec-

tion. Of course, many of the nutrients listed are consumed in the diet. Supplementation of sodium, potassium, chloride, fluoride, iodine, and phosphorus is usually not necessary, although additional potassium, about 1 to 2 grams, may be helpful in some cases. Even extra vitamins D and K may not be needed. The precursor of B6 (pyridoxine), pyridoxal-5-phosphate, may actually be more effective than B6 itself, because some people may not be able to easily convert the pyridoxine to its usable form. Both forms of vitamin B3 are used; niacin offers some circulatory stimulation and flushing while niacinamide supports the general neuromuscular relaxation of B3.

I have seen a high rate of success in the improvement and elimination of symptoms in women who change their diets and implement a regular supplement program. I have also heard other gynecologists, family doctors, and nurse practitioners claim that they

Premenstrual Syndrome Nutrient Program**

Nutrient	Amount	Nutrient	Amount
Vitamin A	5,000–10,000 IU	Iodine*	150–300 mcg
Beta-carotene	10,000–20,000 IU	Iron	15–20 mg
Vitamin D	200–600 IU	Magnesium	750–1,500 mg
Vitamin E	400–1,000 IU	Manganese	2.5–15.0 mg
Vitamin K*	150–300 mcg	Molybdenum	150–500 mcg
Thiamin (B1)	50–250 mg	Phosphorus*	800–1,000 mg
Riboflavin (B2)	50–100 mg	Potassium*	2.5–5.0 g
Niacin (B3)	25–100 mg	Selenium	150–300 mcg
Niacinamide (B3)	50–100 mg	Zinc	15–30 mg
Pantothenic acid (B5)	50–500 mg	GLA (gamma-linolenic acid)	3–6 capsules
Pyridoxine (B6)	50–200 mg	EPA and DHA	1–2 capsules
Pyridoxal-5-phosphate	50–150 mg	L-amino acid formula	1,000 mg
Cobalamin (B12)	50–200 mcg	L-tryptophan+	500–1,000 mg
Folic acid	400–800 mcg	(before bed) or 5-HTP	50–100 mg
Biotin	50–400 mcg	L-phenylalanine	500–1,000 mg
Choline	500–1,000 mg	(in 2 doses during the day)	
Inositol	500–1,000 mg		
PABA	50–100 mg		
Vitamin C	1–3 g		
Bioflavonoids	250–500 mg	*These nutrients will not usually be supplemented.	
Calcium	800–1,000 mg	+ Currently L-tryptophan is available through doctors and compounding pharmacists.	
Chromium	200–400 mcg	** Digestive enzymes, herbs, and glandulars may also be helpful in reducing PMS problems.	
Copper	1–2 mg		

see nearly an 80% success rate with a good program. Of course, learning to deal better with life stresses, relationships, and sexual issues further increases the likelihood of success. Acupuncture can often be helpful for many women's problems, including PMS. Of course, managing stress, diet, and exercise provides the basis for good health, along with proper sleep.

In 1994, the *Diagnostic and Statistical Manual IV* (DMS-IV) sanctioned the diagnostic term premenstrual dysphoric disorder (PMDD). Although this term has been more and more widely used in the world of mental health, not only for classification of problems but also for insurance reimbursement and drug approval (Prozac, for example, is approved for use with PMDD), it is only beginning to catch on in the broader health-care world. PMDD is closest to the PMS-D variant, but long-term acceptance of PMDD as a category of mental health diagnosis is unclear at this point in time.

29. PRE- AND POST-SURGERY (AND INJURIES)

This pre- and post-surgery program, although it is simple, can really make a difference—a few changes and supplements can lessen stress, improve healing, and prevent infections after surgery. I have done my own independent research through the years, suggesting a program similar to this for my patients who have had elective surgery, and they have routinely told me that "the doctors and nurses couldn't believe how fast I healed and was up and about." Invariably there were no, or minimal, complications. In addition, many medical studies reviewing postsurgical healing time and morbidity, particularly from infections, have shown that with a few basic nutritional supplements—namely, vitamin A, vitamin C, and zinc—healing time speeds up. There are also fewer difficulties, and people are out of bed and out of the hospital sooner.

Many doctors, particularly surgeons, resist these findings, however. I do not know whether this is due to economics or because they just do not want to believe that taking nutrients in higher dosages than normal is necessary. Having patients follow a few basic nutritional suggestions would improve both doc-

tor and patient success, I believe. A good nourishing diet and additional vitamin C, vitamin A, and zinc with adequate fluid intake will usually do it. More recently, I have had patients scheduled for elective surgery tell me that their surgeons suggested they take additional supplements starting 2 weeks before their operations, and there appears to be some progress regarding nutrition in the general medical profession.

Anyone having elective surgery should follow this program for 3 to 4 weeks before and 4 to 6 weeks after surgery. With emergency or urgent surgery, it is wise to begin taking the extra supplements as soon as possible and to eat the most nutritious diet available. This program will also work to support tissue healing following an injury, burn, or other trauma or with an infection or sickness that causes tissue damage, and is designed to increase the reuniting of collagen fibers, facilitate protein metabolism, and strengthen the immune system.

General measures important to healing include proper rest and sleep, fluid intake, and, of course, a nutritious and balanced diet high in fiber and low in fats (but adequate in healthy oils) and junk foods. High-quality protein foods (fish, poultry, eggs, nuts, and seeds) are essential because tissue healing requires protein synthesis, so the body needs all of the important amino acids. A healthy intestinal flora is also important to health and healing. Additional *Lactobacillus acidophilus* culture may help replenish the colon. The diet should contain adequate amounts of high-fiber foods (whole grains, vegetables, and legumes), calcium foods (greens, grains, nuts, and small amounts of dairy products), and foods containing essential fatty acids (some nuts, seeds, or vegetable oils). Congestive foods (excess dairy products, sweets, and baked goods) and fatty foods (fried foods, heavy meats, and ham and other cured meats) should be avoided. Fresh vegetable juices in particular help to hydrate and nourish the tissues before and after surgery.

Minimizing and handling stress is also essential to keeping the immune system strong, which is in turn important for preventing infections and supporting healing. It is wise to stay away from steroid drugs, both topical and systemic, as they suppress the immune system. Doctors tend to overprescribe (and patients to overuse) these steroid medicines. Smoking should be stopped or minimized if possible before surgery. Avoiding stimulating drugs (such as coffee and cocaine) and sedating drugs (such as alcohol and marijuana) before elective surgery is also a wise idea. I usually do not recommend that people fast or make any major diet revisions before surgery; rather, they should maintain a nutritious diet with some shifts toward healthier practices. If possible, people should be close to, or just above, their ideal weight for surgery. Obesity increases surgical risks (infection, poor healing), while underweight people often do not have sufficient energy reserves to heal rapidly.

Of course, I recommend a healthy diet all of the time, but it is a good idea to begin increasing protein intake and adding the healing nutrients a few weeks before surgery to build up both the strength and the tissues. Usually, the diet can be a little lighter a few days before surgery, emphasizing more fruits, vegetables, and liquids along with the nutritional supplements. This will help lessen digestive organ stress.

Recovery from surgery takes time. The diet should be a little lighter initially, and low in fats and heavy foods. With any abdominal surgery, often a liquid or soft diet is necessary for a while. This is where protein and/or nutrient powders are useful. There are also more healthful suggestions than the bouillon, Jell-O, coffee, and colas that might be served. Some examples are vegetable and meat broths, fresh juices, light soups, and pureed carrots, squash, potatoes, bananas, apples, or other fruits and vegetables, progressing to oatmeal, cream of rice cereal, and richer soups. After surgery, it is sensible to eat foods as tolerated and as suggested by a nutritionally aware practitioner, gradually resuming the nourishing, pre-surgery diet. Then after 2 or 3 months, when most tissue healing is complete and the body is stronger, a mild cleansing and detoxification may be initiated, especially if general anesthesia was used during the surgery or other potentially toxic drugs were used afterward.

This fine art of administering potentially lethal drugs to reduce pain, induce unconsciousness, and yet maintain life has progressed significantly in the past century. Many procedures are possible now that were only fantasies generations ago. Yet many people realize that the anesthesia is often more difficult to recover from postsurgically than the actual cutting of tissues. Thus I suggest using the least amount of drugs and the simplest anesthetic procedure possible. Clearly the toxicity of anesthesia can be worse with suboptimal nutrition. Local anesthesia is a big advance in medicine of recent years. Before general anesthesia, it is wise for people to nourish themselves well with a high-nutrient diet containing good-quality protein foods and by taking supportive supplements to strengthen tissues and create nutrient reserves. The antioxidant nutrients (vitamins C and A, selenium, zinc, and L-cysteine) are suggested. Vitamin E can be taken but in lower doses (100–200 IU) so that it does not affect blood clotting or tissue healing.

Most books on medical dietetics include many specific diets for various types of surgery. The program suggested here is more general and, I assure you, more healthful. The current hospital diet might make more economic sense, but it is not in the best interest of the patients. Rather, our hospitals need to provide more nutrient-rich, healing diets, with more wholesome (and vital) foods and liquids to help revitalize and nourish (and heal) the patients so that they can return to their normal lives as quickly as possible. Hospitals should also provide a hypoallergenic (low in wheat, yeast, corn, eggs, and milk) and low-chemical (no additives, binders, or artificial colors) diet.

If, as many doctors and dieticians believe, we do not need supplements if we eat a balanced diet, they should then clearly provide a chemical-free, hypoallergenic, and wholesome diet. However, the minimum dietary needs to prevent nutrient deficiencies do not apply to hospitalized and surgical patients; these people need more of most nutrients because of the stress and possible inadequate digestion and assimilation. In addition, the Dietary Reference Intakes (DRIs) do not include many important nutrients, such as boron and vanadium. Hospital diets should also be providing supplemental electrolyte powders to provide additional magnesium, and protein powders to support patients' healing and to prevent muscle wasting. I suggest that people take their own nutritional supplements to the hospital; bring (or have family and friends bring them) good food, drinking water, and fresh juices; and encourage hospitals to provide more natural foods prepared with little or no saturated fats, salts, and chemicals or preservatives.

Another reminder for improved healing from surgery is to become active and involved in the healing process as soon as possible. Most surgeons and nurses are supportive of this practice and will provide encouragement. Often called "think and feel healing," this requires the patient know, believe, and see (through internal visual imagery) that complete recovery is taking place.

Several specific nutrients are particularly important in the pre- and post-surgery program. Vitamin A in the retinol form helps in tissue healing and immune support. The beta-carotene form, provitamin A, adds further vitamin A and has an antioxidant effect. Vitamin C also improves collagen tissue healing and is needed in regular and frequent amounts to replenish the increased amounts of vitamin C used during the stress of surgery and sickness. The bioflavonoids support the beneficial vitamin C effects and aid in tissue healing as well. Zinc is important to tissue healing and immune support through its function in a variety of enzymes. Magnesium also activates many enzymes useful in healing.

The B vitamins are needed, particularly extra riboflavin (B2), which seems to help tissue repair, and pantothenic acid (B5) to deal with the extra stress of surgery. Adequate vitamin K in the diet supports normal blood clotting, which is so important during surgery. Various other vitamins (B1, B3, B6, and B12) and other minerals (selenium, copper, iron, calcium, potassium, manganese, molybdenum, and cobalt) are also important to healing. Of course, with surgical blood loss, more iron may be needed in the recovery stage to build blood cells. Silica is useful to skin and tissues. Bromelain, the pineapple enzyme, has a mild

---

Pre- and Post-surgery Nutrient Program (and for Healing Injuries)

Nutrient	Amount	Nutrient	Amount
Water	2–3 qt	Chromium	200 mcg
Fiber	10–15 g	Copper	2–3 mg**
Protein	70–100 g	Iodine	100–200 mcg
Fat	50–75 g	Iron	20 mg
Vitamin A	10,000–20,000 IU*	Magnesium	500–800 mg
Beta-carotene	15,000 IU	Manganese	10 mg
Vitamin D	400 IU	Molybdenum	800 mcg
Vitamin E	200 IU	Potassium	2–3 g
Vitamin K	300 mcg	Selenium, as selenomethione	200 mcg
Thiamin (B1)	50 mg	Silicon	100–200 mg
Riboflavin (B2)	25–100 mg	Sulfur	400–800 mg
Niacin (B3)	25 mg	Vanadium	150–300 mcg
Niacinamide (B3)	50 mg	Zinc	60–100 mg**
Pantothenic acid (B5)	500–1,000 mg	L-amino acids	1,000 mg
Pyridoxine (B6)	50 mg	L-arginine	500–1,000 mg
Pyridoxal-5-phosphate	25 mg	L-lysine	500–1,000 mg
Cobalamin (B12)	200 mcg	Lactobacillus	2 billion organisms
Folic acid	800 mcg	Bromelain	200–400 mg
Biotin	300 mcg		
Inositol	1,000 mg		
Vitamin C	4–6 g		
Bioflavonoids	500 mg		
Boron	2–3 mg		
Calcium	800–1,200 mg		

* 10,000–20,000 IU vitamin A should only be used for 4 to 6 weeks, beginning 1 or 2 weeks before surgery and continuing 2 to 3 weeks after. At other times, the amount should be limited to about 5,000 IU daily.

**The amount should be higher if more zinc is taken—about a 20:1 ratio of zinc to copper.

anti-inflammatory effect and may be useful after surgery to aid in food digestion as well as to reduce micro blood clots (thrombi). Moderate levels of supplemental L-amino acids can be helpful, and some recent research suggests that additional amounts of L-arginine and L-lysine in particular aid tissue healing as well. The essential fatty acids (omega-3 and omega-6) are also important to wound healing.

Healthy immune function is essential to healing and preventing infections. The antioxidant nutrients are useful in supporting the immune system, but for this program, a lower than usual amount of vitamin E is suggested, usually about 200 IU and definitely not more than 400 IU. Vitamin E has been shown in some studies to slow wound healing time, in contradiction of the popular belief that oral vitamin E and topical E are good for healing tissues; many vitamin E caps have been popped and the oil applied to the skin to help in healing. It would make sense to use vitamin A oil for this purpose, as it is a nutrient known for its tissue healing properties.

Herbs can also be used to support wound healing. Horsetail is high in silica, a mineral that helps strengthen tissues, especially skin, hair, and nails. Goldenseal root is a tonic herb when taken internally and also has mild anti-infection properties. Used locally, it works as an antiseptic. It has been used effectively in helping heal wounds internally and externally, in strengthening mucous membranes, and in ulcer treatment. Comfrey leaf has always been believed to have healing properties when taken internally, although there is not much specific research data to support this observation. It is more often used externally for sprains and bone, muscle, and ligament injuries or internally for broken bones than for healing surgical wounds.

The "Pre- and Post-surgery Nutrient Program" on the opposite page lists the basic nutrients to be taken. Usually, following this program for 2 to 3 weeks before surgery and 4 to 6 weeks after is sufficient. This program may also be used when recovering from wounds, injuries, burns, or infections. It reduces healing time, reduces morbidity secondary to surgery, and lessens the duration of hospital stays.

30. MENTAL HEALTH: DEPRESSION, ANXIETY, AND ATTENTION-DEFICIT/HYPERACTIVITY DISORDER (ADHD)

What is mental health and how can we achieve it? Is it taking a pill, talking to a counselor, daring to change your life in areas you want to improve? How do we get ourselves motivated? Depression and anxiety are commonplace these days, with all the stresses and demands, changes, and challenges of modern life. Mental illnesses include a variety of complex problems (biochemical, emotional, and perceptual) that may generate varying mental and emotional symptoms as well as aberrations in behavior. Because most psychological difficulties are multifaceted, the best approach for understanding and treating them involves an integrated, multidimensional program.

Mood disorders are quite common, as are problems with energy. I differentiate those from mental problems in their scope and persistence. Everyday events, foods, and internal hormonal changes affect our mood—how we feel, as in up or down, or in between. I see often that people and patients are influenced by their diet, and when they improve it, for example when they get off their habits/addictions to substances like sugar, coffee, and alcohol, their moods and energy levels balance out. This can even occur when they take breaks from such foods as wheat and flour products, dairy, soy, or corn syrup. The body is more sensitive (and more durable) than most of us give it credit for, and we can do a great deal to improve our mood and energy level with our lifestyle habits.

In this program for mental health, however, I am talking about more serious and persistent mental issues, specifically depression and anxiety. For mental disorders, standard medical care currently offers psychological counseling and, most commonly, psychoactive pharmaceutical drug therapy as treatment. More innovative therapists may use hypnotherapy, biofeedback, or body therapies (such as massage); they may also realize the importance of orthomolecular nutrient therapy (*orthomolecular* here means the "right molecules in the right amounts," a term coined in 1968 by Nobel prize–winning chemist Linus Pauling), as well as the benefits of a clean, wholesome diet

727

with the elimination of possible food allergens. Many people benefit from a nutritional approach to their psychological problems, especially when some nutritional or allergic causes can be uncovered.

Mental illness encompasses a variety of problems, from mild to severe, and involves many different factors. Milder mental issues can vary from mood swings and premenstrual symptoms to anxiety and phobias; more serious mental illnesses may include paranoia, hyperactivity, obsessive behavior, compulsion, depression, and psychosis. Some of these problems lead to learning disabilities in young people or memory deficits in adults. Many of the milder forms of mental illness tend to be caused by factors other than deep psychological dysfunctions. Brain sensitivity or allergy to various chemicals or foods may play a role. Hyperactive kids, for example, commonly have poor diets and food sensitivities. Blood sugar abnormalities also may create symptoms of anxiety, irritability, confusion, mood swings, depression, and feelings of paranoia; gastrointestinal infestation with the yeast *Candida albicans* may also produce some of these symptoms.

Although people with milder forms of mental illness can usually continue to play an active part in family and community, major mental illnesses seriously affect the ability to function in the world or to relate to others. Mood swings, anxiety, paranoia, depression, and psychosis can become severe, incapacitating problems. Learning disabilities and behavior problems in children may be so extreme as to require separating a child from school and even from family. One major form of mental illness, schizophrenia, is a mysterious and serious psychological problem that has many characteristics; the causes of schizophrenia are not clear, although a genetic link is likely involved. Although nutrition can play a helpful role in the mental health of people with schizophrenia, it is not suggested as the primary treatment but in support of medicinal management.

Symptoms of mental illness may include a variety of internal and external expressions and emotions. Anger, fear, sadness, worry, and even grief may be a part of personal experience; extremes of these emotions, however, are a problem and a cause for concern. Loss of affect (a flat mood) or lack of enthusiasm toward life and low self-esteem are common. Self-involvement, reclusiveness, delusions or hallucinations, aggressive behavior, inappropriate outbursts, and even crime or bizarre behavior are not uncommon in more severe mental conditions. Among the many possible causes that contribute to mental illness are genetics and family dynamics as well as diet and nutritional deficiencies, which can cause or at least aggravate psychological problems. Allergies may be provocative regarding behavior and the psychological state, as discussed in earlier under "Allergies" on page 704. Hypoglycemia and/or hyperglycemia due to excessive use of refined carbohydrate products and sugar may also aggravate mental symptoms. Many other problems result from metabolic and hormonal imbalances or sensitivity to environmental agents or chemicals. Low thyroid levels or imbalances of estrogen and progesterone in women can produce many psychological symptoms.

I believe that many mental problems are indeed organic (physical) rather than purely psychological, especially when we consider the evidence from nutritional medicine. I doubt that most mental illnesses are purely hereditary. **Dealing with food allergies, correcting vitamin and mineral deficiencies, making dietary changes to eliminate sugar, caffeine, or alcohol addictions, and stabilizing blood sugar**

Mental and Related Symptoms of Nutrient Deficiency

Thiamin (B1). Thinking problems, irritability, fear, and depression.

Niacin (B3). Fatigue, anxiety, insomnia, depression, and psychosis.

Pantothenic acid (B5). Fatigue, depression, and irritability.

Pyridoxine (B6). Mood swings and depression.

Cobalamin (B12). Irritability, agitation, depression, and psychosis.

Folic acid. This is often low in mental patients; fatigue.

Vitamin C. Fatigue, allergy, and hyperactivity.

Many minerals. Potassium, magnesium, molybdenum, manganese, chromium, zinc, copper, iron, and iodine, leading to fatigue, poor concentration, anxiety, apathy, and disorientation.

L- amino acids. Anxiety and depression.

will get many people off the psychological roller coaster and back toward a more stable life. I have seen enough people with mental symptoms respond well to supportive nutrient therapy—and not just at "megavitamin" levels—to know that a nutritional approach to mental disorders has much to offer the patients and their families. This does not mean that patients may not need some counseling or drug therapy as well, but it is likely that this approach can reduce the need for them as well as prevent hospitalization.

Allergy and addiction problems can be an important factor to uncover for mental health. As discussed under "Allergies" on page 704, some of these problems can be masked until the offending foods are eliminated. Many of the symptoms they cause are psychological, ranging from fatigue, irritability, anxiety, and depression to full-blown psychosis and hallucinations. Isolating the problem foods and clearing them from the diet, along with a good anti-allergy nutrient program (such as vitamins A, E, C, B3, B5, and B6), can help reduce many of these symptoms over time.

The most common offending foods are those that contribute to what are termed "cerebral allergies," and may include wheat, corn, milk, food chemicals, and sugar and alcohol, as well as many environmental allergens and chemicals. This term does not mean that the brain is literally allergic to these foods. Rather, it relates to the idea that some of us may show immune, digestive, and nervous system reactions from the routine consumption of these foods. For this reason, just avoiding these agents for from 1 to 3 weeks may greatly decrease brain reactions and many mental symptoms.

Not all mental illness is nutritionally and biochemically caused, of course, but still I believe a complete biochemical and nutritional workup should be done for most mental patients as early as possible. Besides food allergy testing, a basic physical and biochemical exam should be done. A test for diabetes and glucose tolerance for hypoglycemia will show positive findings in many patients. Blood vitamin and blood and hair mineral levels should be checked for essential nutrients as well as toxic heavy metals, such as lead and mercury. Food reaction (allergy) testing and avoidance may be helpful in some patients, and a stool evaluation for an overgrowth of the yeast *Candida albicans* and the occurrence of parasites may be positive. Immune and direct gastrointestinal reactions to these organisms are often associated with a variety of mental symptoms.

Dietary therapy for people with psychological problems should work to improve the overall diet by eliminating depleting substances such as refined-sugar and refined-flour products while increasing the nutritious foods. Sometimes a lower-carbohydrate diet than usual is helpful for mental patients, possibly because of gluten (wheat, rye, oat, and barley) sensitivity and reactions to high-carbohydrate foods may alter brain metabolism. In addition to minimizing refined foods, chemicals and food additives should be eliminated or at least greatly reduced. Intake of drugs and stimulants, particularly caffeine-containing drinks, white sugar, tobacco, and alcohol, should also be minimized. There may be allergies to any of these substances. Because of allergic potential and nutrient needs, a variety of foods should be eaten on a rotational basis. Occasionally, fasting or detoxification diets can be helpful to clear symptoms and bring greater individual insight into what is happening nutritionally.

Good nutrition is most likely going to lead to good physical, mental, and emotional energy; however, nutrition means more than just eating wholesome food. To nourish means to provide or receive nurturing love and support on an emotional and psychological level. Isolation and loneliness are like nutritional deficiencies in generating other mental-emotional symptoms. Often a good meal prepared with love not only feeds us physically but nourishes the heart and soul as well. Nutrient therapy can be helpful in the treatment of psychological disorders and is usually much safer than drug therapy. Of course, it is important to uncover the etiology or cause of the problem rather than to just use large amounts of vitamins. But when an organic cause is not identified, additional optimum level or orthomolecular nutrient supplementation can be useful.

All of the B vitamins are needed in above-average amounts, as they support the mechanisms for dealing with psychological and physical stress symptoms as well as correcting depletions. Not only do deficiencies in many of the B vitamins produce mental symptoms, in higher levels than average, certain B vitamins may provide functions that support better brain and body chemistry, such as restoring important neurotransmitter functions. Therapy with vitamin B3 as niacin or niacinamide has been helpful to many schizophrenic and other mental patients. Drs. Abram Hoffer and the late Humphrey Osmond, pioneers in the field of orthomolecular psychiatry, have suggested beginning patients at 100 mg daily and building up their niacin intake to 1,500 mg or even 3,000 mg. In addition, intravenous niacinamide has sometimes been helpful where oral was not. It is clear that deficiencies of B3 can lead to psychological symptoms, but it is not fully known what the positive effects of an increased level will be or how niacin actually works in this regard. More research is needed on niacin and other orthomolecular therapies.

Pyridoxine (B6) is often useful, especially for women with premenstrual water retention. Vitamin B12 has been beneficial for many mental patients, especially those with fatigue. Pantothenic acid aids the adrenals and helps handle the stress of increased mental intensity. Folic acid, PABA, inositol, and choline (which helps in production of the neurotransmitter acetylcholine) are also supportive B vitamins. Dimethylglycine (DMG), a precursor to pangamic acid, has been helpful to some people and may turn out to be useful in children with such problems as autism or hyperactivity.

Vitamin C is also commonly used in mental patients, especially in people with schizophrenia; it has a number of positive effects that may help in reducing symptoms. This antioxidant provides cell membrane protection and counteracts some of the negative biochemical responses to stress; its mild antihistamine effect can also reduce some allergic symptoms. Other antioxidant nutrients—such as vitamin E, selenium, beta-carotene, lipoic acid, and the amino acid L-cysteine—can help reduce toxicity and protect cells and tissues.

Many minerals may have some direct ties to mental condition. Except for increased copper and low zinc, or heavy metal toxicity such as with lead or mercury, there is not much evidence to directly associate mineral deficiencies or toxicities with overt mental disease. Many of these minerals are needed, however, to support good mental and neurological function. Low zinc levels affect the emotions, blood carbon dioxide levels, and general affect. Magnesium or potassium deficiency may be associated with fatigue and depression. Iron deficiency anemia can produce other mental symp-

toms and increase general fatigue and irritability. Manganese has been used by some clinicians in the treatment of schizophrenics, on the basis of the theory that it helps the synthesis of dopamine, a neurotransmitter in the brain. A deficiency of manganese has also been associated with hyperactivity. Deficient body copper, as well as high copper levels, may also be related to mental symptoms.

Iodine is needed for proper thyroid function; deficient iodine can lead to hypothyroidism, which can then cause mental symptoms. Extra calcium is beneficial, especially with a higher intake of vitamin C, which can chelate some of the usable calcium. Vitamins A and D, phosphorus, magnesium, protein, and adequate stomach acid levels to support digestion are also needed for best calcium assimilation and function. Many diets are too high in phosphorus, and this can lead to imbalances in calcium metabolism. It is important to maintain balance in all of these calcium-related nutrients, such as magnesium and zinc. Thus in the person with mental symptoms all of these macro- and microminerals need to be evaluated and supplemented where required.

Normal fatty acid metabolism and many amino acids are also supportive of mental health. The essential fatty acids, such as linoleic acid, are involved in prostaglandin production. the fish oils EPA and DHA are important for brain and nervous system health as well as their development in young people. Fatty acid deficiency can produce a number of possible psychological symptoms, such as hyperactivity or learning disorders. Problems in fatty acid metabolism have also been seen in many cases of schizophrenia.

The L-amino acids that may be correlated with mental conditions include phenylalanine, tyrosine, and tryptophan, and possibly methionine and glutamic acid. Deficiencies of any or all of these have been tied in some way to depression. L-tyrosine, another dopamine precursor, has been helpful in depressed patients. L-tryptophan and 5-HTP (5-hydroxytryptophan) are precursors of serotonin (the uplifting and antidepressant, sleep-supportive neurotransmitter) and are quite helpful for people with insomnia, depression, and anxiety as well as for women in menopause or with depression from menstrual problems. The dosages of the more available 5-HTP are between 50 and 200 mg at bedtime; some people also take it during the day for anxiety dominant depression. L-tryptophan is available through doctors and compounding pharmacists, and that dosage is 10 times the 5-HTP amount, or between 500 and 2,000 mg taken at bedtime.

Be careful about excess intake of amino acids, especially glutamic and aspartic acid. These 2 amino acids are classified as excitatory and generally stimulate nerves and muscles. Some of the problems related to intake of MSG (monosodium glutamate), for example, may be related to the excitatory function of this amino acid. The same can be said for routine high intake of the sweetener Nutrasweet (aspartame), because it partly breaks down into aspartic acid and phenylalanine in the body. A balanced L-amino acid formula may also help to provide energy and stability and a more positive outlook in many mental patients. In certain instances, a blood or urine amino acid profile can reveal specific metabolic imbalances and/or deficiencies. Another test that may even be more helpful is a neurotransmitter evaluation done on urine by a specialty lab like NeuroSciences (see Appendix A, "Laboratories and Clinical Nutrition Tests"). It measures serotonin, dopamine, norepinephrine, and others. It helps health-care specialists design the appropriate treatment for problems like depression and anxiety, the most common mental/medical issues seen today.

Two other relatively common problems of depression and anxiety include postpartum depression (after childbirth) and post-traumatic stress disorder (PTSD). You can apply the nutritional approaches in this program to these conditions as well.

A number of herbs may also be helpful for various mental conditions, although the choice would depend on energy level and other symptoms. Ginseng, ginger, and gotu kola have all been used to support mental faculties. A number of nerve tonics—such as oat straw, skullcap, vervain, and wood betony—can be helpful in reducing some mental symptoms. If hyperactivity, anxiety, or irritability are predominant, such nerve relaxant herbs as hops, valerian, passionflower, chamomile, black cohosh, or lavender may be more beneficial.

Hyperactivity/ADHD

Hyperactivity in children is usually conditioned early and related to many factors; however, some researchers are looking for genetic links. With hyperactivity, there are often associated mental symptoms and some subsequent learning difficulties. The primary problem, I think, is based in nutrition and metabolism; hyperactivity is definitely helped with a good diet and supplement program. Hyperactivity is much more common in boys than in girls, in a ratio of about 3 to 1. Although genetics and personality may be factors, there are definitely strong correlations with poor diet and the overuse of salt, sugar, sodas and other beverages containing caffeine, refined foods, and food chemicals. There may be food allergies or hypersensitivities, and often there are deficiencies in minerals, such as potassium, zinc, magnesium, and manganese, as well as some of the B vitamins.

Nutritionally based treatments can be helpful for youngsters (and adults) with attention-deficit/hyperactivity disorder (ADHD). Regarding food reactions, hyperactivity is usually viewed as a positive stimulatory reaction of the food addiction phase of allergy, as a response to repeated intake of foods or chemicals. During withdrawal phases, there is a temporary, further stimulation or depression; with clinical improvement, the hyperactive state can be duplicated with positive food tests to "challenge" the child. I believe that most hyperactivity problems are related at least in part to these allergy-addiction states. The late Dr. Benjamin Feingold, a pediatric allergist, also connected the presence of poor diet and allergies in many of his cases of hyperactivity in children. His evaluation of food allergies, nutrient deficiencies, lead and other metal toxicity, and sensitivity to sugar, food colorings and preservatives, and salicylates gave him the insight to create a special diet plan that has been effective for many patients.

Common food allergy reactions associated with hyperactivity are to wheat, corn, milk, and eggs, and sometimes the other gluten-containing grains, including rye, oats, and barley. All of these foods are avoided with the Feingold diet, as are soft drinks; sugar and processed foods; foods containing chemicals, especially coloring agents and in particular Yellow No. 5 (also known as tartrazine); and fruits and vegetables that are high in natural salicylates, which include peaches, plums, prunes, nectarines, grapes, raisins, cherries, currants, apples, apricots, strawberries, tomatoes, asparagus, and cucumbers. This special diet also calls for an increase in quality protein and a decrease in refined carbohydrates along with orthomolecular nutrient therapy. The nutritional approach to hyperactivity focuses on the B vitamins, particularly niacin, pyridoxine, and

---

Nutritional Impact on ADD/ADHD: A Natural Treatment Approach

What to Avoid: A Trial Approach

Refined sugar—cane sugar and corn syrup

Cow's milk

Wheat and wheat products as a trial

Craved and habit foods

Other possible food reactions—peanuts, citrus, eggs, soy, chocolate

Artificial coloring agents

Additives that affect neurological function— MSG

Aspartame

Artificial flavors

What to Include as Diet and Supplements

Multivitamin/mineral

Magnesium

Fish oils—EPA and DHA

Lecithin—choline and inositol

Vitamin C

Probiotics (healthy bacteria)

Elimination diet

Food challenges

Testing to Consider

Food reaction tests—antibody levels or cell reactions

Stool test for yeast—with culture and sensitivity

Digestive analysis for function and ecology

Urine test for yeast and bacterial metabolites (organic acid test)

Blood cell mineral measurement for magnesium, potassium, and more

Hair analysis for lead and mercury toxicity

---

pantothenic acid, along with extra vitamins C and E, zinc, manganese, magnesium, calcium, and chromium. L-amino acids may be helpful. Herbal texts suggest red clover blossom tea as a good calming herb for children with this condition. Ritalin, a stimulant drug, apparently has a paradoxical calming effect in hyperactive children, but it has many side effects and is definitely the treatment of last resort.

Depression

Depression could be described as a mood, a state of being, or energy level that includes a lack of motivation, a sense of hopelessness, and a lack of physical energy. It is an emotional state that can result from many aspects of life. Depression may be associated with a variety of nutritional deficiencies; it is a common symptom in many people, from the young to the elderly. It is not always simply an emotional or psychological condition, although it commonly includes emotional components. Depressive reactions may be associated with such problems as fatigue, obesity, headaches, or poor digestion.

In standard medicine, most doctors label depression and then prescribe 1 or more of a wide variety of antidepressant drugs. However, in an integrated approach to medicine, I ask why a problem is present and look at all the factors that contribute to it to achieve an understanding of its existence. Then, I can correct and clear those areas that may be generating the difficulty. For depression, this could involve diet and substance intake, exercise activity, your biochemical and mental states, and how you feel about all areas of your life, such as job, relationships, and family. The first important step involves determining if your depression is short-term or chronic . . . and if it is mild, moderate, or severe. Do some careful self-analysis: How often do you feel depressed? Most people experience some level of depression occasionally; it is just part of our biorhythm of emotional and mental activity, and seasonal sensitivities. If you are depressed right now, how long has this been going on? Is it linked to a stressful external cause—a life event at work or in a relationship? Or does the depression seem to follow you most of the time, like your own personal dark cloud? A state of constant depression may suggest persistent stress or a biochemical imbalance.

There are varying degrees of depression, from mild to severe, from acute to long-term. Physicians often define a condition as chronic if it has persisted more than 1 or 2 months. In the case of depression, if you have experienced an ongoing low for more than 3 months, it is likely a chronic condition and definitely warrants a consultation with a capable, insightful psychiatrist or therapist (or a nutritionally oriented practitioner if you wish to be guided in a natural approach). Antidepressant drugs are clearly another solution and have been helpful to millions. Mild depression is often situational and may come and go. Clinical depression can be a major psychological problem and may include repressed fear, anger, or rage; however, biochemical, metabolic, and nutritional imbalances, including food allergies, may be intimately involved. Along with grief, depression has been correlated with a higher incidence of cancer and may even be responsible for its genesis, as it may affect immune function. Depression can affect us deeply and basically as a lack of enthusiasm for life or even a lack of concern about living. Of course, when we lose our desire to live (and to love), the dying process takes greater hold and grows.

Depression has many causes as well. Western medicine categorizes depression as endogenous (coming from within) and exogenous (coming from outside influences). Exogenous depression comes from reactions to life events and daily stresses, such as loss of a loved one, job problems, or family crises. We also may experience depression from inner conflict, or we may feel overwhelmed by responsibilities. Many drugs can cause mild to moderate levels of depression; these include blood pressure medications, estrogens as in birth control pills, steroids, and antianxiety drugs, like the benzodiazepines (Valium, Xanax, or Ativan). The remedy for many cases of exogenous depression often involves clearing the causative factor or doing some counseling to better integrate our life experiences. Endogenous depression could also be called *biochemical depression*. It tends to run in families, in genetics, and is generated by brain chemistry and imbalances of serotonin (one of the "feel-good" hormones that helps us sleep) or other neurotransmitters. Most of the antidepressant medications currently prescribed are chemicals that maintain or improve serotonin levels. Even the natural approach that uses diet, herbs, and amino acids is geared toward raising serotonin levels.

One of the most commonly prescribed classes of drugs is the selective serotonin reuptake inhibitors (SSRIs)—those substances like Prozac, Paxil, Zoloft, and Effexor. These medicines slow the clearing of this important brain chemical, thus leaving more serotonin available to brain function. This then improves the mood and motivation of its consumer. The problem is that there are many possible, often likely, side effects of these drugs rather than the "side benefits" of a natural approach. Common side effects of the SSRI drugs include weight gain, loss of sexual energy, and bouts of anger or anxiety.

In place of or in addition to drug therapy, many other treatments can be useful. Counseling and psychological support as well as nutritional therapy may be helpful for depression. The nutritional program is threefold—a good diet, devoid of chemicals and junk food; micronutrient support, particularly with the B vitamins niacin, pyridoxine, B_{12}, and folic acid, vitamin C, zinc, and manganese; and nutrients that support the production of neurotransmitter substances. Among this last group, choline helps to generate acetylcholine; L-phenylalanine and L-tyrosine improve dopamine synthesis (and thyroid hormone, also a factor in depression); and L-tryptophan and 5-HTP stimulate serotonin production. All of these substances facilitate nerve conduction, but phenylalanine is usually avoided in patients with hypertension. Methionine and other methyl-containing nutrients including choline, trimethylglycine (TMG), dimethylglycine (DMG), and methylsulfonylmethane (MSM) are also interesting with respect to depression and nerve activity, because one of the "get up and go" nerve substances—epinephrine (formally know as adrenaline)—cannot be produced without the help of these nutrients. The role of these methyl nutrients has become important enough to have generated a whole hypothesis about metabolism and depression, called the *undermethylation hypothesis*.

With depression, it is also important to isolate and eliminate food allergies/reactions. Depression can be created or exacerbated by food addiction and its related allergies, even during "withdrawal" phases. The elimination of chemicals, sugar, and refined foods is important to help many people with bad moods and depression. Regular, moderate exercise will help depressed people feel more "up," as will the avoidance of stimulants such as caffeine, tobacco, and alcohol.

A hidden problem that contributes to depression is hypothyroidism, both the classically low thyroid function that any physician can discover and so-called subclinical hypothyroidism, which is based on body-mind symptoms and body temperature. If you are sluggish, have a slow metabolism, feel cold all the time, are losing hair, and experience constipation and some depression, you may have low thyroid function. Your thyroid numbers may be okay, but you could benefit from low-dose thyroid support, just as some people who are stressed and fatigued feel much better with adrenal support.

As suggested, for mild to moderate depression, it is wise to try a course of natural therapies. For severe or persistent depression, I suggest seeing a conventional or orthomolecular psychiatrist for evaluation and treatment. An integrated approach to any medical problem involves three areas of care: lifestyle (behaviors), natural remedies (diet and supplements), and pharmaceutical drugs as a last resort or for more acute and serious problems.

Orthomolecular Medicine

The approach to psychiatry that incorporates the use of nutrients to rebalance brain chemistry is described as *orthomolecular therapy*. Readers can obtain referrals to trained orthomolecular psychiatrists and physicians in the United States and Canada by calling Orthomolecular Health Medicine in San Francisco at 415-922-6462. Many physician members of the American College for the Advancement of Medicine (ACAM) and most naturopathic practitioners also have training in the treatment of depression using nutritional supplements and herbs. ACAM referrals can be obtained by following the instructions at 800-532-3688.

SELF-CARE FOR DEPRESSION

My general philosophy suggests that behavior involves motivation and attitude, both of which affect how we care for ourselves, such as whether we make healthy food choices or create and maintain a regular exercise program. My approach in medicine, and I think the highest calling of a physician (a philosopher-physician

of the ancient Chinese tradition) is to inspire and educate patients to care for themselves—to live in a way that generates health rather than have a lifestyle that causes disease.

Meditation is a tool of ultimate and major significance. Practiced in moderation, meditation can be a meaningful adjunct to any medical regimen. Our inner dialogue is also important to our emotional health. Most people can learn or relearn how to talk and think more positively. Like anything, this may take some practice; quieting the mind and sitting peacefully is a good beginning. Appreciation is another key to reestablishing joy. I encourage each of us to assess and appreciate what we have and who we are. We can acknowledge the challenges we face and do everything in our power to identify and correct the medical and lifestyle approaches that decrease our depression. Doing this with a counselor is most helpful. Self-image and self-love are important unconscious motivators that affect how we treat ourselves and whether we make the effort to maintain healthy habits. Self-image, our view of our self, has a lot to do with behavior and depression. If we feel unworthy of love, particularly self-love, we may not treat ourselves with respect, or with healthy habits. If we can feel proud of ourselves and believe that we can improve and heal and grow, we may be more able to rise out of our blues. It is common for people with depression to feel withdrawn and to look down, often with a hunched-over back. Sit up, look up, breathe, and embrace life!

EXERCISE AND DEPRESSION

Exercise activity is one way to prevent and chase away depression. Studies show that regular exercisers feel better and have a better mood and attitude toward life than those who do not. Cleansing of toxins from the blood and the body is one positive way that exercise could moderate depression. In addition, there are positive effects on the brain chemicals from exercise, such as an increase in the uplifting endorphins. Work toward a balanced combination of activities that includes aerobic exercise 3 to 5 times per week for 30 to 45 minutes, weight training to improve strength and tone, and stretching to ensure flexibility. It takes an effort to organize your time despite the busyness and demands of modern life. However, it is surely worth it.

I realize that it may be difficult to begin, especially if you feel depressed, but once your routine is established, it will build and potentially moderate some of the depressed state naturally over the course of couple of weeks. Try a 15-minute walk; swing your arms in rhythm with your breathing.

Fatigue, and sometimes anxiety and insomnia, frequently accompany depression. In these cases, it will challenge your creativity to work exercise into your life. Yoga and tai chi, taking classes or perhaps using a video, can be helpful and require less energy. Walking continues to be among the forms of exercise found by patients, doctors, and research to be the most beneficial. If you are too tired to exercise, be sure to seek the care of a health-care professional. Explore some form of sitting qigong or tai chi, such as that used by cancer patients in China with reported benefit, or explore simple yoga postures and deep breathing.

If we can gather the motivation to exercise regularly, it is usually energizing and helps bring about an improved sense of peace and optimism. Beginning with hikes in Nature, walking with the head up and the shoulders back, along with deep breathing of fresh air, will definitely change our energy. Several studies are showing regular exercise to reduce depression and improve mood and outlook on life.

DIET AND DEPRESSION

Foods and moods have been written about many times, and it is clear to me that individual foods as well as various types of diets contribute to how we feel. Food nutrients and chemicals (natural food and synthetic contaminants and additives) affect brain function and neurotransmitter levels, and this leads to experiences such as depression and anxiety, fatigue, or insomnia. Food reactions, allergies, and hypersensitivities also affect energy levels, moods, and mental faculties. My book *The False Fat Diet* describes a broad range of mechanisms involving food reactivity, which can clearly contribute to and alter mental, physical, and emotional states. Many patients and readers of my books have improved their mental states and cleared up depressive states using the programs from *The New Detox Diet* and *The False Fat Diet*. Remember that sugars—especially refined sugars and sweet foods like sodas and candies—alter the glycemic index and are

---

> ## Diet Guidelines to Prevent and Reduce Mild to Moderate Depression
>
> Get all the appropriate nutrients from wholesome foods and supplements.
> Avoid chemicals and junk foods as much as possible.
> Rotate your foods and avoid your reactive foods.
> Watch your sugar and refined-foods intake.
> Minimize your use of caffeine and alcohol.
> Eat adequate proteins along with fresh vegetables.
> Consume fresh fruits and some nuts and seeds.
> Eat whole grains and legumes and some sprouts.

often associated with rapid mood changes and depression. See additional information on the glycemic index on page 35 in chapter 2, Carbohydrates.

SUPPLEMENTS AND DEPRESSION

There is a wide range of vitamins, minerals, amino acids, and herbs that can help alleviate depression. Many of them support brain function and specifically serotonin levels. Others support normal hormone balance, specifically of the thyroid and adrenal glands.

Let's start with the B vitamins and a few minerals. The most important is pyridoxine, vitamin B6. It assists many brain and neurotransmitter functions. You might use this along with a general B complex formula, 50 to 100 mg twice daily after meals. Vitamin B12 along with folic acid supports nerve structure and functions, while pantothenic acid and vitamin C aid the adrenal glands and energy. Choline and inositol aid the brain. Calcium and magnesium allow relaxation and better sleep when taken at night, and iodine supports normal thyroid function. Extra zinc and manganese as well as the L-amino acids can improve energy. Such oil formulas as primrose and flaxseed oils can increase prostaglandin E1 production and thus may also be helpful. In general then, a good quality multivitamin/mineral product is a good start.

Amino acid support may be a valuable key to clearing or reducing depression. Adequate protein in the diet is a good beginning for obtaining needed levels of amino acids. In addition, several specific ones may be helpful. Phenylalanine seems to improve endorphin levels and reduce pain. Tyrosine is energizing and is needed for proper thyroid function; 500 to 1,000 mg can be taken in the morning and after lunch. Tryptophan is the most important because it directly makes serotonin and this substance seems to be low in most people suffering from depression. Tryptophan is currently available through compounding pharmacists with your doctor's prescription, or a precursor to tryptophan, namely 5-HTP (5-hydroxytryptophan), can be obtained at health food stores. The amount to start with is 50 to 100 mg taken at night, as it aids sleep, with an additional 50 to 100 mg in the morning. This is also helpful for those suffering from fibromyalgia (as is magnesium malate or malic acid).

Another related amino acid that appears to provide some benefit to people with depression is s-adenosylmethionine (SAM). Although the mechanism is not clearly known, a dosage of 100 to 200 mg once or twice daily shows some improvement for those suffering from mild or moderate depression. Possible benefits of SAM for depression have been shown as recently as 2004 in research conducted at the AIDS Community Research Initiative of America in New York City. Some people also experience mild side effects. Adding other lifestyle activities and support from the "10 Tips for Preventing and Treating Depression" on this page may provide greater benefits for depression.

There are several herbs that may be helpful in improving depression. St. John's wort, or hypericum as the active ingredient, has been helpful both in research studies and in clinical practice. It needs to be taken consistently for 1 or 2 months to see the benefits and usually 3 times daily using 300 mg capsules of 0.3% hypericum. Other herbs can be used to handle other symptoms that go with depression. This might include valerian and hops for insomnia, kava kava for anxiety, ginseng (panax) for energy, and Siberian ginseng for stress. For women with PMS or menopause, or for men with libido changes, different herbal combinations might be beneficial. Some other herbs that may be helpful in depression are damiana, kola nut (a stimulant), skullcap, lavender, valerian, vervain, and rosemary. These can help to strengthen the nervous system, to improve the attitude, and to tolerate stress.

Consider an integrated approach drawing on the experience of a naturally oriented physician who can

10 Tips for Preventing and Treating Depression

1. **Keep a positive attitude toward life.** Challenges are opportunities to improve your entire being. Learn to turn negatives into positives. Look up (not down) at life with enthusiasm.

2. **Create a regular exercise program** that includes stretching, weights, and aerobic activity. It is difficult to feel depressed when you are creating those motivating endorphins.

3. **Learn ways** to access and talk about your feelings and frustrations with friends or loved ones. If that option is not available, or if you are hesitant to air out your personal issues, find a compatible counselor.

4. **Eat a wholesome and balanced diet,** because having all the right nutrients—vitamins, minerals, amino acids, and essential fatty acids—supports your mental, physical, and emotional health.

5. **Take a regular multivitamin/mineral** appropriate to your needs to ensure adequate levels of all of your required nutrients.

6. **Avoid any regular use of substances** that may alter your moods. This includes sugar, caffeine, alcohol, and many food additives, such as synthetic food colorings and flavorings, MSG, aspartame, and others.

7. **Watch out for food reactions** that can affect your mood and energy—from such foods as sugar, wheat products, and cow's milk.

8. **Try natural remedies** that are known to help with depression, which might include St. John's wort (300 mg 3 times daily) or SAM (200 mg twice daily).

9. **If those do not work** adequately, try the antidepressant amino acids, such as L-tryptophan (500–1,000 mg at night) or its variant, 5-HTP (50–100 mg at night). Both of these improve serotonin levels, which helps with sleep and feeling positive. L-tyrosine is another, more-energizing, antidepressant amino acid.

10. **If all this does not work,** of if the depression is severe, consult with your physician or therapist, and try an antidepressant medication.

help you sort out your options. You may be able to get acceptable results without the use of prescription drugs. Acupuncture could be helpful, as could the use of homeopathic remedies. Massage and relaxation therapies may likewise offer improvement. Meditation can be of great value, as can regular exercise. As with so many diseases, feeling empowered by getting involved in your own program and finding a way to make things right, and to make them work for you (becoming your own best doctor), is likely the highest art in health care. Seek wisdom and guidance from those trained to help you make the best decisions for you. For your long-term care, develop a working partnership with your practitioner. A multifaceted approach typically holds the greatest promise.

Postpartum depression (PPD) occurs fairly commonly in women during the several months after giving birth. This may be a result of hormonal changes, although many authors feel that nutrient depletions are at its heart. Folic acid deficiency is likely the most common in postpartum women; B12 and iron are also usually depleted. Good intake of iron, zinc, B6, B12, magnesium, and protein are all important to alleviate the fatigue, mood swings, and depression that may occur. PPD can be helped with lifestyle support as well. Exercise and massage offer comfort, psychotherapy and meditation can provide benefit, and dietary changes and supplements can be helpful. Taking B vitamins and magnesium for relaxation is important in dealing with stress and PPD.

The "General Program for Mental Health" on page 738 offers a general program for a variety of the mental problems discussed in this section. The amounts listed are daily levels to be taken in several portions. Where ranges are shown, these represent varying amounts that can be used in treating mild to more severe problems. Building from lower to higher amounts can support individual adaptation. Remember, some changes may be slow or subtle, so using the treatment program for several months will give it the best chance. Improvement may occur very rapidly, however. Many of these ranges depend on sensitivity and need. For example, the higher amounts of niacinamide can be taken for anxiety and for sleep, as can the tryptophan products. With more anxiety, the higher amounts of magnesium, B vitamins, and L-tyrosine can be utilized.

RESEARCH AND DEPRESSION

A number of important nutrients are being used to treat depression. Below I highlight the range of approaches that has been reviewed in the medical literature since the mid-1990s.

Hypericum. The active component of St. John's wort, hypericum is considered a promising supplement for the treatment of depression, so promising that the National Institutes of Health has initiated a major clinical trial to evaluate its potential effectiveness. A thorough review of the research on St. John's wort was conducted in Germany by top researchers known for their work on homeopathy. This is what they found:

- The researchers narrowed the data down to 10 studies that compared hypericum with other antidepressant or sedative drugs. The studies included 1,123 participants with "mild to moderately severe depressive disorders."

- The hypericum preparations were found to be about 2.5 times more effective than the placebo (supplements that contained no hypericum).

- They were equally effective as single-preparation antidepressants and 1.5 times as effective as combination antidepressants.

- Among patients taking the hypericum, about a fourth had side effects.

- Almost half (45%) of the patients taking standard antidepressants had side effects.

SAM (SAM-e). A 10-week study at Massachusetts General Hospital in Boston looked at the benefits of SAM in the treatment of depression. They found significant decreases in depression scores—the scores went from more than 19 (very depressed) to less than 11. However, it is important to note that 8 out of the 21 patients dropped out due to uncomfortable physical symptoms, such as diarrhea and increased anxiety. Like many other forms of treatment, the last word is still not in. The potential helpfulness of SAM makes sense, however, because the adrenal glands cannot make epinephrine (one of our "get going" nerve substances) unless SAM is readily available.

General Program for Mental Health

Eat a hypoallergenic, chemical-free diet.

Nutrient	Amount	Nutrient	Amount
Water	2–3 qt	Magnesium	400–800 mg
Protein	50–75 g	Manganese	10–25 mg
Fiber	10–15 g	Molybdenum	500 mcg
Vitamin A	5,000 IU	Potassium	500–2,000 mg
Beta-carotene	20,000 IU	Selenium	200–400 mcg
Vitamin D	400 IU	Zinc	60–100 mg
Vitamin E	400–800 IU	Hydrochloric acid	1–2 tablets with meals
Vitamin K	300 mcg	Digestive enzymes	2–3 tablets after meals
Thiamin (B1)	100–250 mg	L- amino acids	1,500 mg (take 3
Riboflavin (B2)	50–100 mg		500 mg portions
Niacinamide (B3)	200–2,000 mg		after meals)
Niacin (B3)	100–1,000 mg	DL-phenylalanine	500–1,000 mg
Pantothenic acid (B5)	250–1,500 mg	L-tyrosine++	500–1,500 mg
Pyridoxine (B6)	50–200 mg	L-tryptophan+++	500–1,500 mg
Pyridoxal-5-phosphate	25–100 mg	or 5-HTP at bed	50–200 mg
Cobalamin (B12)*	100–500 mcg	Essential fatty acids or	
Folic acid	800–2,000 mcg	flaxseed oil	4–6 capsules
Biotin	300–1,000 mcg		or 2–4 teaspoons
Choline	500–1,500 mg	Evening primrose oil	6–8 capsules
Inositol	500–1,500 mg		(200–400 mg GLA)
PABA	50–500 mg	Lactobacillus acidolphilus	1–2 billion
Vitamin C	2–20 g		
Bioflavonoids	250–500 mg		
Calcium	800–1,200 mg		
Chromium	200 mcg		
Copper+	1–5 mg		
Iodine	150 mcg		
Iron	10–18 mg		

* Can also be taken in 500 mcg. Injections twice weekly.

+ Only if copper levels are normal, and the amount taken varies with zinc.

++ Higher amounts (3–6 g daily, taken in 2–3 portions during the day) for depression.

+++ Used for irritability or insomnia, usually once in the evening if available.

The role of serotonin and treatment using 5-HTP. The connection between pain and low serotonin levels is emphasized in a review on fibromyalgia, "a musculoskeletal pain and fatigue disorder manifested by diffuse myalgia, localized areas of tenderness, fatigue, lowered pain thresholds, and non-restorative sleep." The first step in treatment suggested is to identify low serum tryptophan and serotonin levels through testing. The review also indicates that supplementing the "serotonin substrate" through either L-tryptophan (available only through compounding pharmacists) or through 5-HTP (5-hydroxytryptophan) has been shown to improve symptoms of depression, anxiety, insomnia, and somatic pains.

Genetic links to depression. Research suggests possible indirect genetic links to depression. A study of the effects of exercise on depression and hormone output evaluated 82 healthy male volunteers (ages 18 to 26 years old), who used an exercise bicycle to achieve maximum exertion. The volunteers were tested regarding their mood using the Beck Depression Inventory, an anxiety scale, stress scale, and self-efficacy scale. Blood samples were tested to measure growth hormone, cortisol, and testosterone. The finding: Exercise increases your hormones. The researchers noted, "In the majority of subjects, physical exercise induced remarkable increases in blood levels of the hormones." However, in the participants with test scores that reflected some depression, "growth hormone response was virtually absent." This suggests both a role for growth hormone in stabilizing mood and a possible genetic link between individuals with low growth hormone output and the tendency to depression.

Thyroid. For more information on the possible role of thyroid in depression and how practitioners are approaching treatment, see the website of the Cognitive Enhancement Research Institute (CERI) at www.ceri.com. To order the newsletter, call 1-650-321-CERI.

THE FUTURE OF NUTRITIONAL MEDICINE

This book is all about nutritional medicine, and nutritional medicine is already the future—becoming present to more and more open-minded and health-based practitioners and the public. Addressing causes of ill health and correcting them is the future. To treat symptoms and diseases that are the end result of many of these causes is very superficial medicine in my opinion—and poor nutrition is among the main causes of poor health, and these persistent poor choices lead to many problems over time. A diet that is out of balance for us leads to an imbalance in the body and the single primary disease that has many results. That single disease is cellular malfunction and this has 2 main causes—deficiency and toxicity—not enough of the needed vitamins, minerals, amino acids, fatty acids, and phytonutrients to function optimally, as well as exposure to the many toxins from the air, water, food, and our own body that stress our cells and damage them, not allowing them to function optimally. (This is addressed thoroughly in my friend Raymond Francis's book *Never Get Sick Again*.)

The key to the future of nutritional medicine is the understanding, the balance, the ability to assess thoroughly, and the knowledge to know how to rebalance the ACID-ALKALINE chemistry of the cells, tissues, and body. Much of chronic disease is a result of overly acidic tissues from chemicals and refined foods, excess protein in the diet, overeating and eating too many foods at once, and poor digestion and elimination processes. That's why I focus on detoxification and alkaline dietary programs to help rebalance and heal people initially. Also, that's why I focus on lifestyle habit changes and support as a key to keeping people healthier. I want every doctor's office, and every mom and dad, to learn what it takes to live healthy lives.

Eat well and take care of yourself, your loved ones, and our precious planet Earth.

Remember, genetics is not destiny. With the right guidance and health plan, you can delay your predispositions to certain diseases, from heart disease and cancer to depression. Take care of yourself; it is worth it!

Chapter 18

Detoxification and Cleansing Programs

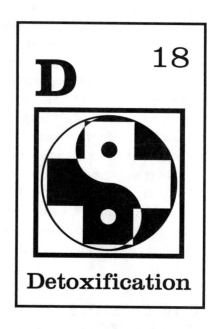

D **18**

Detoxification

So many problems in Western society come from excessive use of foods and drugs. Abuses and addictions touch almost every person's life. This chapter addresses many of the dietary and substance abuses and ways to heal them. We must ask ourselves—as I suggest to people in their initial visit to my clinic—is there anything that we do everyday that we would really miss if we did not have it? If so, this activity is a habit or addiction. Of course, there are positive habits, like exercising, eating good foods, and getting proper sleep. I became hooked on feeling good and having consistent, smooth energy on a daily basis. Yet there are many other habits that may negatively interact with life and health and can lead to a variety of problems—physical, mental, and emotional. Common addictions include sugar, caffeine, alcohol, nicotine, and various drugs (both pharmaceutical and recreational). Most adults have problems with one or more of these substances and may even be aware of their habits/addictions and would like to change them, but they do not, cannot, or will not for various reasons. This chapter deals with the general programs that offer guidance and support for undoing some of these chronic and health-undermining habits. In terms of other habits, we also must be aware of electropollution (see page 483 in chapter 11, Food and the Earth) and what I call "techno traps"—the TVs, phones, computers, VCR, fax machines, microwaves, and other devices that expose us to electrical vibration, including medical testing and exposures while shopping in stores and during transportation, especially on airplanes. We may also have addictions or dependencies to talking or being in love or having sex.

I believe that fasting (and detoxification) is the missing link in the American (and Western) diet, so this is a key chapter regarding personal health, and for that matter, the health of the planet. Taking breaks from things is a good way to assess our true relationship to them and often a way to improve our health. When we treat ourselves with more respect and generate an attitude of self-love, of caring for the body in a positive and loving way, we will choose less polluting ways of living, and this lifestyle will produce less personal and planetary toxicity. Since the original writing of *Staying Healthy with Nutrition*, I have published two books on detoxification: *The Detox Diet: The How-To and When-To Guide for Cleansing the Body* and then the new expanded version entitled *The New Detox Diet:*

The Complete Guide for Lifelong Vitality with Recipes, Menus, and Detox Plans, both published by Celestial Arts, in 1996 and 2004, respectively.

My detoxification books are quite popular, and I believe this is because they are so needed by the public. In these works, I talk about the SNACCs—sugar, nicotine, alcohol, caffeine, and chemicals—and I refer to the SNACC habits on radio shows and in lectures. People relate to this concept, as most everyone has a habit with 1 or more of these substances. Most of us are substance abusers of some form or another, with sugar and caffeine being the most common. Now these are not as problematic as nicotine and alcohol, not to mention amphetamines and heroin, but they still cause problems over time. From questioning my audiences at lectures, it appears that 90% to 95% of the attendees have habits to one or more of these SNACCs.

Because of the popularity of the detox topic and my experience in doing detox groups, which involves taking people through cleanses and various detoxifying programs for 3- to 4-week periods to help them come through with new and improved habits and health, I decided to bring out a new version of *The Detox Diet,* as *The New Detox Diet.* This expanded and updated edition went from 128 to 264 pages and has even more practical guidelines on detoxification, with additional detox programs, patient stories, menu plans, and more than 50 recipes to use in various cleansing programs, including the original detox diet, a smoothie cleanse, and a juice cleanse.

Because *The New Detox Diet* now exists fresh and updated, and because I have included so much new material in this updated edition of *Staying Healthy with Nutrition,* I decided to cut this chapter considerably from the original version. Here I include the primary topics "General Detoxification and Cleansing" (page 741) as well as "Fasting and Juice Cleansing" (page 769). There are brief discussions of sugar, caffeine, alcohol and nicotine in this chapter, but for the more complete and specific programs on detoxification from sugar, nicotine, alcohol, caffeine, and chemicals (and drugs), please refer to *The New Detox Diet.* I regret there is not enough space to cover these topics in-depth within this book.

Much disease, especially degenerative disease, comes from congestion and stagnation in the body (in the organs, tissues, circulation, lymph, and cells), and this congestion/stagnation state can be cleared from the body through cleansing and detoxification.** I have personally experienced it and have seen it in thousands of patients. I believe the processes of detoxification and healing can be synonymous in many instances; of course, this is when applied to the right medical circumstances. **The other side of disease, in simplistic terms and conceptually, originates from depletion and deficiency,** and for people in this state, fasting or cleansing dietary processes are not the answer; in fact, they may make matters worse. These and many other general concepts of detoxification are discussed in the first program, "General Detoxification and Cleansing."

The "Fasting and Juice Cleansing" program on page 769 may take some mind expansion and trust to embrace; however, many people are more than ready for this health information on the art of fasting and concepts of more vital living. Juice fasting/cleansing is a powerful, healing tool—one of the greatest! It is a vehicle to freedom from addiction of all kinds. It helps us open to our true guidance, growth, potentials, and life. Fasting opens us spiritually and emotionally, and supports us in becoming more real in our lives, in doing what we believe and know in our hearts and spirits to be right for us. With that openness and clarity, we can then embrace some of the more spiritual philosophy discussed in the Futureword in "Immortality and Beyond" (page 790).

31. GENERAL DETOXIFICATION AND CLEANSING

Up to this point, so many pages of the book have been devoted to nutrients, foods, diets, and special eating plans to support health and to treat a variety of disease states. Now it is important to emphasize two programs in the category of elimination—the basic processes of detoxification and fasting, which help us cleanse specific common toxins and habits from our lives. It is somewhat difficult to separate the concepts and practices of detoxification from those of fasting or juice cleansing. Fasting (the avoidance of solid food, as I use the term here) is one method of detoxification, probably the most effective, yet extreme, form. There are many other ways to detoxify, however. And I have done many of them. I just completed a 4-day water fast vision quest in the Mohave Desert, away from everything except myself. This was a challenge and stretch for me since I am so used to doing and being active, yet for these four days I was a human "being," not a human "doing." The break from people, talking, electricity, and other normal activities was quite profound with the quiet and the great show of stars. I learned much about myself and more about this cleansing process for my work.

Toxicity is of much greater concern now than ever before. There are many new and stronger chemicals, air and water pollution, radiation, and nuclear power. We ingest new chemicals, use more drugs of all kinds, eat more sugar and refined foods, and daily abuse ourselves with various stimulants and sedatives. The incidence of many toxicity diseases has increased as well. Cancer and cardiovascular disease are two of the main ones. Arthritis, allergies, obesity, and many skin problems are others. In addition, a wide range of symptoms—such as headaches, fatigue, pains, coughs, gastrointestinal problems, and problems from immune weakness—can all be related to toxicity.

Toxicity occurs on two basic levels—external and internal. We can acquire toxins from our environment by breathing them, by ingesting them, or through physical contact with them. Chapter 11, Food and the Earth deals with chemicals in our food supply and how they influence our lives and health. We are exposed to toxins daily. We eat and drink them and impose them upon ourselves repeatedly and regularly. Most drugs, food additives, and allergens can create toxic elements in the body. In fact, any substance can have toxicity—water, sodium, and almost all nutrients can be a problem in certain circumstances. Internally, the body produces toxins through its normal everyday functions. Biochemical, cellular, and bodily activities generate substances that need to be eliminated. The free radicals that have been discussed throughout this book are biochemical toxins. When these substances, molecules, and toxins are not eliminated, they can cause irritation or inflammation of the cells and tissues, blocking normal functions on a cellular, organ, and whole-body level. Microbes of all kinds—intestinal bacteria, foreign bacteria, yeasts, and parasites—produce metabolic

waste products that we must handle. Our thoughts and emotions and stress itself generate increased biochemical toxicity. **The proper level of elimination of these toxins is essential to health. Clearly, a normal-functioning body is able to handle certain levels of toxins; the concern is with excess intake or production of toxins, or a reduction in the processes of elimination.**

A toxin is basically any substance that creates irritating and/or harmful effects in the body, undermining its health or stressing the biochemical or organ functions, or actually damaging tissues and organs. This may result from drugs, which have side effects, or from patterns of physiology that are different from our usual functioning. Recreational drugs also usually have some harmful effects. The free radicals irritate, inflame, age, and cause degeneration of body tissues. Negative "ethers," psychic and spiritual influences, thought patterns, and negative emotions all can be toxins as well—both as stressors and by changing the normal physiology of the body and possibly producing specific symptoms. *Homeostasis* means that the body functions are in balance. This balance is disturbed when we feed ourselves more than we can utilize, or when we partake of specific substances that are toxic. Toxicity may depend on the dosage, frequency, or potency of the toxin. A toxin may produce an immediate or rapid onset of symptoms, as many pesticides and some drugs do; possibly even more commonly, it may cause some long-term negative effect, such as asbestos exposure leading to lung cancer.

Of course, if the body is working well, with good immune and eliminative functions, we can handle

---

The Body's General Detoxification Systems

Gastrointestinal. Liver, gallbladder, colon, and the whole GI tract.
Urinary. Kidneys, bladder, and urethra.
Respiratory. Lungs, bronchial tubes, throat, sinuses, and nose.
Lymphatic. Lymph channels and lymph nodes.
Skin and dermal. Sweat and sebaceous glands and tears.

the basic everyday exposure to toxins. Here I discuss ways to support the elimination of toxins, excessive mucus, congestion, and disease as well as ways to prevent, on a day-to-day basis, the buildup of toxicity. Through detoxification, we clear and filter toxins and wastes and thus allow the body to work on enhancing its basic functions.

The body handles toxins by neutralizing, transforming, and/or eliminating them. As examples, many of the antioxidant nutrients discussed earlier, in chapters 5, 6, and 7 and in the Antiaging program in chapter 16 (pages 588) may neutralize free-radical molecules. The liver helps transform many toxic substances into harmless agents, while the blood carries wastes to the kidneys; the liver also dumps wastes through the bile into the intestines, where much waste is eliminated. We also clear toxins through sweating, from exercise or heat. Our sinuses and skin may also be accessory elimination organs, whereby excess mucus or toxins can be released, as with sinus congestion or skin rashes, respectively.

Detoxification occurs on many other levels as well. Physically, this process can help clear congestions, illnesses, and disease potential. It usually improves energy. Many detox processes help rejuvenate us and prevent degeneration. Mental detoxification is also important. Cleansing our minds of negative thought patterns is essential to health; the physical detoxification also helps this mental process. Emotionally, detoxification helps us uncover and express feelings, especially hidden frustrations, anger, resentments, or fear, and replace them with forgiveness, love, joy, and hope; this then leads more easily to health and success. On a spiritual level, many people experience new clarity and/or an enhancement of their purpose of life during cleansing processes. A light detox over a couple of days can help us feel better, while a longer process and deeper commitment to a new way of life, such as eliminating certain abusive habits and eating a better diet, can help us really change our whole life.

An important topic discussed in *The New Detox Diet* (and a bit in chapter 11, Food and the Earth, on page 483) is **electromagnetic toxicity,** which has become so commonplace in these modern times with our daily exposure to computers, cell phones, and televisions, as well as radiation exposure from airplane travel and medical testing. In some ways, this persistent electrical interaction with our bodies may alter our sensitive cellular, biochemical, immune, and neurological systems. Our bodies are electric and clearly our cells and nerves function and communicate electrically. It makes sense that our bodies pick up and can be altered by these electrical interactions. Thus in addressing toxicity and detoxification, we should be aware of these electromagnetic issues as well. It is also quite possible that excessive electromagnetic stress affects the body's ability to naturally detoxify.

Detoxification is part of a transformational medicine that instills change on many levels. Change and evolution are keys to healing. Enhancing elimination helps us deal with and clear problems from our past— from childhood and parental patterns to recent job or relationship stress. When the body eliminates much of its toxic buildup, we feel lighter and are able to really experience the moment and be open for the future. Detoxification is a relative term. Anything that supports our elimination can be said to help us detoxify. Doing nothing more than drinking an extra quart of water a day helps us eliminate more toxins. Eating more fruits and vegetables—the high-water-content, cleansing foods—and less meat and milk products creates less congestion and more elimination. There are

Excess detox? I do have some concerns about overelimination or overdetoxification, which I see occasionally. Some people go to extremes with fasting, laxatives, enemas, colonics, diuretics, and even exercise and begin to lose essential nutrients. A negative balance can be created in this manner, such as protein or vitamin-mineral deficiencies, although congestion from overintake and underelimination is a more common problem in most modern cultures. I believe that the best and simplest way to perceive symptoms and disease is in terms of excess (congestion) and depletion (deficiency); this is the basis of the traditional Oriental philosophy, as with the idea of yin and yang (opposite energies). Excessive detoxification can be a concern; finding balance is the key for each of us. See *Staying Healthy with the Seasons* and/or *The New Detox Diet* for more information in this area.

> Elimination equals illumination.
> Reduce excesses, but not excessively.
>
> —Bethany Argisle

many levels of the progressive detoxification diets, from making these simple changes to undertaking complete fasting.

Who Should Detoxify?

Almost everyone needs to detox, cleanse themselves, and rest their body functions at times. Cleansing or detoxification is one part of the trilogy of nutritional action—the others being building (toning) and balance (maintenance). With a regular, balanced diet, devoid of excesses, we need less intensive detoxification. The body has a daily elimination cycle, mostly carried out at night and in the early morning, up until breakfast. When we eat a congesting diet higher in fats (such as meats, dairy products, refined foods, and chemicals), detoxification becomes more necessary. **Who needs to detoxify, and when, is based in part on individual lifestyle and needs, which provide clues for deciding how and when to detoxify.** If we have any symptoms or diseases of toxicity and congestion, we will likely benefit more from detoxification practices. It is a vacation for the body and the digestive tract.

More common toxicity symptoms include headache, fatigue, mucus problems, aches and pains, digestive problems, "allergy" symptoms, and sensitivity to such environmental agents as chemicals, perfumes, and synthetics. People who experience these and other symptoms may benefit from diet changes or avoidance of the drug or agent that may be influencing the symptom. It may be important to differentiate allergic symptoms from those of toxicity to determine the appropriate medical care. The diet and detox program outlined in this section is fairly similar to the plan for allergies discussed in chapter 17, Medicaul Treatment Programs (see page 704), and is often helpful in reducing allergic symptoms. The key is to figure out and avoid the allergens from the environment and from our foods. Most of my detox diet plans typically avoid the most common allergens. Fasting can be extremely beneficial for people with allergies. Of course, there may be subtle characteristics of toxicity that differentiate it from other health concerns.

Many common acute and chronic illnesses may be alleviated with a program of detoxification and cleansing, as they are basically created by short- and long-term congestive patterns. People with addictions to any substance may benefit from a detox program, even if it is only the temporary avoidance of the addictive agent or agents. Withdrawal symptoms that commonly occur with many drugs (including sugar, caffeine, and over-the-counter medications) are precipitated by detoxification. **With any serious drug detoxification, I recommend conscious, informed manage-**

Signs and Symptoms of Toxicity

Angina pectoris	Fever	Nausea
Anorexia	Frequent colds*	Nervousness
Anxiety	Headaches	Runny nose
Backaches	High blood fats	Sinus congestion
Bad breath	Hives	Skin rashes*
Circulatory deficits	Immune weakness*	Sleepiness*
Constipation	Indigestion	Sore throat
Cough	Insomnia*	Tight or stiff neck
Depression*	Irritated eyes	Wheezing
Dizziness*	Itchy nose	
Environmental sensitivity	Joint pains	
Fatigue*	Mood changes*	*These symptoms could also result from nutrient deficiencies.

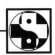

Problems Related to Congestion, Stagnation, and Toxicity

Abscesses	Drug addiction	Mental illness
Acne	Eczema	Migraine headaches
Allergies	Emphysema	Multiple sclerosis
Alzheimer's disease	Fibrocystic breast disease	Obesity
Arthritis	Gallstones	Pancreatitis
Asthma	Gastritis	Parkinson's disease
Atherosclerosis	Gout	Peptic ulcers
Boils	Heart disease	Pneumonia
Bronchitis	Hemorrhoids	Prostate disease
Cancer	Hepatitis	Senility
Cataracts	High cholesterol or triglycerides	Sinusitis
Cirrhosis	Hypertension	Stroke
Colds	Infections by bacteria, fungi,	Tension headaches
Colitis	parasites, viruses, and worms	Thrombophlebitis
Constipation	Kidney disease	Uterine fibroid tumors
Diabetes	Kidney stones	Vaginitis
Diverticulitis	Menstrual problems and PMS	Varicose veins

ment of the detox process by an experienced practitioner. Many of the poisons (toxins) that we ingest or make are stored in the fatty tissues. Obesity is almost always associated with toxicity. When we lose weight, we reduce our fat and thereby our toxic load. **During weight loss, we release more toxins, however, and thus need protection through greater intake of water, fiber, and the antioxidant nutrients, such as vitamins C, E, and beta-carotene, selenium, and zinc.** With exercise we can also turn fat into muscle (over time) and help further detoxification.

Of course, not all of these problems are solely problems of toxicity or completely cured by detoxification. Most of these diseases, and the majority of those factors, have to do with abuses, especially on a nutritional level. Often these problems, many of which are discussed in other sections of this book, are alleviated by eliminating the related toxins and following an appropriate detoxification program.

What Is Detoxification?

Detoxification is the process of clearing toxins from the body or neutralizing or transforming them, as well as clearing excess mucus and congestion. Many of these toxins come from diet, drug use, and environmental exposure, both acute and chronic. Internally, fats (especially oxidized fats and cholesterol), free radicals, and other irritating molecules act as toxins. **Functionally, poor digestion, colon sluggishness and dysfunction, reduced liver function, and poor elimination through the kidneys, respiratory tract, and skin all add to increased toxicity.**

Detoxification involves dietary and lifestyle changes that reduce intake of toxins and improve elimination. Avoidance of chemicals, from food or other sources, refined food, sugar, caffeine, alcohol, tobacco, and many drugs helps minimize the toxin load. Drinking extra water (purified) and increasing fiber by including more fruits and vegetables in the diet are steps in the detoxification process. The effects of dietary detoxification vary. Even mild changes from our current eating plan can produce some responses, while more dramatic dietary shifts can produce a profound cleansing. Shifting from the most congesting foods to the least—eating more fruits, vegetables, grains, nuts, and legumes as well as fewer baked goods, sweets, refined foods, fried foods, and fatty foods as the table on page 746 suggests—can help most of us detoxify somewhat and bring us into better overall balance.

<table>
<tr><th colspan="8" align="center">Most Congesting versus Least Congesting Foods</th></tr>
<tr><th colspan="3">Most Congesting ◄────
(MORE POTENTIALLY TOXIC)</th><th colspan="2"></th><th colspan="3">──────► Least Congesting
(MORE DETOXIFYING)</th></tr>
<tr><td>Drugs</td><td>Fats</td><td>Sweets</td><td>Nuts</td><td>Rice</td><td>Roots</td><td>Fruits</td></tr>
<tr><td>Allergenic foods</td><td>Fried foods</td><td>Milk</td><td>Seeds</td><td>Millet</td><td>Squashes</td><td>Greens</td></tr>
<tr><td>Organ meats</td><td>Refined flours</td><td>Baked goods</td><td>Oats</td><td>Pasta</td><td>Vegetables</td><td>Water</td></tr>
<tr><td>Hydrogenated fats</td><td>Meats</td><td></td><td>Wheat</td><td>Potatoes</td><td></td><td></td></tr>
</table>

Detoxification therapy—particularly fasting and juice cleansing—is the oldest known medical treatment on Earth and a completely natural process. Of the thousands of people I know who have used cleansing programs, the vast majority have experienced positive results. I believe this detoxification process to be a lay therapy for medicine in the twenty-first century and an important first step toward healing the planet. Those who live a healthy lifestyle and eat a more alkaline-based diet will not need to detoxify as often as those who do not. See the "Nontoxic Diet" on page 752. Simply increasing liquid intake and decreasing fats and refined-flour and sugar products will improve elimination and lessen toxin buildup. Increased consumption of filtered water, herb teas, fruits, and vegetables while reducing fats (especially fried foods, red meat, and milk products) will also help us detoxify. A vegetarian diet may be a healthful step for those with some congestive problems. Meats, milk products, breads, and baked goods (especially refined sugar and refined-carbohydrate products) increase body acidity and lead to more mucus production as the body attempts to balance its chemistry. The more alkaline vegetarian foods enhance cleansing. The right balance of acid and alkaline foods for each of us is, of course, the key to detoxification. (See page 394 in chapter 10, Nutritional Habits, and page 503 in chapter 12, The Components of a Healthy Diet, for more information on acid and alkaline.)

The acid-alkaline state is crucial to what scientists call the biological terrain of the body, or the state of the body's tissues and functions. I believe that this terrain affects whether we are healthy. Parasitic, fungal, and other infections are secondary to imbalances of the terrain; diet, stress levels, and other aspects of lifestyle can profoundly influence it. Because animal products, refined foods (sugars and flours), nuts, and seeds are more acidic in their chemical makeup, they create acid residues when metabolized in the body. They contain higher amounts of the minerals phosphorus, sulfur, chlorine, and iodine, while the more alkaline-generating foods contain higher levels of calcium, magnesium, potassium, and sodium. These include most high-water-content fruits and vegetables, as well as some grains and almonds.

From the tracking of body fluids (blood, urine, and saliva), acidic states appear in people with acute and chronic inflammatory and pain syndromes, congestive disorders that include recurrent infections and allergies, and degenerative diseases such as cancer, cardiovascular problems, and diabetes. Once these chronic degenerative diseases have set in, they are more difficult to treat or correct. When I have been able to assess and rebalance an individual's biochemistry, I have seen the lessening of symptoms, the halt of disease progression, and even the reversal of some conditions—and I have witnessed this with thousands of patients.

I want to talk about an important alternative use of the term *detoxification* that can play a helpful role in our understanding of nutrition and health. This use of the word is much more narrow and technical, more scientific and biochemical, than the one I have been using in this chapter thus far. Detoxification can also be used to refer to a specific set of metabolic processes that go on in the liver and other tissues (including our skin and our digestive tract) to neutralize toxins. I am talking about a strictly biochemical level here, where chemical substances get metabolized in the liver cells and other cells. Even though any substance can be toxic, substances that are fat soluble (many of the stronger chemicals) require special handling by our bodies. Because they are not water soluble, they cannot be

Acid-Alkaline: A Key to Health and Longevity

The concepts of congestion/toxicity and deficiency/depletion relate to the duality of balance that includes the acid-alkaline poles. The general ideas about illness and health addressed in this book relate to the relative states of acidity as well as the congestion, irritation, and inflammation that come from this imbalance. The body wants to be more alkaline for best overall health, which is another reason for consuming much more of the alkaline-forming fruits and vegetables and limiting the acid-forming protein foods, refined foods, chemicals, and nonessential fats. I believe the acidic body condition causes the breakdown and degeneration of tissues over time. The consumption of a diet based on animal products creates an acidic state of the tissues, with chronic toxicity as congestion, irritation, inflammation, and degeneration. The endpoint of this process is the many painful and terminal diseases people experience as they age.

My detox diet, initially referred to as the alkaline detoxification diet, consists of steamed vegetables and fresh fruits and water and alkaline drinks to help to balance the body and decrease these acid wastes. The body then lowers its inflammatory and pain states and begins to feel better, more flexible, and more youthful. A diet like this offers great biochemical balancing for the person consuming the typical Western diet—a diet that I have worked diligently to try to change both personally and professionally.

Because many toxins are derived from petroleum, they are fat-soluble and require phase I and II detoxification in the cells and the body. A wide range of toxic substances are included in this class, from food dyes to pesticides to solvent residues, and even to common food additives like sodium benzoate (a preservative). More important, this kind of cellular detoxification requires a constant supply of some specific nutrients. In phase I, these nutrients focus on the antioxidants like vitamin C and E, although other nutrients, like the B complex vitamins, branched-chain amino acids, and some flavonoids, are also important. In phase II, the focus shifts to a collection of molecules that can be easily tacked onto the toxin. Sulfur-containing molecules are especially important here, including glutathione and sulfur itself. Equally essential are the amino acid glycine, glucuronic acid, and a family of molecules known as *methyl donors*. This family includes choline, betaine, and s-adenosylmethionine (SAM, sometimes abbreviated SAM-e). Different clinics around the country specialize in cellular detoxification, and their protocols involve routine supplementation with many of the phase I and phase II nutrients. Perhaps two of the best known are the Environmental Health Center in Dallas, Texas, run by William Rea, MD, and the Institute for Functional Medicine in Gig Harbor, Washington, run by Drs. Jeffrey Bland, PhD, and David Jones, MD.

A simple yet universal way to think about detoxification connects (a bit metaphorically and mostly scientifically) the cell activities and the entire human body. Every day, every moment, the body breathes in air/oxygen and uses nutrients to perform its functions and stay healthy. This basic respiration and metabolism supports life and health. Similarly, nearly every cell in the body does these functions—taking in oxygen and essential nutrients from the blood and breathing out carbon dioxide (like our lungs do) and eliminating waste products (like our kidneys and colon do). This is the daily activity of detoxification that is being done by cells every moment of every day.

We also eat, sleep, and move in a world where our bodies are constantly asked to deal with millions of substances, and our cells must somehow remain themselves and pursue their own functions while at the same time interacting with and accommodating this overwhelming array of substances. They accomplish

eliminated as easily in the sweat or urine or breath. For easy elimination, all of these fat-soluble substances have to be made more water soluble. That is where cellular detox comes in. The cells use enzymes to help activate fat-soluble substances, and once they are activated, other molecules can be attached to them and render them fully water soluble. This two-step process of activation and combination with other molecules happens all the time in the cells. The activation step is usually called *phase I* of detoxification, and the combination step is usually called *phase II*.

Biochemical Detoxification

Phases	Function	Nutrients
Phase I	Activation/ Oxidation	Vitamins C, E, bioflavonoids, B- complex vitamins, glutathione, and branched-chain amino acids (leucine, isoleucine, and valine)
Phase II	Sulfation	Sulfur, in the form of methionine, cysteine, taurine, lipoic acid, glutathione, MSM (methylsulfonylmethane)
	Methylation	Choline, betaine, SAM/SAM-e, (s-adenosylmethionine), DMG (dimethyl-glycine), TMG (trimethylglycine), DMAE (dimethylaminoethanol)
	Glucuronidation	Glucuronic acid
	Glycination (hippuration)	Glycine
	Mercapturation	Glutathione (and NAC)
	Acetylation	Coenzyme A, pantethine

this amazing feat with the help of essential nutrients, and with elaborate procedures for detoxification of substances that could prove harmful. We keep eating, sleeping, breathing, and moving while our cells orchestrate all of the chemical details.

When Is the Best Time to Cleanse or Detoxify?

As we incorporate Nature's cycles with our own cycles, we may notice regular periods of congestion, and we may reduce or prevent these by following a more detoxifying program on a weekly, monthly, or seasonal basis. Whenever we feel congested, the first step is to follow detoxification procedures fine-tuned to our specific needs. I have found personally that when I start to feel congestion or a cold coming on, if I exercise and sweat, sauna or steam, drink loads of fluids, take vitamins C and A, and get a good night's sleep without eating much, almost every time I wake up healed! If I feel my colon requires further cleansing, I take stimulating, laxative-type herbs.

Each of us has a natural cleansing time when the body wants a lighter diet, more liquids, and greater elimination than intake. This occurs daily, usually in the night until midmorning; it may occur weekly but

more commonly for a few days a month. Women, in particular, are aware of this natural cleansing time with their female cycle. In fact, many women do much better premenstrually and during their periods if they follow a cleansing program—more juices, greens, lighter foods, herbs, and so on—in the week before their menstruation. The seasonal cycle is really the most important regarding natural detoxification periods. When we can harmonize with these periods and make appropriate adaptations, we do much to stay healthy. This relationship of the seasons to diet is discussed in other parts of this book as well as in greater detail in my first book, *Staying Healthy with the Seasons*. I explore this further in "Fasting and Juice Cleansing" (page 765).

The seasonal changes are the key stress times in Nature and the times when we most need to lighten up our outer demands and consumptions and turn more within to listen to our inner world, which mirrors the natural cycles. Spring is the key time for detoxification; autumn is also important. At least a 1- to 2-week program is suggested at these times. In spring, we may eat more citrus fruits, fresh greens, and juices or try the Master Cleanser (see page 778) lemonade diet. In autumn we may dine on other harvests, such as apples or grapes, and the many vegetables. An abundance of

Sample Yearlong Detox Program

Spring

For 7–21 days between March 10 and April 15 (or later in the cold or in the northern climates), use one or more of the following plans:

- Spring Master Cleanser (or the "lemonade diet," see page 778).
- Fruits, vegetables, and leafy greens, including blue-green algaes (spirulina, chlorella, and blue-green algae).
- Juices of fruits, vegetables, and greens.
- Herbs with any of the above.
- These plans can be alternated or can include a 3- to 5-day supervised water fast.
- Remember to take time for the transition back to the regular diet (about half as long as the fast itself), which hopefully will have changed for the better.
- Elimination and food testing can also be done at this time. Some people focus on getting off addictions to caffeine, sugar, wheat, dairy, ans so on, to see how they feel, and then later, they can assess what happens when they retry these items—if they even choose to.

Midspring

Take a 3-day cleanse around mid-May as a reminder of healthy habits and as an enhancer of food awareness.

Summer

Try 1 week of fruits and vegetables and/or fresh juices to usher in the warm weather sometime between June 10 and July 4.

Late Summer

Take a 3-day cleanse of fruit and vegetable juices around mid- to late August.

Autumn

Take a 7- to 10-day cleanse between September 11 and October 5, such as:

- Grape fast—whole and juiced—all fresh and preferably organic.
- Apple and lemon juice together, diluted.
- Fresh fruits and vegetables, raw and cooked.
- Fruit and vegetable juices—fruit in the morning, vegetables in the afternoon.
- Juices plus spirulina, algae, or other green chlorophyll powders.
- Whole grains, cooked squashes, and other vegetables (a lighter detox).
- Mixture of the above plans, with garlic as a prime detoxifier.
- Basic low-toxicity diet, with an additional herbal program.
- Colon detox with fiber (psyllium, pectin, and so on), along with enemas or colonics.
- Prepare and plan a new autumn diet, enhancing positive dietary habits.
- An alternative program is to take 3 weeks to change habits by letting go of certain habits, such as the use of sugar or caffeine, or some overconsumed foods that might include dairy and wheat products, corn and corn syrup, or soy to see how you feel, drop weight and some symptoms, and improve overall health.

Midautumn

Take a 3-day cleanse with juices or in-season produce in late October to early November.

Winter

A lighter diet, eaten for 1 or 2 weeks in preparation for the holidays (or as detox from them) can be done between December 10 and January 5.

- Avoid toxins and treats; eat a basic wholesome diet.
- One week of brown rice, cooked vegetables, miso broth, and seaweed. Ginger and cayenne pepper can be used in soups.
- Saunas or steams and massage—you deserve it!
- Hang on until spring!

fresh fruits and vegetables is appropriate when we are going into summer; and legumes, vegetables, soups, and whole grains like brown rice may best simplify our diet in winter.

The "Sample Yearlong Detox Program" on page 749 is designed for a basically healthy person who eats well. It is not appropriate for people with heart problems, extreme fatigue, underweight conditions, or poor circulation (those who experience coldness). More complete, in-depth fasting programs may release even greater amounts of toxins (see "Fasting and Juice Cleansing" on page 769). **Releasing too much toxicity can make sick people sicker; if this happens, they need to increase fluids and eat normally again until they feel better.** People with cancer need to be careful about how they detoxify, and often they need regular, quality nourishment. Fasting should be done only under the care of an experienced physician, usually one who is naturopathically trained—this could be a medical doctor (MD), doctor of osteopathy (DO), naturopathic doctor (ND), doctor of chiropractic (DC), and more. All people should avoid fasting just before surgery and should wait 4 to 6 weeks after surgery before fasting or any strenuous detoxifying. Pregnant or lactating women should avoid heavy detoxification, although they can usually handle mild programs, which should be undertaken only with the guidance of a qualified practitioner.

Where Can We Detoxify?

My focus is to help people detoxify in the midst of their everyday lives, with work, kids, relationships, whatever. When they do this they see that they can make it work within the framework of "real life." Of course, there are many wonderful retreats and spas for detoxification and cleansing programs, and these places make it easier to follow a program and experience results. (And it may be simpler to begin programs, even home programs, when we have at least a few days of less demands.) However, for many I observe, it is quite difficult to take this new lifestyle home with them. Since the most important part of a good program is the follow-through and long-term life change that happens with diet and exercise, putting this into practice in our home world is the ultimate goal.

During basic, simple detoxification programs, most of us can maintain a normal daily routine. In fact, energy, performance, and health often improve. For some, however, the detox process may produce headaches, fatigue, irritability, mucous congestions, or aches and pains for the first few days. Any of the symptoms of toxicity may appear, although usually they do not. Symptoms that have been experienced previously may recur transiently during detoxification; sometimes it is hard to know whether to treat them. Because my approach to medicine is to allow the body to heal itself, I support the natural healing process whenever possible unless the person is uncomfortable or the practitioner is concerned.

It is wise to begin new programs, diets, or lifestyle changes with a few days at home. In time, experience will show what works best. Most of us can maintain a regular work schedule during a cleanse or detox program (and we may even be more productive). However, it might be easier to begin a program on a Friday, as the first few days are usually the hardest. Some of us may be more sensitive during cleansing to the stress of our work environment or to chemical exposures or to relationship challenges. Also, coworkers or family members may provide temptations or challenge our decisions. Having supportive guides or co-cleansers can be a great comfort and source of positive reinforcement when our inner resolve begins to fade. At the end of the first or second day, usually around dinnertime, symptoms like headache and fatigue may begin to appear, and it is good to be able to rest and spend time in familiar, undemanding surroundings. By the third day, we usually feel pretty stable and ready for work, already feeling a bit lighter in our own body. So, day 3 is often the beginning of that cleansing (and healthy, vital) feeling.

Many people like to start new programs on a Monday, knowing that they will do fine, using willpower and visualization to see themselves through. People often feel better than ever and are able to accomplish tasks and meet challenges more easily than usual. In fact, experienced fasters may use fasting during busy work periods to improve their productivity. Preparing and planning, clearing doubts and fears, and keeping a daily journal are all useful during this vital process and are crucial to any successful undertaking.

Why Detoxify?

We detoxify and cleanse for health, vitality, and rejuvenation—to clear symptoms, treat disease, and prevent future problems. A cleansing program is an ideal way to help us reevaluate our lives, make changes, or clear abuses and addictions. Withdrawal happens fairly rapidly, and as cravings are reduced we can begin a new life without the addictive habits or drugs. I cleanse because it makes me feel more vital, creative, and open to emotional and spiritual energies (and because I love to eat and need to balance at times). Many people detox (or, more commonly, fast on water or juices) for spiritual renewal and to feel more alive, awake, and aware. Jesus Christ, Paramahansa Yogananda, Mahatma Ghandi, Dr. Martin Luther King, and many other spiritual and religious teachers have advocated fasting for spiritual and physical health. Detoxification can also be helpful for weight loss, although this is not its primary purpose. I think cleansing is more important as an overall lifestyle and dietary transition. However, just the simplification of the diet can have some detoxifying effects in the body. Anyone eating 4,000 calories daily of fatty, sweet foods in a poorly balanced diet, who begins to eat 2,000 to 2,500 calories daily of more wholesome foods will definitely experience detoxification, weight loss, and improved health simultaneously.

We also cleanse and detoxify to rest or heal our overloaded digestive organs and allow them to catch up on past work and get current. At the same time, we are inspired to cleanse our external life as well, cleaning out rooms, sorting through the piles on our desks, clarifying our personal priorities, or revitalizing our wardrobes. Most often our energy is increased and becomes steadier, motivating us to change both internally and externally.

How Do We Detoxify and Cleanse?

I have already touched on a few ways to detoxify throughout this section, but the remainder focuses on general and specific diet plans, other activities, and supplements, including vitamins, minerals, amino acids, and herbs, to aid in this healing process. There are many levels to this part of the program. The first is to eat a nontoxic diet. When we do this regularly, we have less need for cleansing. If we have not been eating this way, we should detoxify first and then make permanent changes.

Another aspect of the nontoxic diet is avoiding drugs—over-the-counter, prescription, and recreational types—and substituting natural remedies, such as nutrients, herbs, and homeopathic medicines, all of which have fewer side effects. Other natural therapies, such as acupuncture, massage, and chiropractic care may help in treating some problems so that we will not need drugs for them. Avoiding or minimizing exposure to chemicals at home and work is also important. This lessens the total toxic load. Substituting natural cleansers, cosmetics, and clothes for synthetic and chemically based ones is helpful. There are many suggestions for these areas of life in chapter 11, Food and the Earth, and in the "88 Survival Suggestions" on page 785 in the Futureword.

The effects of detoxification diets may vary. Even mild changes from our current plan may produce some responses, while more dramatic dietary shifts can produce a profound cleansing. Shifting from the most congesting foods to the least (see table on page 746)—eating more fruits, vegetables, grains, nuts, and legumes and fewer baked goods, sweets, refined foods, fried foods, and fatty foods—will help most of us detoxify somewhat and bring us into better balance, with more vitalized cells, organs, and body.

Benefits from Cleansing

Prevent disease	To be more:
Reduce symptoms	Organized
Treat disease	Creative
Cleanse body	Motivated
Rest organs	Productive
Purification	Relaxed
Rejuvenation	Energetic
Weight loss	Clear
Clear skin	Conscious
Slow aging	Inwardly attuned
Improve flexibility	Spiritual
Improve fertility	Environmentally attuned
Enhance the senses	Relationship focused

The Nontoxic Diet

- **Eat** organic foods whenever possible.
- **Drink** filtered water.
- **Rotate** foods, especially common allergens, such as milk products, eggs, wheat, and yeast foods.
- **Practice** food combining.
- **Eat** natural, seasonal, and local cuisine.
- **Include** fruits, vegetables, whole grains, legumes, nuts and seeds, and, for omnivarians, some low-fat dairy products as well as fresh fish (not shellfish) and organic poultry.
- **Cook** in iron, stainless steel, glass, or porcelain.
- **Avoid** or minimize red meats, cured meats, organ meats, refined foods, canned foods, sugar, salt, saturated fats, coffee, alcohol, and nicotine.
- **Avoid** toxic relationships and toxic media.

Maintaining the same diet but adding certain supplements can also stimulate detoxification. Fiber, vitamin C, other antioxidants, chlorophyll, and glutathione, mainly as the amino acid L-cysteine, will all help (see the nutritional supplement program on page 768 following this discussion). Such herbs as garlic, red clover, echinacea, or cayenne may also induce some detoxification. Saunas, sweats, and niacin therapy have been used to cleanse the body. Simply increasing liquids and decreasing fats will shift the balance strongly toward improved elimination and less toxin buildup. Increased consumption of filtered water, herb teas, fruits, and vegetables and reducing fats, especially most fried food, red meats, and milk products will also help detoxification. This is a more structured, basic diet, but for most average Westerners, it is a major shift to a cleaner diet. A vegetarian diet would also be a healthful step toward detoxification for those with some congestive problems. In general, moving from an acid-generating diet to a more alkaline one will aid the process of detoxification. Acid-forming foods, such as meats, milk products, breads and baked goods, and especially refined-sugar and refined-carbohydrate products, will increase body acidity and lead to more mucus production and congestion to attempt to balance the body chemistry, whereas the more alkaline,

wholesome vegetarian foods enhance cleansing and clarity in the body. The right balance of acid and alkaline foods for each of us is, of course, the key. Review the above discussion on page 746 on acid-alkaline eating.

For most people, a simple detoxifying diet is made up exclusively of fresh fruits, fresh vegetables (either raw or steamed or roasted), and whole grains (both cooked and sprouted), plus some raw seeds or sprouted seeds or legumes, eaten fresh in salads. No breads or baked goods, animal foods or dairy products, alcohol, or nuts are used. This diet keeps fiber and water intake up and hence helps colon detoxification. Most people can handle this quite easily and make the shift from their regular diet with only a few days' transition. Others might prefer a brown rice cleansing diet (a more macrobiotic approach) for 1 or 2 weeks, eating 3 to 4 bowls of rice daily along with such liquids as green or herbal teas. Vegetable and miso soups can also be consumed, and I would add leafy green vegetables, both raw and steamed.

An even deeper level of detoxification involves a diet consisting solely of fruits and vegetables—all cleansing foods. The green vegetables, especially the chlorophyllic and high-nutrient leafy greens, support purification of the gastrointestinal tract. Another fulfilling detox diet is the raw foods diet, which yields high energy and quality nutrition. It uses sprouted greens from seeds and grains such as wheat, buckwheat, sunflower, alfalfa, and clover; sprouted beans such as mung or garbanzo; soaked or sprouted raw nuts; and fresh fruits and vegetables. Cooked food is not allowed with this diet, as eating foods raw maintains the highest concentrations of vitamins, minerals, and important enzymes. Many people feel that this is their best diet, and it can be supportive over quite some time if it is properly balanced. Most people tolerate this diet better in the warmer weather or tropical climates.

Detox-healing diets are also available, specifically for such problems as yeast overgrowth or food allergies. See chapter 17, Medical Treatment Programs, for an antiyeast diet (page 698) and an antiallergy (hypoallergenic) diet (page 704). They involve aspects of detoxification and balance. The liquid cleanses or fasts move beyond the alkalinizing detoxification and fruit-and-vegetable diets. Juices, vegetable broths, and teas can be used to purify the body during fasting. Miso soup, made from a paste of fermented soybeans, also provides many nutrients and supports colon function by aiding the intestinal bacteria. Spirulina (an algae powder) or other blue-green freshwater algae can also be helpful to fasters who experience fatigue by providing amino acids for protein building (add to juices for best flavor).

Water fasting is more intense than fasting with juices, and often results in more sickness and less energy. Paavo Airola, one of the pioneers of fasting in America, has written in his book *How to Get Well*, "Systematic undereating and periodic fasting are the two most important health and longevity factors." **I do not recommend water fasting other than under direct medical supervision.** However, consuming fresh as well as diluted juices from various fruits and vegetables can be a safe and helpful approach for many conditions. Juices help to eliminate wastes and dead cells while building new tissue with the easily accessible nutrients. Review "Fasting and Juice Cleansing" (page 769) for more information.

The key to proper treatment is to individualize your program. For example, in my practice I look at the patient's general health, physiological balance, energy level, and current lifestyle in order to set up the right program. If you are unsure, start with the basic diet and

---

The Levels of Dietary Detoxification

- Basic diet.
- Reduce toxins daily, ingesting fewer congesting foods and more nourishing ones (see table on page 746); for example, decrease drugs, sugar, fried foods, meats, dairy, and so on. Take 1 to 7 days.
- Fruits, vegetables, whole grains, seeds, and legumes.
- Raw foods.
- Fruits and vegetables.
- Fruit and vegetable juices.
- Specific juice diets, the Master Cleanser (see page 778 for the recipe), apple, carrot, and greens, and so on.
- Water.

---

gradually intensify toward juice fasting and see how you feel. Take a couple of days for each step, and if you feel fine, move to the next level as described below in "The Levels of Dietary Detoxification."

SNACC Detoxification—Clearing Sugar, Nicotine, Alcohol, Caffeine, and Chemicals

As I stated in the introduction to this chapter, the most common and consistent toxins/irritants/stressors that many of us have the biggest problems with are our self-chosen exposures, the SNACCs. And that's mostly because we do them so much and with such daily consistency. Sugar and caffeine are definitely the most common stimulating habits for much of the world. And for many, ranging from young to old, these two substances become abuses and even addictive when used on a daily basis to function. When this level of intake is so great, not having regular caffeine or sugary foods makes people feel sick. In this case it often takes a few days to go through minor withdrawals before they start to feel better and more balanced.

Alcohol and nicotine are the next level of problematic substances, with many more symptoms of excessive, habitual use. Alcohol is used more socially and not everyone who drinks does so excessively. When we begin to drink every day, or we need alcohol to get through the days and our difficulties, it becomes a problem. Help may often be required. Nicotine is its own story. People who smoke become addicted very easily. As much as the tobacco industry would still love to deny the addictive nature of nicotine intake, medical practitioners like myself, and therapists who work with behavior, know how difficult it is for people to free themselves from tobacco addiction.

The use of drugs for health problems is commonplace these days; increased advertising and mass drug pushing by the powerful pharmaceutical industry is supported by the medical profession and the whole Western medical approach. We so easily turn to over-the-counter medicines and prescriptions to deal with health issues rather than pursue an integrated medical approach of sorting out and addressing the underlying causes for the whys and wherefores of these problems, which often come from dietary choices, lack of exercise or sleep, excessive stress, and our emotional states—and from the drugs that we are taking. Addressing lifestyle first, and then working with natural remedies before drugs unless we are acutely ill, where drug medicine has its most effective and important use, is a wiser way to approach health care. I discuss this briefly a few pages above, and I've included a small chart of some of the natural medicine substitutes, taken from *The New Detox Diet,* to help guide you in alternative—or really common sense—and traditional medical approaches to improved health. I encourage you to try a natural remedy the next time you experience a problem, unless of course, you believe your condition to be serious or dangerous. Many of the common problems can be lessened or prevented with detoxification programs and nutritional/herbal supplements.

SUGAR

For most of us, sugar is a symbol of love and nurturance because as infants, our first food is mother's milk, which contains lactose, or milk sugar. Overconsumption and daily use of sugar is the first compulsive habit for most everyone with addictions later in life. Simple sugar, or glucose, is what our body, our cells, and our brain use as fuel for energy. Yet, most of us use it too much, and the problem is more with the refined sugars and the more recent high-fructose corn syrup, which I believe is the greatest factor in the obesity epidemic. I sense the body does not use it as readily and turns more of it into fat.

Sugar and sweeteners have so pervaded our food manufacturing and restaurant industries that it is almost impossible to find prepackaged products that are unsweetened. Consequently, the only way to avoid sweeteners is to avoid packaged products whenever possible. Fruits contain natural fructose, in balance with other nutrients; honey and maple syrup are more highly concentrated natural sugars and are appropriate for most of us in moderation.

Sugar and Health

Many nutritional authorities feel that the high use of sugar in our diet is a significant underlying cause of disease. Too much sweetener in any form can have a negative effect on our health; this includes not only refined sugar, but also corn syrup, honey, and fruit juices, and treats such as sodas, cakes, and candies. Because sugary foods satisfy our hunger, they often replace more nutritious foods and weaken our tissues' health and disease resistance.

A quick look at the yearly statistics gives the impression that we are eating fewer sweets, because our sugar consumption has dropped from about 100 pounds per person to 64. Sounds good. However, our yearly intake of corn sweeteners has gone from about 20 pounds per person to more than 80. Our total intake of sweeteners is now about 150 pounds a year per person—almost 0.5 pound of sweets per day.

Reducing sweeteners in our diet is a very real, positive step each of us can take. It requires an effort, but reducing our dietary load of sugar and sweeteners is of key importance for our health and our children's health.

And the main artificial sweeter, aspartame (NutraSweet), is not a worthy replacement. This substance can be a neurological irritant and can affect users' mood and energy. I have seen many people who do not tolerate this nonsugar sweetener, much like the common reaction to MSG (monosodium glutamate, the flavor enhancer used commonly in Chinese cooking).

Sorbitol may be better tolerated and safer. However, alcohol sweeteners such as sorbitol and mannitol are not well absorbed by the intestines so they may cause gas and loose stools. Stevia is a natural, alternative sweetener that is now widely available. At present it remains an unapproved food additive according to the FDA and is therefore found only in pure form, as a powder or liquid extract and is identified as a dietary supplement. However, it is an herb that most diabetics can use without risk of raising blood sugar levels. There is continuing debate over the health safety of stevia, but the research so far is much less alarming than the research on other currently legal food additives, like saccharin.

Sugar Detox

Although sugar addiction is common, sugar withdrawal is usually physically mild, with periodic strong cravings. The most difficult part for many is making the decision to stop sugar use, and this is because of the emotional attachments to sugar. For those who are sensitive to refined sugar or sweeteners, or who consume it in large amounts, genuine symptoms of abuse and withdrawal may also occur. Some of these symptoms include fatigue, anxiety and irritability, depression and detachment, rapid heart rate and palpitations, and poor sleep. Most symptoms, if they do occur, last only a few days.

We can decide to cut down on or eliminate sugar quite easily by simply avoiding many of the sweet foods. There are plenty of nutritious nibbles to replace sugary snacks or treats—review the chart below for suggestions. We should clear our cupboards of unhealthy sweetened foods. Once sugar has been removed from the diet, it is still possible to use it once in a while, as it is not as re-addicting as many stronger drugs. Most people who have kicked the sugar habit find that they no longer tolerate sugar very well.

Problems Associated with Sugar Intake*

- Tooth decay
- Obesity and its increased risk of diabetes, cancer, and other diseases
- Nutritional deficiency—including anemia and protein and mineral deficiencies
- Hypoglycemia and carbohydrate imbalance
- Chronic dyspepsia and digestive problems
- Immune dysfunction and problems such as recurrent infections
- Menstrual irregularities and premenstrual symptoms (PMS)
- Yeast overgrowth and its many subsequent problems, including craving sweets and carbohydrates
- Hyperactivity and difficulty concentrating
- Alcoholism—a potential link as it is associated with hypoglycemia and abnormal carbohydrate metabolism
- Mood swings, anxiety, depression
- Heart disease

*There is much evidence that eating too many sweets eventually causes disease. If these conditions occur in either your personal or family history, it is important to seriously consider a dietary change for your health's sake.

Good Foods to Replace Sugar Treats

Fresh fruit	Vegetable sticks	Granola (unsweetened)	Salads
Yogurt*	Popcorn	Almonds	Peanuts
Almond butter	Peanut butter	Mixed nuts	Sunflower seeds
Protein smoothies	Edamame (soy)	Pumpkin seeds	Muesli (unsweetened)

* Plain yogurt without the sweeteners is a healthful snack. Fresh fruit can be added along with seasonings such as vanilla, cinnamon, or nutmeg. If dried fruits, such as raisins, are used, consuming them with a few nuts or seeds makes the snack less sugary and lower on the glycemic index.

A diet that is rich in whole grains and other complex carbohydrates, vegetables, and protein foods can also help stabilize blood sugar and minimize the desire for sugar. Many people who are protein-deficient seem to crave sugars and carbohydrate foods. Conversely, eating a diet that focuses on protein and vegetables is a good way to minimize sugar cravings. If you don't tolerate sugars and sweet foods well, fruits should also be minimized and fruit juice avoided.

There are many nutrients that can help reduce sugar craving and the symptoms of sugar withdrawal. These include the B vitamins, vitamin C, zinc, the trace mineral chromium, and the amino acid L-glutamine. Chromium is the central molecule of glucose tolerance factor, which helps insulin work more efficiently in removing sugar from the blood and nourishing the cells. L-glutamine, which can be used directly by the brain, is also helpful in reducing sugar (and alcohol) cravings. A specific nutrient program can be found in *The New Detox Diet*.

Children can also benefit from a nutritional supplement program that includes some of the nutrients mentioned, of course in lower dosages than for adults. Use of a good quality children's multi-vitamin/mineral, additional B vitamins to support the nervous system and general development, vitamin C at about 250 mg twice daily, and extra chromium (50–100 mcg 1–2 times daily) all help to minimize sugar cravings and to transition from sugar and sweetened foods. The supplement plan for children applies to ages 6 to 11; amounts may vary from less to more depending on the age and size of the child. These vitamins are water soluble and basically nontoxic. However, if your child has a special problem or is below the age of 6, you should check with your pediatrician or health-care provider for specific recommendations.

The use of sugar in our culture sometimes resembles the use of a drug, and can be treated as such. Make a clear plan for withdrawal, while working emotionally to eliminate the habit. Responses to flavors, certain food compulsions, and the feelings we get from them are usually conditioned. Self-reflection can be valuable. To change our habits, to stop and see things clearly, or to talk them through helps us transition from compulsion to the safe and balanced use of foods, sugar, and sweetened foods, as well as other substances we may use in our life.

NICOTINE

Cigarette smoking, our primary method of using nicotine, is the single greatest cause of preventable disease and probably creates the most difficult addiction to deal with. The statistics are shocking: Worldwide, 2.5 million people a year die of tobacco-related diseases. In the United States alone, cigarette smoking causes over 1,000 deaths per day and is responsible for about 25% of cancer deaths and 30% to 40% of coronary heart disease deaths.

It also increases the incidence of atherosclerosis, strokes, and peripheral vascular disease. Diseases of the respiratory tract—colds, acute bronchitis, pneumonia, chronic obstructive pulmonary diseases (COPD) such as emphysema and chronic bronchitis, and lung cancer—are all more common in smokers. Infections and allergies are also prevalent in smokers, as is rapid aging of the body, especially facial skin, which results from the poor oxygenation of tissues and other associated chemical effects.

The addiction of many children to cigarettes is the saddest part of the nicotine story. We must insist on more stringent laws to better regulate sales and

High Risk Smokers

Pregnant women

Nursing mothers

Diabetics

Women using birth control pills

Those with family history of heart disease

People with high blood pressure

People with high cholesterol

Heavy smokers

Obese people

Very thin people

Alcoholics or alcohol abusers (daily users)

People with existing smoker's diseases

People who work with toxic chemicals

People having surgery

Ulcer patients

Type A personalities

Problems Associated with Smoking

Cough	Allergies	Cancers
Hoarseness	Rhinitis/sinusitis	lung
Headaches	Lowered immunity	mouth and tongue
Anxiety	Other infections	larynx
Fatigue	Blood disorders	esophagus
Leg pains	Nutrient deficiencies	bladder
Cold hands and feet	Acute bronchitis	cervix
Memory loss	Chronic bronchitis	pancreas
Senility	Emphysema	kidney
Alzheimer's disease	Increased cholesterol	Surgical complications
Rapid skin aging	Atherosclerosis	Increased pregnancy risks
Teeth and finger stains	Hypertension	Increased infant mortality
Periodontal disease	Angina pectoris	Burns from fires
Low libido	Circulation insufficiency	Increased caffeine use
Impotence	Heart and artery disease	Increased alcohol use
Heartburn	Heart attacks and strokes	More job and home changes
Peptic ulcers	Varicose veins	Higher insurance and
Hiatal hernia	Osteoporosis	medical fees

advertising, along with better education to help curtail this problem. Chewing tobacco is also of concern.

The highly addictive nature of nicotine is revealed by the fact that many strong-minded and strong-willed people cannot stop smoking, even if they are otherwise health conscious. Over 80% of smokers say that they want to stop. In my years working in hospitals, I saw lung cancer and emphysema patients smoking between ventilator treatments and patients with tubes in their necks from tracheostomies putting cigarettes into the tubes to inhale.

How Do We Detoxify from Nicotine?

A detoxifying diet to help the body be more alkaline supports the elimination of smoking toxins and reduces cravings. A more acidic diet causes more nicotine cravings See the chart on page 758 for information on acid-alkaline foods and *The New Detox Diet* for a more complete nicotine detox program. A good air filter is also an important preventive measure and can be very effective in removing toxins from the air; a

basic multiple vitamin-mineral and antioxidant formula will help protect us internally. The daily program should include a simple nutrient plan, such as in the following chart.

Smoker's Simple Nutrient Plan

Vitamin C	1,000–2,000 mg, up to 6–8 grams daily
Mixed carotenoids*	15,000–25,000 IU, up to 50,000 IU
Vitamin A	5,000–10,000 IU
Zinc	15–30 mg
Selenium	200 mcg
Vitamin E	400 IU

* Even though beta-carotene did not fare well in recent studies for smokers when used solely, I believe its action within a complete antioxidant formula is still warranted based on a number of other positive studies. Here, the mixed carotenoids are likely more helpful.

Stop-Smoking Diet

Increase Alkaline Foods		Reduce Acid Foods	
Eat more:		Eat less:	
fruits	figs	meats	beef
vegetables	raisins	sugar	chicken
greens	carrots	wheat	eggs
lima beans	celery	bread	milk
millet	almonds	baked goods	cheese

10 Suggestions for Helping with Smoking Cessation

1. **Cut down on other addictive substances,** such as caffeine, sugar, and alcohol, all of which can increase the desire to smoke.
2. **Get another smoker to stop** with you or, even better, get an ex-smoker to support you while you stop.
3. **Tell empathetic friends or family** and ask for their support—that is, go public with your plan to stop.
4. **Stay busy** to prevent boredom and to keep your mind off smoking.
5. **Exercise regularly** to decrease withdrawal, increase motivation, and increase relaxation. Include your favorite aerobic sport and try to do it outdoors.
6. **Create rewards** for being successful and implement them daily.
7. **Get plenty of rest.**
8. **Drink fluids** and use water for therapy by taking showers, baths, saunas, or hot tubs, or by going swimming.
9. **Change daily patterns** to avoid stimulating old smoking conditioning. This may include staying away from bars, alcohol, and coffee, and avoiding friends who smoke.
10. **If cravings arise,** find ways to deal with them: Take a short break, a walk, or a shower, drink tea, or do things with your hands, such as sketching or doodling, working a crossword puzzle, or making a shopping list. Breathe and relax, and be thankful you are not smoking.

ALCOHOL

Even though alcohol is enjoyed worldwide and has been used for thousands of years, its regular overconsumption poses a serious health hazard. As with caffeine, occasional or moderate use is often pleasurable and is no cause for concern except for people with allergic reactions to alcohol or diseases of the liver, gastrointestinal tract, kidneys, brain, or nervous system. Habitual alcohol overconsumption, however, can lead to addiction, emotional problems, and a number of specific degenerative processes including obesity, gastritis and ulcers, hepatitis, cirrhosis, pancreatitis, hypoglycemia and diabetes, gout, nerve and brain dysfunction, cancer, nutritional deficiencies, immune suppression, accidental injury, and death.

Alcohol does have some positive physiological effects. It stimulates the appetite and relieves stress, although not as much as exercise. It acts as a vasodilator, improving blood flow. Alcohol may also effect a slight increase in HDL "good" cholesterol levels; however, it also raises total blood fats. Small to moderate amounts (1–2 drinks daily) may also lessen the progression of atherosclerosis and heart disease. Some studies have shown a lower number of heart attacks in moderate drinkers over nondrinkers of the same age, possibly due to increased HDL cholesterol levels, and reduced atherosclerosis. Higher amounts of alcohol, however, increase blood pressure and heart disease risk. More research is needed to understand the real link between alcohol and heart disease before prescribing it as a preventative measure. Certainly, regular physical activity and nurturing personal relationships are better health supporters and stress reducers than alcohol.

Calorie Content of Alcoholic Beverages

Amount to Provide about 0.5 oz of Alcohol	Type of Beverage	Calories
1 oz	100 or 110 proof liquor	80
1.5 oz	80 proof liquor	90–110
5 oz	8% to 10% wine (French, German)	100–125
4 oz	12% to 14% wine (most American)	95
3 oz	17% to 20% wine (sherry, port)	80
2.5 oz	18% dessert wine	120
8 oz	6% to 7% dark beer (stout, porter)	150
12 oz	4.5% regular beer	140
12 oz	light beer	90
6 oz	mixed drinks (various juices, sodas, sweeteners)	100–250

Source: USDA National Nutrient Database for Standard Reference, Release 18 (2005), Agricultural Research Service, Beltsville, Maryland, and other standardized nutrient databases. Average estimates based upon the USDA National Nurient Database.

Risks of Alcohol

The risk levels of alcohol are directly related to the amount consumed and the time period over which it is used, although individual reactions may vary. High-risk use involves more than 5 drinks daily; moderate-risk use, 3 to 5 drinks daily; and low-risk, 1 or 2. Social drinking of a few drinks a week offers minimal risk.

Those with diabetes, hypertension, or heart disease, and pregnant or nursing mothers, or those planning pregnancy should not drink alcohol at all. People with blood sugar problems, liver disorders (especially hepatitis), ulcers and gastritis, viral diseases, yeast problems, mental confusion, fatigue, or hypersensitive reactions to alcoholic beverages should also avoid it.

- **Symptoms from drinking** include dizziness, delayed reflexes, slowed mental functions, memory loss, poor judgment, emotional outburst, aggressive behavior, lack of coordination, and loss of consciousness.

- **Symptoms of hangover** include mouth dryness, thirst, headache, throbbing temples, nausea, vomiting, stomach upset, fatigue, and dizziness. Alcohol dehydrates the cells, removes fluid from the blood, swells the cranial arteries, and irritates the gastrointestinal tract. Hangovers are more common with stronger, distilled alcohol drinks but can still occur with red and white wines, champagne, and beer.

- **Symptoms of withdrawal** include alcohol craving, nausea, vomiting, gastrointestinal upset, abdominal cramps, anorexia, fatigue, headache, anxiety, irritability, dizziness, fevers, chills, depression, insomnia, tremors, weakness, hallucinations, and seizures.

- **Drinking can put us at risk** of inadvertently harming ourselves or others. Alcohol is involved in the more than 25,000 auto accidents deaths yearly. About 20% of home accidental deaths are attributed to alcohol.

- **Since alcohol converts to fat,** obesity (especially abdominal obesity, the most dangerous area) also often occurs with high alcohol use.

- **95% of alcohol consumed must be metabolized** in the liver, taking precedence over other functions. Fat metabolism slows and fat builds up in the liver.

- **Chronic use can swell, scar, and shrink the liver** until only a small percentage is functional. Complications also include ascites (fluid build-up in the abdomen), hemorrhoids, varicose veins, and bleeding disorders. More serious liver disease such as hepatitis and cirrhosis, when the liver becomes inflamed or enlarged, are also the result of chronic alcohol use. Usually more than half the liver must be destroyed before its work is significantly impaired (but it can regenerate if drinking is stopped).

- **Gastrointestinal disorders** include gastritis, abdominal pain, eating difficulties, gastric ulcers, duodenal ulcers, deficiency of hydrochloric acid and digestive enzymes, "leaky gut" syndrome, esophagitis (irritation of the esophagus), varicose veins, pancreatitis, gallstones, and gallbladder disease.

- **Nervous system disorders,** including polyneuritis (nerve inflammations), premature senility, and encephalopathy (chronic degenerative brain syndrome) can also result from chronic alcohol use.

- **Alcohol intake and abuse** is damaging to the heart and blood vessels and leads to cardiovascular diseases and dysfunctions. These include a decrease in heart function, heart muscle action, and electrical conductivity, congestive heart failure, cardiac arrythmias, and an enlarged heart.

- **Carbohydrate metabolism** is affected by alcohol and can lead to hypoglycemia and diabetes. Alcohol is a simple sugar that is rapidly absorbed and has a tendency to weaken glucose tolerance with chronic use. Impaired glucose metabolism can cause mood swings, depression, emotional outbursts, or anxiety. Furthermore, increased calories from alcohol can lead to weight gain and increased body fat resulting in obesity as alcohol converts to fat unless it is balanced by exercise and a good diet.

- **Nutritional deficiencies** from alcohol use potentially include impaired absorption of nutrients, particularly B vitamins and minerals; liver impairment from reduced absorption of the fat-soluble vitamins A, D, E, and K; loss of nutrients like potassium and magnesium from alcohol's diuretic effect; reduced liver stores of alcohol-metabolizing vitamins B_1 and B_3; anemia due to deficiency of folic acid, vitamin B_{12}, and iron; increased risk of osteoporosis from low vitamin D and poor calcium absorption; lack of appetite, causing deficiencies in vitamin B_2, B_6, A, and C, essential fatty acids, methionine, or really any nutrient that comes from a good and wholesome diet.

- **Alcohol increases levels of the liver enzyme** that breaks down testosterone. In teenage boys, the reduction of testosterone may delay sexual maturity. Alcohol's depressant effect on the nervous system can reduce sexual performance or cause impotence despite reduced inhibitions and increased desire.

- **Alcohol has been implicated in malignancies** of the mouth, esophagus, pancreas, and breasts.

- **Other health problems** include a red swollen nose, dilated blood vessels, gout, yeast vaginitis, PMS, and a suppressed immune system.

- **Regular alcohol use and abuse** can create social problems in personal relationships and career, and economic adversity in regard to lost work and medical costs.

Nutritional Support for Drinkers

The basic support plan for active drinkers resembles that which is used during complete alcohol detox. A generally balanced and nutritious diet will help minimize some of the potential problems from alcohol, although even the best diet and supplement program will not fully protect us from ethanol's toxic effects. When our liver is metabolizing alcohol, it is helpful to avoid fried foods, rancid or hydrogenated fats, and other drugs, all of which are hard on the liver. Alphalipoic acid may help protect the liver against some of the toxicity, as can milk thistle herb.

Alcohol users need more nutrients than most people to protect them from malnutrition. Obviously, basic multivitamin and antioxidant formulas are important. Part, or possibly most, of the toxic effects of alcohol may be caused by the production of free radicals. Higher-than-DRI (dietary reference intake) levels of vitamins A, C, and E, mixed carotenes, and the minerals selenium, zinc, manganese, and magnesium are suggested. Commonly deficient nutrients also need extra support. Thiamin, riboflavin, and niacin

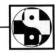

help circulation and blood cleansing and can reduce the effects of hangovers. I recommend folic acid in an amount more than twice the DRI; leafy greens and whole grains, both rich in this vitamin, should be added to the diet. Water and other nonalcoholic liquids are needed to counteract the dehydrating effects of alcohol. Glutathione helps prevent fat buildup in the liver through its enzymatic activities, so the tripeptide glutathione (or L-cysteine, which forms glutathione in the body) may be supplemented along with basic L-amino acids. Additional L-glutamine will enhance brain cell function.

Social Drinking

I recommend that social drinkers use a lighter version of this program, as they still need protection against alcohol's toxicity. A good diet is, of course, essential, plus vitamins B1, B2, and B3, folic acid, and B12. These, along with zinc (15–30 mg), magnesium (300–500 mg), and vitamin C (1,000 mg) should be taken with some food before drinking. In general, drinking should be limited to 2 drinks per day.

A number of things can help prevent drunkenness and hangover. Our alcohol blood level is affected by how much and how fast we drink and absorb. Drink slowly. If we drink fast on an empty stomach, absorption is immediate. Ideally, it is best to have some food in the stomach, or to limit consumption to one drink before eating. Food also prevents us from getting sick. I recommend low-salt complex carbohydrates such as bread, crackers, or vegetable sticks, because carbohydrates delay alcohol absorption. Fat and protein snacks such as milk or cheese will also decrease alcohol absorption, thus reducing drunkenness and hangovers. Some people even drink a little olive oil before parties to coat their stomachs before drinking. A few capsules of evening primrose oil will have a similar effect. Women seem to be more readily affected by alcohol than men, even when body weight is equal.

Once alcohol is ingested, it just takes time to clear it from the blood. With heavy drinking, extra coffee and exercise do not really help; however, with mild intoxication they can increase alertness. Definitely avoid other psychoactive drugs when drinking alcohol, including tranquilizers, narcotics, sedatives, anti-histamines, and marijuana, all of which may increase alcohol's effect.

Overall, we need to monitor our drinking and not let alcohol use turn into abuse and addiction. We also need to pay special attention to children and teenagers and offer them education regarding alcohol and drugs and provide them with good role models in ourselves. Let us all live as examples of how we would like the world to be.

CAFFEINE

Caffeine is a worldwide ubiquitous drug. Used originally in most cultures for ceremonies, it has become an overused energy stimulant in the Western world with the United States among the leaders in coffee and caffeine use. Europeans are drinking more coffee than ever. Germans consume over 16 pounds per person each year and the Swedes lead in consumption with 30 pounds per person per year. The global production of coffee was 7 million tons (14 billion pounds) in 2002 alone, and 2.5 billion pounds of that was consumed in the U.S.

Coffee, brewed from the ground coffee bean (*Coffea arabica*), is the major vehicle for caffeine consumption. In this country, more than 500 million cups are consumed daily, with most people drinking 2 or more cups a day. More than 10 pounds of coffee per person are consumed yearly. This food/drug mixture—often combined with sugar and/or milk—is among the most freely marketed addictive substances in the world.

Physiologically, caffeine is a central nervous system (CNS) stimulant. It is a member of the class of methylxanthine chemicals/drugs. Xanthines (specifically theophylline) are commonly used in medicine to aid in breathing. Theobromine, another xanthine derivative, is found in cocoa and tea. Methylxanthines are found in many other plants, including the kola nut originally used to make cola drinks.

A dosage of 50 to 100 mg caffeine, the amount in 1 cup of coffee, will produce a temporary increase in mental clarity and energy levels while simultaneously reducing drowsiness. It also improves muscular coordination, including work activities like typing. That is why employers love to provide free coffee breaks to their employees. Through its CNS stimulation, caffeine increases brain activity; however it also stimulates the cardiovascular system, raising blood pressure and heart rate. It generally speeds up our body by increasing our basal metabolic rate (BMR), which burns more calories. Initially, caffeine may lower blood sugar; however, this can lead to increased hunger or cravings for sweets. After adrenal stimulation, blood sugar rises again. Caffeine also increases respiratory rates, and for people with tight airways, it can open breathing passages (as do the other xanthine drugs). Caffeine is also a diuretic and a mild laxative.

The amount of caffeine needed to produce stimulation increases with regular use, as is typical of all addictive drugs. Larger and more frequent doses are needed to achieve the original effect, and symptoms can develop if we do not get our "fix." Eventually, we need the drug to function; without it, fatigue, drowsiness, and headaches can occur. Caffeine withdrawal produces tension headaches in almost everyone for 1 to 2 days.

Overall, addiction to caffeine is not as harmful as addiction to most other drugs. Usually, the slower the tapering of caffeine use, the easier the withdrawal. After complete withdrawal and detoxification from caffeine, it is possible to use it in moderation, but care must be taken as it can be re-addicting. For healthier detoxification, a more alkaline diet is helpful, as is drinking plenty of water and doing regular exercise. Since many people appreciate the mild laxative effect of coffee, care must be taken with diet, fiber, and even herbal laxatives to prevent constipation, which worsens any detoxification picture.

Some Common Negative Effects of Caffeine

- Excess nervousness, irritability, insomnia, "restless legs," dizziness, and subsequent fatigue

- Headaches

- General anxiety (even panic attacks)

- Hyperactivity and bed-wetting in children who consume caffeine

- Increased heartburn from stomach hydrochloric acid production (clearly bad for people with existing ulcers or gastritis)

Caffeine Levels* in Common Substances**

Coffee and Other Drinks/6 oz cup	Amount of Caffeine (mg)
Drip	120–150
Percolated	80–110
Instant	60–70
Decaf	3–10
Espresso (1 oz shot)	75
Caffe latte	70
Cappuccino	70
Caffe mocha	80
Black tea	50–60
Earl Grey	50
English breakfast	50
Green tea	30–40
Jasmine tea	20
Cocoa	10–30
Chocolate milk	10–15
Cocoa (dry, 1 oz)	40–50
Chocolate (dry, 1 oz)	5–10
Soft drink, per 12 oz serving	
colas	30–65
Mountain Dew	50
Over-the-counter medicines	
NoDoz	100
Vivarin	200
Dexatrim	200
Cafergot	100
Excedrin	65
Fiorinal	40
Anacin	30
Vanquish	35
Aqua-Ban	100
Midol	30

*These caffeine levels and caffeine equivalents may depend on length of brewing time or amount of product used. The levels given are approximate.

** Information gathered and integrated from multiple sources, including the National Coffee Association, National Soft Drink Association, Tea Council of the USA, and USDA National Nutrient Database for Standard Reference, Release 18 (2005), Agricultural Research Service, Beltsville, Maryland.

- Loss of minerals such as potassium, magnesium, and zinc, and vitamins including the B vitamins, particularly thiamin, and vitamin C

- Reduced absorption of iron and calcium (especially when caffeine is consumed around mealtime)

- Osteoporosis

- Interrupted growth in children and adolescents

- Diarrhea

- Increased blood pressure and hypertension, especially in atherosclerosis and heart disease

- Increased cholesterol and triglyceride blood levels

- Heart rhythm disturbances and mild arrhythmias, tachycardia, and palpitations

- Fibrocystic breast disease (study results vary, but it is clear that some women experience an increase in size and number of cysts with increased use of caffeine)

- Birth defects and miscarriages

- Kidney stones, which can occur as a result of the diuretic and chemical effects

- Increased fevers, both as a direct effect and by counteracting the effect of aspirin

- Increased incidence of certain cancers, including bladder cancer (more frequently due to a combination with nicotine), ovarian cancer, and pancreatic cancer

- Prostate enlargement possibly also attributed to increased caffeine intake

- Adrenal exhaustion/stress/fatigue/hypoglycemia syndrome

While caffeine has the overall effect of increasing blood sugar, stress and sugar intake weaken the adrenal function. Recovery from the resulting fatigue requires rest, stress reduction, and sugar avoidance, and even though caffeine can override this fatigue and restimulate the adrenals temporarily, eventually chronic fatigue, adrenal exhaustion, and subsequent inability to handle any stress or sugar will result. Caffeine will then be of little help.

Herbal Caffeine Substitutes

Roasted barley	Cafix
Chicory root	Miso broth
Dandelion root	Duran
Teeccino	Peppermint
Postum	Ginseng root
Pero	Ginger root
Pioneer	Rombouts
Comfrey leaf	Lemon grass
Roastaroma	Red clover
Wilson's Heritage	

UTILIZING DETOXIFICATION FOR HEALTH

When I set up a detox and cleansing program, I evaluate each individual with a history, physical exam, and specific tests that might include biochemistry testing, dietary analysis, mineral levels, food antibody levels, or gastrointestinal tests to measure digestion and look for abnormal microbes. Looking at the patient's current state of health, symptoms, and disease as an outcome of their diet, lifestyle, and inherent/familial patterns, and then considering their health goals, we create the plan together. As is true with any healing process, the plan must be followed, reevaluated, and fine-tuned to make it work to its best potential. If people are deficient in nutrients and/or energy, they may need a higher-nutrient, higher-protein building diet to improve their health rather than a juice cleanse. Fatigue, mineral deficiencies, and low organ functions may call for this more supportive diet. However, even in these circumstances, short cleanses, such as three days, can help eliminate old debris and prepare the body to build with healthier blocks.

Our individual detox programs can change, as our needs often vary with time. My own personal program has changed over the decades. Initially, fasts were powerful for me, transformative and healing. Now I usually notice little effect, although I feel much cleaner most of the time. If I do get congested with different foods, during travel or when under other stresses, a few days of juices or just light eating will make a big difference. I ate a low-protein, high-complex-carbohydrate, vegetarian diet for a number of years. Now a mild detox for me consists of more strengthening protein-vegetable meals. Fresh fish with lots of vegetables (and fewer grains) satisfies and energizes me more now than in the past. The higher-starch meals led me to overeat more to feel nourished. This new diet has let me reduce calories and weight as well as feel stronger and healthier. And this too, I am sure, will change in time. Yes, detoxification is an individual affair, and many personal aspects are involved in devising a complete plan.

Colon cleansing is among the most important parts of detoxification. The large intestine releases many toxins, and sluggish functioning of this organ can rapidly produce general toxicity. During any detox program, most people will incorporate some colon cleansing. Helpful products include herbal or pharmaceutical laxatives, fiber, and colon detox supplements such as psyllium seed husks alone or mixed with other agents (like aloe vera powder, bentonite clay, and acidophilus culture). Enemas using water, herbs, or even diluted coffee (the latter of which stimulates liver cleansing) may also be used. A series of colonic water irrigations (best performed by a trained professional with filtered water and sterile, disposable equipment) can be the focal point of a detox program accompanied by a cleansing diet and fiber supplements. For a complete body and colon cleansing program, I really like Nature's Pure Body program or the Ejuva program (see Appendix B "Nutritional Supplement Companies"). Whatever the method, keeping the bowels moving is key to feeling well during detoxification.

10 Healthy Hygiene Hints

1. **Wash your hands several times daily—** especially after eliminating, before handling food, after handling animals/pets, when you are sick with an upper respiratory problem (coughing, sneezing, or runny nose), or when you are in close physical contact with others. Also, clean up after a public encounter, such as hand shaking, door opening, or using public phones. Some health-conscious consumers carry their own soap with them in a purse or bag for just such purposes.

2. **Bathe or shower at least once daily,** more if you are sweaty or dirty, in a clean tub or shower; also, use environmentally friendly hygiene products and cleansers.

3. **Exercise and sweat regularly** to help cleanse your skin and move the lymphatic fluids. Deep breathing is also detoxifying

4. **Keep your nails clean and cut,** and clear out dirt and germs that may get under them with hydrogen peroxide or a nailbrush.

5. **Do not put used utensils or your hands** into group food, and no "double dipping" at parties.

6. **Blow your nose and rinse out your nose** and sinuses when you are congested. Also, keep your teeth and mouth clean with regular brushing and flossing.

7. **Follow safe sex guidelines,** especially with a new partner. These include using condoms and appropriate birth control.

8. **Make sure your diet and activity level** facilitate at least 1 to 2 good bowel movements a day and clean yourself properly afterward.

9. **Keep your kitchen and refrigerator clean;** wash counters and cutting boards regularly. Do not let germs breed in your trash bins—wash them regularly as well.

10. **Minimize your use of and exposure to chemicals** at home (such as in your yard and laundry) and in the workplace (you have less control but can make healthful suggestions to the decision makers). Do not replace germs and dirt with chemicals.

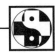

Regular exercise is also important, as it stimulates sweating and encourages elimination through the skin. Exercise also improves general metabolism and helps overall with detoxification. For this reason, regular aerobic exercise is key to maintaining a nontoxic body, especially when we indulge in such substances as sugar or alcohol. Because exercise both produces and releases toxins in the body, it is important to incorporate adequate fluids, antioxidants, vitamins, and minerals. (Also see "Athletes" on page 613, in chapter 16, Performance Enhancement Programs.) Regular bathing cleanses the skin of toxins that have been released and opens the pores for further elimination. It is particularly beneficial during detoxification. Saunas and sweats are commonly used to enhance skin elimination. Dry brushing the skin with an appropriate skin brush before bathing is also suggested to invigorate the skin and cleanse away old cells. Massage therapy (especially lymphatic or deep massage) stimulates elimination and body functions and promotes relaxation. Clearing generalized tensions also makes for a more complete detoxification.

Resting, relaxation, and recharging are also important to this rejuvenation process. During the detox process, we may need more rest, quiet time, and sleep, although more commonly we have more energy and function better on fewer hours of sleep than before. Relaxation exercises help the body rebalance itself as the mind stops interfering with natural homeostasis. The practice of yoga combines quiet yet powerful exercises with breath awareness and regulation, allowing increased flexibility and relaxation.

Certain supplements are appropriate for some detoxification programs. However, general supplementation may be less important in this detox program than with the specific detox plans for alcohol, caffeine, and nicotine, when more nutrients can ease withdrawal symptoms. (These specific substance detoxification programs are discussed in my book *The New Detox Diet*.) For straight juice cleansing or water fasts, I usually do not recommend many supplements; however, I may suggest a couple of nutrients or herbs to stimulate the detoxification process. Examples include potassium, extra fiber with olive oil to clear toxins from the colon, sodium alginate from seaweeds to bind heavy metals, and apple cider vinegar in water (1 tablespoon vinegar in 8 ounces hot water) to help reduce mucus. I have

> ## Simple Supplement for the New Detox Diet
>
> **Multivitamin/mineral (one-a-day type):** 1 tablet or capsule after breakfast.
>
> **Antioxidant combination:** 1 or 2 capsules or tablets twice daily, between meals.
>
> **Vitamin C or buffered powdered C:** with minerals (calcium, magnesium, and potassium). Take 1 tablet or capsule of 500–1,000 mg Vitamin C, or 1/2–1 teaspoon twice daily of powder mixed into liquid.
>
> **Calcium-magnesium capsules or tablets:** 1 to 3 capsules at bedtime or for any muscle cramps to be used if the buffered vitamin C powder is not being used.
>
> **Blue-green algae, spirulina, or chlorella:** 2 to 4 tablets or capsules after breakfast and lunch (double the number of tablets for chlorella because they are smaller).
>
> **Herbal colon tablets of laxative tea:** 1 to 2 tablets twice daily in the morning and evening, or about 1/2 to 1 cup of tea in the morning and at night (varies depending on individual sensitivity).
>
> **Herbal extracts:** These can also be used to support or balance other body systems or to enhance energy. Siberian or other ginsengs are possible, echinacea for immune support, ginger for circulation, and so on. Review the lists of herbs on the next page and on page 767.

used blue-green algae, chlorella, and spirulina, as I and other fasters often feel better and more energetic when we use these nutrient-rich foods. For people who begin with transition diets, I usually suggest a specialized nutrient program to help neutralize toxins and support elimination. With weight loss (for detoxers who are overweight), toxins stored in the fat will need to be mobilized and cleared—more water, fiber, and antioxidant nutrients can help handle this.

The supplement program used for general detoxification (with additional support to reduce nutrient deficiency during detox) is outlined in the table on page 768. It includes a low-dosage multivitamin/mineral supplement to fulfill the basic nutritional requirements

---

Cleansing Herbs

Burdock root. Skin and blood cleanser, diuretic and diaphoretic, improves liver function, antibacterial and antifungal properties.

Cayenne pepper. Blood purifier, increases fluid elimination and sweat.

Chaparral. Strong blood cleanser, with possibilities for use in cancer therapy.

Dandelion root. Liver and blood cleanser, diuretic, filters toxins, a tonic.

Echinacea. Lymph cleanser, improves lymphocyte and phagocyte actions.

Garlic. Blood cleanser, lowers blood fats, natural antibiotic.

Ginger root. Stimulates circulation and sweating.

Goldenseal root. Blood, liver, kidney, and skin cleanser, stimulates detoxification.

Licorice root. A great detoxifier, biochemical balancer, mild laxative.

Oregon grape root. Skin and colon cleanser, blood purifier, liver stimulant.

Parsley leaf. Diuretic, flushes kidneys.

Prickly ash bark. Good for nerves and joints, anti-infectious.

Red clover blossoms. Blood cleanser, good during convalescence and healing.

Sarsaparilla root. Blood and lymph cleanser, contains saponins, which reduce microbes and toxins.

Yellow dock root. Skin, blood, and liver cleanser, contains vitamin C and iron.

Sample Detox Formula

Cayenne pepper	Licorice root
Echinacea	Parsley leaf
Garlic	Yellow dock root
Goldenseal root	

Obtain powders (or ground herb), use equal amounts of all of these herbs except half the cayenne, and put this mixture into 00-size capsules. Take 2 capsules 2 or 3 times daily between meals.

---

during the transitional diet. The B vitamins, particularly niacin, are also important, as are such minerals as zinc, calcium, magnesium, and potassium. The antioxidant nutrients include vitamins C and E, beta-carotene or mixed carotenoids, vitamin A, zinc, and selenium. Some authorities believe that higher amounts of vitamin A (10,000 IU), mixed carotenoids (25,000–50,000 IU), vitamin C (8–12 g), and vitamin E (1,000–1,200 IU) are helpful during detoxification to neutralize the free radicals.

The liver is the most important detoxification organ. The B vitamins, especially B_3 (niacin) and B_6 (pyridoxine), vitamins A and C, zinc, calcium, vitamin E and selenium, and L-cysteine are all also needed to support liver detoxification. Milk thistle herb (often sold as silymarin or *Silybum marianum*) has also been shown to aid liver detoxification and repair. Several amino acids improve or support detoxification, particularly cysteine and methionine, which contain sulfur. L-cysteine supplies sulfhydryl groups that help prevent oxidation and bind such heavy metals as mercury; vitamin C and selenium aid this process as well. Cysteine is the precursor to glutathione—the most important detoxifier—which counters many chemicals and carcinogens. Glutathione is synthesized to form the detoxification enzymes glutathione peroxidase and reductase, which work to prevent peroxidation of lipids and to decrease such toxins as smoke, radiation, auto exhaust, chemicals, drugs, and other carcinogens.

Glycine is a secondary helper. An amino acid that supports glutathione synthesis, glycine decreases the toxicity of such substances as phenols or benzoic acid (a food preservative). Glutamine is also important in helping to heal the gastrointestinal tract as well as reduce cravings for sugar and alcohol, should they occur. Other amino acids that may have mild detoxifying effects are methionine and taurine. For more information on amino acid metabolism and uses, see chapter 3, Proteins.

As mentioned earlier, fiber also supports detoxification. Psyllium seed husks (often combined with other detox nutrients, such as pectin, aloe vera, alginates, and colon herbs) help cleanse mucus along the small intestine, create bulk in the colon, and pull toxins from the gastrointestinal tract. When fiber is combined with 1 or 2 tablespoons of olive oil, it helps bind toxins and reduce the absorption of fats and some basic minerals.

Psyllium husks also reduce absorption of the olive oil itself, which is important in reducing calories and binding any fat-soluble chemicals that may have been released. An option then involves taking 1 to 2 teaspoons each of psyllium husks and bran several times daily (with meals and at bedtime), along with 1 teaspoon of olive oil to help detoxify the colon. Acidophilus and other beneficial bacteria or probiotics in the colon can neutralize some toxins, reduce the metabolism of other microbes, and lessen colon toxicity. Supplemental probiotics can be added to the detox program.

Remember, water should always be used during any type of detox program to help dilute and eliminate toxin accumulations. It is likely the most important detoxifier. It helps clean us through our skin and kidneys, and it improves our sweating with exercise. Drinking 8 to 10 glasses a day (depending on our size and activity level) of clean, filtered water is suggested. Some authorities suggest distilled water for use during detox programs; because of its lack of minerals, it will draw other particles (nutrients and toxins) to it. I think it throws off our bichemical/electrical balance, however, and I prefer regular, purified water (see chapter 1, Water). Drink 2 or 3 glasses of water 30 to 60 minutes before each meal and even at night to help flush toxins during the body's natural elimination time.

A special elimination process has been developed and is used in some clinics to help in the detoxification of chemicals, especially pesticides and even pharmaceutical drugs. This program usually involves several weeks at a center with a therapy including a high fluid and juice intake, exercise, and large amounts of niacin (vitamin B3) with sauna therapies. The saunas are extended and may last for several hours daily, with breaks to drink fluids. The idea is to cleanse the hidden chemicals from the fat through juice cleansing, weight loss, niacin therapy, exercise, and sweats. Niacin is a vasostimulator and vasodilator, aiding circulation.

This "niacin-sauna" program is interesting and definitely has possibilities as an intense, medically supervised detoxification process. However, it is still experimental and does entail risks. Preliminary results are good, especially for people with symptoms caused by exposure to pesticides, such as Agent

---

A General Classification of Herbs Useful in Detoxification*

Blood Cleansers	Laxatives	Diuretics	Skin Cleansers/ Diaphoretics
Echinacea	Cascara sagrada	Parsley	Burdock
Red clover	Buckthorn	Yarrow	Oregon grape root
Dandelion	Dandelion	Cleavers	Yellow dock
Burdock	Yellow dock	Horsetail	Goldenseal
Yellow dock	Rhubarb root	Corn silk	Boneset
Oregon grape root	Senna leaf	Uva ursi	Elder flowers
	Licorice	Juniper berries	Peppermint
			Cayenne pepper
			Ginger root

——— Antibiotics ———		——— Anticatarrhals** ———	
Garlic	Echinacea	Echinacea	Hyssop
Myrrh	Propolis	Boneset	Garlic
Prickly ash	Clove	Goldenseal	Yarrow
Wormwood	Eucalyptus	Sage	

* Not usually for fasting or juice cleansing, but mainly for dietary detoxification—using herbs alone may be the most productive method in some detoxification programs. Consult a naturopathically oriented doctor.

** Anticatarrhals help eliminate mucus.

General Detoxification Nutrient Program

Nutrient	Amount	Nutrient	Amount
Water	2¹/₂–3 qt	Molybdenum	300 mcg
Fiber	20–40 g	Potassium	300–500 mg
Vitamin A	5,000 IU	Selenium	300 mcg
Beta-carotene	15,000–30,000 IU	Silicon	100 mg
Vitamin D	200 IU	Vanadium	300 mcg
Vitamin E	400–800 IU	Zinc	30 mg
Vitamin K	200 mcg		
Thiamin (B₁)	10–25 mg	**Optional**	
Riboflavin (B₂)	10–25 mg	L-amino acids	500–1,000 mg
Niacinamide (B₃)	50 mg	L-cysteine	250–500 mg
Niacin (B₃)	50–2,000 mg*	DL-methionine	250–500 mg
Pantothenic acid (B₅)	250 mg	L-glycine	250–500 mg
Pyridoxine (B₆)	10–25 mg	Psyllium seed	1–2 tsp
Cobalamin (B₁₂)	50–100 mcg	Flaxseed oil	1–2 tsp
Folic acid	400–800 mcg	Olive oil	3–6 tsp
Biotin	200 mcg	Liquid chlorophyll	2–4 tsp
Vitamin C	1–4 g	Apple cider vinegar	1–2 tbsp
Bioflavonoids	250–500 mg	Acidophilus culture	1–2 billion organisms
Calcium	600–850 mg	Detox formula herbs	4–6 capsules
Chromium	200 mcg	(such as echinacea,	
Copper	2 mg	yellow dock, goldenseal,	
Iodine	150 mcg	garlic, parsley, licorice,	
Iron	10–18 mg	cayenne pepper)	
Magnesium	300–500 mg		
Manganese	5–10 mg		

*The higher amounts may be used for special detox programs.

Orange, yet there are some drawbacks. Besides the cost and time required, the extreme detoxification can cause losses of nutrients, especially minerals, creating depletions from which it could take months to recover. Special attention must be given to ensuring proper nutrient restoration during and after this therapy. I think that this program, even short versions of it, can be used to help detoxify from most drugs, especially the recreational types, and daily abuses of alcohol and nicotine. Many of us can do a modified version on our own with the use of a sauna, a few days' juice fast, regular exercise, and supplemental niacin, beginning at 100 to 200 mg and moving up to 2 to 3 grams daily. Be sure to replenish fluids and minerals. If there are medical problems, weakness, or fatigue, I would not suggest doing this without the advice and supervision of a properly trained physician.

Many herbs can support or even create detoxification. In fact, this area is really the strength, I believe, of herbal medicine. There are hundreds of possible herbs to be used for blood cleansing and cleaning the tissues or strengthening the function of specific organs. The old term for blood cleansers is *alteratives,* which is the term used in many standard herbal texts. The "Cleansing Herbs" table on page 766 details some of the more important ones.

The "General Detoxification Nutrient Program," above, ties together many aspects of the detoxification process. The specific supplements to be used should take into account individual circumstances. The program can be carried out for varying lengths of time, from 1 week to 1 or 2 months. Remember to work on all the levels of detoxification and listen within for your true healing information.

The detoxification therapy known as fasting is the oldest treatment known to humans and is a completely natural process. In many cases, as we listen to our inner guidance, as animals do, we may apply this process during many illnesses and states of health and life. Many authorities claim the detox process helps clear wastes and old or dead cells, thus revitalizing the body's natural functions and healing capacities. Of the thousands of people that I know who have used cleansing programs, the vast majority experience positive and incredible results. I believe that fasting/cleansing/detoxification is the missing link in Western nutrition, and if we used this process more often in our daily lives and in the mainstream medical system, we could heal and prevent a great deal of disease. Now is the time for all of us to listen—and to clean and clear our bodies, homes, offices, relationships, towns, cities, countries, and the entire planet—lest we perish from toxicity.

32. FASTING AND JUICE CLEANSING

Fasting is the single greatest natural healing therapy I know. It is nature's ancient, universal remedy for many problems, used instinctively by animals when they are ill and by earlier cultures for healing and spiritual purification. When I first discovered fasting 30 years ago, I felt as if it had saved my life. With my first fast, my stagnant energies began flowing, my allergies, aches, and pains disappeared, and I became more creative and vitally alive. I still find fasting both a useful personal tool and an important therapy for many medical and life problems.

Most of the conditions for which I recommend fasting are ones that result from excess nutrition rather than undernourishment. Dietary abuses generate many chronic degenerative diseases (such as atherosclerosis, hypertension, heart disease, allergies, diabetes, cancer, and substance abuse) that undermine our health and precede the body's breakdown. Fasting is not only therapeutic, but, more important, it acts in preventing many conditions. It often becomes the catalyst for shifting

from unhealthy or abusive habits to a more healthful lifestyle in general. As I use the term here, *fasting* refers to the avoidance of solid food and the intake of liquids only. True fasting would be the total avoidance of anything by mouth. The most stringent form of fasting allows drinking water exclusively; more liberal fasting includes the juices of fresh fruit and vegetables as well as herbal teas. All of these methods generate a high degree of detoxification. Individual experiences with fasting depend on the overall condition of the body, mind, and attitude. Detoxification can be intense and may either temporarily increase sickness or be immediately helpful and uplifting.

Juice fasting is commonly used (rather than water alone) as a mild and effective cleansing plan. Fresh juices are easily assimilated and require minimum digestion, while they supply many nutrients and stimulate the body to clear its wastes. Juice fasting is also safer than water fasting, because it supports the body nutritionally while cleansing and probably even produces a better detoxification and quicker recovery. Fasting (cleansing, detoxification) is 1 part of the trilogy of nutrition; balancing and building (toning) are the others. I believe that fasting is the missing link in the Western diet and lifestyle. And juice cleansing is a true therapeutic program. Most people overeat, eat too often, and eat a high-protein, high-fat, acid-forming, and congesting diet more consistently than is necessary. When we regularly eat a balanced, well-combined, more alkalinizing diet, we will have less need for fasting and toning plans (although both are still highly beneficial, performed throughout the year).

Detoxification is a time when we allow our cells and organs to breathe and restore themselves; it can be a time of rejuvenation. However, we do not necessarily need to fast to experience some cleansing. Even minor dietary shifts—including an increase in fluids, more raw foods, and fewer congesting foods—will initiate and promote better bodily function and improved detoxification. For example, a vegetarian or macrobiotic diet will be cleansing and purifying to someone on a heavier diet. Fasting is a time-proven remedy, with human origins going back many thousands of years. Voluntary abstinence from food has been a tradition in most religions and is still used as a spiritual purification rite. Such religions as Christianity, Judaism, Islam, Buddhism, and Hinduism have encouraged fasting as penance, preparation for cere-mony, purification, mourning, sacrifice, divine union, and to enhance mental and spiritual powers. The Bible is filled with stories of people fasting for purifi-cation and communion with God. The Essenes, authors of the Dead Sea Scrolls, also advocated fasting as a pri-mary method of healing and spiritual revelation, as described in the *Essene Gospel of Peace* (translated by Edmond Bordeaux Szekely from the third-century Aramaic manuscript).

Historically, philosophers, scientists, and physi-cians have fasted as a means to promote life and health after sickness. Socrates, Plato, Aristotle, Galen, Paracel-sus, and Hippocrates all used fasting therapy. Many of today's spiritual teachers recommend fasting as a use-ful tool. In a 1947 lecture entitled "Healing by God's Unlimited Power," Paramahansa Yogananda, spiritual teacher and founder of the Self-Realization Fellowship (known in India as Yogoda Satsanga Society), which is still active today, suggested that fasting increases our natural resistance to disease, stating, "Fasting is a nat-ural method of healing. When animals or savages are sick, they fast. Most diseases can be cured by judicious fasting. Unless one has a weak heart, regular short fasts have been recommended by the yogis as an excel-lent health measure." Yogananda also referred to a doc-tor who had treated many patients successfully with fasting therapy for such disorders as asthma, skin dis-eases, digestive problems, and early stages of athero-sclerosis and hypertension.

Through the centuries, physicians and heal-ers have treated a variety of maladies with fast-ing, acknowledging that ignorance of how to live in accordance with Nature may be our greatest disease. Our inherent knowledge of how to live according to the natural laws and spiritual truths leads to the sacred wisdom of life and subsequent good health. Knowing when and how long to fast is part of this knowledge. Through fasting, we can turn our energies inward, where we can use them for healing, clarity, and change.

Physicians with a spiritual orientation tend to be more inclined than others to employ fasting, both per-sonally and in their practices. Many of my own life tran-sitions were stimulated and supported through fasting; when I felt blocked or needed creative energy in my writing, fasting has been useful. In *Spiritual Nutrition*

and the Rainbow Diet, physician and spiritual teacher Gabriel Cousens, MD, includes an excellent chapter on fasting in which he describes his theories and his own 40-day regime. According to Cousens, "Fasting in a larger context, means to abstain from that which is toxic to mind, body, and soul. A way to understand this is that fasting is the elimination of physical, emotional, and mental toxins from our organism, rather than sim-ply cutting down on or stopping food intake. Fasting for spiritual purposes usually involves some degree of removal of oneself from worldly responsibilities. It can mean complete silence and social isolation during the fast, which can be a great revival to those of us who have been putting our energy outward."

From a medical point of view, I believe that fast-ing is not used often enough. We take vacations from work to relax, recharge, and gain new perspectives on our life—why not take occasional breaks from food? (Or, for that matter, from excessive activity or televi-sion and other electronics?) To break the habit of eat-ing three meals a day is a challenge for most of us. When we stop and let our stomach remain empty, the body goes into an elimination cycle, and most people will experience some withdrawal symptoms, especially when toxicity exists. Symptoms include headaches, irritability, and fatigue. As with all allergy-addictions, eating again assuages these symptoms.

Fasting is a useful therapy for so many condi-tions and people. Those who tend to develop con-gestive symptoms do well with fasting; congestive acidic conditions include colds, flus, bronchitis, mucus con-gestion, and constipation (see the list of symptoms and medical conditions that may benefit from detoxification in the chart on the opposite page). If not addressed, such conditions can lead to headaches, chronic intes-tinal problems, skin conditions, and more severe ail-ments. Most of us living in Western, industrialized nations suffer from both overnutrition and undernu-trition. We take in excessive amounts of potentially toxic nutrients, such as fats, sugars, and chemicals, and inadequate amounts of many essential vitamins and minerals. The resulting congestive diseases are char-acterized by excess mucus and sluggish elimination; deficiency problems result from either poor nourish-ment or ineffective digestion and assimilation. Juice fasting supplies nutrients while still allowing for the elimination of toxins.

The general detoxification and cleansing program discussed a number of symptoms and diseases of toxicity that can be alleviated by detoxification. Juice fasting is mentioned as part of the treatment plans for many other programs. It can be used to detoxify from drugs or whenever we want to embark on a new plan or life transition, provided that there are no contraindications to fasting. Short-term fasting is versatile and generally fairly safe; however, when it is used in the treatment of medical conditions, proper supervision should be employed, including monitoring of physical changes and biochemistry values. Many doctors, clinics, acupuncturists, nutritionists, and chiropractors feel comfortable overseeing people during cleansing and detox programs, and I encourage you to seek them out if your condition warrants supervision.

The use of **fasting as a treatment for fevers** is controversial, but it should not be. Consuming liquids generates less heat, which helps to cool the body. With fever, we need more liquids than usual. Some cases of fatigue respond well to fasting, particularly when the fatigue results from congested organs and stalled energy. With fatigue that results from chronic infection, nutritional deficiency, or serious disease, added nourishment is probably called for as opposed to fasting.

Back pain caused by muscular tightness and stress (rather than from bone disease or osteoporosis) is usually alleviated with a lighter diet or juice fasting. Much tightness and soreness along the back results from colon or other organ congestion; in my experience, **poor bowel function and constipation are commonly associated with back pain.**

Patients with mental illness ranging from anxiety to schizophrenia may be helped by fasting. Although this may sound sensational, fasting's purpose here is not to cure these problems but rather to help understand the relationship of foods, chemicals, and drugs with mental functioning. Additional allergies and environmental reactions are not at all uncommon in people with mental illness. True, the release of toxins or lack of nourishment during fasting may worsen psychiatric problems; if, however, the patient is strong and congested, fasting may be helpful. The supervision of a health-care provider is important for patients with mental illness.

Conditions for Which Fasting May Be Beneficial	
Angina pectoris	Epilepsy
Asthma	Fatigue
Atherosclerosis	Fever
Back pains	Flus
Bronchitis	Food allergies
Cancer	Headaches
Colds	Hypertension
Constipation	Indigestion
Coronary artery disease	Insomnia
Diabetes	Mental illness
Diarrhea	Obesity
Environmental allergies	Skin conditions

People often attempt to remedy obesity by fasting, although it is not the best use of this healing technique. Fasting is actually too temporary an approach for overweight dieters and may even generate feasting reactions in people coming off the fast. A better solution would be a more gradual change of diet with a longer-term weight-reduction plan—something that will replace old dietary habits and food choices with new ones. However, a short 5- to 10-day fast can motivate people to make the necessary dietary changes and renewed commitments to proper eating.

Some obese patients who have needed to shed weights of 100 pounds or more have been on month-long water fasts supervised in hospitals. Other patients have had their jaws wired shut, allowing them to only ingest fluids through straws. Still others have surgery to shrink their stomach size. Newer fasting programs substitute a variety of protein-rich powders for meals. These are also usually medically supervised, and are for people who are at least 30 to 50 pounds overweight. These prepackaged high-protein, low-calorie diets allow patients to burn more fat. Although these programs are not nearly as healthful as vital juice fasts, they are more nutritionally supportive over a longer period of time and can be used on an outpatient basis fairly safely if people are monitored regularly. They provide all the needed vitamins, minerals, and amino acids to sustain life while helping many people lower their weight, blood fats, blood pressure, and blood sugars. However, as with any weight-loss program, success depends on participant motivation to change personal diets and habits permanently, as fluctuating weights may actually be more harmful than just remaining overweight. Many obese people are deficient in nutrients because they eat a highly refined, fatty, sweet diet. They are often fatigued and need to be nourished first before they will do well on any fast. A well-balanced, low-calorie (yet high-nutrient) diet with lots of exercise is still the best way to reduce and maintain a good weight and figure.

Fasting to treat cancer is a controversial topic but is used by many alternative clinics outside the United States. Because of cancer's extremely debilitating effects, this may not be wise. Juice fasting may be helpful in the early stages of cancer and is definitely a preventive measure as it reduces toxicity. Anyone with cancer needs adequate nourishment, however; adding fresh juices to an already wholesome diet can promote mild detoxification and enhance overall vitality.

The Process and Benefits of Fasting

Although the process of fasting may generate various results depending on the individual condition of the faster, there are clearly a number of common metabolic changes and experiences. First, fasting is a catalyst for change and an essential part of transformational medicine. It promotes relaxation and energization of the body, mind, and emotions and supports a greater spiritual awareness. Many fasters feel a letting go of past actions and experiences and develop a positive attitude toward the present. Having energy to get things done and clean up old areas, both personal and environmental, without the usual procrastination is also a common response to the cleansing process. Fasting clearly improves motivation and creative energy; it also enhances health and vitality and lets many of the body systems rest.

Fasting is a multidimensional experience, affecting people physically, mentally, emotionally, and spiritually. Breaking down stored or circulating chemicals is its basic process; the blood and lymph also have the opportunity to be cleaned of toxins as their eliminative functions are alleviated. Each cell has the opportunity to catch up on its work; with

Some Benefits of Fasting
Antiaging effects
Better attitude
Better resistance to disease
Better sleep
Change of habits
Clearer planning
Clearer skin
Creativity
Diet changes
Drug detoxification
Improved senses (vision, hearing, taste)
Inspiration
More clarity (mentally and emotionally)
More energy
More relaxation
New ideas
Purification
Reduction of allergies
Rejuvenation
Rest for digestive organs
Revitalization
Right use of will
Spiritual awareness
Weight loss

fewer new demands, cells can repair themselves and eliminate wastes. Most fasters experience a new vibrancy of their skin and clarity of mind and body. Most important, the liver can spend more time detoxifying the body and creating new essential substances. Drinking 2 to 3 quarts of water and juices daily (or even more in some people) is optimal during fasting to cleanse and support the body.

Metabolically, fasting initially reduces caloric intake to the point where the liver converts stored glycogen to glucose and energy. Body fat and fatty acids can be used for energy (ATP); however, the brain and central nervous system need direct glucose. With fasting, some protein breakdown occurs (less if calories are provided by juices). When glycogen stores are low, the body can convert protein to amino acids and to energy—specifically the amino acids alanine and serine can be used to produce glucose. Fatty acids can also

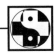

be a source of energy during fasting, as they convert to ketones, which can be used by the body to prevent protein loss. With juice fasting, there is less ketosis (disrupted carbohydrate metabolism), and the simple carbohydrates provided by the juices are easily used for energy and cellular function. **High-protein (fasting) diets and other weight-loss programs may burn more fat and generate more ketosis, but they also add more toxins and may create other health concerns.**

Fasting increases the process of elimination and the release of toxins from the colon, kidneys and bladder, lungs and sinuses, and skin. This process can generate discharge such as mucus from the gastrointestinal tract, respiratory tract, sinuses, or in the urine. This is helpful to clear out the problems that have arisen from overeating and a sedentary lifestyle. **Much of aging and disease, I believe, results from biochemical suffocation, where the cells do not get enough oxygen and nutrients or cannot adequately eliminate their wastes.** Fasting helps us decrease this suffocation by allowing the cells to eliminate and catch up with current processes.

This physiological rest and concentration on cleanup can also generate a number of toxicity symptoms. Hunger is usually present for 2 or 3 days and then departs, leaving many people with a surprising feeling of deep abdominal peace; yet others may feel really hungry. It is good to ask ourselves, "What am I hungry for?" Fasting is an excellent time to work on our psychological connections to consumption.

As far as fasting symptoms, headache is not at all uncommon during the first 1 or 2 days. Fatigue or irritability may arise at times, as may dizziness or light-headedness. Our sensitivity is usually increased. Everyday sounds like the television, music, and that which emanates from the refrigerator may irritate us more now. The sense of smell is also exaggerated, both positively and negatively; I have had whole meals of smells while fasting. The tongues of most people will develop a thick white or yellow furry coating, which can be scraped or brushed off. Bad breath and displeasing tastes in the mouth or foul-smelling urine or stools may occur. Skin odor or skin eruptions (such as small spots or painful boils) may also appear, depending on the state of toxicity. Digestive upset, mucous stools, flatulence, or even

nausea and vomiting may occur during fasting. Some people experience insomnia or bad dreams as their bodies release poisons during the night. (Wild dreams about weird foods are not uncommon.)

The mind may put up resistance, sending messages of doubt or fear that fasting is not right. This can be exaggerated by listening to other people's fears about your fasting. If you are looking for excuses not to fast, they are everywhere. Most symptoms occur early on (if at all) and pass. Generally, energy levels are good, although energy may go down every 2 or 3 days as the body excretes more wastes. It is at these times that resistance and fears (as well as new symptoms) may arise; if symptoms occur, it is wise to drink more fluids. However, most people will feel cleaner, better, and more alive most of the time.

The natural-therapy term for periods of cleansing and symptoms is *crisis,* or *healing crisis.* Old symptoms or patterns from the past may arise during fasts—again usually transiently—or new symptoms of detoxification may appear. This periodic cleansing is not predictable and often raises doubts and questions—is this a new problem or part of the healing process? Generally, time and the healing process will sort things out. Use Hering's Law of Cure to guide you in making these judgment calls: Healing happens from the inside out, from the top down, from more important organs to less important ones, and from the most recent to the oldest symptoms. Most healing crises pass within 1 or 2 days, although some cleansers experience several days of "cold" symptoms or sinus congestion. If any symptom lasts longer than 2 or 3 days, it should be considered a side effect or new problem and should be addressed accordingly. If a problem worsens or causes concern (such as fainting, heart arrhythmias, or bleeding), the fast should be stopped and a doctor consulted.

Medical supervision (from a doctor or knowledgeable practitioner) is important for anyone in poor health or without fasting experience. If the fast is extended for more than 3 or 4 days, regular monitoring, including physical examinations and blood work, should be done weekly (particularly if there is any cause for concern). Fasting may reduce blood protein levels and will definitely lower blood fats. Uric acid levels may rise due to protein breakdown, while levels of some minerals such as potassium, sodium, calcium, or magnesium may drop. Iron levels are usually lower, and the red blood cell count may also drop slightly during this time. Lowered mineral levels can result in fatigue or muscle cramps; if these should occur, additional minerals (particularly calcium, magnesium, and potassium) should be taken, ideally in a powered form for easy assimilation.

Nutritionally, fasting helps us appreciate the more subtle aspects of our diet, as less food and simple flavors will become more satisfying (even food aromas can be fulfilling). Mentally, fasting improves clarity and attentiveness; emotionally, it may make us more sensitive and aware of our feelings. I have seen individuals gain the clarity to make important decisions during this therapy, particularly regarding jobs and relationships. Fasting definitely supports the transformational, evolutionary process. Juice fasting offers a lesson in self-restraint and control of passions. This new and empowering sense of self-discipline can be highly motivating. Fasters who were once spectators suddenly become doers. Fasting is a simple process of self-cleansing. We do not need any special medicines to do it; our body knows how. Provided that we are basically well nourished, systematic undereating and fasting are likely the most important contributors to health and longevity. Fasting is even more important to balance the autointoxication that results from common dietary and drug indiscretions.

I look at fasting as taking a week off work to handle the other aspects of life for which there is often little time. With fasting we can take time to nurture ourselves and rest. Fasting is also like turning off and cleaning a complex and valuable machine so that it will function better and longer. Resting the gastro-intestinal tract, letting the cells and tissues repair themselves, and allowing the lymph, blood, and organs to clear out old, defective, or diseased cells and unneeded chemicals all lead to less degeneration and sickness. As healthy cell growth is stimulated, so is our level of vitality, immune function, and disease resistance as well as our potential for greater longevity.

Fasting Examples

J.R. did a 67-day fast on juices at age 20 when he joined a fasting and health food–oriented community. He describes feeling great and very light. He lost a lot of weight during the fast. His only problems were skin sores that would not heal. These were of course, seen as a detox process. Medically, they could be attributed to protein/nutrient deficiency as well. This long fast on juice nutrients was a major transitional period for J.R. to change his diet to raw foods and strict vegetarianism. It also helped change his beliefs and motivation for life.

S.R. was very overweight and in a family relationship that was not supporting her growth. She clearly longed for spiritual unfoldment. She was strong and had loads of energy and various congestive symptoms—a prime candidate for fasting. After she began her fast, she decided to go 30 days on the Master Cleanser (see page 778) with my support. She did wonderfully, lost 24 pounds, and was not through yet. For the next 30 days, she did the 7-food diet I helped her choose (apples, lemons, alfalfa sprouts, brown rice, carrots, almonds, and broccoli), picking 7 primary foods to make up her diet, thus continuing her willpower and diet focus. After that, S.R. did another 30-day fast on with the Master Cleanser lemonade and other juices. She did well. During these months she moved from bookkeeping and typing into the healing arts. She left her husband and moved to the Midwest to take a job assisting a well-known physician in her healing research.

Another fasting approach is chronicled by the experience B.D. and C.D., a father-and-son team. B.D. (46) and his son C.D. (15) attended a recent fasting group. B.D. was 50 pounds overweight, at 231 pounds and 5 feet 9 inches, and had high blood pressure. On exam, B.D.'s cholesterol was 214. He had in the past followed a low-fat, Pritikin-like diet and felt better. He was ready for a change and wanted to fast. He wanted me to see his son to evaluate whether he also could join the fasting group. C.D. was an overweight teenager, at 181 pounds and 5 feet 9 inches, on a typical teenage diet but inspired toward health.

B.D. did incredibly well on the Master Cleanser for 10 days, feeling fine and energetic and dropping his weight to 213. His new diet plan became more vegetarian, wholesome, and low fat, and included 1- to 2-day fasts weekly, plus a weeklong fast every few months. A follow-up 4 months later found him well and busy in a new job. B.D.'s weight had gotten to a low of 195 and he stabilized at about 202 with his diet. He realized that he could be in control of his diet. He was in much better shape and his self-esteem was much higher; of course, he could see his feet and the ground again as his pants size dropped from 42 inches to 36.

C.D. dropped his weight from 182 to 171 with the fast and was an inspiration to the fasting group. His body and face changed dramatically. New activities and exercise were added to his regimen, and he now is a serious bicyclist. C.D.'s diet also changed dramatically to enjoying salads and fruits and some grains, as well as fish and poultry. He got away from the sweets, sodas, salty snacks, and fried foods he was eating before. Now at 165 pounds, he feels great!

Hazards of Fasting

If fasting is overused, it may create depletion and weakness in the body, lowering resistance and increasing susceptibility to disease. Although fasting does allow the organs, tissues, and cells to rest and handle excesses, the body needs the nourishment provided by food to function after it has used up its stores. **Malnourished people should definitely not fast, nor should some overweight people who are undernourished.** Others who should not fast include people with fatigue resulting from nutrient deficiency, those with chronic degenerative disease of the muscles or bones, or those who are underweight. Diseases associated with clogged or toxic organs respond better to fasting. Sluggish individuals who retain water or whose weight is concentrated in their hips and legs often do worse. Those with low daytime energy and more vitality at night (more yin or alkaline types) may not enjoy fasting either.

I do not recommend fasting for pregnant or lactating women, or for people who have weak hearts, or weakened immunity. (I have, however, seen women use short juice cleanses during their menstrual cycle to help ease pain and other symptoms.) Before or after surgery is not a good time to fast, as the body needs its nourishment to handle the stress and healing demands of the operation. Although some nutritional therapies for cancer include medically supervised fasting, I do not recommend it for cancer patients, particularly those with advanced problems. Ulcer disease is not something for which I usually suggest fasting, either, although fasting may be bene-

ficial for other conditions present in a patient whose ulcer is under control.

Some clinics and fasting practitioners believe in fasting as a treatment for ulcers. In the first test case of the Master Cleanser, Stanley Burroughs, one of the first natural healers to publish a cleansing protocol in the early 1940s, claims to have cured a patient with an intractable ulcer. The two key ingredients of the Master Cleanser, citrus and cayenne pepper, are substances that all the physicians had suggested this patient avoid; Burroughs deduced they might be the only things left to heal the ulcer, however, and perhaps he was right. The fasting process itself is helpful for ulcers as it reduces stomach acid and aids in tissue healing. Cayenne pepper, although hot, heals mucous membranes and is commonly recommended for ulcers in herbal medicines. So even though peptic ulcers are on the contraindication list, many people with inflammation in their digestive tissues may be helped by fasting, especially with cabbage juice, greens, and other fresh vegetable juices.

As with any therapy, fasting has some potential hazards. Clearly, excessive weight loss and nutritional deficiencies may occur—a response more marked with longer water fasts and less likely with juices, as they provide some calories and nutrients. Weakness may occur, or muscle cramps may result from mineral deficits. Sodium, potassium, calcium, magnesium, and phosphorus losses occur initially but diminish after a week. Blood pressure drops, and this can lead to dizziness (especially when changing position from lying to sitting or from sitting to standing). Uric acid levels may rise without adequate fluid intake, although this is rare. All of these problems can be minimized with adequate fluid intake.

Contraindications for Fasting

Cancer	Nursing
Cardiac arrhythmias	Nutritional deficiencies
Cold weather	Peptic ulcers
Fatigue	Pregnancy
Low blood pressure	Pre- and postsurgery
Low immunity	Underweight
Mental illness	Weak heart

Some research reports hormone level changes while fasting. The level of thyroid hormone falls initially, but it rises again in association with protein-sparing ketosis. Female hormone levels fall, possibly as a result of protein malnutrition, and this can lead to a lessening or loss of menstrual flow. Cessation of periods in women is also seen in longtime vegetarians, particularly those who exercise extensively, arising from nutrient depletion. This will usually rebalance with proper diet and nourishment.

Cardiac problems such as arrhythmias can occur with prolonged fasting, especially when there are pre-existing problems. Extra beats, both ventricular and atrial, have been seen, and there have even been deaths from serious ventricular arrhythmias (the latter of which occur most often during long water fasts). Similar problems have turned up in people using any nutrient-deficient protein powders, without supervision, as a weight-loss tool. All of these risks are minimized with juice fasts of no more than 2 weeks duration, or when basic minerals (potassium, calcium, and magnesium) are supplemented during water fasts. **Having our progress monitored through physical exams, blood tests, and even electrocardiograms is another way to protect ourselves from fasting's potential hazards.**

Another side effect (really a "side benefit") of fasting is the way it affects and changes our personal lives. Often we resist inner guidance, feelings, and desires to do something new or get out of a bad situation, but fasting brings them to the fore. Divorce, job changes, and residential moves are all more likely after fasts, as they stimulate self-realization, enhance our potential, and help us focus on the future. During fasting, many people have new sensitivity and renewed awareness of their job, mate, and home. It helps when couples do programs together. I usually warn fasters before they begin of the great potential for change, especially when I sense that they lack commitment or belief in what they are doing. Even though these insights and changes may be traumatic initially, I believe they are ultimately positive and help us follow our true nature.

How to Fast

In the thousands of people I have observed during fasting and detox programs, the complications have been negligible, provided that proper procedures have been followed and attention paid to the ongoing body changes. Usually people feel fine, even euphoric after a few days, although there may be ups and downs or various symptoms. Overall, in my experience, the changes are positive. People commonly state that they feel clearer and less stiff, they sleep better, and they are amazed at how little food they need to feel good. The general plan for fasting is progressive, usually taking a moderate approach for new fasters and unhealthy subjects and leading to a stricter program for the more experienced. It is important to build slowly and take time to transition. Although many people do fine even when making extreme changes, such abruptness clearly maximizes the risks of fasting.

A sensible daily plan mixes fasting with eating. Each day can include a 12- to 14-hour period of fasting from early evening through the night, as indeed breakfast was given that name to denote the time where we break the fast of the night. Many people eat lightly or not at all in the early morning to extend their daily fast; this is more important if dinner or snacking extends into the later evening. If dinner is at an early time, however, a good breakfast can be consumed after water intake and some stretching and exercise.

In preparation for our first day of fasting, we may want to take some time (a few days to a week) to eliminate unhealthy foods or habits from the diet. Abstaining from alcohol, nicotine, caffeine, and sugar is helpful before fasting. Red meats and other animal foods, including milk products and eggs, as well as wheat and baked goods, could be avoided for 1 or 2 days before fasting, thus easing the transition. **Intake of most nutritional supplements should also be curtailed, as these are usually not recommended during a fast.** Many people prepare for their fasts by consuming only fruit and vegetable foods for 3 or 4 days. These slowly detoxify the body so that the actual fast will be less intense.

An initial 1-day fast gives us a chance to see what a short fast can be like. Most of us find that it is not so very difficult and does not cause major distress. Food is abstained from for 36 hours, from 8 p.m. at night

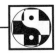

until 8 a.m. 2 days later. Most people will feel a little hungry and may experience a few mild symptoms such as a headache or irritability by the end of the fasting day, usually around dinnertime. **The first two days are generally challenging for everyone.** Take a walk, take a nap, cut your nails, read a book, pray, and bathe instead of eating. Feeling great usually begins around day 3, so longer cleansing is really needed for the grand experience.

One of the ironies of fasting is that it can be the most difficult for those who need it the most; in these cases, people must start with the subtle diet changes just discussed. One transition protocol is the 1-meal-a-day plan. The meal is usually eaten around 3 p.m.; water, juices, teas, and some fresh fruit or vegetable snacks can be eaten at other times. It is important that the wholesome meal be neither excessive nor rich. I suggest a protein and vegetable meal (such as fish and salad or steamed vegetables) or a starch and vegetable meal (such as brown rice and mixed steamed greens, carrots, celery, and zucchini). People on this plan start to detoxify slowly, lose some weight, and after a few days feel pretty sound. The chance of any strong symptoms developing during this transition time or during a subsequent fast is greatly minimized. The next goal for those who have done a 1-meal-a-day program is a 1-day fast. The fasting then progresses to 2- and 3-day fasts, with 1 or 2 days between them when light foods and more raw fruits and vegetables are consumed. This allows us to build up to longer-lasting 5- to 10-day fasts. When the transition is made this slowly, even water fasting can be less intense (although I usually recommend juice fasts).

To avoid being excessively impatient, we need to make and adhere to a plan. It is important to continually observe and listen to your body and keep notes in a journal. Get to know yourself and your nature. Once we have fasted successfully, we can continue to do 1-day fasts weekly or a 3-day fast every month if we need it. This experience helps us to reconnect with ourselves and to work toward a goal of optimum health. Meditation, exercise, fresh air and sunshine, massage, and baths are all essential and nourishing during this and any cleansing period.

A juice cleanse, which I usually recommend, can be longer and is much easier for most people. Most fasting clinics and practitioners recommend the fresh juices of raw fruits and vegetables. They provide calories and nutrients on which to function and build new cells, and they also provide the inherent enzymes contained in these vital foods. (Food enzyme theories, discussed throughout the twentieth century and getting even more popular currently, have been described in such books as *Enzyme Nutrition,* by Edward Howell, MD, and *MicroMiracles: Discover the Healing Power of Enzymes,* by Ellen Cutler, MD, DC.) Raw foods are considered the healing force in the diet because they contain active enzymes, which are broken down when foods are cooked. Many health enthusiasts consider a raw-food diet the most healing and nutritious diet.

In a more adventurous mode, many people, even some who have never fasted, begin with a 7- to 10-day or even longer cleanse using primarily fresh juices. I recommend this for most people who have any of the indications and none of the contraindications discussed in this program. People planning these longer fasts, especially inexperienced fasters who have been eating a random diet, should spend a period about equal in length to the planned fast preparing for it. During this preparatory period, we can follow some of the previous suggestions, such as eliminating sugar and refined foods, fatty foods, chemicals, and drugs from the diet and reducing consumption of meats and other acid-forming foods. We can then move into several days of consuming primarily fruits and vegetables and more fluids. This will lead into an easier and more energizing fast.

Timing of Fasts

The two key times for natural cleansing are the times of transition into spring and autumn. In Chinese medicine, the transition time between the seasons is considered to be about 10 days before and after the equinox or solstice. For spring, this period is about March 10 through April 1; for autumn, it is from about September 11 through October 2. In cooler climates, where spring weather begins later and autumn earlier, the fasting can be scheduled appropriately, as it is easier to do in warmer weather. With fasting, the body tends to cool down. In the general detoxification program on page 741, there is also a complete yearly cycle for cleansing with a variety of ideas and options. For spring, I usually suggest lemon and/or greens as the

---

Master Cleanser

2 tbsp fresh lemon or lime juice

1 tbsp pure maple syrup (up to 2 tbsp if you want
　to drop less weight)

1/10 tsp cayenne pepper

8 ounces spring water

Mix and drink 8 to 12 glasses throughout the day.
Eat or drink nothing else except water, laxative
herb tea, and peppermint or chamomile tea. Keep
the lemonade in a glass container (not plastic) or
make it fresh each time. Rinse your mouth with
water after each glass to prevent the lemon juice
from hurting the enamel of your teeth.

---

focus of the cleansing. Diluted lemon water, lemon
and honey, or (my favorite) the Master Cleanser, could
be used.

Fresh fruit or vegetable juices diluted with an equal
amount of water also stimulate cleansing. Some good
vegetable choices are carrots, celery, beets, and greens.
Soup broths can also be used. Juices with blue-green
algae, spirulina, or chlorella provide more energy, as
they contain quality protein (amino acids) and are easily assimilated. Fasting can also be done in other seasons. Summer, with the warm weather, is a good time
to do 10 days. Winter can be one day a month or longer
cleansing, but with a warming diet, such as brown rice,
vegetables, and miso soup. This can be done for 2 to
3 weeks. In autumn, a fast of at least 3 to 5 days can be
done, using either water or a variety of juices. Juices
could include the Master Cleanser, apple and/or freshly
made grape juice (usually mixed with a little lemon
and water to reduce sweetness), vegetable juices, and
warm broths.

How Do We Know How Long to Fast?

To decide how long to fast, we can either follow a
specific time schedule or listen closely to our own
individual cycles and needs. Paying attention to our
energy level and degree of congestion, and observing of our tongue and its coating will offer helpful
cleansing guidelines. As we gain some fasting expe-

rience, we will become more attuned to specific
times when we need to strengthen or lighten our
diet and when we need to cleanse. If we are under
stress, have been overindulging, or develop some
congestive symptoms, we need to lighten our diet
and possibly cleanse. The odor of our urine, breath,
and sweat are telltale signs of cleansing in action.

Breaking a Fast

Ending or stopping a fast and beginning to eat again
also takes some monitoring. Things to watch include
energy level, weight, detox symptoms, tongue coating,
and degree of hunger. If our energy falls for more than
a day or if our weight gets too low, we should come off
the fast. If symptoms are particularly intense or sudden, it is possible that we need food. Generally, the
tongue is a good indicator of our state of toxicity or clarity. With fasting, the tongue usually becomes coated
with a white, yellow, or gray film. This signals the
body's cleansing process, and it will usually clear when
the detox cycle is complete. However, tongue observation is not a foolproof indicator. Some people's
tongues may coat very little, while others will remain
coated even after cleansing. If in doubt, it is better to
make the transition back to food and then cleanse
again later. Hunger is another sign of readiness to move
back into eating, as it is often minimal during cleansing times. Occasionally people are hungry throughout
a fast, but most lose interest in food from day 3 to 7 and
then experience real, deep-seated hunger once again.
This is a sign to eat carefully.

**Breaking a fast must be well planned and exe-
cuted slowly and carefully to prevent the creation
of symptoms and sickness.** It is wise to make a gradual transition into a regular diet, rather than just going
out to dinner after a week of fasting. It is suggested that
we take half of our total cleansing time to move back
into our regular diet, which is hopefully now better
planned and more healthful. The digestion has been
at rest, so we need to chew our foods well. If we have
fasted on water alone, we need to prepare the digestive tract with diluted juices, perhaps beginning with
a few teaspoons of fresh orange juice in a glass of
water and progressing to stronger mixtures throughout the day. Diluted fresh grape or orange juice stimulates the digestion. Arnold Ehret, a European fasting

---

Autumn Rejuvenation Ration

Contributed by Bethany Argisle

3 cups spring water

1 tbsp ginger root, chopped

1–2 tbsp miso paste (do not boil)

1–2 stalks green onion, chopped

cilantro, to taste, chopped

1–2 pinches cayenne pepper

2 tsp extra virgin olive oil

juice of half a lemon

Boil water. Add ginger root. Simmer 10 minutes. Stir in miso paste to taste. Turn off burner. Then add green onion, some cilantro, cayenne, olive oil, and lemon juice. Remove and cover to steep for 10 minutes. You may vary ingredient portions to satisfy your palate. Enjoy.

---

expert and proponent of the "mucusless" diet, suggests that fruits and fruit juices should not be used right after a meat eater's first fast because they may coagulate intestinal mucus and cause problems. A meat eater's colon bacteria are probably different from a vegetarian's. Consequently, fruit sugars like those in the juices may not be tolerated well; instead, the active gram-positive anaerobic bacteria in the meat eater will produce more toxins. Extra acidophilus supplements continued on a regular basis help shift colon ecology in meat eaters and can even be used during cleanses.

With juice fasting, it is easier to transition back to food. A raw or cooked low-starch vegetable, such as spinach or other greens, is quite appropriate. A little sauerkraut also helps to stimulate the digestive function. A laxative-type meal including grapes, cherries, or soaked or stewed prunes can also be used to initiate eating, as they keep the bowels moving. Some experts say that the bowels should move within 1 or 2 hours after the first meal and, if not, an enema should be used. Some people do a saltwater flush before their first day of food by drinking 1 quart of water containing 2 teaspoons of dissolved sea salt. Be careful, however; see more on colon cleansing on page 781. Our individual transit times vary in response to laxatives and saltwater.

However you make the transition, go slowly, chew well, and do not overeat or mix too many foods at any meal. Start with simple vegetable meals, such as salads or steamed veggies. Fruit should be eaten alone. Soaked prunes or figs are helpful. Well-cooked, watery brown rice or millet is handled well by most people by the second day. From there, progress slowly through grains and vegetables. Some nuts, seeds, or legumes can be added, and then richer protein foods, if these are desired. Returning to food is a crucial time for learning individual responses or reactions. **Self-observation gives us an opportunity to see destructive dietary habits and discover specific food intolerances.** You may wish to keep notes at this time. If you respond poorly to a food, avoid it for a week or so, and then eat it alone to see how it feels. This is when food reactions may be revealed.

Juice Specifics

Some juices work better for certain people or conditions. In general, diluted fresh juices of raw organic fruits and vegetables are best. Canned and frozen juices should be avoided. Some bottled juice may be used, but freshly squeezed or extracted is best, as long as it is used soon after processing. Lemon juice, wheatgrass juice, or a little ginger or garlic juice can be added to drinks for vitality and to stimulate cleansing.

Water and other liquids increase waste elimination. Lemon tends to loosen and draw out mucus and is especially useful for liver cleansing. Diluted lemon juice with or without a little honey, or the Master Cleanser lemonade, loosens mucus quickly, so if this is used, we need to cleanse the bowels regularly to prevent getting sick. Most vegetable juices are milder than lemon juice. Each juice has a unique nutritional composition and probable physiological actions (although these have been studied very little). Fresh juices may be more easily digested, especially if they contain digestive enzymes that are able to maintain activity in the digestive tract. (But once again, there has been minimal research in this area.) In general, some juices are more caloric than others. For example, the juices of apples, grapes, oranges, and carrots are good cleansing juices but might be minimized for weight loss as they are high in calories. Juices more helpful for weight loss include grapefruit, lemon, cucumber, and greens

---

Juices and the Organs or Conditions They Help Heal

Fruit Juices

Apple. Liver, intestines.

Black cherry. Colon, menstrual problems, gout.

Citrus. Cardiovascular disease (CVD), obesity, hemorrhoids, varicose veins.

Grape. Colon, anemia.

Lemon. Liver, gallbladder, allergies, asthma, CVD, colds.

Papaya. Stomach, indigestion, hemorrhoids, colitis.

Pear. Gallbladder.

Pineapple. Allergies, arthritis, inflammation, edema, hemorrhoids.

Watermelon. Kidneys, edema.

Vegetable Juices

Beet greens. Gallbladder, liver, osteoporosis.

Beets. Blood, liver, menstrual problems, arthritis.

Cabbage. Colitis, ulcers.

Carrots. Eyes, arthritis, osteoporosis.

Celery. Kidneys, diabetes, osteoporosis.

Comfrey. Intestines, hypertension, osteoporosis.

Cucumber. Edema, diabetes.

Garlic. Allergies, colds, hypertension, CVD, high fats, diabetes.

Greens. Cardiovascular disease, skin, eczema, digestive problems, obesity, breath.

Jerusalem artichokes. Diabetes.

Parsley. Kidneys, edema, arthritis.

Potatoes. Intestines, ulcer.

Radish. Liver, high fats, obesity.

Spinach. Anemia, eczema.

Watercress. Anemia, colds.

Wheatgrass. Anemia, liver, intestines, breath.

(such as lettuce, spinach, or parsley). Watermelon juice with a bit of ginger is tasty and cleansing. A variety of juices can be used in a fast, prepared fresh daily. Keep recipes of your favorite new combinations.

These juices may be helpful for particular organs or illnesses, based on my experience as well as information contained in *How to Get Well,* by the experienced naturopath Paavo Airola. To prepare juices, we want to start with the freshest and most chemical-free fruits and vegetables possible (using organic will avoid chemical herbicides and pesticides). They should be cleaned or soaked and stored properly. If not organic, they should be peeled, especially if they are waxed. With root vegetables like carrots or beets, the above-ground ends should be trimmed. Some people drop their vegetables into a pot of boiling water for a minute or so to clean them before juicing. The right juicer is important. The rotary-blade juicers (Champion brand) are good at squeezing the juice with minimum molecular irritation and are medium in price range. The centrifuge juicers are also fine, but they waste juice left in pulp. The best juicers are the compressors (Norwalk brand), which are more expensive. Blenders are not really juicers (what they produce is more like liquid salad) but can be used to puree soups or make smoothies. These drinks can also be used for a fast because they are high in fiber and nutrients. I once did a energizing weeklong fast with two blender drinks a day—fruits in the morning and vegetables in the late afternoon—with teas and water in between.

Other Aspects of Healthy Fasting

Healthy fasting is not only about juices and digestive cleanses, however. Changes in our everyday habits can be critical, especially if a balanced lifestyle is not part of our weekly routine. Each of the items on the following list is important for success when fasting:

- **Fresh air.** Plenty is needed to support cleansing and oxygenation of the cells and tissues.

- **Sunshine.** This is needed to revitalize the body; but avoid excessive exposure.

- **Water.** Bathing is important to cleanse the skin at least twice daily. Steams and saunas are also good for giving warmth as well as supporting detoxification.

- **Skin brushing.** Do this with a dry, soft brush before bathing; this will help clear toxins from the skin. This is a good year-round practice as well.

- **Exercise.** This is important to support the cleansing process. It helps to relax the body, clear wastes, and prevent toxicity symptoms. Walking, bicycling, swimming, or other usual exercises can usually be done during a fast, although more dangerous or contact sports might be avoided.

• **No drugs.** None should be used during fasts except mandatory prescription drugs. Particularly, avoidance of alcohol, nicotine, and caffeine is imperative.

• **Vitamin supplements. These are not typically used during fasting; thus there is no table of nutrients with this program.** Occasionally, I recommend a small amount of powdered nutrients; there are new ones out, such as Ola Loa, a multinutrient formula created by orthomolecular physician Richard Kunin, MD. I also use daily a packet of Emergen-C Lite, which provides vitamin C with some B vitamins and minerals. Some supplemental fiber, such as psyllium husks, can be part of a colon detox program. Special chlorophyll and amino acid containing foods/nutrients, such as green barley, chlorella, and spirulina, may also be vitality enhancers and purifiers during cleanses. Occasionally, some mineral support, especially potassium, calcium, and magnesium, or vitamin C will be suggested, usually in powdered or liquid forms (pills are not suggested as they are not easily processed without eating) to help in preventing cramps if there is a lot of physical activity, sweating, and fluid and mineral losses, or for an extended fast. Some people even use amino acid powders and other vitamin powders with some benefit during cleanses. In general, most of these supplemental nutrients are best used with foods.

• **Colon cleansing.** An essential part of healthy fasting, some form of bowel stimulation is recommended. Colonic irrigations with water performed by a trained therapist with modern equipment are the most thorough. These can be done at the beginning, midpoint, and end of the fast. It is suggested that enemas be used at least every other day, especially if they are the primary cleansing method. Fasting clinics often suggest that enemas be used daily or several times a day. With these, water alone is used to flush the colon of toxins. It may be helpful for an enema or laxative preparation to be used the day before the fast begins, to lessen initial toxicity. Herbal laxatives are commonly taken orally during fasting, and many formulas are available either as capsules or for making tea. These include cascara sagrada, senna leaves, licorice root, buckthorn, rhubarb root, aloe vera, and other prepared formulas. The saltwater flush (drinking 1 quart of warm water with 2 teaspoons of sea salt dissolved in it) can be used first thing in the morning on alternate days throughout the fast to flush the entire intestinal tract, although this does not work well for everyone. **It is not recommended for salt-sensitive or water-retaining people or for those with hypertension.**

• **Work and be creative.** Make plans for your life! Staying busy is helpful in breaking our ties to food. We also need time for ourselves. Most fasters experience greater work energy and more creativity and, naturally, find lots to do.

• **Clean up.** A motto during fasting. As we clean the body, we want to clean our room, desk, office, closet, and home—just like spring cleaning. Fasting clearly brings us into harmony with the cleansing process of nutrition. If we want to get ready for the new, we need to make space by clearing out the old.

• **Join others in fasting.** This can generate strong bonds and provide an added spiritual lift. It opens up new supportive relationships and new levels of existing ones. It also provides support if we feel down or want to quit. Most people feel better as their fast progresses—more vital, lighter, less blocked, more flexible, clearer, and more spiritually attuned. For many, it is nice to have someone with whom to share this.

• **Avoid negative influences of others.** Some people may not understand or support you in your fast. There are many fears and misconceptions about fasting. We need to listen to our own inner guidance and not to others' limitations, but we also need to maintain awareness and insight into any problems should they arise. Being in contact with fasters will provide us with the positive support we need.

• **The economy of fasting.** Fasting allows us to save time, money, and future health-care costs. Although we may be worried about not having enough, we may already have too much. Many of us are inspired to share more of ourselves when we are freed from food.

• **Meditation and relaxation.** These are also important aspects of fasting to help attune us to deeper levels of ourselves and clear the stresses that we have carried.

• **Spiritual practice and prayer.** These will affirm our positive attitude toward ourselves and life in general. This supports our meditation and relaxation and provides us with the inner fuel to carry on life with purpose and passion.

Conclusion

Fasting can easily become a way of life and an effective dietary practice. Over a period of time we can go from symptom cleansing to preventive fasting. We should support ourselves regularly with a balanced, wholesome diet, and fast at specific times to treat symptoms and/or to enhance our vitality and spiritual practice. If we could devote one day a week to purification and a cleansing diet, the path of health would be smooth indeed. See the yearly cleansing schedule on page 749 for ideas on how to incorporate a seasonal detoxification approach into your life. We all overdo it with foods or other substances at different times and then may need fasting more frequently. We all need to return to the cycle of a daily fast of 12 to 14 hours overnight until our morning "break fast" and then find our own natural pattern of food consumption. This usually means one main meal and two lighter ones. For low-weight, high-metabolism people, two larger or three moderately sized meals are probably needed. If we eat a heavier evening meal, we need only a light breakfast, and vice versa. Through awareness and experience, we can find our individual nutritional needs and fulfill them by listening to that inner nutritionist—the body.

Choosing healthy foods, chewing well, and maintaining good colon function all minimize the need for fasting. However, if we do get out of balance, we can employ one of the oldest treatments known to humans, the instinctive therapy for many illnesses, Nature's doctor, therapist, and tool for preventing disease—FASTING!

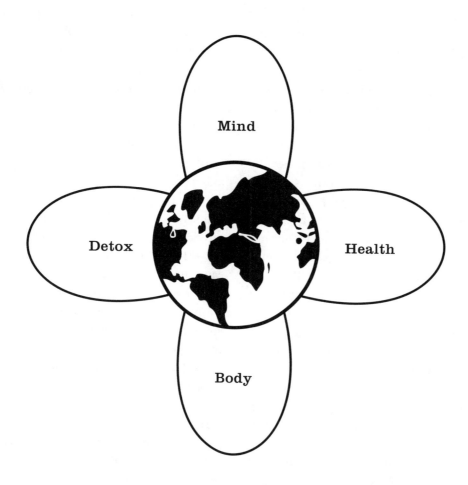

Futureword: Survival, Vitality Now, and Health Forever

Speculating about the future and living idealistically with an "immortal" philosophy are important topics to consider. Both were a part of the first edition of *Staying Healthy with Nutrition*. In this new edition, these ideas appear separately here in this Futureword as a philosophical exploration on how we can live more optimally now to protect both our planet and our health. Review these programs when you need a lift. Blessings to you and your family.

PERSONAL AND PLANETARY SURVIVAL IN THE 21ST CENTURY

The use of certain chemicals has been a great boon to the technological age; it has also been a great detriment to the ecology and health of Mother Earth and her people. Chemistry has changed the balance of life. I am a naturalist at heart and appreciate the beauty and purity of Nature more than almost anything else. It is sad to think that Earth has been violated, which we can sense in the hidden dangers in the planet's water, soil, air, and the food that we eat.

The chemistry of today and the many man-made chemicals include a large amount of both safe and harmful substances. Food additives, for instance, include a wide range of substances—from natural vitamins, minerals, and salts to more disturbing preservatives and artificial colors and flavors. But our chemical concerns are not all related to food. Occupational and industrial uses of chemicals, most of them affecting the food chain in some way, pose additional problems. Home use of potentially toxic chemicals increases yearly and is a large part of total chemical exposure.

It may seem harmless to spray some bugs or kill some weeds to make our home "safer" or more beautiful or, more commonly, to improve the yield of commercial crops. Chemicals can be used in food help protect it and usually lengthen its storage time or shelf life. These factors figure into the profit motive of the agricultural and chemical industries and are affected by the politics of our society. A side effect of this laissez-faire capitalism, however, is that the emphasis on profits and return on the dollar invested in many cases supersedes concerns for the health and well-being of the people and the environment. In the past, it appeared that only a few alarmed citizens and government employees had been looking at the global cost of pollution. Today, each of us must face that responsibility, which inevitably requires cleaning up our mess. This will probably cost more than the profits that were made in the first place. And we will pay for it, possibly with our lives. More citizens planet than ever before are showing concern about the pollution of the planet. But the problem has escalated and will continue to worsen until stronger measures are taken to stop this chemical obsession.

Chemicals are both an outcome of technology and a factor contributing to its development. Chemistry has made life easier in many ways. Plastics products facilitate basic daily tasks, creating less expensive and more durable toys and kitchenware, for example. Some impressive medical advances have resulted from applied chemistry. Foods can be processed more simply in the factory and the kitchen, and we have new taste treats and more edible products every year, as well as more chemicals and drugs, diseases, and extinctions. In the terms of testing and use, however, I believe the government underplays potential toxicity, both the immediate and long-term effects and especially the possible interactions with the environment or other chemicals in use. Synthetic chemicals are used that are not found naturally anywhere on Earth, and neither Earth nor the human body knows how to break down these substances. The organochloride pesticides such as aldrin and dieldrin are examples. (See chapter 11, Food and the Earth, page 432.)

The latency period between exposure to carcinogenic industrial chemicals and cancer may be as long as twenty to thirty years, and the chemicals may last even longer in our environment. Realistically, it is difficult to test for carcinogenicity unless we postpone the use of various chemicals for decades of testing or find more sophisticated methods of predictive testing. Often it is an increased cancer rate in a certain population exposed to a carcinogen, such as asbestos, that alerts us to its danger. Because chemical use is expanding so rapidly, it is unlikely that everything can be studied thoroughly (or that the integrity of the chemical industry executives can be trusted), so life experience must ultimately be our teacher on what works safely. Industrial and home use of chemicals has increased nearly 10,000 times since 1945. More than 33,000 chemicals are in use, and nearly 1,000 are added yearly out of the many thousands presented to the Environmental Protection Agency (EPA) and other government agencies.

Currently, there are several hundred chemicals on the EPA's hazardous list. And every year, the Agency for Toxic Substances and Disease Registry (ATSDR) makes its CERCLA Priority List (Comprehensive Environmental Response, Compensation, and Liability Act) of 275 substances posing the most significant potential threat to human health. In 2003, the CERCLA list was topped by arsenic, lead, mercury, and vinyl chloride, with pesticides, solvents, and vehicle emission toxins rounding out most of the top 25. These substances cause cancer and/or are poisonous in some other way. Many are hydrocarbon petrochemicals, made through the chemical processing of petroleum. They include the aromatic amines, such as dyes and epoxies (glues), the chlorinated olefins (hydrocarbons), such as many plastics and pesticides, and the alkyl halide solvents, such as trichloroethylene (TCE).

What makes these industrial chemicals so harmful is the damage or irritation they can cause on a cellular level, whether immediate or over time. **Most of these chemicals inflict damage in 1 of 5 ways. First, they can be directly genotoxic, meaning they can do direct damage to our genes and genetic material.** They can create breaks in the DNA strands (called *single-strand breaks*). They can link 2 DNA strands together when the 2 are not meant to

be linked (called *cross-linking*). They can insert information where it does not belong, or remove information where it is needed (known as *nucleotide pair insertion* and *deletion*). All categories of toxins have been shown to contain genotoxic substances, including pesticides (like pentachlorophenol), heavy metals (like lead or mercury), and common GRAS-listed (Generally Recommended as Safe) additives (like the preservative sodium bisulfite).

A second route of damage involves the shutdown (or lessening) of energy production. Most of our cells contain key energy production devices called *mitochondria*. The form of energy made by the mitochondria is ATP (adenosine triphosphate). Many toxic substances prevent the mitochondria from making ATP or severely compromise their ability to do so. The plasticizers (like MEHP or DEHP) can have this effect, as can styrene (found in Styrofoam), many pesticides (including DDT), and a long list of common food additives (including BHA and BHT).

Increasing our oxidative stress is another surefire consequence of excess exposure to food toxins. A basic problem here is the formation of too many free radicals, the third area of concern. Free radicals are highly reactive forms of common, everyday molecules. If too many are present in an area of the cell, they are likely to damage some structures. If it is the cell membrane, that is what gets damaged. If it is the cell nucleus (where our genes are housed), that is where the damage occurs. (Excess free-radical formation is usually considered to be a hallmark of oxidative stress, a metabolic imbalance in which oxygen-containing molecules become too unwieldy for the body to handle. Free radicals and oxidative stress are related because many free radicals contain at least 1 oxygen atom.) **Oxidative damage is considered to be a key component of many chronic diseases, including many cancers, heart attacks, the aging process in general, cataracts, Parkinson's disease, inflammatory bowel disease, and others.** The list of food toxins that can increase the risk of oxidative stress is equally long. Included are the heavy metals (cadmium, lead, and mercury), many pesticides, many solvents, asbestos, and aluminum.

Fourth on the list of damaging processes is distortion of chemical signals sent between cells.

Residues from plastic packaging are particularly problematic in this respect, as are solvents like benzene and toluene and heavy metals like cadmium and lead.

The fifth and final route of damage is all too often overlooked, even by nutritionists. Toxic substances have to be detoxified in the body. Our cells are usually up to this task, but the process requires a fairly rich supply of many nutrients. Directly or indirectly, we need a healthy reserve of the minerals sulfur, zinc, and copper; the B vitamins choline, folate, B6 and B12; the amino acids cysteine, taurine, glycine, and glutamine; plus the tripeptide glutathione to detox food additives. **Overexposure to additives puts us at risk of depleting these nutrient reserves.** If we do not have enough of these nutrients to begin with, we are likely to have food additives (toxins) in our bodies much longer than desired. One of the reasons so many of us just feel run down or lacking vitality is because we have used up too much energy and nutrient reserves trying to process out toxic chemicals, including food additives.

Chemical use is now part of all aspects of life; chemistry is here to stay. The question is, "Do we have better living through chemistry?" Learning to live with chemicals and to use them appropriately so that they do not destroy us before our time is my fervent hope. This involves maintaining a healthy immune system, a positive attitude, and a high purpose. Protecting ourselves by reducing chemical usage and exposure, I believe, will greatly reduce our chances of disease, cancer, and early death. This is important for everyone, but especially for the chemically sensitive, infants and young children, the elderly, and invalids—all of whom are more susceptible to chemical toxicity. **Making changes and a commitment to living as chemically free as possible is a strong investment in our personal and collective life insurance plan.**

> Don't give me anything for free, I can't afford it.
> —Edward Spritzer,
> Bethany Argisle's wise father

Four Laws of Ecology by Barry Commoner

1. **Everything is connected to everything else.** We cannot do something in one area of the environment without affecting the rest of it.

2. **Everything must go somewhere.** In Nature, all waste products nourish something else. We now use materials that Nature has no mechanisms to break down.

3. **Nature knows best.** Human advances that violate Nature are detrimental to us all.

4. **There is no such thing as a free lunch.** Many of the gains in productivity are achieved at the expense of the ecosystem in the form of pollution. A price will be paid for this somewhere down the line beyond mere money. Many people are paying the price now in the form of chronic illness caused by artificially synthesized new chemicals

---

88 SURVIVAL SUGGESTIONS

Here I offer 88 suggestions, including activities, ideas, and changes, that each of us can implement to benefit ourselves, our families, and our friends. Further suggestions are offered by Charles T. McGee, MD, in *How to Survive Modern Technology*.

Foods

1. Eat moderately on a regular basis. Overeating stresses the body, and being overweight may result in further health complications.

2. Avoid processed foods, particularly those that contain highly refined ingredients.

3. Reduce or eliminate chemical food additives, particularly preservatives, artificial colors and flavors, and artificial sweeteners.

4. Read package labels to learn about what additives the foods contain. Do not be confused by "natural" or "no preservatives" on the label.

5. Eat more high-fiber foods: vegetables, fruits, and moderate amounts of whole grains.

6. Eat more wholesome, natural foods as they come from Nature—primarily fruits, vegetables, and whole grains, plus some nuts, seeds, and beans.

7. Buy and use organic foods grown without chemical fertilizers and pesticides, and those that are not genetically modified. This action supports the organic food industry and the consciousness of cleaner food. Much produce is contaminated with fumigants and fungicides even after it is harvested.

8. Wash appropriate foods. Know how to clean contaminated foods, with baking soda or a natural wash.

9. Buy more foods at local farmers' markets, where you can find out directly how and where the food is grown. This supports small or family farms. Also, the food sold at such markets is probably fresher, less expensive, and less chemically treated. Or join a subscription farm through a community supported agriculture (CSA) program in your area.

10. Refrigerate or store food appropriately as soon as possible to prevent spoilage.

11. Drink clean water. Use a water filter, buy purified water, or drink well water that has been analyzed regularly (every 1–2 years) and shown to be free of chemicals and germs. Avoid tap water!

12. Avoid red meats—beef, pork, and lamb. Raising livestock on a vast scale is destructive to any natural environment. Overconsumption of these products is unhealthy for most people.

13. Especially avoid chemically treated red meats. Whenever possible, buy the meats of range-fed animals, free of antibiotics and hormones. Do not consume lunch meats or other nitrate- or nitrite-cured meats.

14. Reduce total saturated fat intake to a maximum of 5–10% of total calories in the diet. Consumption of saturated fat is related to the increased incidence of cardiovascular disease and cancer.

15. Limit total fat intake to 20% to 30% of dietary calories. This range is based on climate and personal needs and includes saturated fats (animal products, dairy products, and eggs), monounsaturated (such as olive oil), and polyunsaturated fats (vegetable oils). **The monounsaturated fats are the healthiest category, and flaxseed oil has a good balance of omega-3 and omega-6 oils.** The majority of our fat intake should be with essential (required) fatty acids from raw nuts and seeds as well as from quality fresh vegetable oils.

16. Increase the dietary ratio of polyunsaturated to saturated fats, focusing on the omega-3 polyunsaturated fatty acids like those found in oily fish such as salmon (wild salmon and not farm-raised, which may contain more chemicals and antibiotics, depending on how it was raised). This reduces the risk of cardiovascular disease.

17. Use cold-pressed vegetable oils. These are not extracted with chemical solvents. Olive oil, a monounsaturated fat, may be the best for cooking because it is more stable to heat and air than its polyunsaturated counterparts. Store out of the light.

18. Avoid all organ meats, such as liver, heart, and brain (unless certified organic). These can be high in accumulated chemicals.

19. Buy organic poultry and eggs from range-fed chickens, if you eat such foods. These are not treated with antibiotics or hormones or fed highly chemical feeds.

20. Eat deep-sea fish. Of the animal foods, fish may be the best. Unfortunately, mercury contamination has become a problem with many fish, including tuna, halibut, shark, swordfish, and king mackerel. Farmed salmon can also be problematic, as can albacore tuna. Pacific wild salmon is probably going to stay at the top of my "desirable" list, along with some of the specialty canned tunas that are much lower in mercury and preserve many more of the natural omega-3 fatty acids.

21. Use low-fat or nonfat (ideally organic) milk products if you use milk at all. It is not recommended that cow's milk be consumed either regularly or in large amounts; goat's and sheep's milk products, plain yogurt, kefir, or some cheeses are probably better.

22. Minimize use of soft drinks, with their high amounts of sugar and high-fructose corn syrup. Substitute water or a combination of fruit juice and carbonated mineral water.

23. Minimize use of sugar, particularly sucrose, or white sugar. Try natural sweeteners, such as date sugar, rice or malt syrup, honey, maple syrup, or agave nectar, probably in that order of preference. Stevia is an herbal (naturally occurring) noncaloric sweetener.

24. Avoid waxed fruits and vegetables. The paraffin covering is potentially harmful.

25. Avoid aluminum and Teflon cookware; use glass, Pyrex, iron, or stainless steel. By the way, avoidance of aluminum includes all of the anodized aluminum nonstick pans, even though migration of aluminum from this material is far less than from conventional aluminum cookware.

26. Eat more cruciferous vegetables (organically grown is preferable). This includes cabbage, broccoli, cauliflower, and brussels sprouts.

27. Rotate foods to avoid allergic/sensitivity reactions. Eating most foods only every 3 or 4 days helps reduce this potential.

28. Eat simple meals. This allows better digestion and utilization and makes it easier to isolate any food reactions. Food-combining is a beneficial practice as is chewing well, which supports best digestion.

29. Use a pulse test to see whether food reactions occur. Check the pulse before eating and again 10 and 20 minutes after. If the pulse rate increases by more than 20% (usually 15–20 beats per minute), 1 of the foods eaten may be causing a reaction.

30. Eliminate any reactive food completely for 1 month, then reintroduce it, eating it no more than once every 4 days; if there is a repeated reaction, avoid it.

31. Do occasional cleansing or fasting, as appropriate to the season or your health condition. Detoxification is important for health for most of us in these modern times.

32. Use an additive-free general nutritional supplement and even a hypoallergenic one if you have food or chemical sensitivities.

33. Avoid cheap, colored vitamin pills, as they may contain petroleum products, hydrocarbons, artificial colors or flavors, BHA, BHT, or sugars—all potentially toxic chemicals.

34. Take additional antioxidant nutrients, which may help minimize chemical irritations. These include beta-carotene and vitamins A, C, and E as well as zinc and selenium.

35. Minimize consumption of microwave-cooked foods. Researchers do not really know what the long-term effects are.

36. Do not use irradiated foods. The effects are unknown. These may include pork, some herbs, and now possibly various fruits and vegetables. Keep your eyes and ears open to the progress (or actually the regress) of food irradiation.

37. Minimize barbequing or broiling with gas, as the benzopyrenes created may be hazardous.

38. Avoid genetically modified foods. Researchers know they are unhealthy for the environment, and they are likely unhealthy for us as well. Protect our monarch butterflies and other important species.

Lifestyle Habits

39. Avoid smoking, both primary and secondary smoking. If you do not smoke, ask others to refrain. If you do smoke, try to stop—and succeed!

40. Reduce or avoid alcohol use. Alcohol depresses the senses and reduces immune resistance. Chemicals are used in processing most alcohol products.

41. Use organic wines or beers if drinking for social celebration. Beside supporting growers and manufacturers who avoid chemical use, this helps avoid the common sulfites, solvents, defoamers, and chemical pesticides found in many alcohol products.

42. Create a good exercise program. This includes weight-training exercises, stretching, and at least 30 minutes of vigorous (aerobic) activity several times a week.

43. Avoid excessive sun exposure. With the depletion of the ozone layer and the effect of ultraviolet light, the risks now outweigh the benefits. However, it is still healthful to have some exposure on our skin for vitamin D production and overall health.

44. Practice some form of stress reduction daily. Meditate, lie down without sleeping, or just sit with your eyes closed, breathe deeply, and relax for at least 15 to 20 minutes. There are many teachers and tapes to help in these life-rebalancing processes. Draw pictures, sing, drum, laugh!

45. Minimize your overall use of drugs, particularly over-the-counter drugs and unnecessary prescription drugs.

46. Reduce the use of carcinogenic drugs, such as the antiparasitic drugs metronidazole (Flagyl); estrogens; and the antifungal griseofulvin.

47. Try alternatives to drugs and surgery whenever possible. These include herbs and nutrition, homeopathy, acupuncture, and chiropractic, to name a few possibilities. Educate yourself about health options.

48. Avoid habitual drug (substance) use, such as the consumption of caffeine in coffee, tea, or colas and regular sugar use.

Not just Survive, live life Alive.

—Bethany Argisle

---

49. Minimize or avoid the use of recreational drugs, such as cocaine, sedatives, alcohol, and marijuana. They all have negative effects, especially in the long term.

50. Avoid cosmetics with warnings of certain dangerous ingredients, such as antiperspirant sprays containing aluminum. Also, if you believe in animal rights, avoid using products from companies who conduct experimental testing on animals.

51. Drink more clean water and less soda, coffee, juice, and alcoholic beverages.

52. Wear more natural-fiber clothes, especially if you are sensitive to synthetic materials. Cotton, rayon, hemp, and silk are more comfortable to many people and do not hold and conduct static electricity.

53. Avoid X-rays whenever possible. They may weaken tissues and increase cancer risk.

Positive Changes at Home

54. Keep all chemicals and toxic products away from children and vice versa.

55. Keep the house clean and put food away to avoid unwanted pests and the growth of infectious microorganisms.

56. Try more natural pest-control practices, such as herbs, powders, and fragrant oils that help fight insects and rodents. Avoid using pesticides and other strong chemicals at home whenever possible.

57. Avoid chemical cleaning agents whenever possible. Use more natural products, such as low-phosphate and unscented soaps, baking soda, borax, vinegar, and lemon. Do not replace dirt with chemicals.

58. Avoid using aerosols, artificial scents, and toilet bowl colorings. Use herbs and naturally fragrant oils instead.

59. Use unscented and uncolored paper products, such as toilet paper, paper towels, and napkins, to avoid unnecessary chemicals. Try recycled

paper products whenever possible; their quality has improved in recent years.

60. Try natural drain cleaners, such as hot water with vinegar or baking soda.

61. Wash fruits and vegetables with water. Especially for store-bought, nonorganic produce, use a vegetable brush to scrub firmer-skinned produce, and soak the softer produce for a few minutes. Rinse everything after soaking or scrubbing. Also, remove the outer leaves of vegetables when appropriate.

62. Recycle waste products whenever possible. Organic waste, such as food scraps, can be used in the garden as compost. Glass can be reused or recycled and so can aluminum and newspaper. All this saves energy and materials.

63. Avoid living near toxic industry, such as chemical plants, refineries, toxic dump sites, or water-treatment plants.

64. Avoid living near power lines and electrical plants and any excessive electrical exposure, all of which may pose some health risks. Remember, the body is electromagnetic in nature.

Positive Changes at Work

65. Avoid traveling in rush-hour traffic, if possible, or behind buses and trucks, to reduce carbon monoxide and hydrocarbon gas exposure.

66. Obtain natural lighting or full-spectrum lights at work. If possible, work by a window; if not, full-spectrum fluorescent lighting is worth the small investment.

67. Create good air circulation. Try to get a desk by an operable window or invest in an air purifier for your area. Circulation of good-quality air is vital to health. Breathe freely and often.

68. Avoid tobacco smoke around you. Put a sign on your door or desk and demand a smoke-free area at work. This is less necessary now as indoor smoking has been greatly curtailed (banned by law in most cases).

69. Have good drinking water available in the office. If there is no purified water cooler, bring your own water.

70. Minimize synthetic fibers at work, in rugs and furniture, for example. Hardwood floors are better, especially for the chemically sensitive person.

71. Avoid chemical use at your desk. This involves typewriter correction fluid, glue, and toxic art supplies. Use nontoxic supplies such as staples or paper clips, erasers, or a self-correcting typewriter, now more likely a computer.

72. Take regular breaks from a computer if you use one. Walk and stretch, drink water, and get fresh air. Rest your eyes and move your body, especially your head, neck, and shoulders.

73. Avoid occupational carcinogenic and/or hazardous chemicals at work. Learn more about what substances are used and their potential effects on you.

Learning New Activities

74. Carefully think about the previous suggestions and decide whether there are any you can initiate in your life.

75. Make a list of foods that you have in your refrigerator and cupboards, and the specific chemicals they contain. See if any of these foods can be or should be avoided; find more healthful substitutes for them. (See chapter 11, Food and the Earth, for help in this area.)

76. Learn to listen to your body's messages so you become more adaptable and sensitive to your true nature. This is an important part of staying healthy.

77. Consult a counselor if you experience anxiety or emotional difficulties or are unable to decide what to do regarding any area of your life.

78. Learn to meditate so that you can become your own stress counselor and can be more attuned to your inner nature. Be aware of your own cycles of energy, emotions, and so forth, in

> Be simple, simply be.
>
> —Bethany Argisle

your lifelong process of getting to know your-self more deeply.

79. Have faith and a positive outlook on life. Often, what you see is what you get. The more you visualize what is right for you and your family and environment, the more it becomes part of your life.

80. Learn to prepare healthy foods and to be able to nourish yourself and others, and reap the enjoyment of doing so.

81. Carry your own food and water with you if you have special requirements so that you need not accept whatever is around. Make choices in your best health interest.

82. Learn some healing arts, such as massage, herbal therapy, and nutrition for yourself and others. Touch is an important healing language.

83. Learn about local healing plants for use in day-to-day care and nourishment and for future survival should you need them.

84. Learn to sprout and eat seeds and beans. These are nutritious and wonderful survival foods. (See "Sprouts" on page 323 in chapter 8, Foods.)

Preparing for the Future

85. Plant a garden and grow your own food. This will give you the freshest, chemical-free foods. If you own land, plant fruit and nut trees, which can provide food for many years. Even in cities, flower and vegetable boxes can sur-round your home. If you live in an apartment or condo, you still have space for herbs, toma-toes, lemons, lettuce, and edible flowers.

86. Prepare your home and family for disaster. Whether it is for flood, snow, or earthquakes, gather the essentials. Know where the gas and electric lines are and how to turn them off.

87. Store water, food, and supplies. Keep extra water in durable containers. Store additional nonperishable food, such as grains, beans, dried fruits, and vegetables. Refrigerate nuts and seeds for best storage. Keep extra supplies like rain gear, warm clothes, flashlights, a life raft, and so on, depending on the requirements of your area.

88. Join with neighbors for preparation and plan-ning. Know what to do and how to be. Believe in survival. Love one another.

Give thanks you made it until now and read all 88. Keep your Staying Healthy date!

IMMORTALITY AND BEYOND

This piece is a bit of indulgence in my idealistic phi-losophy of human potential and perfection. I believe that many of these lofty and spiritual concepts can be practically applied to our daily lives. I began writing this original program some time ago, with these words from the *Daily Word,* a spiritual publication of the Unity Church, in mind: "I am a spiritual being, ageless and eternal. The idea that the older one gets, the more one slows down may be a widely accepted belief, but I do not accept it. I am a spiritual being, expressing the age-less, eternal life of God. I do not look upon sickness as something that is synonymous with accrued age. I erase from my mind every thought and belief that would age or idle me either physically or mentally."

This section is not a discussion of death and dying per se, although that is an important topic, especially in this day of artificially prolonged life and unnatural, difficult death. The way in which I view death, which is also how it is described by those who claim to have died and returned, is that the spirit and the body separate, the body remaining on Earth and the spirit moving toward Heaven, with complete awareness of the spiritual world from whence it came, full of timeless consciousness and life. This discussion of immortality and optimum life obvi-ously cannot be easily separated from religion and spirituality. This program is, in fact, about the spiri-tual awareness, or the "essence of things," existing in human life. It addresses many aspects of optimum lifestyle and consciousness.

What is immortality? It is usually defined as eternal life or exemption from death. In Western culture, it seems to have more to do with fame, with one's actions in life being planted deeply in the memory of subsequent generations—leaving a legacy. Spiritual immortality arises from the ability to carry on life simply and to nourish ourselves, our family, and our world. Fame, however, may be more a matter of material immortality through monuments, books, and recordings. Movie and rock stars, writers, musicians, and political leaders seem to lead the lists of famous immortals (or once mortals). Although fame may catapult some people into mass immortality, we all are immortal insofar as our lives have touched others and are remembered through our family genealogies and our careers, as our work, children, and influences on others leave part of us with them. Our greatest sense of immortality may lie in our bonds with our children, grandchildren, and future generations—and our care of the Earth. Many of these circumstances of notoriety, fame, or remembrance may last hundreds or even thousands of years; however, that does not make them truly eternal or immortal. "I dance for life, and death is something I am sure to live through," Bethany Argisle, has wisely said, and continues, "To live in the hearts of those we leave behind is not to die."

For most of us, immortality is the sense that "something," some essence of ourselves, lives on after our death. Many people believe that the spirit is eternal, that it never dies, while death of the body is inevitable. We accept death as natural, like birth. Native Americans believe in the awareness of the right time to die, which then opens the way for the new beings to populate Earth, and to feed the Earth back with our body's nutrients. Many cultures also believe in the possibility of a future existence, when our spiritual being may again enter a physical form and carry on the evolution of consciousness. Some of us remember (experience "re-memories" of) previous lives that may influence us in our current life. Although science cannot easily prove or disprove this concept, this philosophy of reincarnation is prevalent in many religions and spiritual paths.

An Immortalist Philosophy

Our personal beliefs regarding death or eternal life may deeply affect our daily existence, attitudes, ideology, and activities. **In regard to an "immortalist" philosophy, the question of whether we live forever in our physical body is not the issue here, but feeling as if we do allows us to live every day with a loving attitude.** We may be more relaxed, be less limited, overcome challenges more easily, feel more motivation and responsibility to our world, be more courageous and enthusiastic about learning new skills or trades (even in later years), forgive and let go of past experiences, and generally take life less seriously with a sense of being part of a greater universe.

Our ego seems attached to our physical form. Our spiritual nature or consciousness is what will live on eternally. Immortalists believe that awareness and consciousness, knowledge and wisdom, and harmonizing with the natural and universal laws are all part of our eternal path. When we believe that life is a continuum of growth and evolution of our being, we become more responsible for our thoughts, actions, and health. We also believe in karmic patterns—that all of our actions create waves in the cosmic energy that affect the entire universe and ourselves again at some time. The Golden Rule is the essence here: "Do unto others as you would have them do unto you." Perhaps even more appropriate for today is the rule "Do not do unto others as you would not have them do unto you." Or as the Dalai Lama suggests, the simple law of cause and effect is not always immediate or apparent, thus many people do not see or acknowledge its affects. Karma can also be seen as a balancing force in the universe. Even supposedly evil acts may be programmed through some karmic patterns. With ignorance and unconsciousness still part of the Earth's energy vibration, we attract both light and dark experiences and cycles.

Being immortalist in concept and action enhances our responsibility for life—our planet, our children, our own bodies, and each other. We must serve life and do the best we can to care for our human body, supporting and allowing it to be a clean, clear temple of the living Spirit. We want to live at the peak of our potential and express our purpose. Most of us begin with health, vitality, full life potential, and a clean temple and then interfere with it by our lifestyle (and environment), which affects our thoughts and actions and subsequently our outcome and experience, or that of our children, who must deal with our actions. When we are not in touch with or do not believe in a spiritual, "immortal" philosophy, we may then generate and perpetuate an acceptance of a more "deathist" philosophy, where we treat our body with self-abusive habits, as if it matters very little, appearing as if we would just as soon destroy it and get out of here as fast as possible; this seems to correlate with a consciousness that also supports war or destructive relationships of any type—getting the most out of a situation rather than giving the most, or better yet, seeking balance and harmony.

Believing in death as an ominous presence and an end, as many people do, allows other feelings—such as fear, helplessness, apathy, limitation, and self-deception—to enter, as described in *Rebirthing: The Science of Enjoying All of Your Life,* by Jim Leonard and Phil Laut. We then have no choice in life but to live as if it will be over sooner or later, so why try to be our best or create optimum health? The "death" that is hidden in each of our cells then affects our health, life, and consciousness. Accepting death (or illness or aging) is like accepting the concept that 3 meals a day is right or that consuming animal meats is necessary for health. That has been most people's experience and beliefs, yet if we do not allow other possibilities, we can never know for sure or may limit potential new experiences. Those with a deathist philosophy may actually develop an urge to die, become judgmental, and resist change. Many deathists struggle inwardly with life and its issues and challenges. Others live more through their children, whom they may see as life, than through their own capabilities, purpose, and potentials.

With this deathist philosophy, we can more easily accept destructive health- and life-destroying habits, eat dead (nonvital or processed) foods, drive recklessly, and take dangerous devitalizing drugs— because we are going to die anyway. In the Bible and many other religious and spiritual writings, disease represents sin and the presence of Satan in the body. *The Essene Gospel of Peace,* as translated by Edmond Szekely more than a half century ago suggests that fasting can clear Satan (here representing negative think-

ing, disease, and death) and sin from the body and shine new light on life. After 3 days of fasting, Satan starves and we start to feel more alive and positive (although we may meet our own shadow and darkness during those healing days). And then we can begin to live fully every day beyond fear of death or "the end." We realize that there is no end, that life is eternal, consciousness is a forever-moving force of which we are its key vehicle. We are of it, and it is of us. Feeling more immortal than mortal can actually help us be even more involved with and grateful for life and enjoy it with greater abundance, grace, and success because we can look beyond the shortcomings and problems, handle stress, and be positive and motivated toward our future. I am currently and continually learning to live each day as if it could be my last, embracing and feeling life more fully and seeking to hold love in my heart and say yes as much as possible. It feels good to live with the sense that life, relationships, and what we do with our energy and resources are precious.

Much that I have written in this book is supportive of optimum life, vitality, and longevity. How we feed ourselves influences all of these by-products and also may provide the basis for our attitudes and activities in life. **Remember, good foods, good thoughts, good actions—and in that order.** Feeling good about ourselves, loving ourselves, generates the desire for good foods and loving moods. Breathing provides our primary nutrition, oxygen, and is at the center of life experience, attitude, and feeling immortal, eternal, and connected to Spirit. Some breathing techniques may help us better deal with life and move away from degenerative and death activities. Rebirthing (or conscious breathing) is such a technique. It is said to help us open up to memories, both of this life and possibly of other lifetimes, to experience total recall. Some body therapies or certain therapists or healers may also help us release memory patterns stored in our body tissues. There may even be, as some advanced therapists suggest, specific acupuncture points connected to these energies.

Many teachers believe that unpleasant memories are what create disease, or at least contribute to stress and poor health. Past negative or painful experiences that still live inside us and generate emotions of anger, frustration, fear, isolation, and hate must be handled. Forgiveness and integration of the past is essential to living totally and healthfully in the present. Individual psychotherapy may offer us some healing as well. Remembering and processing these past experiences in a loving, supportive way helps heal aspects of our life that may have been painful and generated some death-ist attitudes. Until we become aware of previous experiences, we cannot really deal with them. As we release these patterns, the emotions that have been blocked can be integrated more easily and clearly. The process of moving from disease to healing requires bridging the subconscious-conscious separations through reacquiring self-knowledge. Re-memory that comes from breathing, therapy, and meditation allows us to listen and learn and helps us to gain access to our subconscious while we are conscious. **Within ourselves, we already know everything we need to know to heal and guide us through our life.**

Although immortalists may do all they can to carry on life, support health, and bring about healing in and around them, paradoxically they may have little or no attachment to the physical form. So they care and they do not care—that is, they care about spiritual values more than about the body. These values actually motivate deeper concern for the physical condition; the body is a vehicle to carry out their purpose and expression. Their beliefs may allow them to lay their life on the line and be capable of going all the way to serve their "divine mission." This state of being usually follows a feeling of being tapped for a special purpose. Truly, we each have a special purpose, yet usually this becomes more significant when it goes beyond the self. The bigger Self is humanity and the spiritual realm, or God.

St. Francis of Assisi attempted to bring unity to his followers and those around him. He wanted people to come together toward a greater vision, to stay connected, and to build together—a church, a community, and a spiritually bonded life. He found this difficult, as most were involved in their own "path" or reality. This message is likewise important today, in this new "Aquarian Age," where larger families merge together for greater vision, grander feats, and greater service. This might include new community living styles of co-housing and multiple family dwellings sharing and conserving resources with communal kitchens as well as parenting and educational support for the young. It makes sense to many these days from both an eco-nomic and a spiritual viewpoint as well as the emotional and family support where people commonly live away from biological families and still have very busy lives. Yet, many of us live alone or in nuclear families and are too busy to take the time to join with others to create new models for our future that might go beyond our "self" world. Living in the small "nuclear family" homes is quite inefficient and wasteful of energy use, plus there is a different kind of tribal and worldly perspective that children receive when they are raised in larger groups with many adults providing care and guidance.

To reach a new level of connection and commitment to immortalism, we must often experience some ego death (even going through a near-physical-death experience), where our spiritual sense becomes dominant. The love emotion then enters all aspects of our being and life. As important Judeo-Christian commandments begin "Love thy God with all thy heart" and "Love thy neighbor as thyself," it is clear that listening for and to our spiritual guidance and others' well-being are top priorities in a devoted life. One practicing immortalist, Marilena Silbey, told me, "We create immortality every time we express love."

To fully understand immortality, we must look at the duality of the universe. Even love has its opposite expressions, such as hate or aggression. Immortality in one sense is the opposite of death, although when we speak of the essence or oneness—the Tao or God that exists beyond duality—that itself is immortal or eternal. Immortality in a deeper sense offers us greater spiritual power, vitality, and wisdom. The subsequent longevity grows forth as we support love, attract light, and approach and affirm unity within and outside us. Death itself is a duality; it may represent an end, yet it may be a doorway to our future and other dimensions. (We'll all find out eventually.) In the truest sense, even peace and war are dualities. On a personal level, most of us prefer peace and light and love, the positive aspects of life. Yet in a universal dimension, the dark or negative side may dominate at times, expressing itself as violence and war, even natural disasters. Darkness and light need each other to exist; this is the nature of duality.

The simple symbol of the tai chi, or universal unity, represented by the yin-yang circle, reveals a spot of light in the darkness and a spot of darkness in the light. Nothing exists exclusively as light or dark on the Earth plane. At the extremes, they become their opposite. This dual nature of the world also is relevant in our individual search or struggle for healing and optimum health. Oftentimes, in seeking more light, we struggle with our shadow or dark side, which wants to exist also. Even the healthiest people have symptoms, illnesses, or personal struggles they must handle. **Balance here is the key; integrating both sides is essential.**

Our spiritual essence, however, takes us beyond this duality to discover the power and rhythm of the universe. Many people find this solace and their own sense of peace in meditation, religion, or chanting of spiritual words or songs. Part of the human challenge is to ascend beyond or above this earthly duality and associate with the spiritual level. Being a "carrier of the light" allows us to illuminate our individual and collective paths. As we go beyond our awareness of light and dark and the dealings with our personal doubts, fears, and life struggles (the specific interactions of light and dark), as well as our ego and desires, we may then reach that point of nothingness and eternity together (a touch or feeling of the immortal essence). Yet, even as we might experience this advanced state for a moment, we must still live in and care for our body and our life, thus integrating our divinity with our humanity.

Historically, the science of alchemy understood this interplay of duality and the earthly challenge to rise above a mundane existence. This polarity was represented by the light and dark, masculine and feminine, yang and yin, and sun and moon. **The path toward unity takes us from the struggles and stresses we experience toward greater peace and harmony in our current lives.** This unity, termed the "mystical marriage" of the inner male and female aspects, brought in the spiritual nature of life, great wisdom, power, and health. The "gold" or most brilliant prize was attained through the continued balance of our duality and the unification of our levels of body, mind, heart, and spirit.

In this day and age, politics deals with the basic issues of duality. To go beyond politics, we must deal with the basic nature of ego orientation, competition, and preconceived values. At some level, religion and politics represent duality, as the church and government have historically. On another dimension, religious or spiritual disciplines are what may help us rise above, in concept at least, this basic struggle we encounter in life. Experiencing love for God, self, parents, neighbors, nation, and world is the beginning of a new dimension of spiritual responsibility and immortalism. (I appreciate the Earth/Cosmos connection, the great creation, and the great creator. I also embrace evolution. Yet, a deeper discussion of religion I will save for religious philosophers and scholars.) Doing what is needed physically, psychologically, and emotionally to attain this level of love in life is essential to reaching our spiritual truths. At times, our inner journey may help awaken us from unconsciousness and align us with our true eternal relationships. In a sense, ignorance—meaning unconsciousness here, not the lack of school learning—is the darkness, disease, and demise of life.

In the beautiful book of wisdom *The Medicine of the Sun and Moon,* by insightful metaphysician Manly P. Hall, one paragraph states:

> Thus, to the Chinese, health is the natural or normal state of all living things. To become sick, man must destroy his own health, and this can be done either objectively or collectively. Sickness is a symptom, a symbol of ignorance, neglect, or the disturbance of natural processes by intemperance. To the Chinese mind, therefore, moderation of action is considered the best defense against sickness. The individual who is uncertain should adjust his own life to natural patterns and try not to disturb universal processes. His concept of health should not be a victory over sickness, but rather a victory over his own shortcomings. The person who follows nature in all things is a healthy person.

Following a natural diet and eating mainly wholesome and vital foods is the basis of this entire book, offering one way to support body health and a base for more spiritual purity. My book *Staying Healthy with the Seasons* provides much guidance for living within the laws of Nature and her cycles. Knowledge is essentially wisdom and knowing of truth from the spiritual-universal realm. As I have said, listening within is a way to gain access to this knowledge. Being attentive to Nature's ways and to interactions with people can provide many insights into "natural law." There are also many things to do to elevate our vibrations or consciousness and to live in an immortalist way. Let us now look at applying these aspects of lifestyle to enhance our daily existence.

Enhancing Our Daily Existence

There are many things we can do to feel greater power, spirituality, connectedness to Heaven and Earth, and health and vitality. This is the immortality program. To begin with, a harmony between the mind and heart that allows us to know and do what we believe and feel within will support our physical and psychological health. We also maintain balance and composure, not becoming angry or upset over stresses. This is not necessarily easy in this day and age, yet when we know how to center ourselves, it is possible much of the time.

We can view immortality as optimizing each moment of life and maximizing our life span, portraying an idealistic lifestyle with an avoidance of stress and strain (but not avoiding hard work) and a pursuit of natural living, being in "harmony with the universe." This involves a separation from much of modern technology, pollution, and city living, going back to more pioneering days but maintaining the knowledge about health that society has acquired over the past century.

Although we probably cannot find any pollution-free environments anymore, there are many relatively clean places still left on the planet where we can be nourished with good light, air, and water to vitalize our being. This "utopian" environment provides a home of natural elements, avoiding such synthetic materials as chemicals, plastics, and so on. Energy is generated by solar power, waterpower, or windmills—whichever would be most appropriate for our geographic area, of course with respect for the Earth and our neighbors. There are no big power lines, which are now known to have negative effects on health. Minimum electricity (primarily generated naturally) and/or natural gas is needed for some refrigeration, lighting, cooking, or listening to or playing music, while more affluent functions, such as television, microwaves, or other high-tech services, are avoided. This also reduces local radioactivity. We may maintain our computers to keep up with life, emails, writing, and handling business, unless of course we drop out and minimize electro-

magnetics completely, living more primitively, awakening, working, and sleeping within the light and dark cycles of life.

Our connection to Earth is essential. We work and nourish Earth in planting food, and Earth nourishes us with its bounty. Besides working the soil and getting fresh air and exercise much of the day, we walk in Nature often. Avoid driving in cars, especially on freeways and in traffic. We are not totally isolated, though, and may live in supportive communities where commodities are shared and where help is available in time of need. Human relationships and sharing feelings, love, and family seem necessary for most human beings. We are mainly a tribal species; living alone (lonely) or having a feeling of isolation is correlated with more disease and more rapid demise. Sharing personal dreams connects the community and supports personal healing.

Maintaining a positive attitude toward life with a wonderful self-image and avoiding worry and embracing low-stress plans are all helpful. The natural stresses arising from feeding ourselves, protecting our families, and dealing with Nature's changes and turmoil are sufficient survival stresses for inner motivation and bodily function. Embracing life and living it fully, letting our troubles wash clean with laughter and tears, hard work, and an inner attitude of faith, purpose, and immortality, exist in our essential core. Handling changes, making progress, and accepting and making transitions through our various life stages are important.

Many people may struggle with aging and act as they were, and not as they are. Immortality does not necessarily mean that the physical body does not age, although with healthy living, we can minimize that. It is our essential nature and spirit that are immortal. This guides the body, and immortality is enhanced as we follow our inner core (soul) path and do what we

---

Immortal Argisle-izm

Through birth is all life attained
Through the breath of love,
that which is eternal is sustained.

—Bethany Argisle

are here to do. Acknowledging changes at different ages is one of our many challenges. It is essential to accept and enhance change in age, function, forces, and vitality with the grace, joy, and dance of life, as blessings and guides in our life rather than the discords of our destruction.

Flexibility is the key to immortality in body, emotion, and spirit. This flexibility in regard to changes of weather, relationships to others, and our own internal attitudes or beliefs is important to continued positive evolution and to minimizing the stress incurred in daily life. Many of us may struggle with the common minor everyday experiences; this is not necessary or helpful, and it can be avoided with an open mind, faith in life, and a feeling of spiritual guidance surrounding our existence.

Often, the limits or viewpoints of our own mind or those of our family, friends, or chance opinions may hold us back. It may be a great challenge or struggle to see clearly in these situations and progress beyond them. We often manifest these conflicts as a reflection of our own inner questioning. As in Nature, where there are stresses at the transition or shift points between seasons, so there are for us at our life changes. The evolutionary process of life is among the threads that tie us all together.

Many people may measure themselves in comparison to the accomplishments or values of others or of the world at large. Essential to life is acknowledging our own unique true nature. **Learning who we are and expressing this identity to others, feeling good about ourselves, is the process of growing.** The challenges that are presented to us help us to fine-tune our perceptions, beliefs, and identity. Yet those truths that are at our essential core will remain and shine forth as all the illusions about life are dissolved. From this core wisdom, a true knowledge may arise and be a strong guide in our life.

Acknowledging our true nature is helpful in creating our diet. From an immortalist viewpoint, life and death is really not a moral issue. This is true in regard to food. Carrots and apples have measurable life force, although different from a cow or chicken. We are really dealing with the vibrations of matter and the effects of and needs for certain foods. At different times, we may want and need to eat animal foods; at other instances, we may be vegetarians. (Clearly, though, being vege-

tarian is more ecological in terms of precious resources and worldwide nutrition.) Some people are more inclined to a certain diet for various reasons and stay with that for many years. However, as I have discussed throughout this book, there are many diets, and we may change regularly in terms of the foods we eat, as our seasonal diet and availability of foods are a basic component of what we may or may not eat in our natural lifestyle and over the seasons of our years.

In terms of diet, why not eat the Ideal Diet I have defined in chapter 13 for optimum health and vitality? Let me reemphasize its basic nutritional components that apply to immortality and longevity. First, we must eat simply and not excessively, avoiding too much or too many different foods and sauces at one meal. During my detox and cleansing groups, it is amazing how many participants come to the same realization: "It is awesome to discover how little food we really need to feel our best." For optimum vitality, we eat a high amount of raw foods and possibly an almost exclusively raw diet at certain periods and at warmer times of the year. If we want to support life, we eat more live or close-to-living foods—that is, fresh foods (fruits, vegetables, and sprouted legumes and grains) close to the state in which Nature grows them. If we eat more overcooked or dead (like animal flesh), low-vibration foods, we will potentiate our death sooner. At colder times, however, more heated foods and richer foods, even some of the animal proteins, may be desired and useful, much like a log in the fireplace to warm our home, our body. **The immortalist diet is therefore seasonally based.** No refined foods are used. It is primarily a vegetarian diet, with a focus on complex carbohydrates and vegetables, legumes, and raw, organic nuts and seeds. Grains are used whole or freshly ground for the baking of breads, biscuits, or other goods.

As we garden outside, the kitchen becomes our indoor garden to nourish us within. Sprouting seeds and legumes provides optimum foods—the foods with the highest vibration, vitality, and quality from a nutritional standpoint. Sprouts are also helpful to the gastrointestinal tract in that they provide fiber, chlorophyll, and many vitamins, minerals, and proteins. Foods that may be sprouted include hard wheat, alfalfa seeds, sunflower seeds, radish seeds, chia seeds, buckwheat, mung beans, lentils, and garbanzos, as well as black and aduki beans. (See "Sprouts" on page 323 in chapter 8, Foods.)

In the areas of the world where people commonly live beyond a 100 years, the environment is much cleaner. People work the land and have clean air, water, and food. They exercise as they work and live, have less stress, and take care of the elders who need a positive self-image and purpose (to feel connected and needed, not isolated) to want to continue living. The diet of these "peoples of longevity" tends to be lower in calories, fats, and protein than that of the Western world. They eat unprocessed fresh foods or, in the colder seasons, well-stored foods. And their activity levels are more connected to the natural daily and seasonal cycles. When we live attuned to Nature, we perpetuate and manifest in ourselves its strength, vitality, endurance, and reverence for life.

Our diet also supports our spiritual practice. The first level of the golden rule applies to Mother Earth. When we nurture her soil and create beauty with growing foods, she nourishes each of us and our families. Light eating is important for our times of spiritual seeking. Periodic fasting, especially in the midst of good nutrition, also supports the spiritual connection and reverence for all life.

In this immortality program, we are not supported by extra vitamin pills unless they are helpful for specific medical conditions or we need to counterbalance soil depletions or support detoxification programs, or just for occasional insurance to enhance our levels of vitamins, minerals, or oils in the diet. However, we have cleared out many of the stresses and abuses for which we needed these extra insurance pills and are now supported by nutritionally vital foods and healthy digestion. We eat a variety of foods that will supply us with our full range of specific nutrients. Instead of supplements, we can use more concentrated, high-nutrient foods, such as vegetable juices, nutritional yeast, bee pollen, raw nuts and seeds, various herbs, and sprouts. These foods support us to stay healthy, so that we will not require more concentrated supplements or medicines.

Our day-to-day life is our basic exercise. This immortalist-longevity plan does not find us working the world of business with the hustle and bustle of meetings and constant time-pressure stress, but in the world of smaller communities and in Nature. Our gardening, building, and caretaking helps us in our physical conditioning. Other exercises and aerobic activities keep us even more fit. Dancing, hill walking, bicycling, cross-country skiing, and swimming are all good activities. Some community sports, such as soccer and volleyball, may inspire others. Exercise, however, should not be extreme or overdone, and heavy competition and intense contact sports are not necessary. When we do these activities purely in the spirit of developing our personal performance or coordinating team or group functions rather than for winning, they may fit in with our immortalist-spiritual values of less competition, more cooperation.

A key to immortal vitality can be found in the subtle Eastern exercises like yoga, qi gong, and tai chi, which promote flexibility and mind-body integration. They unite stretching, coordination, balance, strength, mental discipline, and harmonious breathing. They are also more replenishing and stimulating to our energy level than many other activities, yet they are helpful in general stress reduction and tend to relax and loosen our muscles rather than tighten them. Both yoga and tai chi also help open up the internal energy circulation in the body, which is essential to good health.

Other aspects of lifestyle philosophy focus on inner attunement and evolution of our being. **Learning to listen to our body as well as to Nature is essential here.** Adapting to the changes around us and within us, with awareness of both our inner life needs and our food needs, is important. Our personal cycles fit within Nature's, and although we eat a healthy, vital diet, we do have special fast times to uplift us and feast times to help us to slow down, nourish us, and rest more deeply. Our basic sleep cycle should be attuned to Nature as well. We go early to bed so that we can arise with the light of day or just before to meditate and open to the light and spirit coming into our daily life. Writing and being creative, which are so important to life also, come out of this inner silence and depth.

Of course, the "antsy" personality may go through levels of resistance and readjustment to achieve this grace of quiet knowingness. In truth, the ego and will of the human being must submit to the powers of Nature and the universe for the benefit of all. We learn from these larger forces. Our meditation or "receptive quietude" is the greatest power we have in attuning to the wisdom of the universe. If we wish to understand our relationship to people or events around us or when we have questions about other areas of our life, "we need no books to teach us the answers, because if we are quiet, in our hearts we will know," as Manly Hall has written in *The Medicine of the Sun and the Moon.* He continues:

Only when we disobey the quiet reaction of our own inner lives do we get into trouble. If we merely follow the gratification of our emotions, we may be wrong; if we follow the inclinations of our intellects, we may be in error. But if we are very quiet in the presence of need, a light in us suddenly moves us to the solution of this need.

Some basic concepts for the natural laws of our life and body are described in the book *Rays of the Dawn,* by Thurman Fleet, a popular writer about natural health; my adaptations of Mr. Fleet's four natural laws follow:

- **The first law is proper nourishment.** This includes eating a living-food diet, more alkaline than acid. Fleet categorizes our foods as cleansers, builders, and congestors. We want mostly the cleansing fruits and vegetables, some building proteins, and few congestors—that is, refined or sweetened foods, excess starches, or too much of the building foods, such as cheese, meats, or even nuts, seeds, and beans. A vital, more raw-food diet is suggested.

- **The second law is proper movement.** Exercise is the distribution process of our nourishment. It aids the assimilation, utilization, and elimination of foods. Moving every joint every day will maintain flexibility and function. We want to be active enough to keep muscles toned and maintain a strong heart.

- **The third law is proper rest and recuperation.** This balances out our activity. It includes sleep, rest, relaxation, and recreation, particularly important to help us destress. Having playful, enjoyable hobbies and laughing a lot are important to feeling good about ourselves and our life. If we feel this way, it is easier to laugh and play.

- **The fourth law is proper cleanliness, both outer and inner.** Cleaning our skin through regular bathing is important. Sweating helps cleanse the blood of impurities. A wholesome, high-fiber diet allows the bowels to keep elimination current. Order and cleanliness in our surroundings both prevent disease and support creativity. Being clean and organized allows us to be "current" in our life and awareness.

Viewing our actions in regard to both their immediate and their long-term effects is a key to overall health for everyone. This is part of the immortalist philosophy. The contrary view and action for profit motives primarily often cause more pollution of our beautiful planet and our dreams to live in health. Economy has taken precedence over Nature's dance. We may think only of what we can get to fulfill our immediate needs without being concerned about the polluting effects on the environment. We accept that what we need now is most important and, because we are not going to be here, let those who come later deal with the consequences of our actions and how they affect future generations. With the number of toxic chemicals and amount of radiation in use today, a single little mistake can be the only one we are ever allowed.

Many companies are oriented to acquiring profits by producing such products as chemicals and plastics and releasing their wastes, many of them toxic, into the environment (the local air, rivers, or lakes) or storing them underground, where they can leak and pollute soil and groundwater. Many of the products that are being made these days using toxic materials in their creation are not really needed or are toxic themselves. Even though all of these new plastics in particular have become the mainstay of the technological age, we wonder whether this is indeed evolution. Many new and old products are being manufactured more efficiently and with less pollution with greater forethought and concern for continued environmental balance; many are also helpful economically, such as hemp products, organic herbs and produce, and natural dyes.

> Beyond compromise is cooperation.
> —Bethany Argisle

In 1,000 years, people will look back on the twenty-first century as one of the most disastrous, from an immortalist viewpoint, in its long-range effects on the planet. Although some technological progress has been made, more-conscious people are beginning to realize that the cost to Earth and its inhabitants is greater than the short-term profits generated by the productivity, or the extra convenience of the products themselves. Unless we now use our technological skills to clean up the planet, we will be in even bigger trouble in the near future. (See chapter 11, Food and the Earth, for more ideas on this cleanup as well as "88 Survival Suggestions," on page 785.)

Pollution has affected the ozone layer in our stratosphere and the level of radiation in the air. This might give a new image of immortality from the deathist viewpoint—such as surviving while wearing special suits and eyeglasses to protect us from the sun and wearing masks to filter the air. Or, worse yet, we may need to live in underground cities. In a civilization where economy and greed take precedence over the dance of peaceful, evolutionary existence, death takes over. But we will not accept this. I believe solutions to these pollution problems are yet to be revealed; however, healing must begin in our time! (See chapters 1, Water, and 11, Food and the Earth, for discussions on cleaning up our waters and our food supplies.)

We want care for the planet—to live with the sunshine, breathing clean air, having good water to drink, and being able to walk in Nature, to talk to the trees and animals. So let's wake up now! Our health has to do with building the future and keeping the planet healthy. We want to keep alive and extend life by better health practices, medicine, and technology. Let us focus more on our appreciation of life, Nature, and those other beings around us.

Releasing the past is essential to healthy living. Sickness lives in our memories, especially the painful or negatively charged ones we carry around. Live now in preparation for the future, creating with enthusiasm, vitality, and purpose. Utilizing and vitalizing our mind (especially our untapped areas) through meditation and all the aspects of a healthy lifestyle that I have mentioned in this book are ways to keep attuned to the pulse of life around us and to understand the universal laws. This helps us to become more conscious in our

> We suffer to learn until we learn that we do not have to suffer to learn. Then we can recognize that we are choosing the intensity of our experiences. Remaining conscious through inner listening is the tool to learning without suffering. Loving and forgiving ourselves and others is the key to inner peace.
>
> —Marilena Silbey, an immortalist friend

thoughts and words, allowing us to be more creative with our lives. Sensitivity and heartfelt experience give understanding and guide us to correct the aspects of civilization and humanity that may need renewal.

Macromedicine and Micromedicine: Earth, Humanity, and Personal Care

Macromedicine deals with the care of humanity; micromedicine deals with the care of the individual. Let us incorporate both aspects of this knowledge into healing and our health-care system. Caring for ourselves individually and as families can easily extend to populations and the Earth itself. For long-term health, it is important to learn to care for the body in relationship to the world from an early age. Much of the basic information in this book and much of my future life is dedicated to teaching young people the importance of good habits in creating lifelong health.

It is also essential to correct problems early and not let long-term negligence lead to chronic disease or emergencies. Most health emergencies are a result of neglecting little issues and details of health or trying to remain unconscious and resist inner guidance and awareness. In *The Medicine of the Sun and Moon,* author Hall states:

> Health rests upon the simple concept that there is a universal harmony, which can be found everywhere and in everything. Man, by his indiscretions, deprives himself of the natural benefits which heaven bestows. The individual who breaks the rules does not destroy rhythms of infinite life but inhibits the supply of vitality moving through his own body, thereby depriving himself of his proper share of this universal energy.

Learning preventive measures early is important, and treating current mild diseases effectively probably lessens the likelihood of chronic illness and enhances longevity. Stress both arises from and influences physical health. When physical health is poor, greater psychological and emotional stresses may occur. It is important to handle these early to avoid the vicious cycle of poor health, stress, lack of vitality, use of stimulants, more stress, and poorer health.

In terms of basic medical care, nutritional and botanical medicines are the core healers and preventive measures. Homeopathy practice is a fascinating science with many supporters, and it seems to be a useful natural therapeutic approach. Herbs and diet can help rebalance us and heal specific problems, especially when handled early. Foods and herbs are also aligned with seasonal medicine. The changes of season affect the availability of certain foods and plants, and naturally they correlate with our cyclical needs. The spring cleansers and tonics are the many greens and roots. The summer rejuvenators are the fruits, vegetables, and flowers. In the autumn and winter, more roots and building foods are available, which provide more heat to feed the body's furnace and protect us from the changing season. It all fits together perfectly as we let it.

Healing has to do with integrating the body, mind, and spirit and allowing the full energy flows in the body. Pain is held in place by resistance generated by anger, frustration, or fear of the worst—be it disease or death. Increasing tensions lead to increasing tissue disease, which is then harder to heal. Problems can even go beyond healing potential, especially when surgery is done and organs are removed. Pain and limitation lead to much disease. We need to handle this early. Acupuncture, both by needle and electrical stimulation, can help move energy/pain and reestablish homeostasis. Many body therapies can be an important mode of treatment, close in importance to foods and botanicals. The laying on of hands with love and openness can allow these body resistances and pains to be released. Massage, acupressure, chiropractic therapy, and many other modalities can all provide natural healing. Allowing the energy channels to open again will allow our life force to flow freely and create health and vitality. Have people around who understand and are supportive of this process—that of living life healthfully and attuned to the natural!

In our ideal life, we want to associate ourselves with a philosopher-physician who can connect with the entire family and provide preventive and therapeutic care, knowledge of natural medicine, and guidance in harmonious living. If sickness requires stronger medicines or surgery, the doctor provides these or recommends a specialist in the appropriate field. Knowing the limits of our own knowledge is essential to effective treatment, as is getting our ego out of the way and letting our intuition guide us in the best approach for healing. Doctors should know that they are servants of both Nature and God. We are here to support healing and create health; ultimately we all must begin with ourselves. We do this by turning to our spiritual essence and developing our communion with our inner guidance and God. An appreciation of the Heavenly Father, or Spirit, and the Heavenly Mother, or Earth, is inherent in this reverence for life. When we live within the natural laws of the universe, we approach immortality, and our spirit is enhanced. In an article called "Healing Ourselves and Healing Our Planet," the wise spiritual/religious leader Robert Muller suggests that our spiritual development allows us to be in greater harmony with—in this order—

> the planet,
> the heavens,
> the time cycles,
> others and our family,
> and our own self.

Spiritual development arises from listening within and allows us to gain wisdom and elevate our consciousness. As immortalists, we believe that anything is possible. With Jesus' 40-day fast, he was allowed access to all planes of travel—horizontally through people, vertically between God and Earth, inwardly through his depths, and interdimensionally through time and truth. Christ continues to be present as he lives on immortally in the hearts and minds of many of his followers, as do other saintly beings who have ascended from the bonds of Earth, such as Buddha, Lao-tzu, Gandhi, and those who have become immortal in our hearts. To Christians, however, Christ lived on another level above these earthly saints who may have attained greater enlightenment over the typical human, yet they were not the "true son of God." With that, they hold Christ in their hearts as their personal savior, and this supports them to live a life aligned with the great laws of life. I just ask that we apply the great laws of the body such that religious people also treat themselves, their bodies, as a temple of the Holy Spirit, and live more purely without the common everyday abuses that exist all over the planet as well as in our relationships with our children and our future here on Earth.

We, too, can live with this sense of immortality with our individual spiritual development. Understanding Nature and the universe, we know that order and discipline are important to this spiritual path. Yet with the pursuit and enfoldment of our individual path within the harmony of the universe, we can create both a healthy body and life as well as a healthy, vital, and eternal world. Healing the planet begins with each of us and our commitment to being the best and healthiest person that we can be. Peace be in you.

The Earth: Our Food Source

Let's Clean It Up and Keep It Clean!

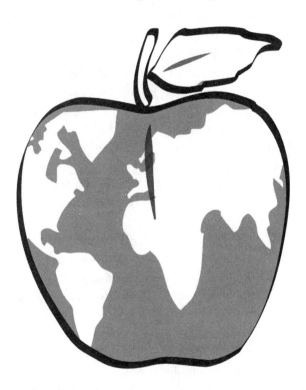

The environment is not a political issue, it is a health issue.
Having clean and nutritious food is essential to good life and health.

An organic apple a day keeps the doctor (bill) away.

Appendix A: Laboratories and Clinical Nutrition Tests

There are medical labs in most cities and within hospitals. There is concern, however, about the accuracy, consistency, and "normal" values of many of these laboratories, and continuous, rigorous quality control is important. In this appendix, I have compiled a list of some of the clinical and/or functional (looking at physiological balance) medicine laboratories that provide the specialized tests I use in my own practice; some other labs that I do not use or use infrequently are also included because of particular nutritional interest. Most of the labs on this list are approved by the CLIA (Clinical Laboratory Improvement Amendments—a certification program for regulating laboratory testing within the United States under the Department of Health and Human Services). There are, of course, many other laboratories all over the United States that provide basic or specialized testing. I have no financial interest in any of these labs, nor did any of them pay to be listed in this book; rather, I include them here only to help spread the word about nutritional and functional medicine.

AAL Reference Laboratories, Inc.
(Antibody Assay Labs)
1826 Kramer Lane, Suite F
Austin, TX 78758
800-522-2611
www.aalrl.com

Provides a wide range of services, including immunology, such as testing for natural killer cells; infectious disease antibodies, as with Epstein-Barr virus and chronic fatigue evaluation; blood nutrient values; and male and female hormonal testing for initial evaluation and replacement monitoring.

Aeron LifeCycles Clinical Laboratories
1933 Davis Street, Suite 310
San Leandro, CA 94577
800-631-7900
www.aeron.com

This specialty laboratory primarily focuses on saliva testing for hormones and is a fully licensed clinical lab in all 50 states, taking a variety of insurances. They are one of the original saliva testing labs and they also do a urine pyrilinks test as a bone loss marker. See a copy of their saliva hormone panel on page 811.

Berkeley Heart Lab
839 Mitten Road
Burlingame, VT 94010
877-454-7437
www.berkeleyheartlab.com

This innovative lab runs an in-depth cardiovascular risk profile and will bill most insurance companies.

Cell Science Systems, Ltd.
1239 E. Newport Center Drive, Suite 101
Deerfield Beach, FL 33442
954-426-2304 or 800-881-2685
www.alcat.com

This lab runs a specialized food reaction test, the ALCAT test (antigen leukocyte cellular antibody test), which does not measure antibody levels but looks at blood cellular reactions to foods. The ALCAT test is a more objective, reproducible, computerized analysis than the once-popular yet less well-accepted cytotoxic test. They also run hormone saliva hormone tests.

Diagnos-Techs, Inc.

6620 South 192nd Place, Building J
Kent, WA 98032
800-878-3787
www.diagnostechs.com

With medical director Elias Ilyia, PhD, this lab runs unusual and helpful saliva adrenal testing called ASI (adrenal stress index), other saliva hormone testing, and digestive analyses that include microbial and digestive markers.

Doctor's Data

3755 Illinois Avenue
St. Charles, IL 60174
800-323-2784
www.doctorsdata.com

This is a specialized lab for mineral levels, both essential (nutritional) and toxic minerals, which can be assessed in the blood (whole blood, plasma, or red blood cells), urine, feces, and hair. Levels of minerals in water can also be measured if there is some concern over excessive quantities of metals. Doctor's Data also performs a specific amino acid profile. Mineral balances are important for optimum body function and tissue health. Adequate levels in the body are also a result of a good diet and effective digestion and assimilation. Measuring at least whole blood and hair levels is part of the nutritional fine-tuning that I like to do for patients. Looking for deficiencies of such minerals as zinc, copper, magnesium, or manganese, as well as excessive levels of lead, mercury, or cadmium helps me to individualize the food and supplemental needs of each patient. (See the Whole Blood Elements test and the Hair Element analysis report, pages 809 and 810.) Doctor's Data also runs stool tests for microbes and other markers.

ELISA/ACT Biotechnologies

14 Pidgeon Hill Drive, Suite 300
Sterling, VA 20165
800-553-5472
www.elisaact.com

This lab directed by Russell M. Jaffe, MD, specializes in immune system reactions to pesticides, as well as measurement of food and chemical allergies through the new ELISA/ACT test (enzyme-linked immunosorbent assay/activated cell test).

Great Smokies Diagnostic Laboratory/Genovations

63 Zillicoa Street
Asheville, NC 28801
800-522-4762 or 828-253-0621
www.gsdl.com

Great Smokies does two of my favorite tests—the comprehensive digestive stool analysis (CDSA) and now the comprehensive parasitology test to evaluate all microbes living in the intestinal tract. The CDSA test evaluates the function and ecology of the digestive tract with more than 20 tests, including food components remaining in the stool, the biochemistry of the stool, and cultures for yeasts (fungi) and bacteria, followed up with antibiotic (for both natural and pharmaceutical antibiotics) sensitivity testing for any abnormal organisms. (See the sample test following this list of laboratories.) Great Smokies also does additional general and specific tests for digestive integrity and other concerns. See an example of their Detoxification Profile and their CDSA printout on pages 806–808.

Hunter Laboratories, Inc.

2605 S. Winchester Boulevard
Campbell, CA 95008
800-762-9722
www.hunterlabs.com

This is a general medical lab in California that provides wonderful service to doctor's offices in measuring blood count, chemistries, liver function, hormones, and cultures for infections. Every practice needs a good laboratory for their basic medical testing.

Immuno Laboratories, Inc.
6801 Powerline Road
Fort Lauderdale, FL 33309
800-231-9197
www.immunolabs.com

This lab's "food allergy" test measures antibody levels (IgG) of more than 100 foods. This test is helpful for the food-reactive or allergic patient or for those looking for health tuning because it provides all of the measurable reactions together. Elimination of these foods may then help relieve related symptoms. Food allergy testing is still a relatively controversial subject in medicine.

Immunosciences Lab, Inc.
8693 Wilshire Boulevard, Suite 200
Beverly Hills, CA 90211
800-950-4686
www.immunoscienceslab.com

This diagnostic and research facility specializes in microbiology and immunology laboratory testing. Directed by Dr. Aristo Vojdani, tests are provided in the following categories: allergy, autoimmune diseases, cancer and its early diagnosis, chronic fatigue syndrome, immunology and serology, immunotoxicology, and intestinal health.

Laboratory Corporation of America (LabCorp)
10930 Bigge Street
San Leandro, CA 94577
800-888-1113
www.labcorp.com

This is another licensed general medical laboratory that also does specialty testing in genetics, immune function, viral antibodies, and much more. LabCorp also took over Immunodiagnostics (IDL) Labs, whom I used for many years for immune testing and other special studies.

Meridian Valley Laboratory
801 SW 16th Street, Suite 126
Renton, WA 98055
425-271-8689
www.meridianvalleylab.com

A specialized nutritional medicine laboratory with well-known practitioner, author, and educator Jonathan Wright, MD, as medical director, this lab performs many progressive tests, such as 24-hour urine for steroid hormones, blood hormones, fatty acid profiles (both the essential fatty acids and their metabolites), IgG/IgE combined food antibodies, and stool tests for microbes and digestive markers.

Metametrix Clinical Laboratory
4855 Peachtree Industrial Boulevard, Suite 201
Norcross, GA 30092
800-221-4640
www.metametrix.com

This pioneering lab has developed nutritional, metabolic, and toxicant analyses, doing testing since the mid-1980s. Some of their important tests are for food antibodies, amino acids, essential fatty acids, nutrient and toxic elements, and organic acids (urine byproducts of metabolism).

NeuroScience, Inc.
373 280th Street
Osceola, WI 54020
888-342-7272

This lab is directed by Gottfried Kellerman, PhD (in biochemistry). They are known for measuring urinary neurotransmitters such as serotonin and epinephrine, as well as saliva testing for adrenal and other hormones.

Pacific Toxicology Laboratories
9348 De Soto Avenue
Chatsworth, CA 91311
800-328-6942
www.pactox.com

This lab specializes in measuring blood, urine, and adipose tissue for toxic industrial and environmental chemicals, including organochlorine and organophosphate pesticides, chlorinated and aromatic solvents and their metabolites, PCBs and PBBs, as well as petroleum distillates and heavy metals like lead and mercury. They also have a clinical lab and drug screen lab.

Preventive Medicine Center of Marin
(Dr. Elson Haas's office)
25 Mitchell Boulevard, Suite 8
San Rafael, CA 94903
415-472-2343
www.elsonhaas.com

Many doctor's offices will do some specific tests, from blood counts to blood chemistries to X-rays. In my office, some of the tests I perform include urinalyses and electrocardiograms, as well as drawing blood for many different laboratory tests, sending it to the more than a dozen labs I use for evaluations, such as most of the ones in this list. I also provide many kits that patients can use at home to collect stool, urine, and saliva samples to ship to labs for testing.

Quest Diagnostics
Quest Diagnostics Corporate Headquarters
1 Malcolm Avenue
Teterboro, NJ 07608
800-222-0446
www.questdiagnostics.com

Many doctors and other labs refer to this reliable laboratory for specialized tests, such as hormonal, immunological, and metabolic assessment. This lab has 1,700 patient service centers throughout the United States.

Sanesco
1200 Ridgefield Boulevard, Suite 200
Asheville, NC 28806
866-670-5705
www.sanesco.net

This relatively new lab does innovative functional testing of blood, urine, and saliva for hormones and neurotransmitters. The very experienced and brilliant physician Denise R. Mark, MD, is the medical director of Sanesco. See a sample copy of their neurotransmitter profile on page 812.

SpectraCell Laboratories
10401 Town Park Drive
Houston, TX 77072
800-227-5227
www.spectracell.com

SpectraCell Laboratories is CLIA-approved and specializes in functional intracellular testing. Their tests offer many clinical conditions, including cardiovascular risk, immunological disorders, metabolism measurements, and nutritional analysis.

Vitamin Diagnostics, Inc.
Route 35 and Industrial Drive
Cliffwood Beach, NJ 07735
732-583-7773
www.vitamindiagnostics.com

This lab, with offices in the United States, Australia, and the Netherlands, offers specialized assessment of blood and urine for many nutrients, including vitamins, minerals, fatty acids, amino acids, hormones, and catecholamines.

ZRT Laboratory
1815 NW 169th Place, Suite 5050
Beaverton, OR 97006
503-466-2445
www.salivatest.com

This specialty lab provides thorough saliva testing for hormones, such as female and male sex hormones and adrenal function, as well as bloodspot testing for thyroid specifically.

Note: The following pages of tests are examples of the new medicine assessment of body states: nutritional and detoxification integrity, hormonal and neurotransmitter status, and digestive health. The intent is not to interpret these test results here, but to familiarize you with the various types of testing available. Many of the labs in this Appendix can refer you to a practitioner in your area who can support your individual needs.

Detoxification Profile (Comprehensive)

Great Smokies Diagnostic Lab

63 Zillicoa Street
Asheville, NC 28801-1074
© Genova Diagnostics

Patient: **SAMPLE PATIENT**

Age: 50
Sex: F
MRN:

Order Number:
Completed:
Received:
Collected:

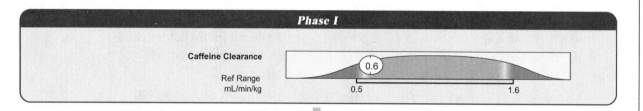

Phase I

Caffeine Clearance

Ref Range mL/min/kg

0.6

0.5   1.6

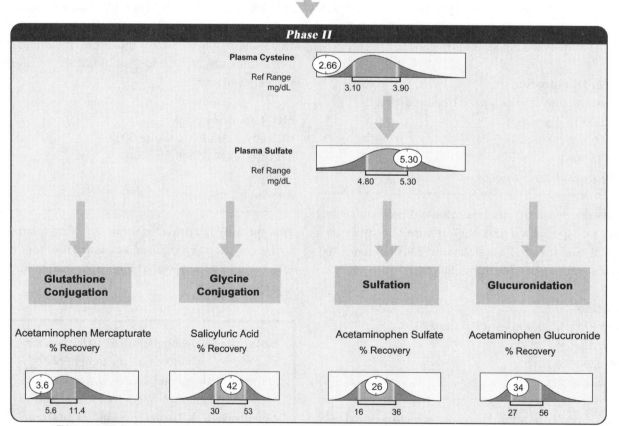

Phase II

Plasma Cysteine

Ref Range mg/dL

2.66

3.10   3.90

Plasma Sulfate

Ref Range mg/dL

5.30

4.80   5.30

Glutathione Conjugation	Glycine Conjugation	Sulfation	Glucuronidation
Acetaminophen Mercapturate	Salicyluric Acid	Acetaminophen Sulfate	Acetaminophen Glucuronide
% Recovery	% Recovery	% Recovery	% Recovery
3.6	42	26	34
5.6 11.4	30 53	16 36	27 56

This test was developed and its performance characteristics determined by GSDL, Inc. It has not been cleared or approved by the U.S. Food and Drug Administration.

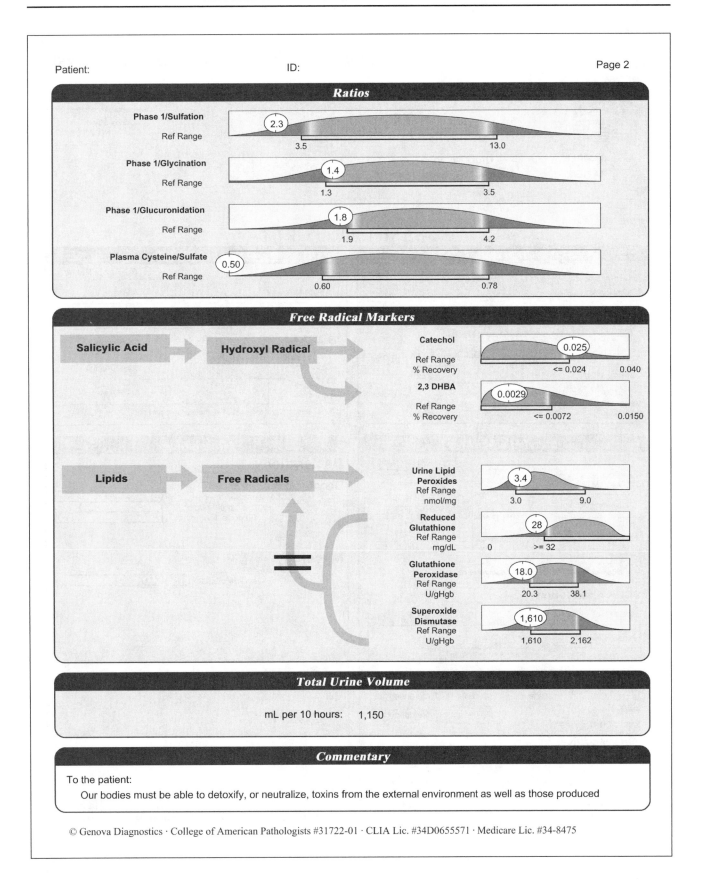

Patient: ID: Page 2

Ratios

Phase 1/Sulfation	2.3	Ref Range 3.5 – 13.0
Phase 1/Glycination	1.4	Ref Range 1.3 – 3.5
Phase 1/Glucuronidation	1.8	Ref Range 1.9 – 4.2
Plasma Cysteine/Sulfate	0.50	Ref Range 0.60 – 0.78

Free Radical Markers

Salicylic Acid → Hydroxyl Radical →

Catechol — 0.025 — Ref Range % Recovery <= 0.024   0.040

2,3 DHBA — 0.0029 — Ref Range % Recovery <= 0.0072   0.0150

Lipids → Free Radicals →

Urine Lipid Peroxides — 3.4 — Ref Range nmol/mg 3.0 – 9.0

Reduced Glutathione — 28 — Ref Range mg/dL 0   >= 32

Glutathione Peroxidase — 18.0 — Ref Range U/gHgb 20.3 – 38.1

Superoxide Dismutase — 1,610 — Ref Range U/gHgb 1,610 – 2,162

Total Urine Volume

mL per 10 hours: 1,150

Commentary

To the patient:

Our bodies must be able to detoxify, or neutralize, toxins from the external environment as well as those produced

© Genova Diagnostics · College of American Pathologists #31722-01 · CLIA Lic. #34D0655571 · Medicare Lic. #34-8475

Comprehensive Digestive Stool Analysis

63 Zillicoa Street
Asheville, NC 28801-1074
© Genova Diagnostics

Patient: **SAMPLE PATIENT**

Age: 39
Sex: M
MRN:

Order Number:

Completed: April 06, 2004
Received: April 06, 2004
Collected: April 06, 2004

SAMPLE REPORT

Digestion

		Reference Range
Chymotrypsin	3.1	0.9-26.8 U/g
Putrefactive SCFAs (Total*)	2.0	1.3-8.6 micromol/g

* Total values equal the sum of all measurable parts.

	Inside	Outside	Reference Range
Meat Fibers	None		None
Vegetable Fibers	Few		None - Few

Absorption

		Reference Range
Tryglycerides	1.1	0.4-5.5 mg/g
Long Chain Fatty Acids	2.2	1.7-51.5 mg/g
Cholesterol	1.5	0.6-5.9 mg/g
Phospholipids	0.2	0.2-1.8 mg/g
Fecal Fat (Total*)	5.0	5.1-59.9 mg/g

* Total values equal the sum of all measurable parts.

Metabolic Markers

		Reference Range
Beneficial SCFAs (Total*)	5.4	>= 13.6 micromol/g
n-Butyrate	3.1	>= 2.5 micromol/g
Beta-Glucuronidase	5,047	406-12,072 U/g
pH	7.1	6.1-7.9

* Total values equal the sum of all measurable parts.

SCFA distribution

		Reference Range
Acetate %	33.4	44.5-72.4 %
Propionate %	9.5	<= 32.1 %
n-Butyrate %	57.4	10.8-33.5 %

Immunology

	Inside	Outside	Reference Range
Fecal Lactoferrin		Positive	Negative

Macroscopic

	Inside	Outside	Reference Range
Color	Brown		Brown
Mucus	Negative		Negative
Occult blood		Positive	Negative

Microbiology

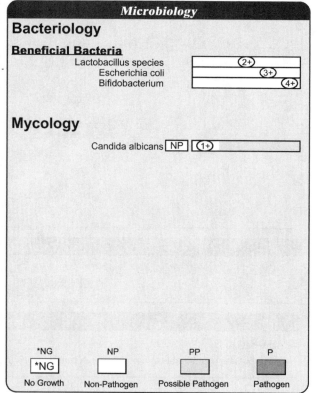

Bacteriology

Beneficial Bacteria

Lactobacillus species	2+
Escherichia coli	3+
Bifidobacterium	4+

Mycology

Candida albicans	NP 1+

*NG	NP	PP	P
*NG			
No Growth	Non-Pathogen	Possible Pathogen	Pathogen

g,rp,cdsa,042904

WHOLE BLOOD ELEMENTS

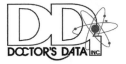

LAB#: B000000-0000-1
PATIENT: Sample Patient
SEX: Female
AGE: 67

CLIENT#: 12345
DOCTOR:
Doctor's Data, Inc.
3755 Illinois Ave.
St. Charles, IL 60174

NUTRIENT ELEMENTS

ELEMENTS	RESULT µg/g	REFERENCE RANGE	PERCENTILE
Calcium	45.0	38- 60.0	
Magnesium	29.4	28- 44.0	
Sodium	75.0	76- 98.0	
Potassium	39.0	33- 51.0	
Phosphorus	322	300- 440	
Copper	0.805	0.61- 1.28	
Zinc	4.96	4.2- 8.1	
Manganese	0.005	0.005-0.017	
Lithium	0.0014	.0003- 0.02	
Strontium	0.011	0.006-0.031	
Sulfur	1200	1010- 1600	
Molybdenum	0.0011	.0007-.0056	

Percentile columns: 2.5th, 16th, 50th, 84th, 97.5th

POTENTIALLY TOXIC ELEMENTS

TOXIC ELEMENTS	RESULT µg/g	REFERENCE RANGE	PERCENTILE
Bismuth	<0.0001	< 0.005	
Cadmium	0.001	< 0.014	
Lead	0.019	< 0.055	
Mercury	<0.0009	< 0.013	
Nickel	<0.005	< 0.019	
Uranium	<0.0001	< 0.006	

Percentile columns: 95th, 99th

SPECIMEN DATA

Comments:
Date Collected: 5/29/2002
Date Received: 5/30/2002
Date Completed: 6/5/2002

Methodology: ICP-MS
µg/g = ppm

V10.00

HAIR ELEMENTS

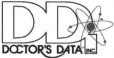

LAB#: H000000-0000-1
PATIENT: Sample Patient
SEX: Female
AGE: 48

CLIENT#: 12345
DOCTOR:
Doctor's Data, Inc.
3755 Illinois Ave.
St. Charles, IL 60174

POTENTIALLY TOXIC ELEMENTS

TOXIC ELEMENTS	RESULT µg/g	REFERENCE RANGE	PERCENTILE 68th / 95th
Aluminum	3.8	< 7.0	
Antimony	< 0.01	< 0.05	
Arsenic	< 0.01	< 0.06	
Beryllium	< 0.01	< 0.02	
Bismuth	0.014	< 0.1	
Cadmium	0.015	< 0.1	
Lead	0.05	< 1.0	
Mercury	2.1	< 1.1	
Platinum	< 0.003	< 0.005	
Thallium	< 0.001	< 0.01	
Thorium	< 0.001	< 0.005	
Uranium	0.035	< 0.06	
Nickel	0.14	< 0.4	
Silver	0.01	< 0.15	
Tin	0.45	< 0.3	
Titanium	0.85	< 1.0	
Total Toxic Representation			

ESSENTIAL AND OTHER ELEMENTS

ELEMENTS	RESULT µg/g	REFERENCE RANGE	PERCENTILE 2.5th / 16th / 50th / 84th / 97.5th
Calcium	2450	300 - 1200	
Magnesium	330	35 - 120	
Sodium	170	12 - 90	
Potassium	33	8.0 - 38	
Copper	9.5	12 - 35	
Zinc	150	140 - 220	
Manganese	0.35	0.15 - 0.65	
Chromium	0.3	0.2 - 0.4	
Vanadium	0.008	0.018 - 0.065	
Molybdenum	< 0.01	0.028 - 0.056	
Boron	0.3	0.3 - 2.0	
Iodine	0.14	0.25 - 1.3	
Lithium	0.18	0.007 - 0.023	
Phosphorus	176	160 - 250	
Selenium	0.73	0.95 - 1.7	
Strontium	34	0.5 - 7.6	
Sulfur	43600	44500 - 52000	
Barium	4.2	0.26 - 3.0	
Cobalt	0.046	0.013 - 0.05	
Iron	8.7	5.4 - 14	
Germanium	0.056	0.045 - 0.065	
Rubidium	0.028	0.007 - 0.096	
Zirconium	0.054	0.02 - 0.42	

SPECIMEN DATA

COMMENTS:
Date Collected: 4/12/2002
Date Received: 6/11/2002
Date Completed: 6/12/2002

Methodology: ICP-MS

Sample Size: 0.191 g
Sample Type: Head
Hair Color: Grey
Treatment:
Shampoo: Otc

V06.99

RATIOS

ELEMENTS	RATIOS	EXPECTED RANGE
Ca/Mg	7.42	4 - 30
Ca/P	13.9	1 - 12
Na/K	5.15	0.5 - 10
Zn/Cu	15.8	4 - 20
Zn/Cd	> 999	> 800

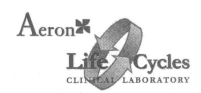

Aeron Accession Number: **0AA008**

Angela R Jones MD
1111 Her Street
Her Town XX   99999

Gail L Smith
999 Any Street
Any Town, XX   99999

Collection: Date	01/30/06	02/10/06	Assay Value Ranges*	
Time	08:00 am	09:00 am	Female	Male
Estradiol	0.5 pg/ml	3.2 pg/ml	Premenopausal 0.5 - 8.0 pg/ml Postmenopausal <1.5 pg/ml Transdermal 10 - 50 pg/ml	<1.5 pg/ml
Estrone	3.2 pg/ml	4.0 pg/ml	Premenopausal 2.6 - 5.4 pg/ml Postmenopausal 2.6 - 5.4 pg/ml	2.6 - 5.4 pg/ml
Estriol	4.8 pg/ml	5.3 pg/ml	Premenopausal 4.4 - 8.3 pg/ml Postmenopausal 3.0 - 11.8 pg/ml Transdermal 300 - 500 pg/ml	4.7 - 7.1 pg/ml
Progesterone	< .05 ng/ml	6.50 ng/ml	Premenopausal 0.1 - 0.5 ng/ml Postmenopausal <0.05 ng/ml Transdermal 1 - 10 ng/ml	<0.05 ng/ml
Testosterone	15.0 pg/ml	32.0 pg/ml	A.M. 17 - 52 pg/ml P.M. 10 - 20 pg/ml	A.M. 26 - 145 pg/ml P.M. 15 - 100 pg/ml
DHEA	50.0 pg/ml	140.0 pg/ml	33 - 300 pg/ml	37 - 336 pg/ml
Cortisol	1.40 ng/ml	1.60 ng/ml	A.M. 1.0 - 8.0 ng/ml P.M. 0.1 - 1.0 ng/ml	A.M. 1.0 - 8.0 ng/ml P.M. 0.1 - 1.0 ng/ml

*See back for expected ranges based on age, gender, menopausal status, phase of cycle, and treatment.

Signed: _____
Charles M. Dollbaum Ph.D., M.D.

Aeron Biotechnology Inc.

Date: _____02/14/06_____

Aeron LifeCycles Laboratory, 1933 Davis St., Suite 310, San Leandro, CA 94577 (800) 631-7900 Fax (510) 729-0383
Internet: http://www.aeron.com

Page 1 of 3

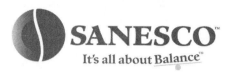

SANESCO™
It's all about Balance™

1200 Ridgefield Blvd Ste 200 Asheville, NC 28806
P 866.670.5705   F 828.670.5805
www.sanesco.net

HPA Profile
Sample Report

Patient Name: Jane Schmoe   Patient ID: 123456   Gender: F   Age: 49

Doctor Name: Anybody, MD   Doctor ID: 789012

Date Collected: Date Received: Lab Final: Report Final:
9/20/2005   9/23/2005   9/28/2005   9/29/2005

Neurotransmitters

Test	Patient Results	Reference Range/Units
Serotonin	48.3 (L)	50-250 mcg/gCr
Dopamine	258.1 (H)	50-250 mcg/gCr
Epinephrine	8.1	3-20 mcg/gCr
Norepinephrine	48.0 (H)	10-45 mcg/gCr
GABA	0.9 (L)	2-10 mcg/gCr
Glutamate	45.6 (H)	5-35 mcg/gCr
Norepi/Epi Ratio	5.9	4-10
Creatinine, Urine	98.3	

Hormones

Test/Time		
Cortisol (07:20)	20.1	13-24 nM
Cortisol (11:05)	4.2 (L)	5-8 nM
Cortisol (15:00)	3.1 (L)	4-7 nM
Cortisol (20:00)	0.9 (L)	1-3 nM
DHEAs (07:20)	11.60 (H)	2-10 ng/ml
DHEAs (15:00)	11.90 (H)	2-10 ng/ml

Definitions

The Reference Range is a statistical calculation derived by measuring levels in an established reference population. The reference range for one population may vary from other populations. This is further complicated by the fact that approximately 70% of the US population exhibit symptoms that are considered to be abnormal and are related to neurotransmitter imbalances.

Norepinephrine to Epinephrine Ratio: The norepi/epi ratio is calculated for the patient to determine if norepinephrine is being converted to epinephrine at a sufficient rate. There are several factors that effect the conversion: low cortisol, low P450 enzymes, magnesium deficiency and an insufficient number of methyl donors are a few of these factors.

Appendix B: Nutritional Supplement Companies

This list of nutritional supplement companies offers the most up-to-date contact information as well as a brief note about the products. If there is a toll-free number, I have given that one instead of the local number. Almost all of these companies are wholesale in nature and prefer, first, written requests, and second, calls for information and catalogs. Or view their website, which should answer many questions about products. Obviously, they prefer interest from stores and practitioners rather than individual consumers, although most companies will answer important questions about their products. There are literally hundreds of companies nationwide; I have included here as many as I could access or that I know about and/or use. Other companies that wish to be reviewed for future editions of this book, please contact me.

To the consumer: I suggest that you use your supplements wisely and be aware of the effects they may have on you; I am sure the companies would appreciate hearing from you about their products' effectiveness. Please note that there is no financial involvement between me and any of these companies. I am a customer of some of these companies and am familiar with many of their products.

A. C. Grace Company

1100 Quitman Road, P.O. Box 570
Big Sandy, TX 75755
903-636-4368 or 800-833-4368 (orders)
www.acgraceco.com

This company carries only one product, one of the best and most active vitamin E supplements, called Unique E, a mixed tocopherol concentrate.

Advanced Medical Labs

2040 Alameda Padre Serra, Suite 101
Santa Barbara, CA 93103
800-366-6056
www.advancedmedicallabs.com

They offer an extensive line of nutritional products through practitioners with a focus on the immune system, hormonal balancing, and aging.

Agape Health Products

4431 Corporate Center Drive, Suite 125
Los Alamitos, CA 90720
800-767-4776
www.perfect7.org

They are the distributor of Perfect 7, one of the better fiber-based intestinal cleansers, as well as a senna herbal laxative.

Alacer Corporation

80 Icon
Foothill Ranch, CA 92610
800-854-0249
www.alacer.com

They are the makers of Emergen-C, a popular electrolyte with powdered vitamin C, and other fine products. I often use and recommend Emergen-C.

Allergy Research Group/Nutricology

2300 North Loop Road
Alameda, CA 94502
800-545-9960
www.allergyresearchgroup.com (for practitioners)
www.nutricology.com (for stores and retail customers)

A company created by Dr. Stephen Levine, ARG sells many innovative and high-quality products for the clinical nutrition practice. Their Nutricology line of products, in contrast to the ARG line, is sold directly in natural food stores.

American Health
2100 Smithtown Avenue
Ronkonkoma, NY 11779
800-445-7137
www.americanhealthvitamins.com

They carry vitamins and supplements under their American Health line, and have a chemical- and animal-free beauty care line called Home Health; all of these are available in natural food stores.

Apex Energetics
16592 Hale Avenue
Irvine, CA 92606
800-736-4381
www.apexenergetics.com

They carry the Futureplex homeopathic and homeo-energetic products as well as flower essences and nutritional supplements, which are sold mainly to practitioners.

ApotheCure, Inc.
4001 McEwen Road, Suite 100
Dallas, TX 75244
800-969-6601
www.apothecure.com

This compounding pharmacy makes a variety of supplements and difficult-to-find medicines.

Arizona Natural Products
12815 North Cave Creek Road
Phoenix, AZ 85022
800-255-2823
www.arizonanatural.com

They carry innovative products using garlic and desert plants, such as yucca, chaparral, and other herbals.

Bezwecken, Inc.
12535 SW Third Street
Wilsonville, OR 97070
800-743-2256
www.bezwecken.com

They carry herbally based natural hormone products for women, sold exclusively through health practitioners. Their products contain actual hormones as well, such as Isocort with some cortisol in each tablet.

Biologic Homeopathic Industries (BHI)/Heel Inc.
10421 Research Road SE
Albuquerque, NM 87123
800-621-7644

The exclusive distributor of Heel homeopathics, BHI also distributes special formulas following the work of the eminent homeopathic physician H. H. Reckeweg.

Biotec Foods
5152 Bolsa Avenue, Suite 101
Huntington Beach, CA 92649
800-331-5888
www.biotecfoods.com

They create special high-potency, enteric-coated antioxidant enzyme formulas, including superoxide dismutase and glutathione peroxidase.

Biotics Research Corporation
6801 Biotics Research Drive
Rosenberg, TX 77471
800-231-5777
www.bioticsresearch.com

They carry a professional line with many products that deal with a wide range of health concerns from candida and digestive issues to inflammatory problems.

Boericke & Tafel, Inc. (see Nature's Way)

Known as "America's oldest and largest homeopathic pharmaceutical firm," they make a full line of traditional and special homeopathics.

Botanical Laboratories (see also, Herbs for Kids and Zand)

1441 West Smith Road

Ferndale, WA 98248

800-232-4005

www.botlab.com

This company carries a wide range of nutritional and herbal products under the company names Zand, Herbs for Kids, Symtec, and Natrabio. They sell to doctors, stores, and consumers.

Bronson Laboratories

350 South 400 West, Suite 102

Lindon, UT 84042

800-235-3200

www.bronsonlabs.com

This longtime nutritional supplement company carries a complete line of supplements for the entire family at a reasonable cost; popular items include their vitamin C crystals and prenatal formula.

Cardiovascular Research

106-B Shary Circle

Concord, CA 94518

800-888-4585

www.ecologicalformulas.net

Created by Jonathon Rothschild, they carry an advanced nutritional medicine line with effective formulas for such areas as immune support, yeast problems, and allergies, sold through practitioners and retail outlets.

College Pharmacy

3505 Austin Bluffs Parkway, Suite 101

Colorado Springs, CO 80918

800-888-9358

http://collegepharmacy.com

This compounding pharmacy creates many natural hormone products and other innovative supplies.

Country Life Vitamins

180 Vanderbilt Motor Parkway

Hauppauge, NY 11788

800-645-5768

www.country-life.com

This common line of supplements sold in natural food stores covers multiple formulas and sports products. They also distribute Biochem and Irontek products, and Long Life teas.

DaVinci Laboratories

20 New England Drive

Essex Junction, VT 05453

800-325-1776

www.davincilabs.com

This lab creates a complete line of nutritional supplements, including Gluconic DMG (N-N-dimethylglycine), for health-care practitioners.

Designs for Health

2 North Road

East Windsor, CT 06088

800-847-8302

www.designsforhealth.com

This professional line is one of my favorites and focuses on nutritional medical therapies including hormonal and metabolic support, digestion, detoxification, and weight control.

Douglas Laboratories

600 Boyce Road

Pittsburgh, PA 15205

888-368-4522 or 800-245-4440

www.douglaslabs.com

This full line of nutritional and herbal products can carry your label or theirs. They also have taken on the Amni line of nutritional products, which includes the Basic Preventive series.

Earthrise Nutritionals, LLC
2151 Michelson Drive, Suite 258
Irvine, CA 92612
800-949-7473
www.earthrise.com and www.supergreenfood.com

In the California desert, Earthrise grows and produces high quality spirulina products that are available in most natural food stores. Their products are high in antioxidants and some are helpful with detoxification.

Eclectic Institute, Inc.
36350 SE Industrial Way
Sandy, OR 97055
888-799-4372
www.eclecticherb.com

Founded by Ed Alstat, ND, they carry unique freeze-dried herbal products, extracts using organic alcohol, and therapeutic vitamin/mineral formulas.

Ecological Formulas (See Cardiovascular Research/Ecological Formulas)

Ejuva
P.O. Box 2716
Lake Arrowhead, CA 92352
866-463-5882
www.ejuva.com

A monthlong herbal detoxification program using high-quality and easy-to-take products within a program that incorporates dietary guidelines as well.

Emerson Ecologics/Karuna (See Karuna)
www.emersonecologics.com

Enzymatic Therapy/PhytoPharmica
825 Challenger Drive
Green Bay, WI 54311
800-558-7372
www.enzy.com

They carry a wide range of high-quality naturopathic products—nutritional, herbal, and glandular—for the store, practitioner, and consumer. See PhytoPharmica for the practitioner's line.

Flora, Inc.
805 E. Badger Road
Lynden, WA 98264
800-446-2110
www.florahealth.com

This company imports and distributes the German-made Floradix products, liquid herbal extracts of vitamins and minerals, as well as a particularly well-tolerated and bioavailable iron formula. These products are found in most health food stores and natural pharmacies.

Food Science Laboratories
20 New England Drive
Essex Junction, VT 05453
800-874-9444
www.foodscienceofvermont.com

This is the retail line of products (and is the similar line of Da Vinci Labs), with specialty DMG supplements.

Freeda
36 E. 41st Street
New York, NY 10017
800-777-3737
www.freeda.com

This company offers a wide range of very clean nutritional formulas (no aluminum, coal tar dyes, gluten, or yeast in their products) for all age groups, with many completely vegetarian products. They also distribute many products and sell to online customers.

Gaia Herbs
108 Island Ford Road
Brevard, NC 28712
888-917-8269
www.gaiaherbs.com

Gaia grows and produces certified organic herbs in Oregon; their high-quality extracts are available in natural food stores. They also have liquid phyto caps available.

Green Foods
2220 Camino del Sol
Oxnard, CA 93030
800-777-4430
www.greenfoods.com

This "green" company produces and markets wonderfully purifying and nourishing barley grass, green food combinations, and vegetable powders to use for smoothies and as nutritional supplements. Great for travelers, too.

Health Concerns
8001 Capwell Drive
Oakland, CA 94621
800-233-9355
www.healthconcerns.com

Founded and directed by herbalist Andrew Gaeddart, this specialty company offers many quality products (both both individual and combination formulas) in the field of Chinese herbology.

Healthy N Fit Nutritionals
435 Yorktown Road, Route 129
Croton-on-Hudson, NY 10520
800-338-5200
www.behealthynfit.com

They carry a special line of nutrient formulas for specific health conditions available to practitioners.

Heel Inc./Biologic Homeopathic Industries (BHI)
P.O. Box 11280
Albuquerque, NM 87192
800-621-7644, 503-293-3843
www.heelusa.com

This company carries a variety of homeopathic remedies that can be found in natural food stores and doctors' offices, with especially good natural products for pain and inflammation, as well as many other health conditions.

Herb Pharm
P.O. Box 116
Williams, OR 97544
800-348-4372
www.herb-pharm.com

They offer a fine line of organically grown, custom wild-crafted herbal extracts, sold through practitioners and stores.

Herbs for Kids (See Botanical Laboratories)

Herbs for Kids provides a line of alcohol-free, good-tasting herbal formulas geared toward children.

Herbs of Light
P.O. Box 1648
High Springs, FL 32655
800-313-3001
www.herbsoflight.com

This company is dedicated to the creation of a wide variety of high-quality and enhanced vibrational herbal extracts.

Intensive Nutrition, Inc.
1972 Republic Avenue
San Leandro, CA 94577
800-333-7414
www.intensivenutrition.com

Dr. Bela Balough and staff provide many excellent powdered, readily usable nutritional metabolic products, including amino acid formulas, multiples, sublingual high-potency folic acid (Folixor) and Tanalbit, one of my favorite natural antimicrobial products.

J. R. Carlson Laboratories, Inc.
15 College Drive
Arlington Heights, IL 60004
888-234-5656
www.carlsonlabs.com

They offer a complete line of nutritional supplements, specializing in high-quality vitamin E and fish oil products.

Jarrow Formulas, Inc.
1824 S. Robertson Boulevard
Los Angeles, CA 90035
800-726-0886
www.jarrow.com

This popular company offers a wide range of nutritional products popular in many health food stores.

Karuna Corporation/Emerson Ecologics, Inc.
7 Commerce Drive
Bedford, NH 03110
800-654-4432
www.emersonecologics.com

The Karuna Corporation, now distributed through Emerson Ecologics, has some of my favorite powdered multiples, the Maxxum series, and a variety of effective nutrient and herbal products. Emerson also has a wide line of nutritional products sold in stores and direct to consumers, whereas Karuna products are sold through practitioners.

Key Company
1313 W. Essex Avenue
St. Louis, MO 63122
800-325-9592
www.thekeycompany.com

They offer some basic, good-quality yet inexpensive supplements and, for MDs and DOs, injectables for use in the nutritional practice.

King Bio
3 Westside Drive
Asheville, NC 28806
800-543-3245
www.kingbio.com

They carry a line of liquid (bioenergetically enhanced, water-based) homeopathic formulas for special clinical needs. They have a consumer's line in stores and a new licensed practitioner line called SafeCare Rx, all liquid sprays.

Kroeger Herb Products
805 Walnut Street
Boulder, CO 80301
303-443-0261 or 800-225-8787
www.kroegerherb.com

They offer a line of special herbal medicinal products developed by Hanna Kroeger, including parasite cleansing and cardiovascular support.

Legere Pharmaceuticals
7326 E. Evans Road
Scottsdale, AZ 85260
800-528-3144

This company provides a variety of products to the practitioner, including oral and injectable drugs as well as vitamins and minerals.

Longevity Plus
708 East Highway 260, Suite C2
Payson, AZ 85541
800-580-7587
wwww.longevityplus.com

This company, founded and directed by medical maverick Garry Gordon, MD, has advanced products for cardiovascular health and aging. They sell to everyone.

Maitake Products, Inc.
22 Bergen Turnpike
Ridgefield Park, NJ 07660
800-747-7418
www.maitake.com

They sell maitake mushroom products for health and immune support.

Mayway Corporation
1338 Mandela Parkway
Oakland, CA 94607
800-262-9929
www.mayway.com

They carry a wide collection of herbal products imported from China and the Orient, sold primarily to practitioners.

MegaFood
P.O. Box 325
Derry, NH 03038
800-848-2542
www.megafood.com

They offer "food-grown" and extracted supplements, which have become popular in recent years.

Metabolic Products
17A Everberg Road
Woburn, MA 01801
800-292-4343
www.prostex.com

Metabolic Products sells Prostex, a prostate support product.

Metagenics, Inc.
100 Avenida La Pata
San Clemente, CA 92673
800-692-9400
www.metagenics.com

Offering a wide range of innovative and top-quality products, this company follows the current research closely and provides special educational seminars for clinical nutrition–oriented practitioners. They sell only through practitioners.

Natren
3105 Willow Lane
Westlake Village, CA 91361
800-992-3323
www.natren.com

They focus on quality probiotic formulas sold mainly through stores and online.

Naturally Vitamins
4404 East Elwood Street
Phoenix, AZ 85040
800-899-4499
www.naturallyvitamins.com

This company has a specialty line of products that deal with enzyme nutrients for inflammation, in particular the well known Wobenzym enzyme from Germany.

Nature's Answer
75 Commerce Drive
Hauppauge, NY 11788
800-439-2324
www.naturesanswer.com

They provide quality liquid herbal/nutrient extracts, including maitake mushroom, sold primarily in natural food stores.

Nature's Herbs
600 East Quality Drive
American Fork, UT 84003
800-437-2257
www.naturesherbs.com

This is a full line of herbal products sold primarily through natural food stores.

Nature's Life/Nutraceutical Corporation
900 Larkspur Landing Circle, Suite 105
Larkspur, CA 94939
800-854-6837
www.natureslife.com

Their wide line of quality supplements is popular in health food stores.

Nature's Plus/Natural Organics
548 Broadhollow Road
Melville, NY 11747
800-645-9500 or 631-293-0030
www.naturesplus.com

This is a well-known line of nutritional supplements sold in natural food stores, including Source of Life multivitamins and Spirutein, a protein supplement/meal replacement.

Nature's Secret/Irwin Naturals/Aromavera
5310 Beethoven Street
Los Angeles, CA 90066
800-669-9514
www.naturessecret.com

Nature's Secret offers a good selection of nutrient/herbal products for detoxification and health. Irwin Naturals is another line of all-liquid gel caps for body wellness, and Aromavera provides skin care and essential oils. All are available in natural food stores.

Nature's Sunshine Products, Inc.
P.O. Box 19005
Provo, UT 84605
800-223-8225
www.naturessunshine.com

This company has been around for many decades and has hundreds of nutritional and herbal products that it sells by direct marketing, or person-to-person networking. They have many detox and cleansing products, colloidal minerals, and Thai-Go, an antioxidant drink for energy and health.

Nature's Way (see also Boericke & Tafel, Inc.)
1375 North Mountain Spring Parkway
Springville, UT 84663
800-9-NATURE or 800-926-8883
www.naturesway.com

This is a complete line of nutritional and herbal supplements and the Boericke & Tafel line of homeopathic remedies.

New Chapter Vitamins
22 High Street
Brattleboro, VT 05301
800-543-7279
www.newchapter.info

They offer a line of fine-quality formulas (many organic) for women and men, sold primarily in natural food stores and through practitioners.

NF Formulas/Integrative Therapeutics, Inc.
825 Challenger Drive
Green Bay, WI 54311
800-917-3696 or 800-931-1709
www.integrativeinc.com

They offer clinically useful naturopathic products, including echinacea–vitamin C tablets.

Nordic Naturals
94 Hangar Way
Watsonville, CA 95076
800-662-2544
www.nordicnaturals.com

This company specializes in high-quality oil products, primarily omega-3 oils from fish.

NutriBiotic
P.O. Box 238
Lakeport, CA 95453
800-225-4345
www.nutribiotic.com

They offer some good quality, powdered supplement products, free of common allergens. Their main product is Citricidal, a natural antimicrobial grapefruit seed extract.

Nutrilite (Quixtar)
7575 E. Fulton Street
Ada, MI 49355
800-253-6500
www.quixtar.com

This multilevel distributor offers a line of fine-quality, food-extracted nutritional supplements, sold from person to person.

Pharmanex/Nu Skin
1 Nu Skin Plaza
Provo, UT 84601
800-487-1000
www.pharmanexusa.com

They offer high-quality, multilevel nutritional supplements and skin products. They use the best ingredients from Nature and use science to back their products, which are more costly than many other products unless you distribute.

PhysioLogics

10701 Melody Drive, Suite 515
Northglenn, CO 80234
1-800-765-6775
www.physiologics.com

They are committed to high quality and low prices, and they focus on cardiovascular health, joints, and immune products.

Phyto-Pharmica/Integrative Therapeutics

825 Challenger Drive
Green Bay, WI 54311
800-553-2370 or 800-917-3696 (for practitioners)
www.phytopharmica.com

Nutritional and herbal supplements are sold mainly to the naturopathic practitioner, but many of their quality products are also available to the public through the Enzymatic Therapy line in health food stores.

Power Organics

P.O. Box 1626
Mt. Shasta, CA 96067
800-327-1956
www.powerorganics.com

This company sells a variety of blue-green algae products from Klamath Lake, plus a special earth salt called Miracle Crystal Salt.

Professional Botanicals

5688 E. 2200 North
Eden, UT 84310
800-824-8181
www.profbot.com

They offer a fine line of special herbal formulas for specific physiological effects and treatment of certain disease processes.

Pure Body Institute

230 S. Olive Street
Ventura, CA 93001
800-952-7873
www.pbiv.com

They produce and supply a popular herbal detox product called Nature's Pure Body Program, as well other detox products for liver and kidneys, and many others.

Purity Products

139 Haven Avenue
Port Washington, NY 11050
800-718-2003
www.purityproducts.com

This mail-order company sells direct to consumers a wide variety of their own products and others they distribute for other companies, all at a discount.

Quantum, Inc.

754 Washinton Street
Eugene, OR 97401
800-448-1448
www.quantumhealth.com

They have a line of nutritional supplements including Super Lysine-Plus that are available through stores and their catalog.

Rainbow Light Nutritional Systems

125 McPherson Street
Santa Cruz, CA 95060
800-635-1233
www.rainbowlight.com

They provide a fine line of food-grown nutrient supplements, found in many natural food stores.

Schiff Nutrition

2002 South 5070 West
Salt Lake City, UT 84104
800-526-6251
www.schiffvitmains.com

This longtime mainstay of the nutritional market has a full line of products available in many health food stores.

Solgar Vitamin & Herb
1170 Valley Brook Avenue
Lyndhurst, NJ 07071
800-645-2246
www.solgar.com

This is a longtime company in the natural food industry, with many quality, tableted formulas.

Source Naturals/Threshold Enterprises
23 Janis Way
Scotts Valley, CA 95066
800-777-5677
www.sourcenaturals.com

This is a quality vegetarian line of nutritional support and therapeutic supplements, such as the Wellness Formula, which is is popular in natural food stores for supporting healthy immune function.

Standard Homeopathic Company/
Hyland's Homeopathic Medicines
P.O. Box 61067
Los Angeles, CA 90061
800-624-9659 or 800-456-7818
www.hylands.com

This company has provided top-quality homeopathics for decades, including the Hyland's Homeopathic Combination Medicines, such as Hyland's Calm Forte for adults and kids, helping with calming and sleep.

Standard Process
1200 W. Royal Lee Drive
P.O. Box 904
Palmyra, WI 53156
800-848-5061
www.standardprocess.com

This extensive, longtime line of special glandular supplements is popular with naturopathic practitioners. Zypan is an excellent nonvegetarian digestive formula.

Sun Chlorella USA
3305 Kashiwa Street
Torrance, CA 90505
800-829-2828
www.sunchlorella.com

They are the makers and distributors of the fabulous Sun Chlorella powder and tablets.

Superior Trading Company
837 Washington Street
San Francisco, CA 94108
415-495-7988
www.superiortrading.com

They offer a variety of Oriental herbal products, such as ginseng, dong quai, and royal jelly.

Supernutrition/Forever Young
100 Santa Rosa Avenue
Pacifica, CA 94044
800-453-0219
www.supernutritionusa.com

I have used these advanced, potent products for 25 years. They are ideal for the active individual interested in high performance. My favorites are tableted vitamin C (Big Rose Hips) and the Energy Caps for stress, and their popular multi is called Opti Pack, all found in natural food stores. ON Balance is the professional line for these products.

Systemic Formulas
1877 West 2800 South
Ogden UT 84401
800-445-4647
www.systemicformulas.com

This specific line of clinically applicable formulas was designed by master herbalist A. S. Wheelwright. They are sold only health practitioners.

Thorne Research, Inc.
P.O. Box 25
Dover, ID 83825
800-228-1966
www.thorne.com

Thorne manufactures an extensive practitioner line of nutritional, hypoallergenic products.

TIDhealth
2015 West Park Avenue, Suite 4
Redlands, CA 92373
800-824-2434
www.tidhealth.com

This is a great distribution company for a wide variety of companies' nutritional and herbal supplements for health professionals.

Twinlab, Inc.
150 Motor Parkway, Suite 210
Hauppauge, NY 11788
800-645-5626
www.twinlabs.com

This extremely thorough line of primarily powdered, easily assimilable products is for the entire family, from basic supplements to bodybuilding formulas for sports nutrition. Their products are mainly handled through their distribution network to health food stores and practitioners.

Tyler Encapsulations/Integrative Therapeutics, Inc.
825 Challenger Drive
Green Bay, WI 54311
800-917-3696 or 800-931-1709
www.integrativeinc.com

They offer a wide variety of quality products specializing in digestive function and detoxification, all in capsules as well.

UAS Labs/DDS Acidophilus
9953 Valleyview Road
Eden Prairie, MN 55343
800-422-3371
www.uaslabs.com

They are the primary developer and distributor of the high-potency *Lactobacillus acidophilus* culture DDS-1.

Vitaline Formulas/Integrative Therapeutics, Inc.
825 Challenger Drive
Green Bay, WI 54311
800-917-3696
www.integrativeinc.com

I have used this good-quality yet relatively inexpensive line of products for years in my practice. I find that patients tolerate the Vitaline products very well. Their CoQ10 products are especially good and have been used in studies.

Vitamin Research Products
4610 Arrowhead Dr.
Carson City, NV 89706
800-877-2477 or 775-884-1300
www.vrp.com

This is an extensive line of well-researched products that can be sold through practitioners. They have a focus on antioxidants and aging with many of their products.

Wakunaga of America
23501 Madero
Mission Viejo, CA 92691
800-421-2998
www.kyolic.com

They are the makers and distributors of Kyolic, an odorless garlic extract formula, and Kyogreen, a barley grass extract, found in natural food stores.

Wellness Health Pharmaceuticals
3401 Indepedence Drive, Suite 231
Birmingham, AL 35209
800-227-2672 or 205-879-6551
www.wellnesshealth.com

This distribution network for many fine nutritional and pharmaceutical products distributes pure nystatin powder and some of the aforementioned supplement lines, for both the practitioner and the consumer. They are also a compounding pharmacy.

Werum Enterprises, Inc.
P.O. Box 903
Shingle Springs, CA 95682
800-822-6193

Werum carries a wide range of nutritional and herbal specialty products that include the Atrium line, R&D Formulations, and R&A Homeopathics, all sold only to health practitioners.

Women's International Pharmacy (WIP)
12012 North 111th Avenue
Youngtown, AZ 85363
800-279-5708
www.womensinternational.com

This experienced compounding pharmacy is used by many physicians' offices to support their patients with bioidentical hormones. They prepare micronized-oil oral capsules with dosages of one or more hormones as directed by the doctor's prescription.

Yerba Prima, Inc.
740 Jefferson Avenue
Ashland, OR 97520
800-421-9972
www.yerba.com

This line of high-quality herbal products are known as "herbs to live by." They can be found in many natural food stores.

Appendix C: Nutrition Educational Organizations and Institutions

ALTERNATIVE SCHOOLS FOR THE STUDY OF NUTRITION AND NATUROPATHY

This group of schools and institutions includes schools with on-campus training and degrees as well as distance learning. Most of these have partly alternative nutrition programs and well as standard studies of nutrition and biochemisty. Many are part of the NANP organization, which is working to create more unified national education standards and certifications.

National Association of Nutrition Professionals (NANP)

P.O. Box 1172
Danville, CA 94526
800-342-8037
www.nanp.org

NANP is a nonprofit business league representing holistically trained nutrition professionals. They enhance the integrity of the holistic nutrition profession by providing self-governance, educational standards, a rigorous code of ethics, and professional registration of holistic nutritionists. Many of the schools on this list are members of NANP.

American Health Sciences University (AHSU) and
National Institute of Nutrition Education (NINE)

1010 S. Joliet #107
Aurora, CO 80012
800-530-8079
www.ahsu.edu

This combined school offers distance education degrees and certificates, such as a master's degree in Nutrition Science and Certified Nutritionist (CN).

American University of Complimentary Medicine

11543 Olympic Boulevard
Los Angeles, CA 90064
310-914-4116
www.aucm.org

This school offers both on-site and distance learning degrees (associate in arts, master's, and PhD) in many areas of study, including classical Chinese medicine, homeopathy, and ayurveda, plus certificate programs in holistic health, herbology, nutritional medicine, and various bodywork therapies.

Bauman College

P.O. Box 940, 10151 Main Street, Suite 128
Penngrove, CA 94951
800-987-7530 or 707-795-1284
www.baumancollege.org

This northern California school offers nutrition certification and culinary arts programs to support careers in nutritional counseling and healthy food preparation.

Clayton College of Natural Health (CCNH)

2140 11th Avenue South, Suite 305
Birmingham, AL 35205
800-659-8274 or 800-995-4590 (admissions)
www.ccnh.edu

This popular distance-learning college offers many degrees in holistic nutrition and naturopathy, as well as graduate degrees. They use this book and other good books and teachers as their faculty.

Hawthorn Health & Nutrition Institute

P.O. Box 275

Whitethorn, CA 95589

800-845-2234

www.hawthorninstitute.org

This state-licensed school has online learning programs for such degrees as nutrition consultant, and a masters of science in holistic nutrition. Their Applied Clinical Nutrition Program is directed toward health professionals who already incorporate nutrition into their practices.

Huntington College of Health Sciences

1204-D Kenesaw

Knoxville, TN 37919

800-290-4226 or 865-524-8079

www.hchs.edu

This distance-learning college offers degrees and diplomas in nutrition and other health sciences.

Institute of Integrative Nutrition

3 East 28th Street, 12th Floor

New York, NY 10016

212-730-5433

www.integrativenutrition.com

This is an active and progressive school in New York City that offers training in Nutrition and Dietary Therapies as well as Holistic Health.

Nutrition Therapy Institute

1574 York Street #100

Denver, CO 80206

866-377-3974 or 303-377-3974

www.instituteofnutrition.com

This Denver school offers both on-site and distance-learning programs in many areas of nutritional studies, including a diploma as a certified nutrition therapist (CNT).

University of Bridgeport

126 Park Avenue

Bridgeport, CT 06604

800-392-3582 or 203-576-4552

www.bridgeport.edu

A progressive international school offering many advanced degrees in the nutritional sciences, naturopathic medicine, acupuncture, and more, the University of Bridgeport has a strong faculty and beautiful campus. They also provide distance learning for people around the globe.

REGIONALLY ACCREDITED COLLEGES AND UNIVERSITIES

Several fully accredited colleges and universities have made a special effort to establish whole, natural foods and ecologically based eating as parts of their curriculum. A few are listed here.

Bastyr University

14500 Juanita Drive NE

Kenmore, WA 98028-4966

425-823-1300

www.bastyr.edu

Located just north of Seattle, Washington, Bastyr University is a regionally accredited, pioneering academic center for the study of natural medicine and related sciences. It offers undergraduate and graduate degrees in the field of nutrition with an emphasis on whole foods and a natural health viewpoint, with accredited ND degrees as well. The university also offers a didactic program in dietetics (DPD) and dietetic internship (DI) that meet the training requirements for registered dietitians (RDs). This aspect of the nutrition program makes it one of the few in the country to provide dietitian training, which includes placement in a fully integrative natural-health center.

Teachers College, Columbia University
Program in Nutrition
525 West 120th Street, Box 137
New York, NY 10027
212-678-3950
www.tc.columbia.edu/hbs/Nutrition

Ecological food choices are part of the focus in the nutrition program at Teacher's College, Columbia University. The scope of the overall program is broad, however, in keeping with an almost 100-year history. The college also offers a dietetic internship program, and facilitates completion of the prior academic training required for registered dietitians.

Tufts University
The Friedman School of Nutrition Science
150 Harrison Avenue
Boston, MA 02111
617-636-6719
http://nutrition.tufts.edu

The Agriculture, Food, and Environment (AFE) program housed within the Friedman School of Nutrition Science at Tufts University may be the only program of its kind in the country, offering master's and doctoral degrees in nutrition that teach evaluation of ecological, political, economic, and social aspects of food production and distribution.

University of Arizona
Program in Integrative Medicine
P.O. Box 245153
Tucson, AZ 85724
http://integrativemedicine.arizona.edu

Thanks to the pioneering work of Dr. Andrew Weil, the University of Arizona is able to offer fellowships to physicians that provide comprehensive training in integrative medicine. Several online courses that carry CME (continuing medical education) credit for physicians are also offered through the University's program in integrative medicine.

University of California at Davis
Sustainable Agriculture Research and
Education Program
One Shields Avenue
Davis, CA 95616
www.sarep.ucdavis.edu

Although technically situated outside of the university's degree programs in nutrition, the Sustainable Agriculture Research and Education Program (SAREP) at the University of California at Davis is an outstanding example of a major state university narrowing the gap between the fields of nutrition and ecology. SAREP offers conferences, workshops, and courses (including online courses) in many areas of sustainability and organics.

NUTRITION-RELATED CERTIFICATION PROGRAMS FOR HEALTH PRACTITIONERS

Several organizations have established certification programs for health-care practitioners wanting to focus on nutrition in their practice. These certification programs typically do not provide their graduates with any legal standing in any state to practice nutrition, but they do often involve training, examination, and continuing education for maintenance of certification. Here are a few.

American College of Nutrition
300 S. Duncan Avenue, Suite 225
Clearwater, FL 33755
727-446-6086
www.amcollnutr.org

Fellowships granted by the American College of Nutrition provide the recipient with the title FACN (fellow of the American College of Nutrition). All fellows must first hold a doctoral degree from an institution recognized by an accrediting board authorized by the U.S. Department of Education, or from a foreign institution with equivalent standards, and have demonstrated expertise in patient care, research, and/or the teaching of nutrition. Specific standards are set for demonstration of excellence, including the authoring of five or more nutrition-related publications in peer-reviewed medical journals.

A certification board set up by the American College of Nutrition (www.cert-nutrition.org/CertificationProcess.htm) provides individuals with existing advanced degrees (master's, doctoral, or professional level) the designation CNS (certified nutrition specialist) upon completion of certification requirements, including formal examination.

The American College for Advancement in Medicine (ACAM)

23121 Verdugo Drive, Suite 204
Laguna Hills, CA 92653
949-583-7666 or 800-532-3688
http://acam.org/conferences.htm

The American College for Advancement in Medicine is a not-for-profit medical society that provides education for physicians and other health-care professionals in preventive and nutritional medicine.

International and American Associations of Clinical Nutritionists (IAACN)

15280 Addison Road, Suite 130
Addison, TX 75001
972-407-9089
www.iaacn.org

This certifying organization provides recognition of nutrition specialization through the awarding of the title CCN (certified clinical nutritionist). A training program and examination are required, in addition to documentation of continuing education once the certification has been issued.

The Intersociety Professional Nutrition Education Consortium (IPNEC)
American Board of Physician Nutrition Specialists (ABPNS)
University of Alabama at Birmingham

439 Susan Mott Webb Nutrition Sciences Building
1675 University Boulevard
Birmingham, AL 35294
205-996-2513
http://main.uab.edu/ipnec/show.asp?durki=35204

This consortium seeks to increase physician knowledge about the role of nutrition in prevention and treatment of disease through a certification program that identifies a physician as a physician nutrition specialists (PNS) following completion of consortium requirements. As of 2006, a minimum of 1,000 hours of mentored clinical nutrition experience is required as part of the certification process.

Appendix D: Recommended Reading and Reference Books

Aero, R., and S. Rick. *Vitamin Power.* New York: Harmony Books, 1987.

Airola, P. *The Airola Diet and Cookbook.* Phoenix, AZ: Health Plus Publishers, 1981.

———. *How to Get Well.* Scottsdale, AZ: Health Plus Publishers, 1988.

Ballentine, R. *Diet and Nutrition: A Holistic Approach.* Honesdale, PA: Himalayan International Institute, 1978.

Baumel, S. *Dealing with Depression Naturally: Alternatives and Complementary Therapies for Restoring Emotional Health.* New York: McGraw-Hill, 2000.

Becker, R. *The Body Electric: Electromagnetism and the Foundation of Life.* New York: HarperCollins, 1998.

———. *Cross Currents: The Promise of Electromedicine, the Perils of Electropollution.* Los Angeles: Jeremy P. Tarcher, 1991.

Berger, S. *The Immune Power Diet.* New York: New American Library, 1985.

Bernstein, R. *The Diabetes Diet.* New York: Little, Brown and Co., 2005.

Berry, L. *Internal Cleansing: Rid Your Body of Toxins and Return to Vibrant Good Health.* Rocklin, CA: Prima Publishing, 1997.

Blaylock, R. *Excitotoxins: The Taste That Kills.* Santa Fe: Health Press, 1997.

Braly, J. *Dr. Braly's Optimum Health Program: For Permanent Weight Loss and a Longer Healthier Life.* New York: Time Books, 1985.

Braly, J. and P. Holford. *The H Factor Solution: Homocysteine, the Best Single Indicator of Whether You Are Likely to Live Long or Die Young.* Bergen, NJ: Basic Health Publications, 2003.

Braverman, E., with C. Pfeiffer. *The Healing Nutrients Within.* New Canaan, CT: Keats, 1987.

Brody, J. *Nutrition Book.* New York: Bantam Books, 1982.

Brown, E. E. *Tassajara Recipe Book: Favorites of the Guest Season.* Boston: Shambala Publications, 1985.

Campbell, T. Collin, with T. Campbell II. *The China Study: Startling Implications for Diet, Weight Loss, and Long-Term Health.* Dallas: BenBella Books, 2005.

Cass, H. and K. Barnes. *8 Weeks to Vibrant Health: A Woman's Take-Charge Program to Correct Imbalances, Reclaim Energy, and Restore Well-Being.* New York: McGraw Hill, 2004.

Castleman, M. *Nature's Cures.* Emmaus, PA: Rodale, 1996.

Center for Science in the Public Interest. *The Household Pollutants Guide.* New York: Anchor Books, 1978.

Chen J., T.C. Campbell, J. Li, and R. Peto. *Diet, Lifestyle, and Mortality in China.* Ithaca, NY: Cornell University Press, 1990.

Chopra, D. *Perfect Health.* Rev. ed. New York: Harmony Books, 2001.

———. *Quantum Healing : Exploring the Frontiers of Mind/Body Medicine.* New York: Bantam Books, 1989.

Cloutier, M., and E. Adamson. *The Mediterranean Diet.* Rev. ed. New York: Avon Books, 2004.

Colbin, A. *The Book of Whole Meals: A Seasonal Guide to Assembling Balanced Vegetarian Breakfasts, Lunches, and Dinners.* New York: Ballantine Books, 1985.

———. *Food and Healing.* New York: Ballantine Books, 1986.

Commoner, B. *Closing Circle: Confronting the Environmental Crisis.* Woodstock, NY: Beekman Publishing, 1973.

Cousens, G. *Conscious Eating.* Berkeley, CA: North Atlantic Books, 2000.

———. *Spiritual Nutrition and the Rainbow Diet.* De Pere, WI: Cassandra Press, 1987.

Crook, W., *The Yeast Connection Handbook.* Jackson, TN: Professional Books, 1996.

Crook, W. and C. Dean. *The Yeast Connection and Women's Health.* 2nd ed. Jackson, TN: Professional Books, 2005.

Crook, W. and M. Jones, *The Yeast Connection Cookbook.* Jackson, TN: Professional Books, 1987.

Cutler, E. with J. Kaslow. *MicroMiracles: Discover the Healing Power of Enzymes.* New York: Rodale Books, 2005.

D'Adamo, P. *Eat Right for Your Type.* New York: G.P. Putnam's Sons, 1996.

Dadd, D. L. *Home Safe Home.* New York: Tarcher/Putnam, 1996.

———. *The Nontoxic Home.* Los Angeles: Tarcher, 1986.

————. *The Nontoxic Home and Office.* New York: Tarcher/Putnam, 1992.

Dufty, W. *Sugar Blues.* New York: Warner Books, 1986.

Eaton, B., M. Shostak, and M. Konner. *The Paleolithic Prescription: A Program of Diet and Exercise and a Design for Living.* New York: HarperCollins, New York, 1989.

Emsley, J. *The Elements.* 3rd ed. Oxford: Clarendon Press, 1998.

Fallon, S., with M. Enig. *Nourishing Traditions: The Cookbook That Challenges Politically Correct Nutrition and the Diet Dictocrats.* Winon Lake, IN: New Trends Publishing, 1999.

Fleet, T. *Rays of the Dawn.* San Antonio, TX: Concept-Therapy Institute, 2000.

Francis, R. *Never Be Sick Again.* Deerfield Beach, FL: Health Communications, 2002.

Gittleman, A. L. *The Fat Flush Plan.* New York: McGraw-Hill, 2002.

Goldbeck, N., and D. Goldbeck. *Nikki and David Goldbeck's American Wholefoods Cuisine.* 10th anniversary ed. Woodstock, NY: Ceres Press, 1993.

Goldberg, B. *Alternative Medicine: The Definitive Guide.* Berkeley, CA: Celestial Arts, 2002.

Green, J. *The Herbal Medicine Maker's Handbook.* Berkeley, CA: Crossing Press, 2000.

Gussow, J., and P. Thomas, eds. *The Nutrition Debate: Sorting Out Some Answers.* Boulder, CO: Bull Publishing, 1987.

Haas, E. *A Cookbook for All Seasons.* Berkeley, CA: Celestial Arts, 2000.

————. *Seasonal Food Guide Poster.* Berkeley, CA: Celestial Arts, 2001.

————. *The Staying Healthy Shopper's Guide.* Berkeley, CA: Celestial Arts, 1999.

————. *Staying Healthy with the Seasons.* Berkeley, CA: Celestial Arts, 2003.

Haas, E., with Daniella Chase. *The New Detox Diet.* Berkeley, CA: Celestial Arts, 2004.

Haas, E., and Cameron Stauth. *The False Fat Diet: The Revolutionary 21-Day Program for Losing the Weight You Think Is Fat.* New York: Ballentine Books, 2001.

Hall, M. P. *The Medicine of the Sun and Moon.* Los Angeles: Philosophical Research Society, 1999.

Hendler, S. *The Complete Guide to Anti-aging Nutrients.* New York: Simon and Schuster, 1985.

Hobbs, C., and Haas, E. *Vitamins for Dummies.* Foster City, CA: IDG Books, Worldwide, 1999.

Holford, Patrick. *The New Optimum Nutrition Bible.* Rev. ed. Berkeley, CA: Crossing Press, 2004.

Howell, E. *Enzyme Nutrition.* Twin Lakes, WI: Lotus Press, 1986.

Hull, J. S. *Sweet Poison: How the World's Most Popular Artificial Sweetener Is Killing Us.* Far Hills, NH: New Horizon Press, 1999

Hull, J. S., with L. T. Dealey. *Splenda: Is It Safe or Not?* Dallas, TX: The Pickle Press, 2005

Hyman, M., and M. Liponis. *UltraPrevention: The 6-Week Plan That Will Make You Healthy for Life.* New York: Atria Books, 2003.

Ivker, R., R. Anderson, and L. Trivieri Jr. *The Complete Self-Care Guide to Holistic Medicine: Treating Our Most Common Ailments.* New York: Tarcher/Putnam, 1999.

Jensen, B. *Dr. Jensen's Nutrition Handbook: A Daily Regimen for Healthy Living.* 2nd ed. New York: McGraw-Hill, 2000.

————. *Foods That Heal.* Rev. ed. New York: Avery Books, 1988.

Khalsa, D. *Food as Medicine.* New York: Atria Books, 2003.

Khalsa, D., with C. Stauth. *Brain Longevity: The Breakthrough Medical Program That Improves Your Mind and Memory.* New York: Warner Books, 1999.

————. *The Pain Cure.* New York: Warner Books, 1999.

Kushi, A., with A. Jack. *Complete Guide to Macrobiotic Cooking for Health, Harmony, and Peace.* New York: Warner Books, 1985.

Kushi, M. *The Cancer Prevention Diet.* New York: St. Martin's, 1994.

Krohn, J., and F. Taylor. *Finding the Right Treatment: Modern and Alternative Medicine.* Point Roberts, WA: Hartley & Marks, 2002.

————. *Natural Detoxification: The Complete Guide to Clearing Your Body of Toxins.* Point Roberts, WA: Hartley and Marks Publishers, 2000.

Kulvinskas, V. *Sprouts for the Love of Every Body.* Woodstock Valley, CT: 21st Century Publications, 1988.

Kulvinskas, V., and R. Tasca Jr. *Survival into the Twenty-First Century.* Woodstock Valley, CT: 21st Century Publications, 1975.

Lamothe, D. *The Taming of the Chew: A Holistic Guide to Stopping Compulsive Eating.* New York: Penguin Books, 2002.

Lappé, F. *Diet for a Small Planet.* New York: Ballantine Books, 1982.

Lark, S. *PMS Self Help Book.* Berkeley, CA: Celestial Arts, 1984.

Leonard, J., and P. Laut. *Rebirthing: The Science of Enjoying All of Your Life.* St. Paul, MN: Trinity Publishing House, 1983.

Lesser, M. *The Brain Chemistry Diet.* New York: Putnam, 2001.

————. *Nutrition and Vitamin Therapy.* New York: Bantam Books, 1983.

Levin, J., and N. Cedarquist. *Vibrant Living: A Live Foods Resource and Recipe Book.* La Jolla, CA: Glo, Inc., 2001.

MacEachern, D. *Save Our Planet.* New York: Dell, 1990.

Makower, J. *Office Hazards.* Oakland, CA: Tilden Press, 1981.

Martin, J. M., and Z. Rona. *Complete Candida Yeast Guidebook: Everything You Need to Know about Prevention, Treatment, and Diet.* 2nd rev. ed. Rocklin, CA: Prima, 2000.

McGee, C. T. *How to Survive Modern Technology.* Alamo, CA: Ecology Press, 1979.

McGraw, P. *The Ultimate Weight Solution: The 7 Keys to Weight Loss Freedom.* New York: Free Press, 2003.

Menzel, P., and F. D'Aluisio. *Hungry Planet: What the World Eats.* Berkeley, CA: Ten Speed Press, 2005.

Meyerwitz, S. *Juice Fasting and Detoxification.* Great Barrington, MA: Sproutman Productions, 2002.

————. *The Organic Food Guide.* Guilford, CT: Globe Pequot Press, 2004.

Miller, P. *Life Extension Revolution: The New Science of Growing Older without Aging.* New York: Bantam Dell, 2005.

Mowrey, D. B. *The Scientific Validation of Herbal Medicine.* Rev. ed. New York: McGraw-Hill, 1998.

Murray, M., and J. Pizzorno. *Encyclopedia of Natural Medicine.* 2nd rev. ed. New York: Three Rivers Press, 1998.

Murray, M., and J. Pizzorno with Lara Pizzorno. *Encyclopedia of Healing Foods.* New York: Atria, 2005.

Nestle, M. *Food Politics: How the Food Industry Influences Nutrition and Health.* Berkeley, CA: University of California Press, 2002.

Nichols, T., and N. Faass. *Optimal Digestion: A Complete Guide.* Rochester, VT: Healing Arts Press, 2005.

Ornish, D. *Dr. Dean Ornish's Program for Reversing Heart Disease: The Only System Scientifically Proven to Reverse Heart Disease without Drugs or Surgery.* New York: Ivy Books, 1995.

————. *Stress, Diet, and Your Heart.* New York: New American Library, 1984.

Pearson, D., and S. Shaw. *Life Extension.* New York: Warner Books, 1987.

Pennington, J. A., A. D. Bowes, and H. N. Church. *Food Values of Portions Commonly Used.* 17th ed. Hagerstown, MD: Lippincott, Williams, and Wilkins, 1998.

Perlmutter, D., and C. Colman. *The Better Brain Book: The Best Tools for Improving Memory and Sharpness and Preventing Aging of the Brain.* New York: Riverhead Books, 2004.

Pfeiffer, C. C. *Mental and Elemental Nutrients: A Physician's Guide to Nutrition and Health Care.* New Canaan, CT: Keats Publishing, 1976.

Pitchford, P. *Healing with Whole Foods: Oriental Traditions and Modern Nutrition.* Rev. ed. Berkeley, CA: North Atlantic Books, 1993.

Pollan, M. 2002. "This Steer's Life." *New York Times Magazine* Section 6, page 50.

Price, W. *Nutrition and Physical Degeneration: A Comparison of Primitive and Modern Diets and Their Effects.* San Diego: Price-Pottenger Foundation, 1970.

Randolph, T. G., and R. Moss. *An Alternative Approach to Allergies: The New Field of Clinical Ecology Unravels the Environmental Causes of Mental and Physical Ills.* New York: HarperCollins, 1990.

Rapp, D. *Is This Your Child's World?* New York: Bantam Books, 1996.

————. *Our Toxic World: A Wake-Up Call.* Buffalo, NY: Environmental Medical Research Foundation, 2004.

Reuben, D. *Everything You Always Wanted to Know About Nutrition.* New York: Avon Books, 1978.

Robbins, J. *Diet for a New America. How Your Food Choices Affect Your Health, Happiness and the Future of Life on Earth.* Tiburon, CA: H. J. Kramer, 1998.

————. *The Food Revolution: How Your Diet Can Help Save Your Life and Our World.* Boston: Conari Press, 2001.

Roberts, H. J. *Aspartame (Nutrasweet): Is It Safe?* Philadelphia: The Charles Press, 1990.

Robertson, L., C. Flinders, and B. Ruppenthal. *The New Laurel's Kitchen: A Handbook for Vegetarian Cookery and Nutrition.* Berkeley, CA: Ten Speed Press, 1996.

Rogers, S. *Depression Cured at Last.* Sarasota, FL: SK Publishing, 1997.

Rosenbaum, M., and D. Bosco. *Super Fitness Beyond Vitamins: The Bible of Super Supplements.* New York: New American Library, 1987.

Samuels, M., and H. Z. Bennett. *Well Body, Well Earth.* San Francisco: Sierra Club Books, 1983.

Schlosser, E. *Fast Food Nation.* New York: Houghton Mifflin, 2001.

Schwartz, G. R. *In Bad Taste: The MSG Symptom Complex.* Santa Fe: Health Press, 1999.

Scott, D., and P. Byrne. *Seasonal Salads from Around the World.* Pownal, VT: Garden Way Publishing, 1986.

Seelig, M. S., and A. Rosanoff. *The Magnesium Factor.* New York: Avery, 2003.

Shames, Richard L., and Karilee H. Shames. *Feeling Fat, Fuzzy, or Frazzled: A 3-Step Program to Beat Hormone Havoc, Restore Thyroid, Adrenal, and Reproductive Balance, and Feel Better Fast.* New York: Hudson Street Press, 2005.

———. *Thyroid Power: Ten Steps to Total Health.* New York: HarperResource, 2002.

Shomon, M. *Living Well with Chronic Fatigue Syndrome and Fibromyalgia: What Your Doctor Doesn't Tell You . . . That You Need to Know.* New York: HarperResource, 2004.

Shulman, M. S. *Fast Vegetarian Feasts.* New York: Dolphin Books, 1986.

Siegel, B. S. *Love, Medicine, and Miracles.* New York: Perennial Currents, HarperCollins, 1990.

———. *Peace, Love, and Healing.* New York: HarperCollins, 1990.

Smith, Jeffrey M. *Seeds of Deception.* Fairfield, IA: Yes! Books, 2003.

Smith, T. J. *Renewal: The Anti-aging Revolution.* Emmaus, PA: Rodale, 1998.

Smith-Jones, S. *Unleash the Power of NatureFoods.* Orem, UT: Fine Living Books, 2006.

Somer, E., and R. Garrison Jr. *Nutrition Desk Reference.* 3rd ed. New York: McGraw-Hill, 1998.

Strohecker, N., and J. Strohecker, eds. *Natural Healing for Depression: Solutions from the World's Great Health Traditions and Practitioners.* New York: Perigee Books, 1999.

Szekely, E. B., trans. *Essene Gospel of Peace.* Nelson, British Columbia: International Biogenic Society, 1981.

Teitelbaum, J. *From Fatigued to Fantastic: A Proven Program to Regain Vibrant Health, Based on a New Scientific Study Showing Effective Treatment for Chronic Fatigue and Fibromyalgia.* New York: Avery, 2001.

Tierra, M. *Healing with the Herbs of Life.* Berkeley, CA: Crossing Press, 2003.

———. *The Way of Herbs.* Rev. ed. New York: Pocket Books, 1998.

Truss, C. O. *The Missing Diagnosis.* Birmingham, AL: Missing Diagnosis, 1985.

Tucker, E., with B. Enloe. *The Artful Vegan: Fresh Flavors from Millennium Restaurant.* Berkeley, CA: Ten Speed Press, 2003.

Turner, K. *The Self-Healing Cookbook: A Macrobiotic Primer for Healing Body, Mind, and Moods with Whole, Natural Foods.* Grass Valley, CA: Earthtones Press, 1988.

Weil, A. *Eating Well for Optimal Health: The Essential Guide to Food, Diet, and Nutrition.* New York: Knopf, 2000.

———. *Healthy Aging: A Lifelong Guide to Your Physical and Spiritual Well-Being.* New York: Knopf, 2005.

———. *The Healthy Kitchen.* New York: Knopf, 2003.

Wharton, C. *Metabolic Man: Ten Thousand Years from Eden.* Orlando, FL: WinMark Publishing, 2001.

Wigmore, A. *The Hippocrates Diet and Health Program.* Garden City Park, NY: Avery Publishing Group, 1984.

Willcox, B. J., D. Willcox, and M. Suzuki. *The Okinawa Program: How the World's Longest-Lived People Achieve Everlasting Health—And How You Can Too.* New York: Three Rivers Press, 2001.

Wolfe, D. *The Sunfood Diet Success System.* San Diego, CA: Maui Brothers Publishing, 2000.

Young, J. L. *Tropic Cooking.* Berkeley, CA: Ten Speed Press, 1987.

Bibliography

CHAPTER 1: WATER

Aynsley-Green, A. 1985. "Metabolic and Endocrine Interrelations in the Human Fetus and Neonate." *American Journal of Clinical Nutrition* 41 (suppl 2): 399–417.

Bihl, G., and A. Meyers. 2001. "Recurrent Renal Stone Disease—Advances in Pathogenesis and Clinical Management." *Lancet* 358 (9282): 651–56.

Bissenden, J. G., P. H. Scott, S. Milner, S. Doughty, L. Ratnapala, and B. A. Wharton. 1979. "The Biochemistry of Amniotic Fluid with Poor Fetal Growth." *British Journal of Obstetrics and Gynaecology* 86 (7): 540–47.

Brewster, D. 2002. "Dehydration in Acute Gastroenteritis." *Journal of Paediatrics and Child Health* 38 (3): 219–22.

Buddington, R. K. 1994. "Nutrition and Ontogenetic Development of the Intestine." *Canadian Journal of Physiology and Pharmacology* 72 (3): 251–59.

Engel, R. R., and A. H. Smith. 1994. "Arsenic in Drinking Water and Mortality from Vascular Disease: An Ecologic Analysis in Thirty Counties in the United States." *Archives of Environmental Health* 49 (5): 418–27.

Environmental Working Group (EWG). 2002. "Consider the Source: Farm Runoff, Chlorination By-Products, and Human Health." EWG, Washington, D.C.

———. 1997. "Tough to Swallow: How Pesticide Companies Profit from Poisoning America's Tap Water." EWG, Washington, D.C.

———. 1997. "Weedkillers by the Glass Study." EWG, Washington, D.C.

Garrity, M. 2002. "Salmon Migration Report Card." American Rivers, Washington, D.C.

Halden, R. U., A. M. Happel, and S. R. Schoen. 2001. "Evaluation of Standard Methods for the Analysis of Methyl Tert-Butyl Ether and Related Oxygenates in Gasoline-Contaminated Groundwater." *Environmental Science and Technology* 35 (7): 1469–74.

Iggulden, H. 1999. "Dehydration and Electrolyte Disturbance." *Elder Care* 11 (3): 17–22; quiz 23.

King, S. R., W. L. Hickerson, and K. G. Proctor. 1991. "Beneficial Actions of Exogenous Hyaluronic Acid on Wound Healing." *Surgery* 109 (1): 76–84.

Kleiner, S. M. 1999. "Water: An Essential but Overlooked Nutrient." *Journal of the American Dietetic Association* 99 (2): 200–6.

Klurfeld, D. M. 1999. "Nutritional Regulation of Gastrointestinal Growth." *Frontiers in Bioscience* (March 15): D299–D302.

Legge, M., P. S. Benny, A. J. Parker, and D. R. Aickin. 1984. "Amniotic Fluid Endocrine Changes during Maternal Hyperalimentation." *JPEN. Journal of Parenteral and Enteral Nutrition* 8 (4): 433–37.

Lucas, A., S. R. Bloom, and A. A. Green. 1985. "Gastrointestinal Peptides and the Adaptation to Extrauterine Nutrition." *Canadian Journal of Physiology and Pharmacology* 63 (5): 527–37.

Magee, M. F., and B. A. Bhatt. 2001. "Management of Decompensated Diabetes: Diabetic Ketoacidosis and Hyperglycemic Hyperosmolar Syndrome." *Critical Care Clinics* 17 (1): 75–106.

"Magnesium in Drinking Water and Death from Acute Myocardial Infarction." 1996. *American Journal of Epidemiology* 143 (5): 456–62.

Meier, J. R. 1988. "Genotoxic Activity of Organic Chemicals in Drinking Water." *Mutation Research* 196: 211–46.

Meyer, L. J., and R. Stern. 1994. "Age-Dependent Changes of Hyaluronan in Human Skin." *Journal of Investigative Dermatology* 102 (3): 385–89.

Miller, A. L. 2001. "The Etiologies, Pathophysiology, and Alternative/Complementary Treatment of Asthma." *Alternative Medicine Review* 6 (1): 20–47.

Millette, J. R., P. J. Clark, J. Stober, and others. 1983. "Asbestos in Water Supplies of the United States." *Environmental Health Perspectives* 53: 45–48.

Parfit, M. 1993. "Sharing the Wealth of Water." *National Geographic* (November): 20–88.

Powledge, F. 1982. *Water: The Nature, Uses, and Future of Our Most Precious and Abused Resource.* New York: Farrar, Straus, and Giroux.

Rubenowitz, E., G. Axelsson, and R. Rylander. 1999. "Magnesium and Calcium in Drinking Water and Death from Acute Myocardial Infarction in Women." *Epidemiology* 10 (1): 31–36.

Rubenowitz, E., I. Molin, G. Axelsson, and R. Rylander. 2000. "Magnesium in Drinking Water in Relation to Morbidity and Mortality from Acute Myocardial Infarction." *Epidemiology* 11 (4): 416–21.

Rylander, R. 1996. "Environmental Magnesium Deficiency as a Cardiovascular Risk Factor." *Journal of Cardiovascular Risk* 3 (1): 4–10.

Rylander, R., H. Bonevik, and E. Rubenowitz. 1991. "Magnesium and Calcium in Drinking Water and Cardiovascular Mortality." *Scandinavian Journal of Work, Environment, and Health* 17 (2): 91–94.

Shaffer, M. 1998. "Waste Lands: The Threat of Toxic Fertilizer." California Public Interest Group Charitable Trust, San Francisco. Article available online at www.calpirg.org.

Sheehy, C. M., P. A. Perry, and S. L. Cromwell. 1999. "Dehydration: Biological Considerations, Age-Related Changes, and Risk Factors in Older Adults." *Biological Research for Nursing* 1 (1): 30–37.

Smith, A. H., C. Hopenhayn-Rich, M. N. Bates, and others. 1992. "Cancer Risks from Arsenic in Drinking Water." *Environmental Health Perspectives* 97: 259–67.

Suffet, I. 1999. "Sorption for Removing Methyl Tertiary Butyl Ether from Drinking Water." *Proceedings of the Annual Conference of the American Water Works Association.* Denver, Colorado: AWWA, 319–36.

Sullivan, A. 1999. "Hydration for Adults." *Nursing Standard* 14 (8): 44–46.

Svensjo, T., B. Pomahac, F. Yao, J. Slama, and E. Eriksson. 2000. "Accelerated Healing of Full-Thickness Skin Wounds in a Wet Environment." *Plastic and Reconstructive Surgery* 106 (3): 602–12; discussion 613–44.

Taylor, H. R. 1999. "Epidemiology of Age-Related Cataract." *Eye* (June 13, part 3b): 445–48.

U.S. Environmental Protection Agency (EPA). 2000. *Estimated Per Capita Water Ingestion in the United States.* Office of Water, EPA 822–R–00–008. Washington, D.C.: Government Printing Office.

———. 1998. *National Water Quality Inventory: 1998 Report to Congress.* EPA 841-R-00-001. Washington, D.C.: Government Printing Office.

Volkman, J. 1997. "A River in Common: The Columbia River, the Salmon Ecosystem, and Water Policy." Report to the Western Water Policy Review Advisory Commission. Washington, D.C.

Western Water Policy Review Commission. 1998. *Water in the West: Challenge for the Next Century.* U.S. Department of the Interior. Washington, D.C: Government Printing Office.

Wirthlin Worldwide. 2002. "February National Quorum Findings." Wirthlin Worldwide, New York.

CHAPTER 2: CARBOHYDRATES

Annison, G., and D. L. Topping. 1994. "Nutritional Role of Resistant Starch: Chemical Structure versus Physiological Function." *Annual Review of Nutrition* 14: 297–320.

Asp, N. G. 1997. "Resistant Starch: An Update on Its Physiological Effects." *Advanced Experimental Medical Biology* 427: 201–10.

Behall, K. M., and J. C. Howe. 1995. "Contribution of Fiber and Resistant Starch to Metabolizable Energy." *American Journal of Clinical Nutrition* 62 (suppl 5): 1158S–1160S.

Bornet, F. R., and F. Brouns. 2002. "Immune-Stimulating and Gut Health–Promoting Properties of Short-Chain Fructo-Oligosaccharides." *Nutrition Review* 60: 326–34.

Brown, I. 1996. "Complex Carbohydrates and Resistant Starch." *Nutrition Review* 54 (11 part 2): S115–S119.

Buddington, R. K., K. Kelly-Quagliana, K. K. Buddington, and others. 2002. "Non-Digestible Oligosaccharides and Defense Functions: Lessons Learned from Animal Models." *British Journal of Nutrition* 87 (suppl 2): S231–S239.

Carson, L, and V. M. Doctor. 1990. "Mechanism of Potentiation of Antithrombin III and Heparin Cofactor II Inhibition by Sulfated Xylans." *Thrombosis Research* 58: 367–81.

Coulston, A. M. 1999. "The Role of Dietary Fats in Plant-Based Diets." *American Journal of Clinical Nutrition* 70: 512S–515S.

Dai, D., N. N. Nanthkumar, D. S. Newburg, and others. 2000. "Role of Oligosaccharides and Glycoconjugates in Intestinal Host Defense." *Journal of Pediatric Gastroenterology and Nutrition* 30 (suppl 2): S23–S33.

Delves, P. J. 1998. "The Role of Glycosylation in Autoimmune Disease." *Autoimmunity* 27 (4): 239–53.

Duncan, C. J., N. Pugh, D. S. Pasco, and S. A. Ross. 2002. "Isolation of a Galactomannan That Enhances Macrophage Activation from the Edible Fungus Morchella Esculenta." *Journal of Agriculture Food Chemistry* 50: 5683–85.

Dykman, K. D., and R. McKinley. 1998. "The Effects of Glyconutritional Supplementation on Autistic Children." *Proceedings of the Annual Meeting of the Pavlovian Society.* Düsseldorf, Germany, October 30–November 1.

Ebringerova, A., A. Kardosova, Z. Hromadkova, A. Malovikova, and V. Hribalova. 2002. "Immunomodulatory Activity of Acidic Xylans in Relation to Their Structural and Molecular Properties." *International Journal of Biological Macromolecules* 30: 1–6.

Englyst, H. N., and J. H. Cummings. 1990. "Non-Starch Polysaccharides (Dietary Fiber) and Resistant Starch." *Advances in Experimental Medicine and Biology* 270: 205–25.

Fernandez-Real, J. M., and W. Ricart. 1999. "Insulin Resistance and Inflammation in an Evolutionary Perspective: The Contribution of Cytokine Genotype/Phenotype to Thriftiness." *Diabetologia* 42: 1367–74.

Fischer, K., P. C. Colombani, W. Langhans, and C. Wenk. 2002. "Carbohydrate to Protein Ratio in Food and Cognitive Performance in the Morning." *Physiology and Behavior* 75 (3): 411–23.

Franz, G. 1989. "Polysaccharides in Pharmacy: Current Applications and Future Concepts." *Planta Medicine* 55 (6): 493–97.

Gallaher, D. D., C. M. Gallaher, G. J. Mahrt, and others. 2002. "A Glucomannan and Chitosan Fiber Supplement Decreases Plasma Cholesterol and Increases Cholesterol Excretion in Overweight Normocholesterolemic Humans." *Journal of the American College of Nutrition* 21: 428–33.

Gordon, M., B. Bihari, E. Goosby, R. Gorter, and others. 1998. "A Placebo-Controlled Trial of the Immune Modulator, Lentinan, in HIV-Positive Patients: A Phase I/II Trial." *Journal of Medicine* 29 (5–6): 305–30.

Hamano, K., H. Gohra, T. Katoh, and others. 1999. "The Preoperative Administration of Lentinan Ameliorated the Impairment of Natural Killer Activity after Cardiopulmonary Bypass." *International Journal of Immunopharmacology* 21 (8): 531–40.

Hissin, P. J., E. Karnieli, I. A. Simpson, L. B. Salans, and S. W. Cushman. 1982. "A Possible Mechanism of Insulin Resistance in the Rat Adipose Cell with High-Fat/Low-Carbohydrate Feeding: Depletion of Intracellular Glucose Transport Systems." *Diabetes* 31 (7): 589–92.

Institute of Medicine. 2002. *Dietary Reference Intakes for Energy, Carbohydrate, Fiber, Fat, Fatty Acids, Cholesterol, Protein, and Amino Acids (Macronutrients).* Washington, D.C: National Academy of Sciences, National Academy Press.

Jacobasch, G., D. Schmiedl, M. Kruschewski, and K. Schmehl. 1999. "Dietary Resistant Starch and Chronic Inflammatory Bowel Diseases." *International Journal of Colorectal Disease* 14 (4–5): 201–11.

Kagawa, R., N. Nakayama, T. Yamaguchi, and others. 2002. "Postoperative Adjuvant Immunochemotherapy Using Lentinan for Advanced Gastric Carcinoma Patients with Metastasis in the Regional Lymph Nodes and Serosal Invasion." *Gan to Kagaku Ryoho* (Tokyo) 29 (11): 1989–94.

Kaltner, H., and B. Stierstorfer. 1998. "Animal Lectins as Cell Adhesion Molecules." *Acta Anatomica* (Basel) 161 (1–4): 162–79.

Kiho, T., S. Itahashi, M. Sakushima, and others. 1997. "Polysaccharides in Fungi. XXXVIII. Anti-diabetic Activity and Structural Feature of a Galactomannan Elaborated by Pestalotiopsis Species." *Biological and Pharmaceutical Bulletin* 20: 118–21.

Kim, S. H., J. Mauron, R. Gleason, and R. Wurtman. 1991. "Selection of Carbohydrate to Protein Ratio and Correlations with Weight Gain and Body Fat in Rats Allowed Three Dietary Choices." *International Journal for Vitamin and Nutrition Research* 61 (2): 166–79.

Komiyama, N., T. Kaneko, A. Sato, and others. 2002. "The Effect of High Carbohydrate Diet on Glucose Tolerance in Patients with Type 2 Diabetes Mellitus." *Diabetes Research and Clinical Practice* 57: 163–70.

Kritchevsky, D. 1995. "Epidemiology of Fibre-Resistant Starch and Colorectal Cancer." *European Journal of Cancer Prevention* 4 (5): 345–52.

Liu, F., V. E. Ooi, and S. T. Chang. 1997. "Free Radical Scavenging Activities of Mushroom Polysaccharide Extracts." *Life Science* 60 (10): 763–71.

Luettig, B., C. Steinmuller, G. E. Gifford, and others. 1989. "Macrophage Activation by the Polysaccharide Arabinogalactan Isolated from Plant Cell Cultures of *Echinacea purpurea*." *Journal of the National Cancer Institute* 81 (9): 669–75.

Matsuoka, H., Y. Seo, H. Wakasugi, T. Saito, and others. 1997. "Lentinan Potentiates Immunity and Prolongs the Survival Time of Some Patients." *Anticancer Research* 17 (4A): 2751–55.

McCarty, M. F. 2002. "Glucomannan Minimizes the Postprandial Insulin Surge: A Potential Adjuvant for Hepatothermic Therapy." *Medical Hypotheses* 58: 487–90.

Muzzarelli, R. A. 1997. "Human Enzymatic Activities Related to the Therapeutic Administration of Chitin Derivatives." *Cellular and Molecular Life Sciences* 53 (2): 131–40.

Ng, M. L., and A. T. Yap. 2002. "Inhibition of Human Colon Carcinoma Development by Lentinan from Shiitake Mushrooms *(Lentinus edodes)*." *Journal of Alternative and Complementary Medicine* 8 (5): 581–89.

Nunes, F. M., and M. A. Coimbra. 2002. "Chemical Characterization of Galactomannans and Arabinogalactans from Two Arabica Coffee Infusions as Affected by the Degree of Roast." *Journal of Agricultural and Food Chemistry* 50: 1429–34.

Pomeranz, Y. 1992. "Research and Development Regarding Enzyme-Resistant Starch (RS) in the USA: A Review." *European Journal of Clinical Nutrition* 46 (suppl 2): S63–S68.

Reaven, G. M. 1995. "The Pathophysiology of Insulin Resistance in Human Disease." *Physiology Reviews* 75 (3): 473–86.

Riccardi, G., and A. A. Rivellese. 2000. "Dietary Treatment of the Metabolic Syndrome: The Optimal Diet." *British Journal of Nutrition* 83 (suppl 1): S143–S148.

Roberfroid, M., and J. Slavin. 2000. "Nondigestible Oligosaccharides." *Critical Reviews in Food Science and Nutrition* 40: 461–80.

Robertson, M. D., R. A. Henderson, G. E. Vist, and R. D. Rumsey. 2002. "Extended Effects of Evening Meal Carbohydrate-to-Fat Ratio on Fasting and Postprandial Substrate Metabolism." *American Journal of Clinical Nutrition* 75: 505–10.

Roche, H. M. 1999. "Dietary Carbohydrates and Triacylglycerol Metabolism." *Proceedings of the Nutrition Society (London)* 58: 201–7.

See, D. M, P. Cimoch, S. Chou, and others. 1998. "The In Vitro Immunomodulatory Effects of Glyconutrients on Peripheral Blood Mononuclear Cells of Patients with Chronic Fatigue Syndrome." *Integrated Physiological and Behavioral Science* 33 (3): 280–87.

Sievenpiper, J. L., A. L. Jenkins, D. L. Whitham, and V. Vuksan. 2002. "Insulin Resistance: Concepts, Controversies, and the Role of Nutrition." *Canadian Journal of Diet and Practical Research* 63: 20–32.

Stern, J. S., P. R. Johnson, B. R. Batchelor, L. M. Zucker, and J. Hirsch. 1975. "Pancreatic Insulin Release and Peripheral Tissue Resistance in Zucker Obese Rats Fed High- and Low-Carbohydrate Diets." *American Journal of Physiology* 228 (2): 543–48.

Tahiri, M., P. Pellerin, J. C. Tressol, and others. 2000. "The Rhamnogalacturonan-II Dimer Decreases Intestinal Absorption and Tissue Accumulation of Lead in Rats." *Journal of Nutrition* 130: 249–53.

Tomoda, M., K. Hirabayashi, N. Shimizu, R. Gonda, N. Ohara, and K. Takada. 1993. "Characterization of Two Novel Polysaccharides Having Immunological Activities from the Root of Panax Ginseng." *Biological and Pharmaceutical Bulletin* 16: 1087–90.

Topping, D. L., and P. M. Clifton. 2001. "Short-Chain Fatty Acids and Human Colonic Function: Roles of Resistant Starch and Nonstarch Polysaccharides." *Physiological Reviews* 81 (3): 1031–64.

Vandenplas, Y. 2002. "Oligosaccharides in Infant Formula." *British Journal of Nutrition* 87 (suppl 2): S293–S296.

Wolever, T. M. 2000. "Dietary Carbohydrates and Insulin Action in Humans." *British Journal of Nutrition* 83 (suppl 1): S97–S102.

———. 1990. "The Glycemic Index." *World Review of Nutrition and Dietetics* 62: 120–85.

Wolever, T. M., and C. Mehling. 2002. "High-Carbohydrate-Low-Glycaemic Index Dietary Advice Improves Glucose Disposition Index in Subjects with Impaired Glucose Tolerance." *British Journal of Nutrition* 87: 477–87.

Wong, C. K., K. N. Leung, K. P. Fung, and others. 1994. "Immunomodulatory and Anti-tumour Polysaccharides from Medicinal Plants." *Journal of International Medical Research* 22 (6): 299–312.

Yamafuji, K., M. Iio, and M. Eto. 1970. "Interaction of Deoxyribonucleic Acid with Xylans Having Antitumor Activity." *Zeitschrift fur Krebsforschung* (Berlin) 75: 55–58.

CHAPTER 3: PROTEINS

Adibi, S. A. 1989. "Glycyl-dipeptides: New Substrates for Protein Nutrition." *The Journal of Laboratory and Clinical Medicine* 113: 665–73.

Bachert, C. 2002. "The Role of Histamine in Allergic Disease: Re-appraisal of Its Inflammatory Potential." *Allergy* 57: 287–96.

Bassit, R. A., L. A. Sawada, R. F. Bacurau, and others. 2002. "Branched-Chain Amino Acid Supplementation and the Immune Response of Long-Distance Athletes." *Nutrition* 18: 376–79.

Bergstrom, J., P. Furst, and E. Vinnars. 1990. "Effect of a Test Meal, without and with Protein, on Muscle and Plasma Free Amino Acids." *Clinical Science* (London) 79: 331–37.

Bonfanti, L., P. Peretto, S. De Marchis, and A. Fasolo. 1999. "Carnosine-Related Dipeptides in the Mammalian Brain." *Progress in Neurobiology* 59: 333–53.

Boucharlat, J., C. Salomon, A. Maitre, J. Pelat, and R. Wolf. 1972. "Clinical Trial of Arginine Aspartate in Secondary Sexual Impotence." *Annales Medico-Psychologiques* (Paris) 1: 394–400.

Deplancke, B., and H. R. Gaskins. 2002. "Redox Control of the Transsulfuration and Glutathione Biosynthesis Pathways." *Current Opinion in Clinical Nutrition and Metabolic Care* 5: 85–92.

Dickinson, D. A, and H. J. Forman. 2002. "Cellular Glutathione and Thiols Metabolism." *Biochemical and Pharmacology* 64: 1019–26.

Filomeni, G., G. Rotilio, and M. R. Ciriolo. 2002. "Cell Signalling and the Glutathione Redox System." *Biochemical Pharmacology* 64: 1057–64.

Food and Agriculture Organization of the United Nations. 1970. *The Amino Acid Content of Foods and Biological Data on Proteins.* Nutritional Study No. 24. Lanham, Maryland: UNIPUB.

Frenhani, P. B., and R. C. Burini. 1999. "Mechanisms of Absorption of Amino Acids and Oligopeptides: Control and Implications in Human Diet Therapy." *Arquivos de Gastroenterologia* (Sao Paulo) 36: 227–37.

Furst, P., K. Pogan, and P. Stehle. 1997. "Glutamine Dipeptides in Clinical Nutrition." *Nutrition* 13: 731–37.

Graz, M., A. Hunt, H. Jamie, G. Grant, and P. Milne. 1999. "Antimicrobial Activity of Selected Cyclic Dipeptides." *Pharmazie* (Berlin) 54: 772–75.

Hanretta, A. T., and J. B. Lombardini. 1987. "Is Taurine a Hypothalamic Neurotransmitter? A Model of the Differential Uptake and Compartmentalization of Taurine by Neuronal and Glial Cell Particles from the Rat Hypothalamus." *Brain Research* 434: 167–201.

Hiroshige, K., T. Sonta, T. Suda, K. Kanegae, and A. Ohtani. 2001. "Oral Supplementation of Branched-Chain Amino Acid Improves Nutritional Status in Elderly Patients on Chronic Haemodialysis." *Nephrology, Dialysis, Transplantation* 16: 1856–62.

Hurson, M., M. C. Regan, S. I. Kirk, and others. 1995. "Maintenance Nitrogen Requirement and Obligatory Nitrogen Losses." *Journal of Nutrition* 110: 1727–35.

Institute of Medicine. 2002. *Dietary Reference Intakes for Energy, Carbohydrate, Fiber, Fat, Fatty Acids, Cholesterol, Protein, and Amino Acids (Macronutrients).* Washington, D.C.: National Academy of Sciences, National Academy Press.

Jackson, A. A. 1983. "Amino Acids: Essential and Nonessential." *Lancet* 1: 1034–37.

Jacobs, E. H., A. Yamatodani, and H. Timmerman. 2000. "Is Histamine the Final Neurotransmitter in the Entrainment of Circadian Rhythms in Mammals?" *Trends in Pharmacological Science* 21: 293–98.

Kao, W. J., and Y. Liu. 2001. "Utilizing Biomimetic Oligopeptides to Probe Fibronectin-Integrin Binding and Signaling in Regulating Macrophage Function In Vitro and In Vivo." *Frontiers in Bioscience* 6: D992–D999.

Klumpp, S., and J. Krieglstein. 2002. "Serine/Threonine Protein Phosphatases in Apoptosis." *Current Opinion in Pharmacology* 2: 458–62.

Leuzzi, V., D. Fois, C. Carducci, I. Antonozzi, and G. Trasimeni. 1997. "Neuropsychological and Neuroradiological (MRI) Variations during Phenylalanine Load: Protective Effect of Valine, Leucine, and Isoleucine Supplementation." *Journal of Child Neurology* 12: 338–40.

Lu, K. P., Y. C. Liou, and X. Z. Zhou. 2002. "Pinning Down Proline-Directed Phosphorylation Signaling." *Trends in Cell Biology* 12: 164–72.

Luo, J. H., and L. Aurelian. 1992. "The Transmembrane Helical Segment but Not the Invariant Lysine Is Required for the Kinase Activity of the Large Subunit of Herpes Simplex Virus Type 2 Ribonucleotide Reductase (ICP10)." *Journal of Biological Chemistry* 267: 9645–53.

Murai, S., H. Saito, E. Abe, Y. Masuda, and T. Itoh. 1992. "A Rapid Assay for Neurotransmitter Amino Acids, Aspartate, Glutamate, Glycine, Taurine and Gamma-aminobutyric Acid in the Brain by High-Performance Liquid Chromatography with Electrochemical Detection." *Journal of Neural Transmission. General Section* 87: 145–53.

Nishimura, M., M. Yoshimura, and H. Takahashi. 2000. "Role of Brain L-Arginine in Central Regulation of Blood Pressure." *Nippon Rinsho. Japanese Journal of Clincal Medicine* (Osaka) 58 (suppl 1): 41–45.

Novaes, M. R., and L. A. Lima. 1999. "Effects of Dietetic Supplementation with L-arginine in Cancer Patients: A Review of the Literature." *Archivos Latinoamericanos de Nutricion* (Caracas) 49: 301–8.

Ohtani, M., K. Maruyama, M. Sugita, and K. Kobayashi. 2001. "Amino Acid Supplementation Affects Hematological and Biochemical Parameters in Elite Rugby Players." *Bioscience, Biotechnology, Biochemistry* 65: 1970–76.

Ohtawa, K., T. Ueno, K. Mitsui, and others. 1998. "Apoptosis of Leukemia Cells Induced by Valine-Deficient Medium." *Leukemia* 12: 1651–52.

Olney, J. W. 2003. "Excitotoxicity, Apoptosis and Neuropsychiatric Disorders." *Current Opinion in Pharmacology* 3: 101–9.

———. 1994. "Excitotoxins in Foods." *Neurotoxicology* 15: 535–44.

Otvos, L., Jr. 2002. "The Short Proline-Rich Antibacterial Peptide Family." *Cellular and Molecular Life Science* 59: 1138–50.

Paolicchi, A., S. Dominici, L. Pieri, E. Maellaro, and A. Pompella. 2002. "Glutathione Catabolism as a Signaling Mechanism." *Biochemical Pharmacology* 64: 1027–35.

Parise, G., and K. E. Yarasheski. 2000. "The Utility of Resistance Exercise Training and Amino Acid Supplementation for Reversing Age-Associated Decrements in Muscle Protein Mass and Function." *Current Opinion in Clinical Nutrition and Metabolic Care* 3: 489–95.

Peters, H., W. A. Border, and N. A. Noble. 1999. "From Rats to Man: A Perspective on Dietary L-arginine Supplementation in Human Renal Disease." *Nephrology, Dialysis, Transplantation* 14: 1640–50.

Prasad, C. 1995. "Bioactive Cyclic Dipeptides." *Peptides* 16: 151–64.

Preli, R. B., K. P. Klein, and D. M. Herrington. 2002. "Vascular Effects of Dietary L-Arginine Supplementation." *Atherosclerosis* 162: 1–15.

Repka-Ramirez, M. S., and J. N. Baraniuk. 2002. "Histamine in Health and Disease." *Clinical Allergy and Immunology* 17: 1–25.

Schousboe, A., C. L. Apreza, H. Pasantes-Morales. 1992. "GABA and Taurine Serve as Respectively a Neurotransmitter and an Osmolyte in Cultured Cerebral Cortical Neurons." *Advances in Experimental Medicine and Biology* 315: 391–97.

Shukla, A., A. M. Rasik, and G. K. Patnaik. 1997. "Depletion of Reduced Glutathione, Ascorbic Acid, Vitamin E, and Antioxidant Defence Enzymes in a Healing Cutaneous Wound." *Free Radical Research* 26: 93–101.

Singh, R. J. 2002. "Glutathione: A Marker and Antioxidant for Aging." *Journal of Laboratory and Clinical Medicine* 140: 380–81.

Skolnick, P., R. T. Layer, P. Popik, G. Nowak, I. A. Paul, and R. Trullas. 1996. "Adaptation of N-methyl-D-aspartate (NMDA) Receptors Following Antidepressant Treatment: Implications for the Pharmacotherapy of Depression." *Pharmacopsychiatry* 29: 23–26.

Snyder, S. H., and P. M. Kim. 2000. "D-amino Acids as Putative Neurotransmitters: Focus on D-serine." *Neurochemical Research* 25: 553–60.

Sochman, J., J. Vrbska, B. Musilova, and others. 1996. "Infarct Size Limitation: Acute N-acetylcysteine Defense (ISLAND Trial): Preliminary Analysis and Report after the First Thirty Patients." *Clinical Cardiology* 19: 94–100.

Taniguchi, K., T. Nonami, A. Nakao, and others. 1996. "The Valine Catabolic Pathway in Human Liver: Effect of Cirrhosis on Enzyme Activities." *Hepatology* 24: 1395–98.

Tomblin, F. A., Jr., and K. H. Lucas. 2001. "Lysine for Management of Herpes Labialis." *American Journal of Health-System Pharmacy* 58: 298–300, 304.

Valencia, E., and G. Hardy. 2002. "Practicalities of Glutathione Supplementation in Nutritional Support." *Current Opinion in Clinical Nutrition and Metabolic Care* 5: 321–26.

Wolosker, H., R. Panizzutti, and J. De Miranda. 2002. "Neurobiology through the Looking-Glass: D-serine as a New Glial-Derived Transmitter." *Neurochemistry International* 41: 327–32.

Young, V. R., and P. L. Pellett. 1994. "Plant Proteins in Relation to Human Protein and Amino Acid Nutrition." *American Journal of Clinical Nutrition* 59 (suppl 5): 1203S–1212S.

Zubay, G. 1993. *Biochemistry.* Third edition. Dubuque, Iowa: William C. Brown, 90–97.

Zwingmann, C., C. Richter-Landsberg, A. Brand, and D. Leibfritz. 2000. "NMR Spectroscopic Study on the Metabolic Fate of [3-(13)C]alanine in Astrocytes, Neurons, and Cocultures: Implications for Glia-Neuron Interactions in Neurotransmitter Metabolism. *Glia* 32: 286–303.

CHAPTER 4: LIPIDS

Andrioli, G., A. Carletto, P. Guarini, and others. 1999. "Differential Effects of Dietary Supplementation with Fish Oil or Soy Lecithin on Human Platelet Adhesion." *Thrombosis and Haemostasis* 82: 1522–27.

Ascherio, A., and W. C. Willett. 1997. "Health Effects of Trans Fatty Acids." *American Journal of Clinical Nutrition* 66: 1006S–1010S.

Benton, D., R. T. Donohoe, B. Sillance, and S. Nabb. 2001. "The Influence of Phosphatidylserine Supplementation on Mood and Heart Rate When Faced with an Acute Stressor." *Nutritional Neuroscience* 4: 169–78.

Buchman, A. L., M. Awal, D. Jenden, M. Roch, and S. H. Kang. 2000. "The Effect of Lecithin Supplementation on Plasma Choline Concentrations during a Marathon." *Journal of the American College of Nutrition* 19: 768–70.

Calder, P. C., P. Yaqoob, F. Thies, F. A. Wallace, and E. A. Miles. 2002. "Fatty Acids and Lymphocyte Functions." *British Journal of Nutrition* 87 (suppl 1): S31–S48.

Craig-Schmidt, M. C. 2001. "Isomeric Fatty Acids: Evaluating Status and Implications for Maternal and Child Health." *Lipids* 36: 997–1006.

Denke, M. A. 1994. "Role of Beef and Beef Tallow, an Enriched Source of Stearic Acid, in a Cholesterol-Lowering Diet." *American Journal of Clinical Nutrition* 60 (suppl 6): 1044S–1049S.

Fickova, M., P. Hubert, G. Cremel, and C. Leray. 1998. "Dietary (n-3) and (n-6) Polyunsaturated Fatty Acids Rapidly Modify Fatty Acid Composition and Insulin Effects in Rat Adipocytes." *Journal of Nutrition* 128: 512–19.

Gauvreau, G. M., R. M. Watson, and P. M. O'Byrne. 1999. "Protective Effects of Inhaled PGE2 on Allergen-Induced Airway Responses and Airway Inflammation." *American Journal of Respiratory and Critical Care Medicine* 159: 31–36.

Gorski, J., A. Dobrzyn, and M. Zendzian-Piotrowska. 2002. "The Sphingomyelin-Signaling Pathway in Skeletal Muscles and Its Role in Regulation of Glucose Uptake." *Annals of the New York Academy of Sciences* 967: 236–48.

Grundy, S. M. 1994. "Influence of Stearic Acid on Cholesterol Metabolism Relative to Other Long-Chain Fatty Acids." *American Journal of Clinical Nutrition* 60 (suppl 6): 986S–990S.

Grundy, S. M., N. Abate, and M. Chandalia. 2002. "Diet Composition and the Metabolic Syndrome: What Is the Optimal Fat Intake?" *American Journal of Medicine* 113 (suppl 9B): 25S–29S.

Grundy, S. M., and M. A. Denke. 1990. "Dietary Influences on Serum Lipids and Lipoproteins." *Journal of Lipid Research* 31: 1149–72.

Hartner, A., A. Pahl, K. Brune, and M. Goppelt-Struebe. 2000. "Upregulation of Cyclooxygenase-1 and the PGE2 Receptor EP2 in Rat and Human Mesangioproliferative Glomerulonephritis." *Inflammation Research* 49: 345–54.

Holm, T., A. K. Andreassen, P. Aukrust, and others. 2001. "Omega-3 Fatty Acids Improve Blood Pressure Control and Preserve Renal Function in Hypertensive Heart Transplant Recipients." *European Heart Journal* (London) 22: 428–36.

Jorissen, B. L., F. Brouns, M. P. Van Boxtel, and W. J. Riedel. 2002. "Safety of Soy-Derived Phosphatidylserine in Elderly People." *Nutritional Neuroscience* 5: 337–43.

Khosla, P., and K. Sundram. 1996. "Effects of Dietary Fatty Acid Composition on Plasma Cholesterol." *Progress in Lipid Research* 35: 93–132.

Kim, H.Y., and J. Hamilton. 2000. "Accumulation of Docosahexaenoic Acid in Phosphatidylserine Is Selectively Inhibited by Chronic Ethanol Exposure in C-6 Glioma Cells." *Lipids* 35: 187–95.

Kolesnick, R. 2002. "The Therapeutic Potential of Modulating the Ceramide/Sphingomyelin Pathway." *Journal of the Clinical Investigator* 110: 3–8.

Kris-Etherton, P. M., and S. Yu. 1997. "Individual Fatty Acid Effects on Plasma Lipids and Lipoproteins: Human Studies." *American Journal of Clinical Nutrition* 65 (suppl 5): 1628S–1644S.

Kritchevsky, D. 1994. "Stearic Acid Metabolism and Atherogenesis: History." *American Journal of Clinical Nutrition* 60 (suppl 6): 997S–1001S.

Kumar, R., H. M. Divekar, V. Gupta, and K. K. Srivastava. 2002. "Antistress and Adaptogenic Activity of Lecithin Supplementation." *Journal of Alternnative and Complementary Medicine* 8: 487–92.

Li, D., A. Ng, N. J. Mann, and A. J. Sinclair. 1998. "Contribution of Meat Fat to Dietary Arachidonic Acid. *Lipids* 33: 437–40.

Meydani, M. 2000. "Omega-3 Fatty Acids Alter Soluble Markers of Endothelial Function in Coronary Heart Disease Patients. *Nutrition Review* 58: 56–59.

Mori, T. A., D. Q. Bao, V. Burke, I. B. Puddey, G. F. Watts, and L. J. Beilin. 1999. "Dietary Fish as a Major Component of a Weight-Loss Diet: Effect on Serum Lipids, Glucose, and Insulin Metabolism in Overweight Hypertensive Subjects." *American Journal of Clinical Nutrition* 70: 817–25.

Parodi, P. W. 1997. "Cows' Milk Fat Components as Potential Anticarcinogenic Agents." *Journal of Nutrition* 127: 1055–60.

Pamplona, R., M. Portero-Otin, C. Ruiz, and others. 2000. "Double Bond Content of Phospholipids and Lipid Peroxidation Negatively Correlate with Maximum Longevity in the Heart of Mammals." *Mechanisms in Ageing and Development* 112 (3): 169–83.

Rivellese, A. A., A. Maffettone, C. Iovine, and others. 1996 "Long-Term Effects of Fish Oil on Insulin Resistance and Plasma Lipoproteins in NIDDM Patients with Hypertriglyceridemia." *Diabetes Care* 19: 1207–13.

Severus, W. E., A. B. Littman, and A. L. Stoll. 2001. "Omega-3 Fatty Acids, Homocysteine, and the Increased Risk of Cardiovascular Mortality in Major Depressive Disorder." *Harvard Review of Psychiatry* 9: 280–93.

Simopoulos, A. P. 2001. "N-3 Fatty Acids and Human Health: Defining Strategies for Public Policy." *Lipids* 36 (suppl): S83–S89.

———. 1997. "Omega-6/Omega-3 Fatty Acid Ratio and Trans Fatty Acids in Non-insulin-dependent Diabetes Mellitus." *Annals of the New York Academy of Sciences* 827: 327–38.

———. 1996. "The Role of Fatty Acids in Gene Expression: Health Implications." *Annals of Nutrition and Metabolism* 40: 303–11.

———. 1990. "Omega-3 Fatty Acids in Health and Disease." *Progress in Clinical and Biological Research* 326: 129–56.

Simopoulos, A. P., A. Leaf, and N. Salem Jr. 1999. "Workshop on the Essentiality of and Recommended Dietary Intakes for Omega-6 and Omega-3 Fatty Acids." *Journal of the American College of Nutrition* 18: 487–89.

Stoll, B. A. 1998. "Essential Fatty Acids, Insulin Resistance, and Breast Cancer Risk." *Nutrition and Cancer* 31: 72–77.

Taber, L., C. H. Chiu, and J. Whelan. 1998. "Assessment of the Arachidonic Acid Content in Foods Commonly Consumed in the American Diet." *Lipids* 33: 1151–57.

Tanaka, T., K. Kouda, M. Kotani, and others. 2001. "Vegetarian Diet Ameliorates Symptoms of Atopic Dermatitis through Reduction of the Number of Peripheral Eosinophils and of PGE2 Synthesis by Monocytes." *Journal of Physiological Anthropology and Applied Human Science* 20: 353–61.

Valenzuela, A., and N. Morgado. 1999. "Trans Fatty Acid Isomers in Human Health and in the Food Industry." *Biological Research* 32: 273–87.

Watkins, B. A., Y. Li, H. E. Lippman, and M. F. Seifert. 2001. "Omega-3 Polyunsaturated Fatty Acids and Skeletal Health." *Experimental Biology and Medicine* 226: 485–97.

Wilson, T. A., C. M. Meservey, and R. J. Nicolosi. 1998. "Soy Lecithin Reduces Plasma Lipoprotein Cholesterol and Early Atherogenesis in Hypercholesterolemic Monkeys and Hamsters: Beyond Linoleate." *Atherosclerosis* 140: 147–53.

Wilson, T. A., M. McIntyre, and R. J. Nicolosi. 2001. "Trans Fatty Acids and Cardiovascular Risk." *Journal of Nutrition, Health, and Aging* 5: 184–87.

Yamaji-Hasegawa, A., and T. Kobayashi. 2002. "Proteins Which Recognize Sphingomyelin." *Tanpakushitsu Kakusan Koso. Protein, Nucleic Acid, Enzyme* (Tokyo) 47: 519–25.

Yamashita, S. 1993. "Studies on Changes of Colonic Mucosal PGE2 Levels and Tissue Localization in Experimental Colitis." *Gastroenterologia Japonica* (Tokyo) 28: 224–35.

Yanagi, S., M. Yamashita, and S. Imai. 1993. "Sodium Butyrate Inhibits the Enhancing Effect of High Fat Diet on Mammary Tumorigenesis." *Oncology* 50: 201–4.

CHAPTER 5: VITAMINS

Vitamin A

Blaner, W. S. 1989. "Retinol-Binding Protein: The Serum Transport Protein for Vitamin A." *Endocrine Review* 10 (3): 308–16.

Chetyrkin, S. V. 2000. "Transport and Metabolism of Vitamin A." *Ukrainskii Biokhimicheskii Zhurnal* (Kiev) 72 (3): 12–24.

Kato, S. 2000. "Transcriptional Control by Nuclear Vitamin A/D Receptors." *Tanpakushitsu Kakusan Koso* (Tokyo) 45 (suppl 9): 1534–45.

Maden, M. 2000. "The Role of Retinoic Acid in Embryonic and Post-Embryonic Development." *Proceedings of the Nutrition Society* 59 (1): 65–73.

Moriwaki, H., M. Okuno, R. Nishiwaki, and Y. Shiratori. 1999. "Retinol-Binding Protein (RBP)." *Nippon Rinsho* (Osaka) 57 (suppl): 279–81.

Smith, J., and T. L. Steinemann. 2000. "Vitamin A Deficiency and the Eye." *International Ophthalmology Clinics* 40 (4): 83–91.

Sundaram, M., A. Sivaprasadarao, and J. B. Findlay. 1998. "Expression and Mutagenesis of Retinol-Binding Protein." *Methods in Molecular Biology* 89: 141–53.

West, C. E. 2000. "Meeting Requirements for Vitamin A." *Nutrition Review* 58 (11): 341–45.

Whiting, S. J., and B. Lemke. 1999. "Excess Retinol Intake May Explain the High Incidence of Osteoporosis in Northern Europe." *Nutrition Review* 57 (6): 192–95.

Wolf, G. 1998. "Release of Stored Retinol from Adipocytes." *Nutrition Review* 56 (1 Pt 1): 29–30.

Zhang, D., W. F. Holmes, S. Wu, and others. 2000. "Retinoids and Ovarian Cancer." *Journal of Cellular Physiology* 185 (1): 1–20.

Carotenoids

Agarwal, S., and A. V. Rao. 2000. "Carotenoids and Chronic Diseases." *Drug Metabolism and Drug Interactions* 17 (1–4): 189–210.

Burri, B. J. 2000. "Carotenoids and Gene Expression." *Nutrition* 16 (7–8): 577–78.

Delgado-Vargas, F., A. R. Jimenez, and O. Paredes-Lopez. 2000. "Natural Pigments: Carotenoids, Anthocyanins, and Betalains—Characteristics, Biosynthesis, Processing, and Stability." *Critical Reviews in Food Science and Nutrition* 40 (3): 173–289.

Handelman, G. J. 2001. "The Evolving Role of Carotenoids in Human Biochemistry." *Nutrition* 17 (10): 818–22.

Krinsky, N. I. 2001. "Carotenoids as Antioxidants." *Nutrition* 17 (10): 815–17.

Young, A. J., and G. M. Lowe. 2001. "Antioxidant and Prooxidant Properties of Carotenoids." *Archives of Biochemistry and Biophysics* 385 (1): 20–27.

Vitamin D

Buckley, L. M., and others. 1996. "Calcium and Vitamin D3 Supplementation Prevents Bone Loss in the Spine Secondary to Low-Dose Corticosteroids in Patients with Rheumatoid Arthritis." *Annals of Internal Medicine* 125: 961–68.

Dawson-Hughes, B., G. E. Dallal, E. A. Krall, and others. 1991. "Effect of Vitamin D Supplementation on Wintertime and Overall Bone Loss in Healthy Postmenopausal Women." *Annals of Internal Medicine* 115 (7): 505–12.

Garland, C. F., F. C. Garland, and E. D. Gorham. 1999. "Calcium and Vitamin D: Their Potential Roles in Colon and Breast Cancer Prevention. *Annals of the New York Academy of Sciences* 889: 107–19.

Hunter, D., P. Major, N. Arden, and others. 2000. "A Randomized Controlled Trial of Vitamin D Supplementation on Preventing Postmenopausal Bone Loss and Modifying Bone Metabolism Using Identical Twin Pairs." *Journal of Bone and Mineral Research* 15: 2276–83.

Lipkin, M., and H. L. Newmark. 1999. "Vitamin D, Calcium, and Prevention of Breast Cancer: A Review." *Journal of the American College of Nutrition* 18 (5): 392S–397S.

Lipkin, M., B. Reddy, H.L. Newmayc, and others. 1999. "Dietary Factors in Human Colorectal Cancer." *Annual Review of Nutrition* 19: 545-86.

Lips, P., W.C. Graafmans, M.E. Ooms, and others. 1996. "Vitamin D Supplementation and Fracture Incidence in Elderly Persons." *Annals of Internal Medicine* 124 (4): 400-6.

Vitamin E

Azzi, A., and A. Stocker. 2000. "Vitamin E: Non-antioxidant Roles." *Progressive Lipid Research* 39 (3): 231–55.

Bendich, A., and L. J. Machlin. 1988. "Safety of Oral Intake of Vitamin E." *American Journal of Clinical Nutrition* 48: 612–19.

Blumberg, J. B. 2002. "An Update: Vitamin E Supplementation and Heart Disease." *Nutrition in Clinical Care* 5: 50–55.

Butterfield, D. A., A. Castegna, J. Drake, G. Scapagnini, and V. Calabrese. 2002. "Vitamin E and Neurodegenerative Disorders Associated with Oxidative Stress." *Nutritional Neuroscience* 5: 229–39.

Chow, C. K., and C. B. Hong. 2002. "Dietary Vitamin E and Selenium and Toxicity of Nitrite and Nitrate." *Toxicology* 180: 195–207.

Darr, D., S. Dunston, H. H. Faust, and others. 1996. "Effectiveness of Antioxidants (Vitamin C and E) with and without Sunscreens as Topical Photoprotectants." *ACTA Dermato-Venereologica* (Oslo) 76: 264–68.

Fleshner, N. E. 2002. "Vitamin E and Prostate Cancer." *Urology Clinics of North America* 29: 107–13, ix.

Liu, L., and M. Meydani. 2002. "Combined Vitamin C and E Supplementation Retards Early Progression of Arteriosclerosis in Heart Transplant Patients." *Nutrition Review* 60: 368–71.

Mascio, P. D., M. E. Murphy, and H. Sies. 1991. "Antioxidant Defense Systems: The Role of Carotenoids, Tocopherols, and Thiols." *American Journal of Clinical Nutrition* 53 (suppl 1): 194S–200S.

Packer, L. 1994. "Vitamin E is Nature's Master Antioxidant." *Scientific American* (March–April): 54–63.

Packer, L., and G. Valacchi. 2002. "Antioxidants and the Response of Skin to Oxidative Stress: Vitamin E as a Key Indicator." *Skin Pharmacology and Applied Skin Physiology* 15: 282–90.

Packer, L., S. U. Weber, and G. Rimbach. 2001. "Molecular Aspects of Alpha-tocotrienol Antioxidant Action and Cell Signaling." *Journal of Nutrition* 131 (2): 369S–373S.

Sokol, R. J. 1984. "Vitamin E Deficiency in Adults." *Annals of Internal Medicine* 100: 769.

Vitamin K

Autret-Leca, E., and A. P. Jonville-Bera. 2001. "Vitamin K in Neonates: How to Administer, When, and to Whom." *Paediatric and Perinatal Drug Therapy* 3: 1–8.

Berkner, K. L. 2000. "The Vitamin K-Dependent Carboxylase." *Journal of Nutrition* 130: 1877–80.

Hey, E. 2003. "Vitamin K—What, Why, and When." *Archive of Diseases in Childhood. Fetal and Neonatal Edition.* 88: F80–83.

Nelsestuen, G. L., A. M. Shah, and S. B. Harvey. 2000. "Vitamin K-dependent Proteins." *Vitamins and Hormones* 58: 355–89.

Rambeck, W. A., and H. B. Stahelin. 2001. "Emerging Scientific Evidence. Vitamin K and Bone Metabolism: Effects of Vitamins on Behaviour and Cognition." *Bibliotheca Nutritio et Dieta* (Basel) 55: 206–8.

Ross, J. A., and S. M. Davies. 2000. "Vitamin K Prophylaxis and Childhood Cancer." *Medical and Pediatric Oncology* 34: 434–37.

Sakagami, H., K. Satoh, Y. Hakeda, and M. Kumegawa. 2000. "Apoptosis-Inducing Activity of Vitamin C and Vitamin K." *Cellular and Molecular Biology* (Noisy-le-Grand, France) 46: 129–43.

Saxena, S. P., E. D. Israels, and L. G. Israels. 2001. "Novel Vitamin K–Dependent Pathways Regulating Cell Survival." *Apoptosis* 6: 57–68.

Vermeer, C., and L. J. Schurgers. 2000. "A Comprehensive Review of Vitamin K and Vitamin K Antagonists." *Hematology/Oncology Clinics of North America* 14: 339–53.

Vermeer, C., H. H. Thijssen, and K. Hamulyak. 2001. "Vitamin K and Tissue Mineralization." *Bibliotheca Nutritio et Dieta* (Basel) 55: 159–70.

Weber, P. 2001. "Vitamin K and Bone Health." *Nutrition* 17: 880–87.

Zittermann, A. 2001. "Effects of Vitamin K on Calcium and Bone Metabolism." *Current Opinion in Clinical Nutrition and Metabolic Care* 4: 483–87.

Vitamin B1

Cascante, M., J. J. Centelles, R. L. Veech, W. N. Lee, and L. G. Boros. 2000. "Role of Thiamin (Vitamin B-1) and Transketolase in Tumor Cell Proliferation." *Nutrion and Cancer* 36: 150–54.

Gibson, G. E, H. Ksiezak-Reding, K. F. Sheu, V. Mykytyn, and J. P. Blass. 1984. "Correlation of Enzymatic, Metabolic, and Behavioral Deficits in Thiamin Deficiency and Its Reversal." *Neurochemical Research* 9: 803–14.

Leevy, C. M. 1982. "Thiamin Deficiency and Alcoholism." *Annals of the New York Academy of Sciences* 378: 316–26.

Liang, C. C. 1977. "Bradycardia in Thiamin Deficiency and the Role of Glyoxylate." *Journal of Nutritional Science and Vitaminology* (Tokyo) 23: 1–6.

Parkhomenko, I. M., G. V. Donchenko, and Z. S. Protasova. 1996. "The Neural Activity of Thiamine: Facts and Hypotheses." *Ukrainski Biokhimicheski Zhurnal* 68: 3–14.

Pohl, M., B. Lingen, and M. Muller. 2002. "Thiamin-Diphosphate-Dependent Enzymes: New Aspects of Asymmetric C-C Bond Formation." *Chemistry* 8: 5288-95.

Suter, P. M., and W. Vetter. 2000. "Diuretics and Vitamin B1: Are Diuretics a Risk Factor for Thiamin Malnutrition?" *Nutrition Review* 58: 319–23.

Weidmann, S. 1994. "'Action Substances' of Peripheral Nerve Re-Visited." *Experientia* 50: 342–45.

Yoshioka, K., H. Nishimura, M. Himukai, and A. Iwashima. 1985. "The Inhibitory Effect of Choline and Other Quaternary Ammonium Compounds on Thiamine Transport in Isolated Rat Hepatocytes." *Biochimica et Biophysica ACTA/General Subjects* (Amsterdam) 815: 499–504.

Vitamin B2

Bacher, A., S. Eberhardt, W. Eisenreich, and others. 2001. "Biosynthesis of Riboflavin." *Vitamins and Hormones* 61: 1–49.

Bacher, A., S. Eberhardt, M. Fischer, K. Kis, and G. Richter. 2000. "Biosynthesis of Vitamin B2 (Riboflavin)." *Annual Review of Nutrition* 20: 153–67.

Belko, A. Z. 1983. "Effects of Exercise on Riboflavin Requirements of Young Women." *American Journal of Clinical Nutrition* 37: 509–17.

Bender, D. A. 1992. *Nutritional Biochemistry of the Vitamins.* New York: Cambridge University Press.

Beutler, E. 1989. "Nutritional and Metabolic Aspects of Glutathione." *Annual Review of Nutrition* 9: 287–302.

Feinman, L., and C. S. Lieber. 1990. "Nutrition and Liver Disease." *Hospital Medicine* (April): 150–66.

Goodrich, R. P. 2000. "The Use of Riboflavin for the Inactivation of Pathogens in Blood Products." *Vox Sang* 78 (suppl 2): 211–15.

Manore, M. M. 2000. "Effect of Physical Activity on Thiamine, Riboflavin, and Vitamin B-6 Requirements." *American Journal of Clinical Nutrition* 72: 598S–606S.

Massey, V. 2000. "The Chemical and Biological Versatility of Riboflavin." *Biochemical Society Transactions* (London) 28: 283–96.

Merrill, A. H., J. D. Lambeth, D. E. Edmonson, and others. 1981. "Formation and Mode of Flavoproteins." *Annual Review of Nutrition* 1: 281–317.

Stahmann, K. P., J. L. Revuelta, and H. Seulberger. 2000. "Three Biotechnical Processes Using Ashbya Gossypii, Candida Famata, or Bacillus Subtilis Compete with Chemical Riboflavin Production." *Applied Microbiology and Biotechnology* 53: 509–16.

Vitamin B3

Alvarsson, M., and V. Grill. 1996. "Impact of Nicotinic Acid Treatment on Insulin Secretion and Insulin." *Scandinavian Journal of Clinical and Laboratory Investigation* (Oxford) 56 (6): 563-70.

Ames, B. N. 1999. "Micronutrient Deficiencies: A Major Cause of DNA Damage." *Annals of the New York Academy of Sciences* 889: 152–56.

Capuzzi, D. M., J. M. Morgan, O. A. Brusco Jr., and C. M. Intenzo. 2000. "Niacin Dosing: Relationship to Benefits and Adverse Effects." *Current Atherosclerosis Reports* 2: 64–71.

DiPalma, J. R., and W. S. Thayer. 1991. "Use of Niacin as a Drug." *Annual Review of Nutrition* 11: 169–87.

Henderson, L. M. 1983. "Niacin." *Annual Review of Nutrition* 3: 289–307.

Jacobson, E. L., W. M. Shieh, and A. C. Huang. 1999. "Mapping the Role of NAD Metabolism in Prevention and Treatment of Carcinogenesis." *Molecular and Cellular Biochemistry* 193 (1–2): 69–74.

Kamanna, V. S., and M. L. Kashyap. 2000. "Mechanism of Action of Niacin on Lipoprotein Metabolism." *Current Atherosclerosis Report* 2: 36–46.

Pieper, J. A. 2002. "Understanding Niacin Formulations." *American Journal of Managed Care* 8: S308–S314.

Sugiyama, K., A. Ohishi, H. Siyu, and others. 1989. "Effects of Methyl-Group Acceptors on the Regulation of Plasma Cholesterol Level in Rats Fed High Cholesterol Diets." *Journal of Nutritional Science and Vitaminology* (Tokyo) 35 (6): 612–26.

Tavintharan, S., and M. L. Kashyap. 2001. "The Benefits of Niacin in Atherosclerosis." *Current Atherosclerosis Reports* 3: 74–82.

Vitamin B5

Fox, H. M. 1984. "Pantothenic Acid." In L. J. Machlin, ed., *Handbook of Vitamins.* New York: Marcel Dekker, 437.

Glusman, M. 1947. "The Syndrome of Burning Feet (Nutritional Melalgia) as Manifestation of Nutritional Deficiency." *American Journal of Medicine* 3: 211–23.

Robishaw, J. D., and J. R. Neely. 1985. "Coenzyme A Metabolism." *American Journal of Physiology* 248: E1–E9.

Rokitzki, L., A. Sagredos, F. Reuss, and others. 1993. "Pantothenic Acid Levels in Blood of Athletes at Rest and after Aerobic Exercise." *Zeitschrift für Ernährungswissenschaft* (Heidelberg) 32 (4): 282–88.

Tahiliani, A. G., and C. J. Beinlick. 1991. "Pantothenic Acid in Health and Disease." *Vitamins and Hormones* 46: 165–227.

Tannenbaum, S. R., and V. R. Young. 1985. "Vitamins and Minerals." In O. R. Fennema, ed., *Food Chemistry.* Second edition. New York: Marcel Dekker, 512.

van den Berg, H. 1997. "Bioavailability of Pantothenic Acid." *European Journal of Clinical Nutrition* 51 (suppl 1): S62–S63.

Yasuda, K., and M. Hiraoka. 1999. "Pantothenic Acid." *Nippon Rinsho.* [Japanese Journal of Clincal Medicine] (Osaka) (suppl): 131–34.

Vitamin B6

Coleman, M., S. Sobel, H. N. Bhagavan, and others. 1985. "A Double-Blind Study of Vitamin B6 in Down's Syndrome Infants: Part 1—Clinical and Biochemical Results." *Journal of Mental Deficiency Research* 29: 233-40.

Effersoe, H. 1954. "The Effect of Topical Application of Pyridoxine Ointment on the Rate of Sebaceous Secretion in Patients with Seborrheic Dermatitis." *ACTA Dermato-Venereologica* (Oslo) 3: 272–77.

Gvozdova, L. G., E. G. Paramanova, E. V. Goriachenkova, and others. 1966. "The Content of Pyridoxal Coenzymes in the Blood Plasma of Patients with Coronary Atherosclerosis on a Background of Therapeutic Diet and after Supplemental Intake of Vitamin B6." *Voprosy pitaniia* (Moscow) 25: 40–44.

Institute of Medicine. 1998. *Dietary Reference Intakes: Thiamin, Riboflavin, Niacin, Vitamin B6, Vitamin B12, Pantothenic Acid, Biotin, and Choline.* Washington, D.C.: National Academy of Sciences, National Academy Press, 390–422.

Korpela, T. K., and P. Christen, eds. 1987. "Biochemistry of Vitamin B6." In volume 2 of *The Proceedings of the Seventh International Congress on Chemical and Biological Aspects of Vitamin B6 Catalysis.* Basel: Birkhauser Verlag.

Leklem, J. E. 1991. "Vitamin B6." In L. J. Machlin, ed., *Handbook of Vitamins.* Second edition. New York: Dekker, 341–92.

Schaumberg, H., J. Kaplan, A. Windebank, and others. 1983. "Sensory Neuropathy from Pyridoxine Abuse: A New Megavitamin Syndrome." *New England Journal of Medicine* 309: 445–48.

Yates, A. A., S. A. Schlicker, and C. W. Suitor. 1998. "Dietary Reference Intakes: The New Basis for Recommendations for Calcium and Related Nutrients, B Vitamins, and Choline." *Journal of the American Dietetic Association* 98: 699–706.

Vitamin B12

Areekul, S., S. Pattanamatum, and others. 1990. "The Source and Content of Vitamin B12 in the Tempehs." *Journal of the Medical Association of Thailand* (Bangkok) 73 (3): 152–56.

Carmel, R. 1997. "Cobalamin, the Stomach, and Aging." *American Journal of Clinical Nutrition* 66 (4): 750–59.

Clementz, G. L., and S. G. Schade. 1990. "The Spectrum of Vitamin B12 Deficiency." *American Family Physician* 41 (1): 150–62.

Davis, R. E. 1984. "Clinical Chemistry of Vitamin B12." *Advanced Clinical Chemistry* 24: 163–216.

Delpre, G., P. Stark, and Y. Niv. 1999. "Sublingual Therapy for Cobalamin Deficiency as an Alternative to Oral and Parenteral Cobalamin Supplementation." *Lancet* 354 (9180): 740–41.

Dharmarajan, T. S., G. U. Adiga, and E. P. Norkus. 2003. "Vitamin B12 Deficiency: Recognizing Subtle Symptoms in Older Adults." *Geriatrics* 58: 30–34, 37–38.

Lovblad, K., G. Ramelli, and others. 1997. "Retardation of Myelination Due to Dietary Vitamin B12 Deficiency: Cranial MRI Findings." *Pediatric Radiology* 27 (2): 155–58.

Martens, J. H., H. Barg, M. J. Warren, and D. Jahn. 2002. "Microbial Production of Vitamin B12." *Applied Microbiology and Biotechnology* 58: 275–85.

Miller, J. W. 2002. "Vitamin B12 Deficiency, Tumor Necrosis Factor-Alpha, and Epidermal Growth Factor: A Novel Function for Vitamin B12?" *Nutrition Review* 60: 142–44.

Selhub, J. 2002. "Folate, Vitamin B12, and Vitamin B6, and One Carbon Metabolism." *Journal of Nutrition, Health, and Aging* 6: 39–42.

Spalla, C., A. Grein, and others. 1997. "Microbial Production of Vitamin B12." Chapter 15 in H. Bickel and Y. Schultz, eds., *Digestion and Absorption of Nutrients, International Journal of Vitamin and Nutrition Research.* Supplement 25. Bern: Hans Huber Publications, 257–84.

Ward, P. C. 2002. "Modern Approaches to the Investigation of Vitamin B12 Deficiency." *Clinics in Laboratory Medicine* 22: 435–45.

Warren, M. J., E. Raux, H. L. Schubert, and J. C. Escalante-Semerena. 2002. "The Biosynthesis of Adenosylcobalamin (Vitamin B12)." *Natural Products Report* 19: 390–412.

Biotin

Attwood, P. V., and J. C. Wallace. 2002. "Chemical and Catalytic Mechanisms of Carboxyl Transfer Reactions in Biotin-Dependent Enzymes." *Accounts of Chemical Research* 35: 113–20.

Bonjour, J. P. 1991. "Biotin." In L. J. Machlin, ed., *Handbook of Vitamins.* Second edition. New York: Dekker, 393–427.

Marquet, A., B. T. Bui, and D. Florentin. 2001. "Biosynthesis of Biotin and Lipoic Acid." *Vitamins and Hormones* 61: 51–101.

McMahon, R. J. 2002. "Biotin in Metabolism and Molecular Biology." *Annual Review of Nutrition* 22: 221–39.

Mock, D. M. 1989. "Biotin." In M. Brown, ed., *Present Knowledge in Nutrition.* Sixth edition. Washington, D.C.: International Life Sciences Institute, 189–207.

Pacheco-Alvarez, D., R. S. Solorzano-Vargas, and A. L. Del Rio. 2002. "Biotin in Metabolism and Its Relationship to Human Disease." *Archives of Medical Research* 33: 439–47.

Said, H. M. 2002. "Biotin: The Forgotten Vitamin." *American Journal of Clinical Nutrition* 75: 179–80.

Sauberlich, H. E. 1980. "Interactions of Thiamin, Riboflavin, and Other B-Vitamins." *Annals of the New York Academy of Sciences* 355: 80.

Zempleni, J., and D. M. Mock. 2000. "Marginal Biotin Deficiency Is Teratogenic." *Proceedings of the Society for Experimental Biology and Medicine* 223: 14–21.

———. 2000. "Utilization of Biotin in Proliferating Human Lymphocytes." *Journal of Nutrition* 130: 335S–337S.

Choline

Arnesen, E., H. Refsum, K. H. Bonaa, and others. 1995. "Serum Total Homocysteine and Coronary Heart Disease." *International Journal of Epidemiology* 24: 704–9.

Brandner, C. 2002. "Perinatal Choline Treatment Modifies the Effects of a Visuo-spatial Attractive Cue upon Spatial Memory in Naive Adult Rats." *Brain Research* 928: 85–95.

Etienne, P., S. Gauthier, D. Dastoor, and others. 1979. "Alzheimer's Disease: Clinical Effects of Lecithin Treatment." Chapter 5 in A. Barbeau, J. H. Growdon, and R. J. Wurtman, eds., *Nutrition and the Brain.* New York: Raven Press, 389–96.

Hirsch, M. J., J. H. Growdon, and R. J. Wurtman. 1978. "Relations between Dietary Choline or Lecithin Intake, Serum Choline Levels, and Various Metabolic Indices." *Metabolism* 27: 953–60.

Holm, P. I., O. Bleie, P. M. Ueland, and others. 2004. "Betaine as a Determinant of Postmethionine Load Total Plasma Homocysteine before and after B-vitamin Supplementation." *Arteriosclerosis, Thrombosis, and Vascular Biology* 24(2): 301-7.

Holmes, G. L., Y. Yang, Z. Liu, and others. 2002. "Seizure-Induced Memory Impairment Is Reduced by Choline Supplementation before or after Status Epilepticus." *Epilepsy Research* 48: 3–13.

Institute of Medicine. 1998. *Dietary Reference Intakes: Thiamin, Riboflavin, Niacin, Vitamin B6, Vitamin B12, Pantothenic Acid, Biotin, and Choline.* Washington, D.C.: National Academy of Sciences, National Academy Press, 390–422.

James, S. J., and L. Yin. 1989. "Diet-Induced DNA Damage and Altered Nucleotide Metabolism in Lymphocytes from Methyl-Donor-Deficient Rats." *Carcinogen* 10 (7): 1209–14.

Paredes, S. R., P. A. Kozicki, and A. M. Battle. 1985. "S-adenosyl-methionine a Counter to Lead Intoxication?" *Comparative Biochemistry and Physiology. B: Comparative Biochemistry* 82 (4): 751–57.

Tang, F., S. Nag, S. Y. Shiu, and S. F. Pang. 2002. "The Effects of Melatonin and Ginkgo Biloba Extract on Memory Loss and Choline Acetyltransferase Activities in the Brain of Rats Infused Intracerebroventricularly with Beta-amyloid 1-40." *Life Science* 71: 2625–31.

Zeisel, S. H. 2000. "Choline: Needed for Normal Development of Memory." *Journal of the American College of Nutrition* 19: 528S–531S.

Folic Acid

Bower, C., F. J. Stanley, and D. J. Nicol. 1993. "Maternal Folate Status and the Risk for Neural Tube Defects: The Role of Dietary Folate." *Annals of the New York Academy of Sciences* 678: 146–55.

Coombs, G. F. 1992. *The Vitamins.* San Diego: Academic Press, 357–76.

Fernstrom, J. D. 2000. "Can Nutrient Supplements Modify Brain Function?" *American Journal of Clinical Nutrition* 71 (suppl 6): 1669S–1675S.

Gregory, J. F., III, and E. P. Quinlivan. 2002. "In Vivo Kinetics of Folate Metabolism." *Annual Review of Nutrition* 22: 199–220.

Halsted, C. H., J. A. Villanueva, and A. M. Devlin. 2002. "Folate Deficiency, Methionine Metabolism, and Alcoholic Liver Disease." *Alcohol* 27: 169–72.

Kaluski, D. N., Y. Amitai, A. Haviv, R. Goldsmith, and A. Leventhal. 2002. "Dietary Folate and the Incidence and Prevention of Neural Tube Defects: A Proposed Triple Intervention Approach in Israel." *Nutrition Review* 60: 303–7.

Little, J., and L. Sharp. 2002. "Colorectal Neoplasia and Genetic Polymorphisms Associated with Folate Metabolism." *European Journal of Cancer Prevention* 11: 105–10.

Mason, J. B., and T. Levesque. 1996. "Folate: Effects on Carcinogenesis and the Potential for Cancer Chemoprevention." *Oncology* 10 (11): 1727–43.

Miller, J. W. 2002. "Homocysteine, Folate Deficiency, and Parkinson's Disease." *Nutrition Review* 60: 410–13.

Molloy, A. M. 2002. "Folate Bioavailability and Health." *International Journal for Vitamin and Nutrition Research* 72: 46–52.

Montes, L. F., M. L. Diaz, J. Lajous, and others. 1992. "Folic Acid and Vitamin B12 in Vitiligo: A Nutritional Approach." *Cutis* 50: 39–42.

Morris, M. S. 2002. "Folate, Homocysteine, and Neurological Function." *Nutrition in Clinical Care* 5: 124–32.

Onicescu, D., A. Marin, and L. Mischiu. 1978. "Folate Metabolism in Normal Human Gingiva and in Chronic Marginal Periodontitis." *Revista de Chirurgie, Oncologie, Radiologie, O.R.L., Oftamologie, Stomatologie. Chirurgie* (Bucharest) 25 (4): 257–64.

Pancharuniti, N., C. A. Lewis, H. E. Sauberlich, and others. 1994. "Plasma Homocyst(e)ine, Folate, and Vitamin B12 Concentrations and Risk for Early-Onset Coronary Artery Disease." *American Journal of Clinical Nutrition* 59: 940–48.

Ristow, K. A., J. F. Gregory, and B. L. Damron. 1982. "Thermal Processing Effects on Folacin Bioavailability in Liquid Model Food Systems, Liver, and Cabbage." *Journal of Agricultural Food Chemistry* 30 (5): 801–6.

Scholl, T. O., and W. G. Johnson. 2000. "Folic Acid: Influence on the Outcome of Pregnancy." *American Journal of Clinical Nutrition* 71 (suppl 5): 1295S–1303S.

Selhub, J. 2002. "Folate, Vitamin B12, and Vitamin B6 and One Carbon Metabolism." *Journal of Nutrition, Health, and Aging* 6: 39–42.

Steinberg, S. E. 1984. "Mechanisms of Folate Homeostasis." *American Journal of Physiology* 246: G319–G324.

Ubbink, J. B., W. J. Vermaak, A. van der Merwe, and P. J. Becker. 1993. "Vitamin B-12, Vitamin B-6, and Folate Nutritional Status in Men with Hyperhomocysteinemia." *American Journal of Clinical Nutrition* 57 (1): 47–53.

Zimmerman, M. B., and B. Shane. 1993. "Supplemental Folic Acid." *American Journal of Clinical Nutrition* 58: 127–28.

Inositol

Agranoff, B. W., and S. K. Fisher. 2001. "Inositol, Lithium, and the Brain." *Psychopharmacology Bulletin* 35: 5–18.

Barker, C. J., I. B. Leibiger, B. Leibiger, and P. O. Berggren. 2002. "Phosphorylated Inositol Compounds in Beta-cell Stimulus-Response Coupling." *American Journal of Physiology, Endocrinology, and Metabolism* 283: E1113–E1122.

Cockcroft, S., and M. A. De Matteis. 2001. "Inositol Lipids as Spatial Regulators of Membrane Traffic." *Journal of Membrane Biology* 180: 187–94.

"Inositol Hexaphosphate. Monograph." 2002. *Alternative Medicine Review* 7: 244–48.

Martelli, A. M., L. Manzoli, I. Faenza, R. Bortul, A. Billi, and L. Cocco. 2002. "Nuclear Inositol Lipid Signaling and Its Potential Involvement in Malignant Transformation." *Biochimica et Biophysica Acta/General Subjects* (Amsterdam) 1603: 11–17.

Phillippy, B. Q. 2003. "Inositol Phosphates in Foods." *Advanced Food Nutrition Research* 45: 1–60.

York, J. D., S. Guo, A. R. Odom, B. D. Spiegelberg, and L. E. Stolz. 2001. "An Expanded View of Inositol Signaling." *Advances in Enzyme Regulation* 41: 57–71.

Vitamin C

Carr, A. C., and B. Frei. 1999. "Toward a New Recommended Dietary Allowance for Vitamin C Based on Antioxidant and Health Effects in Humans." *American Journal of Clinical Nutrition* 69 (6): 1086–107.

Englard, S., and S. Seifter. 1986. "The Biological Functions of Ascorbic Acid." *Annual Review of Nutrition* 6: 365–406.

Hunt, J. V., M. A. Bottoms, and M. J. Mitchinson. 1992. "Ascorbic Acid Oxidation: A Potential Cause of the Elevated Severity of Atherosclerosis in Diabetes Mellitus?" *FEBS Letters* (Amsterdam) 311 (2): 161–64.

Levine, M. 1986. "New Concepts in Biology and Biochemistry of Ascorbic Acid." *New England Journal of Medicine* 314: 892–902.

Levine, M., C. C. Cantilena, and K. R. Dhariwal. 1995. "Determination of Optimal Vitamin C Requirements in Humans." *American Journal of Clinical Nutrition* 62 (suppl): 1347S–1356S.

Medeiros, D. M., M. A. Bock, C. Raab, and others. 1989. "Vitamin and Mineral Supplementation Practices of Adults in Seven Western States." *Journal of the American Dietetic Association* 89 (3): 383–86.

Reaven, P. D., and J. L. Witztum. 1996. "Oxidized Low Density Lipoproteins in Atherogenesis: Role of Dietary Modification." *Annual Review of Nutrition* 16: 51–71.

Subar, A., and G. Block. 1990. "Use of Vitamin and Mineral Supplements." *American Journal of Epidemiology* 132: 1091-101.

Worthington-Roberts, B., and M. Breskin. 1984. "Supplementation Patterns of Washington State Dietitians." *Journal of the American Dietetic Association* 84 (7): 795–800.

Vitamin P (Flavonoids)

Birt, D. F., S. Hendrich, and W. Wang. 2001. "Dietary Agents in Cancer Prevention: Flavonoids and Isoflavonoids." *Pharmacology and Therapeutics* 90: 157–77.

Di Carlo, G., N. Mascolo, A. A. Izzo, and F. Capasso. 1999. "Flavonoids: Old and New Aspects of a Class of Natural Therapeutic Drugs." *Life Science* 65: 337–53.

Fuhrman, B., and M. Aviram. 2001. "Flavonoids Protect LDL from Oxidation and Attenuate Atherosclerosis." *Current Opinions in Lipidology* 12: 41–48.

Hodek, P., P. Trefil, and M. Stiborova. 2001. "Flavonoids— Potent and Versatile Biologically Active Compounds Interacting with Cytochromes P450." *Chemico-Biological Interactions* (Limerick) 139: 1–21.

Horvathova, K., A. Vachalkova, and L. Novotny. 2001. "Flavonoids as Chemoprotective Agents in Civilization Diseases." *Neoplasma* 48: 435–41.

Le Marchand, L. 2002. "Cancer Preventive Effects of Flavonoids—A Review." *Biomedicine and Pharmacotherapy* 56: 296–301.

Manthey, J. A., B. S. Buslig, and M. E. Baker. 2002. "Flavonoids in Cell Function." *Advances in Experimental Medicine and Biology* 505: 1–7.

Martinez-Florez, S., J. Gonzalez-Gallego, J. M. Culebras, and M. J. Tunon. 2002. "Flavonoids: Properties and Antioxidizing Action." *Nutricion Hospitalaria* (Madrid) 17: 271–78.

Mojzisova, G., and M. Kuchta. 2001. "Dietary Flavonoids and Risk of Coronary Heart Disease." *Physiology Research* 50: 529–35.

Ross, J. A., and C. M. Kasum. 2002. "Dietary Flavonoids: Bioavailability, Metabolic Effects, and Safety." *Annual Review of Nutrition* 22: 19–34.

Terao, J. 1999. "Dietary Flavonoids as Antioxidants In Vivo: Conjugated Metabolites of (-)-Epicatechin and Quercetin Participate in Antioxidative Defense in Blood Plasma." *Journal of Medical Investigation* 46: 159–68.

Williamson, G., A. J. Day, G. W. Plumb, and D. Couteau. 2000. "Human Metabolic Pathways of Dietary Flavonoids and Cinnamates." *Biochemical Society Transactions* (London) 28: 16–22.

Wiseman, H. 1999. "The Bioavailability of Non-nutrient Plant Factors: Dietary Flavonoids and Phyto-oestrogens." *Proceedings of the Nutrition Society* (London) 58: 139–46.

Youdim, K. A., J. P. Spencer, H. Schroeter, and C. Rice-Evans. 2002. "Dietary Flavonoids as Potential Neuroprotectants." *Biological Chemistry* 383: 503–19.

CHAPTER 6: MINERALS

General

Dror, Y., F. Stern, Y. N. Berner, and others. 2001. "Micronutrient (Vitamins and Minerals) Supplementation for the Elderly, Suggested by a Special Committee Nominated by the Ministry of Health." *Harefuah* (Tel Aviv) 140: 1062–67, 1117.

Nielsen, F. H. 2000. "Evolutionary Events Culminating in Specific Minerals Becoming Essential for Life." *European Journal of Nutrition* 39: 62–66.

Nishimuta, M. 2000. "The Concept of Intracellular-, Extracellular- and Bone-Minerals." *Biofactors* 12: 35–38.

Pandya, D. P. 2002. "Oxidant Injury and Antioxidant Prevention: Role of Dietary Antioxidants, Minerals, and Drugs in the Management of Coronary Heart Disease (Part II)." *Comprehensive Therapy* 28: 62–73.

Sandberg, A. S. 2002. "Bioavailability of Minerals in Legumes." *British Journal of Nutrition* 88 (suppl 3): S281–S285.

Speich, M., A. Pineau, and F. Ballereau. 2001. "Minerals, Trace Elements, and Related Biological Variables in Athletes and during Physical Activity." *Clinica Chimica Acta* (Amsterdam) 312: 1–11.

Worthington, V. 1998. "Effect of Agricultural Methods on Nutritional Quality: A Comparison of Organic with Conventional Crops." *Alternative Therapies* 4 (1): 58–69.

Calcium

Bell, L., C. E. Halstenson, C. J. Halstenson, and others. 1992. "Cholesterol-Lowering Effects of Calcium Carbonate in Patients with Mild to Moderate Hypercholesterolemia." *Archives of Internal Medicine* 152: 2441–44.

Bostick, R. M., L. Fosdick, G. A. Grandits, and others. 2000. "Effect of calcium supplementation on serum cholesterol and blood pressure." *Archives of Family Medicine* 9: 31–39.

Buckley, L. M., E. S. Leib, K. S. Cartularo, and others. 1996. "Calcium and Vitamin D3 Supplementation Prevents Bone Loss in the Spine Secondary to Low-Dose Corticosteroids in Patients with Rheumatoid Arthritis." *Annals of Internal Medicine* 125: 961–68.

Cappuccio, F. P., P. Elliott, P. S. Allender, and others. 1995. "Epidemiologic Association between Dietary Calcium Intake and Blood Pressure: A Meta-Analysis of Published Data." *American Journal of Epidemiology* 142: 935–45.

Cook, J. D., S. A. Dassenko, and P. Whittaker. 1991. "Calcium Supplementation: Effect on Iron Absorption." *American Journal of Clinical Nutrition* 53: 106–11.

Garland, C. F., F. C. Garland, and E. D. Gorham. 1999. "Calcium and Vitamin D: Their Potential Roles in Colon and Breast Cancer Prevention." *Annals of the New York Academy of Sciences* 889: 107–19.

Hallberg, L. 1998. "Does Calcium Interfere with Iron Absorption?" *American Journal of Clinical Nutrition* 63: 3–4.

Lee, S. J., and J. A. Kanis. 1994. "An Association between Osteoporosis and Premenstrual Symptoms and Postmenopausal Symptoms." *Bone and Mineral* 24: 127–34.

Miller, J. Z., D. L. Smith, L. Flora, and others. 1988. "Calcium Absorption from Calcium Carbonate and a New Form of Calcium (CCM) in Healthy Male and Female Adolescents." *American Journal of Clinical Nutrition* 48: 1291–94.

Minihane, A. M., S. J. Fairweather-Tait, and others. 1998. "Effect of Calcium Supplementation on Daily Nonheme-Iron Absorption and Long-Term Iron Status." *American Journal of Clinical Nutrition* 68: 96–102.

Sakhaee, K., T. Bhuket, B. Adams-Huet, and others. 1999. "Meta-Analysis of Calcium Bioavailability: A Comparison of Calcium Citrate with Calcium Carbonate." *American Journal of Therapeutics* 6: 313–21.

Thys-Jacobs, S., P. Starkey, D. Bernstein, and J. Tian. 1998. "Calcium Carbonate and the Premenstrual Syndrome: Effects on Premenstrual and Menstrual Symptoms. Premestrual Syndrome Study Group." *American Journal of Obstetrics and Gynecology* 179 (2): 444–52.

Weaver, C. M., W. R. Proulx, and R. Heaney. 1999. "Choices for Achieving Adequate Dietary Calcium with a Vegetarian Diet." *American Journal of Clinical Nutrition* 70 (suppl): 543S–548S.

Chlorine/Chloride

Devuyst, O., and W. B. Guggino. 2002. "Chloride Channels in the Kidney: Lessons Learned from Knockout Animals." *American Journal of Physiology. Renal Physiology* 283: F1176–F1191.

Jentsch, T. J., V. Stein, F. Weinreich, and A. A. Zdebik. 2002. "Molecular Structure and Physiological Function of Chloride Channels." *Physiology Review* 82: 503–68.

Nilius, B., and G. Droogmans. 2003. "Amazing Chloride Channels: An Overview." *Acta Physiologica Scandinavica* (Oxford) 177: 119–47.

Thevenod, F. 2002. "Ion Channels in Secretory Granules of the Pancreas and Their Role in Exocytosis and Release of Secretory Proteins. *American Journal of Physiology. Cell Physiology* 283: C651–C672.

Magnesium

Abbott, L. G., and R. K. Rude. 1993. "Clinical Manifestations of Magnesium Deficiency." *Mineral and Electrolyte Metabolism* 19: 314–22.

Bengtsson, B. L. 1969. "Effect of Blanching on Mineral and Oxalate Content of Spinach." *Journal of Food Technology* 4: 141–45.

Firoz, M., and M. Graber. 2001. "Bioavailability of U.S. Commercial Magnesium Preparations." *Magnesium Research* 14 (4): 257–62.

Institute of Medicine. 1997. *Dietary Reference Intakes for Calcium, Phosphorus, Magnesium, Vitamin D, and Fluoride.* Washington, D.C.: National Academy of Sciences, National Academy Press, 190–249.

Iseri, L. K., and J. H. French. 1984. "Magnesium: Nature's Physiologic Calcium Blocker." *American Heart Journal* 108: 188–93.

Lindberg, J. S., M. M. Zobitz, J. R. Poindexter, and others. 1990. "Magnesium Bioavailability from Magnesium Citrate and Magnesium Oxide." *Journal of the American College of Nutrition* 9: 48–55.

Meiners, C. R., N. L. Derise, H. C. Lau, and others. 1976. "The Content of Nine Mineral Elements in Raw and Cooked Mature Dry Legumes." *Journal of Agricultural and Food Chemistry* 24: 1126–30.

Pearson, H. A., V. Campbell, N. Berrow, and others. 1994. "Modulation of Voltage-Dependent Calcium Channels in Cultured Neurons." *Annals of the New York Academy of Sciences* 747: 325–35.

Shils, M. E. 1994. "Magnesium." In M. E. Shils, J. A. Olson, and M. Shike, eds., *Modern Nutrition in Health and Disease.* Eighth edition. Philadelphia: Lea and Febiger, 164–84.

Wester, P. O. 1987. "Magnesium." *American Journal of Clinical Nutrition* 45 (suppl): 1305–12.

Phosphorus

Cashman, K. D., and A. Flynn. 1999. "Optimal Nutrition: Calcium, Magnesium and Phosphorus." *Proceedings of the Nutrition Society* (London) 58: 477–87.

Heaney, R. P. 2001. "Constructive Interactions among Nutrients and Bone-Active Pharmacologic Agents with Principal Emphasis on Calcium, Phosphorus, Vitamin D, and Protein." *Journal of the American College of Nutrition* 20: 403S–409S, discussion on 417S–420S.

Isaeva, B. A., I. A. Alekseeva, N. V. Blazheevich, and V. B. Spirichev. 1979. "Experimental Vitamin D Deficiency with Different Dietary Calcium- Phosphorus Ratios." *Voprosy meditsinskoi khimii* (Moscow) 25: 86–92.

Kuschel, C. A., and J. E. Harding. 2001. "Calcium and phosphorus supplementation of human milk for preterm infants." *Cochrane Database of Systematic Reviews* CD003310.

Root, A. W. 2000. "Genetic Disorders of Calcium and Phosphorus Metabolism." *Critical Reviews in Clinical Laboratory Sciences* 37: 217–60.

Sax, L. 2001. "The Institute of Medicine's 'Dietary Reference Intake' for Phosphorus: A Critical Perspective." *Journal of the American College of Nutrition* 20: 271–78.

Slatopolsky, E., A. Dusso, and A. J. Brown. 1999. "The Role of Phosphorus in the Development of Secondary Hyperparathyroidism and Parathyroid Cell Proliferation in Chronic Renal Failure." *American Journal of Medical "Science* 317: 370–76.

Potassium

Cutler, J. A. 1999. "The Effects of Reducing Sodium and Increasing Potassium Intake for Control of Hypertension and Improving Health." *Clinical and Experimental Hypertension* 21: 769–83.

Debska, G., A. Kicinska, J. Skalska, and A. Szewczyk. 2001. "Intracellular Potassium and Chloride Channels: An Update." *Acta Biochimica Polonica* (Warsaw) 48 (1): 137–44.

Fedida, D., and J. C. Hesketh. 2001. "Gating of voltage-dependent potassium channels." *Progress in Biophysics and Molecular Biology* 75 (3): 165–99.

Griffith, L. C. 2001. "Potassium Channels: The Importance of Transport Signals." *Current Biology* 11 (6): R226–R228.

He, F. J., and G. A. MacGregor. 2001. "Fortnightly Review: Beneficial Effects of Potassium." *British Medical Journal* 323 (7311): 497–501.

Sigworth, F. J. 2001. "Potassium Channel Mechanics." *Neuron* 32 (4): 555–56.

Sobey, C. G. 2001. "Potassium Channel Function in Vascular Disease." *Arteriosclerosis, Thrombosis, and Vascular Biology* 21 (1): 28–38.

Sodium

Alderman, M. H., and H. W. Cohen. 2002. "Impact of Dietary Sodium on Cardiovascular Disease Morbidity and Mortality." *Current Hypertension Reports* 4: 453–57.

Buemi, M., M. Senatore, F. Corica, and others. 2002. "Diet and Arterial Hypertension: Is the Sodium Ion Alone Important?" *Medicinal Research Reviews* 22: 419–28.

Cohen, H. W., and M. H. Alderman. 2002. "Low Sodium Diet after DASH: Has the Situation Changed? Dietary Approaches to Stop Hypertension." *Current Hypertension Reports* 4: 329–32.

Cutler, J. A. 1999. "The Effects of Reducing Sodium and Increasing Potassium Intake for Control of Hypertension and Improving Health." *Clinical and Experimental Hypertension* 21: 769–83.

Hummler, E. 2003. "Epithelial Sodium Channel, Salt Intake, and Hypertension." *Current Hypertension Reports* 5: 11–18.

Tobian, L. 1997. "Dietary Sodium Chloride and Potassium Have Effects on the Pathophysiology of Hypertension in Humans and Animals." *American Journal of Clinical Nutrition* 65: 606S–611S.

Sulfur

Di Buono, M., L. J. Wykes, R. O. Ball, and P. B. Pencharz. 2001. "Total Sulfur Amino Acid Requirement in Young Men as Determined by Indicator Amino Acid Oxidation with L-[1-13C]phenylalanine." *American Journal of Clinical Nutrition* 74: 756–60.

Di Buono, M., L. J. Wykes, D. E. Cole, R. O. Ball, and P. B. Pencharz. 2003. "Regulation of Sulfur Amino Acid Metabolism in Men in Response to Changes in Sulfur Amino Acid Intakes." *Journal of Nutrition* 133: 733–39.

Grimble, R. F. 1994. "Sulphur Amino Acids and the Metabolic Response to Cytokines." *Advances in Experimental Medicine and Biology* 359: 41–49.

Komarnisky, L. A., R. J. Christopherson, and T. K. Basu. 2003. "Sulfur: Its Clinical and Toxicologic Aspects." *Nutrition* 19: 54–61.

Lapenna, D., S. de Gioia, E. Porreca, and others. 1999. "Vascular Non-protein Thiols: Prooxidants or Antioxidants in Atherogenesis?" *Free Radical Research* 31: 487–91.

Matthews, J. O., L. L. Southern, and T. D. Bidner. 2001. "Estimation of the Total Sulfur Amino Acid Requirement and the Effect of Betaine in Diets Deficient in Total Sulfur Amino Acids for the Weanling Pig." *Journal of Animal Science* 79: 1557–65.

Parcell, S. 2002. "Sulfur in Human Nutrition and Applications in Medicine." *Alternative Medicine Review* 7: 22–44.

Chromium

Anderson, R. A. 2000. "Chromium in the Prevention and Control of Diabetes." *Diabetes and Metabolism* 26 (1): 22–27.

Han, C., X. Zhao, X. Zhang, Z. Gao, and Q. Zhu. 2000. "Formation, Photodissociation and Structure of Chromium/Phosphorus Binary Cluster Ions." *Rapid Communications in Mass Spectrometry* 14: 1255–59.

Kobla, H. V., and S. L. Volpe. 2000. "Chromium, Exercise, and Body Composition." *Critical Reviews in Food Science and Nutrition* 40 (4): 291–308.

Kumpulainen, J. T. 1992. "Chromium Content of Foods and Diets." *Biology and Trace Element Research* 32: 9–18.

Kuritzky, L., G. P. Samraj, and D. M. Quillen. 2000. "Improving Management of Type 2 Diabetes Mellitus: 6. Chromium." *Hospital Practice (Office Edition)* 35 (2): 113–16.

Vincent, J. B. 2000. "The Biochemistry of Chromium." *Journal of Nutrition* 130 (4): 715–18.

———. 2000. "Elucidating a biological role for chromium at a molecular level." *Accounts of Chemical Research* 33 (7): 503–10.

Cobalt

Barceloux, D. G. 1999. "Cobalt." *Journal of Toxicology. Clinical Toxicology* 37: 201–6.

Olson, P. A., D. R. Brink, D. T. Hickok, and others. 1999. "Effects of Supplementation of Organic and Inorganic Combinations of Copper, Cobalt, Manganese, and Zinc above Nutrient Requirement Levels on Postpartum Two-Year-Old Cows." *Journal of Animal Science* 77: 522–32.

Stangl, G. I., D. A. Roth-Maier, and M. Kirchgessner. 2000. "Vitamin B-12 Deficiency and Hyperhomocysteinemia Are Partly Ameliorated by Cobalt and Nickel Supplementation in Pigs." *Journal of Nutrition* 130: 3038–44.

Stangl, G. I., F. J. Schwarz, and M. Kirchgessner. 1999. "Cobalt Deficiency Effects on Trace Elements, Hormones, and Enzymes Involved in Energy Metabolism of Cattle." *International Journal for Vitamin and Nutrition Research* 69: 120–26.

Copper

Burkitt, M. J. 2001. "A Critical Overview of the Chemistry of Copper-Dependent Low Density Lipoprotein Oxidation: Roles of Lipid Hydroperoxides, Alpha-tocopherol, Thiols, and Ceruloplasmin." *Archives of Biochemistry and Biophysics* 394 (1): 117–35.

Harris, E. D. 2001. "Copper Homeostasis: The Role of Cellular Transporters." *Nutrition Review* 59 (9): 281–85.

Harris, E. D, Y. Qian, E. Tiffany-Castiglioni, and others. 1998. "Functional Analysis of Copper Homeostasis in Cell Culture Models: A New Perspective on Internal Copper Transport." *American Journal of Clinical Nutrition* 67: 988S-995S.

Institute of Medicine. 2001. *Dietary Reference Intakes for Vitamin A, Vitamin K, Arsenic, Boron, Chromium, Copper, Iodine, Iron, Manganese, Molybdenum, Nickel, Silicon, Vanadium, and Zinc.* Washington, D.C.: National Academy of Sciences, National Academy Press.

Nath, R. 1997. "Copper Deficiency and Heart Disease: Molecular Basis, Recent Advances, and Current Concepts." *International Journal of Biochemistry and Cell Biology* 29(11): 1245-54.

Strausak, D., J. F. Mercer, H. H. Dieter, and others. 2001. "Copper in Disorders with Neurological Symptoms: Alzheimer's, Menkes, and Wilson Diseases." *Brain Research Bulletin* 55 (2): 175–85.

Waggoner, D. J., T. B. Bartnikas, and J. D. Gitlin. 1999. "The Role of Copper in Neurodegenerative Disease." *Neurobiology of Disease* 6 (4): 221-30.

Iodine

Delange, F. 2000. "The Role of Iodine in Brain Development." *Proceedings of the Nutrition Society* (London) 59 (1): 75–79.

Dunn, J. T., and A. D. Dunn. 2001. "Update on Intrathyroidal Iodine Metabolism." *Thyroid* 11 (5): 407–14.

Feldt-Rasmussen, U. 2001. "Iodine and Cancer." *Thyroid* 11 (5): 483–86.

Institute of Medicine. 2001. *Dietary Reference Intakes for Vitamin A, Vitamin K, Arsenic, Boron, Chromium, Copper, Iodine, Iron, Manganese, Molybdenum, Nickel, Silicon, Vanadium, and Zinc.* Washington, D.C.: National Academy of Sciences, National Academy Press.

Roti, E., and E. D. Uberti. 2001. "Iodine Excess and Hyperthyroidism." *Thyroid* 11 (5): 493–500.

Ruwhof, C., and H. A. Drexhage. 2001. "Iodine and Thyroid Autoimmune Disease in Animal Models." *Thyroid* 11 (5): 427–36.

Spitzweg, C., A. E. Heufelder, and J. C. Morris. 2000. "Thyroid Iodine Transport." *Thyroid* 10 (4): 321–30.

Venturi, S., F. M. Donati, A. Venturi, and others. 2000. "Role of Iodine in Evolution and Carcinogenesis of Thyroid, Breast, and Stomach." *Advanced Clinical Pathology* 4 (1): 11–17.

Iron

Beard, J. L. 2001. "Iron Biology in Immune Function, Muscle Metabolism, and Neuronal Functioning." *Journal of Nutrition* 131 (2S–2): 568S–579S, discussion 580S.

Chiueh, C. C. 2001. "Iron Overload, Oxidative Stress, and Axonal Dystrophy in Brain Disorders." *Pediatric Neurology* 25 (2): 138–47.

Emerit, J., C. Beaumont, and F. Trivin. 2001. "Iron Metabolism, Free Radicals, and Oxidative Injury." *Biomedicine and Pharmacotherapy* 55 (6): 333–39.

Hallberg, L. 2001. "Perspectives on Nutritional Iron Deficiency." *Annual Review of Nutrition* 21: 1–21.

Institute of Medicine. 2001. *Dietary Reference Intakes for Vitamin A, Vitamin K, Arsenic, Boron, Chromium, Copper, Iodine, Iron, Manganese, Molybdenum, Nickel, Silicon, Vanadium, and Zinc.* Washington, D.C.: National Academy of Sciences, National Academy Press.

Leung, A. K., and K. W. Chan. 2001. "Iron Deficiency Anemia." *Advanced Pediatrics* 48: 385–408.

Lieu, P. T., M. Heiskala, P. A. Peterson, and Y. Yang. 2001. "The Roles of Iron in Health and Disease." *Molecular Aspects of Medicine* 22 (1–2): 1–87.

Rouault, T. A. 2001. "Systemic Iron Metabolism: A Review and Implications for Brain Iron Metabolism." *Pediatric Neurology* 25 (2): 130–37.

Roy, C. N., and N. C. Andrews. 2001. "Recent Advances in Disorders of Iron Metabolism: Mutations, Mechanisms, and Modifiers." *Human Molecular Genetics* 10 (20): 2181–86.

Thompson, K. J., S. Shoham, and J. R. Connor. 2001. "Iron and Neurodegenerative Disorders." *Brain Research Bulletin* 55 (2): 155–64.

Manganese

Aschner, M. 2000. "Manganese: Brain Transport and Emerging Research Needs." *Environmental Health Perspectives* 108 (suppl 3): 429–32.

Crowley, J. D., D. A. Traynor, and D. C. Weatherburn. 2000. "Enzymes and Proteins Containing Manganese: An Overview." *Metal Ions in Biological Systems* 37: 209–78.

Institute of Medicine. 2001. *Dietary Reference Intakes for Vitamin A, Vitamin K, Arsenic, Boron, Chromium, Copper, Iodine, Iron, Manganese, Molybdenum, Nickel, Silicon, Vanadium, and Zinc.* Washington, D.C.: National Academy of Sciences, National Academy Press.

Keen, C. L., J. L. Ensunsa, and M. S. Clegg. 2000. "Manganese Metabolism in Animals and Humans Including the Toxicity of Manganese." *Metal Ions in Biological Systems* 37: 89–121.

Yoder, D. W., J. Hwang, and J. E. Penner-Hahn. 2000. "Manganese Catalases." *Metal Ions in Biological Systems* 37: 527–57.

Molybdenum

Aupperle, H., H. A. Schoon, and A. Frank. 2001. "Experimental Copper Deficiency, Chromium Deficiency, and Additional Molybdenum Supplementation in Goats—Pathological Findings." *Acta Veterinaria Scandinavica* (Copenhagen) 42: 311–21.

Barceloux, D. G. 1999. "Molybdenum." *Journal of Toxicology. Clinical Toxicology* 37: 231–37.

Chan, S., B. Gerson, and S. Subramaniam. 1998. "The Role of Copper, Molybdenum, Selenium, and Zinc in Nutrition and Health." *Clinics in Laboratory Medicine* 18: 673–85.

Failla, M. L. 1999. "Considerations for Determining 'Optimal Nutrition' for Copper, Zinc, Manganese, and Molybdenum." *Proceedings of the Nutrition Society* (London) 58: 497–505.

Gengelbach, G. P., and J. W. Spears. 1998. "Effects of Dietary Copper and Molybdenum on Copper Status, Cytokine Production, and Humoral Immune Response of Calves." *Journal of Dairy Science* 81: 3286–92.

Hunt, C. D., and S. L. Meacham. 2001. "Aluminum, Boron, Calcium, Copper, Iron, Magnesium, Manganese, Molybdenum, Phosphorus, Potassium, Sodium, and Zinc: Concentrations in Common Western Foods and Estimated Daily Intakes by Infants; Toddlers; and Male and Female Adolescents, Adults, and Seniors in the United States." *Journal of the American Dietetic Association* 101: 1058–60.

Turnlund, J. R. 2002. "Molybdenum Metabolism and Requirements in Humans." *Metal Ions in Biological Systems* 39: 727–39.

Turnlund, J. R., C. M. Weaver, S. K. Kim, and others. 1999. "Molybdenum Absorption and Utilization in Humans from Soy and Kale Intrinsically Labeled with Stable Isotopes of Molybdenum." *American Journal of Clinical Nutrition* 69: 1217–23.

Vyskocil, A., and C. Viau. 1999. "Assessment of Molybdenum Toxicity in Humans." *Journal of Applied Toxicology* 19: 185–92.

Selenium

Abrams, C. K., S. M. Siram, C. Galsim, and others. 1992. "Selenium Deficiency in Long-Term Total Parenteral Nutrition." *Nutrition in Clinical Practice* 7: 175–78.

Badmaev, V., M. Muhammed, and R. A. Passwater. 1996. "Selenium: A Quest for Better Understanding." *Alternative Therapies* 2 (4): 59–67.

Diplock, A. T. 1992. "Selenium, Antioxidant Nutritions, and Human Diseases." *Biological Trace Element Research* 33: 155–56.

Finley, J. W., L. Matthys, T. Shuler, and others. 1996. "Selenium Content of Foods Purchased in North Dakota." *Nutrition Research* 16: 723–28.

Ge, K., and G. Yang. 1993. "The Epidemiology of Selenium Deficiency in the Etiological Study of Endemic Diseases in China. *American Journal of Clinical Nutrition* 57: 259S–263S.

Lane, H. W., C. A. Lotspeich, C. E. Moore, and others. 1987. "The Effect of Selenium Supplementation on Selenium Status of Patients Receiving Chronic Total Parenteral Nutrition." *JPEN. Journal of Parenteral and Enteral Nutrition* 11: 177–82.

Mascio, P. D., M. E. Murphy, and H. Sies. 1991. "Antioxidant Defense Systems: The Role of Carotenoids, Tocopherols, and Thiols." *American Journal of Clinical Nutrition* 53: 194S–200S.

Meiners, C. R., N. L. Derise, H. C. Lau, and others. 1976. "The Content of Nine Mineral Elements in Raw and Cooked Mature Dry Legumes." *Journal of Agricultural and Food Chemistry* 24: 1126–30.

Moriarty, P. M., M. F. Picciano, J. Beard, and others. 1993. "Iron Deficiency Decreases Se–GPX MRNA Level in the Liver and Impairs Selenium Utilization in Other Tissues." *FASEB Journal* 7: A277.

Nishiyama, S., Y. Futagoishi-Suginohara, M. Matsukura, and others. 1994. "Zinc Supplementation Alters Thyroid Hormone Metabolism in Disabled Patients with Zinc Deficiency." *Journal of the American College of Nutrition* 13: 62–67.

Olin, K. L., R. M. Walter, and C. L. Keen. 1994. "Copper Deficiency Affects Selenoglutathione Peroxidase and Selenodeiodinase Activities and Antioxidant Defense in Weanling Rats." *American Journal of Clinical Nutrition* 59: 654–58.

Pedersen, B., and B. O. Eggum. 1983. "The Influence of Milling on the Nutritive Value of Flour from Cereal Grains. Part 2. Wheat." *Qualification of Plant Foods in Human Nutrition* 33: 51–61.

Stone, J., A. Doube, D. Dudson, and others. 1997. "Inadequate Calcium, Folic Acid, Vitamin E, Zinc, and Selenium Intake in Rheumatoid Arthritis Patients: Results of a Dietary Survey." *Seminars in Arthritis and Rheumatism* 27 (3): 180–85.

Silicon

Jugdaohsingh, R., S. H. Anderson, K. L. Tucker, and others. 2002. "Dietary Silicon Intake and Absorption." *American Journal of Clinical Nutrition* 75: 887–93.

Seaborn, C. D., M. Briske-Anderson, and F. H. Nielsen. 2002. "An Interaction between Dietary Silicon and Arginine Affects Immune Function Indicated by Con-A-induced DNA Synthesis of Rat Splenic T-lymphocytes." *Biological Trace Element Research* 87: 133–42.

Seaborn, C. D., and F. H. Nielsen. 2002. "Dietary Silicon and Arginine Affect Mineral Element Composition of Rat Femur and Vertebra." *Biological Trace Element Research* 89: 239–50.

———. 2002. "Silicon Deprivation Decreases Collagen Formation in Wounds and Bone, and Ornithine Transaminase Enzyme Activity in Liver." *Biological Trace Element Research* 89: 251–61.

Shenkin, A. 2003. "Dietary Reference Values for Vitamin A, Vitamin K, Arsenic, Boron, Chromium, Copper, Iodine, Iron, Manganese, Molybdenum, Nickel, Silicon, Vanadium, and Zinc." *Journal of Human Nutrition and Dietetics* 16: 199–200.

Trumbo, P., A. A. Yates, S. Schlicker, and M. Poos. 2001. "Dietary Reference Intakes: Vitamin A, Vitamin K, Arsenic, Boron, Chromium, Copper, Iodine, Iron, Manganese, Molybdenum, Nickel, Silicon, Vanadium, and Zinc." *Journal of the American Dietetic Association* 101: 294–301.

Zinc

Boyle, P., G. Severi, and G. G. Giles. 2003. "The Epidemiology of Prostate Cancer." *Urology Clinics of North America* 30: 209–17.

Chandra, R. K. 1990. "Micronutrients and Immune Functions." *Annals of the New York Academy of Sciences* 587: 9–16.

Dunn, M. A., T. L. Blalock, and R. J. Cousins. 1987. "Metallothionein." *Proceedings of the Society for Experimental Biology and Medicine* 187: 107–19.

Festa, M. D., H. L. Anderson, R. P. Dowdy, and others. 1985. "Effect of Zinc Intake on Copper Excretion and Retention in Men." *American Journal of Clinical Nutrition* 41: 285–92.

Forbes, R. M., and J. W. Erdman Jr. 1983. "Bioavailability of Trace Mineral Elements." *Annual Review of Nutrition* 2: 213–31.

Hambridge, K. M., C. E. Casey, and N. F. Krebs. "Zinc." In W. Mertz, ed., *Trace Elements in Human and Animal Nutrition.* Fifth edition, volume 2. Orlando, Florida: Academic Press.

Neuhouser, M. L., A. R. Kristal, R. E. Patterson, P. J. Goodman, and I. M. Thompson. 2001. "Dietary Supplement Use in the Prostate Cancer Prevention Trial: Implications for Prevention Trials." *Nutrition and Cancer* 39: 12–18.

Patterson, R. E., E. White, A. R. Kristal, M. L. Neuhouser, and J. D. Potter. 1997. "Vitamin Supplements and Cancer Risk: The Epidemiologic Evidence." *Cancer Causes and Control* 8: 786–802.

Prasad, A. S., A. O. Cavdar, G. J. Brewer, and others. 1983. *Zinc Deficiency in Human Subjects.* New York: Alan R. Liss.

Solomons, N. W., and R. J. Cousins. 1984. "Zinc." In N. W. Solomons and I. H. Rosenberg, eds., *Absorption and Malabsorption of Mineral Nutrients.* New York: Alan R. Liss.

Spencer, H. 1986. "Minerals and Mineral Interactions in Human Beings." *Journal of the American Dietetic Association* 86: 864–67.

Wada, L., and J. C. King. 1986. "Effect of Low Zinc Intakes on Basal Metabolic Rate, Thyroid Hormones, and Protein Utilization in Adult Men." *Journal of Nutrition* 116: 1045–53.

Wu, F. Y. H., and C. W. Wu. 1987. "Zinc in DNA Replication and Transcription." *Annual Review of Nutrition* 7: 251–72.

Boron

Coughlin, J. R. 1998. "Sources of Human Exposure: Overview of Water Supplies as Sources of Boron." *Biological Trace Element Research* 66: 87–100.

Groziak, M. P. 2001. "Boron Therapeutics on the Horizon." *American Journal of Therapeutics* 8: 321–28.

Hunt, C. D. 1998. "Regulation of Enzymatic Activity: One Possible Role of Dietary Boron in Higher Animals and Humans." *Biological Trace Element Research* 66: 205–25.

Naghii, M. R. 1999. "The Significance of Dietary Boron, with Particular Reference to Athletes." *Nutrition and Health* 13: 31–37.

Nielsen, F. H. 2000. "The Emergence of Boron as Nutritionally Important throughout the Life Cycle." *Nutrition* 16: 512–14.

———. 1998. "The Justification for Providing Dietary Guidance for the Nutritional Intake of Boron." *Biological Trace Element Research* 66: 319–30.

Penland, J. G. 1998. "The Importance of Boron Nutrition for Brain and Psychological Function." *Biological Trace Element Research* 66: 299–317.

Rainey, C. J., L. A. Nyquist, R. E. Christensen, P. L. Strong, B. D. Culver, and J. R. Coughlin. 1999. "Daily Boron Intake from the American Diet." *Journal of the American Dietetic Association* 99: 335–40.

Samman, S., M. R. Naghii, P. M. Lyons Wall, and A. P. Verus. 1998. "The Nutritional and Metabolic Effects of Boron in Humans and Animals." *Biological Trace Element Research* 66: 227–35.

Fluoride

Hillier, S., C. Cooper, S. Kellingray, G. Russell, D. Coggon, and others. 2000. "Fluoride in Drinking Water and Risk of Hip Fracture in the UK: Case-Control Study." *Lancet* 355 (January): 265–269 (ref 27).

Lau, K. H, C. Goodwin, M. Arias, S. Mohan, and D. J. Baylink. 2002. "Bone Cell Mitogenic Action of Fluoroaluminate and Aluminum Fluoride but Not That of Sodium Fluoride Involves Upregulation of the Insulin-like Growth Factor System." *Bone* 30: 705–11.

Li, Y., C. K. Liang, B. P. Katz, E. J. Brizendine, and G. K. Stookey. 1995. "Long-Term Exposure to Fluoride in Drinking Water and Sister Chromatid Exchange Frequency in Human Blood Lymphocytes." *Journal of Dental Research* 74 (8): 1468–74

Luoma, H., A. Aromaa, S. Helminen, H. Murtomaa, L. Kiviluoto, S. Punsar, and P. Knekt. 1983. "Risk of Myocardial Infarction in Finnish Men in Relation to Fluoride, Magnesium, and Calcium Concentration in Drinking Water." *Acta Medica Scandinavica* 213 (3): 171–76, 33 references.

Ramesh, N., A. S. Vuayaraghavan, B. S. Desai, M. Natarajan, P. B. Murthy, and K. S. Pillai. 2001. "Low Levels of P53 Mutations in Indian Patients with Osteosarcoma and the Correlation with Fluoride Levels in Bone." *Journal of Environmental Pathology, Toxicology, and Oncology* 20: 237–43.

Smith, G. E. 1988. "Fluoride and Fluoridation." *Social Science and Medicine* 26 (4): 451–62.

Swenberg, J. A., M. S. Bogdanffy, A. Ham, and others. 1999. "Formation and Repair of DNA Adducts in Vinyl Chloride–and Vinyl Fluoride–Induced Carcinogenesis." *IARC Scientific Publications* (Lyon) 150: 29–43.

Takahashi, K., K. Akiniwa, and K. Narita. 2001. "Regression Analysis of Cancer Incidence Rates and Water Fluoride in the U.S.A. Based on IACR/IARC (WHO) Data (1978–1992). International Agency for Research on Cancer." *Journal of Epidemiology* 11: 170–79.

Yang, C. Y., M. F. Cheng, S. S. Tsai, and C. F. Hung. 2000. "Fluoride in Drinking Water and Cancer Mortality in Taiwan." *Environmental Research* 82: 189–93.

Germanium

Fujii, A., N. Kuboyama, J. Yamane, S. Nakao, and Y. Furukawa. 1993. "Effect of Organic Germanium Compound (Ge-132) on Experimental Osteoporosis in Rats." *General Pharmacology* 24: 1527–32.

Gerber, G. B., and A. Leonard. 1997. "Mutagenicity, Carcinogenicity, and Teratogenicity of Germanium Compounds." *Mutation Research* 387: 141–46.

Schauss, A. G. 1991. "Nephrotoxicity in Humans by the Ultratrace Element Germanium." *Renal Failure* 13: 1–4.

Seaborn, C. D., and F. H. Nielsen. 1994. "Effects of Germanium and Silicon on Bone Mineralization." *Biological Trace Element Research* 42: 151–64.

Tao, S. H., and P. M. Bolger. 1997. "Hazard Assessment of Germanium Supplements." *Regulatory Toxicology and Pharmacology* 25: 211–19.

Unakar, N. J., M. Johnson, J. Tsui, M. Cherian, and E. C. Abraham. 1995. "Effect of Germanium-132 on Galactose Cataracts and Glycation in Rats." *Experimental Eye Research* 61: 155–64.

Yu, B., J. Wu, and X. Zhou. 1995. "Interference of Selenium, Germanium, and Calcium in Carcinogenesis of Colon Cancer." *Zhonghua Wai Ke Za Zhi* (Beijing) 33: 167–69.

Lithium

Agranoff, B. W., and S. K. Fisher. 2001. "Inositol, Lithium, and the Brain." *Psychopharmacology Bulletin* 35: 5–18.

Coppen, A. 1967. "The Biochemistry of Affective Disorders." *British Journal of Psychiatry* 113: 1237–64.

Coppen, A., C. Swade, S. A. Jones, R. A. Armstrong, J. A. Blair, and R. J. Leeming. 1989. "Depression and Tetrahydrobiopterin: The Folate Connection." *Journal of Affective Disorders* 16: 103–7.

Nabrzyski, M., and R. Gajewska R. 2002. "Content of Strontium, Lithium, and Calcium in Selected Milk Products and in Some Marine Smoked Fish." *Nahrung* (Berlin) 46: 204–8.

Phiel, C. J., and P. S. Klein. 2001. "Molecular Targets of Lithium Action." *Annual Review of Pharmacology and Toxicology* 41:789–813.

Romero, J. R., A. Rivera, A. Monari, G. Ceolotto, A. Semplicini, and P. R. Conlin. 2002. "Increased Red Cell Sodium-Lithium Countertransport and Lymphocyte Cytosolic Calcium Are Separate Phenotypes in Patients with Essential Hypertension." *Journal of Human Hypertension* 16: 353–58.

Sattin, A., S. S. Senanayake, and A. E. Pekary. 2002. "Lithium Modulates Expression of TRH Receptors and TRH-related Peptides in Rat Brain." *Neuroscience* 115: 263–73.

Wang, H. Y., G. P. Johnson, and E. Friedman. 2001. "Lithium Treatment Inhibits Protein Kinase C Translocation in Rat Brain Cortex." *Psychopharmacology* (Berlin) 158: 80–86.

York, J. D., S. Guo, A. R. Odom, B. D. Spiegelberg, and L. E. Stolz. 2001. "An Expanded View of Inositol Signaling." *Advances in Enzyme Regulation* 41: 57–71.

Zhen, X., C. Torres, and E. Friedman. 2002. "Lithium Regulates Protein Tyrosine Phosphatase Activity In Vitro and In Vivo." *Psychopharmacology* (Berlin) 162: 379–84.

Nickel

Barceloux, D. G. 1999. "Nickel." *Journal of Toxicology. Clinical Toxicology* 37: 239–58.

Berg, T., A. Petersen, G. A. Pedersen, J. Petersen, and C. Madsen. 2000. "The Release of Nickel and Other Trace Elements from Electric Kettles and Coffee Machines." *Food Additives and Contaminants* 17: 189–96.

Cangul, H., L. Broday, K. Salnikow, and others. 2002. "Molecular Mechanisms of Nickel Carcinogenesis." *Toxicology Letters* 127: 69–75.

Costa, M. 2002. "Molecular Mechanisms of Nickel Carcinogenesis." *Biology and Chemistry* 383: 961–67.

Costa, M., K. Salnikow, J. E. Sutherland, and others. 2002. "The Role of Oxidative Stress in Nickel and Chromate Genotoxicity." *Molecular and Cellular Biochemistry* 234–35, 265–75.

Denkhaus, E., and K. Salnikow. 2002. "Nickel Essentiality, Toxicity, and Carcinogenicity." *Critical Review of Oncology and Hematology* 42: 35–56.

Nielsen, G. D., U. Soderberg, P. J. Jorgensen, and others. 1999. "Absorption and Retention of Nickel from Drinking Water in Relation to Food Intake and Nickel Sensitivity." *Toxicology and Applied Pharmacology* 154: 67–75.

Stangl, G. I., D. A. Roth-Maier, and M. Kirchgessner. 2000. "Vitamin B-12 Deficiency and Hyperhomocysteinemia Are Partly Ameliorated by Cobalt and Nickel Supplementation in Pigs." *Journal of Nutrition* 130: 3038–44.

Ysart, G., P. Miller, M. Croasdale, and others. 2000. "1997 UK Total Diet Study—Dietary Exposures to Aluminium, Arsenic, Cadmium, Chromium, Copper, Lead, Mercury, Nickel, Selenium, Tin, and Zinc." *Food Additives and Contaminants* 17: 775–86.

Rubidium

Canavese, C., E. DeCostanzi, L. Branciforte, and others. 2001. "Rubidium Deficiency in Dialysis Patients." *Journal of Nephrology* 14: 169–75.

Dranitzki, Z., C. Shenberg, and R. Gale. 1993. "Rubidium: Essential Trace Element or Random Companion?" *Harefuah* (Tel Aviv) 124: 422–24.

Selin, E., and V. Teeyasoontranont. 1991. "Rubidium: A Companion of Potassium or an Essential Trace Element of Its Own? *Beitrage zur Infusionstherapie* (Basel) 27: 86–103.

Sopranzi, N. 1993. "Chronic Administration of Lithium and Rubidium in Rats: General Behavior, Explorative Behavior, and Electric Activity of the Brain." *Clinica Terapeutica* (Rome) 142: 211–18.

Wang, H., and D. G. Grahame-Smith. 1992. "The Effects of Rubidium, Caesium, and Quinine on 5-HT-mediated Behaviour in Rat and Mouse—1. Rubidium." *Neuropharmacology* 31: 413–19.

Yokoi, K., M. Kimura, and Y. Itokawa. 1996. "Effect of Low Dietary Rubidium on Plasma Biochemical Parameters and Mineral Levels in Rats." *Biological Trace Element Research* 51: 199–208.

Strontium

Cabrera, W. E., I. Schrooten, M. E. De Broe, and P. C. D'Haese. 1999. "Strontium and Bone." *Journal of Bone and Mineral Research* 14: 661–68.

Cohen-Solal, M. 2002. "Strontium Overload and Toxicity: Impact on Renal Osteodystrophy." *Nephrology, Dialysis, Transplantation* (Berlin) 17 (suppl 2): 30–34.

Delannoy, P., D. Bazot, and P. J. Marie. 2002. "Long-Term Treatment with Strontium Ranelate Increases Vertebral Bone Mass without Deleterious Effect in Mice." *Metabolism* 51: 906–11.

Dijkgraaf-Ten Bolscher, M., J. C. Netelenbos, R. Barto, and W. J. van Der Vijgh. 2000. "Strontium as a Marker for Intestinal Calcium Absorption: The Stimulatory Effect of Calcitriol." *Clinical Chemistry* 46: 248–51.

Marie, P. J., P. Ammann, G. Boivin, and C. Rey. 2001. "Mechanisms of Action and Therapeutic Potential of Strontium in Bone." *Calcified Tissue International* 69: 121–29.

Morohashi, T., T. Sano, K. Harai, and S. Yamada. 1995. "Effects of Strontium on Calcium Metabolism in Rats. II. Strontium Prevents the Increased Rate of Bone Turnover in Ovariectomized Rats." *Japanese Journal of Pharmacology* (Kyoto) 68: 153–59.

Ozgur, S., H. Sumer, and G. Kocoglu. 1996. "Rickets and Soil Strontium." *Archive of Diseases in Childhood. Fetal and Neonatal Edition* 75: 524–26.

Sips, A. J., W. J. van der Vijgh, R. Barto, and J. C. Netelenbos. 1996. "Intestinal Absorption of Strontium Chloride in Healthy Volunteers: Pharmacokinetics and Reproducibility." *British Journal of Clinical Pharmacology* 41: 543–49.

Tin

Beynen, A. C., H. L. Pekelharing, and A. G. Lemmens. 1992. "High Intakes of Tin Lower Iron Status in Rats." *Biological Trace Element Research* 35: 85–88.

Biego, G. H., M. Joyeux, P. Hartemann, and G. Debry. 1999. "Determination of Dietary Tin Intake in an Adult French Citizen." *Archives of Environmental Contamination and Toxicology* 36: 227–32.

Jin, K. W. 1989. "Pathological Survey of Lung Cancer Induced by Tin Mine Dust in Yunnan." *Zhonghua Bing Li Xue Za Zhi* (Beijing) 18: 204–6.

Nagy, L., A. Szorcsik, and K. Kovacs. 2000. "Tin Compounds in Pharmacy and Nutrition." *Acta Pharmaceutica Hungarica* (Budapest) 70: 53–71.

Pekelharing, H. L., A. G. Lemmens, and A. C. Beynen. 1994. "Iron, Copper, and Zinc Status in Rats Fed on Diets Containing Various Concentrations of Tin." *British Journal of Nutrition* 71: 103–9.

Rader, J. I. 1991. "Anti-nutritive Effects of Dietary Tin." *Advances in Experimental Medicine and Biology* 289: 509–24.

Reicks, M., and J. I. Rader. 1990. "Effects of Dietary Tin and Copper on Rat Hepatocellular Antioxidant Protection." *Proceedings of the Society for Experimental Biology and Medicine* 195: 123–28.

Yokoi, K., M. Kimura, and Y. Itokawa. 1990. "Effect of Dietary Tin Deficiency on Growth and Mineral Status in Rats." *Biological Trace Element Research* 24: 223–31.

Ysart, G., P. Miller, M. Croasdale, and others. 2000. "1997 UK Total Diet Study—Dietary Exposures to Aluminium, Arsenic, Cadmium, Chromium, Copper, Lead, Mercury, Nickel, Selenium, Tin, and Zinc." *Food Additives and Contaminants* 17: 775–86.

Yu, S., and A. C. Beynen. 1995. "High Tin Intake Reduces Copper Status in Rats through Inhibition of Copper Absorption." *British Journal of Nutrition* 73: 863–69.

Vanadium

Basak, R., and M. Chatterjee. 2000. "Combined Supplementation of Vanadium and 1alpha,25-dihydroxyvitamin D3 Inhibit Placental Glutathione S-transferase Positive Foci in Rat Liver Carcinogenesis." *Life Science* 68: 217–231.

Cam, M. C., R. W. Brownsey, and J. H. McNeill. 2000. "Mechanisms of Vanadium Action: Insulin-Mimetic or Insulin-Enhancing Agent?" *Canadian Journal of Physiology and Pharmacology* 78: 829–47.

Crans, D. C. 2000. "Chemistry and Insulin-like Properties of Vanadium(IV) and Vanadium(V) Compounds." *Journal of Inorganic Biochemistry* 80: 123–31.

Goldwaser, I., D. Gefel, E. Gershonov, M. Fridkin, and Y. Shechter. 2000. "Insulin-like Effects of Vanadium: Basic and Clinical Implications." *Journal of Inorganic Biochemistry* 80: 21–25.

Poggioli, R., R. Arletti, A. Bertolini, C. Frigeri, and A. Benelli. 2001. "Behavioral and Developmental Outcomes of Prenatal and Postnatal Vanadium Exposure in the Rat." *Pharmacology Research* 43: 341–47.

Sakurai, H. 2002. "A New Concept: The Use of Vanadium Complexes in the Treatment of Diabetes Mellitus." *Chemical Record* 2: 237–48.

Shafrir, E., S. Spielman, I. Nachliel, M. Khamaisi, H. Bar-On, and E. Ziv. 2001. "Treatment of Diabetes with Vanadium Salts: General Overview and Amelioration of Nutritionally Induced Diabetes in the Psammomys Obesus Gerbil." *Diabetes and Metabolism Research Review* 17: 55–66.

Trumbo, P., A. A. Yates, S. Schlicker, and M. Poos. 2001. "Dietary Reference Intakes: Vitamin A, Vitamin K, Arsenic, Boron, Chromium, Copper, Iodine, Iron, Manganese, Molybdenum, Nickel, Silicon, Vanadium, and Zinc." *Journal of the American Dietetic Association* 101: 294–301.

Willsky, G. R., A. B. Goldfine, P. J. Kostyniak, and others. 2001. "Effect of Vanadium(IV) Compounds in the Treatment of Diabetes: In Vivo and In Vitro Studies with Vanadyl Sulfate and Bis(maltolato)oxovanadium(IV)." *Journal of Inorganic Biochemistry* 85: 33–42.

Aluminum

Baylor, N. W., W. Egan, and P. Richman. 2002. "Aluminum Salts in Vaccines—U.S. Perspective." *Vaccine* 20 (suppl 3): S18–S23.

Jugdaohsingh, R., D. M. Reffitt, C. Oldham, and others. 2000. "Oligomeric but Not Monomeric Silica Prevents Aluminum Absorption in Humans." *American Journal of Clinical Nutrition* 71: 944–49.

Keith, L. S., D. E. Jones, and C. H. Chou. 2002. "Aluminum Toxicokinetics Regarding Infant Diet and Vaccinations." *Vaccine* 20 (suppl 3): S13–S17.

Lopez, F. E., C. Cabrera, M. L. Lorenzo, and M. C. Lopez. 2002. "Aluminum Levels in Convenience and Fast Foods: In Vitro Study of the Absorbable Fraction." *Science of the Total Environment* (Amsterdam) 300: 69–79.

Nayak, P. 2002. "Aluminum: Impacts and Disease." *Environmental Research* 89: 101–15.

Pratico, D., K. Uryu, S. Sung, S. Tang, J. Q. Trojanowski, and V. M. Lee. 2002. "Aluminum Modulates Brain Amyloidosis through Oxidative Stress in APP Transgenic Mice." *FASEB Journal* 16: 1138–40.

Rondeau, V. 2002. "A Review of Epidemiologic Studies on Aluminum and Silica in Relation to Alzheimer's Disease and Associated Disorders." *Reviews on Environmental Health* (Tel Aviv) 17: 107–21.

Soni, M. G., S. M. White, W. G. Flamm, and G. A. Burdock. 2001. "Safety Evaluation of Dietary Aluminum." *Regulatory Toxicology and Pharmacology* 33: 66–79.

Arsenic

Calderon, J., M. E. Navarro, M. E. Jimenez-Capdeville, and others. 2001. "Exposure to Arsenic and Lead and Neuropsychological Development in Mexican Children." *Environmental Research* 85: 69–76.

Cooney, C. A. 2001. "Dietary Selenium and Arsenic Affect DNA Methylation." *Journal of Nutrition* 131: 1871–72.

Llobet, J. M., G. Falco, C. Casas, A. Teixido, and J. L. Domingo. 2003. "Concentrations of Arsenic, Cadmium, Mercury, and Lead in Common Foods and Estimated Daily Intake by Children, Adolescents, Adults, and Seniors of Catalonia, Spain." *Journal of Agriculture Food Chemistry* 51: 838–42.

McDorman, E. W., B. W. Collins, and J. W. Allen. 2002. "Dietary Folate Deficiency Enhances Induction of Micronuclei by Arsenic in Mice." *Environmental and Molecular Mutagenesis* 40: 71–77.

Perez-Granados, A. M., and M. P. Vaquero. 2002. "Silicon, Aluminium, Arsenic, and Lithium: Essentiality and Human Health Implications." *Journal of Nutrition, Health, and Aging* 6: 154–62.

Pesch, B., U. Ranft, P. Jakubis, and others. 2002. "Environmental Arsenic Exposure from a Coal-Burning Power Plant as a Potential Risk Factor for Nonmelanoma Skin Carcinoma: Results from a Case-Control Study in the District of Prievidza, Slovakia." *American Journal of Epidemiology* 155: 798–809.

Prestera, T., W. D. Holtzclaw, Y. Zhang, and P. Talalay. 1993. "Chemical and Molecular Regulation of Enzymes That Detoxify Carcinogens." *Proceedings of the National Academy of Sciences* 90: 2965–69.

Quig, D. 1998. "Cysteine Metabolism and Metal Toxicity." *Alternative Medicine Review* 3: 262–70.

Shenkin, A. 2003. "Dietary Reference Values for Vitamin A, Vitamin K, Arsenic, Boron, Chromium, Copper, Iodine, Iron, Manganese, Molybdenum, Nickel, Silicon, Vanadium, and Zinc." *Journal of Human Nutrition and Dietetics* 16: 199–200.

Smith, A. H., P. A. Lopipero, M. N. Bates, and C. M. Steinmaus. 2002. "Public Health: Arsenic Epidemiology and Drinking Water Standards." *Science* 296: 2145–46.

Trumbo, P., A. A. Yates, S. Schlicker, and M. Poos. 2001. "Dietary Reference Intakes: Vitamin A, Vitamin K, Arsenic, Boron, Chromium, Copper, Iodine, Iron, Manganese, Molybdenum, Nickel, Silicon, Vanadium, and Zinc." *Journal of the American Dietetic Association* 101: 294–301.

Ysart, G., P. Miller, M. Croasdale, and others. 2000. "1997 UK Total Diet Study—Dietary Exposures to Aluminium, Arsenic, Cadmium, Chromium, Copper, Lead, Mercury, Nickel, Selenium, Tin, and Zinc." *Food Additives and Contaminants* 17: 775–86.

Cadmium

Brzoska, M. M., and J. Moniuszko-Jakoniuk. 2001. "Interactions between Cadmium and Zinc in the Organism." *Food and Chemical Toxicology* (Oxford) 39: 967–80.

Himeno, S., T. Yanagiya, S. Enomoto, Y. Kondo, and N. Imura. 2002. "Cellular Cadmium Uptake Mediated by the Transport System for Manganese." *Tohoku Journal of Experimental Medicine* 196: 43–50.

Satarug, S., J. R. Baker, S. Urbenjapol, and others. 2003. "A Global Perspective on Cadmium Pollution and Toxicity in Non-occupationally Exposed Population." *Toxicology Letters* 137: 65–83.

Shukla, A., G. S. Shukla, and R. C. Srimal. 1996. "Cadmium-Induced Alterations in Blood-Brain Barrier Permeability and Its Possible Correlation with Decreased Microvessel Antioxidant Potential in Rats." *Human Experimental Toxicology* 15: 400–5.

Skoczynska, A., R. Poreba, A. Sieradzki, R. Andrzejak, and U. Sieradzka. 2002. "The Impact of Lead and Cadmium on the Immune System." *Medycyna Pracy* (Warsaw) 53: 259–64.

Takeda, A., M. Suzuki, and N. Oku. 2002. "Possible Involvement of Plasma Histidine in Differential Brain Permeability to Zinc and Cadmium." *Biometals* 15: 371–75.

Thevenod, F. 2003. "Nephrotoxicity and the Proximal Tubule: Insights from Cadmium." *Nephron Physiology* 93: 87–93.

Verougstraete, V., D. Lison, and P. Hotz. 2003. "Cadmium, Lung, and Prostate Cancer: A Systematic Review of Recent Epidemiological Data." *Journal of Toxicology and Environmental Health Part B: Critical Reviews* 6: 227–55.

Zalups, R. K., and S. Ahmad. 2003. "Molecular Handling of Cadmium in Transporting Epithelia." *Toxicology and Applied Pharmacology* 186: 163–88.

Lead

de la Fuente, H., D. Portales-Perez, L. Baranda, and others. 2002. "Effect of Arsenic, Cadmium, and Lead on the Induction of Apoptosis of Normal Human Mononuclear Cells." *Clinical and Experimental Immunology* 129: 69–77.

Flora, S. J. 2002. "Lead Exposure: Health Effects, Prevention, and Treatment." *Journal of Environmental Biology* 23: 25–41.

Harris, S., and B. L. Harper. 2001. "Lifestyles, Diets, and Native American Exposure Factors Related to Possible Lead Exposures and Toxicity." *Environmental Research* 86: 140–48.

He, L., A. T. Poblenz, C. J. Medrano, and D. A. Fox. 2000. "Lead and Calcium Produce Rod Photoreceptor Cell Apoptosis by Opening the Mitochondrial Permeability Transition Pore." *Journal of Biology and Chemistry* 275: 12175–84.

Houston, D. K., and M. A. Johnson. 2000. "Does Vitamin C Intake Protect against Lead Toxicity?" *Nutrition Review* 58: 73–75.

Kalcher, K., W. Kern, and R. Pietsch. 1993. "Cadmium and Lead in the Smoke of a Filter Cigarette." *Science of the Total Environment* (Amsterdam) 128: 21–35.

Lidsky, T. I., and J. S. Schneider. 2003. "Lead Neurotoxicity in Children: Basic Mechanisms and Clinical Correlates." *Brain* 126: 5–19.

Oberto, A., N. Marks, H. L. Evans, and A. Guidotti. 1996. "Lead (Pb+2) Promotes Apoptosis in Newborn Rat Cerebellar Neurons: Pathological Implications." *Journal of Pharmacology and Experimental Therapeutics* 279: 435–42.

Piomelli, S. 2002. "Childhood Lead Poisoning." *Pediatric Clinics of North America* 49: 1285–304, vii.

Qian, Y., and E. Tiffany-Castiglioni. 2003. "Lead-Induced Endoplasmic Reticulum (ER) Stress Responses in the Nervous System." *Neurochemical Research* 28: 153–62.

Quig, D. 1998. "Cysteine Metabolism and Metal Toxicity." *Alternative Medicine Review* 3: 262–70.

Sanborn, M. D., A. Abelsohn, M. Campbell, and E. Weir. 2002. "Identifying and Managing Adverse Environmental Health Effects: 3. Lead Exposure." *Canadian Medical Association Journal* 166: 1287–92.

Shabani, A., and A. Rabbani. 2000. "Lead Nitrate Induced Apoptosis in Alveolar Macrophages from Rat Lung." *Toxicology* 149: 109–14.

Torrence, K. M., R. L. McDaniel, D. A. Self, and M. J. Chang. 2002. "Slurry Sampling for the Determination of Arsenic, Cadmium, and Lead in Mainstream Cigarette Smoke Condensate by Graphite Furnace–Atomic Absorption Spectrometry and Inductively Coupled Plasma-Mass Spectrometry." *Annales de Biologie Clinique* (Paris) 372: 723–31.

Mercury

Ahlqwist, M., C. Bengtsson, L. Lapidus, I. A. Gergdahl, and A. Schutz. 1999. "Serum Mercury Concentration in Relation to Survival, Symptoms, and Diseases: Results from the Prospective Population Study of Women in Gothenburg, Sweden." *Acta Odontologica Scandinavica* (Oslo) 57: 168–74.

Andre, J., A. Boudou, F. Ribeyre, and M. Bernhard. 1991. "Comparative Study of Mercury Accumulation in Dolphins (Stenella Coeruleoalba) from French Atlantic and Mediterranean Coasts." *Science of the Total Environment* (Amsterdam) 104: 191–209.

Aschner, M., and S. J. Walker. 2002. "The Neuropathogenesis of Mercury Toxicity." *Molecular Psychiatry* 7 (suppl 2): S40–S41.

Bernard, S., A. Enayati, H. Roger, T. Binstock, and L. Redwood. 2002. "The Role of Mercury in the Pathogenesis of Autism." *Molecular Psychiatry* 7 (suppl 2): S42–S43.

Burger, J., C. Dixon, C. S. Boring, and M. Gochfeld. 2003. "Effect of Deep-Frying Fish on Risk from Mercury." *Journal of Toxicology and Environmental Health* 66: 817–28.

Chapman, L., and H. M. Chan. 2000. "The Influence of Nutrition on Methyl Mercury Intoxication." *Environmental Health Perspectives* 108 (suppl 1): 29–56.

Choy, C. M., C. W. Lam, L. T. Cheung, C. M. Briton-Jones, L. P. Cheung, and C. J. Haines. 2002. "Infertility, Blood Mercury Concentrations, and Dietary Seafood Consumption: A Case-Control Study." *BJOG: An International Journal of Obstetrics and Gynecology* (London) 109: 1121–25.

Gundacker, C., B. Pietschnig, K. J. Wittmann, and others. 2002. "Lead and Mercury in Breast Milk." *Pediatrics* 110: 873–78.

Hood, E. 2003. "A Diet Rich in Fish: High-End Consumers Face More Mercury Risks." *Environmental Health Perspectives* 111: A233.

Inasmasu, T., A. Ogo, M. Yanagawa, and others. 1986. "Mercury Concentration Change in Human Hair after the Ingestion of Canned Tuna Fish." *Bulletin of Environmental Contamination and Toxicology* 37: 475–81.

Kales, S. N., and R. H. Goldman. 2002. "Mercury Exposure: Current Concepts, Controversies, and a Clinic's Experience." *Journal of Occupational and Environmental Medicine* 44: 143–54.

Llobet, J. M., G. Falco, C. Casas, A. Teixido, and J. L. Domingo. 2003. "Concentrations of Arsenic, Cadmium, Mercury, and Lead in Common Foods and Estimated Daily Intake by Children, Adolescents, Adults, and Seniors of Catalonia, Spain." *Journal of Agriculture Food Chemistry* 51: 838–42.

Louie, H. W., D. Go, M. Fedczina, K. Judd, and J. Dalins. 1985. "Digestion of Food Samples for Total Mercury Determination." *Journal—Association of Official Analytical Chemists* 68: 891–93.

Nakagawa, R., Y. Yumita, and M. Hiromoto. 1997. "Total Mercury Intake from Fish and Shellfish by Japanese People." *Chemosphere* 35: 2909–13.

Patrick, L. 2002. "Mercury Toxicity and Antioxidants: Part 1: Role of Glutathione and Alpha-lipoic Acid in the Treatment of Mercury Toxicity." *Alternative Medicine Review* 7: 456–71.

Pilgrim, W., L. Poissant, and L. Trip. 2000. "The Northeast States and Eastern Canadian Provinces Mercury Study: A Framework for Action: Summary of the Canadian Chapter." *Science of the Total Environment* (Amsterdam) 261: 177–84.

Schober, S. E., T. H. Sinks, R. L. Jones, and others. 2003. "Blood Mercury Levels in U.S. Children and Women of Childbearing Age, 1999–2000." *Journal of the American Medical Association* 289: 1667–74.

Storelli, M. M., and G. O. Marcotrigiano. 2001. "Total Mercury Levels in Muscle Tissue of Swordfish (Xiphias Gladius) and Bluefin Tuna (Thunnus Thynnus) from the Mediterranean Sea (Italy)." *Journal of Food Protection* 64: 1058–61.

Tollefson, L., and F. Cordle F. 1986. "Methylmercury in Fish: A Review of Residue Levels, Fish Consumption, and Regulatory Action in the United States." *Environmental Health Perspectives* 68: 203–8.

van Veizen, D., H. Langenkamp, and G. Herb. 2002. "Review: Mercury in Waste Incineration." *Waste Management Research* 20: 556–68.

Watanabe, C. 2002. "Modification of Mercury Toxicity by Selenium: Practical Importance?" *Tohoku Journal of Experimental Medicine* 196: 71–77.

Yoshida, M. 2002. "Placental to Fetal Transfer of Mercury and Fetotoxicity." *Tohoku Journal of Experimental Medicine* 196: 79–88.

Ysart, G., P. Miller, M. Croasdale, and others. 2000. "1997 UK Total Diet Study—Dietary Exposures to Aluminium, Arsenic, Cadmium, Chromium, Copper, Lead, Mercury, Nickel, Selenium, Tin, and Zinc." *Food Additives and Contaminants* 17: 775–86.

CHAPTER 7: SPECIAL SUPPLEMENTS

Aloe

Afzal, M., M. Ali, R. A. H. Hassan, and others. 1991. "Identification of Some Prostanoids in Aloe Vera Extracts." *Planta Medica* 57: 38–40.

Danhoff, I. E., and B. H. McAnally. 1983. "Stabilised Aloe Vera, Its Effect on Human Skin Cells." *Drugs in the Cosmetics Industry* 133: 52–196.

Davis, R. H., J. M. Kabbani, and N. P. Moro. 1987. "Aloe Vera and Wound Healing." *Journal of the American Podiatric Medical Association* 77 (4): 165–69.

Heggers, J. P. 1996. "Beneficial Effect of Aloe on Wound Healing in an Excisional Wound Healing Model." *Journal of Alternative and Complementary Medicine* 2 (2): 271–77.

Hu, Y., J. Xu, and Q. Hu. 2003. "Evaluation of Antioxidant Potential of Aloe Vera (Aloe Barbadensis Miller) Extracts." *Journal of Agriculture Food Chemistry* 51: 7788–91.

Lambert, R. J., P. N. Skandamis, P. J. Coote, and G. J. Nychas. 2001. "A Study of the Minimum Inhibitory Concentration and Mode of Action of Oregano Essential Oil, Thymol, and Carvacrol." *Journal of Applied Microbiology* 91 (3): 453–62.

Lee, K. Y., S. T. Weintraub, and B. P. Yu. 2000. "Isolation and Identification of a Phenolic Antioxidant from Aloe Barbadensis." *Free Radical Biology and Medicine* 28: 261–65.

Lorenzetti, L. J., R. Salisbury, J. L. Beal, and others. 1964. "Bacteriostatic Property of Aloe Vera." *Journal of the Pharmaceutical Society* 53: 1287–90.

Obata, M., S. Ito, H. Beppu, and others. 1993. "Mechanisms of Anti-inflammatory and Anti-thermal Burn Action of Carboxypeptidase from Aloe Aborescens Miller, Natalensis Berger in Rats and Mice." *Physiotherapy Research* 7 (special issue): 530–33.

"Oral Ulcers Remedy Gets FDA Clearance." 1994. *Journal of the American Dental Association* 125 (10): 1308, 1310.

Sheets, M. A., B. A. Unger, G. F. Giggleman, and others. 1991. "Studies of the Effect of Ace Mannan on Retrovirus Infections, Clinical Stabilisation of Feline Leukemia Virus Infected Cats." *Molecular Biothermy* 3: 41–45.

Sims, P., M. Ruth, and E. R. Zimmerman. 1971. "Effect of Aloe Vera on Herpes Simplex and Herpes Virus (Strain Zoster)." *Aloe Vera of American Archives* 1: 239–40.

———. 1971. "The Effects of Aloe Vera on Mycotic Organism (Fungi)." *Aloe Vera of American Archives* 1: 237–38.

Strickland, F. M., R. P. Pelley, M. L. Kripke, and others. 1993. "Prevention of Ultraviolet Radiation and Induced Suppression of Contact and Delyed Hypersensitivity by Aloe Barbadensis Gel Extract." *Journal of Investigative Dermatology* 9 (6): 197–204.

Vogler, B. K., and E. Ernst. 1999. "Aloe Vera: A Systematic Review of Its Clinical Effectiveness." *British Journal of General Practice* 49 (447): 823–28.

Winters, W. D. 1993. "Immuno-reactive Lectins in Leaf Gel Form from Aloe Barbadensis Miller. *Phytotherapy Research* 7: S23–S25.

Arabinogalactan

Currier, N. L., D. Lejtenyi, and S. C. Miller. 2003. "Effect over Time of In-Vivo Administration of the Polysaccharide Arabinogalactan on Immune and Hemopoietic Cell Lineages in Murine Spleen and Bone Marrow." *Phytomedicine* 10: 145–53.

Grieshop, C. M., E. A. Flickinger, and G. C. Fahey Jr. 2002. "Oral Administration of Arabinogalactan Affects Immune Status and Fecal Microbial Populations in Dogs." *Journal of Nutrition* 132: 478–82.

Kelly, G. S. 1999. "Larch Arabinogalactan: Clinical Relevance of a Novel Immune-Enhancing Polysaccharide." *Alternative Medicine Review* 4: 96–103.

Kim, L. S., R. F. Waters, and P. M. Burkholder. 2002. "Immunological Activity of Larch Arabinogalactan and Echinacea: A Preliminary, Randomized, Double-Blind, Placebo-Controlled Trial." *Alternative Medicine Review* 7: 138–49.

"Larch Arabinogalactan." 2002. *Alternative Medicine Review* 5: 463–66.

Taguchi, I., H. Kiyohara, T. Matsumoto, and H. Yamada. 2004. "Structure of Oligosaccharide Side Chains of an Intestinal Immune System Modulating Arabinogalactan Isolated from Rhizomes of Atractylodes Lancea DC." *Carbohydrate Research* 339: 763–70.

Artichoke

Agarwal, R., and H. Mukhtar. 1996. "Cancer Chemoprevention by Polyphenols in Green Tea and Artichoke." *Advances in Experimental Medicine and Biology* 401: 35–50.

Gebhardt, R. 1997. "Antioxidative and Protective Properties of Extracts from Leaves of the Artichoke (Cynara Scolymus L.) against Hydroperoxide-Induced Oxidative Stress in Cultured Rat Hepatocytes." *Toxicology and Applied Pharmacology* 144: 279–86.

Pittler, M. H., C. O. Thompson, and E. Ernst. 2002. "Artichoke Leaf Extract for Treating Hypercholesterolaemia." *Cochrane Database of Systematic Reviews* CD003335.

Wegener, T., and V. Fintelmann. 1999. "Pharmacologyogical Properties and Therapeutic Profile of Artichoke (Cynara Scolymus L.)." *Wiener Medizinische Wochenschrift* (Vienna) 149: 241–47.

Ashwaganda

Bhattacharya, S. K., and A. V. Muruganandam. 2003. "Adaptogenic Activity of Withania Somnifera: An Experimental Study Using a Rat Model of Chronic Stress." *Pharmacology, Biochemistry, and Behavior* 75: 547–55.

Davis, L., and G. Kuttan. 2002. "Effect of Withania Somnifera on Cell Mediated Immune Responses in Mice." *Journal of Experimental Clinical Cancer Research* 21: 585–90.

Gupta, S. K., A. Dua, and B. P. Vohra. 2003. "Withania Somnifera (Ashwagandha) Attenuates Antioxidant Defense in Aged Spinal Cord and Inhibits Copper Induced Lipid Peroxidation and Protein Oxidative Modifications." *Drug Metabolism and Drug Interactions* 19: 211–22.

Jayaprakasam, B., Y. Zhang, N. P. Seeram, and M. G. Nair. 2003. "Growth Inhibition of Human Tumor Cell Lines by Withanolides from Withania Somnifera Leaves." *Life Science* 74: 125–32.

Mishra, L. C., B. B. Singh, and S. Dagenais. 2000. "Scientific Basis for the Therapeutic Use of Withania Somnifera (Ashwagandha): A Review." *Alternative Medicine Review* 5: 334–46.

Berberine-Containing Herbs (Goldenseal, Oregon Grape, Barberry)

Kaneda, Y., T. Tanaka, and T. Saw. 1990. "Effect of Berberine: A Plant Alkaloid on the Growth of Anaerobic Protozoa in Axenic Culture." *Tokai Journal of Experimental Clinical Medicine* 15 (6): 417–23.

Kaneda, Y., M. Torrii, T. Tanaka, and others. 1991. "In Vitro Effects of Berberine Sulfate on the Growth of Entamoeba Histolytica, Giardia Lamblia, and Tricomonas Vaginalis." *Annals of Tropical Medicine and Parasitology* 85: 417–25.

Kumazawa, Y., A. Itagaki, M. Fukumoto, and others. 1984. "Activation of Peritoneal Macrophages by Berberine-Type Alkaloids in Terms of Induction of Cytostatic Activity." *International Journal of Immunopharmacology* 6 (6): 587–92.

Sun, D., H.S. Courtney, E. H. Beachey, and others. 1988. "Berberine Sulfate Blocks Adherence of Streptococcus Pyogenes to Epithelial Cells, Fibronectin, and Hexadecane." *Antimicrobial Agents and Chemotherapy* 32 (9): 1370–74.

Beta-Sitosterol

Drexel, H., C. Breier, H. J. Lisch, and S. Sailer. 1981. "Lowering Plasma Cholesterol with Beta-sitosterol and Diet." *Lancet* 1: 1157

Nair, P. P., N. Turjman, G. Kessie, B. Calkins, G. T. Goodman, H. Davidovitz, and G. Nimmagadda. 1984. "Diet, Nutrition Intake, and Metabolism in Populations at High and Low Risk for Colon Cancer. Dietary Cholesterol, Beta-sitosterol, and Stigmasterol." *American Journal of Clinical Nutrition* 40: 927–30.

van Rensburg, S. J., W. M. Daniels, J. M. van Zyl, and J. J. Taljaard. 2000. "A Comparative Study of the Effects of Cholesterol, Beta-sitosterol, Beta-sitosterol Glucoside, Dehydroepiandrosterone Sulphate, and Melatonin on In Vitro Lipid Peroxidation." *Metabolic Brain Disease* 15: 257–65.

Weisweiler, P., V. Heinemann, and P. Schwandt. 1984. "Serum Lipoproteins and Lecithin: Cholesterol Acyltransferase (LCAT) Activity in Hypercholesterolemic Subjects Given Beta-sitosterol." *International Journal of Clinical Pharmacology and Therapeutics Toxicology* 22: 204–6.

Butylated Hydroxytoluene (BHT)

Freeman, D. J., G. Wenerstrom, and S. L. Spruance. 1985. "Treatment of Recurrent Herpes Simplex Labialis with Topical Butylated Hydroxytoluene." *Clinical Pharmacology and Therapeutics* 38: 56–59.

Keith, A. D., D. Arruda, W. Snipes, and P. Frost. 1982. "The Antiviral Effectiveness of Butylated Hydroxytoluene on Herpes Cutaneous Infections in Hairless Mice." *Proceedings of the Society for Experimental Biology and Medicine* 170: 237–44.

Richards, J. T., M. E. Katz, and E. R. Kern. 1985. "Topical Butylated Hydroxytoluene Treatment of Genital Herpes Simplex Virus Infections of Guinea Pigs." *Antiviral Research* 5: 281–90.

Bilberry

Canter, P. H., and E. Ernst. 2004. "Anthocyanosides of Vaccinium Myrtillus (Bilberry) for Night Vision—A Systematic Review of Placebo-Controlled Trials." *Survey of Opthamology* 49: 38–50.

Cignarella, A., M. Nastasi, E. Cavalli, and L. Puglisi. 1996. "Novel Lipid-Lowering Properties of Vaccinium Myrtillus L. Leaves, a Traditional Antidiabetic Treatment, in Several Models of Rat Dyslipidaemia: A Comparison with Ciprofibrate." *Thrombosis Research* 84: 311–22.

Fraisse, D., A. Carnat, and J. L. Lamaison. 1996. "Polyphenolic Composition of the Leaf of Bilberry." *Annales Pharmaceutiques Francaises* (Paris) 54: 280–83.

Katsube, N., K. Iwashita, T. Tsushida, K. Yamaki, and M. Kobori. 2003. "Induction of Apoptosis in Cancer Cells by Bilberry (Vaccinium Myrtillus) and the Anthocyanins." *Journal of Agriculture Food Chemistry* 51: 68–75.

Kay, C. D., and B. J. Holub. 2002. "The Effect of Wild Blueberry (Vaccinium Angustifolium) Consumption on Postprandial Serum Antioxidant Status in Human Subjects." *British Journal of Nutrition* 88: 389–98.

Muth, E. R., J. M. Laurent, and P. Jasper. 2000. "The Effect of Bilberry Nutritional Supplementation on Night Visual Acuity and Contrast Sensitivity." *Alternative Medicine Review* 5: 164–73.

Taulavuori, E., E. K. Hellstrom, K. Taulavuori, and K. Laine. 2001. "Comparison of Two Methods Used to Analyse Lipid Peroxidation from Vaccinium Myrtillus (L.) during Snow Removal, Reacclimation and Cold Acclimation." *Journal of Experimental Botany* 52: 2375–80.

Black Currant Oil

Crozier, G. L., M. Fleith, and P. A. Finot. 1987. "Effects of Feeding Black Currant Seed Oil on Fatty Acid Composition of Lipid Classes in the Guinea Pig Liver." *International Journal for Vitamins and Nutrition Research* 57: 343.

Crozier, G. L., M. Fleith, H. Traitler, and P. A. Finot. 1989. "Black Currant Seed Oil Feeding and Fatty Acids in Liver Lipid Classes of Guinea Pigs." *Lipids* 24: 460–66.

Diboune, M., G. Ferard, Y. Ingenbleek, P. A. Tulasne, B. Calon, M. Hasselmann, P. Sauder, D. Spielmann, and P. Metais. 1992. "Composition of Phospholipid Fatty Acids in Red Blood Cell Membranes of Patients in Intensive Care Units: Effects of Different Intakes of Soybean Oil, Medium-Chain Triglycerides, and Black-Currant Seed Oil." *Journal of Parenteral and Enteral Nutrition* 16: 136–41.

Hirschberg, Y., A. Shackelford, E. A. Mascioli, V. K. Babayan, B. R. Bistrian, and G. L. Blackburn. 1990. "The Response to Endotoxin in Guinea Pigs after Intravenous Black Currant Seed Oil." *Lipids* 25: 491–96.

Tate, G. A., and R. B. Zurier. 1994. "Suppression of Monosodium Urate Crystal-Induced Inflammation by Black Currant Seed Oil." *Agents and Actions* 43: 35–38.

Wu, D., M. Meydani, L. S. Leka, Z. Nightingale, G. J. Handelman, J. B. Blumberg, and S. N. Meydani. 1999. "Effect of Dietary Supplementation with Black Currant Seed Oil on the Immune Response of Healthy Elderly Subjects." *American Journal of Clinical Nutrition* 70: 536–43.

Borage Seed Oil

Bahmer, F. A., and J. Schafer. 1992. "Treatment of Atopic Dermatitis with Borage Seed Oil (Glandol)—A Time Series Analytic Study." *Kinderarztliche Praxis* (Leipzig) 60: 199–202.

Borrek, S., A. Hildebrandt, and J. Forster. 1997. "Gamma-Linolenic-Acid-Rich Borage Seed Oil Capsules in Children with Atopic Dermatitis: A Placebo-Controlled Double-Blind Study." *Klinische Padiatrie* (Stuttgart) 209: 100–4.

Harvey, R. G. 1999. "A Blinded, Placebo-Controlled Study of the Efficacy of Borage Seed Oil and Fish Oil in the Management of Canine Atopy." *Veterinary Record* 44: 405–7.

Boswellia

Adelakun, E. A., E. A. Finbar, S. E. Agina, and A. A. Makinde. 2001. "Antimicrobial Activity of Boswellia Dalziellii Stem Bark." *Fitoterapia* (Milan) 72: 822–24.

Badria, F. A., B. R. Mikhaeil, G. T. Maatooq, and M. M. Amer. 2003. "Immunomodulatory Triterpenoids from the Oleogum Resin of Boswellia Carterii Birdwood." *Zeitschrift für Naturforschung* (Tübingen) 58: 505–16.

"Boswellia Serrata." 1998. *Alternative Medicine Review* 3: 306–7.

Gerhardt, H., F. Seifert, P. Buvari, H. Vogelsang, and R. Repges. 2001. "Therapy of Active Crohn Disease with Boswellia Serrata Extract H 15." *Zeitschrift fur Gastroenterologie* (Munich) 39: 11–17.

Gupta, I., V. Gupta, A. Parihar, S. Gupta, R. Ludtke, H. Safayhi, and H. P. Ammon. 1998. "Effects of Boswellia Serrata Gum Resin in Patients with Bronchial Asthma: Results of a Double-Blind, Placebo-Controlled, Six-Week Clinical Study." *European Journal of Medical Research* 3: 511–14.

Gupta, I., A. Parihar, P. Malhotra, S. Gupta, R. Ludtke, H. Safayhi, and H. P. Ammon. 2001. "Effects of Gum Resin of Boswellia Serrata in Patients with Chronic Colitis." *Planta Medicine* 67: 391–95.

Gupta, I., A. Parihar, P. Malhotra, G. B. Singh, R. Ludtke, H. Safayhi, and H. P. Ammon. 1997. "Effects of Boswellia Serrata Gum Resin in Patients with Ulcerative Colitis." *European Journal of Medical Research* 2: 37–43.

Kimmatkar, N., V. Thawani, L. Hingorani, and R. Khiyani. 2003. "Efficacy and Tolerability of Boswellia Serrata Extract in Treatment of Osteoarthritis of Knee—A Randomized Double Blind Placebo Controlled Trial." *Phytomedicine* 10: 3–7.

Reichling, J., H. Schmokel, J. Fitzi, S. Bucher, and R. Saller. 2004. "Dietary Support with Boswellia Resin in Canine Inflammatory Joint and Spinal Disease." *Schweizer Archiv fur Tierheilkunde* (Zurich) 146: 71–79.

Bromelain

Gaspani, L., E. Limiroli, P. Ferrario, and M. Bianchi. 2002. "In Vivo and In Vitro Effects of Bromelain on PGE(2) and SP Concentrations in the Inflammatory Exudate in Rats." *Pharmacologyogy* 65: 83–86.

Maurer, H. R. 2001. "Bromelain: Biochemistry, Pharmacology, and Medical Use." *Cellular and Molecular Life Science* (Basel) 58: 1234–45.

Taussig, S. J., and S. Batkin. 1988. "Bromelain, the Enzyme Complex of Pineapple (Ananas Comosus) and Its Clinical Application: An Update." *Journal of Ethnopharmacology* 22: 191–203.

Carnosine

Boldyrev, A., and H. Abe. 1999. "Metabolic Transformation of Neuropeptide Carnosine Modifies Its Biological Activity." *Cellular and Molecular Neurobiology* 19: 163–75.

Bonfanti, L., P. Peretto, S. De Marchis, and A. Fasolo. 1999. "Carnosine-Related Dipeptides in the Mammalian Brain." *Progress in Neurobiology* 59: 333–53.

Decker, E. A., S. A. Livisay, and S. Zhou. 2000. "A Re-Evaluation of the Antioxidant Activity of Purified Carnosine." *Biochemistry* (Moscow) 65: 766–70.

Gariballa, S. E., and A. J. Sinclair. 2000. "Carnosine: Physiological Properties and Therapeutic Potential." *Age and Ageing* (Oxford) 29: 207–10.

Hipkiss, A. R. 2000. "Carnosine and Protein Carbonyl Groups: A Possible Relationship." *Biochemistry* (Moscow) 65: 771–78.

———. 1998 "Carnosine, a Protective, Anti-ageing Peptide?" *International Journal of Biochemistry and Cell Biology* 30: 863–68.

Hipkiss, A. R., and C. Brownson. 2000. "A Possible New Role for the Anti-ageing Peptide Carnosine." *Cellular and Molecular Life Sciences* 57: 747–53.

Severina, I. S., O. G. Bussygina, and N. V. Pyatakova. 2000. "Carnosine as a Regulator of Soluble Guanylate Cyclase." *Biochemistry* (Moscow) 65: 783–88.

Stuerenburg, H. J. 2000. "The Roles of Carnosine in Aging of Skeletal Muscle and in Neuromuscular Diseases." *Biochemistry* (Moscow) 65: 862–65.

Stvolinsky, S. L., and D. Dobrota. 2000. "Anti-ischemic Activity of Carnosine." *Biochemistry* (Moscow) 65: 849–55.

Trombley, P. Q., M. S. Horning, and L. J. Blakemore. 2000. "Interactions between Carnosine and Zinc and Copper: Implications for Neuromodulation and Neuroprotection." *Biochemistry* (Moscow) 65: 807–16.

Wang, A. M., C. Ma, Z. H. Xie, and F. Shen. 2000. "Use of Carnosine as a Natural Anti-senescence Drug for Human Beings." *Biochemistry* (Moscow) 65: 869–71.

Carotenoids

Bast, A., G. R. Haenen, R. van den Berg, and H. van den Berg. 1998. "Antioxidant Effects of Carotenoids." *International Journal for Vitamin and Nutrition Research* 68: 399–403.

Krinsky, N. I. 1998. "The Antioxidant and Biological Properties of the Carotenoids." *Annals of the New York Academy of Sciences* 854: 443–47.

Packer, L. 1993. "Antioxidant Action of Carotenoids In Vitro and In Vivo and Protection against Oxidation of Human Low-Density Lipoproteins." *Annals of the New York Academy of Sciences* 691: 48–60.

Palace, V. P., N. Khaper, Q. Qin, and P. K. Singal. 1999. "Antioxidant Potentials of Vitamin A and Carotenoids and Their Relevance to Heart Disease." *Free Radical Biology and Medicine* 26: 746–61.

Rock, C. L., R. A. Jacob, and P. E. Bowen. 1996. "Update on the Biological Characteristics of the Antioxidant Micronutrients: Vitamin C, Vitamin E, and the Carotenoids." *Journal of the American Dietetic Association* 96: 693–702; quiz 703–4.

Young, A. J., and G. M. Lowe. 2001. "Antioxidant and Pro-oxidant Properties of Carotenoids." *Archives of Biochemistry and Biophysics* 385: 20–27.

Catalase

Kohen, R., A. Kakunda, and A. Rubinstein. 1992. "The Role of Cationized Catalase and Cationized Glucose Oxidase in Mucosal Oxidative Damage Induced in the Rat Jejunum." *Journal of Biological Chemistry* 267: 21349–54.

Nayak, M. S., M. Kita, and M. F. Marmor. 1993. "Protection of Rabbit Retina from Ischemic Injury by Superoxide Dismutase and Catalase." *Investigative Ophthalmology and Visual Science* 34: 2018–22.

Cayenne/Capsaicin

Bari, F., D. Paprika, G. Jancso, and F. Domoki. 2000. "Capsaicin-Sensitive Mechanisms Are Involved in Cortical Spreading Depression-Associated Cerebral Blood Flow Changes in Rats." *Neuroscience Letters* 292: 17–20.

Charkoudian, N., B. Fromy, and J. L. Saumet. 2001. "Reflex Control of the Cutaneous Circulation after Acute and Chronic Local Capsaicin." *Journal of Applied Physiology* 90: 1860–64.

Gonzalez, R., R. Dunkel, B. Koletzko, V. Schusdziarra, and H. D. Allescher. 1998. "Effect of Capsaicin-Containing Red Pepper Sauce Suspension on Upper Gastrointestinal Motility in Healthy Volunteers." *Digestive Diseases and Sciences* 43: 1165–71.

Kawada, T., K. Hagihara, and K. Iwai. 1986. "Effects of Capsaicin on Lipid Metabolism in Rats Fed a High Fat Diet." *Journal of Nutrition* 116: 1272–78.

Kiraly, A., G. Suto, J. Czimmer, O. P. Horvath, and G. Mozsik. 2001. "Failure of Capsaicin-Containing Red Pepper Sauce Suspension to Induce Esophageal Motility Response in Patients with Barrett's Esophagus." *Journal de Physiologie* (Paris) 95: 197–200.

Lee, C. Y., M. Kim, S. W. Yoon, and C. H. Lee. 2003. "Short-Term Control of Capsaicin on Blood and Oxidative Stress of Rats In Vivo." *Phytotherapy Research* 17: 454–58.

Lee, S. S., and K. A. Sharkey. 1993. "Capsaicin Treatment Blocks Development of Hyperkinetic Circulation in Portal Hypertensive and Cirrhotic Rats." *American Journal of Physiology* 264: G868–G873.

Mitchell, J. A., F. M. Williams, T. J. Williams, and S. W. Larkin. 1997. "Role of Nitric Oxide in the Dilator Actions of Capsaicin-Sensitive Nerves in the Rabbit Coronary Circulation." *Neuropeptides* 31: 333–38.

Munce, T. A., and W. L. Kenney. 2003. "Age-Specific Skin Blood Flow Responses to Acute Capsaicin." *Journals of Gerontology. Series A, Biological Sciences and Medical Sciences* 58: 304–10.

Sambaiah, K., and M. N. Satyanarayana. 1980. "Hypocholesterolemic Effect of Red Pepper and Capsaicin." *Indian Journal of Experimental Biology* 18: 898–99.

Chamomile

Kobayashi, Y., Y. Nakano, K. Inayama, A. Sakai, and T. Kamiya. 2003. "Dietary Intake of the Flower Extracts of German Chamomile (Matricaria Recutita L.) Inhibited Compound 48/80–Induced Itch-Scratch Responses in Mice." *Phytomedicine* 10: 657–64.

Kyokong, O., S. Charuluxananan, V. Muangmingsuk, O. Rodanant, K. Subornsug, and W. Punyasang. 2002. "Efficacy of Chamomile-Extract Spray for Prevention of Post-operative Sore Throat." *Journal of the Medical Association of Thailandl* 85 (suppl 1): S180–S185.

Smolinski, A.T., and J. J. Pestka. 2003. "Modulation of Lipopolysaccharide-Induced Proinflammatory Cytokine Production In Vitro and In Vivo by the Herbal Constituents Apigenin (Chamomile), Ginsenoside Rb(1) (Ginseng) and Parthenolide (Feverfew)." *Food and Chemical Toxicology* (Oxford) 41: 1381–90.

Uteshev, B. S., I. L. Laskova, and V. A. Afanas'ev. 1999. "The Immunomodulating Activity of the Heteropolysaccharides from German Chamomile (Matricaria Chamomilla) during Air and Immersion Cooling." *Eksperimental'naia i Klinicheskaia Farmakologiia* (Moscow) 62: 52–55.

Chlorella

Halperin, S. A., B. Smith, C. Nolan, J. Shay, and J. Kralovec. 2003. "Safety and Immunoenhancing Effect of a Chlorella-Derived Dietary Supplement in Healthy Adults Undergoing Influenza Vaccination: Randomized, Double-Blind, Placebo-Controlled Trial." *Canadian Medical Association Journal* 169: 111–17.

Lee, H. S., C. Y. Choi, C. Cho, and Y. Song. 2003. "Attenuating Effect of Chlorella Supplementation on Oxidative Stress and NFkappaB Activation in Peritoneal Macrophages and Liver of C57BL/6 Mice Fed on an Atherogenic Diet. *Bioscience, Biotechnology, and Biochemistry* 67: 2083–90.

Merchant, R. E., and C. A. Andre. 2001. "A Review of Recent Clinical Trials of the Nutritional Supplement Chlorella Pyrenoidosa in the Treatment of Fibromyalgia, Hypertension, and Ulcerative Colitis." *Alternative Therapies in Health and Medicine* 7: 79–91.

Merchant, R. E., C. A. Andre, and D. A. Sica. 2002. "Nutritional Supplementation with Chlorella Pyrenoidosa for Mild to Moderate Hypertension." *Journal of Medicinal Food* 5: 141–52.

Shibata, S., Y. Natori, T. Nishihara, K. Tomisaka, K. Matsumoto, H. Sansawa, and V. C. Nguyen. 2003. "Antioxidant and Anti-cataract Effects of Chlorella on Rats with Streptozotocin-Induced Diabetes." *Journal of Nutritional Science and Vitaminology* (Tokyo) 49: 334–39.

Cinnamon

Otsuka, H., S. Fujioka, T. Komiya, E. Mizuta, and M. Takamoto. 1982. "Studies on Anti-inflammatory Agents. VI. Anti-inflammatory Constituents of Cinnamomum Sieboldii Meissn." (trans.) *Yakugaku zasshi. Journal of the Pharmaceutical Society of Japan* (Tokyo) 102: 162–72.

Ouattara, B., R. E. Simard, R. A. Holley, G, J. Piette, and A. Begin. 1997. "Antibacterial Activity of Selected Fatty Acids and Essential Oils against Six Meat Spoilage Organisms." *International Journal of Food Microbiology* 37: 155–62.

Quale, J. M., D. Landman, M. M. Zaman, S. Burney, and S. S. Sathe. 1996. "In Vitro Activity of Cinnamomum Zeylanicum against Azole Resistant and Sensitive Candida Species and a Pilot Study of Cinnamon for Oral Candidiasis." *American Journal of Chinese Medicine* 24: 103–9.

Takenaga, M., A. Hirai, T. Terano, Y. Tamura, H. Kitagawa, and S. Yoshida. 1987. "In Vitro Effect of Cinnamic Aldehyde, a Main Component of Cinnamomi Cortex, on Human Platelet Aggregation and Arachidonic Acid Metabolism." *Journal of Pharmacobiodynamics* 10: 201–8.

VanderEnde, D. S., and J. D. Morrow. 2001. "Release of Markedly Increased Quantities of Prostaglandin D2 from the Skin In Vivo in Humans after the Application of Cinnamic Aldehyde." *Journal of the American Academy of Dermatology* 45: 62–67.

Cod Liver Oil

Benedek, T. G. 1998. "Treatment of Systemic Lupus Erythematosus: From Cod-Liver Oil to Cyclosporin." *Lancet* 352: 901–2.

Brox, J., K. Olaussen, B. Osterud, E. O. Elvevoll, E. Bjornstad, G. Brattebog, and H. Iversen. 2001. "A Long-Term Seal- and Cod-Liver-Oil Supplementation in Hypercholesterolemic Subjects." *Lipids* 36: 7–13.

Brustad, M., T. Sandanger, T. Wilsgaard, L. Aksnes, and E. Lund. 2003. "Change in Plasma Levels of Vitamin D after Consumption of Cod-Liver and Fresh Cod-Liver Oil as Part of the Traditional North Norwegian Fish Dish 'Molje.'" *International Journal of Circumpolar Health* 62: 40–53.

Gruenwald, J., H. J. Graubaum, and A. Harde. 2002. "Effect of Cod Liver Oil on Symptoms of Rheumatoid Arthritis." *Advances in Therapy* 19: 101–7.

Olafsdottir, A. S., K. H. Wagner, I. Thorsdottir, and I. Elmadfa. 2001. "Fat-Soluble Vitamins in the Maternal Diet, Influence of Cod Liver Oil Supplementation and Impact of the Maternal Diet on Human Milk Composition." *Annals of Nutrition and Metabolism* 45: 265–72.

Rajakumar, K. 2003. "Vitamin D, Cod-Liver Oil, Sunlight, and Rickets: A Historical Perspective." *Pediatrics* 112: E132–E135.

Stene, L. C., and G. Joner. 2003. "Use of Cod Liver Oil during the First Year of Life Is Associated with Lower Risk of Childhood-Onset Type 1 Diabetes: A Large, Population-Based, Case-Control Study." *American Journal of Clinical Nutrition* 78: 1128–34.

Codonopsis

Chen, S., Z. Zhou, S. Sun, and others. 1998. "The Effect of Codonopsis Pilosula (Franch.) Nannf. on Gastric Acid, Serum Gastrin, and Plasma Somatostatin Concentration in Dogs." *Zhongguo Zhong Yao Za Zhi.* (Beijing) 23 (5): 299–301, 320.

Grey-Wilson, C. 1990. "A Survey of the Genus Codonopsis." *Plantsman* 12 (2): 65–99.

Wang, Xu. 1993. "Two New Species of Codonopsis from China." *Acta Phytotax Sinica* (Tokyo) 31 (2): 184–87.

Wang, Z.T., and others. 1996. "Immunomodulatory Effect of a Polysaccharide-Enriched Preparation of Codonopsis Pilosula Roots." *General Pharmacology* 27 (8): 1347–50.

Coenzyme Q

Burke, B. E., R. Neuenschwander, and R. D. Olson. 2001. "Randomized, Double-Blind, Placebo-Controlled Trial of Coenzyme Q10 in Isolated Systolic Hypertension." *Southern Medical Journal* 94: 1112–17.

Folkers, K., P. Langsjoen, R. Willis, P. Richardson, L. J. Xia, C. Q. Ye, and H. Tamagawa. 1990. "Lovastatin Decreases Coenzyme Q Levels in Humans." *Proceedings of the National Academy of Sciences* 87: 8931–34.

Ghirlanda, G., A. Oradei, A. Manto, S. Lippa, L. Uccioli, S. Caputo, A. V. Greco, and G. P. Littarru. 1993. "Evidence of Plasma CoQ10-Lowering Effect by HMG-coA Reductase Inhibitors: A Double-Blind, Placebo-Controlled Study." *Journal of Clinical Pharmacology* 33: 226–29.

Karlsson, J., B. Diamant, K. Folkers, and B. Lund. 1991. "Muscle Fibre Types, Ubiquinone Content, and Exercise Capacity in Hypertension and Effort Angina." *Annals of Medicine* 23: 339–44.

Karlsson, J., S. Gunnes, and B. Semb. 1996. "Muscle Fibers, Ubiquinone, and Exercise Capacity in Effort Angina." *Molecular and Cellular Biochemistry* 156: 179–84.

Karlsson, J., L. Lin, S. Gunnes, C. Sylven, and H. Astrom. 1996. "Muscle Ubiquinone in Male Effort Angina Patients. *Molecular and Cellular Biochemistry* 156: 173–78.

Malm, C., M. Svensson, B. Ekblom, and B. Sjodin. 1997. "Effects of Ubiquinone-10 Supplementation and High Intensity Training on Physical Performance in Humans." *Acta Physiologica Scandinavica* (Oxford) 161: 379–84.

Singh, R. B., M. A. Niaz, S. S. Rastogi, P. K. Shukla, and A. S. Thakur. 1999. "Effect of Hydrosoluble Coenzyme Q10 on Blood Pressures and Insulin Resistance in Hypertensive Patients with Coronary Artery Disease." *Journal of Human Hypertension* 13: 203–8.

Spigset, O. 1994. "Coenzyme Q10 (Ubiquinone) in the Treatment of Heart Failure: Are Any Positive Effects Documented?" *Tidsskrift for den Norske Laegeforening* (Oslo) 114: 939–42.

Coleus/Forskoklin

Buschmans, E., D. J. Hearse, and A. S. Manning. 1985. "Forskolin: Effects on Cyclic AMP and Contractile Function in the Isolated Rat and Guinea Pig Heart." *Canadian Journal of Cardiology* 1: 385–94.

Fujita, A., T. Takahira, M. Hosono, and K. Nakamura. 1992. "Improvement of Drug-Induced Cardiac Failure by NKH477, a Novel Forskolin Derivative, in the Dog Heart-Lung Preparation." *Japanese Journal of Pharmacology* 58: 375–81.

Hearse, D. J., R. Zucchi, E. Buschmans, and A. S. Manning. 1986. "Forskolin and Myocardial Function in the Normal, Ischemic, and Reperfused Rat Heart." *Canadian Journal of Cardiololgy* 2: 303–12.

Ishizuka, O., M. Hosono, and K. Nakamura. 1992. "Profile of Cardiovascular Effects of NKH477, a Novel Forskolin Derivative, Assessed in Isolated, Blood-Perfused Dog Heart Preparations: Comparison with Isoproterenol." *Journal of Cardiovascular Pharmacology* 20: 261–67.

Mulieri, L. A., B. J. Leavitt, B. J. Martin, J. R. Haeberle, and N. R. Alpert. 1993. "Myocardial Force-Frequency Defect in Mitral Regurgitation Heart Failure Is Reversed by Forskolin." *Circulation* 88: 2700–4.

Neumann, J., S. Bartel, T. Eschenhagen, A. Haverich, S. Hirt, P. Karczewski, E. G. Krause, W. Schmitz, H. Scholz, B. Stein, and M. Thoenes. 1999. "Dissociation of the Effects of Forskolin and Dibutyryl cAMP on Force of Contraction and Phospholamban Phosphorylation in Human Heart Failure." *Journal of Cardiovascular Pharmacology* 33: 157–62.

Sonoki, H., Y. Uchida, M. Masuo, T. Tomaru, A. Katoh, and T. Sugimoto. 1986. "Effects of Forskolin on Canine Congestive Heart Failure." *Nippon Yakurigaku Zasshi* (Kyoto) 88: 389–94.

Williams, J. L., Jr, and K. J. Malik. 1990. "Forskolin Stimulates Prostaglandin Synthesis in Rabbit Heart by a Mechanism That Requires Calcium and Is Independent of Cyclic AMP." *Circulation Research* 67: 1247–56.

Creatine

Koons, S., and R. Cooke. 1986. "Function of Creatine Kinase Localization in Muscle Contraction." *Advances in Experimental Medicine and Biology* 194: 129–37.

Kushmerick, M. J. 1998. "Energy Balance in Muscle Activity: Simulations of Atpase Coupled to Oxidative Phosphory-lation and to Creatine Kinase." *Comparative Biochemistry and Physiology. B: Comparative Biochemistry* 120: 109–23.

Mesa, J. L., J. R. Ruiz, M. M. Gonzalez-Gross, A. Gutierrez Sainz, and M. J. Castillo Garzon. 2002. "Oral Creatine Supplementation and Skeletal Muscle Metabolism in Physical Exercise." *Sports Medicine* 32: 903–44.

Rawson, E. S., and J. S. Volek. 2003. "Effects of Creatine Supplementation and Resistance Training on Muscle Strength and Weightlifting Performance." *Journal of Strength and Conditioning Research* 17: 822–31.

Wallimann, T., and W. Hemmer. 1994. "Creatine Kinase in Non-muscle Tissues and Cells." *Molecular and Cellular Biochemistry* 133–34: 193–220.

Wyss, M., and T. Wallimann. 1994. "Creatine Metabolism and the Consequences of Creatine Depletion in Muscle." *Molecular and Cellular Biochemistry* 133–34: 51–66.

Dehydroepiandrosterone (DHEA)

Arlt, W., F. Callies, I. Koehler, J. C. Van Vlijmen, M. Fassnacht, C. J. Strasburger, M. J. Seibel, D. Huebler, M. Ernst, M. Oettel, M. Reincke, H. M. Schulte, and B. Allolio. 2001. "Dehydroepiandrosterone Supplementation in Healthy Men with an Age-Related Decline of Dehydroepiandros-terone Secretion." *Journal of Clinical Endocrinology and Metabolism* 86: 4686–92.

Buvat, J. 2003. "Androgen Therapy with Dehydroepiandros-terone." *World Journal of Urology* 21: 346–55.

Carlson, L. E., M. Speca, K. D. Patel, and E. Goodey. 2004. "Mindfulness-Based Stress Reduction in Relation to Quality of Life, Mood, Symptoms of Stress and Levels of Cortisol, Dehydroepiandrosterone Sulfate (DHEAS) and Melatonin in Breast and Prostate Cancer Outpatients." *Psychoneuroendocrinology* 29: 448–74.

Dhatariya, K. K., and K. S. Nair. 2003. "Dehydroepiandros-terone: Is There a Role for Replacement?" *Mayo Clinic Proceedings* 78: 1257–73.

Hirshman, E., E. Wells, M. E. Wierman, B. Anderson, A. Butler, M. Senholzi, and J. Fisher. 2003. "The Effect of Dehydro-epiandrosterone (DHEA) on Recognition Memory Deci-sion Processes and Discrimination in Postmenopausal Women." *Psychonomic Bulletin and Review* 10: 125–34.

Legrain, S., and L. Girard. 2003. "Pharmacologyogy and Ther-apeutic Effects of Dehydroepiandrosterone in Older Subjects." *Drugs and Aging* 20: 949–67.

Maayan, R., G. Shaltiel, M. Poyurovsky, E. Ramadan, O. Morad, A. Nechmad, A. Weizman, and G. Agam. 2004. "Chronic Lithium Treatment Affects Rat Brain and Serum Dehydroepiandrosterone (DHEA) and DHEA-sulphate (DHEA-S) Levels." *International Journal of Neuropsychopharmacology* 7: 71–75.

Rigaud, A. S., and J. Pellerin. 2001. "Neuropsychic Effects of Dehydroepiandrosterone." *Annales de Medecine Interne* (Paris) 152 (suppl 3): IS43–IS49.

Spark, R. F. 2002. "Dehydroepiandrosterone: A Springboard Hormone for Female Sexuality." *Fertility and Sterility* 77 (suppl 4): S19–S25.

Strous, R. D., R. Maayan, R. Lapidus, R. Stryjer, M. Lustig, M. Kotler, and A. Weizman. 2003. "Dehydroepiandrosterone Augmentation in the Management of Negative, Depres-sive, and Anxiety Symptoms in Schizophrenia." *Archives of General Psychiatry* 60: 133–41.

Dimethylglycine (DMG)

Allen, R. H., S. P. Stabler, and J. Lindenbaum. 1993. "Serum Betaine, N,n-dimethylglycine, and N-methylglycine Levels in Patients with Cobalamin and Folate Deficiency and Related Inborn Errors of Metabolism." *Metabolism* 42: 1448–60.

Bolman, W. M., and J. A. Richmond. 1999. "A Double-Blind, Placebo-Controlled, Crossover Pilot Trial of Low Dose Dimethylglycine in Patients with Autistic Disorder." *Journal of Autism and Developmental Disorders* 29: 191–94.

Hariganesh, K., and J. Prathiba. 2000. "Effect of Dimethyl-glycine on Gastric Ulcers in Rats." *Journal of Pharmacy and Pharmacology* 52: 1519–22.

Kendall, R. V. 1994. "Comment: N,n-dimethylglycine and L-carnitine as Performance Enhancers in Athletes." *Annals of Pharmacotherapy* 28: 973.

Kern, J. K., V. S. Miller, P. L. Cauller, P. R. Kendall, P. J. Mehta, and M. Dodd. 2001. "Effectiveness of N,n-dimethyl-glycine in Autism and Pervasive Developmental Disor-der." *Journal of Child Neurology* 16: 169–73.

Liet, J. M., V. Pelletier, B. H. Robinson, M. D. Laryea, U. Wen-del, S. Morneau, C. Morin, G. Mitchell, and J. Lacroix. 2003. "The Effect of Short-Term Dimethylglycine Treat-ment on Oxygen Consumption in Cytochrome Oxidase Deficiency: A Double-Blind Randomized Crossover Clinical Trial." *Journal of Pediatrics* 142: 62–66.

Dimethyl Sulfoxide (DMSO)

Ali, B. H. 2001. "Dimethyl Sulfoxide: Recent Pharmacological and Toxicological Research." *Veterinary and Human Toxi-cology* 43: 228–31.

Brayton, C. F. 1986. "Dimethyl Sulfoxide (DMSO): A Review." *Cornell Vet* 76: 61–90.

Santos, N. C., J. Figueira-Coelho, J. Martins-Silva, and C. Saldanha. 2003. "Multidisciplinary Utilization of Dimethyl Sulfoxide: Pharmacological, Cellular, and Mol-ecular Aspects." *Biochemical Pharmacology* 65: 1035–41.

Echinacea

Barrett, B. 2003. "Medicinal Properties of Echinacea: A Critical Review." *Phytomedicine* 10: 66–86.

Barrett, B., M. Vohmann, and C. Calabrese. 1999. "Echinacea for Upper Respiratory Infection." *Journal of Family Practice* 48: 628–35.

Bauer, R. 2002. "New Knowledge Regarding the Effect and Effectiveness of Echinacea Purpurea Extracts." *Wiener Medizinische Wochenschrift* (Vienna) 152: 407–11.

Block, K. I., and M. N. Mead. 2003. "Immune System Effects of Echinacea, Ginseng, and Astragalus: A Review." *Integrative Cancer Therapies* 2: 247–67.

Ernst, E. 2002. "The Risk-Benefit Profile of Commonly Used Herbal Therapies: Ginkgo, St. John's Wort, Ginseng, Echinacea, Saw Palmetto, and Kava." *Annals of Internal Medicine* 136: 42–53.

Giles, J. T., C. T. Palat III, S. H. Chien, Z. G. Chang, and D. T. Kennedy. 2000. "Evaluation of Echinacea for Treatment of the Common Cold." *Pharmacotherapy* 20: 690–97.

Glanville, I. 2003. "Echinacea: Immune Effects Need More Research." *Advance for Nurse Practitioners* 11: 25–26.

Li, J. R., Y. Y. Zhao, and T. M. Ai. 2002. "Advances in the Study of the Chemical Constituents and Biological Activities of 3 Species of Echinacea." *Zhongguo Zhong Yao Za Zhi.* (Beijing) 27: 334–47.

Mark, J. D., K. L. Grant, and L. L. Barton. 2001. "The Use of Dietary Supplements in Pediatrics: A Study of Echinacea." *Clinical Pediatrics* 40: 265–69.

Melchart, D., K. Linde, P. Fischer, and J. Kaesmayr. 2000. "Echinacea for Preventing and Treating the Common Cold." *Cochrane Database of Systematic Reviews* CD000530.

Percival, S. S. 2000. "Use of Echinacea in Medicine." *Biochemical Pharmacology* 60: 155–58.

Evening Primrose Oil

Belch, J. J., and A. Hill. 2000. "Evening Primrose Oil and Borage Oil in Rheumatologic Conditions." *American Journal of Clinical Nutrition* 71: 352S–356S.

Blommers, J., E. S. De Lange-De Klerk, D. J. Kuik, P. D. Bezemer, and S. Meijer. 2002. "Evening Primrose Oil and Fish Oil for Severe Chronic Astalgia: A Randomized, Double-Blind, Controlled Trial." *American Journal of Obstetrics and Gynecology* 187: 1389–94.

Joe, L. A., and L. L. Hart. 1993. "Evening Primrose Oil in Rheumatoid Arthritis." *Annals of Pharmacotherapy* 27: 1475–77.

Kerscher, M. J., and H. C. Korting. 1992. "Treatment of Atopic Eczema with Evening Primrose Oil: Rationale and Clinical Results." *The Clinical Investigator* 70: 167–71.

Puri, B. K. 2004. "The Clinical Advantages of Cold-Pressed Non-raffinated Evening Primrose Oil over Refined Preparations." *Med Hypotheses* 62: 116–18.

Williams, H. C. 2003. "Evening Primrose Oil for Atopic Dermatitis." *British Medical Journal* 327: 1358–59.

Yoon, S., J. Lee, and S. Lee. 2002. "The Therapeutic Effect of Evening Primrose Oil in Atopic Dermatitis Patients with Dry Scaly Skin Lesions Is Associated with the Normalization of Serum Gamma-interferon Levels." *Skin Pharmacology and Applied Skin Physiology* 15: 20–25.

Flavonoids

Borissova, P., S. Valcheva, and A. Belcheva. 1994. "Antiinflammatory Effect of Flavonoids in the Natural Juice from Aronia Melanocarpa, Rutin and Rutin-Magnesium Complex on an Experimental Model of Inflammation Induced by Histamine and Serotonin." *Acta Physiologica et Pharmacologica Bulgarica* (Sofia) 20: 25–30.

Bors, W., C. Michel, and K. Stettmaier. 1997. "Antioxidant Effects of Flavonoids." *Biofactors* 6: 399–402.

Carlotti, M. E., M. Gallarate, M. R. Gasco, and others. 1994. "Inhibition of Lipoperoxidation of Linoleic Acid by Five Antioxidants of Different Lipophilicity." *Pharmazie* (Berlin) 49 (1): 49–52.

Catapano, A. L. 1997. "Antioxidant Effect of Flavonoids." *Angiology* 48: 39–44.

Korkina, L. G., and I. B. Afanas'ev. 1997. "Antioxidant and Chelating Properties of Flavonoids." *Advanced Pharmacology* 38: 151–63.

Manthey, J. A. 2000. "Biological Properties of Flavonoids Pertaining to Inflammation." *Microcirculation* 7: S29–S34.

Manthey, J. A., K. Grohmann, and N. Guthrie. 2001. "Biological Properties of Citrus Flavonoids Pertaining to Cancer and Inflammation." *Current Medicinal Chemistry* 8: 135–53.

Middleton, E., Jr., C. Kandaswami, and T. C. Theoharides. 2000. "The Effects of Plant Flavonoids on Mammalian Cells: Implications for Inflammation, Heart Disease, and Cancer." *Pharmacology Review* 52: 673–751.

Nair, S., and R. Gupta. 1996. "Dietary Antioxidant Flavonoids and Coronary Heart Disease." *Journal of the Association of Physicians of India* (Bombay) 44: 699–702.

Rotelli, A. E., T. Guardia, A. O. Juarez, N. E. De La Rocha, and I. E. Pelzer. 2003. "Comparative Study of Flavonoids in Experimental Models of Inflammation." *Pharmacology Research* 48: 601–6.

Flaxseed Oil

Allman, M. A., M. M. Pena, and D. Pang. 1995. "Supplementation with Flaxseed Oil versus Sunflowerseed Oil in Healthy Young Men Consuming a Low Fat Diet: Effects on Platelet Composition and Function." *European Journal of Clinical Nutrition* 49: 169–78.

Cunnane, S. C., M. J. Hamadeh, A. C. Liede, L. U. Thompson, T. M. Wolever, and D. J. Jenkins. 1995. "Nutritional Attributes of Traditional Flaxseed in Healthy Young Adults." *American Journal of Clinical Nutrition* 61: 62–68.

"Flaxseed Oil: Healthful or Harmful for Men?" 2003. *Harvard Men's Health Watch* 8: 5–6, 8.

Francois, C. A., S. L. Connor, L. C. Bolewicz, and W. E. Connor. 2003. "Supplementing Lactating Women with Flaxseed Oil Does Not Increase Docosahexaenoic Acid in Their Milk." *American Journal of Clinical Nutrition* 77: 226–33.

Kurzer, M. S., J. W. Lampe, M. C. Martini, and H. Adlercreutz. 1995. "Fecal Lignan and Isoflavonoid Excretion in Premenopausal Women Consuming Flaxseed Powder." *Cancer Epidemiology, Biomarkers, and Prevention* 4: 353–58.

Mantzioris, E., M. J. James, R. A. Gibson, and L. G. Cleland. 1995. "Nutritional Attributes of Dietary Flaxseed Oil." *American Journal of Clinical Nutrition* 62: 841–42.

Nesbitt, P. D., and L. U. Thompson. 1997. "Lignans in Home-made and Commercial Products Containing Flaxseed." *Nutrition and Cancer* 29: 222–27.

Nestel, P. J., S. E. Pomeroy, T. Sasahara, T. Yamashita, Y. L. Liang, A. M. Dart, G. L. Jennings, M. Abbey, and J. D. Cameron. 1997. "Arterial Compliance in Obese Subjects Is Improved with Dietary Plant N-3 Fatty Acid from Flaxseed Oil Despite Increased LDL Oxidizability." *Arteriosclerosis, Thrombosis, and Vascular Biology* 17: 1163–70.

Schuman, B. E., E. J. Squires, and S. Leeson. 2000. "Effect of Dietary Flaxseed, Flax Oil and N-3 Fatty Acid Supplement on Hepatic and Plasma Characteristics Relevant to Fatty Liver Haemorrhagic Syndrome in Laying Hens." *British Poultry Science* 41: 465–72.

Utsunomiya, T., S. R. Chavali, W. W. Zhong, and R. A. Forse. 1994. "Effects of Continuous Tube Feeding of Dietary Fat Emulsions on Eicosanoid Production and on Fatty Acid Composition during an Acute Septic Shock in Rats." *Biochimica et Biophysica Acta/General Subjects* (Amsterdam) 1214: 333–39.

Garlic

Ali, M., M. Thomson, and M. Afzal. 2000. "Garlic and Onions: Their Effect on Eicosanoid Metabolism and Its Clinical Relevance." *Prostaglandins, Leukotrienes, and Essential Fatty Acids* 62 (2): 55-73.

Bianchini, F. and H. Vainio. 2001. "Allium Vegetables and Organosulfur Compounds: Do They Help Prevent Cancer?" *Environmental Health Perspectives* 109 (9): 893-902.

Boyle, S. P., V. L. Dobson, S. J. Duthie, J. A. Kyle, and A. R. Collins. 2000. "Absorption and DNA Protective Effects of Flavonoid Glycosides from an Onion Meal." *European Journal of Nutrition* 39 (5): 213-223.

Challier, B., J. M. Perarnau, and J. F. Viel. 1998. "Garlic, Onion, and Cereal Fibre as Protective Factors for Breast Cancer: A French Case-Control Study." *European Journal of Epidemiology* 14 (8): 737-747.

Dorant, E., P. A. Van Den Brandt, and R. A. Goldbohm. 1996. "A Prospective Cohort Study on the Relationship between Onion and Leek Consumption, Garlic Supplement Use and the Risk of Colorectal Carcinoma in the Netherlands." *Carcinogenesis* 17 (3): 477-84.

———. 1995. "Allium Vegetable Consumption, Garlic Supplement Intake, and Female Breast Carcinoma Incidence." *Breast Cancer Research and Treatment* 33 (2): 163-70.

———. 1994. "A Prospective Cohort Study on Allium Vegetable Consumption, Garlic Supplement Use, and the Risk of Lung Carcinoma in the Netherlands." *Cancer Research* 54 (23): 6148-53.

Dorant, E., P. A. Van Den Brandt, R. A. Goldbohm, and F. Sturmans. 1996. "Consumption of Onions and a Reduced Risk of Stomach Carcinoma." *Gastroenterology* 110 (1): 12-20.

Fukushima S., N. Takada, T. Hori, and H. Wanibuchi. 1997. "Cancer Prevention by Organosulfur Compounds from Garlic and Onion." *Journal of Cellular Biochemistry. Supplement* 27: 100-105.

Keiss, H. P., V. M. Dirsch, T. Hartung, and others. 2003. "Garlic (Allium Sativum L.) Modulates Cytokine Expression in Lipopolysaccharide-Activated Human Blood Thereby Inhibiting NF-KappaB Activity." *Journal of Nutrition* 133 (7): 2171–75.

O'Reilly, J. D., A. I. Mallet, G. T. McAnlis, and others. 2001. "Consumption of Flavonoids in Onions and Black Tea: Lack of Effect on F2-isoprostanes and Autoantibodies to Oxidized LDL in Healthy Humans." *American Journal of Clinical Nutrition* 73 (6): 1040-1044.

Pinto, J. T., and R. S. Rivlin. 2001. "Antiproliferative Effects of Allium Derivatives from Garlic." *Journal of Nutrition* 131 (3s): 1058S–1060S.

Thomson, M., and M. Ali. 2003. "Garlic [Allium Sativum]: A Review of Its Potential Use as an Anti-cancer Agent." *Current Cancer Drug Targets* 3 (1): 67–81.

Wattenberg, L. W., V. L. Sparnins, and G. Barany. 1989. "Inhibition of N-nitrosodiethylamine Carcinogenesis in Mice by Naturally Occurring Organosulfur Compounds and Monoterpenes." *Cancer Research* 49 (10): 2689-92.

Germanium

Fujii, A., N. Kuboyama, J. Yamane, S. Nakao, and Y. Furukawa. 1993. "Effect of Organic Germanium Compound (Ge-132) on Experimental Osteoporosis in Rats." *General Pharmacology* 24: 1527–32.

Gerber, G. B., and A. Leonard. 1997. "Mutagenicity, Carcinogenicity, and Teratogenicity of Germanium Compounds." *Mutation Research* 387: 141–46.

Goodman, S. 1988. "Therapeutic Effects of Organic Germanium." *Medical Hypotheses* 26: 207–15.

Schauss, A. G. 1991. "Nephrotoxicity in Humans by the Ultratrace Element Germanium." *Renal Failure* 13: 1–4.

Seaborn, C. D., and F. H. Nielsen. 1994. "Effects of Germanium and Silicon on Bone Mineralization." *Biological Trace Element Research* 42: 151–64.

Tao, S. H., and P. M. Bolger. 1997. "Hazard Assessment of Germanium Supplements." *Regulatory Toxicology and Pharmacology* 25: 211–19.

Unakar, N. J., M. Johnson, J. Tsui, M. Cherian, and E. C. Abraham. 1995. "Effect of Germanium-132 on Galactose Cataracts and Glycation in Rats." *Experimental Eye Research* 61: 155–64.

Ginger

Erler, J., and others. 1988. "Essential Oils from Ginger (Zingiber Officinalis Roscoe)." *Zeitschrift für Lebensmitteluntersuchung und -forschung A* (Berlin) 186 (3): 231–34.

Harvey, D. J. 1981. "Gas Chromatographic and Mass Spectrometric Studies of Ginger Constituents. Identification of Gingerdiones and New Hexahydrocurcumin Analogues." *Journal of Chromatography* 212 (1): 75–84.

Park, K. K., K. S. Chun, J. M. Lee, S. S. Lee, and Y. J. Surh. 1998. "Inhibitory Effects of [6]-gingerol, a Major Pungent Principle of Ginger, on Phorbol Ester-Induced Inflammation. *Cancer Letters* 129 (2): 139–44.

Xiong, H. X. 1986. "Changes in Multihormones in Treating Male Sterility with Acupuncture and Indirect Moxibustion Using Ginger Slices on the Skin." *Zhong Xi Yi Jie He Za Zhi* (Beijing) 6: 726–27, 708.

Ginkgo

Akiba, S., T. Kawauchi, T. Oka, T. Hashizume, and T. Sato. 1998. "Inhibitory Effect of the Leaf Extract of Ginkgo Biloba L. on Oxidative Stress-Induced Platelet Aggregation." *Biochemistry and Molecular Biology International* 46 (6): 1243-48.

Akisu, M., N. Kultursay, I. Coker, and A. Huseyinov. 1998. "Platelet-Activating Factor Is an Important Mediator in Hypoxic Ischemic Brain Injury in the Newborn Rat. Flunarizine and Ginkgo Biloba Extract Reduce PAF Concentration in the Brain." *Biology Neonate* 74 (6): 439–44.

"Ginkgo Biloba and Peripheral Artery Disease." 2000. *Harvard Heart Letter* 10 (10): 4–5.

Kose, K., and P. Dogan. 1995. "Lipoperoxidation Induced by Hydrogen Peroxide in Human Erythrocyte Membranes. 1. Protective Effect of Ginkgo Biloba Extract (EGB 761)." *Journal of International Medical Research* 23 (1): 1–8.

Lamant, V., G. Mauco, P. Braquet, H. Chap, and L. Douste-Blazy. 1987. "Inhibition of the Metabolism of Platelet Activating Factor (PAF-Acether) by Three Specific Antagonists from Ginkgo Biloba." *Biochemical Pharmacology* 36 (17): 2749–52.

Lenoir, M., E. Pedruzzi, S. Rais, K. Drieu, and A. Perianin. 2002. "Sensitization of Human Neutrophil Defense Activities through Activation of Platelet-Activating Factor Receptors by Ginkgolide B, a Bioactive Component of the Ginkgo Biloba Extract EGB 761." *Biochemical Pharmacology* 63 (7): 1241–49.

Letzel, H., and W. Schoop. 1992. "Gingko Biloba Extract EGB 761 and Pentoxifylline in Intermittent Claudication: Secondary Analysis of the Clinical Effectiveness." *VASA. Zeitschrift fur Gefasskrankheiten* 21 (4): 403–10.

Maitra, I., L. Marcocci, M. T. Droy-Lefaix, and L. Packer. 1995. "Peroxyl Radical Scavenging Activity of Ginkgo Biloba Extract EGB 761." *Biochemical Pharmacology* 49 (11): 1649–55.

Oyama, Y., P. A. Fuchs, N. Katayama, and K. Noda. 1994. "Myricetin and Quercetin, the Flavonoid Constituents of Ginkgo Biloba Extract, Greatly Reduce Oxidative Metabolism in Both Resting and Ca(2+)-Loaded Brain Neurons." *Brain Research* 635 (1-2): 125–29.

Pittler, M. H., and E. Ernst. 2000. "Ginkgo Biloba Extract for the Treatment of Intermittent Claudication: A Meta-analysis of Randomized Trials." *American Journal of Medicine* 108 (4): 276–81.

Sastre, J., A. Millan, J. Garcia de la Asuncion, and others. 1998. "A Ginkgo Biloba Extract (EGB 761) Prevents Mitochondrial Aging by Protecting against Oxidative Stress." *Free Radical Biology and Medicine* 24 (2): 298–304.

Smith, P. F., K. Maclennan, and C. L. Darlington. 1996. "The Neuroprotective Properties of the Ginkgo Biloba Leaf: A Review of the Possible Relationship to Platelet-Activating Factor (PAF)." *Journal of Ethnopharmacology* 50 (3): 131–39.

Stucker, O., C. Pons, J. P. Duverger, K. Drieu, P. D'Arbigny. 1997. "Effect of Ginkgo Biloba Extract (EGB 761) on the Vasospastic Response of Mouse Cutaneous Arterioles to Platelet Activation." *International Journal of Microcirculation, Clinical and Experimental* 17 (2): 61–66.

Wei, Z., Q. Peng, B. H. Lau, and V. Shah. 1999. "Ginkgo Biloba Inhibits Hydrogen Peroxide-Induced Activation of Nuclear Factor Kappa B in Vascular Endothelial Cells." *General Pharmacology* 33 (5): 369–75.

Yan, L. J., M. T. Droy-Lefaix, and L. Packer. 1995. "Ginkgo Biloba Extract (EGB 761) Protects Human Low Density Lipoproteins against Oxidative Modification Mediated by Copper." *Biochemical and Biophysical Research Communications* 212 (2): 360–66.

Glucosamine Sulfate/Chondroitin Sulfate

Angermann, P. 2003. "Glucosamine and Chondroitin Sulfate in the Treatment of Arthritis." *Ugeskrift for Laeger* (Copenhagen) 165: 451–54.

Brief, A. A., S. G. Maurer, and P. E. Di Cesare. 2001. "Use of Glucosamine and Chondroitin Sulfate in the Management of Osteoarthritis." *Journal of the American Academy of Orthopedic Surgeons* 9: 71–78.

Deal, C. L., and R. W. Moskowitz. 1999. "Nutraceuticals as Therapeutic Agents in Osteoarthritis: The Role of Glucosamine, Chondroitin Sulfate, and Collagen Hydrolysate." *Rheumatic Diseases Clinics of North America* 25: 379–95.

Hungerford, D. S., and L. C. Jones. 2003. "Glucosamine and Chondroitin Sulfate Are Effective in the Management of Osteoarthritis." *Journal of Arthroplasty* 18: 5–9.

Kelly, G. S. 1998. "The Role of Glucosamine Sulfate and Chondroitin Sulfates in the Treatment of Degenerative Joint Disease." *Alternative Medicine Review* 3: 27–39.

Schenck, R. C., Jr. 2000. "New Approaches to the Treatment of Osteoarthritis: Oral Glucosamine and Chondroitin Sulfate." *Instructional Course Lectures* 49: 491–94.

Setnikar, I., and L. C. Rovati. 2001. "Absorption, Distribution, Metabolism, and Excretion of Glucosamine Sulfate: A Review." *Arzeneimittel-Forschung* (Aulendorf, Germany) 51: 699–725.

Glutamine

Akobeng, A. K., V. Miller, A. G. Thomas, and K. Richmond. 2000. "Glutamine Supplementation and Intestinal Permeability in Crohn's Disease." *JPEN. Journal of Parenteral and Enteral Nutrition* 24(3): 196.

Gore, D. C., and R. R. Wolfe. 2003. "Metabolic Response of Muscle to Alanine, Glutamine, and Valine Supplementation during Severe Illness." *JPEN. Journal of Parenteral and Enteral Nutrition* 27: 307–14.

Miskovitz, P. 2002. "Glutamine Supplementation in Critically Ill and Elective Surgical Patients: Does the Evidence Warrant Its Use?" *Critical Care Medicine* 30: 2152–53.

Novak, F., D. K. Heyland, A. Avenell, J. W. Drover, and X. Su. 2002. "Glutamine Supplementation in Serious Illness: A Systematic Review of the Evidence." *Critical Care Medicine* 30: 2022–29.

Peng, X., H. Yan, Z. You, P. Wang, and S. Wang. 2004. "Effects of Enteral Supplementation with Glutamine Granules on Intestinal Mucosal Barrier Function in Severe Burned Patients." *Burns* 30: 135–39.

Rathmacher, J. A., S. Nissen, L. Panton, R. H. Clark, P. Eubanks May, A. E. Barber, J. D'Olimpio, and N. N. Abumrad. 2004. "Supplementation with a Combination of Beta–hydroxy-beta-methylbutyrate (HMB), Arginine, and Glutamine Is Safe and Could Improve Hematological Parameters." *JPEN. Journal of Parenteral and Enteral Nutrition* 28: 65–75.

Savy, G. K. 2002. "Glutamine Supplementation. Heal the Gut, Help the Patient." *Journal of Infusion Nursing* 25: 65–69.

Tubman, T. R., and S. W. Thompson. 2001. "Glutamine Supplementation for Prevention of Morbidity in Preterm Infants." *Cochrane Database of Systematic Reviews* CD001457.

Yeh, S. L., Y. N. Lai, H. F. Shang, M. T. Lin, and W. J. Chen. 2004. "Effects of Glutamine Supplementation on Innate Immune Response in Rats with Gut-Derived Sepsis." *British Journal of Nutrition* 91: 423–29.

Yoshida, S., A. Kaibara, N. Ishibashi, and K. Shirouzu. 2001. "Glutamine Supplementation in Cancer Patients." *Nutrition* 17: 766–68.

Glutathione/N-acetyl cysteine (NAC)

Breuille, D., and C. Obled. 2000. "Cysteine and Glutathione in Catabolic States. *Nestle Nutrition Workshop Series. Clinical and Performance Programme* 3: 173–91; discussion 191–97.

Dickinson, D. A., and H. J. Forman. 2002. "Cellular Glutathione and Thiols Metabolism." *Biochemical Pharmacology* 64: 1019–26.

Droge, W. 1999. "Cysteine and Glutathione in Catabolic Conditions and Immunological Dysfunction." *Current Opinion in Clinical Nutrition and Metabolic Care* 2: 227–33.

Droge, W., V. Hack, R. Breitkreutz, E. Holm, and others. 1998. "Role of Cysteine and Glutathione in Signal Transduction, Immunopathology and Cachexia." *Biofactors* 8: 97–102.

Filomeni, G., G. Rotilio, and M. R. Ciriolo. 2002. "Cell Signalling and the Glutathione Redox System." *Biochemical Pharmacology* 64: 1057–64.

Singh, R. J. 2002. "Glutathione: A Marker and Antioxidant for Aging." *The Journal of Laboratory and Clinical Medicine* 140: 380–81.

Valencia, E., and G. Hardy. 2002. "Practicalities of Glutathione Supplementation in Nutritional Support." *Current Opinion in Clinical Nutrition and Metabolic Care* 5: 321–26.

Glutathione Peroxidase

Michelson, A. M. 1998. "Selenium Glutathione Peroxidase: Some Aspects in Man." *Journal of Environmental Pathology, Toxicology, and Oncology* 17: 233–39.

Neve, J. 1995. "Human Selenium Supplementation as Assessed by Changes in Blood Selenium Concentration and Glutathione Peroxidase Activity." *Journal of Trace Elements in Medicine and Biology* 9: 65–73.

Tarp, U. 1994. "Selenium and the Selenium-Dependent Glutathione Peroxidase in Rheumatoid Arthritis." *Danish Medical Bulletin* 41: 264–74.

Vitoux, D., P. Chappuis, J. Arnaud, M. Bost, M. Accominotti, and A. M. Roussel. 1996. "Selenium, Glutathione Peroxidase, Peroxides, and Platelet Functions." *Annales de Biologie Clinique* (Paris) 54: 181–87.

Goldenseal

Hwang, B. Y., S. K. Roberts, L. R. Chadwick, C. D. Wu, and A. D. Kinghorn. 2003. "Antimicrobial Constituents from Goldenseal (the Rhizomes of Hydrastis Canadensis) against Selected Oral Pathogens." *Planta Medica* 69: 623–27.

Mahady, G. B., S. L. Pendland, A. Stoia, and L. R. Chadwick. 2003. "In Vitro Susceptibility of Helicobacter Pylori to Isoquinoline Alkaloids from Sanguinaria Canadensis and Hydrastis Canadensis." *Phytotherapy Research* 17: 217–21.

Periera Da Silva, A., R. Rocha, C. M. Silva, L. Mira, M. F. Duarte, and M. H. Florencio. 2000. "Antioxidants in Medicinal Plant Extracts: A Research Study of the Antioxidant Capacity of Crataegus, Hamamelis, and Hydrastis." *Phytotherapy Research* 14: 612–16.

Rehman, J., J. M. Dillow, S. M. Carter, J. Chou, B. Le, and A. S. Maisel. 1999. "Increased Production of Antigen-Specific Immunoglobulins G and M Following In Vivo Treatment with the Medicinal Plants Echinacea Angustifolia and Hydrastis Canadensis." *Immunology Letters* 68: 391–95.

Scazzocchio, F., M. F. Cometa, L. Tomassini, and M. Palmery. 2001. "Antibacterial Activity of Hydrastis Canadensis Extract and Its Major Isolated Alkaloids." *Planta Medica* 67: 561–64.

Grapefruit Seed Extract

Heggers, J. P., J. Cottingham, J. Gusman, and others. 2002. "The Effectiveness of Processed Grapefruit-Seed Extract as an Antibacterial Agent: II. Mechanism of Action and In Vitro Toxicity." *Journal of Alternative and Complementary Medicine* 8 (3): 333–40. Erratum in *Journal of Alternative and Complementary Medicine* 8 (4): 521.

Green Tea

Baltaziak, M., E. Skrzydlewska, A. Sulik, W. Famulski, and M. Koda. 2004. "Green Tea as an Antioxidant Which Protects against Alcohol Induced Injury in Rats: A Histopathological Examination." *Folia Morphologica* (Warsaw) 63: 123–26.

Henning, S. M., C. Fajardo-Lira, H. W. Lee, A. A. Youssefian, V. L. Go, and D. Heber. 2003. "Catechin Content of Eighteen Teas and a Green Tea Extract Supplement Correlates with the Antioxidant Capacity." *Nutrition and Cancer* 45: 226–35.

Higashi-Okai, K., M. Yamazaki, H. Nagamori, and Y. Okai. 2001. "Identification and Antioxidant Activity of Several Pigments from the Residual Green Tea (Camellia Sinensis) after Hot Water Extraction." *Journal of the University of Occupational and Environmental Health* 23: 335–44.

Katiyar, S. K. 2003. "Skin Photoprotection by Green Tea: Antioxidant and Immunomodulatory Effects." *Current Drug Targets. Immune, Endocrine, and Metabolic Disorders* 3: 234–42.

Skrzydlewska, E., J. Ostrowska, A. Stankiewicz, and R. Farbiszewski. 2002. "Green Tea as a Potent Antioxidant in Alcohol Intoxication." *Addiction Biology* 7: 307–14.

Thiagarajan, G., S. Chandani, C. S. Sundari, S. H. Rao, A. V. Kulkarni, and D. Balasubramanian. 2001. "Antioxidant Properties of Green and Black Tea, and Their Potential Ability to Retard the Progression of Eye Lens Cataract." *Experimental Eye Research* 73: 393–401.

Vayalil, P. K., C. A. Elmets, and S. K. Katiyar. 2003. "Treatment of Green Tea Polyphenols in Hydrophilic Cream Prevents UVB-Induced Oxidation of Lipids and Proteins, Depletion of Antioxidant Enzymes and Phosphorylation of MAPK Proteins in SKH-1 Hairless Mouse Skin." *Carcinogenesis* 24: 927–36.

Hawthorn

Bahorun, T., E. Aumjaud, H. Ramphul, M. Rycha, A. Luximon-Ramma, F. Trotin, and O. I. Aruoma. 2003. "Phenolic Constituents and Antioxidant Capacities of Crataegus Monogyna (Hawthorn) Callus Extracts." *Nahrung* (Berlin) 47: 191–98.

Bahorun, T., F. Trotin, J. Pommery, J. Vasseur, and M. Pinkas. 1994. "Antioxidant Activities of Crataegus Monogyna Extracts." *Planta Medica* 60: 323–28.

Guo, J., X. Zhao, and G. Liu. 1999. "The Antioxidant Activity of Wild Jujubi, Crataegus, and Grape in Vitro." *Wei Sheng Yan Jiu* (Shanghai) 28: 108–10.

Kirakosyan, A., E. Seymour, P. B. Kaufman, S. Warber, S. Bolling, and S. C. Chang. 2003. "Antioxidant Capacity of Polyphenolic Extracts from Leaves of Crataegus Laevigata and Crataegus Monogyna (Hawthorn) Subjected to Drought and Cold Stress." *Journal of Agriculture Food Chemistry* 51: 3973–76.

Periera Da Silva, A., R. Rocha, C. M. Silva, L. Mira, M. F. Duarte, and M. H. Florencio. 2000. "Antioxidants in Medicinal Plant Extracts: A Research Study of the Antioxidant Capacity of Crataegus, Hamamelis, and Hydrastis." *Phytotherapy Research* 14: 612–16.

Rakotoarison, D. A., B. Gressier, F. Trotin, C. Brunet, T. Dine, M. Luyckx, J. Vasseur, M. Cazin, J. C. Cazin, and M. Pinkas. 1997. "Antioxidant Activities of Polyphenolic Extracts from Flowers, In Vitro Callus and Cell Suspension Cultures of Crataegus Monogyna." *Pharmazie* (Berlin) 52: 60–64.

Shahat, A. A., P. Cos, T. De Bruyne, S. Apers, F. M. Hammouda, S. I. Ismail, S. Azzam, M. Claeys, E. Goovaerts, L. Pieters, D. Vanden Berghe, and A. J. Vlietinck. 2002. "Antiviral and Antioxidant Activity of Flavonoids and Proanthocyanidins from Crataegus Sinaica." *Planta Medica* 68: 539–41.

Horse Chestnut

Calabrese, C., and P. Preston. 1993. "Report of the Results of a Double-Blind, Randomized, Single-Dose Trial of a Topical 2% Escin Gel versus Placebo in the Acute Treatment of Experimentally-Induced Hematoma in Volunteers." *Planta Medica* 59: 394–97.

Diehm, C., H. J. Trampish, S. Lange, and others. 1996. "Comparison of Leg Compression Stocking and Oral Horse Chestnut Seed Extract Therapy in Patients with Chronic Venous Insufficiency." *Lancet* 347: 292–94.

Guillaume, M., and F. Padioleau. 1994. "Venotonic Effect, Vascular Protection, Anti-inflammatory, and Free Radical Scavenging Properties of Horse Chestnut Extract." *Arzneimittel-Forschung* (Berlin-Heidelberg) 44: 25–35.

Pittler, M. H., and E. Ernst. 1998. "Horse Chestnut Seed Extract for Chronic Venous Insufficiency: A Criteria-Based Systematic Review." *Archives of Dermatology* 134: 1356–60.

Wilhelm, K., and C. Felmeier. 1977. "Thermometric Investigations about the Efficacy of Beta-escin to Reduce Postoperative Edema." *Medizinische Klinik* (Munich) 72: 128–34.

Ipriflavone

Acerbi, D., G. Poli, and P. Ventura. 1998. "Comparative Bioavailability of Two Oral Formulations of Ipriflavone in Healthy Volunteers at Steady-State. Evaluation of Two Different Dosage Schemes." *European Journal of Drug Metabolism and Pharmacokinetics* 23: 172–77.

Alexandersen, P., A. Toussaint, C. Christiansen, and others. 2001. "Ipriflavone in the Treatment of Postmenopausal Osteoporosis: A Randomized Controlled Trial." *Journal of the American Medical Association* 285: 1482–88.

Avioli, L. V. 1997. "The Future of Ipriflavone in the Management of Osteoporotic Syndromes." *Calcified Tissue International* 61 (suppl 1): S33–S35.

Gennari, C. 1997. "Ipriflavone: Background." *Calcified Tissue International* 61 (suppl 1): S3–S4.

Head, K. A. 1999. "Ipriflavone: An Important Bone-Building Isoflavone." *Alternative Medicine Review* 4: 10–22.

Kass-Annese, B. 2000. "Alternative Therapies for Menopause." *Clinical Obstetrics and Gynecology* 43: 162–83.

Makita, K., and H. Ohta. 2002. "Ipriflavone in the Treatment of Osteoporosis." *Nippon Rinsho. Japanese Journal of Clincal Medicine* (Osaka) 60 (suppl 3): 359–64.

Messina, M., and V. Messina. 2000. "Soyfoods, Soybean Isoflavones, and Bone Health: A Brief Overview." *Journal of Renal Nutrition* 10: 63–68.

Kava

Assemi, M. 2001. "Herbs Affecting the Central Nervous System: Gingko, Kava, St. John's Wort, and Valerian." *Clinical Obstetrics and Gynecology* 44: 824–35.

Bilia, A. R., S. Gallon, and F. F. Vincieri. 2002. "Kava-Kava and Anxiety: Growing Knowledge about the Efficacy and Safety." *Life Science* 70: 2581–97.

Denham, A., M. Mcintyre, and J. Whitehouse. 2002. "Kava—The Unfolding Story: Report on a Work-in-Progress. *Journal of Alternative and Complementary Medicine* 8: 237–63.

Ernst, E. 2002. "The Risk-Benefit Profile of Commonly Used Herbal Therapies: Ginkgo, St. John's Wort, Ginseng, Echinacea, Saw Palmetto, and Kava. *Annals of Internal Medicine* 136: 42–53.

Kinder, C., and M. J. Cupp. 1998. "Kava: An Herbal Sedative." *Nurse Practitioner* 23: 14, 156.

Nowakowska, E., A. Ostrowicz, and A. Chodera. 1998. "Kava-Kava Preparations—Alternative Anxiolytics." *Polski Merkuriusz Lekarski* (Warsaw) 4: 179–180a.

Pepping, J. 1999. "Kava: Piper Methysticum." *American Journal of Health-System Pharmacy* 56: 957–58, 960.

Pittler, M. H., and E. Ernst. 2002. "Kava Extract for Treating Anxiety." *Cochrane Database of Systematic Reviews* CD003383.

Singh, Y. N., and N. N. Singh. 2002. "Therapeutic Potential of Kava in the Treatment of Anxiety Disorders." *CNS Drugs* 16: 731–43.

Teschke, R., W. Gaus, and D. Loew. 2003. "Kava Extracts: Safety and Risks Including Rare Hepatotoxicity." *Phytomedicine* 10: 440–46.

Lactoferrin

Baveye, S., E. Elass, J. Mazurier, G. Spik, and D. Legrand. 1999. "Lactoferrin: A Multifunctional Glycoprotein Involved in the Modulation of the Inflammatory Process." *Clinical Chemistry and Laboratory Medicine* 37: 281–86.

Cavestro, G. M., A. V. Ingegnoli, G. Aragona, V. Iori, N. Mantovani, N. Altavilla, N. Dal Bo, A. Pilotto, A. Bertele, A. Franze, F. Di Mario, and L. Borghi. 2002. Lactoferrin: Mechanism of Action, Clinical Significance, and Therapeutic Relevance." *Acta Bio-Medica de L'Ateneo Parmense* (Parma) 73: 71–73.

Conneely, O. M. 2001. "Antiinflammatory Activities of Lactoferrin." *Journal of the American College of Nutrition* 20: 389S–395S; discussion 396S–397S.

Dial, E. J., and L. M. Lichtenberger. 2002. "Effect of Lactoferrin on Helicobacter Felis Induced Gastritis." *Biochemistry and Cell Biology* 80: 113–17.

Kanyshkova, T. G., V. N. Buneva, and G. A. Nevinsky. 2001. "Lactoferrin and Its Biological Functions." *Biochemistry* (Moscow) 66: 1–7.

Kruzel, M. L., and M. Zimecki. 2002. "Lactoferrin and Immunologic Dissonance: Clinical Implications." *Archivum Immunologiae et Therapiae Experimentalis* (Warsaw) 50: 399–410.

Van Der Strate, B. W., L. Beljaars, G. Molema, M. C. Harmsen, and D. K. Meijer. 2001. "Antiviral Activities of Lactoferrin." *Antiviral Research* 52: 225–39.

Licorice

Fukai, T., A. Marumo, K. Kaitou, T. Kanda, S. Terada, and T. Nomura. 2002. "Anti-helicobacter Pylori Flavonoids from Licorice Extract." *Life Science* 71: 1449–63.

Matsumoto, T., M. Tanaka, H. Yamada, and J. C. Cyong. 1996. "Effect of Licorice Roots on Carrageenan-Induced Decrease in Immune Complexes Clearance in Mice." *Journal of Ethnopharmacology* 53: 1–4.

Palagina, M. V., N. S. Dubniak, I. N. Dubniak, and P. S. Zorikov. 2003. "Correction of Respiratory Organ Impairment with Ural Licorice Preparations in Chronic Skin Diseases." *Terapevticheskii Arkhiv* (Moscow) 75: 63–65.

Shibata, S. 2000. "A Drug over the Millennia: Pharmacognosy, Chemistry, and Pharmacology of Licorice." *Yakugaku zasshi. Journal of the Pharmaceutical Society of Japan* (Tokyo) 120: 849–62.

Suzuki, F., D. A. Schmitt, T. Utsunomiya, and R. B. Pollard. 1992. "Stimulation of Host Resistance against Tumors by Glycyrrhizin, an Active Component of Licorice Roots." *In Vivo* 6: 589–96.

Takagi, K., and M. Harada. 1969. "Pharmacologyogical Studies on Herb Paeony Root. II. Anti-Inflammatory Effect, Inhibitory Effect on Gastric Juice Secretion, Preventive Effect on Stress Ulcer, Antidiuretic Effect of Paeoniflorin and Combined Effects with Licorice Component FM 100." *Yakugaku zasshi. Journal of the Pharmaceutical Society of Japan* (Tokyo) 89: 887–92.

Takagi, K., and Y. Ishii. 1967. "Peptic Ulcer Inhibiting Properties of a New Fraction from Licorice Root (FM 100). I. Experiental Peptic Ulcer and General Pharmacology." *Arzneimittel-Forschung* (Aulendorf, Germany) 17: 1544–47.

Takagi, K., S. Okabe, K. Kawashima, and T. Hirai. 1971. "The Therapeutic Effect of FM100, a Fraction of Licorice Root, on Acetic Acid Ulcer in Rats." *Japanese Journal of Pharmacology* 21: 832–33.

Watanabe, S. I., X. Y. Chey, K. Y. Lee, and T. M. Chang. 1986. "Release of Secretin by Licorice Extract in Dogs." *Pancreas* 1: 449–54.

Lutein

Granado, F., B. Olmedilla, and I. Blanco. 2003. "Nutritional and Clinical Relevance of Lutein in Human Health." *British Journal of Nutrition* 90: 487–502.

Iannone, A., C. Rota, S. Bergamini, A. Tomasi, and L. M. Canfield. 1998. "Antioxidant Activity of Carotenoids: An Electron-Spin Resonance Study on Beta-carotene and Lutein Interaction with Free Radicals Generated in a Chemical System." *Journal of Biochemical and Molecular Toxicology* 12: 299–304.

Krinsky, N. I., J. T. Landrum, and R. A. Bone. 2003. "Biologic Mechanisms of the Protective Role of Lutein and Zeaxanthin in the Eye." *Annual Review of Nutrition* 23: 171–201.

Kruger, C. L., M. Murphy, Z. Defreitas, F. Pfannkuch, and J. Heimbach. 2002. "An Innovative Approach to the Determination of Safety for a Dietary Ingredient Derived from a New Source: Case Study Using a Crystalline Lutein Product." *Food and Chemical Toxicology* (Oxford) 40: 1535–49.

Landrum, J. T., and R. A. Bone. 2001. "Lutein, Zeaxanthin, and the Macular Pigment." *Archives of Biochemistry and Biophysics* 385: 28–40.

Mares-Perlman, J. A., A. E. Millen, T. L. Ficek, and S. E. Hankinson. 2002. "The Body of Evidence to Support a Protective Role for Lutein and Zeaxanthin in Delaying Chronic Disease. Overview." *Journal of Nutrition* 132: 518S–524S.

Sies, H., and W. Stahl. 2003. "Non-nutritive Bioactive Constituents of Plants: Lycopene, Lutein and Zeaxanthin." *International Journal for Vitamin and Nutrition Research* 73: 95–100.

Van Den Berg, H. 1998. "Effect of Lutein on Beta-Carotene Absorption and Cleavage." *International Journal for Vitamin and Nutrition Research* 68: 360–65.

Lysine

Flodin, N. W. 1997. "The Metabolic Roles, Pharmacology, and Toxicology of Lysine." *Journal of the American College of Nutrition* 16 (1): 7–21.

Gurfinkel, E. P., R. Altman, A. Scazziota, and others. 2000. "Fast Platelet Suppression by Lysine Acetylsalicylate in Chronic Stable Coronary Patients. Potential Clinical Impact over Regular Aspirin for Coronary Syndromes." *Clinical Cardiology* 23 (9): 697–700.

Seidlin, M., and S. E. Straus. 1984. "Treatment of Mucocutaneous Herpes Simplex Infections." *Clinical Dermatology* 2 (2): 100–16.

Tomblin, F, A., Jr., and K. H. Lucas. 2001. "Lysine for Management of Herpes Labialis. *American Journal of Health-System Pharmacy* 58 (4): 298–300, 304.

Methylsulfonylmethane (MSM)

Barrager, E., and A. G. Schauss. 2003. "Methylsulfonylmethane as a Treatment for Seasonal Allergic Rhinitis: Additional Data on Pollen Counts and Symptom Questionnaire." *Journal of Alternative and Complementary Medicine* 9: 15–16.

Barrager, E., J. R. Veltmann Jr., A. G. Schauss, and R. N. Schiller. 2002. "A Multicentered, Open-Label Trial on the Safety and Efficacy of Methylsulfonylmethane in the Treatment of Seasonal Allergic Rhinitis." *Journal of Alternative and Complementary Medicine* 8: 167–73.

Ebisuzaki, K. 2003. "Aspirin and Methylsulfonylmethane (MSM): A Search for Common Mechanisms, with Implications for Cancer Prevention." *Anticancer Research* 23: 453–58.

Gaby, A. R. 2002. "Methylsulfonylmethane as a Treatment for Seasonal Allergic Rhinitis: More Data Needed on Pollen Counts and Questionnaire." *Journal of Alternative and Complementary Medicine* 8: 229.

"Methylsulfonylmethane (MSM). Monograph." 2003. *Alternative Medicine Review* 8: 438–41.

Milk Thistle

Ahmad, N., H. Gali, S. Javed, and R. Agarwal. 1998. "Skin Cancer Chemopreventive Effects of a Flavonoid Antioxidant Silymarin Are Mediated via Impairment of Receptor Tyrosine Kinase Signaling and Perturbation in Cell Cycle Progression." *Biochemical and Biophysical Research Communications* 247: 294–301.

Jiang, C., R. Agarwal, and J. Lu. 2000. "Anti-angiogenic Potential of a Cancer Chemopreventive Flavonoid Antioxidant, Silymarin: Inhibition of Key Attributes of Vascular Endothelial Cells and Angiogenic Cytokine Secretion by Cancer Epithelial Cells." *Biochemical and Biophysical Research Communications* 276: 371–78.

Kohno, H., T. Tanaka, K. Kawabata, Y. Hirose, S. Sugie, H. Tsuda, and H. Mori. 2002. "Silymarin, a Naturally Occurring Polyphenolic Antioxidant Flavonoid, Inhibits Azoxymethane-Induced Colon Carcinogenesis in Male F344 Rats." *International Journal of Cancer* 101: 461–68.

Singh, R. P., and R. Agarwal. 2002. "Flavonoid Antioxidant Silymarin and Skin Cancer." *Antioxidants and Redox Signaling* 4: 655–63.

Soto, C., R. Recoba, H. Barron, C. Alvarez, and L. Favari. 2003. "Silymarin Increases Antioxidant Enzymes in Alloxan-Induced Diabetes in Rat Pancreas." *Comparative Biochemistry and Physiology. C, Comparative Pharmacology and Toxicology* 136: 205–12.

Vinh, P. Q., S. Sugie, T. Tanaka, A. Hara, Y. Yamada, M. Katayama, T. Deguchi, and H. Mori. 2002. "Chemopreventive Effects of a Flavonoid Antioxidant Silymarin on N-butyl-N-(4-hydroxybutyl)nitrosamine-Induced Urinary Bladder Carcinogenesis in Male ICR Mice." *Japanese Journal of Cancer Research* 93: 42–49.

Zhao, J., M. Lahiri-Chatterjee, Y. Sharma, and R. Agarwal. 2000. "Inhibitory Effect of a Flavonoid Antioxidant Silymarin on Benzoyl Peroxide-Induced Tumor Promotion, Oxidative Stress and Inflammatory Responses in SENCAR Mouse Skin." *Carcinogenesis* 21: 811–16.

Nettle

Bnouham, M., F. Z. Merhfour, A. Ziyyat, H. Mekhfi, M. Aziz, and A. Legssyer. 2003. "Antihyperglycemic Activity of the Aqueous Extract of Urtica Dioica. *Fitoterapia* (Milan) 74: 677–81.

Farzami, B., D. Ahmadvand, S. Vardasbi, E. J. Majin, and S. H. Khaghani. 2003. "Induction of Insulin Secretion by a Component of Urtica Dioica Leave Extract in Perifused Islets of Langerhans and Its In Vivo Effects in Normal and Streptozotocin Diabetic Rats." *Journal of Ethnopharmacology* 89: 47–53.

Gulcin, I., O. I. Kufrevioglu, M. Oktay, and M. E. Buyukokuroglu. 2004. "Antioxidant, Antimicrobial, Antiulcer, and Analgesic Activities of Nettle (Urtica Dioica L.)." *Journal of Ethnopharmacology* 90: 205–15.

Konrad, L., M. H. Muller, C. Lenz, H. Laubinger, G. Aumuller, and J. J. Lichius. 2000. "Antiproliferative Effect on Human Prostate Cancer Cells by a Stinging Nettle Root (Urtica Dioica) Extract." *Planta Medica* 66: 44–47.

Krzeski, T., M. Kazon, A. Borkowski, A. Witeska, and J. Kuczera. 1993. "Combined Extracts of Urtica Dioica and Pygeum Africanum in the Treatment of Benign Prostatic Hyperplasia: Double-Blind Comparison of Two Doses." *Clinical Ther* 15: 1011–20.

Obertreis, B., K. Giller, T. Teucher, B. Behnke, and H. Schmitz. 1996. "Anti-inflammatory Effect of Urtica Dioica Folia Extract in Comparison to Caffeic Malic Acid." *Arzneimittel-Forschung* (Aulendorf, Germany) 46: 52–56.

Randall, C., K. Meethan, H. Randall, and F. Dobbs. 1999. "Nettle Sting of Urtica Dioica for Joint Pain—An Exploratory Study of This Complementary Therapy." *Complementary Therapies in Medicine* 7: 126–31.

Testai, L., S. Chericoni, V. Calderone, G. Nencioni, P. Nieri, I. Morelli, and E. Martinotti. 2002. "Cardiovascular Effects of Urtica Dioica L. (Urticaceae) Roots Extracts: In Vitro and In Vivo Pharmacological Studies." *Journal of Ethnopharmacology* 81: 105–9.

Teucher, T., B. Obertreis, T. Ruttkowski, and H. Schmitz. 1996. "Cytokine Secretion in Whole Blood of Healthy Subjects Following Oral Administration of Urtica Dioica L. Plant Extract." *Arzneimittel-Forschung* (Aulendorf, Germany) 46: 906–10.

Oregano

Akgul, A., and M. Kivanc. 1988. "Inhibitory Effects of Selected Turkish Spices and Oregano Components on Some Foodborne Fungi. *International Journal of Food Microbiology* 6 (3): 263–268.

Force, M., W. S. Sparks, R. A. Ronzio. 2000. "Inhibition of Enteric Parasites by Emulsified Oil of Oregano In Vivo." *Phytotherapy Research* 14 (3): 213–14.

Lagouri, V., and D. Boskou. 1996. "Nutrient Antioxidants in Oregano." *International Journal of Food Sciences and Nutrition* 47 (6): 493–97.

Lambert, R. J., P. N. Skandamis, P. J. Coote, and G. J. Nychas. 2001. "A Study of the Minimum Inhibitory Concentration and Mode of Action of Oregano Essential Oil, Thymol and Carvacrol." *Journal of Applied Microbiology* 91 (3): 453–62.

Takacsova, M., A. Pribela, and M. Faktorova. 1995. "Study of the Antioxidative Effects of Thyme, Sage, Juniper, and Oregano." *Nahrung* (Berlin) 39 (3): 241-43.

Oregon Grape

Bezakova, L., V. Misik, L. Malekova, E. Svajdlenka, and D. Kostalova. 1996. "Lipoxygenase Inhibition and Antioxidant Properties of Bisbenzylisoqunoline Alkaloids Isolated from Mahonia Aquifolium." *Pharmazie* (Berlin) 51: 758–61.

Cernakova, M., and D. Kost'alova. 2002. "Antimicrobial Activity of Berberine—A Constituent of Mahonia Aquifolium." *Folia Microbiologica* (Prague) 47: 375–78.

Cernakova, M., D. Kost'alova, V. Kettmann, M. Plodova, J. Toth, and J. Drimal. 2002. "Potential Antimutagenic Activity of Berberine, a Constituent of Mahonia Aquifolium." *BMC Complementary Alternative Medicine* 2: 2.

Hajnicka, V., D. Kost'alova, D. Svecova, R. Sochorova, N. Fuchsberger, and J. Toth. 2002. "Effect of Mahonia Aquifolium Active Compounds on Interleukin-8 Production in the Human Monocytic Cell Line THP-1." *Planta Medica* 68: 266–68.

Vollekova, A., D. Kost'alova, V. Kettmann, and J. Toth. 2003. "Antifungal Activity of Mahonia Aquifolium Extract and Its Major Protoberberine Alkaloids." *Phytotherapy Research* 17: 834–37.

Vollekova, A., D. Kost'alova, and R. Sochorova. 2001. "Isoquinoline Alkaloids from Mahonia Aquifolium Stem Bark Are Active against Malassezia Spp." *Folia Microbiologica* (Prague) 46: 107–11.

Zeng, X., B. Lao, X. Dong, X. Sun, Y. Dong, G. Sheng, and J. Fu. 2003. "Study on Anti-influenza Effect of Alkaloids from Roots of Mahonia Bealei In Vitro." *Zhong Yao Cai* (Beijing) 26: 29–30.

Peppermint

Belanger, J. T. 1998. "Perillyl Alcohol: Applications in Oncology." *Alternative Medicine Review* 3 (6): 448–57.

Imai, H., K. Osawa, H. Yasuda, H. Hamashima, T. Arai, and M. Sasatsu. 2001. "Inhibition by the Essential Oils of Peppermint and Spearmint of the Growth of Pathogenic Bacteria." *Microbios* 106 (suppl 1): 31–39.

Inoue, T., Y. Sugimoto, H. Masuda, and C. Kamei. 2001. "Effects of Peppermint (Mentha Piperita L.) Extracts on Experimental Allergic Rhinitis in Rats." *Biological and Pharmaceutical Bulletin* (Tokyo) 24 (1): 92–95.

Kline, R. M., J. J. Kline, J. Di Palma, and G. J. Barbero. 2001. "Enteric-Coated, pH-Dependent Peppermint Oil Capsules for the Treatment of Irritable Bowel Syndrome in Children." *Journal of Pediatrics* 138 (1): 125–128.

Liu, J. H., G. H. Chen, H. Z. Yeh, C. K. Huang, and S. K. Poon. 1997. "Enteric-Coated Peppermint-Oil Capsules in the Treatment of Irritable Bowel Syndrome: A Prospective, Randomized Trial." *Journal of Gastroenterology* 32 (6): 765–68.

Pittler, M. H., and E. Ernst. 1998. "Peppermint Oil for Irritable Bowel Syndrome: A Critical Review and Metaanalysis." *American Journal of Gastroenterology* 93 (7): 1131–35.

Samarth, R. M., P. K. Goyal, and A. Kumar. 2001. "Modulatory Effect of Mentha Piperita (Linn.) on Serum Phosphatases Activity in Swiss Albino Mice against Gamma Irradiation." *Indian Journal of Experimental Biology* 39 (5): 479–82.

Spirling, L. I., and I. R. Daniels. 2001. "Botanical Perspectives on Health Peppermint: More Than Just an After-Dinner Mint." *Journal of the Royal Society of Health* 121 (1): 62–63.

Phosphatidylcholine and Phosphatidylserine

Andrioli, G., A. Carletto, P. Guarini, S. Galvani, D. Biasi, P. Bellavite, and R. Corrocher. 1999. "Differential Effects of Dietary Supplementation with Fish Oil or Soy Lecithin on Human Platelet Adhesion." *Thrombosis and Haemostasis* 82: 1522–27.

Benton, D., R. T. Donohoe, B. Sillance, and S. Nabb. 2001. "The Influence of Phosphatidylserine Supplementation on Mood and Heart Rate When Faced with an Acute Stressor." *Nutrition Neuroscience* 4: 169–78.

Buchman, A. L., M. Awal, D. Jenden, M. Roch, and S. H. Kang. 2000. "The Effect of Lecithin Supplementation on Plasma Choline Concentrations during a Marathon." *Journal of the American College of Nutrition* 19: 768–70.

Jorissen, B. L., F. Brouns, M. P. Van Boxtel, R. W. Ponds, F. R. Verhey, J. Jolles, and W. J. Riedel. 2001. "The Influence of Soy-Derived Phosphatidylserine on Cognition in Age-Associated Memory Impairment." *Nutritional Neuroscience* 4: 121–34.

Jorissen, B. L., F. Brouns, M. P. Van Boxtel, and W. J. Riedel. 2002. "Safety of Soy-Derived Phosphatidylserine in Elderly People." *Nutritional Neuroscience* 5: 337–43.

Kim, H. Y., and J. Hamilton. 2000. "Accumulation of Docosahexaenoic Acid in Phosphatidylserine Is Selectively Inhibited by Chronic Ethanol Exposure in C-6 Glioma Cells." *Lipids* 35: 187–95.

Kumar, R., H. M. Divekar, V. Gupta, and K. K. Srivastava. 2002. "Antistress and Adaptogenic Activity of Lecithin Supplementation." *Journal of Alternative and Complementary Medicine* 8: 487–92.

Wilson, T. A., C. M. Meservey, and R. J. Nicolosi. 1998. Soy Lecithin Reduces Plasma Lipoprotein Cholesterol and Early Atherogenesis in Hypercholesterolemic Monkeys and Hamsters: Beyond Linoleate." *Atherosclerosis* 140: 147–53.

Propolis

Boyanova L., S. Derejian, R. Koumanova, and others. 2003. "Inhibition of Helicobacter Pylori Growth In Vitro by Bulgarian Propolis: Preliminary Report." *Journal of Medical Microbiology* 52 (May, part 5): 417–19.

Gregory, S. R., N. Piccolo, M. T. Piccolo, and others. 2002. "Comparison of Propolis Skin Cream to Silver Sulfadiazine: A Naturopathic Alternative to Antibiotics in Treatment of Minor Burns." *Journal of Alternative and Complementary Medicine* 8 (1): 77–83.

Hegazi, A. G., and F. K. Abd El Hady. 2002. "Egyptian Propolis: 3. Antioxidant, Antimicrobial Activities, and Chemical Composition of Propolis from Reclaimed Lands." *Zeitschrift für Naturforschung* (Tübingen) 57 (3–4): 395–402.

Kartal, M., S. Yildiz, S. Kaya, and others. 2003. "Antimicrobial Activity of Propolis Samples from Two Different Regions of Anatolia." *Journal of Ethnopharmacology* 86 (1): 69–73.

Shiitake Mushroom

Fukushima, M., T. Ohashi, Y. Fujiwara, K. Sonoyama, and M. Nakano. 2001. "Cholesterol-Lowering Effects of Maitake (Grifola Frondosa) Fiber, Shiitake (Lentinus Edodes) Fiber, and Enokitake (Flammulina Velutipes) Fiber in Rats." *Experimental Biology and Medicine* 226: 758–65.

Hayakawa, M., and F. Kuzuya. 1985. "Studies on Platelet Aggregation and Cortinellus Shiitake." *Nippon Ronen Igakkai Zasshi* (Tokyo) 22: 151–59.

Jong, S. C., and J. M. Birmingham. 1993. "Medicinal and Therapeutic Value of the Shiitake Mushroom." *Advances in Applied Microbiology* 39: 153–84.

Kabir, Y., M. Yamaguchi, and S. Kimura. 1987. "Effect of Shiitake (Lentinus Edodes) and Maitake (Grifola Frondosa) Mushrooms on Blood Pressure and Plasma Lipids of Spontaneously Hypertensive Rats." *Journal of Nutritional Science and Vitaminology* (Tokyo) 33: 341–46.

Nanba, H., and H. Kuroda. 1987. "Antitumor Mechanisms of Orally Administered Shiitake Fruit Bodies." *Chemical and Pharmaceutical Bulletin* (Tokyo) 35: 2459–64.

Nanba, H., K. Mori, T. Toyomasu, and H. Kuroda. 1987. "Antitumor Action of Shiitake (Lentinus Edodes) Fruit Bodies Orally Administered to Mice." *Chemical and Pharmaceutical Bulletin* (Tokyo) 35: 2453–58.

Takazawa, H., F. Tajima, and C. Miyashita. 1982. "An Antifungal Compound from 'Shiitake' (Lentinus Edodes)." *Yakugaku Zasshi. Journal of the Pharmaceutical Society of Japan* (Tokyo) 102: 489–91.

Takehara, M., K. Mori, K. Kuida, and M. A. Hanawa. 1981. "Antitumor Effect of Virus-like Particles from Lentinus Edodes (Shiitake) on Ehrlich Ascites Carcinoma in Mice." *Archives of Virology* 68: 297–301.

Takehara, M., T. Toyomasu, K. Mori, and M. Nakata. 1984. "Isolation and Antiviral Activities of the Double-Stranded RNA from Lentinus Edodes (Shiitake)." *Kobe Journal of Medical Science* 30: 25–34.

St. John's Wort

Barnes, J., L. A. Anderson, and J. D. Phillipson. 2001. "St John's Wort (Hypericum Perforatum L.): A Review of Its Chemistry, Pharmacology, and Clinical Properties." *The Journal of Pharmacy and Pharmacology* 53: 583–600.

Greeson, J. M., B. Sanford, and D. A. Monti. 2001. "St. John's Wort (Hypericum Perforatum): A Review of the Current Pharmacological, Toxicological, and Clinical Literature." *Psychopharmacology* (Berlin) 153: 402–14.

Kasper, S. 2001. "Hypericum Perforatum—A Review of Clinical Studies." *Pharmacopsychiatry* 34 (suppl 1): S51–S55.

Kumar, V., P. N. Singh, A. V. Muruganandam, and S. K. Bhattacharya. 2000. "Hypericum Perforatum: Nature's Mood Stabilizer." *Indian Journal of Experimental Biology* 38: 1077–85.

Reichling, J., A. Weseler, and R. Saller. 2001. "A Current Review of the Antimicrobial Activity of Hypericum Perforatum L." *Pharmacopsychiatry* 34 (suppl 1): S116–S118.

Rodriguez-Landa, J. F., and C. M. Contreras. 2003. "A Review of Clinical and Experimental Observations about Antidepressant Actions and Side Effects Produced by Hypericum Perforatum Extracts." *Phytomedicine* 10: 688–99.

Verotta, L. 2003. "Hypericum Perforatum: A Source of Neuroactive Lead Structures." *Current Topics in Medicinal Chemistry* 3: 187–201.

Superoxide Dismutase (SOD)

Baker, K., C. B. Marcus, K. Huffman, and others. 1998. "Synthetic Combined Superoxide Dismutase/Catalase Mimetics Are Protective as a Delayed Treatment in a Rat Stroke Model: A Key Role for Reactive Oxygen Species in Ischemic Brain Injury." *Journal of Pharmacology and Experimental Therapeutics* 284 (1): 215–21.

Disilvestro, R. A., J. Marten, and M. Skehan. 1992. "Effects of Copper Supplementation on Ceruloplasmin and Copper-Zinc Superoxide Dismutase in Free-Living Rheumatoid Arthritis Patients." *Journal of the American College of Nutrition* 11: 177–80.

Eldad, A., P. Ben Meir, S. Breiterman , and others. 1998. "Superoxide Dismutase (SOD) for Mustard Gas Burns." *Burns* 24 (2): 114–19.

Lefaix, J. L., S. Delanian, J. J. Leplat, and others. 1993. "Radiation-Induced Cutaneo-Muscular Fibrosis (III): Major Therapeutic Efficacy of Liposomal Cu/Zn Superoxide Dismutase." *Bulletin of Cancer* 80 (9): 799–807.

Mulder, T. P., A. Van Der Sluys Veer, H. W. Verspaget, G. Griffioen, A. S. Pena, A. R. Janssens, and C. B. Lamers. 1994. "Effect of Oral Zinc Supplementation on Metallothionein and Superoxide Dismutase Concentrations in Patients with Inflammatory Bowel Disease." *Journal of Gastroenterology and Hepatology* 9: 472–77.

Theanine

Kakuda, T. 2002. "Neuroprotective Effects of the Green Tea Components Theanine and Catechins." *Biological and Pharmaceutical Bulletin* (Tokyo) 25: 1513–18.

Sadzuka, Y., T. Sugiyama, A. Miyagishima, Y. Nozawa, and S. Hirota. 1996. "The Effects of Theanine, as a Novel Biochemical Modulator, on the Antitumor Activity of Adriamycin." *Cancer Letters* 105: 203–9.

Sadzuka, Y., T. Sugiyama, and T. Sonobe. 2000. "Improvement of Idarubicin Induced Antitumor Activity and Bone Marrow Suppression by Theanine, a Component of Tea." *Cancer Letters* 158: 119–24.

Sugiyama, T., and Y. Sadzuka. 2003. "Theanine and Glutamate Transporter Inhibitors Enhance the Antitumor Efficacy of Chemotherapeutic Agents." *Biochimica et Biophysica Acta/General Subjects* (Amsterdam) 1653 (2): 47–59.

Sugiyama, T., T. Sadzuka, K. Tanaka, and T. Sonobe. 2001. "Inhibition of Glutamate Transporter by Theanine Enhances the Therapeutic Efficacy of Doxorubicin." *Toxicology Letters* 121: 89–96.

Yokogoshi, H., M. Mochizuki, and K. Saitoh. 1998. "Theanine-Induced Reduction of Brain Serotonin Concentration in Rats." *Bioscience, Biotechnology, and Biochemistry* 62: 816–17.

Zhang, G., Y. Miura, and K. Yagasaki. 2002. "Effects of Dietary Powdered Green Tea and Theanine on Tumor Growth and Endogenous Hyperlipidemia in Hepatoma-Bearing Rats." *Bioscience, Biotechnology, and Biochemistry* 66: 711–16.

Zheng, G., K. Sayama, T. Okubo, L. R. Juneja, and I. Oguni. 2004. "Anti-obesity Effects of Three Major Components of Green Tea, Catechins, Caffeine, and Theanine, in Mice." *In Vivo* 18: 55–62.

Turmeric

Kang, B. Y., Y. J. Song, K. M. Kim, Y. K. Choe, S. Y. Hwang, and T. S. Kim. 1999. "Curcumin Inhibits Th1 Cytokine Profile in CD4+T Cells by Suppressing Interleukin-12 Production in Macrophages." *British Journal of Pharmacology* 128(2): 380–84.

Negi, P. S., G. K. Jayaprakasha, L. Jagan Mohan Rao, and K. K. Sakariah. 1999. "Antibacterial Activity of Turmeric Oil: A Byproduct from Curcumin Manufacture. *Journal of Agriculture Food Chemistry* 47 (10): 4297–300.

Phan, T. T., P. See, S. T. Lee, and S. Y. Chan. 2001. "Protective Effects of Curcumin against Oxidative Damage on Skin Cells in Vitro: Its Implication for Wound Healing." *Journal of Trauma* 51 (5): 927–31.

Ramirez-Tortosa, M. C., M. D. Mesa, M. C. Aguilera, and others. 1999. "Oral Administration of a Turmeric Extract Inhibits LDL Oxidation and Has Hypocholesterolemic Effects in Rabbits with Experimental Atherosclerosis." *Atherosclerosis* 147 (2): 371–78.

Shah, B. H., Z. Nawaz, S. A. Pertani, and others. 1999. "Inhibitory Effect of Curcumin, a Food Spice from Turmeric, on Platelet-Activating Factor- and Arachidonic Acid-Mediated Platelet Aggregation through Inhibition of Thromboxane Formation and Ca2+ Signaling." *Biochemistry Pharmacology* 58 (7): 1167–72.

Wuthi-Udomler, M., W. Grisanapan, O. Luanratana, and W. Caichompoo. 2000. "Antifungal Activity of Curcuma Longa Grown in Thailand." *Southeast Asian Journal of Tropical Medicine and Public Health* 31 (suppl 1): 178–82.

Tea Tree Oil

Carson, C. F., and T V. Riley. 2001. "Safety, Efficacy, and Provenance of Tea Tree (Melaleuca Alternifolia) Oil. *Contact Dermatitis* 45 (2): 65–67.

Mantle, D., M. A. Gok, and T. W. Lennard. 2001. "Adverse and Beneficial Effects of Plant Extracts on Skin and Skin Disorders." *Adverse Drug Reactions and Toxicological Reviews* 20 (2): 89–103.

Valerian

Cavadas, C., I. Araujo, M. D. Cotrim, T. Amaral, A. P. Cunha, T. Macedo, and C. F. Ribeiro. 1995. "In Vitro Study on the Interaction of Valeriana Officinalis L. Extracts and Their Amino Acids on GABAA Receptor in Rat Brain." *Arzneimittel-Forschung* (Aulendorf, Germany) 45: 753–55.

Fernandez, S., C. Wasowski, A. C. Paladini, and M. Marder. 2004. "Sedative and Sleep-Enhancing Properties of Linarin, a Flavonoid-Isolated from Valeriana Officinalis." *Pharmacology, Biochemistry, and Behavior* 77: 399–404.

Marder, M., H. Viola, C. Wasowski, S. Fernandez, J. H. Medina, and A. C. Paladini. 2003. "6-Methylapigenin and Hesperidin: New Valeriana Flavonoids with Activity on the CNS." *Pharmacology, Biochemistry, and Behavior* 75: 537–45.

Ortiz, J. G., J. Nieves-Natal, and P. Chavez. 1999. "Effects of Valeriana Officinalis Extracts on [3H]flunitrazepam Binding, Synaptosomal [3H]GABA Uptake, and Hippocampal [3H]GABA Release." *Neurochemical Research* 24: 1373–78.

Plushner, S. L. 2000. "Valerian: Valeriana Officinalis." *American Journal of Health-System Pharmacy* 57: 328, 333, 335.

Wasowski, C., M. Marder, H. Viola, J. H. Medina, and A. C. Paladini. 2002. "Isolation and Identification of 6-Methylapigenin, a Competitive Ligand for the Brain GABA(A) Receptors, from Valeriana Wallichii." *Planta Medica* 68: 934–36.

Vinpocetine

Bereczki, D., and I. Fekete. 2000. "Vinpocetine for Acute Ischaemic Stroke." *Cochrane Database of Systematic Reviews* CD000480.

———. 1999. "A Systematic Review of Vinpocetine Therapy in Acute Ischaemic Stroke." *European Journal of Clinical Pharmacology* 55: 349–52.

Bonoczk, P., B. Gulyas, V. Adam-Vizi, A. Nemes, E. Karpati, B. Kiss, M. Kapas, C. Szantay, I. Koncz, T. Zelles, and A. Vas. 2000. "Role of Sodium Channel Inhibition in Neuroprotection: Effect of Vinpocetine." *Brain Research Bulletin* 53: 245–54.

Hadjiev, D. 2003. "Asymptomatic Ischemic Cerebrovascular Disorders and Neuroprotection with Vinpocetine." *Ideggyogyaszati Szemle* (Budapest) 56: 166–72.

Horvath, S. 2001. "The Use of Vinpocetine in Chronic Disorders Caused by Cerebral Hypoperfusion." *Orvosi Hetilap* (Budapest) 42: 383–89.

Szatmari, S. Z., and P. J. Whitehouse. 2003. "Vinpocetine for Cognitive Impairment and Dementia." *Cochrane Database of Systematic Reviews* CD003119.

Vas, A., B. Gulyas, Z. Szabo, P. Bonoczk, L. Csiba, B. Kiss, E. Karpati, G. Panczel, and Z. Nagy. 2002. "Clinical and Non-Clinical Investigations Using Positron Emission Tomography, Near Infrared Spectroscopy, and Transcranial Doppler Methods on the Neuroprotective Drug Vinpocetine: A Summary of Evidences." *Journal of the Neurological Sciences* 203–4, 259–62.

"Vinpocetine. Monograph." 2002. *Alternative Medicine Review* 7: 240–43.

Wheat Germ Oil/Octacosanol

Consolazio, C. F., L. O. Matoush, R. A. Nelson, and others. 1963. "Physiological and Biochemical Evaluation of Potential Antifatigue Drugs. III. The Effect of Octacosanol, Wheat Germ Oil, and Vitamin E on the Performance of Swimming Rats." *Report. United States. Army Medical Research and Nutrition Laboratory, Denver.* 275: 1–2.

Kato, S., K. Karino, S. Hasegawa, J. Nagasawa, A. Nagasaki, M. Eguchi, T. Ichinose, K. Tago, H. Okumori, K. Hamatani, and A. L. Et. 1995. "Octacosanol Affects Lipid Metabolism in Rats Fed on a High-Fat Diet." *British Journal of Nutrition* 73: 433–41.

Kim, H., S. Park, D. S. Han, and T. Park. 2003. "Octacosanol Supplementation Increases Running Endurance Time and Improves Biochemical Parameters after Exhaustion in Trained Rats." *Journal of Medicinal Food* 6: 345–51.

Norris, F. H., E. H. Denys, and R. J. Fallat. 1986. "Trial of Octacosanol in Amyotrophic Lateral Sclerosis." *Neurology* 36: 1263–64.

Snider, S. R. 1984. "Octacosanol in Parkinsonism." *Annals of Neurology* 16: 723.

Taylor, J. C., L. Rapport, and G. B. Lockwood. 2003. "Octacosanol in Human Health." *Nutrition* 19: 192–95.

CHAPTER 8: FOODS

Fruits

Bhatia, I. S., and K. L. Bajaj. 1972. "Tannins in Black-Plum (Syzygium Cumini L.) Seeds." *Biochemical Journal* (London) 128 (1): 56P.

Canal, J. R., M. D. Torres, A. Romero, and C. Perez. 2000. "A Chloroform Extract Obtained from a Decoction of Ficus Carica Leaves Improves the Cholesterolaemic Status of Rats with Streptozotocin-Induced Diabetes. *Acta Physiologica Hungarica* (Budapest) 87 (1): 71–76.

Collins, B. H., A. Horska, P. M. Hotten, and others. 2001. "Kiwifruit Protects against Oxidative DNA Damage in Human Cells and In Vitro." *Nutrition and Cancer* 39 (1): 148–53.

Culpitt, S. V., D. F. Rogers, P. S. Fenwick, and others. 2003. "Inhibition by Red Wine Extract, Resveratrol, of Cytokine Release by Alveolar Macrophages in COPD." *Thorax* 58: 942–61.

Day, A. P., H. J. Kemp, C. Bolton, and others. 1997. "Effect of Concentrated Red Grape Juice Consumption on Serum Antioxidant Capacity and Low-Density Lipoprotein Oxidation." *Annals of Nutrition and Metabolism* 41 (6): 353–57.

De Amorin, A., H. R. Borba, J. P. Carauta, and others. 1999. "Anthelmintic Activity of the Latex of Ficus Species." *Journal of Ethnopharmacology* 64 (3): 255–58.

Dunjic, B. S., I. Svensson, J. Axelson, and others. 1993. "Green Banana Protection of Gastric Mucosa against Experimentally Induced Injuries in Rats: A Multicomponent Mechanism." *Scandinavian Journal of Gastroenterology* 28 (10): 894–98.

Edwards, A. J., B. T. Vinyard, E. R. Wiley, and others. 2003. "Consumption of Watermelon Juice Increases Plasma Concentrations of Lycopene and Beta-Carotene in Humans." *Journal of Nutrition* 133 (4): 1043–50.

Egbekun, M. K., J. I. Akowe, and R. J. Ede. 1996. "Physicochemical and Sensory Properties of Formulated Syrup from Black Plum (Vitex Doniana) Fruit." *Plant Foods Human Nutrition* 49 (4): 301–6.

Fan, Y., Z. Ding, L. Yang, and others. 1995. "A Preliminary Study on Bioactivity of Orange and Tangerine Peel Extracts against Aphis and Mites." *Zhongguo Zhong Yao Za Zhi.* (Beijing) 20 (7): 397–98, 446.

Freedman, J. E., C. Parker III, L. Li, and others. 2001. "Select Flavonoids and Whole Juice from Purple Grapes Inhibit Platelet Function and Enhance Nitric Oxide Release." *Circulation* 103 (23): 2792–98.

Galati, E. M., M. T. Monforte, S. Kirjavainen, and others. 1994. "Biological Effects of Hesperidin, a Citrus Flavonoid. (Note I): Antiinflammatory and Analgesic Activity." *Farmaco* (Pavia, Italy) 40 (11): 709–12.

Galati, E. M., A. Trovato, S. Kirjavainen, and others. 1996. "Biological Effects of Hesperidin, a Citrus Flavonoid. (Note III): Antihypertensive and Diuretic Activity in Rat." *Farmaco* (Pavia, Italy) 51 (3): 219–21.

Gharagozloo, M., and A. Ghaderi. 2001. "Immunomodulatory Effect of Concentrated Lime Juice Extract on Activated Human Mononuclear Cells." *Journal of Ethnopharmacology* 77 (1): 85–90.

Honow, R., N. Laube, A. Schneider, T. Kessler, and A. Hesse. 2003. "Influence of Grapefruit-, Orange-, and Apple-Juice Consumption on Urinary Variables and Risk of Crystallization." *British Journal of Nutrition* 90 (2): 295–300.

Huang, C., Y. Huang, J. Li, and others. 2002. "Inhibition of Benzo(a)pyrene Diol-epoxide-induced Transactivation of Activated Protein 1 and Nuclear Factor KappaB by Black Raspberry Extracts." *Cancer Research* 62 (23): 6857–63.

Ikken, Y., P. Morales, A. Martinez, and others. 1999. "Antimutagenic Effect of Fruit and Vegetable Ethanolic Extracts against N-nitrosamines Evaluated by the Ames Test." *Journal of Agriculture Food Chemistry* 47 (8): 3257–64.

Joseph, J. A., B. Shukitt-Hale, N. A. Denisova, and others. 1999. "Reversals of Age-Related Declines in Neuronal Signal Transduction, Cognitive, and Motor Behavioral Deficits with Blueberry, Spinach, or Strawberry Dietary Supplementation." *Journal of Neuroscience* 19 (18): 8114–21.

———. 1998. "Long-Term Dietary Strawberry, Spinach, or Vitamin E Supplementation Retards the Onset of Age-Related Neuronal Signal-Transduction and Cognitive Behavioral Deficits." *Journal of Neuroscience* 18 (19): 8047–55.

Kahkonen, M. P., A. I. Hopia, and M. Heinonen. 2001. "Berry Phenolics and Their Antioxidant Activity." *Journal of Agriculture Food Chemistry* 49 (8): 4076–82.

Kalt, W., C. F. Forney, A. Martin, and R. L. Prior. 1999. "Antioxidant Capacity, Vitamin C, Phenolics, and Anthocyanins after Fresh Storage of Small Fruits." *Journal of Agriculture Food Chemistry* 47 (11): 4638–44.

Karadeniz, F., R. W. Durst, and R. E. Wrolstad. 2000. "Polyphenolic Composition of Raisins." *Journal of Agriculture Food Chemistry* 48 (11): 5343–50.

Karakaya, S., S. N. El, and A. A. Tas. 2001. "Antioxidant Activity of Some Foods Containing Phenolic Compounds." *International Journal of Food Science and Nutrition* 52 (6): 501–8.

Kawaii, S., Y. Tomono, E. Katase, and others. 1999. "Antiproliferative Effects of the Readily Extractable Fractions Prepared from Various Citrus Juices on Several Cancer Cell Lines." *Journal of Agriculture Food Chemistry* 47 (7): 2509–12.

Liu, M., X. Q. Li, C. Weber, and others. 2002. "Antioxidant and Antiproliferative Activities of Raspberries." *Journal of Agriculture Food Chemistry* 50 (10): 2926–30.

Maffei Facino, R., M. Carini, G. Aldini, and others. 1997. "Regeneration of Endogenous Antioxidants, Ascorbic Acid, Alpha Tocopherol, by the Oligomeric Procyanide Fraction of Vitus Vinifera L.:ESR Study." *Bollettino Chimico Farmaceutico* (Milano) 136 (4): 340–44.

Mata, L., C. Vargas, D. Saborio, and M. Vives. 1994. "Extinction of Vibrio Cholerae in Acidic Substrata: Contaminated Cabbage and Lettuce Treated with Lime Juice." *Revista de Biologia Tropical* (San Jose, Costa Rica) 42 (3): 487–92.

McGhie, T. K., G. D. Ainge, L. E. Barnett, and others. 2003. "Anthocyanin Glycosides from Berry Fruit Are Absorbed and Excreted Unmetabolized by Both Humans and Rats." *Journal of Agriculture Food Chemistry* 51 (16): 4539–48.

Misra, N., S. Batra, and D. Mishra. 1988. "Fungitoxic Properties of the Essential Oil of Citrus Limon (L.) Burm. against a Few Dermatophytes." *Mycoses* 31 (7): 380–82.

Miyagi, Y., K. Miwa, and H. Inoue. 1997. "Inhibition of Human Low-Density Lipoprotein Oxidation by Flavonoids in Red Wine and Grape Juice." *American Journal of Cardiology* 80 (12): 1627–31.

Miyake, Y., A. Murakami, Y. Sugiyamam, and others. 1999. "Identification of Coumarins from Lemon Fruit (Citrus Limon) as Inhibitors of In Vitro Tumor Promotion and Superoxide and Nitric Oxide Generation." *Journal of Agriculture Food Chemistry* 47 (8): 3151–57.

Nakatani, N., S. Kayano, H. Kikuzaki, and others. 2000. "Identification, Quantitative Determination, and Antioxidative Activities of Chlorogenic Acid Isomers in Prune (Prunus Domestica L.)." *Journal of Agriculture Food Chemistry* 48 (11): 5512–16.

Ogata, S., Y. Miyake, K. Yamamoto, and others. 2000. "Apoptosis Induced by the Flavonoid from Lemon Fruit (Citrus Limon Burm. F.) and Its Metabolites in HL-60 Cells." *Bioscience, Biotechnology, and Biochemistry* 64 (5): 1075–78.

Perez, C., J. R. Canal, J. E. Campillo, and others. 1999. "Hypotriglyceridaemic Activity of Ficus Carica Leaves in Experimental Hypertriglyceridaemic Rats." *Phytotherapy Research* 13 (3): 188–91.

Prior, R. L., S. A. Lazarus, G. Cao, and others. 2001. "Identification of Procyanidins and Anthocyanins in Blueberries and Cranberries (Vaccinium Spp.) Using High-Performance Liquid Chromatography/Mass Spectrometry." *Journal of Agriculture Food Chemistry* 49 (3): 1270–76.

Rakhimov, M. R. 2000. "Pharmacologyogical Study of Papain from the Papaya Plant Cultivated in Uzbekistan." *Eksperimental'naia i klinicheskaia farmakologiia* (Moscow) 63 (3): 55–57.

Rao, N. M. 1991. "Protease Inhibitors from Ripened and Unripened Bananas." *Biochemistry International* 24 (1): 13–22.

Rapisarda, P., A. Tomaino, R. Lo Cascio, and others. 1999. "Antioxidant Effectiveness as Influenced by Phenolic Content of Fresh Orange Juices." *Journal of Agriculture Food Chemistry* 47 (11): 4718–23.

Rauha, J. P., S. Remes, M. Heinonen, and others. 2000. "Antimicrobial Effects of Finnish Plant Extracts Containing Flavonoids and Other Phenolic Compounds." *International Journal of Food Microbiology* 56 (1): 3–12.

Revel, A., H. Raanani, E. Younglai, J. Xu, I. Rogers, R. Han, J. F. Savouret, and R. F. Casper. 2003. "Resveratrol, a Natural Aryl Hydrocarbon Receptor Antagonist, Protects Lung from DNA Damage and Apoptosis Caused by Benzo[a]pyrene." *Journal of Applied Toxicology* 23 (4): 255–61.

Roberti, M., D. Pizzirani, D. Simoni, R. Rondanin, R. Baruchello, C. Bonora, F. Buscemi, S. Grimaudo, and M. Tolomeo. 2003. "Synthesis and Biological Evaluation of Resveratrol and Analogues as Apoptosis-Inducing Agents." *Journal of Medicinal Chemistry* 46 (16): 3546–54.

Rodrigues, A., H. Brun, and A. Sandstrom. 1997. "Risk Factors for Cholera Infection in the Initial Phase of an Epidemic in Guinea-Bissau: Protection by Lime Juice." *American Journal of Tropical Medicine and Hygiene* 57 (5): 601–4.

Sanchez-Moreno, C., G. Cao, B. Ou, and R. L. Prior. 2003. "Anthocyanin and Proanthocyanidin Content in Selected White and Red Wines. Oxygen Radical Absorbance Capacity Comparison with Nontraditional Wines Obtained from Highbush Blueberry." *Journal of Agriculture Food Chemistry* 51 (17): 4889–96.

Seeram, N. P., R. A. Momin, M. G. Nair, and L. D. Bourquin. 2001. "Cyclooxygenase Inhibitory and Antioxidant Cyanidin Glycosides in Cherries and Berries." *Phytomedicine* 8 (5): 362–69.

Solovchenko, A., and M. Schmitz-Eiberger. 2003. "Significance of Skin Flavonoids for UV-B-protection in Apple Fruits." *Journal of Experimental Botany* 54 (389): 1977–84.

Sommerburg, O., J. E. Keunen, A. C. Bird, and F. J. Van Kuijk. 1998. "Fruits and Vegetables That Are Sources for Lutein and Zeaxanthin: The Macular Pigment in Human Eyes." *British Journal of Ophthalmology* 82 (8): 907–10.

Van Der Sluis, A. A., M. Dekker, and G. Skrede. 2002. "Activity and Concentration of Polyphenolic Antioxidants in Apple Juice. 1. Effect of Existing Production Methods." *Journal of Agriculture Food Chemistry* 50 (25): 7211–19.

Walker, A. F., R. Bundy, S. M. Hicks, and others. 2002. "Bromelain Reduces Mild Acute Knee Pain and Improves Well-Being in a Dose-Dependent Fashion in an Open Study of Otherwise Healthy Adults." *Phytomedicine* 9 (8): 681–86.

Wang, S. Y., and H. Jiao. 2000. "Scavenging Capacity of Berry Crops on Superoxide Radicals, Hydrogen Peroxide, Hydroxyl Radicals, and Singlet Oxygen." *Journal of Agriculture Food Chemistry* 48 (11): 5677–84.

Wang, S. Y., and H. S. Lin. 2000. "Antioxidant Activity in Fruits and Leaves of Blackberry, Raspberry, and Strawberry Varies with Cultivar and Developmental Stage." *Journal of Agriculture Food Chemistry* 48 (2): 140–46.

Wills, R. B., F. M. Scriven, and H. Greenfield. 1983. "Nutrient Composition of Stone Fruit (Prunus Spp.) Cultivars: Apricot, Cherry, Nectarine, Peach, and Plum." *Journal of the Science of Food and Agriculture* 34 (12): 1383–89.

Yuan, J. M., D. O. Stram, K. Arakawa, H. P. Lee, and M. C. Yu. 2003. "Dietary Cryptoxanthin and Reduced Risk of Lung Cancer: The Singapore Chinese Health Study." *Cancer Epidemiology, Biomarkers, and Prevention* 12 (9): 890–98.

Zhang, W., M. F. Jin, X. J. Yu, and Q. Yuan. 2001. "Enhanced Anthocyanin Production by Repeated-Batch Culture of Strawberry Cells with Medium Shift." *Applied Microbiology and Biotechnology* 55 (2): 164–69.

Vegetables

Beecher, C. 1994. "Cancer Preventive Properties of Varieties of Brassica Oleracea: A Review." *American Journal of Clinical Nutrition* 59 (suppl): 1166S–1170S.

Bobek, P., S. Galbavy, and M. Mariassyova. 2000. "The Effect of Red Beet (Beta Vulgaris Var. Rubra) Fiber on Alimentary Hypercholesterolemia and Chemically Induced Colon Carcinogenesis in Rats." *Nahrung* (Berlin) 44 (3): 184–87.

Brooks, J. D., V. G. Paton, and G. Vidanes. 2001. "Potent Induction of Phase 2 Enzymes in Human Prostate Cells by Sulforaphane." *Cancer Epidemiology, Biomarkers and Prevention* 10 (9): 949–54.

Cheney, G. 1950. "Anti-Peptic Ulcer Dietary Factor." *Journal of the American Dietetic Association* 26 (1950): 668–72.

Duke, J. A. 1992. *Handbook of Phytochemical Constituents of GRAS Herbs and Other Economic Plants.* Boca Raton, Florida: CRC Press.

Edenharder, R., G. Keller, K. L. Platt, and K. K. Unger. 2001. "Isolation and Characterization of Structurally Novel Antimutagenic Flavonoids from Spinach (Spinacia Oleracea)." *Journal of Agriculture Food Chemistry* 49 (6): 2767–73.

Fowke, J. H., F. L. Chung, F. Jin, D. Qi, Q. Cai, C. Conaway, J. R. Cheng, X. O. Shu, Y. T. Gao, and W. Zheng. 2003. "Urinary Isothiocyanate Levels, Brassica, and Human Breast Cancer." *Cancer Research* 63 (14): 3980–86.

Kapadia, G. J., H. Tokuda, T. Konoshima, and H. Nishino. 1996. "Chemoprevention of Lung and Skin Cancer by Beta Vulgaris (Beet) Root Extract." *Cancer Letters* 100 (1–2): 211–14.

Kawamori, T., T. Tanaka, M. Ohnishi, and others. 1995. "Chemoprevention of Azoxymethane-Induced Colon Carcinogenesis by Dietary Feeding of S-methyl Methane Thiosulfonate in Male F344 Rats." *Cancer Research* 55 (18): 4053–58.

Kurilich, A. C., G. J. Tsau, A. Brown, and others. 1999. "Carotene, Tocopherol, and Ascorbate Contents in Subspecies of Brassica Oleracea." *Journal of Agriculture Food Chemistry* 47 (4): 1576–81.

Kushad, M. M., A. F. Brown, A. C. Kurilich, and others. 1999. "Variation of Glucosinolates in Vegetable Crops of Brassica Oleracea." *Journal of Agriculture Food Chemistry* 47 (4): 1541–48.

Kwak, M. K., P. A. Egner, P. M. Dolan, and others. 2001. "Role of Phase 2 Enzyme Induction in Chemoprotection by Dithiolethiones." *Mutation Research* 480–81: 305–15.

Longnecker, M. P., P. A. Newcomb, R. Mittendorf, and others. 1997. "Intake of Carrots, Spinach, and Supplements Containing Vitamin A in Relation to Risk of Breast Cancer." *Cancer Epidemiology, Biomarkers and Prevention* 6 (11): 887–92.

Michnovicz, J. J., and H. L. Bradlow. 1991. "Altered Estrogen Metabolism and Excretion in Humans Following Consumption of Indole-3-Carbinol." *Nutrition and Cancer* 16 (1): 59–66.

Nyska, A., L. Lomnitski, J. Spalding, and others. 2001. "Topical and Oral Administration of the Natural Water-Soluble Antioxidant from Spinach Reduces the Multiplicity of Papillomas in the Tg.AC Mouse Model." *Toxicology Letters* 122 (1): 33–44.

Seeger, P. G. 1967. "The Anthocyans of Beta Vulgaris Var. Rubra (Red Beets), Vaccinium Myrtillis (Whortleberries), Vinum Rubrum (Red Wine), and Their Significance as Cell Respiratory Activators for Cancer Prophylaxis and Cancer Therapy." *Arztliche Forschung* (Berlin) 21 (2): 68–78.

Steinkellner, H., S. Rabot, C. Freywald, and others. 2001. "Effects of Cruciferous Vegetables and Their Constituents on Drug Metabolizing Enzymes Involved in the Bioactivation of DNA-Reactive Dietary Carcinogens." *Mutation Research* 480–81: 285–97

Stoewsand, G. S. 1995. "Bioactive Organosulfur Phytochemicals in Brassica Oleracea Vegetables—A Review." *Food and Chemical Toxicology* (Oxford) 33 (6): 537–43.

Thimmulappa, R. K., K. H. Mai, S. Srisuma, and others. 2002. "Identification of Nrf2-regulated Genes Induced by the Chemopreventive Agent Sulforaphane by Oligonucleotide Microarray." *Cancer Research* 62 (18): 5196–5203.

Verhoeven, D. T., R. A. Goldbom, G. Van Poppel, and others. 1996. "Epidemiologcal Studies on Brassica Vegetables and Cancer Risk." *Cancer Epidemiology, Biomarkers and Prevention* 5 (9): 773–48.

Yang, Y., E. D. Marczak, M. Yokoo, H. Usui, and M. Yoshikawa. 2001. "Isolation and Antihypertensive Effect of Angiotensin I–Converting Enzyme (ACE) Inhibitory Peptides from Spinach Rubisco." *Journal of Agriculture Food Chemistry* 51 (17): 4897–4902.

Yurtsever, E., and K. T. Yardimci. 1999. "The In Vivo Effect of a Brassica Oleracea Var. Capitata Extract on Ehrlich Ascites Tumors of MUS Musculus BALB/C Mice." *Drug Metabolism and Drug Interactions* 15 (2–3): 215–22.

Grains

Ezeala, D. O. 1985. "Nutrients, Carotenoids, and Mineral Compositions of the Leaf Vegetables, Amaranthus Viridis and Amaranthus Caudatus." *Tropical Agriculture* 62 (2): 95–96.

Johnson, D. L., and S. M. Ward. 1993. "Quinoa." In J. Janick and J. E. Simon, eds., *New Crops.* New York: Wiley, 219–21.

Lorenz, K. 1983. "Tannins and Phytate Content in Proso Millets (*Panicum miliaceum*)." *Cereal Chemistry* 60 (6): 424–26.

Rastrelli, L., R. Aquino, and others. 1998. "Studies on the Constituents of Amaranthus Caudatus Leaves: Isolation and Structure Elucidation of New Triterpenoid Saponins and Ionol-Derived Glycosides." *Journal of Agriculture and Food Chemistry* 46 (5): 1797–1804.

Zhu, N., S. Sheng, D. Li, E. J. Lavoie, M. V. Karwe, and others. 2001. "Antioxidative Flavonoid Glycosides from Quinoa Seeds (*Chenopodium quinoa* willd). *Journal of Food Lipids* 8 (1): 37.

CHAPTER 9: DIETS

Australian Bureau of Statistics. 2002. *Apparent Consumption of Foodstuffs.* Sydney: Australian Bureau of Statistics, Belconnan, Canberra, Australian Capital Territory (ACT).

Boccardo, F., G. L. Lunardi, A. R. Petti, and others. 2003. "Enterolactone in Breast Cyst Fluid: Correlation with EGF and Breast Cancer Risk." *Breast Cancer Research and Treatment* 79 (1): 17–23.

Burroughs, S. *The MasterCleanser.* N.p.: Burroughs Books, 1976.

Campbell, T. C., and J. Chen. 1999. "Energy Balance: Interpretation of Data from Rural China." *Toxicological Sciences* 52: 87–94.

Chen J., T. C. Campbell, J. Li, and others. 1990. *Diet, Lifestyle, and Mortality in China.* Oxford, Ithica and Beijing: Oxford University Press, Cornell University Press, and People's Publishing House.

Covas, M. I., J. Marrugat, M. Fito, and others. 2002. "Scientific Aspects That Justify the Benefits of the Mediterranean Diet: Mild-to-Moderate versus Heavy Drinking." *Annals of the New York Academy of Sciences.* 957 (May): 162–73.

Curtis, B. M., and J. H. O'Keefe Jr. 2002. "Understanding the Mediterranean Diet. Could This Be the New 'Gold Standard' for Heart Disease Prevention?" *Postgrad Medicine* 112 (2): 35–38, 41–45.

Dagnelie, P. C., and van Staveren, W. A. 1994. "Macrobiotic Nutrition and Child Health: Results of a Population-Based, Mixed-Longitudinal Cohort Study in the Netherlands." *American Journal of Clinical Nutrition* 59 (suppl 5): 1187S–1196S.

Dangelie, P. C., W. A. van Staveren, J. G. Hautvast, and others. 1991. "Stunting and Nutrient Deficiencies in Children on Alternative Diets." *Acta Paediatrica Scandinavia* 374: (suppl): 111–18.

Djuric, Z., J. B. Depper, V. Uhley, and others. 1998. "Oxidative DNA Damage Levels in Blood from Women at High Risk for Breast Cancer Are Associated with Dietary Intakes of Meats, Vegetables, and Fruits." *Journal of the American Dietetic Association* 98 (5): 524–28.

Epstein, S. S. 1996. "Unlabeled Milk from Cows Treated with Biosynthetic Growth Hormones: A Case of Regulatory Abdication." *International Journal of Health Services* 26 (1): 173–85.

Flores, R., and A. Ojea-Rodriguez. 2002. "The WCRF Expert Panel Report as a Model for Advice and Policy Analysis for Other (Non-cancer) Chronic Disease, with Specific Note on WHO Technical Report 797 on Diet, Nutrition, and Prevention of Chronic Disease: Summary of Working Group 4." *Asia Pacific Journal of Clinical Nutrition* 11 (suppl 9): S777–S778.

Giovannucci, E. 1999. "Nutritional Factors in Human Cancers." *Advances in Experimental Medicine and Biology* 472: 29–42

Hallmans, G., J. X. Zhang, E. Lundin, and others. 2003. "Rye, Lignans, and Human Health." *Proceedings of the Nutrition Society* (London) 62 (1): 193–99.

Kushi, L. H., J. E. Cunningham, J. R. Hebert, and others. 2001. "The Macrobiotic Diet in Cancer." *Journal of Nutrition* 131 (suppl 11): 3056S–3064S.

Magarey, A. M., L. A. Daniels, and T. J. Boulton. 2001. "Prevalence of Overweight and Obesity in Australian Children and Adolescents: Reassessment of 1985 and 1995 Data against New Standard International Definitions." *Medical Journal of Australia* 174 (11): 561–64.

McCullough, M. L., D. Feskanich, M. J. Stampfer, and others. 2003. "Diet Quality and Major Chronic Disease Risk in Men and Women: Moving toward Improved Dietary Guidance." *American Journal of Clinical Nutrition* 78 (2): 349.

Michaud, D. S., K. Augustsson, E. B. Rimm, and others. 2001. "A Prospective Study on Intake of Animal Products and Risk of Prostate Cancer." *Cancer Causes and Control* 12 (6): 557–67.

Millward, D. J. 1999. "The Nutritional Value of Plant-Based Diets in Relation to Human Amino Acid and Protein Requirements." *Proceedings of the Nutrition Society* (London) 58 (2): 249–60.

National Heart Foundation of Australia. 2003. "Position Statement on Dietary Fat and Overweight/Obesity." *Nutrition and Dietetics* 60: 174–76.

National Institute of Alcohol Abuse and Alcoholism (NIAAA). 2000. *Per Capita Alcohol Consumption, Based on Alcohol Sales Data. Apparent Per Capita Ethanol Consumption for the United States, 1850–2000. [Gallons of Ethanol, Based on Population Age 15 and Older Prior to 1970 and on Population Age 14 and Older Thereafter."* Washington, D.C.: NIAAA.

Parsons, T. J., M. van Dusseldorp, M. van der Vliet, and others. 1997. "Reduced Bone Mass in Dutch Adolescents Fed a Macrobiotic Diet in Early Life." *Journal of Bone Mineral Research* 12 (9): 1486–94.

Perfetti, R., T. A. Brown, R. Velikina, and S. Busselen. 1999. "Control of Glucose Homeostasis by Incretin Hormones." *Diabetes Technology and Therapeutics* 1 (3): 297–305.

Ravnskov, U., C. Allen, D. Atrens, and others. 2002. "Studies of Dietary Fat and Heart Disease." *Science* 295 (5559): 1464–65.

Stark, A. H., and Z. Madar. 2002. "Olive Oil as a Functional Food: Epidemiology and Nutritional Approaches." *Nutrition Review* 60 (6): 170–76.

Stolzenberg-Solomon, R. Z., E. R. Miller III, M. G. Maguire, and others. 1999. "Association of Dietary Protein Intake and Coffee Consumption with Serum Homocysteine Concentrations in an Older Population." *American Journal of Clinical Nutrition* 69: 467–75.

van Dusseldorp, M., J. Schneede, H. Refsum, and others. 1999. "Risk of Persistent Cobalamin Deficiency in Adolescents Fed a Macrobiotic Diet in Early Life." *American Journal of Clinical Nutrition* 69 (4): 664–71.

Wolf-Maier, K., R. S. Cooper, J. R. Banegas, and others. 2003. "Hypertension Prevalence and Blood Pressure Levels in 6 European Countries, Canada, and the United States." *Journal of the American Medical Association* 289: 2363–69.

Young, V. R., and P. L. Pellett. 1994. "Plant Proteins in Relation to Human Protein and Amino Acid Nutrition." *American Journal of Clinical Nutrition* 59 (suppl 5): 1203S–1212S.

Zheng, W., D. R. Gustafson, R. Sinha, and others. 1998. "Well-Done Meat Intake and the Risk of Breast Cancer." *Journal of the National Cancer Institute* 90 (22): 1724–29.

CHAPTER 10: NUTRITIONAL HABITS

American Psychiatric Association (APA). 1994. *Diagnostic and Statistical Manual of Mental Disorders.* Fourth edition. Washington, D.C.: APA.

Hutchinson, A., J. R. Maltby, and C. R. Reid. 1988. "Gastric Fluid Volume and pH in Elective Inpatients. Part I: Coffee or Orange Juice versus Overnight Fast." *Canadian Journal of Anaesthesiology* 35 (1): 12–15.

Intorre, L. S. Bertini, E. Luchetti, and others. 1996. "The Effect of Ethanol, Beer, and Wine on Histamine Release from the Dog Stomach." *Alcohol* 13 (6): 547–51.

Mead, P. S., L. Slutsker, V. Dietz, and others. 1999. "Food-Related Illness and Death in the United States." *Emerging Infectious Dieseases* 5 (5): 607-25.

Sanchez, A. 1973. "Role of Sugars in Human Neutrophilic Phagocytosis." *American Journal of Clinical Nutrition* 26: 1180–84.

Saporito, B. 1994. "Home Cooking Is Off the Boil." *Fortune* 129 (6): 15.

Splinter, W. M., J. A. Stewart, and J. G. Muir. 1990. "Large Volumes of Apple Juice Preoperatively Do Not Affect Gastric pH and Volume in Children." *Canadian Journal of Anaesthesiology* 37 (1): 36–39.

U.S. Department of Agriculture. 2003. *Antibiotic Use in U.S. Livestock Production.* Animal and Plant Health Inspection Service (APHIS), Centers for Epidemiology and Animal Health Center for Emerging Issues, Emerging Health Issues. Antimicrobial Resistance Project, available at: www.aphis.usda.gov/vs/ceah/cei/Emerging AnimalHealthIssues_files/antiresist.antibiouse.pdf.

U.S. Government Accounting Office (GAO). 2004. *Economic Impact of a Ban on the Use of Over-the-Counter Antibiotics in U.S. Swine Rations.* Report to Congressional Requesters. Washington, D.C.: GAO.

CHAPTER 11: FOOD AND THE EARTH

Akerstedt, T., B. Arnetz, G. Ficca, and others. 1999. "A 50-Hz Electromagnetic Field Impairs Sleep." *Journal of Sleep Research* 8 (1): 77–81.

"Aluminium." 1997. *Environmental Health Criteria* 194: 252.

Bernard, B. K., M. R. Osheroff, A. Hofmann, and others. 1990. "Toxicology and Carcinogenesis Studies of Dietary Titanium Dioxide-Coated Mica in Male and Female Fischer 344 Rats." *Journal of Toxicology and Environmental Health* 29 (4): 417–30.

Bhakdi, S., and J. Bohl. 2003. "Prions, Mad Cow Disease, and Preventive Measures: A Critical Appraisal." *Medical Microbiology and Immunology* (Berlin) 192 (3): 117–22.

Brooks, B. O., F. D. Aldrich, G. M. Utter, and others. 1992. "Immune Responses to Pollutant Mixtures from Indoor Sources." *Annals of the New York Academy of Sciences* 641: 199–214.

Brown, D. R., F. Hafiz, L. L. Glasssmith, and others. 2000. "Consequences of Manganese Replacement of Copper for Prion Protein Function and Proteinase Resistance." *European Molecular Biology Organization Journal* 9 (6): 1180–86.

Buss, N. E., A. G. Renwick, K. M. Donaldson, and others. 1992. "The Metabolism of Cyclamate to Cyclohexylamine and Its Cardiovascular Consequences in Human Volunteers." *Toxicology and Applied Pharmacology* 115 (2): 199–210.

Camfield, P. R., C. S. Camfield, J. M. Dooley, and others. 1992. "Aspartame Exacerbates EEG Spike-Wave Discharge in Children with Generalized Absence Epilepsy: A Double-Blind Controlled Study." *Neurology* 42 (5): 1000–3.

Cantor, K. 2003. "Cancer Risk and Exposures to Drinking Water Contaminants." *Crisp Data Base National Institutes of Health [CRISP]* available online at: http://crisp.cit.nih.gov/.

Caplan, L. S., E. R. Schoenfeld, E. S. O'Leary, and others. 2000. "Breast Cancer and Electromagnetic Fields— A Review." *Annals of Epidemiology* 10 (1): 31–44.

Carlborg, F. W. 1985. "A Cancer Risk Assessment for Saccharin." *Food and Chemical Toxicology* (Oxford) 23 (4–5): 499–506.

"Carrageenan." 1983. *IARC Monographs on the Evaluation of the Carcinogenic Risk of Chemicals to Humans* 31: 79–94.

Chiba, T. 1993. "Cell Kinetics of Carcinoma Originating from Rat Colitis Induced by Dextran Sulphate Sodium." *Japanese Journal of Gastroenterology* 90 (4): 774–81.

Cocco, P., E. F. Heineman, and M. Dosemeci. 1999. "Occupational Risk Factors for Cancer of the Central Nervous System (CNS) among U.S. Women." *American Journal of Industrial Medicine* 36 (1): 70–74.

Committee on the Assessment of Asthma and Indoor Air, Division of Health Promotion and Disease Prevention, Institute of Medicine. 2000. *Clearing the Air: Asthma and Indoor Air Exposures.* Washington, D.C.: National Academy of Sciences Press.

Dalsgaard, N. J. 2002. "Prion Diseases: An Overview." *Acta Pathologica, Microbiologica et Immunologica Scandinavica* (Oxford) 110 (1): 3–13.

De Heer, C., H.-J. Schuurman, G. F. Houben, and others. 1995. "The SCID-Hu Mouse as a Tool in Immunotoxicological Risk Assessment: Effects of 2-acetyl-4(5)-tetrahydroxybutyl-imidazole (THI) and Di-n-butyltin dichloride (DBTC) on the Human Thymus in SCID-Hu Mice." *Toxicology* 100 (1–3): 203–11.

Decker, D. S., R. Dinardi, and E. J. Calabrerse. 1984. "Does Chloroform Exposure while Showering Pose a Serious Public Health Concern." *Medical Hypotheses* 15 (2) 119–24.

Dietert, R. R., and A. Hedge. 1996. "Chemical Sensitivity and the Immune System." Fourteenth International Neurotoxicology Conference, Hot Springs, Arkansas, October 13–16. *Neurotoxicology* (Little Rock) 17 (3–4): 253–57.

Diniz, Y. S., A. A. Fernandes, K. E. Campos, and others. 2004. "Toxicity of Hypercaloric Diet and Monosodium Glutamate: Oxidative Stress and Metabolic Shifting in Hepatic Tissue." *Food and Chemical Toxicology* (Oxford) 42 (2): 313–19.

Dunnick, J. K., and R. I. Melnick. 1993. "Assessment of the Carcinogenic Potential of Chlorinated Water: Experimental Studies of Chlorine, Chloramine, and Trihalomethanes." *Journal of the National Cancer Institute* 85 (10): 817–22.

Dutta, S. K. 2000. "Carcinogeneic Substances and Health Efects of Electmagentic Fields." *Crisp Data Base.* National Institutes of Health.

Elefteriou, F., S. Takeda, X. Liu, and others. 2003. "Monosodium Glutamate–Sensitive Hypothalamic Neurons Contribute to the Control of Bone Mass." *Endocrinology* 144 (9): 3842–47.

English, P. B. 2003. "Historic Traffic Exposure Maps for Cancer Studies." *Crisp Data Base.* National Institutes of Health.

Ewen, S. W. and A. Pusztai. 1999. "Effect of Diets Containing Genetically Modified Potatoes Expressing Galanthus Nivalis Lectin on Rat Small Intestine." *Lancet* 354 (9187): 1353–54.

Farnworth, J. J., H. B. Hayes, J. W. Nunn, and others. 1996. "The Use of Beringite to Remove Fulvic Acids (Mutagen Precursors) from Water." *Environmental Technology* 17 (5): 509–16.

Feychting, M and A. Ahlbom. 1993. Magnetic Fields and Cancer in Children Residing near Swedish High-Voltage Power Lines. *American Journal of Epidemiology* 138 (7): 467–81.

"Final Report on the Safety Assessment of Sorbic Acid and Potassium Sorbate." 1988. *Journal of the American College of Toxicology* 7 (6): 837–80.

Freni, S. C., and D. W. Gaylor. 1992. "International Trends in the Incidence of Bone Cancer Are Not Related to Drinking Water Fluoridation." *Cancer* 70 (3): 611–18.

Gales, M. A., and T. M. Nguyen. 2000. "Sorbitol Compared with Xylitol in Prevention of Dental Caries." *Annals of Pharmacotherapy* 34 (1): 98–100.

Garshick, E. 2003. "Diesel Particle Exposure and Lung Cancer." *Crisp Data Base.* National Institutes of Health.

Gomaa, E. A., J. I. Gray, S. Rabie, and others. 1993. "Polycyclic Aromatic Hydrocarbons in Smoked Food Products and Commercial Liquid Smoke Flavourings." *Food Additives and Contaminants* 10 (5): 503–21.

Graham, C., M. R. Cook, M. M. Gerkovich, and others. 2001. "Examination of the Melatonin Hypothesis in Women Exposed at Night to EMF or Bright Light. *Environmental Health Perspectives* 109 (5): 501–7. Erratum in *Environmental Health Perspectives* 109 (7): A304.

Hadnagy, W., R. Stiller-Winkler, H. Idel, and others. 1996. "Immunological Alterations in Sera of Persons Living in Areas with Different Air Pollution." *Toxicology Letters* 88 (1–3): 147–53.

Harlow, B. L., D. W. Cramer, D. A. Bell, and others. 1992. "Perineal Exposure to Talc and Ovarian Cancer Risk." *Obstetrics and Gynecology* 80: 19–26.

Houben, G. F., A. H. Penninks, W. Seinen, and others. 1993. "Immunotoxic Effects of the Color Additive Caramel Color III: Immune Function Studies in Rats." *Fundamental Applied Toxicology* 20 (1): 30–37.

Jickells, S. M., J. W. Gramshaw, L. Castle, and others. 1992. "The Effect of Microwave Energy on Specific Migration from Food Contact Plastics." *Food Additives and Contaminants* 9 (1): 19–27.

Johns, D. R. 1986. "Migraine Provoked by Aspartame." *New England Journal of Medicine* 315 (August 14): 456.

Jones, D. B., P. Slaughter, S. Lousley, and others. 1985. "Low Dose Guar Improves Diabetic Control." *Journal of the Royal Society of Medicine* 78 (7): 546–48.

Kador, P. F., J. W. Lee, S. Fujisawa, and others. 2000. "Relative Importance of Aldose Reductase versus Nonenzymatic Glycosylation on Sugar Cataract Formation in Diabetic Rats." *Journal of Ocular Pharmacology and Therapeutics* 16 (2): 149–60.

Kamei, H., T. Koide, Y. Hashimoto, and others. 1999. "Tumor Cell Growth Suppression by Tannic Acid." *Cancer Biotherapy and Radiopharmaceuticals* 14 (2): 135–38.

Kangsadalampai, K., C. Butryee, and K. Manoonphol. 1997. "Direct Mutagenicity of the Polycylic Aromatic Hydrocarbon-Containing Fraction of Smoked and Charcoal-Broiled Foods Treated with Nitrite in Acid Solution." *Food and Chemical Toxicology* (Oxford) 35 (2): 213.

Kilburn, K. H., and R. H. Warshaw. 1992. "Irregular Opacities in the Lung, Occupational Asthma, and Airways Dysfunction in Aluminum Workers." *American Journal of Industrial Medicine* 21 (6): 845–53.

Koivusalo, M., J. J. K. Jaakkola, T. Vartiainen, and others. 1994. "Drinking Water Mutagenicity and Gastrointestinal Urinary Tract Cancers: An Ecological Study in Finland." *American Journal of Public Health* 84 (8): 1223–28.

Koivusalo, M., E. Pukkala, T. Vartiainen, and others. 1997. "Drinking Water Chlorination and Cancer: A Historical Cohort Study in Finland." *Cancer Causes Control* 8 (2): 192–200.

Kuo, H. W., T. F. Chiang, I. I. Lo, and others. 1998. "Estimates of Cancer Risk from Chloroform Exposure during Showering in Taiwan." *Science of the Total Environment* 218 (1): 1–7.

Leonard, A., and E. D. Leonard. 1989. "Mutagenic and Carcinogenic Potential of Aluminium and Aluminium Compounds." *Toxicological and Environmental Chemistry* 23 (1/4): 27–31.

Levin, B. 1999. *Environmental Nutrition: Understanding the Link between Environment, Food Quality, and Disease.* Vashon Island, Washington: Hingepin Publishing.

Li, C. M., H. Chiang, Y. D. Fu, and others. 1999. "Effects of 50 Hz Magnetic Fields on Gap Junctional Intercellular Communication." *Bioelectromagnetics* 20 (5): 290–94.

Linet, M. 2003. "Studies of Non-ionizing Radiation-Related Cancer." *Crisp Data Base.* National Institutes of Health.

McGeehin, M. A., J. S. Reif, J. C. Becher, and others. 1993. "Case-Control Study of Bladder Cancer and Water Disinfection Methods in Colorado." *American Journal of Epidemiology* 138 (7): 492–501.

McNeal, T. P., and H. C. Hollifield. 1993. "Determination of Volatile Chemicals Released from Microwave-Heat-Susceptor Food Packaging." *Journal of AOAC (Association of Analytical Communities) International* 76 (6): 1268–75.

National Toxicology Program. 1993. *Toxicology and Carcinogenesis Studies of Talc (GAS No 14807-96-6) in F344/N Rats and B6C3F, Mice (Inhalation Studies).* Technical Report Series No. 421. Washington, D.C.: Department of Health and Human Services.

Oishi, S. 2002. "Effects of Parabens on the Male Reproductive System in Rats (2)." *Environmental Sciences: An International Journal of Environmental Physiology and Toxicology* 9 (2–3): 181.

Olney, J. W. 1994. "Excitotoxins in Foods." *Neurotoxicology* 15 (3): 535–44.

Olney, J. W., N. B. Farber, E. Spitznagel, and others. 1996. "Increasing Brain Tumor Rates: Is There a Link to Aspartame?" *Journal of Neuropathology and Experimental Neurology* 55 (11): 1115–23.

Osterman, J. W. 1990. "Evaluating the Impact of Municipal Water Fluoridation on the Aquatic Environment." *American Journal of Public Health* 80 (10): 1230–35.

Purdy, M. 2002. "The Manganese Loaded/Copper Depleted Bovine Brain Fails to Neutralise Incoming Shock Bursts of Low Frequency Infrasound; the Origins of BSE?" *Journal of Cattle Practise (Journal of the British Cattle Veterinary Association)* 10 (4): 311–35.

————. 2000. "Ecosystems Supporting Clusters of Sporadic Tses Demonstrate Excesses of the Radical-Generating Divalent Cation Manganese and Deficiencies of Antioxidant Cofactors Cu, Se, Fe, Zn." *Medical Hypotheses* 54 (2): 278–306.

Putnam, K. P., D. W. Bombick, J. T. Avalos, and others. 1999. "Comparison of the Cytotoxic and Mutagenic Potential of Liquid Smoke Food Flavourings, Cigarette Smoke Condensate and Wood Smoke Condensate." *Food and Chemical Toxicology* (Oxford) 37 (11): 1113–18.

Reed, G. A., M. J. Ryan, and K. S. Adams. 1990. "Sulfite Enhancement of Diolepoxide Mutagenicity: The Role of Altered Glutathione Metabolism." *Carcinogenesis* (Eynsham, England) 11 (9): 1635–40.

"Saccharin and Its Salts." 1999. *IARC Monographs on the Evaluation of Carcinogenic Risks to Humans* 73: 517–624.

Santodonato, J., S. Bosch, W. Meylan, and others. 1985. *Monograph on Human Exposure to Chemicals in the Workplace: Titanium Dioxide.* Report No. SRC-TR-84-804. Syracuse, New York: Center for Chemical Hazard Assessment, Syracuse Research Corporation.

Scher, W, and B. M. Scher. 1992. "A Possible Role for Nitric Oxide in Glutamate (MSG)-Induced Chinese Restaurant Syndrome, Glutamate-Induced Asthma, 'Hot-Dog Headache', Pugilistic Alzheimer's Disease, and Other Disorders." *Medical Hypotheses* 38 (3): 185–88.

Shahandeh, H., M. I. Cabrera, M. E. Sumner, and others. 1992. "Evaluation of Nutrasweet Sludge as a Nitrogen Fertilizer for Corn and Wheat." *Communications in Soil Science and Plant Analysis* 23 (15–16): 1911–21.

Sheth, A. R. 1998. "Aspartame: Is It Really Safe?" *Pharmacy Times* 30 (December 11–14): 27.

Stolze, K., and H. Nohl. 1998. "Erythrocyte Membrane Alterations Induced by the Antioxidant T-butylhydroquinone." Thirty-ninth Spring Meeting of the German Society for Experimental and Clinical Pharmacologyogy and Toxicology, Mainz, Germany, March 17–19. *Naunyn-Schmiedeberg's Archives of Pharmacologyogy* 357 (suppl 4): R123.

Takahashi, K. 1998. "Fluoride-Linked Down Syndrome Births and Their Estimated Occurrence Due to Water Fluoridation." *Fluoride* 31 (2): 61–73.

Takayama, S., S. M. Sieber, R. H. Adamson, and others. 1998. "Long-Term Feeding of Sodium Saccharin to Nonhuman Primates: Implications for Urinary Tract Cancer." *Journal of National Cancer Institute* 90 (1): 19–25.

"Tannic Acid and Tannins." 1976. *IARC Monographs on the Evaluation of Carcinogenic Risk of Chemicals to Man* 10: 253–62.

Tariq, M. 1993. "Reproductive Toxicity of Aluminum." *Reproductive Toxicology* 245–261.

Tassou, C. C., E. H. Drosinos, and G.-J. E. Nychas. 1997. "Short Communication: Weak Antimicrobial Effect of Carob (Ceratonia Siliqua) Extract against Food-Related Bacteria in Culture Media and Model Food Systems." *World Journal of Microbiology and Biotechnology* 13 (4): 479–81.

Tobacman, J. K. 2001. "Review of Harmful Gastrointestinal Effects of Carrageenan in Animal Experiments." *Environmental Health Perspectives* 109: 983–94.

Uhari, M., T. Kontiokari, and M. Niemela. 1998. "Novel Use of Xylitol Sugar in Preventing Acute Otitis Media." *Pediatrics* 102 (10): 879–84.

van Dokkum, H. P., I. H. Hulskotte, and K. J. Kramer. 2004. "Emission, Fate, and Effects of Soluble Silicates (Waterglass) in the Aquatic Environment." *Environmental Science and Technology* 38 (2): 515–21.

Winter, R. 1984. *A Consumer's Dictionary of Food Additives.* New York: Crown.

Woessner, K. M., R. A. Simon, D. D. Stevenson, and others. 1999. "Monosodium Glutamate Sensitivity in Asthma." *Journal of Allergy and Clinical Immunology* 104 (2 part 1): 305–10.

Yabiku, H. Y., M. S. Martins, and M. Y. Takahashi. 1993. "Levels of Benzo(a)pyrene and Other Polycyclic Aromatic Hydrocarbons in Liquid Smoke Flavour and Some Smoked Foods." *Food Additives and Contaminants* 10 (4): 399–405.

Yiamouyiannis, J. A. 1993. "Fluoridation and Cancer: The Biology and Epidemiology of Bone and Oral Cancer Related to Fluoridation." *Fluoride* 26 (2): 83–96.

CHAPTER 12: THE COMPONENTS OF A HEALTHY DIET

Alaimo, K., M. A. McDowell, R. R. Briefel, and others. 1994. "Dietary Intake of Vitamins, Minerals, and Fiber of Persons Ages Two Months and Over in the United States: Third National Health and Nutrition Examination Survey, Phase 1, 1988–91." *Advanced Data* (November 14) (258): 1–28.

Albertson, A. M., and R. C. Tobelmann. 1995. "Consumption of Grain and Whole-Grain Foods by an American Population during the Years 1990 to 1992." *Journal of the American Dietetic Association* 95 (6): 703–4.

Anderson, J. W., T. J. Hanna, X. Peng, and R. J. Kryscio. 2000. "Whole Grain Foods and Heart Disease Risk. *Journal of the American College of Nutrition* 19 (suppl 3): 291S–299S.

Centers for Disease Control and Prevention (CDC). 2004. "Trends in Intake of Energy and Macronutrients—United States, 1971–2000." *MMWR. Morbidity and Mortality Weekly Report* 53 (4): 80–82.

Food Surveys Research Group. 1999. *Pyramid Servings Data. Results from the USDA's 1994096 Continuing Survey of Food Intakes by Individuals (CSFII).* Table Set 9. Beltsville Human Research Center. Beltsville, Maryland: U.S. Department of Agriculture.

Hutchinson, A., J. R. Maltby, and C. R. Reid. 1988. "Gastric Fluid Volume and pH in Elective Inpatients. Part I: Coffee or Orange Juice versus Overnight Fast." *Canadian Journal of Anaesthesiology* 35 (1): 12–15.

Institute of Medicine. 2002. *Dietary Reference Intakes for Energy, Carbohydrate, Fiber, Fat, Fatty Acids, Cholesterol, Protein, and Amino Acids (Macronutrients).* Washington, D.C.: National Academy of Sciences, National Academy Press.

Slesinski, M. J., A. F. Subar, and L. L. Kahle. 1996. "Dietary Intake of Fat, Fiber, and Other Nutrients Is Related to the Use of Vitamin and Mineral Supplements in the United States: The 1992 National Health Interview Survey." *Journal of Nutrition* 126 (12): 3001–8.

Splinter, W. M., J. A. Stewart, and J. G. Muir. 1990. "Large Volumes of Apple Juice Preoperatively Do Not Affect Gastric pH and Volume in Children." *Canadian Journal of Anaesthesiology* 37 (1): 36–39.

Welsh, S., A. Shaw, and C. Davis. 1994. "Achieving Dietary Recommendations: Whole-Grain Foods in the Food Guide Pyramid." *Critical Reviews in Food Science and Nutrition* 34 (5–6): 441–51.

Wright, J. D., C. Y. Wang, J. Kennedy-Stephenson, and others. 2003. "Dietary Intake of Ten Key Nutrients for Public Health, United States: 1999–2000." *Advanced Data* (April 17) (334): 1–4.

CHAPTER 13: THE IDEAL DIET

Beinfield, H., and E. Korngold. 1995. "Chinese Traditional Medicine (C.T.M.): An Introductory Overview." *Alternative Therapies in Health and Medicine* 1 (1): 44–52.

Bhatt, A. D. 2001. "Clinical Research on Ayurvedic Therapeutics: Myths, Realities, and Challenges." *Journal of the Association of Physicians of India* (Bombay) 49 (May): 558–62.

D'Adamo, P. J. 1991. "Gut Ecosystems II: Lectins and Other Mitogens." *The Townsend Letter for Doctors* 124: 1089.

Davidson, P., K. Hancock, D. Leung, and others. 2003. "Traditional Chinese Medicine and Heart Disease: What Does Western Medicine and Nursing Science Know about It?" *European Journal of Cardiovascular Nursing* 2 (3): 171–81.

Elder C. 2004. "Ayurveda for Diabetes Mellitus: A Review of the Biomedical Literature." *Alternative Therapies in Health and Medicine* 10 (1): 44–50.

Ko, K. M., D. H. Mak, P. Y. Chiu, M. K. Poon, and others. 2004. "Pharmacologyogical Basis of 'Yang-Invigoration' in Chinese Medicine." *Trends in Pharmacological Sciences* 25 (1): 3–6.

Nachbar, M. S., and J. D. Oppenheim. 1980. "Lectins in the United States Diet: A Survey of Lectins in Commonly Consumed Foods and a Review of the Literature." *American Journal of Clinical Nutrition* 33: 2338–45.

CHAPTER 15: LIFE STAGE PROGRAMS

Preconception

Koren, G. 1993. "Preconceptional Folate and Neural Tube Defects: Time for Rethinking." *Canadian Journal of Public Health* 84 (3): 207–8.

Summers, L., and R. A. Price. 1993. "Preconception Care: An Opportunity to Maximize Health in Pregnancy." *Journal of Nurse-Midwifery* 38 (4): 188–98.

Infants and Toddlers

Altman J., G. D. Das, and K. Sudarshan. 1970. "The Influence of Nutrition on Neural and Behavioral Development. I. Critical Review of Some Data on the Growth of the Body and the Brain Following Dietary Deprivation during Gestation and Lactation." *Developmental Psychobiology* 3 (4): 281–301.

Pipes, P. L., and C. M. Trahms. 1993. *Nutrition in Infancy and Childhood.* Fifth edition. St. Louis: Mosby.

Adolescence

Baker, J., and B. K. Sandhu. 2000. "Nutrition, Eating, and Gastrointestinal Conditions in Adolescence." *Journal of the Royal College of Physicians* (London) 34 (2): 137–40.

Dimeglio, G. 2000. "Nutrition in Adolescence." *Pediatrics Review* 21 (1): 32–33.

Lifshitz, F., O. Tarim, and M. M. Smith. 1993. "Nutrition in Adolescence." *Endocrinology and Metabolism Clinics of North America* 22 (3): 673–83.

Thakur, N., and F. D'Amico. 1999. "Relationship of Nutrition Knowledge and Obesity in Adolescence." *Family Medicine* 31 (2): 122–27.

Adult Men

Ascherio, A., E. B. Rimm, E. L. Giovannucci, and others. 1992. "A Prospective Study of Nutritional Factors and Hypertension among U.S. Men." *Circulation* 86 (5): 1475–84.

Ballesteros, M. N., R. M. Cabrera, M. S. Saucedo, and others. 2001. "Dietary Fiber and Lifestyle Influence Serum Lipids in Free Living Adult Men." *Journal of the American College of Nutrition* 20 (6): 649–55.

Elahi, V. K., D. Elahi, R. Andres, and others. 1983. "A Longitudinal Study of Nutritional Intake in Men." *Journal of Gerontology* 38 (2): 162–80.

Hawkes, W. C., D. S. Kelley, and P. C. Taylor. 2001. "The Effects of Dietary Selenium on the Immune System in Healthy Men." *Biological Trace Element Research* 81 (3): 189–213.

Hu, F. B., E. B. Rimm, M. J. Stampfer, and others. 2000. "Prospective Study of Major Dietary Patterns and Risk of Coronary Heart Disease in Men." *American Journal of Clinical Nutrition* 72 (4): 912–21.

McCullough, M. L., D. Feskanich, E. B. Rimm, and others. 2000. "Adherence to the Dietary Guidelines for Americans and Risk of Major Chronic Disease in Men." *American Journal of Clinical Nutrition* 72 (5): 1223–31.

Ubbink, J. B., W. J. Vermaak, A. van der Merwe, and others. 1993. "Vitamin B-12, Vitamin B-6, and Folate Nutritional Status in Men with Hyperhomocysteinemia." *American Journal of Clinical Nutrition* 57 (1): 47–53.

Van Dam, R. M., E. B. Rimm, W. C. Willett, and others. 2002. "Dietary Patterns and Risk for Type 2 Diabetes Mellitus in U.S. Men." *Annals of Internal Medicine* 136 (3): 201–9.

Adult Women

American Dietetic Association. 1995. "Women's Health and Nutrition." *Journal of the American Dietetic Association* 95: 362.

Faine, M. P. 1995. "Dietary Factors Related to Preservation of Oral and Skeletal Bone Mass in Women." *Journal of Prosthetic Dentistry* 73 (1): 65–72.

Finn, S. C. 2000. "Women in Midlife: A Nutritional Perspective." *Journal of Women's Health and Gender-Based Medicine* 9 (4): 351–56.

Lukmanji, Z. 1992. "Women's Workload and Its Impact on Their Health and Nutritional Status." *Progress in Food and Nutrition Science* (Oxford) 16 (2): 163–79.

Seibel, M. M. 1999. "The Role of Nutrition and Nutritional Supplements in Women's Health." *Fertility and Sterility* 72 (4): 579–91.

Stephens, F. O. 1999. "The Rising Incidence of Breast Cancer in Women and Prostate Cancer in Men. Dietary Influences: A Possible Preventive Role for Nature's Sex Hormone Modifiers—The Phytoestrogens (Review)." *Oncology Report* 6 (4): 865–70.

Walker, S. P. 1997. "Nutritional Issues for Women in Developing Countries." *Proceedings of the Nutrition Society* (London) 56 (1B): 345–56.

Pregnancy and Lactation

Anderson, A. 1994. "Diet and Pregnancy: What to Advise." *Practitioner* 238 (1542): 607–11.

Antal, M. 1999. "Current Questions Concerning Nutrition during Pregnancy." *Orvosi Hetilap* (Budapest) 140 (45): 2507–11.

Cochrane, W. A. 1965. "Overnutrition in Prenatal and Neonatal Life: A Problem?" *Canadian Medical Association Journal* (Ottawa) 93: 893–99.

Gaby, A. R. 2000. "The Myth of Rebound Scurvy." *Townsend Letter for Doctors* (June): 122.

Klemola, T., T. Vanto, K. Juntunen-Backman, and others. 2002. "Allergy to Soy Formula and to Extensively Hydrolyzed Whey Formula in Infants with Cow's Milk Allergy: A Prospective, Randomized Study with a Follow-up to the Age of 2 Years." *Journal of Pediatrics* 140 (2): 219–24.

Ladipo, O. A. 2000. "Nutrition in Pregnancy: Mineral and Vitamin Supplements." *American Journal of Clinical Nutrition* 72 (suppl 1): 280S–290S.

Lucassen, P. L., W. J. Assendelft, J. W. Gubbels, and others. 2000. "Infantile Colic: Crying Time Reduction with a Whey Hydrolysate: A Double-Blind, Randomized, Placebo-Controlled Trial." *Pediatrics* 106 (6): 1349–54.

Scholl, T. O., and W. G. Johnson. 2000. "Folic Acid: Influence on the Outcome of Pregnancy." *American Journal of Clinical Nutrition* 71 (suppl 5): 1295S–1303S.

Udipi, S. A., P. Ghugre, and U. Antony. 2000. "Nutrition in Pregnancy and Lactation. *Journal of the Indian Medical Association* 98 (9): 548–57.

Weigel, M. M., W. M. Narvaez, A. Lopez, and others. 1991. "Prenatal Diet, Nutrient Intake, and Pregnancy Outcome in Urban Ecuadorian Primiparas." *Archivos Latinoamericanos de Nutricion* (Caracas) 41 (1): 21–37.

Williams, S. R. 1984. *Mowry's Basic Nutrition and Diet Therapy.* St. Louis, Missouri: Times Mirror/Mosby.

Winick, M. 1986. *Nutrition in Health and Disease.* Hoboken, New Jersey: Wiley and Sons.

Worthington-Roberts, B., and S. Williams. 1993. *Nutrition in Pregnancy and Lactation.* Fifth edition. St. Louis, Missouri: Mosby.

Menopause

Albertazzi, P., F. Pansini, G. Bonaccorsi, and others. 1998. "The Effect of Dietary Soy Supplementation on Hot Flushes." *Obstetrics and Gynecology* 91 (1): 6–11.

Brockie, J. 1999. "Dietary and Lifestyle Changes for Menopausal Women." *Community Nurse* 5 (9): 13–14.

Eden, J. 1998. "Phytoestrogens and the Menopause." *Baillieres Clinical Endocrinology and Metabolism* (London) 12 (4): 581–87.

Keller, C., J. Fullerton, and C. Mobley. 1999. "Supplemental and Complementary Alternatives to Hormone Replacement Therapy." *Journal of the American Academy of Nurse Practitioners* 11 (5): 187–98.

Savegh, R. A., and P. G. Stubblefield. 2002. "Bone Metabolism and the Perimenopause Overview, Risk Factors, Screening, and Osteoporosis Preventive Measures." *Obstetrics and Gynecology Clinics of North America* 29 (3): 495–510.

Vincent, A., and L. A. Fitzpatrick. 2000. "Soy Isoflavones: Are They Useful in Menopause?" *Mayo Clinic Proceedings* 75 (11): 1174–84.

Wimalawansa, S. J. 2000. "Prevention and Treatment of Osteoporosis: Efficacy of Combination of Hormone Replacement Therapy with Other Antiresorptive Agents." *Journal of Clinical Densitometry* 3 (2): 187–201.

The Later Years

American Dietetic Association. 2000. "Nutrition, Aging, and the Continuum of Care—Position of ADA." *Journal of the American Dietetic Association* 100: 580–95.

Boyd, J. A., R. J. Hospodka, P. Bustamante, and others. 1991. "Nutritional Considerations in the Elderly." *American Pharmacy* 31 (4): 45–50.

Bunout, D., and C. Fjeld. 2001. "Nutritional Reversion of Cognitive Impairment in the Elderly." *Nestle Nutrition Workshop series. Clinical and performance programme.* (5): 263–77; discussion 277–81.

Charlton, K. E. 1999. "Elderly Men Living Alone: Are They at High Nutritional Risk?" *Journal of Nutrition, Health, and Aging* 3 (1): 42–47.

Dwyer, J. 1994. "Nutritional Problems of Elderly Minorities." *Nutrition Review* 52 (8 Pt 2): S24–S27.

Evans, W. J. 1998. "Exercise and Nutritional Needs of Elderly People: Effects on Muscle and Bone." *Gerodontology* 15 (1): 15–24.

Gariballa, S. E. 2000. "Nutritional Support in Elderly Patients." *Journal of Nutrition, Health, and Aging* 4 (1): 25–27.

High, K. P. 2001. "Nutritional Strategies to Boost Immunity and Prevent Infection in Elderly Individuals." *Clinical Infectious Diseases* 33 (11): 1892–900.

Joosten, E., A. Van Den Berg, R. Riezler, and others. 1993. "Metabolic Evidence That Deficiencies of Vitamin B12 (Cobalamin), Folate, and Vitamin B6 Occur More Commonly in Elderly People." *American Journal of Clinical Nutrition* 58: 468–76.

Klein, S., and R. Rogers. 1990. "Nutritional Requirements in the Elderly." *Gastroenterology Clinics of North America* 19 (2): 473–91.

Lesourd, B. M. 1997. "Nutrition and Immunity in the Elderly: Modification of Immune Responses with Nutritional Treatments." *American Journal of Clinical Nutrition* 66 (2): 478S–484S.

Oesterling, J. E. 1996. "Benign Prostatic Hyperplasia: A Review of Its Histogenesis and Natural History." *Prostate* 6: 67–73.

Sahota, O., and D. J. Hosking. 2001. "The Contribution of Nutritional Factors to Osteopenia in the Elderly." *Current Opinion in Clinical Nutrition and Metabolic Care* 4 (1): 15–20.

Wahlqvist, M. L., T. L. Setter, G. S. Savige, and others. 2001. "Role of Physical Activity in Ensuring Nutritional Well-Being in the Elderly." *World Review of Nutrition and Dietetics* (Basel) 90: 102–9.

CHAPTER 16: PERFORMANCE ENHANCEMENT PROGRAMS

Agarwal, S., and A. V. Rao. 2000. "Carotenoids and Chronic Diseases." *Drug Metabolism and Drug Interactions* 17: 189–210.

Andreassen, A. K., A. Hartmann, J. Offstad, O. Geiran, K. Kvernebo, and S. Simonsen. 1997. "Hypertension Prophylaxis with Omega-3 Fatty Acids in Heart Transplant Recipients." *Journal of the American College of Cardiology* 29: 1324–31.

Bartzokis, G. 2004. "Age-Related Myelin Breakdown: A Developmental Model of Cognitive Decline and Alzheimer's Disease." *Neurobiology of Aging* 25: 5–18; author reply 49–62.

Bauer, V., and F. Bauer. 1999. "Reactive Oxygen Species as Mediators of Tissue Protection and Injury." *General Physiology and Biophysics* (Bratislava, Slovakia) 18 (spec no.): 7–14.

Biesalski, H. K. 2002. "Free Radical Theory of Aging." *Current Opinion in Clinical Nutrition and Metabolic Care* 5: 5–10.

Brennan, P. C., K. Kokjohn, C. J. Kaltinger, and others. 1991. "Enhanced Phagocytic Cell Respiratory Burst Induced by Spinal Manipulation: Potential Role of Substance P." *Journal of Manipulative and Physiological Therapeutics* 14 (7): 399–408.

Chan, S., B. Gerson, and S. Subramaniam. 1998. "The Role of Copper, Molybdenum, Selenium, and Zinc in Nutrition and Health." *Clinics in Laboratory Medicine* 18: 673–85.

Curry, S. J., T. Byers, and M. Hewitt, eds. 2003. *Fulfilling the Potential of Cancer Prevention and Early Detection.* Washington, D.C.: National Research Council, Institute of Medicine, National Academy of Sciences.

Cutler, J. A. 1999. "The Effects of Reducing Sodium and Increasing Potassium Intake for Control of Hypertension and Improving Health." *Clinical and Experimental Hypertension* 21: 769–83.

Digiesi, V., F. Cantini, A. Oradei, G. Bisi, G. C. Guarino, A. Brocchi, F. Bellandi, M. Mancini, and G. P. Littarru. 1994. "Coenzyme Q10 in Essential Hypertension." *Molecular Aspects of Medicine* 15 (suppl): S257–S263.

Djojosubroto, M. W., Y. S. Choi, H. W. Lee, and others. 2003. "Telomeres and Telomerase in Aging, Regeneration, and Cancer." *Molecular Cells* 15: 164–75.

Failla, M. L. 1999. "Considerations for Determining 'Optimal Nutrition' for Copper, Zinc, Manganese, and Molybdenum." *Proceedings of the Nutrition Society* (London) 58: 497–505.

Freeland-Graves, J. H., M. L. Ebangit, and P. J. Hendrikson. 1980. "Alterations in Zinc Absorption and Salivary Sediment Zinc after a Lacto-Ovo-Vegetarian Diet." *American Journal of Clinical Nutrition* 33: 1757–66.

Gao, Y. T. 1996. "Risk Factors for Lung Cancer among Nonsmokers with Emphasis on Lifestyle Factors." *Lung Cancer* 14 (suppl 1): S39–S45.

Ghosh, S. K., E. B. Ekpo, I. U. Shah, and others. 1994. "A Double-Blind, Placebo-Controlled Parallel Trial of Vitamin C Treatment in Elderly Patients with Hypertension." *Gerontology* 40: 268–72.

Goodman, S. 1988. "Therapeutic Effects of Organic Germanium." *Medical Hypotheses* 26: 207–15.

Grimble, R. F. 1997. "Effect of Antioxidative Vitamins on Immune Function with Clinical Applications." *International Journal of Vitamin and Nutrition Research* (Bern) 67: 312–20.

Harman, D. 2003. "The Free Radical Theory of Aging." *Antioxidants and Redox Signaling* 5: 557–61.

Hughes, D. A. 1999. "Effects of Dietary Antioxidants on the Immune Function of Middle-Aged Adults." *Proceedings of the Nutrition Society* (London) 58: 79–84.

Hunt, J. R. 2003. "Bioavailability of Iron, Zinc, and Other Trace Minerals from Vegetarian Diets." *American Journal of Clinical Nutrition* 78: 633S–639S.

Indian Council of Medical Research (ICMR). 2001. "Non-nutrients and Cancer Prevention." *ICMR Bulletin* (New Delhi) 31: 1-9.

Julian, D., and C. Leeuwenburgh. 2004. "Linkage between Insulin and the Free Radical Theory of Aging. *American Journal of Physiology. Regulatory, Integrative and Comparative Physiology* 286: R20–21.

Kar, S., and R. Quirion. 2004. "Amyloid Beta Peptides and Central Cholinergic Neurons: Functional Interrelationship and Relevance to Alzheimer's Disease Pathology." *Progressive Brain Research* 145: 261–74.

Kim, H., S. Park, D. S. Han, and T. Park. 2003. "Octacosanol Supplementation Increases Running Endurance Time and Improves Biochemical Parameters after Exhaustion in Trained Rats." *Journal of Medicinal Food* 6: 345–51.

King, G. D., and R. Scott Turner. 2004. "Adaptor Protein Interactions: Modulators of Amyloid Precursor Protein Metabolism and Alzheimer's Disease Risk?" *Experimental Neurology* 185: 208–19.

Krinsky, N. I. 2001. "Carotenoids as Antioxidants." *Nutrition* 17: 815–17.

McCarron, D. A. 1997. "Role of Adequate Dietary Calcium Intake in the Prevention and Management of Salt-Sensitive Hypertension." *American Journal of Clinical Nutrition* 65: 712S–716S.

Mendez, J. D., and M. P. Hernandez. 1993. "Effect of L-arginine and Polyamines on Sperm Motility." *Ginecologia y obstetricia de Mexico* (Colonia Napoles) 61: 229–34.

Meydani, S. N., and M. G. Hayek. 1995. "Vitamin E and Aging Immune Response." *Clinical Geriatric Medicine* 11: 567–76.

Moriguchi, S. 1998. "The Role of Vitamin E in T-cell Differentiation and the Decrease of Cellular Immunity with Aging." *Biofactors* 7: 77–86.

Moriguchi, S., M. Hamada, K. Yamauchi, and others. 1998. "The Role of Vitamin E in T-cell Differentiation and the Decrease of Cellular Immunity with Aging." *Journal of Medical Investigation* 45: 1–8.

Ngeh, J., and S. Gupta. 2001. "Inflammation, Infection, and Antimicrobial Therapy in Coronary Heart Disease—Where Do We Currently Stand?" *Fundamental Clinical Pharmacology* 15: 85–93.

Noble, M. 2004. "The Possible Role of Myelin Destruction as a Precipitating Event in Alzheimer's Disease." *Neurobiology of Aging* 25: 25–31.

Nofer, J. R., B. Kehrel, M. Fobker, B. Levkau, G. Assmann, and A. Von Eckardstein. 2002. "HDL and Arteriosclerosis: Beyond Reverse Cholesterol Transport." *Atherosclerosis* 161: 1–16.

Ringheim, G. E., and K. Conant. 2004. "Neurodegenerative Disease and the Neuroimmune Axis (Alzheimer's and Parkinson's Disease, and Viral Infections)." *Journal of Neuroimmunology* 147: 43–49.

Scibona, M., P. Meschini, S. Capparelli, C. Pecori, P. Rossi, and G. F. Menchini Fabris. 1994. "L-arginine and Male Infertility." *Minerva Urologica e Nefrologica* (Turin) 46: 251–53.

Srivastava, S., P. Desai, E. Coutinho, and G. Govil. 2000. "Protective Effect of L-arginine against Lipid Peroxidation in Goat Epididymal Spermatozoa." *Physiological Chemistry and Physics and Medical NMR* 32: 127–35.

Sumimoto, H. 2002. "Etiological View of Diseases from Protein Domain—Activation Mechanism of Reactive-Oxygen-Species Producing Phagocyte NADPH Oxidase Important Rule in Host Defence." *Masui* (Japan) 51 (suppl): S63–S71.

Tabira, T. 2004. "Development of Prevention and Treatment of Alzheimer's Disease: A Minireview." *Nippon Ronen Igakkai Zasshi* (Tokyo) 41: 23–25.

Taylor, J. C., L. Rapport, and G. B. Lockwood. 2003. "Octacosanol in Human Health." *Nutrition* 19: 192–95.

Turnlund, J. R. 2002. "Molybdenum Metabolism and Requirements in Humans." *Metal Ions in Biological Systems* 39: 727–39.

Urano, S. 1998. "Vitamin E: Its Role in Aging." *Sub-Cellular Biochemistry* 30: 391–412.

CHAPTER 17: MEDICAL TREATMENT PROGRAMS

Aba-Alkhail, B. A., and F. M. El-Gamal. 2000. "Prevalence of Food Allergy in Asthmatic Patients." *Saudi Medical Journal* 21: 81–87.

Altfas, J. R. 2002. "Prevalence of Attention Deficit/Hyperactivity Disorder among Adults in Obesity Treatment." *BMC Psychiatry* 2: 9.

Anderson, J. A. 1995. "Mechanisms in Adverse Reactions to Food: The Brain." *Allergy* 50: 78–81.

———. 1992. "Chromium, Diabetes Mellitus, and Lipid Metabolism." *Journal of the American College of Nutrition* 11 (5): 607/Abstract 35.

Baldewicz, T., K. Goodkin, D. J. Feaster, N. T. Blaney, M. Kumar, A. Kumar, G. Shor-Posner, and M. Baum. 1998. "Plasma Pyridoxine Deficiency Is Related to Increased Psychological Distress in Recently Bereaved Homosexual Men." *Psychosomatic Medicine* 60: 297–308.

Barrager, E., and A. G. Schauss. 2003. "Methylsulfonylmethane as a Treatment for Seasonal Allergic Rhinitis: Additional Data on Pollen Counts and Symptom Questionnaire." *Journal of Alternative and Complementary Medicine* 9: 15–16.

Bendich, A. 2000. "The Potential for Dietary Supplements to Reduce Premenstrual Syndrome (PMS) Symptoms." *Journal of the American College of Nutrition* 19: 3–12.

Birdsall, T. C. 1997. "Gastrointestinal Candidiasis: Fact or Fiction?" *Alternative Medicine Review* 2 (5): 346–54.

Bischoff, S. C., J. H. Mayer, and M. P. Manns. 2000. "Allergy and the Gut." *International Archives of Allergy and Applied Immunology* (Basel) 121: 270–83.

Boschmann, M., J. Steiniger, U. Hille, and others. 2003. "Water-Induced Thermogenesis." *Journal of Clinical Endocrinology and Metabolism* 88 (12): 6015–19.

Bottiglieri, T., M. Laundy, R. Crellin, B. K. Toone, M. W. Carney, and E. H. Reynolds. 2000. "Homocysteine, Folate, Methylation, and Monoamine Metabolism in Depression." *Journal of Neurology, Neurosurgery, and Psychiatry* 69: 228–32.

Brosnahan, J. 2003. "Supplementation with Key Nutrients Reduced Postoperative Infections and Length of Hospital Stay after Gastrointestinal Surgery." *Evidence-Based Nursing* 6: 47.

Clancy, S. P., D. M. Clarkson, M. E. Decheke, and others. 1994. "Effects of Chromium Picolinate on Beginning Weight Training Students." *International Journal of Sports Nutrition* 2 (4): 343–50.

Fava, M., and others. 1999. "Open Study of the Catechol-O-methyltransferase Inhibitor Tolcapone in Major Depressive Disorder." *Journal of Clinical Psychopharmacology* 19 (4): 329–35.

Flegal, K. M., M. D. Carroll, C. L. Ogden, and C. L. Johnson. 2002. "Prevalence and Trends in Obesity among U.S. Adults, 1999–2000." *Journal of the American Medical Association* 288: 1723–27.

Gaby, A. R. 2002. "Methylsulfonylmethane as a Treatment for Seasonal Allergic Rhinitis: More Data Needed on Pollen Counts and Questionnaire." *Journal of Alternative and Complementary Medicine* 8: 229.

Harro, J., H. Rimm, M. Harro, and others. 1999. "Association of Depressiveness with Blunted Growth Hormone Response to Maximal Physical Exercise in Young Healthy Men." *Psychoneuroendocrinology* 24 (5): 505–17.

Hefle, S. L. 1999. "Impact of Processing on Food Allergens." *Advances in Experimental Medicine and Biology* 459: 107–19.

Hourihane, J. O. 1998. "Prevalence and Severity of Food Allergy—Need for Control. *Allergy* 53: 84–88.

Ikeda, K., Y. Kimura, T. Iwaya, K. Aoki, K. Otsuka, H. Nitta, M. Ogawa, N. Sato, K. Ishida, and K. Saito. 2004. "Perioperative Nutrition for Gastrointestinal Surgery." *Nippon Geka Gakkai Zasshi* (Tokyo) 105: 218–22.

Johnson, S. R. 1998. "Premenstrual Syndrome Therapy." *Clinical Obstetrics and Gynecology* 41: 405–21.

Juhl, J. H. 1998. "Fibromyalgia and the Serotonin Pathway." *Alternative Medicine Review* 3 (5): 367–75.

Kankaanpaa, P., Y. Sutas, S. Salminen, A. Lichtenstein, and E. Isolauri. 1999. "Dietary Fatty Acids and Allergy." *Annals of Medicine* 31: 282–87.

Kim, K. T., and H. Hussain. 1999. "Prevalence of Food Allergy in 137 Latex-Allergic Patients." *Allergy and Asthma Proceedings* 20: 95–97.

Kuczmarski, R. J. 1992. "Prevalence of Overweight and Weight Gain in the United States." *American Journal of Clinical Nutrition* 55: 495S–502S.

Levine, J., Panchalingam, K., Rapoport, A. and others. 2000. "Increased Cerebrospinal Fluid Glutamine Levels in Depressed Patients." *Biological Psychiatry* 47 (7): 586–93.

Linde, K., C. D. Mulrow, M. Berner, and others. 2005. "St John's wort for depression." *Cochrane Database of Systematic Reviews* (2): CD000448.

Loch, E. G., H. Selle, and N. Boblitz. 2000. "Treatment of Premenstrual Syndrome with a Phytopharmaceutical Formulation Containing Vitex Agnus Castus." *Journal of Women's Health and Gender-Based Medicine* 9: 315–20.

McCarty, M. 1991. "The Case for Supplemental Chromium and a Survey of Clinical Studies with Chromium Picolinate." *Journal of Applied Nutrition* 43 (1): 58–66.

Meyers, S. 2000. "Use of Neurotransmitter Precursors for Treatment of Depression." *Alternative Medicine Review* 5 (1): 64–71.

Moreno, L. A., B. Tresaco, G. Bueno, J. Fleta, G. Rodriguez, J. M. Garagorri, and M. Bueno. 2003. "Psyllium Fibre and the Metabolic Control of Obese Children and Adolescents." *Journal of Physiology Biochemistry* 59: 235–42.

Moudgil, H. 2000. "Prevalence of Obesity in Asthmatic Adults." *British Medical Journal* 321: 448.

Mulrow, L. K. 2000. "St John's Wort for Depression." *Cochrane Database of Systematic Reviews* (2): CD000448.

Pelto, L., O. Impivaara, S. Salminen, T. Poussa, R. Seppanen, and E. M. Lilius. 1999. "Milk Hypersensitivity in Young Adults." *European Journal of Clinical Nutrition* 53: 620–24.

Rinkel, H.J. 1963. "The Management of Clinical Allergy. IV. Food and Mold Allergy." *Archives of Otolaryngology* 77: 302-26.

Rinkel, H.J., C. H. Lee, D. W. Brown Jr, and others. 1964. "The Diagnosis of Food Allergy." *Archives of Otolaryngology* 79: 71-9.

Sampson, H. A. 1999. "Food Allergy. Part 1: Immunopathogenesis and Clinical Disorders." *Journal of Allergy and Clinical Immunology* 103: 717–28.

Sellden, E. 2002. "Peri-operative Amino Acid Administration and the Metabolic Response to Surgery. *Proceedings of the Nutrition Society* (London) 61: 337–43.

Stewart, A. 1991. "Vitamin B6 in the Treatment of the Premenstrual Syndrome—Review." *British Journal of Obstetrics and Gynaecology* (Oxford) 98: 329–30.

Sullivan, A. C. 1974. "The Influence of (−) Hydroxycitrate on In Vivo Rates of Hepatic Glycogenesis, Lipogenesis, and Cholesterogenesis." *Federation Proceedings* 33: 656.

Thys-Jacobs, S. 2000. "Micronutrients and the Premenstrual Syndrome: The Case for Calcium." *Journal of the American College of Nutrition* 19: 220–7.

Watson, J. A., M. Fang, and J. M. Lowenstein. 1969. "Tricarballyate and Hydroxycitrate: Substrate and Inhibitor of ATP: Citrate Oxaloacetate Lyase." *Archives of Biochemistry and Biophysics* 135: 200–17.

Wyatt, K. M., P. W. Dimmock, P. W. Jones, and P. M. Shaughn O'Brien. 1999. "Efficacy of Vitamin B-6 in the Treatment of Premenstrual Syndrome: Systematic Review." *British Medical Journal* 318: 1375–81.

CHAPTER 18: DETOXIFICATION AND HEALING PROGRAMS

Aly, K. O., and P. A. Ockerman. 1978. "Fasting and Vegetarian Food—A Therapeutic Alternative." *Lakartidningen* (Stockholm) 75: 2619–22.

Ames, D. A. 1994. "A Comparison of Mental Health Center Operated Detoxification Programs in North Carolina." *Alcohol* 11: 477–80.

Bland, J. S., E. Barrager, R. G. Reedy, and K. Bland. 1995. "A Medical Food-Supplemented Detoxification Program in the Management of Chronic Health Problems." *Alternative Therapies in Health and Medicine* 1: 62–71.

Breslau, N., E. O. Johnson, E. Hiripi, and R. Kessler. 2001. "Nicotine Dependence in the United States: Prevalence, Trends, and Smoking Persistence." *Archives of General Psychiatry* 58: 810–16.

Efimov, A. S., A. V. Shcherbak, P. M. Karabun, L. P. Derevianko, and L. A. Iavorskii. 1987. "Therapeutic Fasting in the Combined Therapy of Obese Patients." *Vrachebnoe Delo* 8: 63–65.

Etter, J. F. 2004. "Associations between Smoking Prevalence, Stages of Change, Cigarette Consumption, and Quit Attempts across the United States." *Preventive Medicine* 38: 369–73.

Grant, B. F. 1994. "Alcohol Consumption, Alcohol Abuse, and Alcohol Dependence: The United States as an Example." *Addiction* 89: 1357–65.

Harwood, H. J., D. Fountain, and G. Fountain. 1999. "Economic Cost of Alcohol and Drug Abuse in the United States, 1992: A Report." *Addiction* 94: 631–35.

Holland, P., and M. Mushinski. 1999. "Costs of Alcohol and Drug Abuse in the United States, 1992. Alcohol/Drugs COI Study Team." *Statistical Bulletin of the Metropolitan Life Insurance Company* 80: 2–9.

Michalsen, A., W. Weidenhammer, D. Melchart, J. Langhorst, J. Saha, and G. Dobos. 2002. "Short-Term Therapeutic Fasting in the Treatment of Chronic Pain and Fatigue Syndromes—Well-Being and Side Effects with and without Mineral Supplements." *Forschende Komplementärmedizin und Klassische Naturheilkunde* (Basel) 9: 221–27.

"Prevalence of Current Cigarette Smoking among Adults and Changes in Prevalence of Current and Some Day Smoking—United States, 1996–2001." 2003. *Journal of the American Medical Association* 289: 2355–56.

"Prevalence of Current Cigarette Smoking among Adults and Changes in Prevalence of Current and Some Day Smoking—United States, 1996–2001." 2003. *MMWR. Morbidity and Mortality Weekly Report* 52: 303–4, 306–7.

Ryan, T., and V. Rothwell. 1997. "Residential Alcohol Detoxification: New Role for Mental Health Nurses." *British Journal of Nursing* 6: 280–84.

Saitz, R., M. F. Lepore, L. M. Sullivan, H. Amaro, and J. H. Samet. 1999. "Alcohol Abuse and Dependence in Latinos Living in the United States: Validation of the CAGE (4M) Questions." *Archives of Internal Medicine* 159: 718–24.

Shwartz, M., R. Saitz, K. Mulvey, and P. Brannigan. 1999. "The Value of Acupuncture Detoxification Programs in a Substance Abuse Treatment System." *Journal of Substance Abuse Treatment* 17: 305–12.

Slesarenko, S. S., G. G. Zhdanov, A. G. Shubin, and A. D. Matveev. 1996. "The Use of Therapeutic Fasting for the Preoperative Preparation of Obesity Patients." *Vestnik khirurgii imeni I. I. Grekova.* (Moscow) 155: 78–80.

Index

F

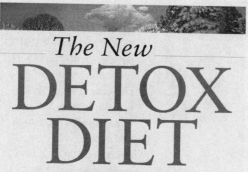
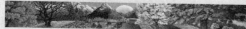
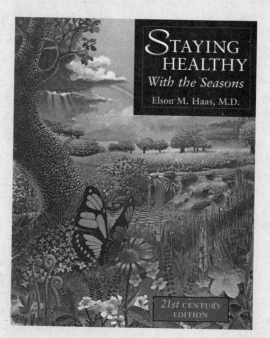
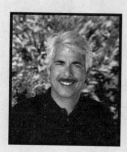